Nuclear Medicine and PET

Technology and Techniques

FIFTH EDITION

Nuclear Medicine and PET

Technology and Techniques

Edited by

PAUL E. CHRISTIAN, BS, CNMT
Manager, PET and Cyclotron Operations
Huntsman Cancer Institute
University of Utah
Salt Lake City, Utah

DONALD BERNIER, CNMT
Formerly Clinical Instructor
Nuclear Medicine Technology
School of Allied Health Professions
Saint Louis University
St. Louis, Missouri

JAMES K. LANGAN, CNMT
Formerly Assistant Administrator
Department of Radiography
The Johns Hopkins Hospital
Baltimore, Maryland

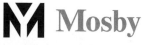
An Affiliate of Elsevier

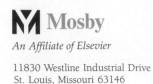

Mosby
An Affiliate of Elsevier

11830 Westline Industrial Drive
St. Louis, Missouri 63146

NOTICE

Nuclear Medicine is an ever-changing field. Standard safety precautions must be followed, but as new research and clinical experience broaden our knowledge, changes in treatment and drug therapy may become necessary or appropriate. Readers are advised to check the most current product information provided by the manufacturer of each drug to be administered to verify the recommended dose, the method and duration of administration, and contraindications. It is the responsibility of the licensed prescriber, relying on experience and knowledge of the patient, to determine dosages and the best treatment for each individual patient. Neither the publisher nor the author assumes any liability for any injury and/or damage to persons or property arising from this publication.

Previous editions copyrighted 1981, 1989, 1994, 1997

Publisher: Andrew Allen
Executive Editor: Jeanne Wilke
Senior Developmental Editors: Linda Woodard, Jennifer Moorhead
Publishing Services Manager: Linda McKinley
Senior Project Manager: Rich Barber
Senior Designer: Mark A. Oberkrom
Cover Art: Christine Hoog

Printed in the United States

Last digit is the print number: 9 8 7 6 5 4 3

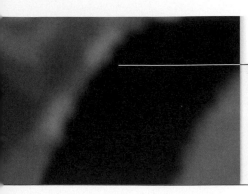

Contributors

Carolyn J. Anderson, PhD
Associate Professor of Radiology
Washington University School of Medicine
Department of Radiology/Division of Radiological Sciences
St. Louis, Missouri

Marcia Boyd, MS, CNMT
Director of Quality Management
Administration
Shelby County Government
Memphis, Tennessee

Paul H. Brown, PhD
Medical Physicist
Professor of Diagnostic Radiology
Oregon Health & Science University
Portland, Oregon

Julia W. Buchanan, BS
Research Associate
Division of Nuclear Medicine
Department of Radiology
The Johns Hopkins Medical Institutions
Baltimore, Maryland

Paul E. Christian, BS, CNMT
Manager, PET and Cyclotron Operations
Huntsman Cancer Institute
University of Utah
Salt Lake City, Utah

R. Edward Coleman, MD
Professor of Radiology
Vice Chairman
Department of Radiology
Duke University Medical Center
Durham, North Carolina

James J. Conway, MD
Attending Radiologist
The Children's Memorial Hospital
Chicago, Illinois

Helen H. Drew, CNMT
Chief Technologist
Nuclear Medicine
The Johns Hopkins Hospital
Baltimore, Maryland

Tracy Faber, PhD
Associate Professor of Radiology
Nuclear Medicine, Emory University Hospital
Atlanta, Georgia

James R. Galt, PhD
Director of Nuclear Medicine Physics
Nuclear Medicine, Emory University Hospital
Emory University
Atlanta, Georgia

Stanley J. Goldsmith, MD
Director, Nuclear Medicine
Professor, Radiology and Medicine
New York Presbyterian Hospital-Weill Cornell Medical
   Center
New York, New York

L. Stephen Graham, PhD, FACR
Radiation Safety Officer/Medical Physicist
VA Greater Los Angeles Healthcare System/
UCLA School of Medicine
Los Angeles, California

William L. Hubble, MA, CNMT, RT (RT)(R)(N)(CT)
Chairman, Nuclear Medicine Technology Program
Assistant Professor
School of Allied Health
Saint Louis University
St. Louis, Missouri

Jonathan M. Links, PhD
Professor
Environmental Health Sciences
Johns Hopkins Bloomberg School of Public Health
Baltimore, Maryland

Leon S. Malmud, MD
Dean Emeritus
Stauffer Professor of Diagnostic Imaging and Professor of
    Medicine
Temple University School of Medicine
Temple University Hospital
Philadelphia, Pennsylvania

Donna Mars, MEd, CNMT, NCT
Assistant Professor, Nuclear Medicine Technology
Baptist College of Health Sciences
Memphis, Tennessee

Marleen M. Moore, MS
Medical Physicist
Radiation Oncology, Fletcher Allen Health Care
Burlington, Vermont

Neeta Pandit, MBBS
Clinical Assistant Physician
Memorial Sloan Kettering Cancer Center
Assistant Professor of Radiology, Weil Medical College of
    Cornell University
Department of Radiology
Memorial Sloan Kettering Cancer Center
New York, New York

David J. Phegley, MBA, CNMT
Assistant Professor
School of Allied Health Professions
Saint Louis University
Saint Louis, Missouri

David F. Preston, MD
Professor Emeritus
Division of Nuclear Medicine
University of Kansas Medical Center
Kansas City, Kansas

Jay K. Rhine, BS, CNMT
Director
Nuclear Medicine Technology Program
The Johns Hopkins Medical Institutions
Division of Nuclear Medicine
Department of Radiology
Baltimore, Maryland

Henry D. Royal, MD
Associate Director of Nuclear Medicine
Mallinckrodt Institute of Radiology
Professor of Radiology
Washington University School of Medicine
St. Louis, Missouri

Sally W. Schwarz, MS, BCNP
Research Instructor in Radiology
Division of Radiological Sciences
Mallinckrodt Institute of Radiology
Washington University School of Medicine
St. Louis, Missouri

Roger H. Secker-Walker, MB, FRCP
Professor Emeritus
College of Medicine
University of Vermont
Burlington, Vermont

Arvind Sinha, MD
Fellow, Nuclear Oncology
Department of Radiology
Memorial Sloan Kettering Cancer Center
New York, New York

Jay Spicer, MS
Director, Nuclear Pharmacy Services
Assistant Professor of Radiology/Pharmacy
University of Kansas Hospital Authority
Kansas City, Kansas

H. William Strauss, MD
Clinical Director
Department of Radiology
Memorial Sloan Kettering Cancer Center
New York, New York

Zsolt Szabo, MD, PhD
Associate Professor of Radiology
The Johns Hopkins Medical Institutions
Baltimore, Maryland

Kathy E. Thompson, MS, CNMT
Chair, Nuclear Medicine Program
Baptist College of Health Sciences
Memphis, Tennessee

Boyd E. Vomocil, MD
Director, PET Imaging and Nuclear Medicine
Huntsman Cancer Institute
University of Utah
Salt Lake City, Utah

Henry N. Wagner Jr., MD
Professor of Environmental Health Sciences
Johns Hopkins Bloomberg School of Public Health
Baltimore, Maryland

Susan C. Weiss, CNMT
Chief Technologist
The Children's Memorial Hospital
Chicago, Illinois

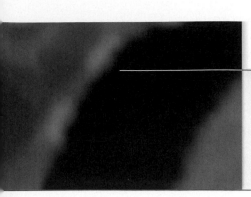

Reviewers

Robin G. Avison, CNMT, RT (N)(MR)
Chief MR Research Technologist
University of Kentucky
Lexington, Kentucky

Bobby R. Brown BS, CNMT
Program Director, Nuclear Medicine Technology
University of Texas Medical Branch
Galveston, Texas

Jeffrey Alan Galen, CNMT, MSEd, BSEd, BHS-NM
Director of Nuclear Medicine Technology
University of Missouri-Columbia
Columbia, Missouri

Raymond E. Robinson, BA, CNMT, RT (N)
Instructor
University of Medicine and Dentistry of New Jersey, School
  of Nuclear Medicine
Newark, New Jersey

Michael Teters, MS, DABR
Program Director/Assistant Professor
University of Medicine and Dentistry of New Jersey
Newark, New Jersey

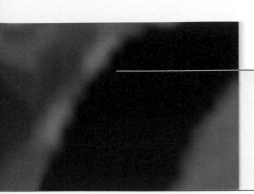

Dedication

This book is dedicated to my co-editors, Don Bernier and Jim Langan, for their friendship and their dedication to nuclear medicine over several decades. Both are now retired and throughout their professional careers demonstrated a concern for quality patient care, teaching, and sharing their knowledge and experience.

I also thank my wife Denise for her support of my continued enthusiasm and passion for this profession.

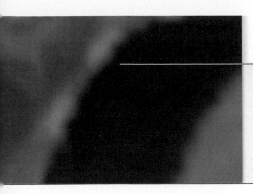

Foreword

The first edition of *Nuclear Medicine Technology and Techniques*, published in 1981, and the subsequent editions have provided the multifaceted information necessary to understand the technology that we work with on a daily basis. These books have been the standard textbooks for the nuclear medicine technology student. In addition, they have been excellent reference materials for practicing nuclear medicine technologists, nuclear medicine residents, and radiology residents. I frequently will use the latest edition to answer a specific question that I have concerning technology and techniques. The editors are to be congratulated on keeping the editions current. The editors are veterans in the production of books for nuclear medicine technologists, and they have used their considerable expertise in providing the latest information related to nuclear medicine technology. The authors include technologists, scientists, and physicians associated with outstanding programs in nuclear medicine. The editors have made sure that the chapters are up-to-date with state-of-the-art images.

This edition has a new title that includes PET. Although PET had been included in some of the chapters in the previous edition, the preeminent role of PET in the nuclear medicine of today is highlighted in this edition. The chapters on the fundamentals of PET address the specific topics of PET instrumentation, image reconstruction, fusion imaging, and other aspects important to PET instrumentation, image acquisition, and image processing. Because the primary utilization of PET is in oncology, a chapter has been added that is devoted to PET in oncology. The reader is pro-

vided an excellent overview of the role of PET in clinical oncology by the contents of the chapter. The chapters related to the brain and cardiovascular system now include more data on the use of PET in those organ systems.

Another important addition to this edition is a new chapter on SPECT imaging. SPECT imaging continues to have an increasing role in nuclear medicine, and it is appropriate to address this topic in more detail. The applications of SPECT in cardiac imaging are obvious to persons working in nuclear medicine/nuclear cardiology. SPECT imaging is now being performed more frequently in bone imaging and is routinely performed in evaluation of parathyroid pathology, monoclonal antibody imaging, and In-111 octreotide imaging. SPECT is now being used for imaging some radiopharmaceuticals that were not routinely used for SPECT imaging including I-131 iodide for thyroid cancer diagnosis and I-131 MIBG imaging for neuroendocrine tumor diagnosis.

The remaining chapters provide an overview of the basic sciences related to nuclear medicine and the clinical applications of nuclear medicine. This book provides an excellent review of the important aspects of nuclear medicine as we move into the era of molecular medicine. Even though we are in a specialty that is rapidly evolving, this book will be current for several years. The fifth edition of *Nuclear Medicine and PET: Technology and Techniques* raises the bar as a standard for a textbook in nuclear medicine.

R. EDWARD COLEMAN, MD

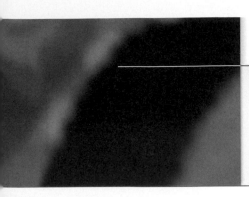

Preface

For more than two decades *Nuclear Medicine: Technology and Techniques* has served the nuclear medicine community as a resource on the procedures and technologies related to this ever-changing imaging specialty. This text may serve as a principle introductory textbook of nuclear medicine for both technologists and physicians, or it may be used as an update on the varied sciences and procedures that unite to form this unique tool to image physiology.

Because PET is being used more as a clinical tool, we have elected to use a more comprehensive title, *Nuclear Medicine and PET: Technology and Techniques* for the fifth edition. Although the field of nuclear medicine has significantly matured since the first edition of this text, nuclear medicine continues to evolve in technology, the number of clinical sites performing nuclear medicine procedures, and in the diversity of applications in medicine continues to expand.

As with previous editions, this book remains divided into two sections: those chapters that present the basic sciences that relate specifically to nuclear medicine and clinical chapters that are organized primarily by organ system. Each clinical chapter continues to review the physiology and anatomy that are important to the particular organ system, followed by the applicable radiopharmaceuticals and procedures. The enhancements made to the previous edition of an outline and learning objectives for this chapter have been retained, because these elements have been helpful in instruction and study of individual chapters.

All chapters represent the state-of-the-art practice of nuclear medicine at this writing and have been updated with new techniques, radiotracers, and procedures. Notable changes have been made to the instrumentation chapter to ensure that material presented here describes general operation and performance of today's devices. Although SPECT imaging is introduced in the chapter on instrumentation, an extensive chapter on SPECT (Chapter 9) has been added to expand in detail the many aspects of this widespread technology. The authors, Drs. James Galt and Tracy Faber, have done a magnificent job of discussing the material in an extremely well organized and easily understood manner. They have also supplemented the chapter with numerous diagrams, photographs, and images to clarify the fine points of this complex technology.

Since the fourth edition, PET applications to oncology, along with reimbursement, has had a profound effect on the growth of the clinical applications to the point that it has become part of the routine workup for many cancer patients. To aid in the understanding of PET technology, significant new material has been added to Chapter 6, Radiochemistry and Radiopharmacology. Detailed descriptions of the production, characteristics, and quality control of the most common PET radiopharmaceuticals have been added by the chapter authors. In addition, two new chapters on PET have been added to this book. Chapter 10, Fundamentals of Molecular Imaging with PET, covers the principles of physics, instrumentation, and radiation safety as they specifically relate to PET. Chapter 11, Clinical PET Oncology, discusses the most common application of this technology. Cardiac and neurological PET studies are found within those respective clinical chapters.

We would like to acknowledge the efforts and contributions of all the chapter authors. They have each been invited to contribute to this text because of their recognized expertise in their fields. It is only through their support, time, and knowledge that this book is possible. In addition, we acknowledge and thank the many people at Mosby who have made this fifth edition a reality.

INSTRUCTOR'S RESOURCE
Evolve—Online Course Management

Evolve is an interactive learning environment designed to work in coordination with *Patient Care*. Instructors may use Evolve to provide an Internet-based course component that reinforces and expands on the concepts delivered in class. Evolve may be used to publish the class syllabus, outlines, and lecture notes; set up "virtual office hours" and email communication; share important dates and information through the online Class Calendar; and encourage student participation through chat rooms and discussion boards. Evolve allows instructors to post exams and manage their grade book online. For more information, visit *http://www.evolve.elsevier.com* or contact an Elsevier sales representative.

PAUL E. CHRISTIAN
DONALD R. BERNIER
JAMES K. LANGAN

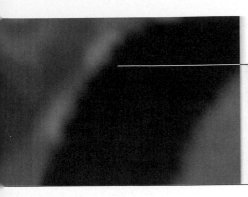

Contents

Nuclear Medicine and PET

Technology and Techniques

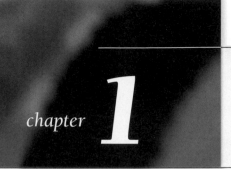

Paul H. Brown

Mathematics and Statistics

Objectives

Use scientific notation in performing algebraic operations.

Use the inverse square law to calculate the intensity of a radiation field at various distances.

Perform radioactive dilution calculations.

Define the units of radioactivity, radiation exposure, radiation absorbed dose, and radiation dose equivalent.

Perform calculations with logarithms and exponents using a calculator.

Discuss numeric accuracy, significant digits, and rounding.

Calculate quantities of radioactivity using the general form of the decay equation and decay factors.

Compute the concentration of ^{99}Mo in ^{99m}Tc.

Compute effective half-life and biologic half-life.

Calculate intensity with half-value layers.

Diagram various types of graphs and graphing techniques.

Discuss curve-fitting techniques.

Define mean, standard deviation, and coefficient of variation.

Discuss Gaussian and Poisson distributions.

State the formula for standard deviation, and perform calculations in the presence of background.

Explain the function of the chi-square test and interpretation of results.

Interpret the results of a chi-square test using a probability table.

Discuss the use and interpretation of *t*-tests.

Describe interpretation of sensitivity, specificity, prevalence, and accuracy.

Nuclear medicine technology occupies a unique position in the allied health sciences because of its strong dependence on quantitative, or mathematical, results. This chapter attempts to provide a sound basis for performing calculations that are typically required of nuclear medicine technologists. The emphasis here is on practical use, not on theoretical principles. Practical examples are provided, and each type of calculation includes a discussion on the use of pocket calculators and rudimentary instructions for the use of Microsoft Excel. This chapter reviews elementary algebra, graphing techniques, and statistical principles, always with an emphasis on practical applications. It is presumed that readers have a working knowledge of high school–level mathematics. The more advanced reader may wish to skip to the pertinent sections of this chapter. The reader who requires a more basic review of algebra may wish to consult another mathematics text.[1]

FUNDAMENTALS

Scientific Notation

Numbers in scientific calculations are often very small, such as 0.0015, or very large, such as 23,000. Scientific notation allows these numbers to be presented in a more convenient notation without cumbersome commas and zeros: 1.5×10^{-3} and $2.3E \times 10^4$. The exponent on the 10 specifies how many places the decimal point in the number is to be shifted to the left (for negative exponents) or shifted to the right (for positive exponents). Sometimes these numbers are alternatively represented as $1.5E - 3$ and $2.3 + 4$, a form found on pocket calculators or in printed tabular data (e.g., in calculations of internal radiation dosimetry), where the superscript is cumbersome to print. Pocket calculators typically have an EE key (for **E**nter **E**xponent), which allows easy entry of data in scientific notation. For example, if it is desired to calculate:

$$(1.5 \times 10^{-3}) \div (2.3 \times 10^4)$$

then the procedure on the calculator would be as follows (Figure 1-1):

1.5	enter value for numerator
EE	*enter exponent* key
±	*change sign* key to make the exponent negative
3	enter the value of the exponent
÷	division key
2.3	enter the value for denominator
EE	*enter exponent* key
4	enter the value of the exponent
=	(see result of 6.5217391E-8 in display)

This is precisely the same result as would be obtained by dividing 0.0015 by 23000 on the calculator.

It is often desirable to use numeric prefixes to represent very small or large numbers (Table 1-1). The value 6.52×10^{-8} grams (g), or 6.52E-8 g, can be more conveniently represented by converting the exponent to one of the exponent values shown in Table 1-1, which are usually exponents divisible by 3 (such as 3, 6, 9, and so on). Thus 6.52×10^{-8} g can be represented as 65.2×10^{-9} g, or in convenient shorthand form as 65.2 nanograms (ng), where the *nano-* stands for 10^{-9}. Notice that the decimal point in the number 6.52×10^{-8} can be shifted to the right by making the exponent smaller by 1 for each right shift of the decimal (e.g., $6.52 \times 10^{-8} = 65.2 \times 10^{-9}$), the object being to have an exponent that is divisible by 3 so that the numeric prefixes in Table 1-1 can be used. Similarly, a number like 2.3×10^4 counts (ct) can be expressed as 23.0×10^3 t, or 23 kct, with the k denoting *kilo,* or thousand.

This type of notation is often used for units of radioactivity, which is measured in Becquerels (Bq). A patient might be injected with 7.4×10^8 Bq of radioactivity, which can be

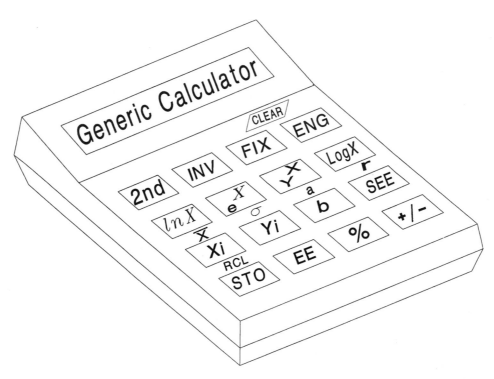

Figure 1-1 Generic scientific calculator demonstrating keys useful in nuclear medicine. The *2nd* key produces function above the key (e.g., *2nd*) and X_i produces the mean n of X_i values. The *INV* key produces functional inverse of the key. For example, *INV* and *lnX* are e^x functions. Most calculators do not have an e^x key if they also offer *INV* and *lnX* keys. The *FIX* key sets number of decimal places to be displaced (e.g., *FIX* and 3) and will display only three decimal places for all subsequent calculation. The *ENG* key causes the calculator to display results in scientific notation. X_i key is used to enter x values to calculate mean $\bar{x}$ and standard deviation σ. X_i and Y_i keys are used to enter x and y values for least squares curve fit (linear regression) to produce straight line with intercept (a), slope (b), correlation (r), and standard error of estimate (SEE). +/− key changes sign of number.

written 0.74×10^9 Bq (the decimal point can be shifted *left* if the exponent is *increased* by 1 for each left shift). So the injected radioactivity could be conveniently represented as 0.74 GBq. Alternatively, the value 7.4×10^8 Bq could be written 740.0×10^6 Bq = 740 MBq (the decimal was shifted two places to the right so the exponent is decreased by 2). Choosing between the two forms is simply a matter of preference. Note that pocket calculators often have an engineering notation key, which controls the scientific notation exponents in the calculator display to always be a power of 3. For example, 7.4×10^8 Bq is displayed as 740E6 on the calculator, which the user understands to be the same as 740 MBq.

Fractions and Percentages

Fractions, such as $\frac{1}{3}$, consist of a numerator (1) that is to be divided by a denominator (3). The value of a fraction may also be expressed decimally, such as $\frac{3}{4} = 0.750$ (a fraction that terminates in a zero digit), or $\frac{4}{3} = 1.3333\ldots$ (a fraction that never terminates in a zero digit). The mathematical manipulation of fractions requires care as to the number of digits and placement of the decimal point. The safest way to handle mathematical manipulation of fractions is to simply use the power of the pocket calculator to perform calculations such as $\frac{1}{3} + \frac{3}{4}$ by first converting the fractions to decimals and then carrying out the other arithmetic:

$$\frac{1}{3} = 0.333$$
$$\frac{3}{4} = 2.250$$
$$\text{sum} = 2.583$$

As a general rule the arithmetic should maintain at least one more digit in each fraction than is necessary in the final result. For example, if it is desired to describe the area of a rectangle (area = width × length) to the nearest centimeter,

Table 1-1	Numeric prefixes	
Abbreviation	**Prefix**	**Numeric value**
a	atto-	10^{-18}, one quintillionth
F	femto-	10^{-15}, one quadrillionth
P	pico-	10^{-12}, one trillionth
N	nano-	10^{-9}, one billionth
μ	micro-	10^{-6}, one millionth
M	milli-	10^{-3}, one thousandth
C	centi-	10^{-2}, one hundredth
D	deci-	10^{-1}, one tenth
Dk	deka-	10^1, ten
K	kilo-	10^3, thousand
M	mega-	10^6, million
G	giga-	10^9, billion
T	tera-	10^{12}, trillion
P	peta-	10^{15}, quadrillion

then measurements of the width and length of the rectangle should be made to the nearest tenth of a centimeter. Use of the pocket calculator generally produces at least eight digits of accuracy, which is more than enough for nuclear medicine calculations.

Percentages are values expressed as a fraction of some whole, entire value: 75% of some number is the same as 0.75 multiplied by that number. This is exemplified in the following:

$$75\% \text{ of } 5\,\text{ml} = 0.75 \times 5\,\text{ml} = 3.75\,\text{ml}$$

Many pocket calculators have a % key, which makes it unnecessary to first convert the percentage to a decimal:

75	enter percent value
%	*percent* key
×	*multiply* key
5	enter 5
=	(see result of 3.75 in display)

Percentages are often used to express percentage change between two values. For example, a patient may have had a kidney function test last month that showed a kidney clearance rate of 42 milliliters per minute (ml/min). The patient returns today and has a kidney clearance rate of 58 ml/min. The patient's kidney function has increased by 38% based on the following:

$$\% \text{ change} = [(\text{new value} - \text{old value})/\text{old value}] \times 100$$
$$= [(58 - 42)/42] \times 100$$
$$= (16/42) \times 100$$
$$= 0.38 \times 100 = 38\%$$

Algebraic Equations and Ratios

Calculations in nuclear medicine often involve expressing a mathematical concept as a ratio. For example, an intensity setting of 240 on a display screen may produce a suitable image for a bar phantom with 500,000 ct in the acquisition. Now it is desired to change to 300,000 ct in the image. The intensity on the screen is known to change linearly with the intensity control setting. What intensity setting should be used for the new 300,000 ct image? This translates mathematically into the following:

$$\frac{x}{300\text{k ct}} = \frac{240 \text{ intensity}}{500\text{k ct}}$$

This is typical of numeric equations in nuclear medicine. First, it is necessary to translate a mathematical concept, expressed in words, into an algebraic equation. The equation generally contains several numbers and one unknown value; here the new intensity setting is the unknown value (x). The object is to solve for the unknown value by rearranging the terms in the equation. In this example the unknown intensity x can be isolated on one side of the equation by multiplying both sides of the equation by 300 k ct. Remember, we can always do any math operation to both sides of an equation without changing the equality. Many students may have learned this technique as cross-multiplying to solve a proportion.

$$300k \text{ ct} \times \left[\frac{(x)}{300k \text{ ct}} \right] = 300k \text{ ct} \times \left[\frac{240 \text{ intensity}}{500k \text{ ct}} \right]$$

The 300 k ct cancels in the left numerator and denominator, so:

$$x = 300k \text{ ct} \times \frac{240 \text{ intensity}}{500k \text{ ct}} = 144 \text{ intensity}$$

Another frequently encountered problem relates to radioactivity concentrations in patient doses. For example, the morning elution of the ^{99}Mo-^{99m}Tc generator yields 943 mCi of ^{99m}Tc radioactivity in 20 ml of saline eluate. What volume should be withdrawn from the eluate vial into a patient syringe to immediately perform a 20 mCi patient scan?

$$\frac{x}{20 \text{ mCi}} = \frac{20 \text{ ml}}{943 \text{ mCi}}$$

$$x = 20 \text{ mCi} \times \frac{20 \text{ ml}}{943 \text{ mCi}} = 0.42 \text{ ml}$$

Inverse Square Law

The radiation exposure from a radioactive point source is governed by a mathematical relationship called the *inverse square law.* This states that the radiation exposure or intensity (I) at a distance (d) from a radioactive source is proportional to the inverse square of the distance. This law holds for a point source (a source that is very small when compared with the large distances from the source involved) that emits radiation not absorbed in the distances involved. A syringe source of x-rays or γ-rays at a distance of 1 meter (m) or more in air would qualify as a point source. Air is only weakly absorbing of x-rays or γ-rays in the energy ranges typically encountered in nuclear medicine. A syringe source for exposure to the hands does not obey the inverse square law because the distance from the syringe to the hands is not large compared with the syringe dimensions. Similarly, the exposure from standing near patients does not follow the simple inverse square law. Mathematically the inverse square law states:

$$I \propto \frac{k}{d^2}$$

where k is a proportionality constant that depends on the type of radioactive source and its activity. The symbol $\propto$ means *is proportional to.* The inverse square law results in the radiation intensity quadrupling if the distance from the source is halved, or the radiation intensity is decreased to one fourth its value if the distance is doubled. Changing the distance by a factor of 3 results in a factor of 9 change in intensity (nine times more intensity for one third the distance, or one ninth the intensity for three times the distance). This is usually stated in a form relating the old

intensity (I_2) at some old distance (d_2) to a new intensity (I_1) at some new distance (d_1).

$$I_1(d_1)^2 = I_2(d_2)^2$$

The intensity of radiation is usually measured in units of Roentgens (R) or milliRoentgens (mR) per hour. For example, a technologist is working 2 m from a small vial of radioactivity that results in an intensity or exposure level of 2.5 mR/hr at this distance. If the technologist moves to a distance of 3 m from the source, what is the new radiation intensity?

$$I_1 \times (3 \text{ m})^2 = (2.5 \text{ mR/hr}) \times (2 \text{ m})^2$$

or

$$I_1 = (2.5 \text{ mR/hr}) \times (2 \text{ m})^2 / (3 \text{ m})^2$$
$$I_1 = (2.5 \text{ mR/hr}) \times (4/9) = 1.1 \text{ mR/hr}$$

The technologist's radiation exposure is more than halved by his moving further from the source. Note that pocket calculators generally have an x^2 key, which facilitates the calculation:

2.5	enter intensity value
×	*multiply* key
2	enter old distance value
x^2	*squaring* key
÷	*division* key
3	enter new distance value
x^2	*squaring* key
=	(see result of 1.1 in display)

In another example, a technologist is working 4 feet (ft) from a point source that results in an intensity of 0.62 mR/hr. Concerns of radiation safety suggest that the intensity should be maintained at no more than 0.25 mR/hr for a safe working environment. To what distance from the source should the technologist move to achieve an exposure level of 0.25 mR/hr?

$$0.25 \text{ mR/hr} \times (d_1)^2 = 0.62 \text{ mR/hr} \times (4 \text{ft})^2$$

$$(d_1)^2 = \frac{(0.62 \text{ mR/hr}) \times (4 \text{ft})^2}{0.25 \text{ mR/hr}}$$

$$(d_1)^2 = \frac{(0.62 \text{ mR/hr}) \times 16 \text{ft}^2}{0.25 \text{ mR/hr}}$$

$$(d_1)^2 = 39.7 \text{ft}^2$$

$$\sqrt{(d_1)^2} = \sqrt{39.7 \text{ft}^2}$$

$$d_1 = 6.3 \text{ft}$$

Again, pocket calculators generally have a square root key ($\sqrt{\ }$), which facilitates calculation:

0.62	enter old intensity value
×	*multiply* key
4	enter old distance value
x^2	*squaring* key
÷	*division* key

0.25   enter new intensity value
=   results of division
$\sqrt{}$ *square root* key (see result of 6.3 in display)

Notice that in solving this problem the left side of the equation contained $(d_1)^2$, but because we wanted to solve for d_1, we took the square root of both sides of the equation. The squaring function and the square root function canceled on the left side of the equation because $x^2 = x$. Functions that have this property are called *inverse functions*. The squaring function $(x)^2$ and the square root function $(\sqrt{})$ are inverse functions.

For example, say a dilute standard solution is made by diluting a 1-ml volume of some standard radioactivity up to a 500-ml volume. This dilute standard, which has a low enough radioactivity to be accurately counted in a well counter, is then counted, and 2 ml of the diluted standard yields 15,346 ct. How many counts were in the original 1 ml of the standard?

$$C_1 V_1 = C_2 V_2$$
$$C_1 \times 1\,\text{ml} = \left(\frac{15,346\,\text{ct}}{2\,\text{ml}}\right) \times 500\,\text{ml}$$
$$C_1 = 3,836,500\,\text{ct/ml}$$

Notice how the units are carefully included with each number.

The dilution principle can also be used to measure an unknown volume. For example, suppose a 2-ml sample of a standard solution produces 647,530 ct per minute (cpm) in a well counter. This standard sample is then injected intravenously into a patient, and a 2-ml sample of patient blood yields 2600 ct in 10 minutes (or 260 cpm). What is the patient's blood volume?

$$C_1 V_1 = C_2 V_2$$
$$\left(\frac{260\,\text{cpm}}{2\,\text{ml}}\right) \times V_1 = \left(\frac{647,530\,\text{cpm}}{2\,\text{ml}}\right) \times 2\,\text{ml}$$
$$V_1 = 4981\,\text{ml}$$

Often it is necessary to inject a patient with a more concentrated solution than can be accurately counted in a well counter to ensure an adequate measure of the patient blood counts, without undue statistical counting noise. In the previous example, for instance, the patient blood counts yielded only 260 cpm/2 ml, which would be subject to a large statistical uncertainty (as discussed in the following section). It would therefore be necessary to obtain more blood counts. This requires increasing the activity in the standard source, which then becomes too concentrated to be accurately counted in the well counter. The problem is either that the standard is too strong or the patient sample is too weak because of the large dilution in the patient blood volume. The answer to the problem is to dilute a portion of the standard and count this diluted standard while the full-strength undiluted standard can be injected into the patient. The standard can be diluted by adding 1 ml of it to a flask, which is then filled to 500 ml. The dilution factor is then 500. For example, a 2-ml sample of the 1 : 500 diluted standard in a well counter might yield 26,835 cpm. Then 5 ml of the undiluted standard is injected into the patient, producing blood plasma counts of 26,500 cpm in 2 ml of plasma. What is the plasma volume?

$$C_1 V_1 = C_2 V_2$$
$$\left(\frac{26,500\,\text{cpm}}{2\,\text{ml}}\right) \times V_1 = \left(500 \times \frac{26,835\,\text{cpm}}{2\,\text{ml}}\right) \times 5\,\text{ml}$$
$$V_1 = 2530\,\text{ml}$$

Notice here that the standard counts had to be multiplied by the dilution factor of 500 to obtain the true standard concentration, which was injected into the patient.

Units

When manipulating numbers, it is critical to always consider the units of the numbers involved. Forgetting to specify whether a patient was injected with 5 µCi or 5 mCi of iodine-131 (^{131}I) radioactivity can have disastrous consequences. It is best to develop a habit of writing down the units for all the numbers in any calculation.

Units are agreed on standard quantities of measurement. They are often composed of some combination of the three fundamental properties of mass, length, and time. These are the properties that can be measured in our physical or biologic world. From these fundamental units we can derive other units, such as speed in m/sec, cm/sec, or ft/sec. These three units of speed are derived from the three different measurement systems that arose many years ago: the meter-kilogram-second, or mks, system of units; the centimeter-gram-second, or cgs, system of units; and the foot-pound-second system of units. Also commonly encountered are energy units of 1 Joule ($1\,\text{kg} \times \text{m}^2/\text{sec}^2$) in the mks system and 1 Erg ($1\,\text{g} \times \text{cm}^2/\text{sec}^2$) of energy in the cgs system. Table 1-2 lists units often encountered in nuclear medicine. In 1977 the three existing unit systems were modified when a worldwide Systeme International d'Unités (SI) was developed. Although the intent of SI units was simplification, both the old units and SI units continue to be in use in the United States. In SI, each unit is named after a person, and numeric factors are not present in the definition of the SI unit. For example, the old temperature scale of centigrade was replaced by Celsius, and the old unit of radioactivity, the Curie (3.7×10^{10} disintegrations per second [dps]), was replaced in SI units by the Bq (1 dps), which has no complicating numeric factor in the definition. The reader should be familiar with both the old units and the SI units shown in Table 1-2. It is often necessary to convert between various systems for consistency in applying mathematics equations. Most common is the necessity to convert between the old units and SI units for radioactivity, radiation exposure, absorbed dose, and dose equivalent. For example, what is the activity in Bq for 20 mCi of a radionuclide? This can be calculated from the conversion factor in Table 1-2 as follows:

Table 1-2	Units			
Measured property	**Old unit**		**SI unit**	**Conversion factor**
Radioactivity	Curie (Ci) = 3.7×10^{10} dps		Becquerel (Bq) = 1 dps	1 Ci = 3.7×10^{10} Bq
				1 Bq = 2.7×10^{-11} Ci
Radiation exposure	Roentgen (R) = 2.58×10^{-4} C/kg		Coulomb/kg (C/kg)	1 R = 2.58×10^{4} C/kg
				1 C/kg = 3.88×10^{3} R
Radiation absorbed dose	rad = 100 Erg/g		Gray (Gy) = 1 Joule/kg	1 rad = 0.01 Gy
				1 Gy = 100 rad
Radiation dose equivalent	rem = QF × rad		Sievert (Sv) = QF × Gy	1 rem = 0.01 Sv
				1 Sv = 100 rem

SI, Systeme Internationale; *QF,* quality factor.

$$\text{Activity in Bq} = 20\,\text{mCi} \times \left(10^{-3}\,\frac{\text{Ci}}{\text{mCi}}\right) \times$$

$$\left(3.7 \times 10^{10}\,\frac{\text{Bq}}{\text{Ci}}\right)$$

$$= 20 \times 10^{-3} \times 3.7 \times 10^{10}\,\text{Bq}$$

$$= 7.4 \times 10^{8}\,\text{Bq} = 740 \times 10^{6}\,\text{Bq}$$

$$= 740\,\text{MBq (or 0.74\,GBq)}$$

So 20 mCi is the same activity as 740 MBq. Notice how all the units except Bq canceled between numerator and denominator in the conversion. Use of the *enter exponent* key for scientific notation on the pocket calculator facilitates such calculations.

Similarly, it might be desired to convert a radiation absorbed dose (rad) of 5 rad into the new SI units of grays (Gy):

$$\text{Absorbed dose} = 5\,\text{rad} \times \frac{1\,\text{Gy}}{100\,\text{rad}} = 0.05\,\text{Gy}$$

$$= 5\,\text{centigray (cGy)}$$

So 5 rad is the same absorbed dose as 5 cGy.

To convert dose equivalent in the new Systeme Internationale (SI) units of 1 cSv into the old unit of rem:

$$\text{Dose equivalent} = 1\,\text{cSv} \times 10^{-2}\,\frac{\text{Sv}}{\text{cSv}} \times \frac{100\,\text{rem}}{\text{Sv}}$$

$$= 1\,\text{rem}$$

So 1 cSv is the same dose equivalent as 1 rem. Again, notice that all the units except the final desired value cancel in numerator and denominator.

Use of the radioactive decay equations discussed in the following section often requires converting between different time units. Suppose it was necessary to convert the time difference between 10:45 AM and 1:20 PM into units of days. The time difference is 155 minutes, which can be converted to days:

$$155\,\text{min} \times \frac{1\,\text{hr}}{60\,\text{min}} \times \frac{1\,\text{day}}{24\,\text{hr}} = 0.108\,\text{day}$$

The process of converting such units consists of repeatedly multiplying by a conversion factor of 1 (expressed as a fraction, such as $^{1\,\text{hr}}/_{60\,\text{min}}$) until the desired final unit result is obtained. For example, to convert the speed of light (3×10^{10} cm/sec) into a speed measured in furlongs ($\frac{1}{8}$ miles [mi]) per fortnight (14 days):

$$\frac{3 \times 10^{10}\,\text{cm}}{\text{sec}}$$

$$\times \frac{\left(\frac{1\,\text{in}}{2.54\,\text{cm}}\right) \times \left(\frac{1\,\text{ft}}{12\,\text{in}}\right) \times \left(\frac{1\,\text{mi}}{5280\,\text{ft}}\right) \times \left(\frac{8\,\text{furlong}}{\text{mi}}\right)}{\left(\frac{1\,\text{min}}{60\,\text{sec}}\right) \times \left(\frac{1\,\text{hr}}{60\,\text{min}}\right) \times \left(\frac{1\,\text{day}}{24\,\text{hr}}\right) \times \left(\frac{1\,\text{fortnight}}{14\,\text{days}}\right)}$$

$$= \frac{(3 \times 10^{10}) \times \left(\frac{1}{2.54}\right) \times \left(\frac{1}{12}\right) \times \left(\frac{1}{5280}\right) \times (8)\,\text{furlong}}{\left(\frac{1}{60}\right) \times \left(\frac{1}{60}\right) \times \left(\frac{1}{24}\right) \times \left(\frac{1}{14}\right)\,\text{fortnight}}$$

$$= \frac{1.49 \times 10^{6}\quad \text{furlong}}{8.27 \times 10^{-7}\quad \text{fortnight}}$$

$$= 1.8 \times 10^{12}\,\text{furlong/fortnight}$$

The conversion factors in the numerator convert centimeters to furlongs, and the conversion factors in the denominator convert seconds to fortnights. Completion of this otherwise silly problem on the calculator provides useful practice in unit conversion and calculator manipulation. Notice how the units in juxtaposed conversion factors always cancel between numerator and denominator until only the final desired units remain.

Lengthy calculations such as this one may best be handled on the calculator by first calculating the numerical value of the numerator and denominator separately. Calculate for the numerator with the following progression of keys:

3
EE
10
÷
2.54

$\div$

12

$\div$

5280

$\times$

8

=   (see result 1.4912909E6 for numerator in display)

Calculate for the denominator with the following progression of keys:

1

$\div$

60

$\div$

60

$\div$

24

$\div$

14

=   (see result of 0.0000008 in display)

EE   put calculator in scientific notation

(see result of 8.2671958E-7 in display)

Notice that the calculator had to be placed in scientific notation for the denominator to observe more than one significant figure in the display. Calculators from various manufacturers might function differently. The calculation is then completed by dividing the numerator by the denominator to obtain the final answer of 1.8×10^{12} furlongs/fortnight. Most scientific calculators have memory locations; you can temporarily store the numerator result in one memory location, with the denominator result stored in another. Then the memory locations can easily be recalled to divide numerator by denominator without having to enter the intermediate results by hand.

Exponent Laws and Logarithms

This section expands the algebra of exponents and logarithms. In general, exponent notation is set up as follows:

$$\text{base}^{\text{exponent}} = \text{number}$$

For example:

$$10^4 = 10,000$$

The exponent notation of 10^4 means the same as 10 multiplied four times:

$$10^4 = 10 \times 10 \times 10 \times 10 = 10,000$$

Generally, we are confronted with exponential calculations involving raising a base of 10, 2, or e to some power. Base 2 problems often arise in computer considerations where it might be required to calculate:

$$2^8 = 2 \times 2 \times 2 \times 2 \times 2 \times 2 \times 2 \times 2 = 256$$

Scientific pocket calculators generally have a Y^x key, meaning raise the base Y to the power x, which facilitates this type of calculation. To find 2^8 using the calculator:

2   enter base value Y

Y^x *exponentiation* key

8   enter exponent value x

=   (see result of 256 in display)

A special case arises when the exponent is zero. By mathematics definition any number (except zero) raised to the zero power is equal to 1:

$$e^0 = 1$$
$$10^0 = 1$$
$$2^0 = 1$$

Negative exponents provide a convenient form for representing small numbers:

$$10^{-4} = \frac{1}{10^4} = 0.0001$$

Notice that this shows how a number in exponent notation can be moved from numerator to denominator simply by changing the sign of the exponent:

$$2^8 = \frac{1}{2^{-8}} = 256$$

The algebra of exponents in equations follows certain rules. *Multiplication:* add the exponents.

$$B^x \times B^y = B^{x+y}$$
$$10^2 \times 10^3 = 10^5$$
$$10^4 \times 10^{-5} = 10^{-1}$$

To find the area of a rectangle multiply width times height:

$$\text{area} = 20\,\text{cm} \times 30\,\text{cm} = 600\,\text{cm}^2$$

Notice how this follows the rule for multiplying exponents:

$$\text{cm}^1 \times \text{cm}^1 = \text{cm}^2$$

Division: subtract the exponents.

$$\frac{B^x}{B^y} = B^{x-y}$$

$$\frac{10^2}{10^3} = 10^{2-3} = 10^{-1}$$

$$\frac{10^4}{10^{-5}} = 10^{4-(-5)} = 10^9$$

$$\frac{2^3}{2^3} = 2^0 = 1$$

A practical problem might involve calculation of the *mass attenuation coefficient* μ_m, which is defined by the quotient of the *linear* attenuation coefficient μ (in units of cm^{-1} or 1/cm) divided by the density ρ (in units of g/cm^3) for some substances such as human soft tissues. For example:

if $\mu = 0.12\,1/cm$, and $\rho = 3.4\,g/cm^3$, then

$$\mu_m = \frac{0.12\,1/cm}{3.4\,g/cm^3}$$

The difficulty here is how to evaluate the units. First eliminate denominator units within each term of the equation—that is, write 1/cm as cm^{-1} and g/cm^3 as $g \times cm^{-3}$, using the rule discussed above for moving from denominator to numerator by changing sign of the exponent. Then:

$$\mu_m = \frac{0.12\,cm^{-1}}{3.4\,g \times cm^{-3}}$$

Now follow the rule above for division of exponents with cm dimensions:

$$\mu_m = \frac{0.12\,cm^{-1-(-3)}}{3.4g} = \frac{0.12\,cm^2}{3.4g} = 0.035\frac{cm^2}{g}$$

Or the units of μ_m might be written as $\mu_m = 0.035\,cm^2 \times g^{-1}$.

Another example is Hertz (Hz), the measure of frequency expressed as the number of waves or cycles per second. For example, if three waves pass by a certain point in space in 1 sec, then the frequency (ν) is given by:

$$\nu = 3\,1/sec, \text{ or } 3\,sec^{-1}, \text{ or } 3\,Hz$$

Taking the root of a number is the inverse of raising to a power. A special case is the square root ($\sqrt{\ }$) of a positive number x, which is defined by:

$$\sqrt{x} \times \sqrt{x} = x$$
$$\text{e.g., } \sqrt{9} \times \sqrt{9} = 3 \times 3 = 9$$

Note that finding the square root is the same as raising a number to the half power: $\sqrt{x} = x^{1/2}$. As mentioned previously, the square root and squaring operation are inverses of each other because:

$$\sqrt{(x^2)} = x$$
$$\text{and } (\sqrt{x})^2 = x$$

Whether the squaring or the square root is performed first, the inverse function always cancels the other operation and simply returns the number x. Other roots can be calculated as the nth root of a number, which is written as $\sqrt[n]{x}$. For example, $\sqrt[3]{64} = 4$, because $4 \times 4 \times 4 = 64$. Some pocket calculators have a root key such as $\sqrt[x]{y}$, or the calculator might have an inverse (INV) key (see Figure 1-1), which is pressed before pressing another function to get the inverse of that function. For example, to calculate $\sqrt[3]{64}$ on the calculator:

64	enter value y to find cube root
INV and Y^x	or root key $\sqrt[x]{y}$, which is same as INV – Y^x
3	enter root value x
=	(see display of result, 4)

The base e ($= 2.718\ldots$) is an irrational number called *Euler's number*, named after Swiss mathematician and physicist Leonhard Euler (1707-1783). Calculations involving e pervade our mathematical, physical, and biological world: radioactive decay, absorption of radiation, growth of bacteria, and radiation damage to cells. Scientific pocket calculators often have a special e^x key that is used for calculations. Some calculators require the user to invoke the e^x function by virtue of the fact that the e^x function and the natural logarithm function ($\ln x$) are inverse of each other. This means that $\ln(e^x) = x$, and $e^{(\ln x)} = x$. For example, a radioactive decay problem might require the following calculation:

$$e^{-0.693} \times 4.5/6.0 = e^{-0.51975} = 0.59$$

This can be performed on the pocket calculator as follows:

0.693	enter value
+/–	*change sign* key
x	multiply
4.5	enter value
÷	
6	enter value
=	(see result of division)
INV and ln x	or e^x key (see result of 0.59 in display)

Logarithms provide another convenient system of notation that can make mathematical problems easier to solve. In nuclear medicine, logarithms can be used to linearize certain graphs (change a curved line into a straight line), solve problems in radioactive decay or radiation absorption, or provide a graphic axis scale capable of using a wide range of numeric values. The pocket calculator quickly computes logarithms so the reader needs to become familiar only with their algebraic properties. The logarithm ($\log_b x$) of a number (x) is the value to which the base (b) must be raised to equal the number:

$$x = b^{\log_b x}$$

For example, for base 10 logarithms the $\log_{10} 1000 = 3$, because $1000 = 10^3$. Note that the expression $\log_{10} 1000$ is read as *the base ten log of 1000*. Some examples follow:

$$\log_{10} 0.01 = -2$$
$$\log_{10} 0.1 = -1$$
$$\log_{10} 1 = 0$$
$$\log_{10} 10 = 1$$
$$\log_{10} 100 = 2$$
$$\log_{10} 10^n = n$$

If a $\log_b x$ is written without any value specified for the base (as $\log x$) then base 10 is understood.

The blackness of a nuclear medicine image on a piece of photographic film is measured by the optical density (OD) of the film, which is defined by shining a beam of light through the film:

$$OD = \log (100\%/\% \text{ transmitted through film})$$

The human eye can generally distinguish optical densities in the 0.25 to 2.25 range; below 0.25 is too dim to be seen, and above 2.25 is too black. The OD corresponds to the percentage of light transmitted through the film.

% light transmitted through film	OD
100	$\log 100/100 = 0$
10	$\log 100/10 = 1$
1	$\log 100/1 = 2$
0.1	$\log 100/0.1 = 3$

Logarithms have certain algebraic properties that can simplify mathematical calculations.

Multiplication: $\log xy = \log x + \log y$
Division: $\log x/y = \log x - \log y$
Exponents: $\log x^n = n \times \log x$

The other frequently encountered base for logarithms is the base e, or the natural logarithm, which is denoted by the special symbol ln:

$$\ln x = \log_e x$$

Pocket calculators usually have an $\ln x$ key, which allows easy calculation. The major use of natural logarithms in nuclear medicine is to solve problems in radioactive decay and radiation absorption, such as the time of decay (t) in the following equation:

$$0.25 = e^{-0.693 \times t/6\,hr}$$

The difficulty here is to solve for *t* by removing it from within the exponent. To eliminate a function (like e^x), we can take the natural logarithm of both sides of the equation:

$$\ln(0.25) = \ln e^{-0.693 \times t/6\,hr}$$

Using the rule above for log of exponents:

$$\ln 0.25 = \left(\frac{-0.693 \times t}{6\,hr}\right) \times \ln e$$

And now using $\ln e = 1$:

$$\ln 0.25 = \frac{-0.693 \times t}{6\,hr}$$

Notice that the minus sign and units are carefully retained. Simply rearranging algebraically to solve for *t* then results in:

$$t = \frac{-6\,hr \times \ln 0.25}{0.693}$$
$$= \frac{-6\,hr \times (-1.386)}{0.693} = +12\,hr$$

The minus from the original equation times the negative value of $\ln 0.25$ results in a + sign.

Numeric Accuracy: Significance and Rounding

The accuracy of mathematical calculations is governed by three concepts: significant *figures, rounding,* and significant *decimal places. Significant figures* refers to the number of digits required to preserve the mathematical accuracy in a number.

Numeric accuracy rule 1. For a number with no leading or trailing zeros, the number of significant figures is the number of digits.

Number	Number of significant figures
3	1
3.45	3

Numeric accuracy rule 2. For a number with leading zeros, the leading zeros are not significant.

Number	Number of significant figures
0.0015	2
−0.0463	3

Notice that expressing a number like 0.0015 in scientific notation as 1.5×10^{-3} eliminates the leading zeros and therefore eliminates the need for rule 2!

Numeric accuracy rule 3. Trailing zeros in a number should be retained only if they are significant, which depends on the context of the problem. Thus a problem may state that a drug costs $37; the cost has two significant figures. Or the problem may state that the drug costs $37.00, which is interpreted as being accurate in both dollars and cents; it has four significant figures. A length expressed as 4 cm has one significant figure; the length was measured to the nearest centimeter. But a length expressed as 4.0 cm has two significant figures; the length was measured more accurately to the nearest millimeter.

Numeric accuracy rule 4. The accuracy of the result in multiplication or division is such that the product or quotient has the number of significant figures equal to that of the term with the smaller number of significant figures.

For example, $2 \times 2.54 = 5$; the correct answer has only one significant figure because the 2 in the calculation has only one significant figure. But $2.00 \times 2.54 = 5.08$; the result has three significant figures because we presume that the trailing zeros in the 2.00 are significant. In another example:

$$\frac{0.061}{12.34} = 0.0049$$

or

$$\frac{6.1 \times 10^{-2}}{12.34} = 4.9 \times 10^{-3}$$

The result has only two significant figures. Note that a calculator display might show 0.0049433 or 4.9432739E-3, but the proper answer to record as a result is 0.0049 or 4.9E-3, with only two significant figures.

It is necessary to properly round off the result from the calculator before recording the result. For example:

$$\frac{0.061}{1.233} = 0.0494728 = 0.049$$

whereas

$$\frac{0.061}{1.232} = 0.0495130 = 0.050$$

Both answers have two significant figures, but the results are different because of rounding. The mechanics of rounding off a number consist of carrying the mathematical calculations to several more digits than are needed in the final answer. Then the final result is rounded off by the following rules.

Numeric accuracy rule 5. If the right-most digits, beyond the significant figures in the final result, are less than 5000, then simply drop the right-most digits. As an example, consider $^{0.061}/_{1.233} = 0.0494728$, which must be rounded to two significant figures (because 0.061 has two significant figures). The right-most digits are 4728, which is less than 5000, so the 0.049 is the correct rounded-off final answer.

Numeric accuracy rule 6. If the right-most digits, beyond the significant figures, are greater than 5000, then increase the least significant figure by 1. As an example, consider $^{0.061}/_{1.232} = 0.0495130$, which again must be rounded to two significant figures (because of the 0.061). The right-most digits are 5130, which is greater than 5000, so the final answer needs to be rounded up by one least significant digit (0.049 + 0.001). The final answer is 0.050, rounded off correctly to two significant figures.

Numeric accuracy rule 7. It may sometimes be necessary to round off a number when the right-most digit is exactly 5. The rule here is to round down the number if the digit to the left of the 5 is even, and round up the number if the digit to the left of the 5 is odd. For example 2.45 is 2.4, rounded to two significant figures; 1.5 is 2, rounded to one significant figure. This rounding scheme for numbers that end in 5 is arbitrary and results in averaging out rounding errors when a large number of calculations are performed.

Numeric accuracy rule 8. For addition and subtraction the final result has the same number of significant *decimal places* (rather than significant figures) as the number in the problem with the least number of significant decimal places. For example:

0.123 + 3.42 = 3.54 (two significant decimal places)
0.1 + 3.42 = 3.5 (one significant decimal place)
1 + 3.42 = 4 (0 significant decimal places)

Sometimes addition and rounding must be employed simultaneously, as in 0.125 + 3.42 = 3.547, which should properly be rounded to 3.55 with only two significant decimal places because the 3.42 has only two significant decimal places.

Scientific pocket calculators often have a key for fixing the number of decimal places to be used in a calculation.

The calculator also does the rounding off, simplifying such calculations.

Calculators and Personal Computers

Examples throughout this chapter have emphasized the use of the pocket scientific calculator. These scientific calculators are available from many manufacturers and should offer, as a minimum, the $\ln x$ and e^x functions. On some calculators, these options may be presented through a combination of $\ln x$ and inverse keys, as discussed in the previous examples. Figure 1-1 shows a typical calculator keyboard that would be useful in nuclear medicine. Generally, a scientific calculator also offers other useful statistical functions such as mean, standard deviation, and linear regression (or least squares curve fitting). Mastering the pocket calculator will greatly speed the results of many common nuclear medicine tests. Calculation of the variability in a nuclear counting system through a chi-square test, for example, can be conveniently derived from the standard deviation function on the pocket calculator.

A programmable calculator allows the user to store the instructions for frequently performed functions in the calculator memory or on a magnetic media program card of some sort that is inserted into the calculator. This would allow the user to program a function such as:

$$GFR = a[1 - e^{-b(c-d)}]$$

into the calculator. Simply entering a, b, c, and d would produce the answer for *GFR*. Other options for calculating such results include using a programming language such as BASIC, FORTRAN, or C, which is sometimes available on imaging computers or on PC-type computers within the nuclear medicine department. Whether using pocket calculator or other computers, the user must master some software to extend the range of user-defined calculations.

Several spreadsheet programs such as Microsoft Excel are now available for personal computers and greatly increase the number of mathematical calculations available to the user. In Excel, for instance, the user could simply enter numeric data values for a, b, c, and d in the above equation for GFR into four data cells (e.g., A1, A2, A3, A4) and then enter the GFR formula in another cell, B1, by clicking on cell B1 and typing in the following:

$$A1*(1 - \exp(-A2*(A3 - A4)))$$

Excel would calculate the GFR and place the answer in cell B1. Note that the symbol exp is a particular language that Excel understands to mean e^x, and the = sign in the equation above is something that Excel interprets as *evaluate the numerical value of this equation, and place the result in cell B1*. The use of PC software, instead of the scientific calculator, also offers several operation advantages: the ability to easily save the data, ability to easily edit the data, and hardcopy printouts and graphing.

PRACTICAL APPLICATIONS

Radioactive Decay

Nuclei that have an unstable balance of neutrons and protons spontaneously undergo radioactive decay to a more stable nuclear configuration. The number of radioactive nuclei that decay per unit time interval defines the radio-activity, which is measured in Curies or Bq (see Table 1-2). A radioactivity level is computed as follows:

$$1\,mCi = \left(1 \times 10^{-3}\,\frac{Ci}{mCi}\right) \times \left(3.7 \times 10^{10}\,\frac{dps}{Ci}\right)$$
$$= 3.7 \times 10^{7}\,dps$$

which means that $3.7 \times 10^{7}\,dps$ occur in the sample of radioactive material. The equation that defines the decay of the activity (A) over time (t) arises from a differential equation, which states that the number of atoms decaying per second is proportional to the number of atoms present. If we double the number of atoms in a sample of radioactive material, then the number of atoms decaying per second is also doubled. Solving the differential equation yields the radioactive decay law:

$$A = A_0 e^{-\lambda t}$$

where

$$A = \text{activity at time t}$$
$$A_0 = \text{activity at starting time}$$
$$\lambda = \text{decay constant}$$
$$t = \text{time since starting time}$$

The decay constant λ is the fraction of atoms that decay per (small) time interval, and has units of 1 over time (e.g., 1/hr) or inverse time (hr^{-1}). The decay constant for ^{99m}Tc, for example, is $0.115\,hr^{-1}$, which means that a fraction of *about* 0.115 (or 11.5%) of the ^{99m}Tc atoms decay per hour.

Note carefully that the verbal *interpretation* of the decay constant λ as the fraction that decays per some time interval is an *approximation* that holds only when the period being considered leads to a very small fractional decay. It is incorrect, for example, to conclude that $\lambda = 0.115\,hr^{-1}$ means that in 6 hours a fraction of 6×0.115 or 69% of the atoms decay (it is really 50%). Even saying 11.5% decay per hour is only approximate (it is really 10.9%). It is advisable to simply use λ for the exact mathematical calculations using the radioactive decay equation and to avoid using the inaccurate verbal interpretation as fractional decay.

The typical radioactive decay calculation required in nuclear medicine specifies three of the four variables (A, A_0, λ, t) in the decay equation, requiring that the fourth unknown variable be solved for. For example, a radiopharmacy delivers a 20.0 mCi dose of ^{99m}Tc ($\lambda = 0.115\,hr^{-1}$) to the nuclear medicine department at 8 AM. What amount of radioactivity would be injected into the patient for an 11 AM nuclear medicine scan?

$$A_0 = 20.0\,mCi, \lambda = 0.115\,hr^{-1}, \text{ and } t = 3.00\,hr$$
$$A = A_0 e^{-\lambda t}$$
$$A = 20.0\,mCi \times e^{-(0.115\,hr^{-1}) \times (3.00\,hr)}$$
$$A = 20.0\,mCi \times e^{-0.345}$$
$$A = 14.2\,mCi$$

To solve this problem on the pocket calculator, it is best to first evaluate the exponential expression and then multiply by 20.

0.115	enter λ value
+/–	*change sign* key to make negative
×	*multiply* key
3	enter t value
=	do the multiplication
INV – ln x	or e^x key
×	*multiply* key
20	enter A_0 value
=	(see result of 14.2 in display)

The radioactive decay law is often expressed in an algebraic form involving the half-life ($t_{1/2}$), rather than the decay constant λ. The $t_{1/2}$, which depends on the radioactive material involved, is that time at which the activity is decreased to half its original value. The radioactive decay law may alternatively be expressed as:

$$A = A_0 e^{-0.693 \times (t/t_{1/2})}$$

The factor 0.693 is actually ln 2, which is commonly written with three significant figures. Each half-life of radioactive decay causes the activity level to drop by 50%. Following is a timeline for radioactivity remaining:

Activity remaining	= 100% →	50% →	25% →	12.5% ...
At time	= 0	$t_{1/2}$	$2t_{1/2}$	$3t_{1/2}$ ...

(See Figure 1-3 for a graph of the radioactive decay law as a function of time for ^{99m}Tc with $t_{1/2} = 6\,hr$.)

Because both forms of the radioactive decay law are valid, we can write:

$$A = A_0 e^{-\lambda t} = A_0 e^{-(0.693) \times (t/t_{1/2})} = A_0 e^{-(0.693/t_{1/2}) \times t}$$

Because the expressions in the exponent e in these equations are equal, we can see that a relationship between λ and $t_{1/2}$ is given by:

$$\lambda = \frac{0.693}{t_{1/2}}$$

The λ and $t_{1/2}$ are inversely proportional to each other: a large λ means a small $t_{1/2}$ and vice versa. Whether to use one form of the radioactive decay law or the other is simply a matter of convenience. Given λ, we can easily calculate $t_{1/2}$ (and vice versa). For example, given that the decay constant λ for ^{99m}Tc is $0.1153\,hr^{-1}$, what is the $t_{1/2}$?

$$t_{1/2} = \frac{0.693}{\lambda} = \frac{0.693}{0.1153\,hr^{-1}} = 6.01\,hr$$

Careful attention to the units is necessary to avoid errors. To make the units clearer this might be restated as:

$$t_{1/2} = \frac{0.693}{0.1153\frac{1}{hr}}$$

To get the units of 1/hr out of the denominator, multiply both numerator and denominator by units of hours (essentially multiply by 1):

$$t_{1/2} = \frac{0.693}{0.1153\frac{1}{hr}}\frac{hr}{hr}$$

The 1/hr and the hr cancel in the denominator, leaving:

$$t_{1/2} = \frac{0.693}{0.1153}hr$$

Here again the common radioactivity problem is to solve for one of the four variables (A, A_0, t, $t_{1/2}$) when the problem specifies three of them.

For example, on Monday at 8 AM, a sample of ^{131}I ($t_{1/2}$ = 8.04 days) is calibrated for radioactivity of 10μCi. What radioactivity will be given to the patient if the dose is administered on the following Friday at 2 PM?

Given: $A_0 = 10\mu$Ci, t = Mon 8 AM $\rightarrow$ Fri 2 PM,

$$t_{1/2} = 8.04\,days$$

Solve for: $A = A_0e^{-(0.693)\times(t/t_{1/2})}$

Here, a digression to discuss units is necessary. Remember the good practice of always writing down the units associated with every number. Any problem involving the e^x function must have a dimensionless number for the value of x, so it is absolutely necessary that identical units be used for both t and $t_{1/2}$. Then the units cancel in the numerator and denominator of $t/t_{1/2}$, making the calculation independent of the units chosen to measure time. In this problem the time of decay (Mon 8 AM $\rightarrow$ Fri 2 PM) is 102 hours, but we have already been given $t_{1/2}$ in days. It would be correct to express the time of decay t as 4.25 days (rather than 102 hr) with the $t_{1/2}$ also in days, or it would be correct to express the $t_{1/2}$ as 193 hr (rather than 8.04 days) with the t also in hours.

$$A = 10\mu Ci \times e^{-0.693} \times (4.25\,days/8.04\,days)$$

or

$$A = 10\mu Ci \times e^{-0.693\times(102\,hr/193\,hr)}$$
$$A = 10\,\mu Ci \times e^{-0.366} = 6.93\mu Ci$$

A quick check of the results of the calculator's answer is also useful, based on the 100% $\rightarrow$ 50% $\rightarrow$ 25% $\rightarrow$ . . . timeline for each half-life. In this example the decay time of 4.25 days is less than one $t_{1/2}$ (8.04 days), so we know the answer should be between 100% and 50% of the initial 10μCi activity. The calculator result of 6.93μCi agrees with our mental check. Inadvertent calculator usage errors can be prevented with these mental checks.

A radionuclide is often calibrated for some activity level on a Friday, but it might have been administered to the patient on the previous Monday. This type of radioactivity problem can be calculated by using negative time values for times that precede the time of A_0 calibration. For example, a radionuclide with a 2-day half-life is calibrated for Friday at noon to be 3 mCi. What activity level is present on the preceding Monday at noon?

Given: $A_0 = 3\,$mCi,

$$t = -96\,hr\,(4\,days),\, t_{1/2} = 2\,days$$
Find: $A = A_0e^{0.693\times(t/t_{1/2})}$
$$A = 3\,mCi \times e^{-0.693\times(-4\,days/2\,days)}$$
$$A = 3\,mCi \times e^{+1.386}\,(notice\,(-)\,times\,(-)\,is\,(+))$$
$$A = 12\,mCi$$

This result is easy to check mentally since the time difference is exactly 2 half-lives; the answer should be that Monday noon has four times the activity of Friday noon, in agreement with our calculator result.

Sometimes a problem concerns only the fraction of remaining radioactivity (A/A_0), rather than with the actual remaining activity in mCi. For example, what fraction of radioactivity is left at a time equal to 3 half-lives? Here, we are given $t = 3t_{1/2}$ and asked to find A/A_0. The radioactive decay law can be algebraically rearranged (dividing both sides of the decay equation by A_0) as:

$$A/A_0 = e^{-0.693\times(t/t_{1/2})}$$
$$A/A_0 = e^{-0.693\times(3t_{1/2}/t_{1/2})}$$
$$A/A_0 = e^{-0.693\times3}$$
$$A/A_0 = e^{-2.079}$$
$$A/A_0 = 0.125$$

A quick mental check confirms the result: in 3 half-lives the radioactivity should decay 100% $\rightarrow$ 50% $\rightarrow$ 25% $\rightarrow$ 12.5%.

Remember that the radioactive decay equation always refers to the *remaining activity,* which is the same as 100% minus the decayed activity. It is important to determine whether the problem is stating the radioactivity remaining, which the decay equation predicts, or the radioactivity that has decayed away. For example, the previous problem showed that only 12.5% of the original radioactivity remains after 3 half-lives. This problem could also state that 87.5% of the radioactivity decays away in 3 half-lives.

Radioactive decay problems can also require you to solve for the t or $t_{1/2}$ value in the radioactive decay law. These values are contained in the decay law as part of the exponent function, so the exponent must be removed. An example might be to calculate the time necessary for 99.9% of a sample of ^{99m}Tc to decay away. Remember that the decay law works with the remaining radioactivity.

Given: $A/A_0 = 0.1\% = 0.001$,

$$t_{1/2} = 6.01\,hr$$

Solve for t in: $A/A_0 = e^{-(0.693) \times (t/t_{1/2})}$

$$0.001 = e^{-0.693 \times (t/6.01 hr)}$$

Taking the natural logarithm of both sides and using $\ln(e^x) = x$ yields:

$$\ln(0.001) = -0.693 \times t/6.01 \, hr$$

Now the t value is out of the exponent and the equation can be simply rearranged algebraically:

$$t = -6.01 \, hr \times \ln(0.001)/0.693$$

Notice how the minus sign and the units are carried correctly. Now using $\ln(0.001) = -6.908$ yields:

$$t = -6.01 \, hr \times (-6.908/0.693) = 59.9 \, hr$$

The two minus signs are multiplied and cancel each other. About 60 hr (or about 10 half-lives) is necessary for the radioactivity of ^{99m}Tc to decay to 1/1000 of its original value. For a radionuclide such as ^{131}I, it is still true that 10 half-lives cause decay to about 1/1000 of the original activity, but for ^{131}I, 10 half-lives is $10 \times 8.04 \, days = 80.4 \, days$.

As another example, an experiment finds that a sample of radioactivity decays to 30% of its original value in 5 hr. What is the $t_{1/2}$?

$$A/A_0 = e^{-0.693 \times (t/t_{1/2})}$$
$$0.30 = e^{-0.693 \times (5hr/t_{1/2})}$$
$$\ln(0.30) = -0.693 \times (5 \, hr/t_{1/2})$$
$$-1.204 = -0.693 \times (5 \, hr/t_{1/2})$$

so

$$t_{1/2} = -0.693 \times \frac{5 \, hr}{-1.204} = 2.9 \, hr$$

Do the mental check. Does this seem a reasonable answer? If 2.9 hr is the correct $t_{1/2}$, then a decay time of 5 hr is not quite 2 half-lives. So the expected answer is that 5 hr of decay with a 2.9 hr $t_{1/2}$ should leave slightly more than 25% of the radioactivity remaining. The problem has sensible results: 30% remaining at time just less than 2 half-lives.

In many practical problems it is necessary to combine radioactive decay calculations with concentration-volume problems. The nuclear medicine department may obtain its radioactivity from a ^{99}Mo-^{99m}Tc generator through an early morning elution of the generator. This eluate decays throughout the day, resulting in a changing concentration (in mCi/ml). For example, a generator is eluted at 7 AM, yielding 900 mCi in 20 ml of eluate solution. What volume should be withdrawn from the eluate vial into a syringe to perform a 15 mCi scan at 2 PM? First calculate the radioactivity remaining in the eluate vial at 2 PM:

$$A = 900 \, mCi \times e^{-0.693 \times (7hr/6.01hr)} = 402 \, mCi$$

(A quick mental check confirms the reasonableness of this answer; slightly less than 50% remaining at a time slightly greater than $t_{1/2}$.) The concentration (radioactivity per volume) in the eluate vial is then $(^{402 \, mCi}/_{20 \, ml})$ at 2 PM. The volume needed to be withdrawn into the syringe for a 15 mCi dose at 2 PM can be calculated from the equation activity = concentration × volume.

$$A = C \times V$$
$$15 \, mCi = \left(\frac{402 \, mCi}{20 \, ml}\right) \times V$$
$$15 \, mCi = \left(\frac{20.1 \, mCi}{ml}\right) \times V$$

so

$$V = \frac{15 \, mCi}{\left(20.1 \frac{mCi}{ml}\right)} = 0.75 \, ml$$

^{99}Mo-^{99m}Tc Radionuclide Generators

Another common problem for radioactive decay is to calculate the ratio of ^{99}Mo ($t_{1/2} = 65.9 \, hr$) activity to ^{99m}Tc activity in generator eluate. The problem is that some ^{99}Mo is also eluted out along with the ^{99m}Tc in the morning elution. The ^{99}Mo is a radionuclidic impurity that is limited by regulatory agencies to be less the 0.15 μCi ^{99}Mo per mCi ^{99m}Tc for injection into a patient. Consider a generator that is eluted at 7 AM and yields an eluate vial containing 30 μCi ^{99}Mo along with 250 mCi ^{99m}Tc. Can this eluate be used for a brain scan at the elution time of 7 AM? Calculate the ratio of ^{99}Mo to ^{99m}Tc activity at 7 AM as:

$$\frac{^{99}Mo}{^{99m}Tc} = \frac{30 \mu Ci \,^{99}Mo}{250 \, mCi \,^{99m}Tc} = 0.12 \frac{\mu Ci \,^{99}Mo}{mCi \,^{99m}Tc}$$

This eluate is less than the regulatory limit (0.15) and may be used.

Could this same eluate be used 6 hr later to prepare a lung scan? Now the ratio of activities at 1 PM is:

$$\frac{^{99}Mo}{^{99m}Tc} = \frac{30 \mu Ci \times e^{-0.693 \times (6hr/65.9hr)}}{250 \, mCi \times e^{-(0.693) \times (6hr/6.01hr)}}$$

$$= \frac{30 \, \mu Ci \times 0.939}{250 \, mCi \times 0.500} = \frac{28.17 \, \mu Ci \,^{99}Mo}{125 \, mCi \,^{99m}Tc}$$

$$= \frac{0.23 \, \mu Ci \,^{99}Mo}{mCi \,^{99m}Tc}$$

This eluate cannot be used, since the ^{99}Mo/^{99m}Tc ratio is greater than the 0.15 regulatory limit. The ^{99}Mo has not changed very much in the 6 hr since generator elution, but the ^{99m}Tc has halved, resulting in a large increase in the ^{99}Mo/^{99m}Tc ratio.

The mathematics of this type of radionuclide generator are governed by the laws of radioactivity[2], relating radionuclides denoted as a parent-daughter-granddaughter-and so on decay chain. The parent radionuclide ^{99}Mo decays to the daughter ^{99m}Tc, which in turn decays to the granddaughter ^{99}Tc, and the decay chain continues. Without dealing with the exponential algebra for this type of decay, it is possible to easily calculate the ^{99m}Tc radioactivity expected to be eluted from the generator by knowing three values:

1. The activity of ^{99}Mo in the generator, which is given by the manufacturer's calibration date and the decay law for ^{99}Mo ($t_{1/2} = 65.9$ hr)
2. The time since the last elution of the generator, which is commonly 24 hr for daily elutions
3. The ratio of ^{99m}Tc to ^{99}Mo in the generator, which depends on the time since the last elution (^{99m}Tc to ^{99}Mo ratios are shown in Table 1-3 as a function of the time since last elution)

For example, a generator is delivered on Saturday and calibrated by the manufacturer for the following Monday at 6 PM to contain 2 Ci of ^{99}Mo. The generator is eluted daily (Monday-Friday) at 7 AM. What activity of ^{99m}Tc is available in the generator at 7 AM on Tuesday? The required data are:

1. ^{99}Mo activity Tuesday 7 AM, 13 hr after calibration time.

$$A = 2\,Ci \times e^{-0.693 \times (13hr/65.9hr)}$$
$$= 1744\,mCi \text{ of } ^{99}Mo \text{ in the generator,}$$
$$\text{Tuesday 7 AM}$$

2. Time since last elution is 24 hr, since the generator is eluted daily.
3. From Table 1-3, the ^{99m}Tc/^{99}Mo ratio is 0.87 for 24 hr since last elution,

so

$$\text{Activity }^{99m}Tc = 0.87 \times \text{Activity }^{99}Mo$$
$$= 0.87 \times 1744\,mCi$$
$$= 1518\,mCi$$

Depending on the quality of the generator, only a percentage of this 1518 mCi of ^{99m}Tc will appear in the eluate. This is known as the elution efficiency of the generator. If the elution efficiency is 95%, then the ^{99m}Tc found in the Tuesday morning eluate would be calculated as $0.95 \times 1518\,mCi = 1442\,mCi$. This is available for patient studies.

Half-life: Biological, Physical, and Effective

In most clinical applications the nuclear medicine gamma camera measures the radioactive counts over an organ of interest in the patient's body. Typically the patient organ excretes the radiopharmaceutical with some biologic half-life t_B while the radioactivity also decays physically with a physical half-life that is denoted as t_P. The biologic half-life is an indicator of the physiologic fate of the radiopharmaceutical. The counts observed by the gamma camera follow an exponential decay law based on the effective half-life t_E, where:

$$\frac{1}{t_E} = \frac{1}{t_P} + \frac{1}{t_B}$$

Table 1-3	Generator ^{99}Mo-^{99m}Tc activity ratio
Time since last elution (HR)	**^{99}Mo-^{99m}Tc ratio**
1	0.094
2	0.18
3	0.25
4	0.32
5	0.39
6	0.44
7	0.49
8	0.54
10	0.61
12	0.68
14	0.73
16	0.78
18	0.80
20	0.83
22	0.85
24	0.87
26	0.88
30	0.91
∞	0.95

or, in a format that is much easier for calculational purposes,

$$t_E = \frac{t_P \times t_B}{(t_P \times t_B)}$$

For example, if the liver excretes a ^{99m}Tc radiopharmaceutical with $t_B = 3$ hr, then the gamma camera over the liver would observe an effective half-life:

$$t_E = \frac{6\,hr \times 3\,hr}{(6\,hr + 3\,hr)} = 2\,hr$$

The effective half-life is always less than or equal to the smaller of t_P or t_B.

Attenuation of Radiation

The calculation of the intensity (I) of x-ray or γ-ray photons transmitted through some thickness (x) of absorbing material follows exactly the same algebra as the equations of radioactive decay. Figure 1-2 shows a beam of monoenergetic x-ray or γ-ray photons striking a thickness of absorbing material. Monoenergetic means that the photons all have the same energy, such as a beam of photons from a ^{99m}Tc radionuclide source that emits photons of energy 140 keV. The initial intensity (number of photons per second) entering the absorbing material is called I_0. The material attenuates, or absorbs, some fraction of the photons, and the photon beam emerges with a transmitted (i.e., not absorbed) intensity I. The intensity of the transmitted radiation is given by:

$$I = I_0 e^{-\mu x}$$

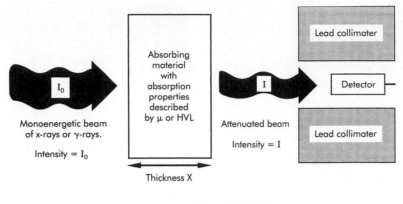

$$I = I_0 e^{-\mu X} = I_0 e^{-0.693\,(X/HVL)}$$

Figure 1-2 Attenuation of radiation in an absorbing medium.

where μ is the linear attenuation coefficient, or the fraction of the beam absorbed in some (very small) thickness x. The linear attenuation coefficient μ is the analog of the decay constant λ in radioactive decay. The linear attenuation coefficient μ depends on the type of absorbing material and the energy of the photons. A large μ value means a strongly absorbing material. For ^{99m}Tc γ-rays the μ value in lead is about $23\,cm^{-1}$, whereas the μ in water is only $0.15\,cm^{-1}$. Lead is a much more strongly absorbing material than water.

A typical calculation deals with the fraction I/I_0 transmitted through a thickness x. For example, what percent of 140 keV photons are transmitted through 10 cm of water ($\mu = 0.15\,cm^{-1}$)?

$$I/I_0 = e^{-\mu x}$$
$$I/I_0 = e^{-0.15cm^{-1} \times 10cm}$$
$$I/I_0 = e^{-1.5} = 0.22, \text{ or } 22\%$$

Because 22% are transmitted, we can also say that 78% are absorbed in 10 cm of water.

Consider a problem that asks what fraction of ^{131}I photons at energy 364 keV is transmitted through a half inch of lead ($\mu = 2.2\,cm^{-1}$ at 364 keV). Your inclination might be to calculate as follows:

$$I/I_0 = e^{-\mu x}$$

but

$$I/I_0 \neq e^{-2.2cm^{-1} \times 0.5in.}$$

The calculation is incorrect because the units in the exponent do not cancel each other. A dimensionless number must be in the exponent to make the result independent of the units used to describe μ and x. We can use any units we choose as long as the units of μ and x are inverse of each other. It is easiest to look up the μ values, from published tables, and then convert the thickness x to the corresponding units, rather than convert the units of μ to correspond with those of x. For this problem convert $x = 0.5$ in to 1.27 cm to obtain:

$$I/I_0 = e^{-2.2cm^{-1} \times 1.27cm} = 0.061$$

So 0.5 in of lead transmits only 6.1% of a beam of 364 keV photons from ^{131}I. This also means that the lead absorbs 93.9% of the photons. The linear attenuation coefficient suffers from the same problem as λ: it is difficult to conceptualize. It is therefore common to follow the method used in radioactive decay and define a *half-value layer (HVL)* as that thickness of material that absorbs 50% of the photons. The HVL is the analog of $t_{1/2}$ in radioactive decay. One HVL transmits 50% of the photons, two HVLs transmit 25% of the original beam, and so on. The absorption line looks like the following:

Photon
intensity $= \rightarrow 100\% \rightarrow 50\% \rightarrow 25\% \rightarrow 12.5\% \ldots$
Thickness $= \quad 0 \quad\quad 1\,HVL \quad 2\,HVL \quad 3\,HVL$

The equation of photon attenuation then can be expressed as:

$$I = I_0 e^{-\mu x} = I_0 e^{-0.693 \times (x/HVL)}$$

and a relationship exists between μ and HVL, given by $\mu = 0.693/HVL$. If we know the HVL or μ value, it is a straightforward calculation to find the other and use whichever attenuation equation is most convenient.

As an example, what percent of 140 keV photons from ^{99m}Tc are attenuated by 10 cm of water? The HVL for 140 photons in water is 4.6 cm.

$$I/I_0 = e^{-0.693 \times (x/HVL)}$$
$$I/I_0 = e^{-0.693 \times (10cm/4.6cm)}$$
$$I/I_0 = 0.22, \text{ or } 22\%$$

Remember the units of x and HVL must be the same, and remember that this equation calculates the *transmitted* intensity. A fraction (0.22) of the photons is transmitted. This is precisely the same result that was obtained previously in this section using the attenuation equation with μ. The problem, however, asks what fraction is *attenuated* by the water, so $1 - 0.22 = 0.78$ is the attenuated fraction; 10 cm of water absorbs 78% of the photons emitted by ^{99m}Tc. This type of calculation can be carried out easily on the pocket scientific calculator.

0.693	enter value
+/−	change sign key
×	*multiply* key
10	enter thickness value
÷	*divide* key
4.6	enter HVL value
=	(see result of division)
INV and ln x	or e^x key
	(see result of 0.22 in display)

Here again a quick mental check of the calculator result is useful. The thickness here (10 cm) is just slightly more than 2 HVLs (since HVL = 4.6 cm), so the attenuation answer should be just slightly less than 25%.

Another problem might require solving the attenuation equation for either x or the HVL, both of which are contained in the exponent in the attenuation equation. Just as in radioactive decay (where we needed to solve for t or $t_{1/2}$), we can eliminate the exponent with the natural logarithm as the inverse function of e^x.

$$I/I_0 = e^{-\mu x} - e^{-0.693 \times (x/HVL)}$$

or

$$\ln(I/I_0) = -\mu x = -0.693 \times (x/HVL)$$

For example, if 10 cm is known to transmit 22% of the photon beam, what is the HVL?

$$\ln(0.22) = -0.693 \times (10\,cm/HVL),$$

so

$$HVL = \frac{-0.693 \times 10\,cm}{\ln(0.22)}$$

$$= \frac{-0.693 \times 10\,cm}{-1.51} = 4.6\,cm$$

Note how the minus signs cancel and how the units are carefully carried. To calculate the HVL on the pocket calculator:

0.693	enter value
+/−	*change sign* key
×	*multiply* key
10	enter x value
÷	*divide* key
0.22	enter fraction value
ln x	*natural logarithm* key
=	(see result of 4.6 cm in display)

One further nuance occurs for attenuation of photons. The μ value, or the corresponding HVL value, for any material also depends on the physical density ρ (g/cm^3): the HVL in water vapor is different from the HVL in liquid water, which is also different from the HVL in ice, and so on. This makes calculations using the μ or HVL values somewhat difficult because the μ values are usually tabulated only for the common physical state of the material in question (e.g., for liquid water). To circumvent this problem, a new parameter is defined as the *mass* attenuation coefficient μ_m (cm^2/g) = μ/ρ. The mass attenuation coefficient is *independent* of the

physical density of the absorber and is therefore easily tabulated. The transmission of photons can then be expressed in one of three equivalent forms:

$$I/I_0 = e^{-\mu x}$$
$$I/I_0 = e^{-0.693 \times (x/HVL)}$$
$$I/I_0 = e^{-\rho \mu_m x}$$

Calculation of a result using the more easily tabulated value of mass attenuation coefficient also requires looking up the density (ρ) of the absorbing material.

It should also be noted that these equations for the transmitted fraction of photons apply only to a situation known as *good geometry,* or narrow-beam geometry, meaning that a very thin, pencil-like beam of photons enters the absorber and is detected by a small collimated detector. Scattered photons (photons not traveling in a straight line between the origin of the photon and the detector) are excluded by the good geometry. In most practical applications, such as photons arising in the patient's heart and being detected by a gamma camera, the geometry is broad-beam. The photons can leave the patient's heart and move toward the thyroid, for example, and then scatter in the thyroid and travel toward the gamma camera to be detected as a photon apparently arising from the thyroid. The scattered photons increase the apparent transmission through the patient's body, and the equation is typically modified by a multiplicative buildup factor B, with B $\geq$ 1. Buildup factors are dependent on the absorbing material, energy of the photon, and geometry. A large patient has a buildup factor greater than that of a thin patient, so in broad beam geometry:

$$I/I_0 = Be^{-\mu x}$$

Specification of the buildup factor, or some other correction for scatter, such as arbitrarily using a smaller μ value, may be necessary for accurate quantification of photons originating inside a patient.

Graphs

The modern technologic world can often inundate us with data. Graphs provide a practical, highly visual way to convey large amounts of information. They can also be used to predict one variable based on another. The most common type of graph uses a linear set of x and y axes in the familiar Cartesian coordinate system. Figure 1-3 shows a graph or plot of the remaining radioactivity level versus time from a sample of radioactive material with $t_{1/2} = 6\,hr$. The x axis (or abscissa) shows the time of each data point (for 0, 2, 6, and 12 hr), and the y axis (or ordinate) shows the activity in milliCuries for each data point. One variable is often considered to depend on another independent variable. The independent variable is generally plotted on the x axis, with the dependent variable on the y axis. In Figure 1-3, time is considered the independent variable on the x axis, and activity level is considered the dependent variable on the y axis.

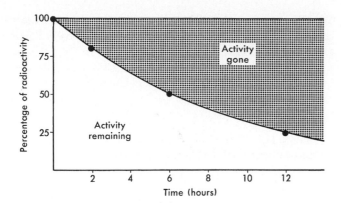

Figure 1-3 Linear plot of radioactive decay for $t_{1/2} = 6\,\text{hr}$.

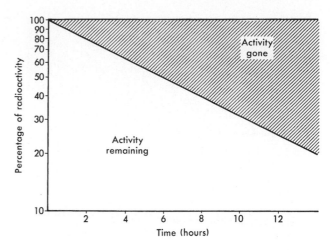

Figure 1-4 Semilog plot of radioactivity for $t_{1/2} = 6\,\text{hr}$. The *y* axis is logarithmic.

Mathematically, activity (*y*) is a function of time, or $y = f(t)$. The data points in Figure 1-3 are called *discrete data points* because a measurement of activity was taken at four discrete, individual data points (0, 2, 6, and 12 hr). Graphs of discrete data points may or may not, at the user's discretion, show the data points joined by smooth curves or a connect-the-dots type of straight line. Our knowledge of the decay process suggests a smooth curve should best represent radioactive decay. On the other hand, a graph of the number of monthly kidney scans might be graphed as discrete data points joined in a connect-the-dots fashion because no reason implies a smoother curve.

Figure 1-3 shows a continuous curve of activity versus time for the radioactive decay equation:

$$A = A_0 e^{-\lambda t}$$

The $t_{1/2}$ for the data in Figure 1-3 is 6 hr because the radioactivity drops 100%, 50%, and 25% in 0, 6, and 12 hr, respectively. If the natural logarithm is taken on both sides of the equation, the curve in Figure 1-3 will simplify into the straight line shown in Figure 1-4 because:

$$\ln A = \ln (A_0 e^{-\lambda t})$$
$$\ln A = \ln A_0 + \ln (e^{-\lambda t})$$
$$\ln A = \ln A_0 - \lambda t$$

or

$$y = a + bt$$

This is the equation of a straight line with *y*-intercept $a = \ln A_0$, and slope $b = -\lambda$. This is an important practical result: the logarithm of radioactive decay data plotted versus time is a straight line graph with negative slope equal to the decay constant. Note that the logarithmic plot of activity still shows the activity dropping by 50% every 6 hr.

A brief review of the graphic interpretation of straight line data seems pertinent. A straight line graph of *y* versus *x* is represented by the general formula:

$$y = a + bx$$

The *y*-intercept, which is the value of *y* at $x = 0$, is represented by *a*. The slope, which represents the steepness of

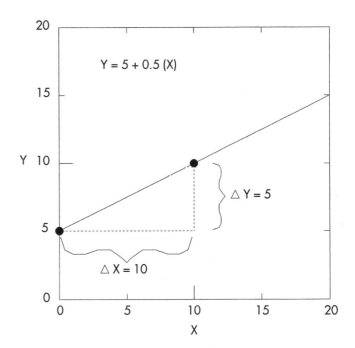

Figure 1-5 Straight line graph with slope = 0.5 and intercept = 5.

the line, is represented by *b*. Figure 1-5 shows a straight line graph with $b = 0.5$ as the slope. The slope is calculated from any two arbitrary points on the line as:

$$\text{Slope} = \frac{\Delta y}{\Delta x} = \frac{(y_2 - y_1)}{(x_2 - x_1)}$$

In Figure 1-5 the slope is calculated from the points $(x_1, y_1) = (0, 5)$ and $(x_2, y_2) = (10, 10)$.

$$\text{Slope} = \frac{(10-5)}{(10-0)} = 0.5$$

For a straight line graph, it does not matter which two points on the line are chosen to calculate the slope; the same answer is obtained. In Figure 1-5 the *y*-intercept *a* equals 5

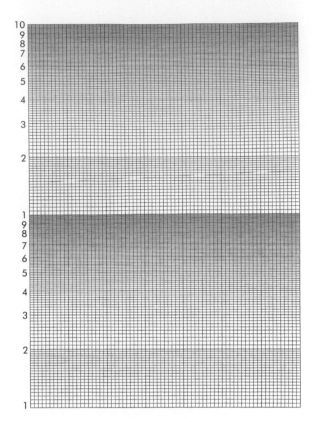

Figure 1-6   Two-cycle semilog graph paper.

because the value of y is 5 at x equals 0. Hence the equation of the straight line in Figure 1-5 is given by:

$$y = 5 + 0.5x$$

Given any x value, the equation can be used to calculate the y value. The sign of the slope merely reflects whether the curve slopes upward (a positive slope) or downward (a negative slope). Straight line curves are generally used in nuclear medicine to prove a direct or linear relationship between two variables or to predict some y variable based on the value of the x variable.

Mathematical relationships or curves that are nonlinear, such as radioactivity versus time, are often transformed by a mathematical operation to make the graph a straight line. For exponential curves such as radioactive decay, taking the natural logarithm of the activity transforms the data into a straight line. The straight line form might be preferred because subsequent interpretation or calculations are simplified. The use of logarithms as a process to transform curvilinear data into straight lines is so common that a special type of graph paper is often used to simplify the process (Figure 1-6). Semilogarithmic graph paper has axes with divisions that are proportional to the logarithm of the y axis, so the y values are simply plotted at the appropriate point without the necessity of calculating the logarithm of the y axis data. Semilogarithmic graph paper is available with a varying number of cycles, or powers of 10, on the y axis. Figure 1-6 shows two-cycle graph paper, which can accommodate y values that span a range of no more than

10^2. The user simply relabels the numeric values on the y axis to correspond to the range of the data involved. For example, the y values could range from 0.23 to 7.9, with the y axis labeled with 0.1 at the bottom, 1.0 in the middle, and 10.0 at the top. Alternatively, the data might fall into the range of 200 to 8000, with the cycles labeled from 100 through 1000 to 10,000.

Measurement of Effective Half-life

A typical procedure with nuclear medicine data is to calculate the effective $t_{1/2}$ of excretion from some organ in the body. As an example, consider a patient who is given a meal of radioactive food to determine the $t_{1/2}$ of emptying of the stomach. The radioactivity counts emanating from the stomach are plotted on semilogarithmic graph paper (Figure 1-7). The $t_{1/2}$ of excretion can be determined by drawing a freehand visual-estimate straight line through the data points. Each data point is contaminated with statistical and systematic noise, or uncertainty, in the actual y value, so the straight line will probably not pass exactly through all, if any, of the data points. Use of this method to determine $t_{1/2}$ relies on the data points being reasonably well represented as a straight line on a semilogarithmic plot. Often the data appear more and more like a straight line at later time values, so these values are used to estimate the straight line fit. After the straight line is drawn, the $t_{1/2}$ can be determined as the interval needed for the straight line to decrease by a factor of $1/2$. Just pick any convenient starting value for y, then read off the graph the time needed to reach $y/2$. In Figure 1-7 the visual-estimate best-fit straight line has a y-intercept (or Y_0) of 7800 cts, and the line falls to 3900 cts ($Y_0/2$) in 12.5 min, so $t_{1/2} = 12.5$ min by the visual-estimate best-fit line.

In some cases the data never decrease by a factor of $1/2$ over the time of the experiment, but it is still desired to calculate the $t_{1/2}$. In this case the proper calculation (remembering radioactive decay follows the equation $\ln Y = \ln Y_0 - \lambda t$) is to find the slope, which is equal to $-\lambda$, and the negative decay constant, based on the counts (y) and time (t) of any two points on the straight line.

$$-\lambda = \frac{[\ln(y_2) - \ln(y_1)]}{[t_2 - t_1]}$$

Then the $t_{1/2}$ is calculated from the $t_{1/2} = 0.693/\lambda$. Note that the equation for the decay constant slope requires calculation of the natural logarithm of the count values in the numerator. The logarithm need not be calculated to *plot* the data (because of the convenience of semilogarithmic graph paper), but calculation of the slope λ *does* require calculation of the logarithm of any two arbitrary points on the straight line. Suppose that the data were acquired through only 10 minutes and that it was desired to still calculate $t_{1/2}$, although the data do not decrease to $Y_0/2$ in only 10 min. Using two points on the estimated best-fit straight line (0, 7800) and (10, 4400) the decay constant is calculated as follows:

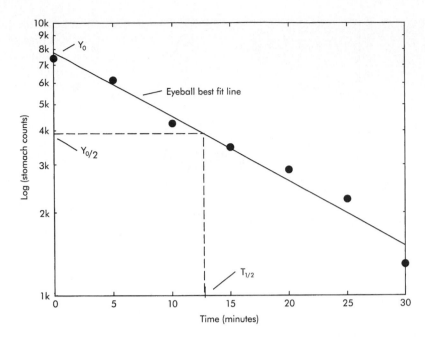

Figure 1-7   Measurement of effective $t_{1/2} = 12.5$ minutes in the stomach by visual estimate of best-fit line on semilog plot.

$$-\lambda = \frac{[\ln(4400) - \ln(7800)]}{[10\,\text{min} - 0\,\text{min}]} = \frac{-0.573}{10\,\text{min}}$$

so

$$\lambda = 0.0573\,\text{min}^{-1}$$

Then $t_{1/2} = 0.693/\lambda$ is calculated as 12.1 min, in close agreement with the graphic method above, which estimated $t_{1/2} = 12.5$ min.

Note that many nuclear medicine procedures yield graphs of counts versus time that do not follow a simple straight line on semilogarithmic plots. Several half-lives or several organs might be excreting a radiopharmaceutical from the body. It is then not correct to calculate a single $t_{1/2}$ from any data that do not appear to follow a straight line. Analysis of multiple half-life data requires other methods, such as curve stripping and nonlinear least squares.

Least Squares Curve Fitting

The technique of visually estimating the best-fit straight line is fraught with inaccuracy and imprecision because each observer's visual estimate line is unique. This could result in different values for the $t_{1/2}$, which is based on the straight line, or in different values for predicting a y value at any x value using the straight line fit to the data. A more mathematically precise method to fit the straight line to the data is the method of least squares, or linear regression.[1] In this technique a set of n data values at the points (x_i, y_i), where $i = 1 \rightarrow n$, is graphed and fitted with a mathematically exact technique. No imprecision occurs; every observer who uses this method obtains exactly same answer. This type of calculation is generally performed to show a linear relationship

between two variables or to predict some y variable based on measurement of some x variable.

Figure 1-8 shows data for x, y values from an experiment involving measurement of cardiac ejection fraction (EF) by two different techniques: a previously used method and the new method, which involves some change in experimental technique. Do these data show that the old method and the new method yield identical results? Or, given some value for ejection fraction by the old method (an x value), what would be the predicted results for ejection fraction by the new method (a y value)? The least squares method, or linear regression, calculates the best-fit values for y-intercept (a) and slope (b) in the best-fit straight line: $y = a + bx$. The intercept and slope parameters define a straight line as discussed previously. The least squares method calculates the a and b that minimizes the sum of the square of the distance in the y direction between the best-fit straight line and the data points. Use of a scientific pocket calculator can greatly speed calculations. Typically, a calculator requires the user to enter the first x value and press some key (e.g., Xi in Figure 1-1), telling the calculator this is x_1, to enter the corresponding first y value and tell the calculator this is y_1 (with the Yi key, see Figure 1-1); and to enter x_2, y_2, and so on, until all n data points have been entered. Then display the intercept and slope. Use of a computer is even simpler: the user enters x, y values in a spreadsheet format and instructs the computer to plot the data and the regression line. Almost all popular spreadsheet and graphics software packages offer linear regression (e.g., a personal computer [PC] spreadsheet program calculates and plots the best-fit line).

Calculation of the regression line by hand is tedious but not really complicated. The first step is the calculation of four sums based on the x, y data values. Then some simple

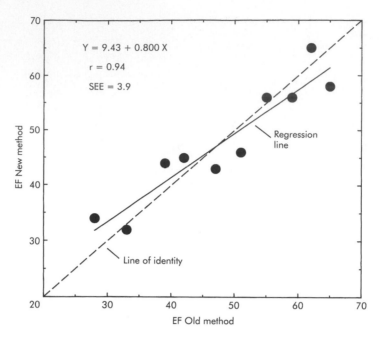

Figure 1-8 Regression analysis or least squares best-fit curve to compare old and new method for calculating ejection fraction *(EF)*.

Table 1-4	Linear regression: comparison of two methods for calculation of ejection fraction*	
Old method: x (%)		**New method: y (%)**
47		43
62		65
39		44
33		32
55		56
42		45
59		56
65		58
28		34
51		46

*$y = 9.43 + 0.800$ x; $r = 0.94$; standard error of the estimate (SEE) = 3.9.

multiplication and division produce the intercept and slope as follows. First calculate the four required sums, using the data for Figure 1-8, as shown in Table 1-4:

$$\Sigma x = x_1 + x_2 + \ldots + x_n$$
$$= 47 + 62 + \ldots + 51 = 481$$
$$\Sigma y = y_1 + y_2 + \ldots + y_n$$
$$= 43 + 65 + \ldots + 46 = 479$$
$$\Sigma xy = x_1y_1 + x_2y_2 + \ldots + x_ny_n$$
$$= 47(43) + 62(65) + \ldots + 51(46) = 24165$$
$$\Sigma x^2 = x_1^2 + x_2^2 + \ldots + x_n^2$$
$$= 47^2 + 62^2 + \ldots + 51^2 = 24543$$

Then the intercept and slope are calculated as:

$$a = \frac{[\Sigma x^2(\Sigma y) - \Sigma x(\Sigma xy)]}{[n(\Sigma x^2) - \Sigma x(\Sigma x)]}$$

$$a = \frac{[24543(479) - 481(24165)]}{[10(24543) - 481(481)]} = 9.43$$

and

$$b = \frac{[n(\Sigma xy) - \Sigma x(\Sigma y)]}{[n(\Sigma x^2) - \Sigma x(\Sigma x)]}$$

$$b = \frac{[10(24165) - 481(479)]}{[10(24543) - 481(481)]} = 0.800$$

The best-fit line is then given by:

$$y = 9.43 + 0.80(x)$$

This line is drawn onto the graph of y versus x by calculating two points at the endpoints of the regression line and then joining these points with a straight line. At $x = 20$ the best-fit line value of y is $9.43 + 0.80(20) = 25$; and at $x = 70$ the best-fit line value of y is $9.43 + 0.8(70) = 65$. The regression line has been drawn in Figure 1-8. Also shown in Figure 1-8 is the line of identity, which is the line with zero y-intercept and slope equal 1, defined by $y = x$. The line of identity is often drawn on regression graphs when the *same* parameter, here the ejection fraction, is being plotted on both the x and y axes. The line of identity facilitates an evaluation of whether the two methods (the x and y axes) are predicting the same result for ejection fraction. If the two methods produce the same value for ejection fraction, then the regression line should be the same as the line of identity. The line of identity is not a useful concept if the particular experiment being considered does not have identical

Table 1-5	Linear correlation coefficient r at a probability of P				

Number of data points	Probability (P)				
	0.10	**0.05***	**0.01**	**0.005**	**0.001**
5	0.805	0.878	0.959	0.974	0.991
10	0.549	0.632	0.765	0.805	0.872
15	0.441	0.514	0.641	0.683	0.760
20	0.378	0.444	0.561	0.602	0.679
30	0.306	0.361	0.463	0.499	0.570

*Minimum value of correlation coefficient for significant correlation is in this column. Larger r values are more highly correlated.

parameters on the x and y axes. A regression of blood pressure versus age, for example, would not use the line of identity.

So what does the regression equation predict in Figure 1-8? The old and new methods do not predict exactly the same ejection fraction since the predicted regression line does not coincide exactly with the line of identity. For any given old method result (the x value), the regression equation or graph can be used to predict what the new method would yield for an ejection fraction result. This prediction of a y value, based on some measured x value, is the goal of regression analysis. Figure 1-8 shows that the new method produces results greater than the old method for ejection fractions below about 47 by the old method because the regression line is above the line of identity. The new method underestimates the ejection fraction, compared with the old method, for ejection fractions greater than 47 by the old method.

Figure 1-8 also lists the value of goodness of fit parameters, which help determine whether it is reasonable that the data points are truly represented by a straight line. The linear correlation coefficient r is calculated from the sums used to find the intercept and slope, along with one additional sum from the data points (Σy^2):

$$r = \frac{n(\Sigma xy) - \Sigma x(\Sigma y)}{[n(\Sigma x^2) - \Sigma x(\Sigma x)]^{1/2}[n(\Sigma y^2) - \Sigma y(\Sigma y)]^{1/2}}$$

The sign of the correlation coefficient is merely the same as the sign of the slope. A correlation $r = 1$ is a perfect fit, with the straight line passing exactly through each data point. The closer r is to 1, the more highly correlated are the x and y data. A chance, or probability (P), always exists that data that are truly not linearly related to each other will randomly appear in a fairly linear fashion. The statistical significance of correlation values less than 1 must be evaluated from statistical tables of probability (Table 1-5). If the correlation value for the n data points shows a P value of less than 0.05 from the statistical tables, then the data are said to be linearly correlated. Figure 1-8 shows $r = 0.94$ for $n = 10$ data points, which from Table 1-5 has $P < 0.001$, so the data are

highly linearly correlated. If the r value was 0.632 or less (the $P = 0.05$ value for $n = 10$ from Table 1-5), then the data are not shown to be linearly correlated and it would not be prudent to suggest a best-fit straight line to the data. A statistically significant correlation (meaning an r-value with $P < 0.05$) merely implies a linear relationship between the x and y variables. This linear correlation or relationship does not necessarily imply that x causes y. A graph, for instance, of number of human babies (y) versus number of stork nests (x) would probably show a high correlation, but this does not mean storks bring babies. More likely, both x and y depend on some other variable, such as the number of people in the house: people have babies, people live in houses, storks build nests on these houses.

The use of Microsoft Excel for linear regression is quite straightforward. If 10 pairs of x,y data are known, as in Table 1-4, just enter these data into a new Excel spreadsheet with x values into column A, and y values into column B. Then click on cell C1 and type in the following:

$$= SLOPE(B1:B10, A1:A10)$$

Click on cell C2 and type in:

$$= INTERCEPT(B1:B10, A1:A10)$$

Click on cell C3 and type in:

$$= CORREL(B1:B10, A1:A10)$$

Note that Excel then calculates slope, intercept, and correlation coefficient into cells C1, C2, C3. You can now print the results, change the x,y data, and so on. If you change the x,y data values, note that the values for slope and other items will also change. You can now also quickly ask Excel to plot the data: highlight the block of cells containing the x,y data by painting a box around them by holding down the left mouse button. Then click on the Chart Wizard icon near the top of the desktop and select XY-Scatter for the type of plot. After the plot appears, you can ask Excel to add the linear regression line to the graph by doing the following: click on the center of the graph, click the word Chart at the top of the display, and then choose Add Trendine. The least-squares line will be added to your graph.

The other plus of fit parameter shown in Figure 1-8 is the standard error of the estimate (SEE), sometimes denoted S_{yx}, which is defined as follows:

$$SEE = [\Sigma(y - a - bx)^2/(n - 2)]^{1/2}$$

The SEE is the root mean square average deviation in the y direction of a data point from the regression line—that is, how far away the average data point is from the regression line in the y direction. In Figure 1-8, SEE = 3.9, so the average data point is about 4 units on the y axis from the regression line. Another interpretation of SEE might be that the old and new ejection fraction methods disagree, on average, by 4. A line that passes exactly through each data point produces $r = 1$ and SEE = 0, for a perfect fit. The SEE grows larger as the data points fall farther from the regression line. There is no easy way to state a P value for whether the SEE is small enough or not small enough to say the fit is statistically acceptable.

Least squares curve fitting could also be used to improve the precision of measurement of effective $t_{1/2}$ of data such as that shown in Figure 1-7. The calculation merely requires using the time as x values, and the ln (counts) as the y values in the regression equations. The best-fit line has a slope that is the decay constant λ, and the half-life is then $t_{1/2} = 0.693/\lambda$. This least squares fit eliminates the imprecision of visual-estimate best-fit lines.

Several other caveats are known regarding least squares curve fitting. The linear correlation coefficient r describes only the degree of *linear* relationship between x and y. Some exact *nonlinear* relationship may in fact exist between x and y that yields a nonsignificant linear correlation. Data generated from the relationship $y = x^2$ ($x = -2, -1, 0, 1, 2$ with corresponding $y = 4, 1, 0, 1, 4$) would produce the straight line fit $y = 0.0 + 2 \times x$, with $r = 0$. An exact relationship in fact exists between x and y, but it is not linear.

The least squares best-fit line intercept and slope values have ± standard error uncertainties, according to formulas available in statistics texts.[3] This results in a range of possible best-fit lines. A statistical uncertainty is actually in the predicted y value for any x value. These uncertainties in the predicted line can be used, for example, to ascertain whether the predicted regression line is really different from the line of identity, or the x and y values can be tested for difference using t-tests, as discussed in the following section.

Other Graphs

Another graph useful in nuclear medicine is a histogram, which is used to display a single list of numbers such as number of tests per month (Figure 1-9). Note that the y axis is displayed with a minimum value of 2000 rather than 0 to accentuate month-to-month differences. Another type of

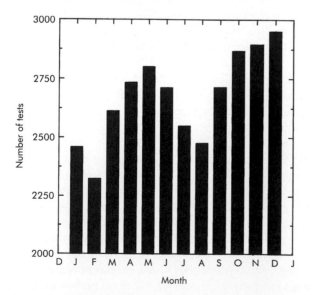

Figure 1-9　Histogram showing monthly variation in number of tests.

graph is the pie chart, which is typically used to present some whole object broken down into its component parts. The width of each slice of the pie is proportional to each component's percentage share.

STATISTICS

Mean and Standard Deviation

Statistical analysis in nuclear medicine allows us to consider such things as how confident we are of the accuracy of some measurement or how confident we are that a patient's test value is different from a normal result. Two concepts that often emerge in statistical considerations are *precision* and *accuracy*. *Precision* refers to the spread, or range, of data values obtained when some parameter is measured many times or in many patients. A small precision means that little variation exists in the data values. *Accuracy,* on the other hand, refers to how close the results are to the true, or "gold standard," result. Suppose that the length of a 96-inch long board is measured twice, obtaining results of 94 in and 98 in. These data could be called accurate because the average (or mean) value of the two yields the correct answer of 96 in. The large range of the data (94 to 98 in), however, would be considered not nearly precise enough for any practical construction measurements. Another person might measure the length of the board and obtain 96.25 and 96.50 in. These results are more precise (smaller range of data) but less accurate (the average is 96.37 in) than the previous measurement. A good measurement is both accurate and precise, but no necessarily fixed relationship exists between accuracy and precision in any experiment. Statistical parameters, such as the mean and standard deviation, allow quantification of the concepts of accuracy and precision.

Suppose that some parameter x is measured n times. Then the mean (or average) of the n values of the parameters x is defined by the symbol $\bar{x}$:

$$\bar{x} = \frac{\Sigma x}{n}$$

The symbol Σx means the sum of all the measurements of x.

As an example, a patient has four measurements of serum thyroxine (T_4, a thyroid hormone) given by 9.5, 9.0, 9.2, and 8.7 µg/dl. The mean value x is as follows:

$$\bar{x} = \frac{(9.5 + 9.0 + 9.2 + 8.7)}{4} = 9.1 \,µg/dl$$

If the true answer for the serum T_4 was known, then the mean value $x = 9.1$ µg/dl could be compared with the true value to discuss the accuracy of the test. The *standard deviation,* a measure of the precision of the data, is given by the symbol σ, defined as:

$$\sigma = [\Sigma(x - \bar{x})^2/(n - 1)]^{1/2}$$

Recall that an exponent of $\frac{1}{2}$ means the same as the square root ($\sqrt{\ }$). The standard deviation is a measure of the deviation or spread of the data points from the mean value. For the thyroid T_4 data above:

$$\sigma = \{[(9.5 - 9.1)^2 + (9.0 - 9.1)^2 + (9.2 - 9.1)^2$$
$$+ (8.7 - 9.1)^2]/[4 - 1]\}^{1/2}$$
$$\sigma = \{(0.16 + 0.01 + 0.01 + 0.16)/3\}^{1/2}$$
$$\sigma = \{0.34/3\}^{1/2} = 0.1133^{1/2} = 0.3366$$
$$\sigma = 0.3\,\mu g/dl, \text{ correctly rounded to one}$$
significant decimal place

The standard deviation is often expressed in a format of the mean value $\pm\sigma$, so this patient has a T_4 test result of $9.1 \pm 0.3\,\mu g/dl$. A large σ value indicates data with a large range and therefore poor precision.

Sometimes it is more useful to express standard deviation as a percentage of the mean value, which is frequently called the percent standard deviation, or *coefficient of variation* (CV):

$$CV = \left(\frac{\sigma}{\bar{x}}\right) \times 100$$

For the thyroid function data above:

$$CV = \left(\frac{0.3367}{9.10}\right) \times 100 = 3.7\%$$

The CV merely shows how large the standard deviation is when compared with the mean value. For example, consider two separate experimental measurements of the length of an object. Both experiments produce the same standard deviation of 2 cm, but the two objects have different mean lengths of 2 m and 2 km. So one experiment has a CV of (2 cm/200 cm) × 100, or 1%, whereas the other experiment has a CV of (2 cm/200,000 cm) × 100, or 0.001%. The standard deviations of the two experiments are the same, but the CVs are vastly different, showing a much better precision in the second experiment (CV = 0.001%) than in the first experiment (CV = 1%).

Microsoft Excel can conveniently be used to calculate statistical parameters. As an example, for the four values of T_4 discussed above, just enter these data values in cells A1, A2, A3, A4 in a new Excel spreadsheet. Then, in cell B1, type:

$$= \text{AVERAGE(A1:A4)}$$

In cell B2 type:

$$= \text{STDEV(A1:A4)}$$

In cell B3 type:

$$= \text{B2/B1}$$

Note the coefficient of variation is calculated in cell B3 as 0.036995, and the user must realize that this is 3.6995%, properly rounded to 3.7%.

As another example, consider two different blueberry farms. Suppose farm A has blueberries of diameter $6 \pm 7\,mm$ and farm B has blueberries of diameter $9 \pm 2\,mm$. From which farm would you rather have blueberries? It depends on what you want. Farm A has a wider range of blueberry diameters. Indeed, some farm A blueberries must be quite small or large to produce such a significant 7 mm standard deviation, but the average blueberry is only 6 mm at Farm A. Farm B has blueberries that are bigger (9 mm) on the average, but the standard deviation for Farm B is smaller, so few really big (or small) blueberries are at Farm B.

The scientific pocket calculator generally has keys for calculation of mean and standard deviation. The user enters the first data value and then pushes the key (e.g. X_i) that tells the calculator this is x_1. Then the second data value is entered and the X_i key is pushed again, telling the calculator this is x_2, and so on up to x_n. Then press the key to display the mean $\bar{x}$ and σ (sometimes denoted on calculators as σ_{n-1}).

Further calculations with statistics require consideration of the *theoretical distribution* of the data values. We may know that a sample of blueberries produces diameters of $9 \pm 2\,mm$, but suppose we want to know how many blueberries have diameters greater than 11 mm or what the probability is of getting a blueberry bigger than 13 mm. The theoretical distribution refers to a theoretical measurement of *all* the blueberries of Farm A, or of the T_4 values in *all* patients and so on. The distribution is a theoretical graph of how many blueberries there are with which diameters or of how many patients there are with a certain value of T_4. What is usually measured in an experiment is not the theoretical distribution but rather *a sample* of data values (say 20 blueberries or 10 patients) that is part of the whole theoretical distribution. Two types of theoretical distributions of data values are important in nuclear medicine: the *Gaussian distribution* and the *Poisson distribution*. Many measurable quantities can be described by a Gaussian distribution, whereas the only thing of interest to nuclear medicine that follows a Poisson distribution is counting statistics.

Gaussian Distributions

The Gaussian distribution is also called the *bell-shaped distribution* or the *normal distribution*.[3] In general, measurements of some parameter might be expected to follow a Gaussian distribution if a reasonably large sample is taken from a very large distribution, where the parameter being measured is expected to vary randomly. For example, the diameters of blueberries in a 1-gallon sample would be expected to follow a Gaussian distribution. The measurement of the decay counts of a sample of several thousand radioactive atoms (sampled from the distribution of about 10^{23} atoms in a small piece of radioactive material) would also be expected to follow a Gaussian distribution. Student scores on an examination might follow a Gaussian distribution. Saying that something follows a Gaussian distribution means that if the number of times a certain value occurs is plotted on the y axis versus the measured numeric value (e.g., blueberry diameter or number of counts) on the x axis, then a graph such as Figure 1-10 is obtained. Analysis

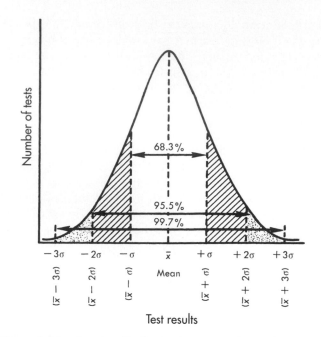

Figure 1-10 Gaussian distribution for test results can be expected to show the results in large population where test value is expected to vary randomly. Note that 68% of all test results are within the mean ±1 standard deviation ($\bar{x} \pm 1\sigma$), 95% of all test results are in the range of $\bar{x} \pm 2\sigma$, and so on.

reveals that a Gaussian distribution has 68% of all results within the range $\bar{x} \pm 1\sigma$, 95% of all results within $\bar{x} \pm 2\sigma$, and 99% within $\bar{x} \pm 3\sigma$. Figure 1-10 shows this distribution. Hence returning to the sample of blueberries, if $\bar{x} = 9\,mm$ and $\sigma = 2\,mm$, then if all the blueberries in the bucket are examined, we would expect the following:

68% within 7-11 mm	($\bar{x} \pm 1\sigma$)
95% within 5-13 mm	($\bar{x} \pm 2\sigma$)
99% within 3-15 mm	($\bar{x} \pm 3\sigma$)

The chance of getting a blueberry less than 5 mm, or greater than 13 mm, is only 5%. This is called *the area in the tails* (the ends) of the distribution. Because 95% are within $\bar{x} \pm 2\sigma$, it must be that only 5% are beyond the range $\bar{x} \pm 2\sigma$.

The properties of the Gaussian distribution are often used in quality control procedures and to determine normal ranges A quality control procedure might measure some daily parameter to determine whether an instrument is working properly. If today's value is beyond the $\bar{x} \pm 2\sigma$ value (based on previous measurements), then the instrument might be considered to be operating improperly because the probability of getting a result beyond $\bar{x} \pm 2\sigma$ is only 5%. This type of quality control, or normal value range determination, uses the 95% confidence interval (the $\bar{x} \pm 2\sigma$ range) as a conventionally accepted range. This means that a 1 in 20 (or 5%) chance exists that we will incorrectly reject what is in fact an acceptable quality control test or that a 5% chance exists that a normal subject would be incorrectly called abnormal. The preponderance of results, 19 out of 20 (95%), will be correctly classified.

Poisson Distributions and Counting Statistics

Counting statistics, meaning the number of counts expected from a sample, follow the Poisson distribution. In the Poisson distribution the standard deviation (σ_C) for any number of counts (C) is fixed at the square root of C:

$$\sigma_c = \sqrt{C}$$

This fixed definition of standard deviation does not exist in Gaussian distributions; essentially only counting statistics are Poisson. One farm could have a Gaussian distribution of blueberries of diameter $9 \pm 2\,mm$ (i.e., mean $\pm \sigma$), and another farm could have blueberries of diameter $9 \pm 4\,mm$. Neither farm has $\sigma = \sqrt{9}$. Any combination of a mean value and a standard deviation is possible in Gaussian data, whereas Poisson counting statistics always have the standard deviation of the counts from a sample equal to the square root of the counts.

EXAMPLE: What is the standard deviation of a sample that produced 10,000 counts?

$$\sigma_c = \sqrt{10,000} = 100\,counts$$

EXAMPLE: What is the coefficient of variation of 10,000 counts?

$$CV = \left(\frac{\sigma_c}{C}\right) \times 100 = \left(\frac{100}{10,000}\right) \times 100\% = 1\%$$

EXAMPLE: What is the σ and CV for 100 counts?

$$\sigma_c = \sqrt{100} = 10\,counts$$
$$CV = \left(\frac{\sqrt{100}}{100}\right) \times 100\% = 10\%$$

These examples show that, as the number of counts increases from 100 to 10,000, the absolute magnitude of the standard deviation goes up (from 10 to 100 counts), but the percent standard deviation or CV goes down (from 10% to 1%). Less relative variability occurs in large count values.

Counting statistics, besides being Poisson, are also described by a Gaussian distribution as long as the number of counts is greater than about 30. Hence given some number of counts C, we automatically know the standard deviation. We also know that 68% of repeat measures of the sample falls within $C \pm \sqrt{C}$ and 95% of repeat measures of the sample fall within $C \pm 2\sqrt{C}$, and so on.

EXAMPLE: A sample with 10,000 counts. What is the 95% confidence interval for this sample?

$$95\% \text{ confidence} = C \pm 2\sigma_c = C \pm 2\sqrt{C}$$
$$= 10,000 \pm 2\sqrt{10,000}$$
$$= 10,000 \pm 200\,counts$$

The 95% confidence interval is then from 9800 to 10,200 counts. If this represents a sample of the counts actually emanating from radioactive material, we can say we are 95% sure that the true counts from this radioactive material are in the 9800 to 10,200 range (or we would expect that 95%

of repeat measurements would be in the range 9800 to 10,200 counts). The number of counts actually emitted by a radioactive source varies from time to time, in a random fashion, according to both Poisson and Gaussian distributions. The variation in the number of counts is often referred to as *counting noise*.

Sometimes this type of problem is expressed by saying that 10,000 counts are needed to be 95% confident that the true count is within 2% of the measured value. The presence of two different percentage values can seem confusing. The 95% confidence interval on 10,000 counts is ±200 counts, and this figure of 200 counts represents 2% of 10,000 counts. The general formula expressing the number of counts needed to be $n\sigma$ sure that the true answer is within some percent (p) of the measured counts is given by:

$$C = \left[\frac{n}{\left(\dfrac{p}{100\%}\right)} \right]^2$$

In this formula n is replaced with a 1 for 68% confidence, a 2 for 95% confidence, and a 3 for 99% confidence.

EXAMPLE: How many counts are needed to be 95% sure that the true answer is within 1% of the measured value? Here $n = 2$ and $p = 1\%$.

$$C = \left[\frac{2}{\left(\dfrac{1\%}{100\%}\right)} \right]^2 = \left[\frac{2}{.01}\right]^2 = 40,000 \text{ counts}$$

If this sample were recounted, then 95% of repeat measurements would be in the range $40,000 \pm 2\sqrt{40,000}$ or $40,000 \pm 400$, which represents a 1% uncertainty (because 400 is 1% of 40,000). Some radiation counters may have a preset count dial labeled as the percent error at the 95% confidence level, rather than a preset count dial actually labeled in number of counts. Setting such a preset count dial at 1% error would be the same as collecting 40,000 counts. Setting such a preset count dial at 5% would mean collecting 1600 counts, since:

$$1600 = \left(\frac{2}{0.05}\right)^2$$

Some problems may deal with the count *rate* R that is obtained by counting a number of counts, C, in time, T:

$$R = \frac{C}{T}$$

The standard deviation in the count rate is σ_R:

$$\sigma_R = \left(\frac{\sqrt{C}}{T}\right)$$

This presumes that no error occurs in measurement of the time T. By using $C = RT$, the σ_R can be alternatively written as the following:

$$\sigma_R = \frac{[\sqrt{(RT)}]}{T} = \sqrt{\left(\frac{R}{T}\right)}$$

EXAMPLE: A sample shows 43,627 counts in 5 minutes. What are the count rate and standard deviation in the count rate?

$$R = \frac{43,627 \text{ counts}}{5 \text{ min}}$$

$$R = \frac{8725 \text{ counts}}{\text{min}} = 8725 \text{ cpm}$$

$$\sigma_R = \frac{(\sqrt{43,627})}{5} = 42 \text{ cpm}$$

Hence the count rate would be expressed as 8725 ± 42 cpm.

EXAMPLE: The count rate is 8765 cpm for a 2-minute count. What range of count rates would be predicted to occur in 68% of repeat measurements? This is simply asking what is the value of σ_R because $1\sigma_R$ is the 68% confidence interval.

$$\sigma_R = \sqrt{(R/T)} = \sqrt{(8765/2)} = \sqrt{4382.5} = 66 \text{ cpm}$$

If the experiment were then repeated, we would predict that 68% of the repeat measurements would be in the range 8765 ± 66 cpm.

Background counts are a problem in most measurements of counts from a radioactive sample. Background arises from natural terrestrial and cosmic sources of radioactivity or from other nearby sources of radioactive material. The sample is usually counted in the presence of some background radiation, yielding a gross count for sample plus background, denoted by the letter C. Then the sample is removed from the counter and the background B is counted. The net, or true counts, which represents the sample only, is denoted by N and given by:

$$N = C - B$$

The standard deviation of the net counts is given by

$$\sigma_N = \sqrt{(C + B)}$$

This is an example of the rules for combinations of errors,[1] which states that for addition or subtraction, errors add in quadrature within the square root:

$$\sigma_N = \sqrt{(\sigma_C^2 + \sigma_B^2)}$$

Additionally, since $\sigma_C = \sqrt{C}$ and $\sigma_B = \sqrt{B}$, we obtain $\sigma_N = \sqrt{(C+B)}$.

EXAMPLE: A sample is counted in the presence of background yielding $C = 1600$ counts. Then the background is counted alone, producing 900 counts. What are the true or net counts and standard deviation?

$$N = C - B = 1600 - 900 = 700 \text{ counts}$$

$$\sigma_N = \sqrt{(1600 + 900)} = \sqrt{2500} = 50 \text{ counts}$$

Hence the net counts can be expressed as 700 ± 50 counts. Note that the presence of background has increased the statistical uncertainty in the results. If there were *no* background, the sample in this example would have produced $N = 700 \pm \sqrt{700} = 700 \pm 26$ counts.

Similar considerations can yield the rules for the net count *rate*:

$$R_N = R_C - R_B = C/T_C - B/T_B$$
$$\sigma_{R_N} = \sqrt{(\sigma_{R_C}^2 + \sigma_{R_B}^2)}$$
$$\sigma_{R_N} = \sqrt{(C/T_C^2 + B/T_B^2)}$$

or

$$\sigma_{R_N} = \sqrt{(R_C/T_C + R_B/T_B)}$$

Chi-Square Tests

Suppose we wish to test the reliability of operation of some counting instrument, as a quality control test, by confirming that the instrument always produces the same counts in a reliable fashion. How can we do this when we now know that the number of counts recorded will vary from measurement to measurement because of the statistical nature of radioactive decay? The answer is to count a sample a reasonable number of times (typically 10 repeat measurements are used) and then determine if the 10 different values show a suitable amount of variation. Too little or too much variation in the repeat measurements indicates a counter that may not be functioning properly. The chi-square (χ^2) test is used to determine an acceptable range of variability in the repeat measurements. The mean $\overline{C}$ of the 10 measurements is determined ($\overline{C} = \Sigma C/n$), and χ^2 is calculated as:

$$\chi^2 = \frac{[\Sigma(C - \overline{C})^2]}{\overline{C}}$$

Table 1-6 shows the calculation of χ^2 for some counter, which yielded a value of 24.7 for χ^2. Is this an acceptable amount of variation between the 10 measurements? The definition of acceptable χ^2 is given by looking up the probability (P) of this χ^2 value for the n (here 10) repeated measures in Table 1-7. Too little variation is shown by a χ^2 smaller than the $P = 0.9$ value; an amount of variation exactly as expected from the statistical nature of the decay process would yield $P = 0.50$; and an unacceptably large χ^2 would yield a P value greater than 0.10:

If $0.90 > (P \text{ of } \chi^2) > 0.10$, detector is OK.
If $(P \text{ of } \chi^2) > 0.90$, the detector shows too little variation.
If $(P \text{ of } \chi^2) < 0.10$, the detector exhibits too much variation.

For the data in Table 1-6, χ^2 was calculated = 24.7. In Table 1-7, this $n = 10$ measurement has a P value < 0.01, so this detector is *not* operating properly; the χ^2 is too large, the detector is showing too much variation in counts. The detector probably needs to be repaired. An acceptable χ^2 for 10 measurements would be in the range: $4.17 < \chi^2 < 14.7$ because this is the $0.90 > P > 0.10$ range. Here again it is only common convention that fixes the $P = 0.90 - 0.10$ range as acceptable. Some laboratories might be willing to accept more variation, or they may be willing to use $0.95 - 0.05$ as the acceptable P range for χ^2.

Notice the similarities in statistical approach for calculating the linear correlation coefficient r and χ^2. Both are calculated from the data based on some equation, and then the P value of the r or χ^2 is determined to assess significance of the result. This is typical of most statistical tests: calculate a parameter and then look up the probability of this result.

Table 1-6	Calculation of Chi-square		
Observation	Counts (C)	Deviation $(C - \overline{C})$	Square $(C - \overline{C})^2$
1	10,324	144.7	20,938.1
2	10,285	105.7	11,172.5
3	9,847	−332.3	110,423.3
4	10,168	−11.3	127.7
5	10,352	172.7	29,825.3
6	10,234	54.7	2,992.1
7	9,986	−193.3	37,364.9
8	10,139	−40.3	1,624.1
9	10,356	176.7	31,222.9
10	10,102	−77.3	5,975.3
	$\Sigma = 101,793$	$\Sigma = 0$	$\Sigma = 251,666$

$\overline{C} = 10179.3$
$\chi^2 = \Sigma(C - \overline{C})^2/\overline{C}$
$\chi^2 = \dfrac{251,666}{10,179.3} = 24.7$
$SD = [\Sigma(C - \overline{C})^2/(n - 1)]^{1/2}$
$SD = (251,666/9)^{1/2} = 167.2$

Table 1-7	Chi-square value at probability P						
Number of sample measurements	Probability (P)						
	0.99	0.95	0.90*	0.50	0.10†	0.05	0.01
5	0.30	0.71	1.06	3.36	7.78	9.49	13.3
10	2.09	3.33	4.17	8.34	14.7	16.9	21.2
15	4.66	6.57	7.79	13.3	21.1	23.7	29.1
20	7.63	10.1	11.7	18.3	27.2	30.1	36.2

*Smallest acceptable χ^2 is in this column.
†Largest acceptable χ^2 is in this column.

Does the result for the data in Table 1-6 seem sensible, that the detector is showing too much variation? Consider that we know that a properly operating detector should have 68% (about seven out of 10) of repeat measurements within the mean count $\pm \sqrt{(\text{mean count})}$. So the deviation $C - \overline{C}$ in Table 1-6 should be less than 1σ, less than $\pm\sqrt{10179.3} = 101$ counts, in seven out of 10 measurements. Examination of Table 1-6 shows that only four of the measurements (instead of the expected seven) have deviations from the mean within $\pm1\sigma$, or within ±101 counts. Too many measurement values are beyond $\pm1\sigma$. The detector is not working properly by this crude visual check, in agreement with the too large a χ^2 value. Similar visual checks can be made to assess that only one out of 20 measurements should have deviations from the mean of more than $\pm2 \times 101$ counts. In fact, Table 1-6 shows that one measure is a deviation of -333 counts (about 3σ) and another is almost 2σ (actually -193 counts), so about two out of 10 are beyond $\pm2\sigma$ in contrast with the predicted one out of 20 measurements with this much variation. The calculated P value of χ^2 will always agree with such common sense data checks.

Lastly, a word about calculating χ^2. Most scientific pocket calculators do not have a calculation function for χ^2, but most calculators can calculate the standard deviation of the repeat count measurements, here denoted as SD:

$$SD = \left[\frac{\Sigma(C - \overline{C})^2}{(n - 1)} \right]^{1/2}$$

This can be algebraically solved for $\Sigma(C - \overline{C})^2$:

$$\Sigma(C - \overline{C})^2 = (n - 1) \times (SD)^2$$

This is simply the numerator of the definition of χ^2, so the equation for χ^2 can be written in terms of the mean and SD as the following:

$$\chi^2 = (n - 1) \times \frac{(SD)^2}{\overline{C}}$$

To calculate χ^2, therefore, the pocket calculator (or the PC computer spreadsheet program) is used as described previously to calculate the SD and the mean, which are then used in the above equation for χ^2. The data in Table 1-6 show $SD = 167.2$ with a mean $\overline{C} = 10179.3$, so:

$$\chi^2 = \frac{(10-1) \times (167.2)^2}{10179.3} = 24.7,$$

exactly as obtained previously in Table 1-6.

To use Microsoft Excel to calculate χ^2, using the data of Table 1-6, just enter the data into cells A1 through A10 in a new Excel spreadsheet. In cell B1, type the number 10, or the number of data points. In cell C1 type:

$$= (B1-1)*STDEV(A1:A10)^\wedge 2/AVERAGE(A1:A10)$$

Excel then places the value of χ^2 in cell C1.

The χ^2 statistic, in other algebraic definitions, has other uses besides a test for stability of counters in nuclear medicine. Chi-squared is commonly used in 2×2 contingency tables,[3] which could consider, for example, the number of persons who are well or ill, tabulated according to being male or female. Alternatively, a categorization could be made of the number of persons with positive or negative imaging tests using gamma cameras from two different manufacturers. A χ^2 calculation would show whether the two gamma cameras find different or same numbers of positive/negative test results.

t-Tests

The *t*-test is used to test for differences between *mean* values.[3] This test is also commonly referred to as the Student *t*-test because the original proposal for this test was published by an author using the pseudonym *Student*. The two forms of the *t*-test are for *independent* samples and *paired* samples.

For independent *t*-tests, two independent groups of data are used. For example, some test result is measured in a group of n_1 ill patients and a group of n_2 well patients. The two groups are completely independent. No relationship or correlation exists between the two groups, typically because the groups represent different patients. The two groups have mean and standard deviations denoted by $\bar{n}_1$, SD_1, $\bar{n}_2$, and SD_2.

The *t*-test is a test of a null hypothesis that the mean values in the two groups are equal. The hypothesis being tested can be abbreviated H_0: $\bar{n}_1 = \bar{n}_2$. The null hypothesis is statistical nomenclature, meaning that no difference is found. This test is called a *two-tailed test* because either group could be equally expected to have the larger mean value. The calculation of the *t*-test requires no new algebraic details from the data; the *t*-test result is simply calculated from the means and standard deviations in the two groups as follows:

$$t = (\bar{x}_1 - \bar{x}_2)/$$

$$\left\{ \frac{[(n_1 - 1) \times SD_1^2 + (n_2 - 1) \times SD_2^2] \times \left(\frac{1}{n_1} \times \frac{1}{n_2} \right)}{n_1 + n_2 - 2} \right\}^{1/2}$$

The calculated t is then compared with tabulated values of the critical *t*-test (Table 1-8) with $n_1 + n_2 - 2$ degrees of freedom (ν) at the $P = 0.05$ level:

If $t \leq t_{n1+n2-2, 0.05}$—then the study does not reject H_0: $\bar{n}_1 = \bar{n}_2$, and no statistically significant difference is shown between the two groups.

$t > t_{n1+n2-2, 0.05}$—then the hypothesis H_0: $\bar{n}_1 = \bar{n}_2$ is rejected, and the difference between the two groups is said to be statistically significant.

EXAMPLE: One group of $n_1 = 6$ patients is given a drug, and their thyroid T_4 levels (8.8, 8.7, 9.2, 8.6, 8.5, 9.0) have $\bar{n}_1 = 8.80$ and $SD_1 = 0.26$. A second group of $n_2 = 5$ patients is given a placebo, and their T_4 results (8.3, 8.5, 8.2, 8.1, 8.4) have $\bar{n}_2 = 8.3$ and $SD_2 = 0.16$. Is there a difference in T_4 levels between the two groups? Did the drug affect T_4 level?

$$t = (8.80 - 8.30)/$$

$$\left\{ \frac{[(6-1) \times (0.26)^2 + (5-1) \times (0.16)^2 \times \left(\frac{1}{6} + \frac{1}{5}\right)]}{(6+5-2)} \right\}^{1/2}$$

$$t = \frac{0.50}{\left\{ \frac{[0.4404] \times (0.3667)}{9} \right\}^{1/2}}$$

$$t = \frac{0.50}{\{0.01794\}^{1/2}} = 3.73$$

From Table 1-8 the critical t value at the 5% or 0.05 level with $n_1 + n_2 - 2 = 9$ degrees of freedom is $t_{9,0.05} = 2.26$. Because calculated t is greater than critical t, we conclude that a statistically significant difference exists between the drug and placebo groups. The drug *did* make a statistically significant difference. In fact, the statistical tables show the critical t statistic at the 1% level $t_{9,0.01} = 3.25$, so we are actually more than 99% confident that a difference exists between the drug group and the placebo group because calculated t is greater than $t_{9,0.01}$. We can also say that less than a 1% likelihood exists that the difference between the drug and placebo groups is the result of a chance occurrence rather than because of the drug.

Most PC-type computer software packages (spreadsheets, statistics software) offer calculation capabilities of t-tests for which the user simply enters two columns of data values and selects an independent or paired t-test. The PC calculates the t-test result and the associated probability, sparing the user from any tedious calculations. In using such software it can be helpful to enter some test data, such as from the examples given here, to insure that the software produces the same t-test and probability value as in the examples given here. Alternatively, the t-test can be performed as in the example here, after first using the pocket calculator to calculate the means and standard deviations of the two groups as discussed above. To use Microsoft Excel for an independent t-test, for the T4 data example above: enter the first group's set of data values in column A (cells A1, A2, ..., A6), enter the number of data points for the first group in cell B1 (i.e., for the T4 example data above, enter the number 6 in cell B1), enter the data values for the second group in cells C1 through C5, enter the number 5 in cell D1 (representing the number of data values in the second group). Then click on cell E1 and type in:

$$= \text{TINV}(E2, B1 + D1-2)$$

Click on cell E2 and type in:

$$= \text{TTEST}(A1:A6, C1:C5, 2, 2)$$

In the Excel equation above for TTEST, the numbers 2, 2 are telling Excel to do an independent two-tailed t-test. Excel then places the t-statistic (3.73) in cell E1, and the probability P (0.00466) for this t-statistic in cell E2. If P is ≤ 0.05, then we reject H_0 and a statistically significant difference becomes evident between the two groups. If $P > 0.05$, then we cannot reject H_0; we failed to find a statistically significant difference between the two groups. In this example, the P value of 0.00466 is < 0.01, so we can say even more stringently that we reject H_0 at the 1% level and that we are more than 99% sure that the differences between the two groups are not caused by chance, just as concluded by our hand calculations above.

A special term, *standard error,* is used when referring to the variability in *mean* values. The standard error (SE) governs the variability of repeated measurements of the *mean* value, whereas the standard deviation (SD) governs the variability of any one *individual* patient measurement. The results of an experiment to measure a mean value usually is expressed as $\bar{x} \pm$ SE, rather than $\bar{x} \pm$ SD, although this is not universal practice and confusion occurs if the specification of SE or SD is not made clear. The SE is given by:

$$\text{SE} = \text{SD}/\sqrt{n}$$

The data in the t-test example above would most commonly be specified as mean ± standard error:

$$\text{Drug group mean} = 8.80 \pm 0.11 \, \mu\text{g/dl}$$
$$\text{Placebo group mean} = 8.30 \pm 0.07 \, \mu\text{g/dl}$$

Stating the data in this manner helps compare the means in the two groups. A graphic representation often shows the individual data values as dots on the graph, with a separate symbol for the mean. The mean symbol on the graph often includes ± standard error bars, drawn as vertical lines of length equal to 1 SE above and below the mean value. The t-test is essentially a measure of how far apart the mean values are, measured in terms of their standard errors.

A paired t-test is used for testing differences between two mean values when the data are from the *same* patient. For example, a group of n patients could have their ventricular ejection fraction measured before (x_1) and after (x_2) taking

Table 1-8	t-Test Value at Probability P			
Degrees of Freedom (ν)	Probability (*P*)			
	0.10	0.05*	0.01	0.001
4	2.13	2.78	4.60	8.61
5	2.01	2.57	4.03	6.87
6	1.94	2.45	3.71	5.96
7	1.89	2.36	3.50	5.41
8	1.86	2.31	3.36	5.04
9	1.83	2.26	3.25	4.78
10	1.81	2.23	3.17	4.59
15	1.75	2.13	2.95	4.07
20	1.72	2.09	2.84	3.85
30	1.70	2.04	2.75	3.65
60	1.67	2.00	2.66	3.46
∞	1.64	1.96	2.58	3.29

*Minimum value of t-test for significant difference is in this column. Larger t values imply a more significant difference.

some drug. The ejection fractions before and after drug administration are correlated; a patient with a large ejection fraction before drug administration could also be expected to have a large ejection fraction after drug administration. What matters in paired data is the difference $d = x_1 - x_2$ between any two values. The difference between the first and second measurement is tabulated in each patient to calculate the mean difference $\overline{d}$:

$$\overline{d} = \frac{\Sigma(x_1 - x_2)}{n}$$

The standard deviation of the difference (SDD) is defined in the following:

$$SDD = \left\{ \frac{\Sigma(d - \overline{d})^2}{(n - 1)} \right\}^{1/2}$$

Note that the algebraic sign, either + or −, of the difference (*d*) in each patient must be carefully used in calculating $\overline{d}$ and SDD. Then the paired *t*-test tests the null hypothesis that no mean difference exists between the first and second measurements, $H_0: \overline{d} = 0$, by comparing the calculated *t*-statistic, $t = \overline{d} / (SDD/\sqrt{n})$, to the critical *t* value at the 0.05 level with $n - 1$ degrees of freedom ($= t_{n-1, 0.05}$). If $t > t_{n-1, 0.05}$, no difference is shown between the two measurements. If $t > t_{n-1, 0.05}$, a statistically significant difference exists between the first and second measurements. If the calculated *t* is just greater than the critical *t* with $n - 1$ degrees of freedom at the *P* confidence level (e.g., $P = 0.05, 0.01, 0.005, 0.001$, and so on), then we say that a difference is shown between the two measurements at the *P* confidence level.

Table 1-9 shows calculation of $\overline{d}$ and SDD for the old versus new ejection fraction data from Table 1-4. Note carefully how the algebraic sign (+ or −) of d and $d - \overline{d}$ is considered in Table 1-9. The null hypothesis being tested is $H_0:$ old EF = new EF. The calculated $t = 0.14$ is much less than the critical *t* value ($t_{9, 0.05} = 2.26$) from Table 1-8, so the conclusion is that no statistically significant difference exists between the old and new EF values; we cannot reject H_0. This is another way of saying that the linear regression line in Figure 1-8 is not statistically different from the line of identity.

To use Microsoft Excel for a paired *t*-test, proceed to enter the data values exactly as described above for using Excel for an independent *t*-test. For the example data of Table 1-8, there would be 10 data values in column A and 10 data values in column C. Cells B1 and D1 would both be entered as 10, but now enter the Excel formulas as follows: Click on cell E1 and enter:

$$=TINV(E2, B1\text{-}1)$$

Click on cell E2 and enter:

$$=TTEST(A1\text{:}A10, C1\text{:}C10, 2, 1)$$

The *2, 1* in the Excel TTEST equation here is telling Excel to do a two-tailed paired *t*-test. Excel places the *t*-statistic (0.14) in cell E1 and the *P* value (0.89) in cell E2. Because *P* is >0.05, we cannot reject the null hypothesis, we failed to find any difference between the two ejection fraction methods, which is exactly as concluded by our hand calculation method above.

Note that a *t*-test (for either independent or paired data) either fails to show a statistically significant difference ($t \geq t$-critical) or does show a statistically significant difference ($t > t$-critical). A *t*-test that fails to show a difference does *not* prove that the two mean values are equal[3], it merely indicates that the data are inadequate to prove a difference exists. A semantic nuance that may be encountered is that independent *t*-tests consider the difference between the means, whereas a paired *t*-test considers the mean of the differences.

If more than two mean values are involved, the simple *t*-test is not appropriate. For example, we might wish to know whether a difference exists between the means of a test value in four independent groups of patients The null hypothesis is ($H_0: \mu_1 = \mu_2 = \mu_3 = \mu_4$). This test requires a method called *analysis of variance (ANOVA)* to most powerfully find differences between the four groups. ANOVA also offers various methods for testing not just for whether all the means are the same but also for testing for differences between pairs of the mean value. Alternatively to ANOVA, but less powerfully for finding differences, the data can be tested for all pairs of differences with a *t*-test using the Bonferroni method, which requires lowering the significant *P* value from 0.05 to 0.05/*n*, where *n* is the number of possible tests. For four groups of patients are six possible *t*-tests: group 1 versus 2,3,4; group 2 versus 3,4; group 3 versus 4. We could do all six *t*-tests and claim a significant difference only between pairs of mean values with a *t* value larger than the critical *t* value at the $0.05/6 = 0.0083$ *P* value.

Table 1-9	Paired *t*-test Data			
EF old method	**EF new method**	**Difference (d = old − new)**	**d − $\overline{d}$**	**(d − $\overline{d}$)²**
47	43	4	3.8	14.44
62	65	−3	−3.2	10.24
39	44	−5	−5.2	27.04
33	32	1	0.8	0.64
55	56	−1	−1.2	1.44
42	45	−3	−3.2	10.24
59	56	3	2.8	7.84
65	58	7	6.8	46.24
28	34	−6	38.44	−6.2
51	46	>5	4.8	23.04
		$\overline{d} = 0.2$		sum = 179.60

SDD = $[\Sigma(d - \overline{d})^2/(n - 1)]^{1/2}$
    = $[179.6/(10 - 1)]^{1/2}$
    = $[19.96]^{1/2} = 4.47$
$t_9 = \overline{d}/(SDD/\sqrt{n})$
    = $0.2/(4.47/\sqrt{10}) = 0.14$

Medical Decision Making

Medical decision making would not be necessary if medical tests always produced a result that correctly identified the patient as either ill or well. Unfortunately, because of the diversity of biologic response, possible statistical noise in data, and other technological deficiencies, a medical test often produces identical results for ill and well patients. Therefore by some, often somewhat arbitrary method, we establish a test result normal range for well people and then say that results outside this normal range indicate illness.

For example, suppose we measure T_4 thyroid hormone in a group of well people and find the mean ±2 SD normal range is from 4 to $12\,\mu g/dl$. We then define any subsequent patient test as normal or euthyroid for $4 \geq T_4 \geq 12$ and hyperthyroid for $T_4 > 12$. However, isn't this a little foolish? A patient with $T_4 = 11.9$ is labeled well, whereas a patient with $T_4 = 12.1$ is labeled ill, even though the difference in the two values may be within the limit of accuracy of the experimental technique. This is because most test values indicate a continuum of results, not a *yes* or *no* answer, as in pregnancy. What about a patient image test that produces an image that looks suspicious—not quite clearly normal but not extremely abnormal? We can call the image test either positive (*yes,* it shows a defect) or negative (*no,* defect is shown). What are the consequences of being a lax image reader (who calls lots of positive studies) versus a strict image reader (who requires very strong abnormal image characteristics before calling an image positive)? These are some of the questions that medical decision making can consider.

A test that finds a result for which the test was performed is called a *positive test.* A positive test for hyperthyroidism would be a $T_4 > 12\,\mu g/dl$. A positive myocardial perfusion imaging test would be a patient image with a cold defect in the heart. A positive ^{99m}Tc bone scan would be a patient image with a hot spot in the bone. The test result might be low, high, cold, or hot, but it is positive for the condition being tested for.

A test that does not show the tested-for result is called a *negative test.* A T_4 result in the euthyroid (normal) range would be a negative test for hyperthyroidism. A myocardial perfusion scan with no defects in the heart image would be a negative scan for coronary artery disease. Note carefully that the positive or negative value refers to the *test* result; positive or negative is not defined by the patient's clinical condition.

The patient condition can be similarly categorized as either well or ill. This categorization must be obtained from some test *other than* the one being considered as the nuclear medicine test with positive or negative results. The patient condition is usually established as well or ill through some other medical test called the *gold standard test.* A patient, for example, could have either a positive or a negative myocardial perfusion imaging test, and the true state of the patient, as well or ill, is usually established from some other clinical

test such as coronary angiography. An imaging phantom study could have an image result that is called either *positive* or *negative,* and the true gold standard result is the known fact about whether the phantom contains an imaging abnormality or defect. Some presentations of this subject material might use the terms normal and abnormal in lieu of well and ill.

Given these definitions, all of the following material relates to placing each patient's test result into one of four categories:

1. *True positive (TP):* persons with a positive test result who are truly ill
2. *False positive (FP):* persons with a positive test result who are not ill
3. *True negative (TN):* persons with a negative test result who are truly well
4. *False negative (FN):* persons with a negative test result who are not well

A woman with a positive pregnancy test who is actually pregnant is called a *TP result.* If the pregnancy test result was negative but the woman is actually pregnant, then the result is an FN result. More typically, in nuclear medicine a decision is made to call an image test positive if the image shows some agreed-on defect. Then patients are categorized as TP, FP, TN, or FN by combining their nuclear medicine image test result with that of some other gold standard clinical test. A patient with a negative myocardial perfusion imaging test (no abnormal defects on the image study) who is known to have coronary artery disease would be called an *FN test* result. A phantom study that calls the image positive, in an area of the phantom where a lesion definitely exists would be a TP result.

Now consider the following test results. A study of imaging tests in 1000 patients produced the following data:

	Test Result	
	(−)	(+)
Well	836 = TN	44 = FP
Ill	26 = FN	94 = TP

From these categorized data we can derive several other parameters that define the usefulness of the test.

The *sensitivity,* or *true positive fraction (TPF),* is the percentage or fraction of ill patients who have a positive test:

$$\text{Sensitivity} = \text{TPF} = \frac{\text{TP}}{(\text{TP} + \text{FN})}$$

For the above data:

$$\text{Sensitivity} = \frac{94}{(94 + 26)} = 78\%$$

meaning that the study found a positive test result in 78% of the ill people. Note the distinction between similar appearing symbols, TP and TPF.

The *specificity,* or *true negative fraction (TNF),* is the percentage or fraction of well patients who have a negative test:

$$Specificity = TNF = \left(\frac{TN}{TN + FP}\right)$$

For the above data:

$$Specificity = \frac{836}{(836 + 44)} = 95\%$$

meaning that the study found a negative test result in 95% of the well people. Again, note the distinction between similar appearing symbols, TN and TNF. (The decision on whether to use the term sensitivity or TPF, and specificity or TNF is purely arbitrary.) The above data show a sensitivity of 78%, less than the specificity of 95%, which means that this test does a better job at correctly diagnosing well people than it does at correctly diagnosing ill people.

The ideal medical test would have sensitivity and specificity both equal 100%. Unfortunately, medical data usually appear as in Figure 1-11, with an overlap between the test results for the well and ill patient populations. Which is more important, a high sensitivity (correctly finding ill people), or a high specificity (correctly finding well people)? The answer to this question is complex, often depending on the medical/economic/social consequences of the test. If the imaging test is intended to detect brain tumors that are known always to be fatal, but for which a simple medical cure with no side effects can be found even in well people, then a high sensitivity might be preferred. The consequences of misdiagnosing an ill person would be death, whereas the consequences of misdiagnosing a well person would be a harmless drug regimen. On the other hand, suppose the consequence of finding a positive result in an imaging scan was immediate total frontal lobotomy, which would prolong the patient's life by only a few months. Given the dire consequences of treatment, a high specificity would be preferred to avoid misdiagnosis in well patients.

Another factor that affects the most desirable sensitivity and specificity of a test is the prevalence of disease. The *prevalence* is the fraction or percentage of ill persons in the study population:

$$Prevalence = \frac{(TP + FN)}{(TP + FN + TN + FP)}$$

The above data had a prevalence of:

$$\frac{(26 + 94)}{(26 + 94 + 836 + 44)} = 12\%$$

meaning that 12% of the study subjects were ill.

The prevalence is characteristic of the patient population; prevalence is not a characteristic of the test itself. Prevalence is shown graphically in Figure 1-11 by the area under the ill curve compared with the area under both the ill and well curves. The relative heights of the ill and well curves show the prevalence, which can vary from one hospital to another. If the prevalence is high, many sick people are present, and the optimum test may be one that gives priority to a high sensitivity at the expense of lowered specificity (we can more easily afford a few FP errors in the small number of well people). To the contrary, a screening test for some rare disease operates in a patient population with a low prevalence, where the optimum test may be one that gives priority to a high specificity at the expense of lowered sensitivity

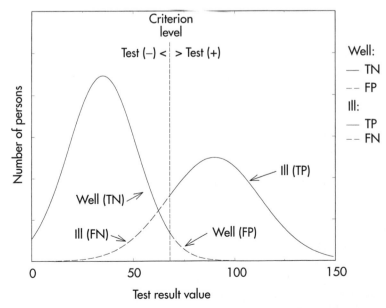

Figure 1-11   Distribution of test results for two groups: well (D–) and ill (D+). Test result is called *negative (T–)* or *positive (T+)* depending on whether it is below or above criterion level. Note that the well and ill populations overlap, creating well persons who are either TN or FP, and ill persons who are either TP or FN.

to avoid a large number of FP results in the preponderance of well people.

A parameter that specifies the total number of correct answers, regardless of being ill or well, is the *accuracy* of the test.

$$Accuracy = \frac{(Total \ number \ correct)}{(Total \ number \ of \ persons)}$$

$$= \frac{(TN + TP)}{(TN + TP + FP + FN)}$$

The above data show an accuracy of:

$$\frac{(836 + 94)}{(836 + 94 + 44 + 26)} = 93\%$$

meaning that the test correctly diagnosed 93% of all patients as ill or well. One problem is that the accuracy of a test depends strongly on the prevalence of disease for the same sensitivity and specificity of a test. This means that the accuracy between two hospitals can be very different for the same test because the prevalence at the two hospitals can be very different. Accuracy can be written specifically in terms of sensitivity, specificity, and prevalence as:

Accuracy = (Sensitivity × Prevalence) +

Specificity × (1 − Prevalence)

where prevalence is expressed as a fraction, not a percent.

Using these parameters for defining the goodness of a test, consider the following situation. A patient has a positive test result on some nuclear medicine study. We know this must be either a TP result in a truly ill person, or an FP result in a truly well person. The referring physician simply wants to know what is the probability of disease, given the positive test result? We can give the referring physician a wealth of parameters about the goodness of our *test*: the sensitivity = 78%, specificity = 95%, prevalence = 12%, accuracy = 93%. However, these parameters do not answer the clinical question at hand: what is the chance that this patient, who had a positive test result, is truly ill? We need a parameter that deals with the clinical usefulness of the test, not just goodness-of-the-test parameters such as sensitivity.

The *positive predictive value,* or *predictive value of a positive test* P(D+ : T+) can be read as the conditional probability of having disease (D+), given a positive test result (T+). This is merely the fraction of persons with positive test results who are truly ill:

$$P(D+:T+) = \frac{TP}{(TP + FP)}$$

For the above data:

$$P(D+:T+) = \frac{94}{(94 + 44)} = 68\%$$

meaning that the answer to the referring physician's question is that only a 68% chance exists that the patient with the positive test result is truly ill. Of course this means that

a 32% chance exists that the patient with this positive nuclear medicine test result is not ill. These considerations are a reflection of a mathematical concept called Bayes theorem, after Thomas Bayes (1702-1761), an English mathematician and theologian. It allows us to recalculate the probability of illness based on the new information of a positive test result. Before the nuclear medicine test, the chance that the patient had disease was simply the prevalence (often referred to as the pre-test probability of disease) of 12%. After a positive test, however, the probability of disease has jumped to a post-test probability of 68%.

Conversely, the *negative predictive value,* or *predictive value of a negative test* P(D− : T−) is the probability P of not having disease (D−), given a negative test result (T−), or the fraction of all persons with a negative test who are truly well:

$$P(D-:T-) = \frac{TN}{(TN + FN)}$$

For the above data P(D− : T−) = 836/(836 + 26) = 97%, meaning that a patient with a negative nuclear medicine test result has a 97% chance of being truly well. Note Bayes theorem at work here. Before the nuclear medicine test, the patient had a (1-prevalence), or 88% chance of being well (the pre-test probability of wellness was 88%). After a negative nuclear medicine test the post-test probability that the patient is truly well has jumped to 97%.

In all of the discussion so far, we have not touched on how the patient's true condition, well or ill, is determined from some gold standard test. Calculation of all the parameters (such as TN, FP, sensitivity, specificity, or accuracy) requires that we know, from some other test, who is truly ill or well. Hence when evaluating the goodness of test results such as sensitivity, it is always necessary to ask what was used for the gold standard to define illness. Two hospitals may have vastly different parameters for sensitivity and specificity, not because of any difference in the nuclear medicine test result, but rather because the two hospitals define illness in different terms. For example, an invasive procedure such as coronary angiography is often used as a gold standard to calculate the sensitivity and other parameters of nuclear medicine myocardial perfusion imaging, but there may be no commonly agreed-on definition of illness in the gold standard test. One hospital might say that the test must show coronary arteries narrowed by only 40% for a diagnosis of illness, but a second hospital might say that a patient is not ill until the gold standard coronary angiography test shows more than 70% narrowing of the coronary arteries. This difference in gold standard conbines with the characteristics of the nuclear medicine test to produce different sensitivities and other parameters at the two hospitals.

When calculating sensitivity, for example, it is necessary to carefully define the test criterion level that characterizes a positive test. One hospital may say a positive test for hyperthyroidism is any $T_4 > 10.5 \, \mu g/dl$, whereas another hospital may say $T_4 > 12.5 \, \mu g/dl$ is a positive test result. Different sensitivity values result. In fact, when we receive information from the diagnostic test, we can operate with any criterion level we choose to define a positive test. A lax criterion level (e.g., calling a nuclear medicine study positive with just a hint of abnormality in the image) leads to high sensitivity and low specificity. If we want a high sensitivity, we can call all tests positive, resulting in sensitivity = 100%. Of course, there would then be no TN tests, so the specificity would be zero. Want a high specificity? Just call every test negative, resulting in specificity = 100% (but sadly, sensitivity = 0).

As the criterion level that defines a negative or positive test result is moved left or right in Figure 1-11, the sensitivity and specificity change accordingly. Sensitivity and specificity then are not parameters fixed as constants in nature, by some inherent property of a test, or by an image reader's skill level. Rather, sensitivity and specificity depend on the gold standard used to define illness *and* on the criterion level that defines a positive test. In Figure 1-11, if we slide the criterion level to the right so that it is stricter in calling a positive test result, the sensitivity decreases while specificity increases. Slide the criterion level to the left so that it becomes more lax in defining a positive test, and the sensitivity improves while specificity worsens. To further guide our thinking in these matters we often plot a *receiver operating characteristic (ROC) curve,* which shows sensitivity and specificity as a function of the criterion level used to call a test positive.

An ROC curve is shown in Figure 1-12. The y axis is the sensitivity, and the x axis is the specificity. Note that the x axis is inverted in the sense that it *decreases* left to right from 100% to 0% specificity. (An alternate labeling for the axes of an ROC curve will have true positive fraction [TPF] from 0 to 1 on the y axis, and false positive fraction [FPF] from 0 to 1 on the x axis.) The ideal point for a test result would be the upper left corner of the ROC curve in Figure 1-12, with sensitivity = 100% and specificity = 100%.

An ROC curve is a graphic representation of the effect of changing the criterion level, just as we moved the criterion level left or right in Figure 1-11. A wealth of information can be gleaned from an ROC curve concerning which sensitivity/specificity is the optimum operating point—that is, what optimum criterion level should be used to call a test positive. No definitive answers may be available, but the ROC curve clearly shows the available options. The ROC curve is still dependent on prevalence and the gold standard test to define illness. Suppose that a planar imaging study is reported in the literature with specificity = 61% and sensitivity = 86%. Another study in the literature reports a tomographic study with specificity = 82% and sensitivity = 64%. Which is the better test: planar or tomographic?

We cannot say which test is better *unless both* sensitivity and specificity are improved in one of the tests. In fact, these data could represent the same test results; the difference could simply be from a changed criterion level for calling a test result positive. The hospital with the planar data could be calling a test result positive with a lower degree of image abnormality, leading to improved sensitivity but worsened specificity. We cannot clearly say which test is better without seeing the entire ROC curve for both the planar and tomographic data.

To form an ROC curve from any data we simply tabulate the TP, FN, TN, and FP results to calculate sensitivity and specificity for each criterion level that defines a positive test. For an in vitro T_4 blood test we just calculate sensitivity and specificity using different criterion levels for a positive test (e.g., calculate sensitivity and specificity for T+ defined as $T_4 \geq 0$, as $T_4 \geq 1$, as $T_4 \geq 2$, and so on). Then a plot of sensitivity versus specificity at the various criterion levels yields the ROC curve. Image data are somewhat different because a quantifiable numeric result for imaging studies is not always available. Hence a rating scale is typically employed to score an image from 1 to 5 as follows:

Image Score	Meaning
1	Definitely normal image
2	Probably normal image
3	Possibly abnormal image
4	Probably abnormal image
5	Definitely abnormal image

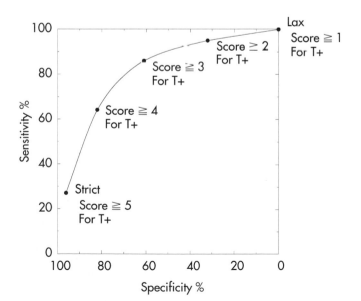

Figure 1-12 ROC curve showing sensitivity and specificity as function of minimum image score needed to call image positive. Note x axis for specificity reads left-to-right, from 100 to 0. A lax reader might call any image with score ≥2 positive, with high sensitivity and low specificity. A strict reader would require high score to call image positive, resulting in low sensitivity and high specificity. Best overall test operates near upper left corner of ROC curve.

Suppose we had an imaging study with 50 patients. From some other gold standard test we know which patients are truly ill or well: 28 are well, and 22 are ill. A reader scores each image as above. The sensitivity and specificity can be calculated from the TN, FP, FN, and TP results for each criterion level as follows:

Positive test = score ≥	TN	FP	FN	TP	Specificity (%)	Sensitivity (%)
1 (lax)	0	28	0	22	0	100
2	9	19	1	21	32	86
3	17	11	3	19	61	86
4	23	5	8	14	82	64
5 (strict)	27	1	16	6	96	27

Figure 1-12 is an ROC curve for these data. The planar and tomographic results above *could* represent just two different operating points on this single ROC curve. The planar test could have been called abnormal for an image score ≥3, whereas the tomographic data may have been called a positive test only for a stricter image score ≥4. Alternatively, a difference in ROC curves could be noted for the planar and tomographic results, but this could be ascertained only from seeing the entire ROC curve for both studies.

A medical test cannot be judged solely on sensitivity and specificity because these parameters are a strong function of the definition of the test criterion level used to call a test positive. The ideal operating point on the ROC curve could be at the upper left corner, with sensitivity equaling 100% and specificity equaling 100%. In general, the test that is closest to this ideal is the better test, so the best operating point (at what score to call a test positive) may be the one that results in an operating point closest to the upper left corner of the ROC curve. Alternatively, as discussed previously, considerations of prevalence of disease and consequences of diagnosis may suggest favoring sensitivity over specificity, or vice versa. It is also common to see two different ROC curves characterized by the area under the ROC curve, denoted by A_z. The highest A_z value is used to define which test is best because a higher A_z value means that the ROC curve is closer to the ideal operating point in the upper left corner of the ROC curve.

REVIEW QUESTIONS (answers appear on p. 598)

1. The radiation intensity from a point source of ^{99m}Tc is 9 mR/hr at 3 m from the source. If the distance is changed to 9 m, what is the new radiation intensity?
   a. 0.5 mR/hr
   b. 1.0 mR/hr
   c. 2.0 mR/hr
   d. 3.0 mR/hr

2. A technologist is sitting near a bone mineral densitometer, which is a point source of x-rays. If the x-ray intensity at 1 m from the x-ray beam is 0.20 mR/hr, what distance from the x-ray beam should the technologist move to decrease total weekly exposure to the occupational limit of 2 mR for a 40-hour workweek?
   a. 0.5 m
   b. 1.5 m
   c. 2.0 m
   d. 2.5 m

3. A radioactivity of 10 mCi is equal to how many Becquerels?
   a. 370 Bq
   b. 370 kBq
   c. 370 MBq
   d. 370 Gbq

4. A radioactivity of 20 mCi is equal to how many Becquerels?
   a. 0.74 GBq
   b. 0.37 GBq
   c. 0.54 GBq
   d. 0.20 Gbq

5. The dose equivalent for occupational whole-body exposure is commonly limited to 50 mSv. How many rem is this?
   a. 5000 rem
   b. 500 rem
   c. 50 rem
   d. 5 rem

6. A source of ^{131}I ($t_{1/2} = 8.05$ d) is delivered to the nuclear medicine department calibrated for 100 mCi at 0800 on Monday. If this radioactivity is injected into a patient at noon on the following Tuesday, what radioactivity will the patient receive?
   a. 80 mCi
   b. 85 mCi
   c. 90 mCi
   d. 95 mCi

7. A patient was injected with ^{131}I on Monday at 10:00 AM. On Tuesday at 10:00 AM the thyroid probe was placed over the thyroid and produced were 100,000 counts. On Thursday at 10:00 AM the probe showed 25,000 counts. What is the effective half-life in this patient's thyroid?
   a. 12 hr
   b. 24 hr
   c. 48 hr
   d. 72 hr

8. A ^{99}Mo/^{99m}Tc generator is eluted Monday at 7:00 AM, producing 1.8 Ci of ^{99m}Tc in the eluate vial, in 20 ml saline. What volume of eluate should be withdrawn from the eluate vial into a syringe in order to inject a patient with 20 mCi of ^{99m}Tc at 3 PM? (Given the $t_{1/2}$ of ^{9m}Tc is 6.02 hr.)
   a. 0.56 ml
   b. 0.66 ml
   c. 0.76 ml
   d. 0.86 ml

9. If the HVL for some radionuclide in lead is 0.30 mm, what thickness of lead shielding is necessary to reduce the radiation exposure from 8 mR/hr to 1 mR/hr?

    a. 0.30 mm
    b. 0.45 mm
    c. 0.60 mm
    d. 0.90 mm

10. The linear attenuation coefficient in lead for ^{99m}Tc gamma rays (140 keV) is 23 cm^{-1}. What percentage of these gamma rays will be absorbed by a lead apron that contains 0.60 mm of lead?

    a. 75%
    b. 50%
    c. 25%
    d. 12.5%

11. A new gamma camera/computer system that uses a new method of calculating cardiac ejection fraction (EF) is installed in a nuclear medicine department. The department decides to calculate EF for the next 25 patients on both the old gamma camera and the new gamma camera before discontinuing the use of the old camera. In the future, if it desired to convert the new EF value to that which would have been obtained on the old gamma camera (e.g., to assess if the patient's EF had changed), the mathematical analysis to be used is called:

    a. Independent t-test
    b. Linear regression
    c. Standard error
    d. Chi-square

12. What is the standard deviation of 40,000 counts?

    a. 4000 counts
    b. 2000
    c. 400
    d. 200

13. What is the coefficient of variation of 40,000 counts?

    a. 2%
    b. 1%
    c. 0.5%
    d. 0.25%

14. How many counts should be acquired into each pixel of a nuclear medicine flood image if we wish to be 95% confident that the true count in each pixel is within 1% of the measured counts in each pixel?

    a. 100,000 counts
    b. 40,000
    c. 10,000
    d. 4000

15. A patient's thyroid is counted with the thyroid probe and produces 8,000 counts. Then the patient is removed and background is found to be 2000 counts. The (net counts) ± (standard deviation in the net counts) in this patient is:

    a. 10,000 ± 100 counts
    b. 10,000 ± 77 counts
    c. 6000 ± 77 counts
    d. 6000 ± 100 counts

16. The gamma camera seems to be producing erratic results. A ^{57}Co flood source is counted 10 times, producing the following count values (1000, 975, 1032, 1096, 982, 997, 1012, 1090, 994, 977). What is the χ^2 value for these counts?

    e. 19.3
    f. 18.3
    g. 17.3
    h. 16.3

17. Which expression describes the operation of the gamma camera in question 16?

    a. Operating properly
    b. Showing too much variation
    c. Showing too little variation
    d. Not enough information to answer the question

18. One group of 20 patients is given a drug that is thought to have an effect on kidney function, and another group of 20 patients is given a placebo (i.e., sugar pill, which is known not have an effect on kidney function). The nuclear medicine gamma camera is used to calculate the glomerular filtration rate (GFR) in these two groups of patients. What would be the proper statistical test to use to test the hypothesis that no difference in GFR exists between these two groups of patients?

    a. Chi-square test
    b. Paired t-test
    c. Independent t-test
    d. Linear regression analysis

19. A nuclear medicine test produces a positive test result in only 80 of the 100 patients known to be ill. Similarly, the test produces a negative test result in only 190 of the 200 patients known to be not ill. Which is correct?

    a. Sensitivity = 80%, specificity = 95%, accuracy = 90%, prevalence = 33%
    b. Sensitivity = 90%, specificity = 95%, accuracy = 90%, prevalence = 33%
    c. Sensitivity = 90%, specificity = 80%, accuracy = 90%, prevalence = 33%
    d. Sensitivity = 90%, specificity = 80%, accuracy = 70%, prevalence = 33%

20. One radiologist is known to be a lax reader compared with another radiologist who is known to be a strict reader. In comparing these radiologists, how would you expect their sensitivity and specificity to compare?

  a. The lax reader would have lower sensitivity and higher specificity
  b. The lax reader would have higher sensitivity and lower specificity
  c. The readers would be expected to have the same sensitivity and specificity
  d. Not enough information to answer the question

REFERENCES

1. Bevington PR: *Data reduction and error analysis for the physical sciences,* New York, 1991, McGraw-Hill.
2. Bushberg JT et al: *The essential physics of medical imaging,* ed 2, Philadelphia, 2002, Lippincott Williams and Wilkins.
3. Colton T: *Statistics in medicine,* Philadelphia, 1975, Lippincott Williams and Wilkins.

chapter **2**

Paul E. Christian

Physics of Nuclear Medicine

Objectives

Describe the properties of electromagnetic radiation.

Describe the structure of the atom and its components and their properties.

Explain the structure of the chart of the nuclides and define the line of stability.

State the relationship of mass and energy in Einstein's equation.

Write the correct form of radionuclide notation.

List the nuclear families and state their characteristics.

Name and describe the primary forms of radioactive decay.

Diagram the schematics of the various radioactive decay processes.

Define decay constant.

Use the general form of the radioactive decay equation to calculate precalibration and postcalibration quantities of radioactivity.

List the radioactive units and define curie and becquerel.

Write the equations for average half-life and effective half-life and calculate effective and biologic half-lives.

Describe the interactions of charged particles with matter.

Discuss the processes of excitation and ionization.

Explain annihilation and the resultant products.

Describe the photoelectric effect and explain the processes.

Describe Compton scattering and explain the resultant products of this process.

Describe pair production and explain the resultant products of this process.

Discuss the production of characteristic x rays.

Describe the process of the production Auger electrons.

Write the general form of the attenuation equation for gamma photons.

Calculate the reduction of gamma radiation using the general attenuation equation.

State the relationship between the linear attenuation coefficient and half-value layer.

Physics is the study both of matter and energy and of the properties, forces, and interactions that influence the behavior of matter. Nuclear medicine applies the principles of physics to all aspects of radioactive decay, to the interaction of radiation and matter, and to the detection and measurement of properties and quantity of radiation and radiation protection. A basic understanding of these principles is critical to the use of radioactive materials and radiation-detecting instrumentation.

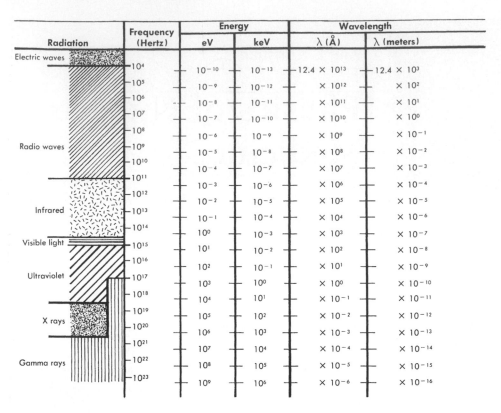

Figure 2-1 Electromagnetic spectrum.

ELECTROMAGNETIC RADIATION

Heat waves, radio waves, infrared light, visible light, ultraviolet light, and x rays and gamma rays are all forms of electromagnetic radiation (Figure 2-1). They differ only in frequency and wavelength. Longer wavelength, lower frequency waves (heat and radio) have less energy than the shorter wavelength, higher frequency waves (visible light, x and gamma rays). The wave properties of light were first shown by Christian Huygens in 1678 in his experiments with the separation of light into the color spectrum. The particulate characteristics of light were not appreciated until the experiments and research of Einstein, Planck, and Milliken in the early 1900s. Although electromagnetic energy has no mass, at very high frequencies it behaves more as a particle does, whereas at lower frequencies it behaves more as a wave does. The best way to think of electromagnetic radiation is as a wave packet called a photon. Photons are chargeless bundles of energy that travel in a vacuum at the velocity of light, c, which is 3×10^{10} cm/sec^{-1} or 186,000 miles/sec^{-1}.

The wave nature of electromagnetic radiation is symbolized by the Greek letter *lambda*, λ. Note that the Greek lambda used to refer to electromagnetic radiation should not be mistaken for the radioactive decay constant, discussed later. Electromagnetic waves, as their name indicates, consist of fluctuating fields of electric and magnetic energy. Figure 2-2 shows the pattern of the wave cycle. Since light travels at a constant velocity, the oscillating electromagnetic field wavelength and frequency are related by the equation:

$$c = \lambda \nu$$

where λ is the wavelength, ν is the frequency, and c is the velocity of light. The time for one wave period, or cycle, is measured in cycles per second, called hertz. Planck described the relationship of the electromagnetic wave frequency to the energy as:

$$E = hf$$

where f represents the frequency of the electromagnetic wave and h is Planck's constant, 6.625×10^{-27} erg.s/cycles. This equation can be manipulated to relate to energy and wavelength as:

$$E = \frac{12.4}{\lambda}$$

This equation expresses the energy in electron volts (eV) to the wavelength measured in angstroms (10^{-8} cm). The relationship indicates that very short wavelength photons have high energy and vice versa.

ATOMS AND MOLECULES

Matter is anything that occupies space and has mass. Ancient Greek philosophers theorized that all matter was composed of small indivisible pieces, which they called atoms. An atom is the smallest quantity of an element (e.g., hydrogen, carbon, oxygen) that retains all the chemical properties of that element. Atoms cannot be broken into smaller particles

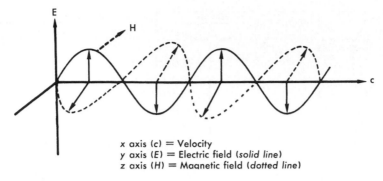

x axis (c) = Velocity
y axis (E) = Electric field (*solid line*)
z axis (H) = Magnetic field (*dotted line*)

Figure 2-2   Component energy fields of electromagnetic wave.

without losing their chemical properties. They are classified by their characteristics of weight, number of subparticles, and chemical properties. Two or more atoms may combine to form a molecule. A molecule is the smallest particle of a chemical compound that retains all the chemical characteristics of that compound. Molecules can have as few as two or as many as hundreds of atoms; therefore tens of thousands of different chemical compounds can be created by changing the number of atoms or the configuration of atoms within the molecule.

The atom is made up of two basic parts, the nucleus and the orbital electrons. A simple representation of an atom is a structure similar to a miniature solar system (Figure 2-3). This elementary model of an atom divides the atom into two portions: nuclear (in the center) and extranuclear (the surrounding area). Three principal types of subatomic particles compose an atom—protons, neutrons, and electrons. The nucleus is composed of two types of these particles—protons and neutrons; hence protons and neutrons are called *nucleons*. The nucleus is a cluster of these particles and gives the atom most of its mass.

The extranuclear region of the atom is the area outside the nucleus and is mostly empty space with electrons that orbit the nucleus like planets revolving around the sun. This region of the atom, especially the outermost electrons, is responsible for all chemical interactions with other atoms, and is the area in which most of the interactions of radiation and matter occur.

In 1960 the International Unions of Pure and Applied Physics and Chemistry set the standard substance physical scale to the carbon 12 (^{12}C) atom, whose mass is defined to be exactly 12.00000 atomic mass units (amu). All other atomic and particle weights are measured from the ^{12}C atom.

Basic discussions of the composition of atoms are limited to the fundamental particles: electrons that orbit the nucleus and the particles in the nucleus, protons, and neutrons. Particle physics describes several families that hold many dozens of subatomic particles. For example, protons and neutrons are in the family called hadrons; electrons and neutrinos are in a family of "light" mass particles called leptons; and photons are in a group called bosons.

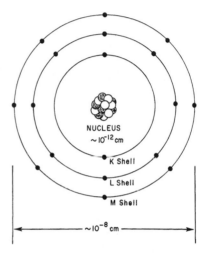

Figure 2-3   Bohr's atomic model with central nucleus surrounded by extranuclear region.

In 1964 Murray Gell-Mann and George Zweig proposed that the hundreds of particles known at that time might be composed of combinations of three simpler fundamental particles that they called "quarks" (Figure 2-4). Experiments since that time have shown that there are actually six quarks that compose subatomic particles.

Fortunately, for our purposes we can describe the composition of the atom and the processes of radioactive decay using the most common particles.

Electrons

Electrons are the smallest of the subatomic particles and are found in the extranuclear region of the atom. Electrons are also called negatrons and are given the symbol e or e^-. They have one negative unit of charge (1.6×10^{-19} coulombs) and a small mass of 9.1×10^{-28} g, or 0.000549 amu, and travel at about one tenth the velocity of light. Because they carry a negative charge, they are deflected by electric or magnetic fields. Their mass allows them to have kinetic energy that is proportional to the square of their velocity. Electrons are

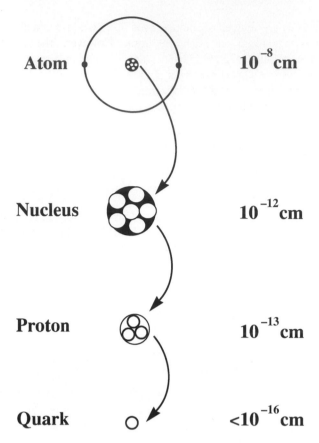

Atom	10^{-8} **cm**
Nucleus	10^{-12} **cm**
Proton	10^{-13} **cm**
Quark	$<10^{-16}$ **cm**

Figure 2-4   Size of the components within an atom.

held in their orbits around the nucleus by binding energy, which in conjunction with their motion and centrifugal force keeps them from being attracted into the positively charged nucleus. An electrically neutral atom has an equal number of protons and electrons.

Protons

Protons are found within the nucleus of an atom and are symbolized by the letter p or p^+. They have one positive unit of charge, which is equal but opposite to the charge of the electron. The protons within the nucleus provide its positive charge. The proton has a mass of 1.67×10^{-24} g, or 1.00759 amu, which is 1835 times that of an electron. The total number of protons is the atomic number, symbolized by the letter Z, and defines the element: for example, one proton is hydrogen, two protons is helium, three protons is lithium.

Neutrons

A neutral particle within the nucleus of the atom had been theorized by Rutherford in 1920, but neutrons were not experimentally found until 1932 by Chadwick. Neutrons are slightly heavier than protons, have no electric charge, and have a mass of 1.00898 amu. For simplification, the mass of a neutron and a proton are considered to be the same—1 amu. Neutrons are symbolized by the letter n.

For our purposes we can consider that a neutron is a combination of a proton and an electron. Neutrons are unstable particles, and break down into the simpler more stable particles of a proton, an electron (beta-minus particle), and a neutrino. This instability of the neutron is the source of one type of radioactive decay. The decay process and the resultant particles are discussed later.

ATOMIC STRUCTURE

The model of the atom described by Neils Bohr in 1913 is one of the most easily understood representations. This miniature solar system has mostly empty space with the electrons in orbit around a small central nucleus. Three subatomic particles are used in this model. The electrons occupy specific orbits, or shells, around the center nucleus. The electron shells are labeled K, L, M, N, O, P, and Q (see Figure 2-3), beginning with the innermost, the K shell. Specific amounts of energy hold each electron in its orbit. The innermost electrons are more tightly bound to the nucleus, and therefore more energy is required to remove them. Outer electrons are more loosely bound and require only smaller amounts of energy to be removed. Electrons can be removed from their orbits only by overcoming the *binding energy* for that shell. Binding energies are greatest for the innermost electrons, and the binding energy of specific electron shells is greater in heavier elements.

The electrons do not actually revolve around the nucleus in circular orbits in one plane; they move around the nucleus in a spherical pattern. Collectively, the electrons swarming about the nucleus form an electron cloud. Individually, the electrons change their distance from the nucleus and can even occasionally pass right through the nucleus.

Remember that the chemical properties of the atom are determined by the outermost electrons. The number of electrons that can occupy each orbit is limited. The formula $2n^2$ defines the number of atoms that can be contained in the major shells, where n is the shell number. For example, the K shell can contain only two electrons; the second shell can contain no more than eight; the third shell may contain 18; the fourth shell 32 electrons, and so on. Each major shell is composed of several subshells.

The nucleus of an atom has an approximate diameter of 10^{-12} cm (see Figure 2-3) and is composed of a cluster of protons and neutrons. Most of the matter in the atom is located here; therefore the density of the nucleus is extremely high. Particles in the nucleus—protons and neutrons—are known as *nucleons*. The simplest atom, hydrogen, consists of one proton, no neutrons, and one orbital electron. The second element, helium, has a nucleus consisting of two protons, two neutrons, and two orbital electrons. More complex atoms have an increased number of protons and neutrons. In approximately the first 20 elements, the ratio of neutrons to protons is 1:1; however, elements with atomic numbers greater than 20 have more neutrons than protons to maintain nuclear stability. Very

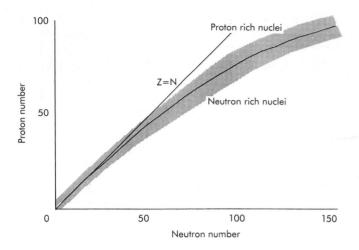

Figure 2-5   Neutron-proton ratio with line of nuclear stability.

large atoms will have a neutron-to-proton ratio of 1.6 : 1 (Figure 2-5).

As with electrons in the extranuclear orbit structure of the atom, the protons and neutrons in the nucleus are bound there with a specific amount of energy. Stability of the nucleus is determined by the total binding energy of nucleons in addition to the number and configuration of the proton-neutron arrangement. Protons and neutrons tend to pair up, creating a more stable nucleus, depending on the neutron-to-proton ratio. Nucleons move about within the nucleus and occupy certain energy states. Some nuclei hold additional energy in a nearly stable, or metastable, state. The nucleus can emit this extra energy in a manner called an isomeric transition, with the emission of electromagnetic radiation (gamma ray).

MASS-ENERGY RELATIONSHIP

In Einstein's equation $E = mc^2$, c represents the velocity of light measured in centimeters per second, m is mass measured in grams, and E is energy measured in ergs. According to this equation, matter can be converted into energy, and conversely, energy can create matter. This equation applies to a mass that is not moving and is therefore termed the *rest mass* of a particle of matter. When matter is converted to energy, the type of energy produced is of a form that is not imparted to or held by matter, such as heat or binding energy. Rather, it is pure energy, electromagnetic radiation.

The rest mass of an electron, 9.1×10^{-28} g, can be found by this equation to be equivalent to 0.511 MeV. Also, the rest mass of a proton can be found to be 931 MeV, and the rest mass of a neutron 939 MeV. This relationship is further defined in the discussions of radioactive decay and the interaction of radiation and matter.

Mass Defect

The relationship between mass and energy can be observed in the strong nuclear forces that exist in the nucleus. The sum of the masses of the nucleons in a ^{12}C atom is defined and measured as 12.00000 amu. However, the mass of a proton is 1.00759 amu; the mass of a neutron is 1.00898 amu; and the mass of an electron is 0.00054 amu. There are six protons, six neutrons, and six electrons in this atom, or a total mass of the individual particles of:

$6 \times 1.00759 = 6.04554$

$6 \times 1.00898 = 6.05388$

$\underline{6 \times 0.00054 = 0.00324}$

12.10266 amu

Since the carbon atom weighs 12.00000 amu, a difference of 0.10266 amu has been converted into binding energy of the particles in the nucleus. The difference in mass of the constituent particles and the total mass is called the **mass defect**. This amount of mass converts to 95.62779 MeV of nuclear binding energy. Particles can be removed from the atom only by expending a force greater than the binding energy.

Nuclear Stability

The number of protons and neutrons that form all possible configurations of the nucleus are graphed in Figure 2-5. Any configuration of protons and neutrons forming an atom is called a **nuclide**. Of the approximately 1500 nuclides, most are unstable and spontaneously release energy or subatomic particles in an attempt to reach a more stable state. This nuclear instability is the basis for the process we call *radioactive decay*. Approximately 280 of the nuclides are in a stable form, comprising only 83 elements. The remainder of the approximately 1500 nuclides are radioactive and are termed *radionuclides*.

The cause of nuclear instability stems from the energy configuration of the protons and neutrons in the nucleus. Although we might think of the structure of the nucleus as being like a cluster of grapes, each nucleon has a certain energy state. For one specific radionuclide there are a specific release of particles and a specific amount of energy released by its unstable atoms in this decay process. For example, ^{131}I always decays by emitting beta-minus (β^-) particles and gamma rays of specific energies. From radioactive decay, each radionuclide has its own "fingerprint" of characteristic radiation.

In Figure 2-5 the approximately 280 stable nuclides follow along the center of the line of stability with radionuclide forms located on either side of this line. Radionuclides above the line of stability represent a region with a relative abundance of protons, termed *proton-rich* (or *neutron-poor*) *nuclei*. Radionuclides in this region achieve nuclear stability primarily by undergoing the decay processes of positron emission or electron capture. Radionuclides below the line of stability in the *neutron-rich (or proton-poor)* area undergo a radioactive decay process called *beta decay* in which a neutron becomes a proton followed by a release of a beta particle from the nucleus.

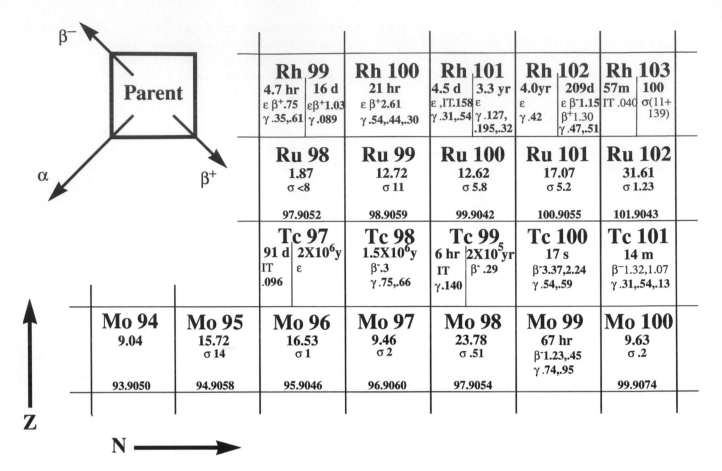

Figure 2-6 Section from the chart of nuclides.

Some radionuclei are in a metastable form. These radionuclides carry a slight amount of excess nuclear energy, which can be emitted as electromagnetic radiation to allow the atom to reach a more stable form.

The plotting of nuclides by their number of protons (vertical axis) and neutron number (horizontal axis) is the basis for the *chart of the nuclides* (Figure 2-6). This chart contains all possible nuclides, both stable and unstable radioactive forms. The chart is useful in identifying daughter decay products from a particular radionuclide or series of decays. Each nuclide is represented in a small square containing information such as the half-life, decay mechanism, and radiation type and energy.

NUCLEAR NOTATION AND NUCLEAR FAMILIES

There is a standard notation in the physical sciences for representing elements with a one- or two-letter chemical name symbol; it is taken primarily from the Greek names of the elements. The generalized symbol form appears as:

$$_Z^A X$$

where X is the chemical symbol; Z is the element's atomic number (number of protons); and A represents the atomic mass number of the atom (protons plus neutrons). Although the number of neutrons can be indicated as a trailing subscript number, it is usually not written because it can be calculated by subtracting Z from A. As an example, carbon with 6 protons and 8 neutrons would be written as C. Because an atom with 6 protons will always be a carbon atom, writing a 6 and C is a duplication of information; therefore by convention, it may be written simply as ^{14}C.

Although early scientists learned much about determining atomic weights and organizing the elements into the periodic chart, they did not immediately understand that there could be different atomic forms of the same element. The same element will always have a specific number of protons, as listed by the atomic number Z, and will have the same chemical properties; however, the number of neutrons can differ. The term *nuclide* refers to any configuration of the atom. The Greek terms *iso*, meaning same, and *topos*, meaning place, indicate the atoms have the same position on the periodic table of elements. The term *isotope*, though sometimes erroneously used interchangeably with nuclide, actually defines a specific element with different forms of that element, each containing different numbers of neutrons. ^{97}Tc, ^{98}Tc, ^{99}Tc, ^{100}Tc, and ^{101}Tc are all isotopes of element 43 (see Figure 2-6) and follow a horizontal line on the chart of the nuclides. Because the periodic chart of the elements is far too small to contain all the different isotopes of each element, the chart of the nuclides is commonly used to list the 1500 isotopes of all the elements. Because the chart is laid out in a pattern following the line of stability listed by the number of protons and neutrons (see Figure 2-5), it is relatively simple to identify the isotopes. Isotopes for each element are found as a horizontal line, since the number of neutrons is plotted horizontally.

Additional families of nuclei are isotones, isobars, and isomers. Isotones are atoms of different elements that have the same number of neutrons, but varying numbers of protons. The following are isotones: $^{98}_{42}Mo$, $^{99}_{43}Tc$, $^{100}_{44}Ru$, and $^{101}_{45}Rh$, all having 56 neutrons and forming a vertical line on the chart of the nuclides (see Figure 2-6). Isobars are nuclides that have equal weights or the same mass number (protons plus neutrons). Examples of isobars are ^{99}Rh, ^{99}Ru, ^{99}Tc, and ^{99}Mo; they are found on a 45-degree angle in Figure 2-6.

Isomers are atoms that have identical physical attributes as far as the number of protons, neutrons, and electrons; however, they contain a different amount of nuclear energy. Isomeric forms of an atom are identified by putting an *m* after the mass number *A*. The *m* means the atom is currently in a metastable form and will emit gamma radiation from the nucleus to achieve the more stable energy configuration. The most commonly used radionuclide in nuclear medicine is an isomer—^{99m}Tc. Technetium 99 (^{99}Tc) is a more stable form with a half-life of 2.13×10^5 years. Other isomers that have been used in nuclear medicine are ^{113m}In and ^{87m}Sr.

The isotones are found in vertical columns on the chart, as the number of protons is represented on a vertical axis. Isobars are found on a 45-degree angle running from the lower right to upper left. Isomers are designated by a vertical line within the square for a specific radionuclide.

Another format for diagramming nuclide information is presented with a hexagonal box for each nuclide, as in Figure 2-7 (the Trilinear Chart), where vertically adjacent neighbors are isobars. Oblique neighbors from upper left to lower right represent isotones, and obliquely adjacent neighbors from lower left to upper right represent isotopes. Isomers are identified with a vertical line through the hexagon. Within each hexagon is a box that identifies the element symbol, atomic number, and mass number. As an example of the information contained in this chart, ^{99}Mo and ^{99}Tc should be carefully examined. In Figure 2-7 molybdenum 99 has a physical half-life of 2.76 days and emits both beta and gamma radiation during radioactive decay. The energy in MeV is listed as 1.230 for beta decay (β^-), and gamma ray emissions are identified. Vertical downward arrows show that 92% of the time, molybdenum decays to the isomeric form of ^{99m}Tc and 8% of the time to ^{99}Tc. The left side of the hexagon representing technetium shows that isomeric transition (discussed later) will occur 100% of the time ^{99m}Tc decays. Also indicated in the left side is the gamma energy of 0.140 MeV (or 140 keV). Technetium 99, as represented on the right half of the box, is radioactive, with a half-life of 2.13×10^5 years. Decay is by beta radiation to its daughter product ruthenium 99, which is a stable

element. Note that the ^{99m}Tc decays first to ^{99}Tc before its decay to stable ruthenium.

DECAY PROCESSES

Alpha Decay

Alpha particles (helium nuclei consisting of two protons and two neutrons) are radioactive decay products from radionuclides having large mass. Using standard nuclear notation, the parent element *M* with atomic number *Z*, and mass number *A* decays by alpha (α) emission as:

$$^A_Z M = ^{A-4}_{Z-2} N + \alpha + energy$$

to the daughter product symbolized by *N*. Because alpha particles have a +2 charge and a large mass of 4 amu, they are very damaging to biologic systems and therefore have no role in diagnostic nuclear medicine.

Beta Decay

The concept of a neutron's being composed of a proton and electron is important in certain types of radioactive decay. A nucleus that is neutron rich becomes stable through the conversion of one of its neutrons by the reaction:

$$n = p + \beta^- + \bar{v} + energy$$

As a result, a proton and an electron (β^-) have been created from the neutron. The mass number of the new nuclei is the same as the parent nuclei, because the masses of a neutron and proton are virtually the same; however, a different element remains. The formation of a different element by a radioactive decay process is called *transmutation*, or *isobaric radioactive decay*. The β^- particle that has been created in the nucleus through this decay process is ejected. In this decay process an antineutrino ($\bar{v}$) is created and carries away part of the energy of this reaction. The laws of conservation of momentum and energy are accounted for by this particle. Neutrinos (v) and antineutrinos have no electrical charge and a mass of almost zero. They travel at the velocity of light and are almost undetectable. The excess energy from the neutron is shared between the beta particle and antineutrino. This sharing of kinetic energy is not equal. Sometimes the electron receives more of the energy, and the neutrino receives less, or vice versa. As a result, the energy of the beta particle varies in a continuous energy spectrum with some maximum energy (E_{max}) that was available from the nucleus (Figure 2-8). The nuclear decay process by this method is termed beta-minus (β^-) or simply beta decay. The parent element M with atomic number *Z* and mass number *A* decays by beta emission as:

$$^A_Z M = ^A_{Z+1} N + \beta^- + \bar{v} + energy$$

The energy released by this process is shared as kinetic (motion) energy by the beta particle and the antineutrino. An example of a beta-emitting radionuclide used in nuclear medicine is ^{131}I, which decays as follows:

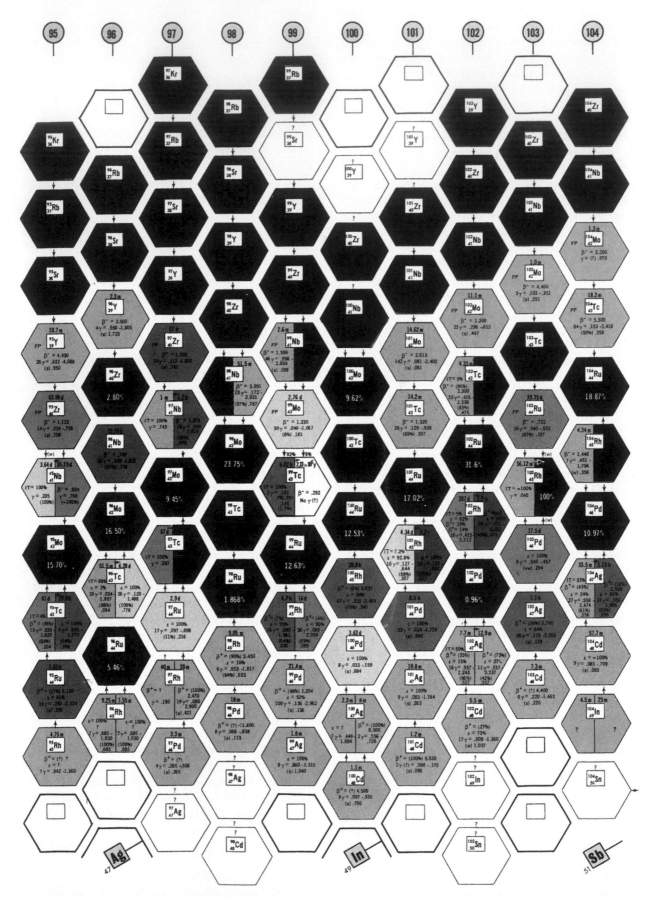

Figure 2-7   Trilinear chart of nuclides. Stable forms (*black background*), instability (*dark- to light-shaded areas*). (Courtesy Mallinckrodt, Inc., St. Louis)

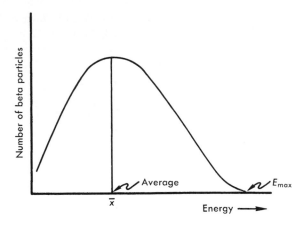

Figure 2-8   Generalized beta particle energy spectrum.

$$^{131}_{53}I = {}^{131}_{54}Xe + \beta^- + \bar{\nu}$$

Positron (β^+) Decay and Electron Capture

A nucleus that is proton rich (neutron poor) reduces its proton surplus by two possible decay processes:

$$p = n + \beta^+ + \nu + energy \quad (positron\ decay)$$

or

$$p + e^- = n + \nu + energy \quad (electron\ capture)$$

The first process is *positron decay,* and the second is *electron capture.*

Positron decay or *emission* results when a proton is converted to a neutron, positron (β^+), neutrino, and energy. In nuclear notation the general form of positron decay is written as:

$$\beta^+ + e^- = \gamma(0.511\ MeV) + \gamma(0.511\ MeV)$$

An example of positron decay is:

$$^{18}_{9}F = {}^{18}_{8}O + \beta^+ + \nu$$

An emitted positron loses kinetic energy through collision with surrounding matter, because it is then moving slowly enough to be attracted to an electron. The positron and negatron spiral in toward each other, forming a temporary "positronium" atom for a brief instant before the two particles undergo annihilation. In the annihilation interaction the mass of each particle (positron and negatron) is converted into electromagnetic energy. The rest mass of each particle results in two 0.511 MeV photons. The two 0.511 MeV photons travel in opposite directions to conserve momentum (Figure 2-9).

Electron capture occurs when an orbital electron travels in the proximity of the nucleus and is captured and combined with a proton to form a neutron. Remember from the cloud model of the atom that electrons can spend a very small amount of their time in the proximity of the nucleus. Electron capture is generalized as:

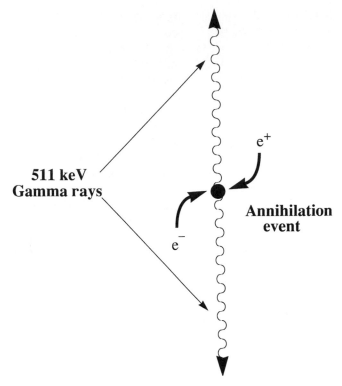

Figure 2-9   Annihilation of a positron and negatron. The resultant pair of 0.511 MeV gamma rays travel 180 degrees apart.

$$^{A}_{Z}M + e^- = {}^{A}_{Z-1}N + \nu + energy$$

An example is the decay of ^{125}I:

$$^{125}_{53}I + e^- = {}^{125}_{52}Te + \nu$$

Electrons involved in electron capture are usually those from the K or L shell. The probability for capture from another energy level is very low. A result of electron capture is ionization of the atom with subsequent relocation of an outer shell electron to fill the vacancy created by the capture.

Proton-rich nuclei can reach stability through either positron emission or electron capture. These are always competing processes; however, the configuration of the nuclei and a high energy content of some nuclei increase the probability of positron emission. If the energy content is less, electron capture occurs. Some atoms can undergo either process with a certain probability.

A commonly used radionuclide in nuclear medicine, ^{67}Ga, undergoes electron capture. In addition to the changes that take place within the nucleus, characteristic x rays are emitted because of energy changes resulting from the electrons filling vacant positions.

Gamma Decay

Gamma ray emission represents a mechanism for an excited nucleus to release energy. The release of energy as a gamma ray (γ) may be part of another decay process, such as alpha or β^-. In addition, it is the process for releasing energy from a metastable nucleus.

Gamma-ray emission usually occurs when there is greater than 100 keV of energy in the excited nucleus. It should be remembered that gamma rays and x rays are characteristically the same, but are named based on their origin, gamma rays being emitted from the nucleus and x rays from the electron shells. The ideal radionuclides for nuclear medicine are those that emit only gamma rays without emitting particulate radiation. These radionuclides thereby provide gamma rays for imaging without increasing patient radiation exposure. With particulate radioactive decay the nucleus is most often left with additional energy, which is released promptly in the form of electromagnetic radiation.

When a metastable nucleus is present, there is a significant amount of time from any previous radioactive decay (such as from ^{99}Mo to ^{99m}Tc) before further release of energy. The release from the metastable state is termed an *isomeric transition*. In this transition the nucleus goes from a higher energy level to a lower energy level through emission of electromagnetic radiation (usually greater than 100 keV); this is sometimes termed *gamma decay*. The equation for an isomeric transition may be written as follows:

$$^A_Z M = {}^A_Z M + \gamma$$

An example of an isomeric transition is:

$$^{99m}_{43} Tc = {}^{99}_{43} Tc + \gamma$$

An alternative process to gamma ray emission in metastable nuclei is termed *internal conversion* and is the transfer of energy from the nucleus to an orbital electron, which is then ejected from the atom (Figure 2-10). Internal conversion reactions usually involve electrons from the K shell, but occasionally involve electrons from the L or M shell. In this process the ejected electron is called a *conversion electron*. This leaves an ionized atom, which follows

normal processes of reshuffling its electrons, resulting in the release of characteristic x rays or Auger electrons.

Metastable nuclei are the most pure sources of gamma rays for nuclear medicine imaging. The isomeric forms for these medically important radionuclides require that they be generator produced within the nuclear medicine laboratory. Technetium-99m has become the most important radionuclide in nuclear medicine imaging.

SCHEMATICS OF RADIOACTIVE DECAY

The various decay processes of radionuclei can be represented diagrammatically to illustrate the relationship of individual processes that take place in radioactive disintegration. This diagram shows the relationship of the parent radionuclide to the daughter nuclide.

The diagrammatic representation of a decay scheme is based on representing the atomic number on the horizontal axis and the energy of the nucleus on the vertical axis (Figure 2-11, *top*). The parent nucleus, being larger, contains more energy and is represented as a horizontal line at the top of the diagram. Through the process of radioactive decay the resulting daughter nucleus has less energy and is

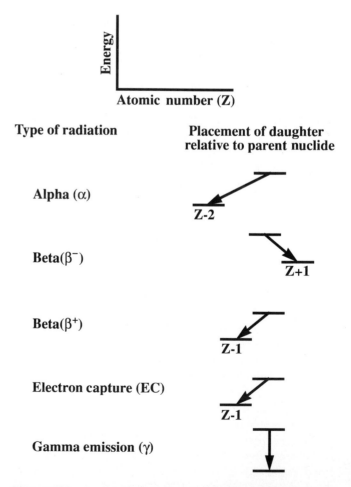

Figure 2-11 Axes (*top*) show directions of increasing energy and atomic number in decay schemes. Directional placement of each daughter nucleus is relative to parent in decay schemes.

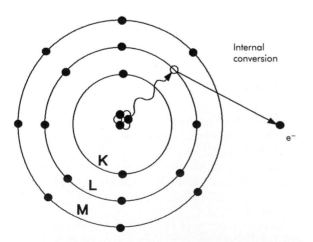

Figure 2-10 Internal conversion of L-shell electron. Energy transfer from nucleus ejecting orbital electron is alternative to gamma-ray emission. Internal conversion electron will have kinetic energy equal to gamma-ray energy minus binding energy.

positioned lower on the diagram. Arrows are used to illustrate the emission of radiation. These arrows show the transition of the nucleus by alpha decay as a decrease in atomic number (Z), shifting to the left, indicating the atomic number is decreased by 2 in the decay process. In β^- decay there is an increase in Z by 1, with a corresponding shift to the right. With positron decay and electron capture there is a decrease in Z by −1. Gamma emission is shown as a vertical down arrow, indicating the release of electromagnetic radiation and resulting only in a decrease in nuclear energy without a change in atomic number. The energy levels of the parent and daughter nuclei are represented as horizontal lines. The parent radionuclide, $_Z^A M$, is shown in general form as the decay process for β^- emission (Figure 2-12) to the daughter product $_{Z+1}^A M$. Two different diagonal arrows in this diagram represent two different energies of beta particle decay. In one case the longer diagonal line represents the emission of a beta particle going directly to the daughter nucleus without any additional energy release. This beta particle energy equals the difference between the parent and daughter energy levels. The shorter arrow represents release of a beta particle of lesser energy to an intermediate state with the prompt release of a gamma ray (vertical down arrow) to the daughter product. One individual atom of the parent radionuclide can release its energy in this beta decay by following either path; therefore one of two beta particles with different energies can be seen in this transition, and only those betas from the lower energy transition are accompanied by a gamma ray.

Figure 2-13 shows a simplified decay scheme for ^{131}I. The actual decay process for ^{131}I has several different beta energies, though only one is prominent (93%). With this beta

particle is the gamma transition releasing 0.364 MeV. Figure 2-14 shows the decay scheme for ^{99}Mo followed by the transitions of ^{99m}Tc and ^{99}Tc to ^{99}Ru. Approximately 82% of the transition from ^{99}Mo to ^{99m}Tc is by one particular beta energy. The radionuclide is then in the metastable form of ^{99m}Tc, which has a half-life of 6 hours. The isomeric transition of ^{99m}Tc is represented as a vertical line downward of a 0.140 MeV gamma ray to the daughter product ^{99}Tc. Technetium 99 has a long half-life (2.2×10^5 years) and by beta decay yields stable ^{99}Ru.

Figure 2-15 shows the decay process for ^{125}I, which is used in radioimmunoassay. The electron capture process is followed by an internal conversion process. The resulting daughter of tellurium, with the electron vacancy left by internal conversion, subsequently emits K-characteristic x rays.

The radioactive decay schemes shown in Figs. 2-11, 2-13, 2-14, and 2-15 have been simplified. Some radionuclides can emit several different gamma-ray energies, as illustrated in Table 2-1 for ^{67}Ga. Gallium 67 decays by electron capture to ^{67}Zn; the zinc nucleus then emits several energies of gamma photons. As indicated in Table 2-1 there is a gamma ray abundance percentage for each ^{67}Ga atom that decays. For every 100 atoms, approximately 38% emit gamma rays at 93.3 keV, and so on. Decay schemes of this nature are helpful in identifying the most abundant peaks for selecting imaging windows. Two, three, or four peaks can be selected for imaging on some instruments. Certain decay schemes have more than one gamma ray emitted for each

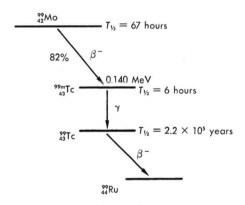

Figure 2-14   Generalized decay scheme for ^{99}Mo.

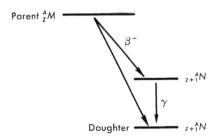

Figure 2-12 Hypothetical decay scheme representing beta particle emission.

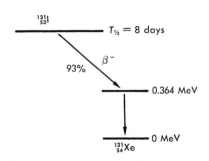

Figure 2-13   Generalized decay scheme for ^{131}I.

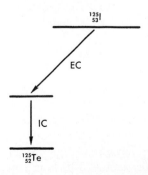

Figure 2-15   Generalized decay scheme for ^{125}I.

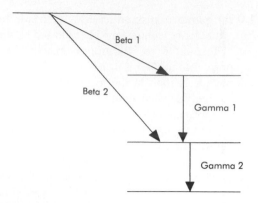

Figure 2-16   Decay by beta 1 is followed by emission of gamma 1 and gamma 2. Emission of higher-energy beta 2 is followed only by single gamma emission, gamma 2. Some radionuclides yield several gamma rays for single disintegration.

Table 2-1	Gallium 67 photon emissions	
Photons	**Abundance percentage**	**Mean energy (keV)**
Gamma 2	38	93.3
Gamma 3	21	184.6
Gamma 5	16	300.2
Gamma 6	4	393.5

atom that decays. Figure 2-16 shows a radionuclide that yields more than one gamma ray for each atom that disintegrates. Decay by beta 1 leaves the daughter nucleus with energy that will be released by gamma 1 and gamma 2. Decay of beta 2 is followed only by gamma 2.

Mathematics of Decay

Individual atoms undergo spontaneous transformations to release energy and form daughter nuclei. There is no way of predicting when that transformation will occur for one specific atom. However, when a large number of atoms are present, a certain probability of radioactive decay is obtained and a mathematical average rate of decay can be determined. A sample that contains N radioactive atoms has on average a certain number of atoms decaying per unit time represented as $\Delta N/\Delta t$. This can be described mathematically as:

$$\frac{\Delta N}{\Delta t} = -\lambda N$$

where λ is the decay constant of the radionuclide. In this equation the minus sign indicates that $\Delta N/\Delta t$ is negative, or decreasing with time. The decay constant λ therefore represents a probability or average percent of atoms present that will decay in a certain time period. The units of λ are 1/time or time^{-1}. A value such as 0.10 hour^{-1} means that in each hour 10% of the atoms undergo radioactive decay. Through

Table 2-2	Decay factors for ^{99m}Tc	
Hours	**Decay factor**	**Precalibration factor**
0	1.000	1.000
$\frac{1}{2}$	0.944	1.059
1	0.891	1.122
2	0.794	1.259
3	0.707	1.414
4	0.630	1.587
5	0.561	1.782
6	0.500	2.000
7	0.445	2.247
8	0.397	2.518
9	0.354	2.824
10	0.315	3.174
11	0.281	3.558
12	0.250	4.000

calculus the above equation is manipulated to derive the number of atoms remaining at any specific time:*

$$N_t = N_0 e^{-\lambda t}$$

where N_t is the number of atoms that remain at any time t, and N_0 is the number of radioactive atoms at the original time zero.

The factor $e^{-\lambda t}$ represents the fraction of radioactive atoms that remain after time t and is called the *decay factor.* The e represents Euler's number, the base of natural logarithms (2.718); it has been raised to the power $-\lambda t$. The decay factor ($e^{-\lambda t}$) is an exponentially decreasing function with time and can be determined using a calculator (see Chapter 1). The decay factors for various time intervals can be calculated; decay factors for ^{99m}Tc are given in Table 2-2.

The number of radioactive atoms (N) is, by the above definition ($\Delta N/\Delta t = -\lambda N$), proportional to the radioactivity (A). This equation can therefore be written to apply to radioactivity. It is called the *general decay equation:*

$$A_t = A_0 e^{-\lambda t}$$

---

*Derivation of the general decay equation.

$$\frac{\Delta N}{\Delta t} = -\lambda N$$

$$\frac{dN}{dt} = -\lambda N$$

$$\frac{dN}{N} = -\lambda dt$$

$$\int \frac{1}{N} dN = -\int \lambda dt$$

$$\frac{N_i}{N_o} = e^{-\lambda t}$$

$$N_i = N_o e^{-\lambda t}$$

It is frequently difficult to work with the decay factor λ; it is much more practical to use another parameter $t_{1/2}$, known as *half-life*. The decay constant λ and $t_{1/2}$ are related by the equation:

$$\lambda = \frac{0.693}{t_{1/2}}$$

where 0.693 is the value of the natural logarithm of 2. This relationship can be derived from the general decay equation by inserting values for the initial activity (A_0) and the activity at the time (t) when the activity (A_t) is at 50% of the activity at time zero. The decay equation may be represented by substituting the relationship of half-life for decay constant and be written as:

$$A_t = A_0 e^{-0.693t/t_{1/2}}$$

where the decay factor (DF) equals the exponential portion of this equation:

$$DF = e^{-0.693t/t_{1/2}}$$

The fraction of elapsed time relative to the half-life can be generated and used for the determining decay factor for any radionuclide, sometimes called the *universal decay table*. The calculation of decay factors is reviewed in Chapter 1. Since the decay factor represents an exponential function, it can be plotted either linearly or semilogarithmically (Figure 2-17). When reviewing this graphic representation, note that the number of atoms remaining is 0.50 at one half-life and observe that the semilogarithmic plot (Figure 2-17, *bottom*) is represented as a straight line where the slope is determined by the decay constant.

RADIOACTIVITY UNITS

Radioactivity is quantitatively measured as the number of atoms that disintegrate per unit time. Two different units can be used to describe a quantity of radioactivity, the *curie* (Ci) and the *becquerel* (Bq). The curie was named in honor of Marie Curie, an early pioneer in the study of radioactivity. It is defined as the amount of radioactivity that decays at a rate of 3.7×10^{10} disintegrations per second (dps). This basic unit can be multiplied by standard mathematical scientific notation to yield larger and smaller multiples of the curie:

kilocurie (kCi)	$= 10^3$	$\times$ Ci $=$	3.7×10^3dps
curie (kCi)	$= 10^0$	$\times$ Ci $=$	3.7×10^{10}dps
millicurie (mCi)	$= 10^{-3}$	$\times$ Ci $=$	3.7×10^7dps
microcurie (μCi)	$= 10^{-6}$	$\times$ Ci $=$	3.7×10^4dps
nanocurie (nCi)	$= 10^{-9}$	$\times$ Ci $=$	3.7×10^1dps
picocurie (pCi)	$= 10^{-12}$	$\times$ Ci $=$	3.7×10^{-2}dps

The Systeme Internationale (SI) defines the other unit of radioactivity, the becquerel (Bq). Henri Becquerel was the first person to identify radioactivity in 1894. One becquerel is the amount of radioactivity contained in a sample that decays at a rate of 1 dps. Because this unit is very small,

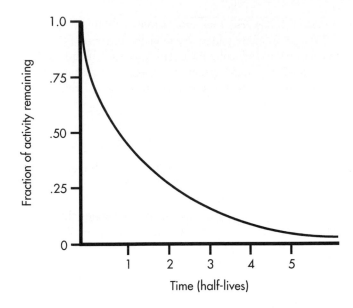

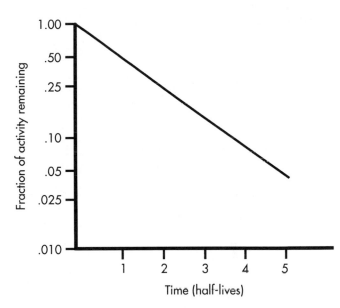

Figure 2-17   Fraction of radioactivity remaining (decay constant) as function of time is shown for a linear plot (*top*) and a semilogarithmic graph (*bottom*). Slope of semilogarithmic straight line is determined by decay constant.

nuclear medicine terminology uses multiples of the becquerel such as kilobecquerels (kBq) and megabecquerels (MBq).

Because most radioactivity in nuclear medicine is administered in doses of millicuries, or megabecquerels, it is important to understand rapid methods of converting between these two units of measure. Multiply the number of millicuries by 37 MBq/mCi to convert to the number of megabecquerels. For example, 20 mCi $\times$ 37 MBq/mCi $=$ 740 MBq. Conversely, covert the number of megabecquerels millicuries by dividing by 37 MBq/mCi, for example, 111 MBq/(37 MBq/mCi) $=$ 3 mCi.

The quantities of radioactivity administered to most patients are on the order of several millicuries (several hundred MBq). The total radioactivity contained in a ^{99}Mo-^{99m}Tc radionuclide generator is on the order of 1 Ci (many tens of thousands of MBq). The quantity of radioactivity contained in patient specimens or assayed in a scintillation well counter is on the order of nanocuries to microcuries (kilobecquerels).

Decay Calculations

Decay factors other than those in decay tables (see Table 2-2) for ^{99m}Tc can be found by multiplying together those that correspond to the decay interval. For example, a 14-hour DF equals the 12-hour DF (0.250) times the 2-hour DF (0.794), or 0.198; or you could multiply the 7-hour DF (0.445) by itself to get 0.198, or any other combination.

Sometimes it is necessary to dispense or use a radiopharmaceutical prior to the calibration time. Precalibration DFs may be calculated from the inverse (1/DF) of the decay factor for the time interval. As an example, the precalibration decay factor for 2 hours equals 1/DF or 1/0.794 = 1.26.

> **EXAMPLE 1:** A vial contains 10 mCi of ^{99m}Tc; how much radioactivity remains after 2 hours?
>
> $$DF \text{ for } 2 \text{ hours} = 0.794$$
> $$10 \text{ mCi} \times 0.794 = 7.94 \text{ mCi}$$
>
> How much radioactivity was present 5 hours before for 10 mCi?
>
> $$\text{Precalibration DF for 5 hours} = 1.782$$
> $$10 \text{ mCi} \times 1.782 = 17.82 \text{ mCi}$$
>
> How much of the 10 mCi remains after 36 hours?
>
> DF for 12 hours is 0.250, which we apply three times.
> $$10 \text{ mCi} \times 0.250 \times 0.250 \times 0.250 = 0.156 \text{ mCi}$$
>
> **EXAMPLE 2:** Using the general decay equation, calculate the activity of 5 mCi/ml of ^{201}Tl after 48 hr ($t_{1/2}$ = 73 hr).
>
> $$A_t = A_0 e^{-0.693t/t_{1/2}}$$
> $$A_t = 5 \text{ mCi/(ml)} \times e^{-0.693t/t_{1/2}}$$
> $$A_t = 5 \text{ mCi/(ml)} \times e^{-0.693 \times (48 \text{ hr})/(73 \text{ hr})}$$
> $$A_t = 5 \text{ mCi/(ml)} \times e^{-0.456}$$
> $$A_t = 3.17 \text{ mCi/(ml)}$$

Average Half-life and Effective Half-life

Average half-life describes the average lifetime of an atom. Mathematically, the average half-life can be calculated as:

$$T_{ave} = 1.44 \times t_{1/2}$$

Although this term represents the average interval for which a group of atoms exists, it has no clinical use in patient dose calculations. The decay constant of a radionuclide represents the physical radioactive decay. It does not indicate the nature of biologic turnover. Because rates are additive, the biologic decay constant can be added to the physical decay constant to give the *effective* decay constant:

$$\lambda_{eff} = \lambda_b + \lambda_p$$

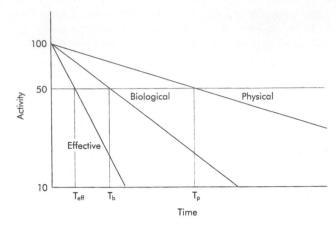

Figure 2-18 Semilogarithmic plot of physical (T_p) and biologic (T_b) half-life components of shorter effective half-life, T_{eff}.

Since $\lambda = 0.693/t_{1/2}$, and dividing by 0.693 this equation can be represented in terms of the half-life:

$$\frac{1}{t_{eff}} = \frac{1}{t_b} + \frac{1}{t_p}$$

where t_{eff} is the *effective half-life* (Figure 2-18), t_b is the biologic half-life, and t_p is the physical half-life.

An example of effective half-life might be the determination of the disappearance of ^{99m}Tc-MAA from the lungs. Assume that the biologic half-life is 3 hours.

$$\frac{1}{t_{eff}} = \frac{1}{(3 \text{ hr})} + \frac{1}{(6 \text{ hr})}$$

The effective half-life (t_{eff}) in the lung is thus 2 hours.

INTERACTIONS

Interactions of Charged Particles with Matter

Electrically charged particles (alpha particles, electrons, and positrons) have a high probability of interacting with the matter through which they move. Their mass and electrical charges interact with the mass of the nucleus and electrical charges of atoms. In addition, the kinetic energy of these particles and the properties of the surrounding matter determine how the particles will interact and how far these particles will travel. The density of matter, its atomic number, and its mass number influence the type and probability of these interactions.

Excitation and Ionization

Excitation is a process of absorbing small amounts of energy temporarily in the outer electron structure of an atom. Energy from a passing charged particle or from an interaction with electromagnetic radiation causes a short-lived or metastable excitement of an outer electron to a slightly higher energy level. The outer electron is not removed from

Table 2-3	Interactions between electromagnetic radiation and matter		
Interaction	**Interaction site**	**Energy range**	**Secondary effects**
Photoelectric	Inner electron shells	Several keV to 0.5 MeV	Photoelectrons, characteristic x rays
Compton	Outer electron shells	Several keV to several MeV	Compton electron, scattered photon
Pair production	Nuclear field	>1.02 MeV	Positron, electron, annihilation photons

the atom, and therefore no ionization occurs. Typically, excitation is very short-lived, and the atom spontaneously gives up the extra energy in the form of electromagnetic radiation.

Ionization of an atom results from the collision of radiation with the electron structure of an atom. Ionization occurs only when there is sufficient energy of the radiation to completely remove an electron from its orbit. The energy must therefore be larger than the binding energy of the particular orbital electron. For example, if the binding energy of an electron were 54 keV and the incident energy were 78 keV, the electron would be ejected from the atom with 24 keV of kinetic energy. Ionization occurs in all forms of matter—solids, liquids, and gases.

Alpha Particles

An alpha particle (α) is the nucleus of a helium atom ($^4_2$He). Alpha particles are produced by radioactive decay in very large, unstable atoms. Their high mass and double-positive electrical charge give them a high ionizing potential in a short pathway in solids, liquids, or gases. They typically have energies between 3 and 8 MeV. Because it takes only about 34 eV to create one ion pair, the high energy of alpha particles along with their high mass and positive charge can create several hundred thousand ion pairs in only a fraction of a millimeter; this is devastating to biologic systems. Radionuclides that emit alpha particles have no use in nuclear medicine.

Beta Particles

The interaction of negatively charged beta particles in the proximity of the nucleus of an atom results in the attraction to the positively charged nucleus. As the beta particle is deflected and slowed in its path, there is a release of energy as x rays, called *bremsstrahlung radiation*. These x rays are released in a continuous spectrum because of the variations in kinetic energy and path geometry of the beta particle. Bremsstrahlung interactions increase in probability with materials that have a high Z number. A beta particle emitting radionuclide, such as ^{32}P, should not be shielded by a high Z material such as lead. It is more appropriate to use a shielding material of low Z, such as plastic, because bremsstrahlung interactions are less likely to occur.

Annihilation

Positively and negatively charged electrons (positrons and negatrons) are antiparticles of each other. When positrons are produced in a decay process and are ejected from an atom, they have enough kinetic energy to travel a maximum of a few millimeters. The positron and an orbital electron from an atom are attracted because of their opposite charges, spiral in toward each other, and interact in a process called *annihilation*. The path distance required for a positron to find an electron for this interaction depends on the positron energy and number of electrons in the immediate area of the atom from which the positron was originally emitted. In the annihilation process the mass of the two particles is converted into energy according to Einstein's equation $E = mc^2$. The rest masses of the positron and negatron are identical (0.511 MeV), giving a total energy of 1.022 MeV. The mass of each particle is converted into a 0.511 MeV gamma ray (see Figure 2-9). The gamma rays travel in opposite directions, 180 degrees from each other, to conform to the law of the conservation of momentum.

$$\beta^+ + e^- = \gamma(0.511 \text{ MeV}) + \gamma(0.511 \text{ MeV})$$

The detection of these two annihilation gamma rays is the foundation for positron emission tomography (PET) imaging.

PHOTONS

Electromagnetic radiation, or photons, is far more penetrating in matter than particulate types of radiation. There is no specific range for these photons, and their interaction with matter is based only on a probability of interaction. In matter, photons may undergo scattering, may have no interaction with matter, or, because they are simply energy, may be completely absorbed and disappear. Although photons are more penetrating than particulate radiation, they demonstrate absorption, which diminishes exponentially with the distance traveled. For photons with energies associated with x rays and gamma rays, three types of interactions occur: photoelectric, Compton, and pair production (Table 2-3).

Photoelectric Effect

The photoelectric effect is an interaction that takes place between an incident photon and an inner orbital electron.

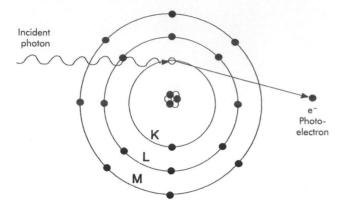

Figure 2-19 In photoelectric effect, incident photon is totally absorbed and transfers all its energy to resultant photoelectron.

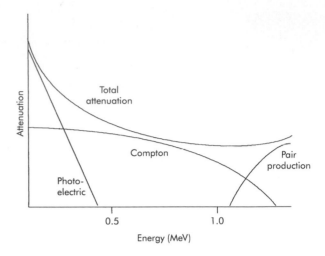

Figure 2-20 Interactions by photoelectric, Compton, and pair production combine to form attenuation coefficient. Probability of attenuation by photoelectric effect is dominant at low energy, but decreases rapidly with increasing photon energy. Interactions through Compton scattering decrease more slowly, and pair production becomes dominant above 1.02 MeV.

For the photoelectric effect to occur, the energy of the incident photon must be greater than the binding energy of the orbital electron. In the photoelectric effect the photon energy is totally absorbed, with some of its energy used to break the bond of the electron in its shell and the remaining energy given to the electron in the form of motion or kinetic energy (Figure 2-19). Therefore a generalized relationship for this interaction can be written as:

Photon energy = Electron binding energy +
electron kinetic energy

The photoelectric effect usually occurs with electrons found in the K or L shell. Since an electron has been removed from the atom, there is no longer an electrically neutral balance between the number of protons and electrons; therefore the atom has been ionized with an inner shell vacancy created. In this interaction an ion pair has been formed—the positively charged atom and negatively charged photoelectron—which leaves the atom.

The electron vacancy can be filled (1) by another orbital electron dropping in to fill a vacancy with the subsequent emission of a characteristic x ray or (2) by an Auger electron (discussed later). The ejected photoelectron is no different from any other free electron in matter and is involved in other interactions, depending on its kinetic energy. The disappearance of the incident photon is important clinically because the energy has been absorbed completely by the patient.

The probability of a photoelectric interaction occurring depends on the energy of the incident gamma ray and the atomic number of the material. Obviously, the photoelectric effect cannot occur unless the photon energy is above the binding energy. As a photon's energy increases, the probability for photoelectric interactions decreases (Figure 2-20). The probability of a photoelectric interaction increases dramatically with the atomic number, that is, photoelectric interactions are unlikely to occur in low Z materials such as water and tissue but are likely to occur in high Z materials such as the iodine in a sodium iodide crystal or in lead. The photoelectric effect is therefore the primary type of inter-

action for detecting gamma rays with nuclear medicine instruments. All the gamma ray energy is given to the crystal material in a thallium-activated sodium iodide crystal. The photoelectric effect is therefore one of the most important interactions for nuclear medicine applications.

Compton Scattering

As its name implies, Compton scattering is an incomplete absorption of gamma rays or scattering of gamma radiation. The Compton effect involves an inelastic interaction of photons with outer orbital electrons. As in the photoelectric effect, there is the emission of an electron that is ejected from the atom; however, not all of the incident gamma ray energy is absorbed, and a scattered photon of lower energy and longer wavelength is emitted. Figure 2-21 illustrates the incident photon at a high energy with short wavelength and a scattered photon with lower energy and longer wavelength. The energy and wavelength of the scattered photon are always lower than those of the incident photon, and the scattered photon's energy also depends on the atomic number of the scattering material, the incident photon's energy, and the angle of scatter. The energy of the scattered photon is related to the angle of deflection. The minimum energy loss of the scattered photon will be at a shallow scatter angle and can be calculated using the relationship:

$$E_{min} = \frac{E_0}{(1 + 2E_0 / 0.511)}$$

where E_0 is the incident photon energy (in MeV). As an example, for a 0.140 MeV gamma ray, E_{min} equals 0.090 MeV, for 0.364 MeV, E_{min} is 0.150 MeV.

The maximum energy E_{max}, or *backscatter energy*, will be at a scatter angle of 180 degrees and can be calculated from:

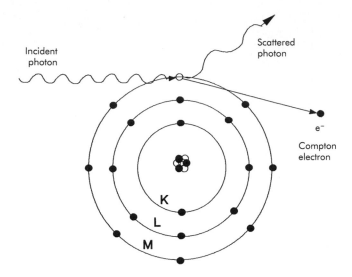

Figure 2-21 Compton scattering occurs in outer-shell electrons, with scattered photons having lower energy and longer wavelength. Ejection of Compton electron leaves ionized atom.

$$E_{max} = \frac{E_0^2}{(E_0 + 0.2555)}$$

This maximum scattered energy for a 0.140 MeV photon is 0.049 MeV and for a 0.364 MeV photon is 0.214 MeV. The maximum scatter energy identifies the sharp increase in scatter on the gamma-ray spectrum, called the Compton edge.

The likelihood of Compton scatter is proportional to the atomic number; therefore there is more Compton scattering in high atomic number materials. Compton interactions are less likely to occur with higher energy photons (see Figure 2-20).

Pair Production

Pair production is an interaction produced when a photon with energy greater than 1.02 MeV passes near the high electric field of the nucleus. The strong electrical force brings about the energy-mass conversion. When the photon comes near the nucleus, it disappears totally and two particles of matter are created, an electron and positron, each possessing the mass equivalence of 0.511 MeV. For this interaction to occur, the initial photon must possess 1.02 MeV or more of energy. Any additional energy of the incident photon is converted into kinetic energy, which is given to the positron and negatron, thus conserving energy and momentum. The photon originally had zero charge, and the offsetting positive and negative charges of the negatron and positron ensure that the net charge remains zero.

The fates of the negatron and positron are the same as if those particles were created by radioactive decay processes. The negatron interacts with surrounding atoms, possibly causing ionization and excitation. The positron loses some of its energy through interactions and ultimately undergoes

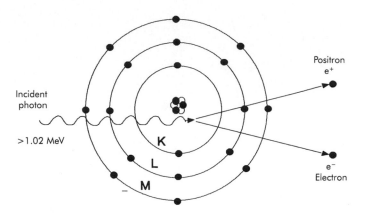

Figure 2-22 In pair production, photons with energy greater than 1.02 MeV may interact with strong forces near nucleus. Positron-electron pair is created with kinetic energy equal to excess above 1.02 MeV. Positron will undergo annihilation with electron.

annihilation with an orbital electron from an atom, producing a gamma ray pair with 0.511 MeV each. Figure 2-22 illustrates the pair production process.

Figure 2-20 shows the dominance of pair production interactions for very-high-energy photons. Note that there can be no pair production interactions below 1.02 MeV.

EXTRANUCLEAR ENERGY RELEASE

Three processes occur in the electron structure of the atom to release energy. These result in the creation of bremsstrahlung radiation, characteristic x rays, and Auger electrons.

Bremsstrahlung Radiation

Bremsstrahlung is a German word that simply means *braking radiation*. Bremsstrahlung is a process of the rapid deceleration of a charged particle as it comes under the intense electric field of the nucleus. The particle, electron or positron, has a very small mass in comparison with the nucleus. The rapidly moving particle is attracted to or repulsed from the nucleus and rapidly decelerated, and its direction changes. In this deflection and deceleration a significant loss of energy is emitted in the form of electromagnetic radiation in the x-ray region (Figure 2-23). In this type of interaction the conservation of energy and momentum must be maintained; therefore the energy of the incident charged particle is equal to the sum of the energy of the particle after deflection and the bremsstrahlung x ray.

The production of bremsstrahlung x rays can increase the total amount of radiation being produced and be more hazardous if thin lead shields are used. The production of bremsstrahlung radiation is not as significant in low atomic number materials, such as plastic; therefore it is better to shield pure beta-emitting radionuclides such as ^{32}P with plastic shielding instead of thin lead.

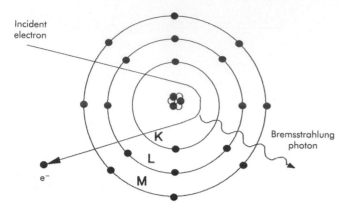

Figure 2-23 Deceleration of a charged particle passing near nucleus results in release of energy in the form of bremsstrahlung x rays.

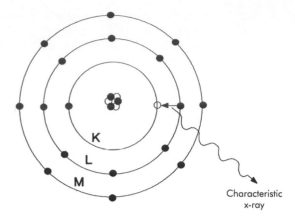

Figure 2-24 Characteristic x rays are produced when electron fills lower shell vacancy. Energy of x ray represents energy difference between two electron shells.

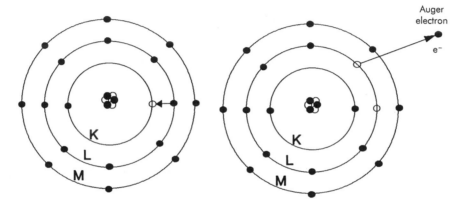

Figure 2-25 Alternative process to production of characteristic x rays is emission of Auger electron. As electron fills lower energy shell (*left*), energy is transferred to release orbital electron. Atom (*right*) is left with two vacancies, which will be filled by outer orbital electrons with subsequent characteristic x rays or additional Auger electron production.

Characteristic X Rays

The production of characteristic x rays occurs in atoms that have electron vacancies in their inner shell electron structure. In the process of filling these inner shells by electrons dropping in from outer orbits, there is a release of electromagnetic energy in the x-ray region (Figure 2-24). The characteristic x-ray energy is determined by the energy shell difference; electrons filling in the K shell are more energetic than those that fill an L shell because of the proximity to the nucleus and the higher binding energy.

Auger Electrons

Characteristic x rays are produced in reducing excess energy when electrons fill vacancies in inner shells. An alternative to characteristic x rays is the Auger (pronounced *oh-zhay*) effect. In this interaction the surplus energy is given to another orbital electron, which is ejected (Figure 2-25). The ejected electron is called an Auger electron, and the atom is now left with two vacancies occurring in the electron structure. These vacancies are filled by additional electrons from outer orbits, followed by the emission of characteristic x rays or secondary Auger electrons. The production of Auger

electrons results in increased radiation exposure when these processes take place within the body tissue.

ATTENUATION AND TRANSMISSION OF PHOTONS

As discussed previously, gamma photons interact with matter through photoelectric, Compton, and pair production processes. These interactions combine into the linear attenuation coefficient, μ. The linear attenuation coefficient is the probability of attenuation per distance traveled through an absorber, therefore μ has the units of 1/distance (cm^{-1}). The general attenuation equation is:

$$I = I_0 e^{-\mu x}$$

where the initial intensity of radiation I_0 is reduced by the exponential function of the linear attenuation coefficient μ and distance traveled x, to give the reduced intensity of the radiation field I.

The linear attenuation coefficient μ is related to the half-value layer (HVL) of the material by:

$$\mu = \frac{0.693}{HVL}$$

The HVL is the thickness of absorber necessary to diminish the intensity of the radiation to half its initial strength.

The general attenuation equation can be rewritten to incorporate the relationship to HVL as:

$$I = I_0 e^{-0.693x/HVL}$$

An example using these equations is the shielding of a source of ^{131}I with lead. The HVL for $364\,keV$ gamma rays is $0.3\,cm$. The value of μ is then calculated to be $2.31\,cm^{-1}$. Assume that we have $0.9\,cm$ of lead and an exposure rate of $5\,mR/hr$. Using the general attenuation equation we calculate:

$$I = 5(mR)/(hr)e^{-2.31 \times 0.9}$$
$$I = 5(mR)/(hr)e^{-2.079}$$
$$I = 5(mR)/(hr) \times 0.125$$
$$I = 0.625(mR)/(hr)$$

Since the thickness of the lead is $3\,HVLs$, an alternative method to more simply solve this problem is to divide the intensity of the radiation field by 2, three times, or:

$$\frac{([(5mR)/(hr)/2]/2)}{2} = 0.635(mR)/(hr)$$

The measure of attenuation can also be done with another parameter, the mass attenuation coefficient, μ_{mass}, which depends on the material's density. The units of this coefficient are cm^2/g. From the following the relationship between these two attenuation coefficients is represented as:

$$\mu_{mass} = \frac{\mu_{linear}}{density}$$

Using these attenuation relationships results in the following expression:

$$cm^2/g = \frac{cm^{-1}}{(g/cm^3)}$$

The mass attenuation coefficient can be broken down into its components for the processes of photoelectric, Compton, and pair production interactions.

L. Stephen Graham, Jonathan M. Links

chapter 3

Instrumentation

Objectives

Describe the construction and operating principles of gas-filled detectors, including ionization chambers and Geiger-Mueller detectors.

Explain the operation of scintillation detectors and photomultiplier tubes.

Describe the mechanisms for performing spectrometry with a scintillation detector.

Diagram the differences between liquid scintillation counting systems and scintillation crystal systems.

Discuss count rate limitations of gas-filled and scintillation detectors relative to dead time, efficiency, geometry, and attenuation.

Diagram an Anger design of a scintillation camera system and explain the function of each component.

Diagram and discuss the properties of various camera collimators.

Discuss spatial resolution and sensitivity of the scintillation camera.

Diagram and describe the function of position logic circuitry for the scintillation camera.

Describe the operation of a pulse height analyzer for energy discrimination.

Explain how images are formed using photographic or digital systems.

Define SPECT and explain the principles behind emission computed tomography.

Describe the relative advantages of multiple detector SPECT cameras.

Describe the operation of positron imaging systems for dedicated PET tomography, PET imaging with SPECT, and coincidence imaging.

Describe quality control procedures required for survey instruments.

List the quality control procedures required for the dose calibrator and how each procedure is performed and results interpreted.

Explain quality control requirements for nonimaging scintillation detectors.

List and discuss quality control procedures required for the scintillation camera system, including SPECT.

Define NEMA standards and their application to nuclear medicine.

Define signal-to-noise ratio and its influence on data quality.

Nuclear medicine is a high-technology discipline. Accordingly, much more emphasis is placed on the design, manufacture, and use of its instruments than in some other fields. The equipment evolves out of a multidisciplinary approach, encompassing basic radiation physics, electronics, detector design, and computers. Although the nuclear medicine technologist does not need to become an expert in all these fields, a basic knowledge of the principles behind the equipment is vital to maximizing a given imaging system's performance. The technologist is the key player, since he or she directly interacts with the equipment. A technologist needs an understanding of how nuclear instrumentation works far beyond knowing "which buttons to push."

This chapter emphasizes the principles of radiation detection, image formation, and tomography. A knowledge of basic mathematics and radiation physics is assumed. References to specific vendors or equipment are specifically avoided; the same general principles apply to all modern nuclear medicine imaging systems.

RADIATION DETECTION

Two main types of detectors are used in nuclear medicine: gas-filled detectors and scintillators. *Gas-filled detectors* are typically used in nonimaging instruments, whereas *scintillators* form the basis of most imaging instruments.

Gas-Filled Detectors

The basic approach of a gas-filled detector is quite simple: radiation is sensed by detecting the ionization of gas molecules produced by deposition of energy during passage of radiation through the gas-filled detector. In essence, a gas-filled detector is a container of gas with two electrodes, one positive (the anode) and one negative (the cathode). When ionizing radiation produces ion pairs in the gas, the resulting free electrons are attracted to the anode and the positively charged gas molecule ions are attracted to the cathode. (An *ion pair* is the positively charged gas molecule ion and the free electron that came from it.) This bulk movement of charge produces an electrical signal from the detector. Commonly used gases include helium, neon, argon, hydrogen, and air. Gases that have a high affinity for electrons, such as oxygen or halogens, are not used, because these would compete with the anode for the free electrons.

Types. There are three main types of gas-filled detectors: ionization chambers, proportional counters, and Geiger-Mueller detectors. Although in practice many factors determine which type a given detector represents, in theory the type is given by the value of the applied voltage across the electrodes in the detector. The curve that relates the applied voltage to the signal from a gas-filled detector is shown in Figure 3-1. The y axis is labeled *number of ion pairs collected per event.* An event refers to one alpha, beta, x ray, or gamma ray passing through the detector and depositing energy in the gas (in the process of ionizing gas molecules). Because

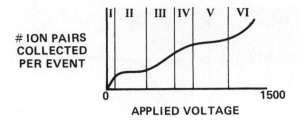

Figure 3-1 Relationship between applied voltage and number of ion pairs collected per event in a gas-filled detector. Curve is divided into six regions: **I**, recombination; **II**, ionization; **III**, proportional; **IV**, limited proportional; **V**, Geiger-Mueller; **VI**, continuous or spontaneous discharge.

the electrodes have a voltage across them, the free electrons are attracted to the anode and the gas molecule ions are attracted to the cathode. This movement of charge produces an electrical signal across the electrodes with a size that is proportional to the numbers of electrons and gas ions (i.e., ion pairs) collected at the electrodes. In general, a gas-filled detector gives one electrical pulse for every alpha, beta, x ray, or gamma ray it detects, with the *size of the pulse* determined by the number of ion pairs collected at the electrodes. The curve in Figure 3-1 is divided into six regions: recombination, ionization, proportional, limited proportional, Geiger-Mueller, and continuous discharge. These divisions imply different operational modes for a gas-filled detector.

When the applied voltage across the electrodes is very low, the gas ions and electrons feel very little attraction toward their respective electrodes. Even though many ion pairs may have been created in the gas by ionizing radiation, these gas ions and electrons are more apt to *recombine* with each other than to be separated and collected at the electrodes. There is reduced signal from a gas-filled detector in the recombination region of operation, thus detectors are not operated with voltages in this region.

If the applied voltage is increased to 100 to 400 V, the electrodes apply sufficient force to overcome the mutual attraction of the gas molecule ions and free electrons. As a result all the ion pairs produced by deposition of energy in the detector are collected. This means that the size of each pulse in this *ionization region* of operation is directly related to the amount of energy deposited in the gas by the ionization event. If the gas is air, ionization chambers can directly measure *exposure* in roentgens.

When the applied voltage is increased to 400 to 800 V, the free electrons gain a significant amount of kinetic energy on their way to the anode. The larger the voltage on the anode, the greater the electron's acceleration and increase in kinetic energy. These electrons now have sufficient energy to cause ionization themselves. As they make their way to the anode, they produce more ion pairs. Most of this additional ionization occurs near the anode, because by this point the electrons have gained the most kinetic energy. Some of these secondary electrons also gain enough kinetic energy to cause further ionization. The end result is that many more ion pairs are collected than were initially produced in the gas by

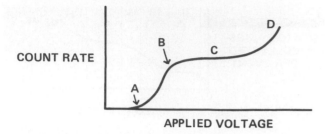

Figure 3-2   Characteristic curve for a Geiger-Mueller detector, showing relationship between applied voltage and observed count rate from a radioactive source. **A,** Starting voltage or threshold; **B,** knee; **C,** plateau region; **D,** region of continuous or spontaneous discharge.

the incoming ionizing radiation. However, the final number of ion pairs collected is still *proportional* to the initial number produced. Thus the size of a pulse from a proportional counter is proportional to the energy deposited in the detector. Because of this *gas amplification* the size is a factor of 100 to 10,000 times the size from an ionization chamber (depending on the particular instrument) for the same energy deposited.

As the voltage across the electrodes is increased above about 800 V, free electrons from initial ionization events gain sufficient kinetic energy to ionize a significant fraction of the gas molecules in the detector. In this *limited proportional region* the detector is approaching its saturation point, such that the number of ion pairs collected (and thus pulse size) is not strictly proportional to the energy deposited. Detectors are not generally operated in this region.

If the applied voltage is increased to 1000 to 1500 V, the free electrons from initial ionization events gain enough kinetic energy to produce an *avalanche* of ionization, resulting in as complete an ionization of the gas in the detector as possible. This can be thought of as the *saturation point*. In this situation the number of ion pairs collected is independent of the initial number formed. Thus the size of the pulse from a detector operating in this *Geiger-Mueller region* is independent of the energy deposited by the ionizing radiation; every event yields the same large size pulse. It is interesting to note that the actual number of gas molecules ionized at saturation is still only a small fraction of the total number of molecules in the detector.

Figure 3-2 shows a characteristic curve for a Geiger-Mueller detector system, in which the observed pulse or count rate from a radioactive source is plotted as a function of applied voltage. Note that this curve has a different y axis than that in Figure 3-1. The y axis in Figure 3-1 refers to the size of a given pulse, whereas that in Figure 3-2 refers to the number of pulses per unit time. This curve has several features: *A,* starting voltage or threshold; *B,* knee; *C,* plateau region; and *D,* region of continuous discharge. This curve is used to characterize the voltage-response function of a particular Geiger-Mueller detector to select the appropriate operating voltage (usually about one third of the way along the plateau).

Increases of more than 1500 V can produce arcing between the electrodes. The actual voltage depends on several factors, including electrode separation distance. This spontaneous electrical discharge will create ion pairs in the same way that a bolt of lightning ionizes the air along its path. The electrical discharge is continuous. Operation in this region is not useful and is harmful to the detector.

Spontaneous discharge can also occur at lower voltages in Geiger-Mueller detectors if not prevented. X rays are released when positive gas molecule ions reach the cathode (the detector wall) and recombine with electrons from the wall. These x rays can produce ionization, leading to another avalanche and the generation of a pulse. This effect will continue indefinitely once started unless it is *quenched*. Quenching is accomplished by using a small concentration of a second polyatomic or halogen quenching gas. The energy released by recombination of the positive ions and electrons is absorbed by the quench gas, causing dissociation. Halogen-quenched detectors have a long life, because the halogen molecules, typically Br_2 or Cl_2, recombine after dissociation. Quenching is not required in ionization chambers or proportional counters because the applied voltage is not high enough to cause sufficient gas amplification for the low-energy x rays to produce a detectable pulse.

A complete detection system consists of the gas-filled detector itself, a high-voltage power supply, a preamplifier (used to shape the pulses by narrowing their width to increase count rate capability), an amplifier (used to linearly increase the size of the pulses), and a readout device that consists of either a scaler (used to actually count the pulses) and a timer (used to control the duration of counting) or a ratemeter. Because it is possible for noise to arise in the electronics that count the pulses, a discriminator is used to eliminate the noise pulses, which are typically of lower amplitude. This discriminator, which is located in the preamplifier or amplifier, is an electronic threshold that only allows pulses above a certain size to pass on to be counted. The presence of this discriminator produces the threshold seen in Figure 3-2. Without it, counts would be observed at a very low applied voltage.

Uses. Gas-filled detectors are most commonly used in nuclear medicine as dose calibrators and survey meters. A *dose calibrator* is used to determine the radioactivity in a test tube, vial, or syringe (Figure 3-3). Dose calibrators are based on ionization chambers filled with argon at a pressure of 22 atmospheres. As such, they directly measure exposure rate. This direct measure of exposure rate can be converted into a measure of the amount of radioactivity present. Exposure is based on the production of a known number of ion pairs in a known volume of air. In a dose calibrator, measured exposure rate is converted to activity by the following equation:

$$A = E\,d^2/G$$

where *A* is the activity of the source, *E* is the measured exposure rate, *d* is the distance between the source and the detec-

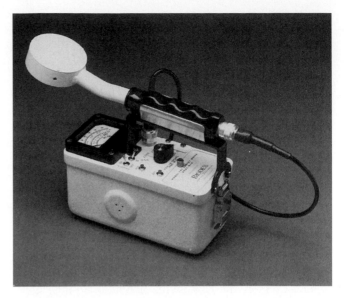

Figure 3-4 Survey instrument used to detect location and relative amount of radioactivity. System is usually based on a Geiger-Mueller counter. (Courtesy of Biodex Medical Systems, Inc., Shirley, New York.)

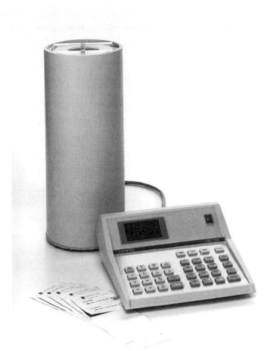

Figure 3-3 Dose calibrator used to assay amount of radioactivity in a vial or syringe. System is based on a calibrated ionization chamber. (Courtesy of Capintec, Inc., Ramsey, New Jersey.)

tor, and G is the specific gamma ray constant. This gamma ray constant expresses the ability of a given amount of activity of a radionuclide to ionize air molecules. This constant is based on the type, number, and energies of emissions from a given radionuclide and is different for each radionuclide. Dose calibrators thus have a selector switch or dial that selects the appropriate constant for that radionuclide, so that actual activity can be displayed on the calibrator's readout.

The second application of gas-filled detectors is as *survey meters* (Figure 3-4). These are used to locate a source of radioactivity and to assess the amount of radioactivity present or the exposure rate from the source. When the location of a radioactive source is not known, Geiger-Mueller detectors are frequently used. These typically read out in units of counts/min and thus indicate the relative amount of radioactivity that is present. They are the most sensitive gas-filled detector for this purpose. When the location of the source is known, an ionization chamber may be used to accurately measure exposure rate in mR/hr. This is particularly useful in estimating the exposure risk from patients, syringes, and packages. Manufacturers can calibrate Geiger-Mueller detectors so that they read out in units of mR/hr. However, these detectors should be used with caution for measurement of exposure rate (e.g., mR/hr), because the calibration is very energy dependent.

It is important to consider the materials used in constructing gas-filled detectors, for their characteristics and thickness will determine what radiations can penetrate the

detector housing and interact in the gas. For example, *thin end-window* Geiger-Mueller detectors have one end of extremely thin mica, which allows counting of low-energy alphas and betas. *Side-window* Geiger-Mueller detectors, on the other hand, have windows that are typically ten times as thick and are only useful for higher energy betas and electromagnetic radiation.

If a detector readout is in units of counts/time or exposure/time, it is called a *ratemeter*. Such a meter responds to changes in activity. The speed with which the meter responds is determined by the meter's *time constant*. A long time constant means that the ratemeter responds sluggishly. If the activity rapidly changes, the meter's reading will lag behind. If the time constant is short, the meter will rapidly respond to changes, even if only due to the statistical nature of radioactive decay rather than to a true change in activity. The choice of a time constant reflects a compromise between the ability to detect true changes in activity and smoothing the rapid meter fluctuations due to statistical variation.

Scintillation Detectors

The most commonly used detector in nuclear medicine is the scintillation detector. This type of detector is based on the property of certain crystals to emit light photons (*scintillate*) after deposition of energy in the crystal by ionizing radiation. To understand how these inorganic scintillators work, the band theory of solids must be considered. In this theory the outer electrons have energy levels that lie in a *valence band*. Above the valence band is a band of electron energy levels called the *conduction band*. The region of energies between the valence and conduction bands is called the *forbidden gap* and represents electron energies that do not exist in a pure crystal. In the crystal's ground energy state, the valence band is completely filled with electrons and the conduction band is empty. If energy is imparted to the crystal, electrons may be raised from the valence band to the conduction band. Because this results in an energetically unstable state, the electrons fall back to the valence band, giving off energy (as electromagnetic radiation) in the process. This electromagnetic radiation represents the difference in energy between the valence band and the conduction band and is usually in the visible light range. In a typical scintillator the light photons have wavelengths between 350 and 500 nanometers. The number of photons emitted is proportional to the energy deposited.

The most commonly used scintillation crystal in nuclear medicine is sodium iodide. This crystal absorbs moisture from the air (it is hygroscopic), so it is hermetically sealed in an aluminum can. Because the aluminum absorbs alphas and betas, sodium iodide detectors are generally used only for detection of x rays and gamma rays. Interactions of x rays or gamma rays will not cause a crystal of pure sodium iodide to fluoresce at room temperature. However, if impurity atoms (usually thallium) are incorporated into the crystal, *luminescence centers* are created in the forbidden gap. Electrons excited during interaction of ionizing radiation are trapped in these centers. As the electrons return to the valence band, light is released in the crystal. In most thallium-activated sodium iodide crystals, about 20 to 30 light photons are released for each keV of energy absorbed.

The light photons are converted to an electrical signal through the use of a *photomultiplier tube* (PMT) that is optically coupled to the crystal. The photomultiplier tube is a vacuum tube with a large potential voltage distributed across a series of intermediate electrodes called *dynodes*. The light photons leave the transparent crystal and impinge on the photosensitive surface (*photocathode*) of the photomultiplier tube. The photocathode is an extremely thin layer of an alloy such as cesium and antimony, or cesium, antimony, sodium, and potassium (in a typical bialkali photomultiplier tube). For every three to five light photons incident on the photocathode, one electron is released by the photoelectric effect.

The photoelectrons are accelerated to the first dynode, which is positively charged and positioned a short distance from the photocathode. For each electron reaching the first dynode, three to four electrons are released. The second dynode has a higher voltage than the first; thus the liberated electrons are accelerated to it. Each of these electrons in turn liberates three or four electrons from this second dynode. This process is repeated at 10 to 14 successive dynodes in the photomultiplier tube, and 10^6 to 10^8 electrons reach the tube's anode for each electron liberated from the photocathode. Electrons collected by the anode are directed into a preamplifier circuit, which forms and shapes a pulse that is then further amplified by a linear amplifier from a few millivolts to a few volts. A diagram of a complete scintillation counting system is shown in Figure 3-5.

Spectrometry

Measurement principles. The size or *height* of each pulse from the photomultiplier tube is proportional to the energy deposited in the crystal by ionizing radiation. As with gas-filled detectors, the number of pulses coming from the detector per unit time is related to the activity of the source. Scintillation spectrometry, or *pulse height analysis,* refers to the use of a scintillation counting system to obtain an energy spectrum from a radioactive source . This energy spectrum is simply a histogram of pulse height (which is proportional to the energy deposited in the crystal) on the x axis versus the number of pulses with a given pulse height on the y axis. This spectrum is a function of the energies of the x rays or gamma rays emitted by the source and the interactions of these radiations in the crystal. This spectrum has two main features: a broad range of energies called the *Compton plateau,* and a peak at the highest pulse heights or energies called the *photopeak.* The broad plateau is produced by Compton scatter interactions in the crystal. The right-most limit of this plateau, called the *Compton edge,* represents Compton interactions in which the incoming x ray or gamma ray is backscattered 180 degrees in the crystal, thus depositing the maximum energy possible in a Compton interaction. The photopeak represents x rays or gamma rays that come directly from the source and deposit all their energy in either a single photoelectric interaction or one or more Compton interactions followed by a photoelectric interaction. Because an x ray or gamma ray cannot lose all its energy in a single Compton scatter event, there is a separation between the Compton plateau and the photopeak. A typical pulse height spectrum for ^{99m}Tc is shown in Figure 3-6.

In an ideal detector the photopeak would be a single vertical line at the pulse height representing the energy of the emitted x ray or gamma ray. In reality the statistical nature of the light emission and the finite energy resolution of a pulse height analyzer smear out this line, producing a bell-shaped photopeak. In nuclear medicine imaging the general term *resolution* can be thought of as the ability of a system to accurately depict two separate events in space, time, or

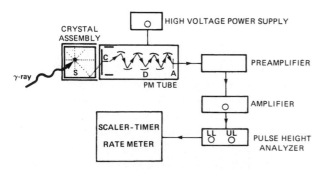

Figure 3-5   Scintillation spectrometry system. **S,** Scintillation event; **C,** photocathode; **D,** dynode; **A,** anode; **LL,** lower level discriminator; **UL,** upper level discriminator.

energy as separate. Resolution can also be thought of as the amount by which a system smears out a single event in space, time, or energy. These two ways of looking at resolution are, of course, related, because the less smearing a system produces, the closer in space, time, or energy two events can be and still be distinguished as being separate. The worse the energy resolution of a pulse height analyzer, the broader the photopeak. Energy resolution can be quantified as the *full width at half maximum* (FWHM) of the photopeak (Figure 3-7). This is measured by first determining the number of counts at the top of the photopeak and then locating the points on either side of the peak where the counts are half of the peak counts. The width of the photopeak in pulse height units is obtained by subtracting the lower pulse height from the upper. Finally, this width is divided by the pulse height (energy) at the apex of the photopeak and multiplied by 100 to produce an energy resolution measurement in percent.

% energy resolution = (FWHM/photopeak center) × 100

The smaller the number, the better the energy resolution. Typical scintillation systems average 7% to 9% for ^{137}Cs; typical camera systems average 8% to 12% for ^{99m}Tc. It is important to note that the time resolution of the scintillation system also plays a role in energy resolution. If two scintillation events occur within the system's time resolution, a single, summed pulse of larger size will be produced. Such pulses can contribute to an apparent widening of the photopeak.

To calibrate a pulse height analyzer to establish the quantitative relationship between energy deposited and pulse height (e.g., 1 pulse height unit = 1 keV), either the applied voltage across the photomultiplier tube or the amplification in the electronics must be adjusted until the photopeak from a known energy source falls at the desired pulse height. Changing the applied voltage across the photomultiplier tube changes the size of pulses coming out of the detector by changing the amplification in the tube. If the voltage across each dynode is increased, electrons liberated from the previous dynode gain more kinetic energy. On striking the next dynode, a larger number of electrons are liberated. This leads to a larger signal from the photomultiplier tube. Changing the amplification in the electronics directly changes the size of each pulse. In any event, a linear proportionality exists between pulse height and energy. Calibrating the analyzer at one energy usually calibrates it for all energies. However, some systems are not perfectly linear. This is especially true at very low energies such as those of the photons from 1 to 125.

Uses. Spectrometry systems are generally used to determine which radionuclides (and their amounts) are present in a mixed sample or to determine how much activity of a known radionuclide is present in a sample. To assay the amount of radioactivity in a test tube, a *well counter* is commonly used (Figure 3-8). This counter consists of a cylindrical lead-shielded sodium iodide detector 1 to 3 inches in diameter, containing a hole passing through the

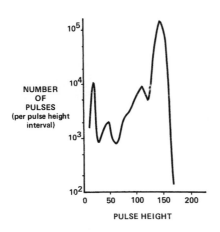

Figure 3-6 Pulse height spectrum of ^{99m}Tc. **A,** Photopeak produced by total absorption of the 140 keV gamma rays, **B,** photopeak produced by lead x rays from a collimator or shield, **C,** photopeak produced by characteristic x rays from Tc-99m.

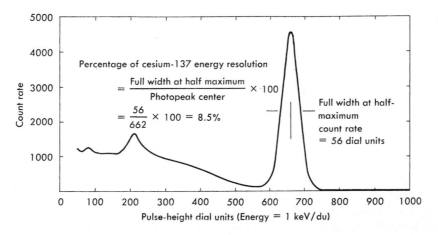

Figure 3-7 Cesium-137 energy spectrum and energy resolution: **du,** Dial or energy units.

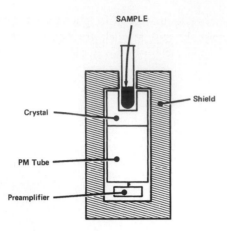

Figure 3-8 Arrangement of a standard well counter for assay of radioactivity. System is based on a crystal scintillator.

lead and part way through the crystal. A test tube containing the radioactive sample can be placed in the "well." Because the crystal surrounds the test tube on all sides except the top, the counting geometry is very close to optimum. To count radioactivity in a person, a *probe system* is often used (Figure 3-9). The probe consists of a sodium, the required electronics, and a collimator. This collimator is a piece of lead with a large hole in it (Figure 3-10). Its purpose is to limit the *field of view* of the crystal so that the probe only detects activity from a defined volume in space in front of it. A major application of these probe systems is in thyroid uptake studies. The probe is used to measure the amount of orally ingested radioiodine that accumulates in the thyroid gland. This requires the use of a *flat-field collimator*. This collimator provides relatively uniform detection sensitivity across the region of the thyroid, while excluding most radioactivity outside the neck from the probe's field of view.

Pulse height analyzers are very important in well counters and probes in two ways. First, they can be used to determine which radionuclides are present in a sample by analysis of the pulse height spectrum. For example, a small sample of the liquid solution that is eluted from the chemical ion exchange column of a radionuclide generator system can be counted in a well counter. The pulse height spectrum from the counter will be a composite of the desired radionuclide's spectrum and spectra from any radioactive impurities in the eluate. Because each radionuclide has a characteristic pulse height spectrum, inspection of the composite spectrum will reveal the presence of impurities as additional photopeaks in the observed spectrum. Their amounts will be indicated by the heights of the peaks relative to the desired radionuclide's photopeak.

The second application of pulse height analyzers is to count a preselected range of energies (Figure 3-11). This is accomplished through the use of a *pulse height window*. The pulse height window is a combination of a lower level discriminator and an upper level discriminator. The lower level discriminator only allows pulses above a certain size to pass

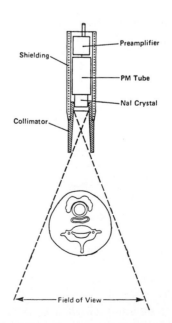

Figure 3-9 Probe/well counting system using scintillation spectrometry. Usually used for iodine or technetium thyroid-uptake studies. The "well" is fastened to the lower frame. The computer has special circuitry and software so that it operates as a multichannel analyzer. (Courtesy of Capintec, Inc., Ramsey, New Jersey.)

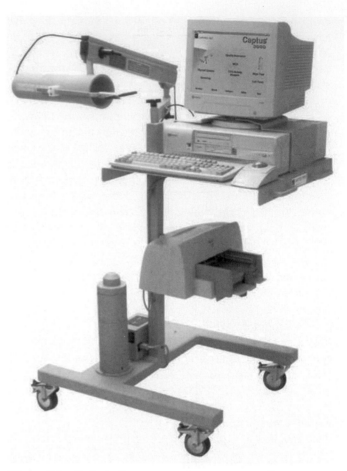

Figure 3-10 Flat-field collimator, which limits probe's field of view to region of interest—in this case, the neck.

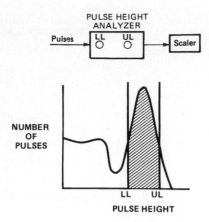

Figure 3-11 Use of pulse height window, defined by lower level and upper level discriminators, to select desired range of energies (usually photopeak energies, representing unscattered events, and small angle scatter).

and be counted, whereas the upper level discriminator allows only pulses below a certain size to pass and be counted. The combination of lower and upper level discriminators in an *anti-coincidence circuit* permits the range of pulses between the lower and upper levels to pass and be counted. The importance of selecting a certain range of pulses, which represents a specific range of energies deposited in the crystal by x rays or gamma rays, is discussed later.

Liquid Scintillation Counting

One special spectrometry technique is liquid scintillation counting. This technique is used to assess the activity of small sources of beta emitters, such as tritium (^{3}H) or carbon 14. In liquid scintillation counting, the radioactive samples are dissolved in a liquid that scintillates, called a *cocktail*. This liquid scintillation cocktail is put into a vial with the sample. Photomultiplier tubes are used to measure the light produced within the scintillation cocktail.

Liquid scintillation cocktails are composed of three main ingredients: an organic solvent, a primary fluor, and a secondary fluor. The *solvent* is used to dissolve the small sample containing the radioactivity, which is usually biologic tissue. The solvent accounts for about 99% of the cocktail's volume. Because of this, most of the interactions of ionizing radiation with the cocktail are with solvent molecules rather than directly with a scintillator. The *primary fluor* scintillates when energy is transferred to it from the solvent. The color of these scintillation photons from the primary fluor is generally not ideal for the photocathode of modern photomultiplier tubes, so a *secondary fluor* (a so-called *wave length shifter*) is usually used. This fluor produces a different color light from the primary fluor when energy is transferred to it from the primary fluor.

The pulses from liquid scintillation counting systems are very small, and electronic noise is a problem. Two techniques are used to reduce this noise. The first is to cool the entire counting system by putting it in a refrigerator. This reduces noise, because stray electrical signals (the source of the noise) originate in the electronics as electrons that are "freed" from atoms by heat (this process is called *thermionic emission*). Reducing the temperature decreases thermionic emissions. The second technique to reduce noise is to use *coincidence counting,* in which two photomultiplier tubes view the vial from opposing sides. A special coincidence circuit determines if a pulse occurs at the same time in both tubes. When a flash of light occurs in the vial, both tubes will generate a pulse and the coincidence circuit will generate a pulse to be counted. In most cases noise pulses will occur in only one photomultiplier tube/electronics stage at a time, so no coincidence circuit pulse will be generated.

An additional problem in liquid scintillation counting is *quenching,* which refers to any undesirable reduction in light output from the scintillation cocktail. (This use of the term *quenching* should not be confused with its completely different meaning in Geiger-Mueller detectors.) There are three main types of quenching. Chemical quenching is caused by the presence of materials in the cocktail that interfere with the transfer of energy from the solvent to the fluor or from the primary fluor to the secondary fluor. Oxygen is a common chemical quench agent. Color quenching is the result of having colored material in the cocktail (e.g., blood) that absorbs light from the primary or secondary fluor. Optical quenching is produced by condensation, fingerprints, or dirt on the vial.

Factors Affecting Count Rate

For both gas-filled and scintillation detectors, the size of each pulse (pulse height) is related to the energy deposited in the detector during the passage of a single ionizing particle or x ray or gamma ray through the detector (except for detectors operated in the Geiger-Mueller region, where the pulses are always the same, large size). The number of pulses produced per unit time (pulse rate) is proportional to the amount of radioactivity in the source. Typically, pulses of certain sizes are counted, and these data are used to represent relative activity. In practice, the observed count rate from a detector is typically less than the actual disintegration or decay rate of the radioactive source.

Time. First, after the deposition of energy in the detector by an alpha, beta, x ray, or gamma ray, it takes a certain amount of time for the detector's response to occur (i.e., for the ions and electrons to travel to the electrodes in a gas-filled detector or for the light to be emitted in a scintillator). Figure 3-12 shows the pulse size of a second event as a function of the time interval between two events for a gas-filled detector. During this time the detector is either not responsive or only partially responsive to the deposition of additional energy. The so-called *resolving time* represents how long it takes to "count" a given event. For a nonparalyzable system its inverse yields the maximum count rate capability

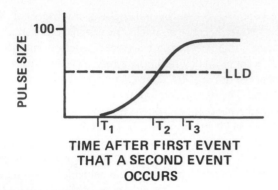

Figure 3-12 Timing characteristics of a detector system, showing relationship between the time after an event that a second event occurs and the pulse size of the second event. T_1, Dead time; T_2, resolving time; T_3, recovery time; **LLD**, lower level discriminator setting.

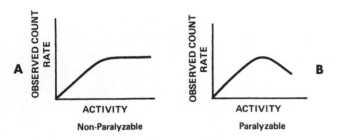

Figure 3-13 Effect of activity on observed count rate. **A**, Nonparalyzable system. **B**, paralyzable system.

of the detector. For example, if a typical counting system has a resolving time of $4\,\mu$sec its maximum count rate will be approximately 250,000 counts/sec.

The effects of timing can be separated into two types of situations: paralyzable and nonparalyzable systems (Figure 3-13). In a *non-paralyzable system,* as the activity increases, the count rate increases, until it reaches a maximum value given by the inverse of the resolving time. No matter how much the activity increases beyond that point the count rate will not increase. However, if the resolving time of the detector is known, comparison of its inverse (1/resolving time) with the observed count rate will indicate whether the detector is operating at an unacceptably high count rate. If so, the activity should be reduced until the count rate is at an acceptable level (i.e., below the maximum or plateau value). In a *paralyzable system,* as the activity increases, the count rate increases to a maximum value and then actually starts decreasing at higher activity levels. In this situation it is not possible to determine if the detector is operating on the ascending or descending portion of the curve. The detector should only be operated in the ascending portion of the curve. Accordingly, the user needs to know ahead of time what activity levels are reasonable to count with the detector. Alternatively, the user can count the activity, dilute it, and then recount the same size aliquot. If the observed count rate decreases after dilution, the detector was initially oper-

ating on the ascending portion of the curve (which is good); if it increases, the detector was on the descending portion (which is unacceptable).

Efficiency. The second factor is the *efficiency* of the detector itself. Not every alpha, beta, x ray, or gamma ray that passes through the detector will deposit energy in the detector material. If no energy is deposited, obviously no pulse will be generated. Gas-filled detectors can approach 100% efficiency for most alphas and betas that enter the detector, but are only about 1% efficient for x rays and gamma rays. Sodium iodide scintillators are approximately 50% efficient for x rays and gamma rays.

Geometry. The third factor is called *geometry* and takes into account the inverse square law. The greater the distance between the source and the detector, the lower the observed count rate. The count rate is changed by the square of the change in distance (e.g., if the distance is doubled, the count rate is reduced by a factor of four). Technically the inverse square relationship only applies when the both the source and detector are point sources. Geometry also takes into account the front cross-sectional area of the detector. The larger the surface of the detector facing the source, the more radioactive emissions that will intersect the detector, and the higher the count rate. Efficiency and geometry are often combined into a single term called *sensitivity.* This term reflects the fraction of radioactive emissions from the source ultimately detected.

Attenuation. The fourth factor is attenuation of the radioactive emissions, either self-attenuation in the source itself or attenuation in the medium between the source and the detector. In either case, radioactive emissions from the source are "removed" from the beam before they can strike the detector, thus lowering the observed count rate.

Random decay. The preceding factors are deterministic in nature. One final factor is the random nature of radioactive decay itself. Radioactive decay is governed by Poisson statistics. In the Poisson distribution the mean and variance are equal. Thus the coefficient of variation decreases as the mean increases. In the case of nuclear medicine the "mean" is the total number of observed decays (i.e., the total acquired counts). The greater this number, the better the statistical precision of the measurement. This statistical nature of decay is also the primary source of image noise.

ANGER SCINTILLATION CAMERAS

The Anger scintillation camera was invented by Hal Anger of Donner Laboratory, University of California at Berkeley, in the late 1950s. Pictures of two modern scintillation cameras are shown in Figure 3-14. Scintillation cameras are the most commonly used imaging instrument in nuclear medicine today. The complete camera system consists of a lead collimator, a 10- to 25-in circular, square,

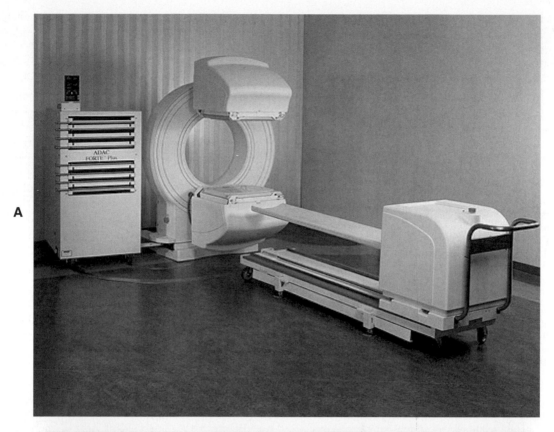

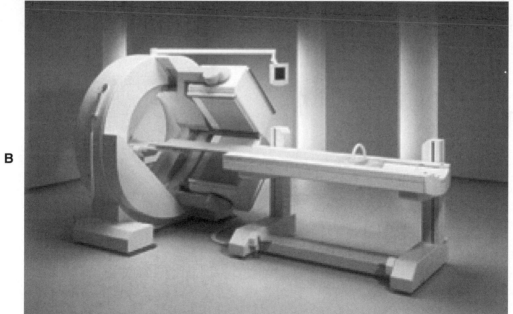

Figure 3-14 Dual detector Anger scintillation cameras. **A,** Philips Forte (Courtesy of Philips Medical Systems, Milpitas, California.) **B,** Siemens E.cam (Courtesy of Siemens Medical Solutions USA, Inc., Hoffman Estates, Illinois.)

or rectangular sodium iodide scintillation crystal, an array of photomultiplier tubes on the crystal, a positioning logic network, a pulse height analyzer, a scaler-timer, and a cathode ray tube (CRT) display. A side view is shown in Figure 3-15.

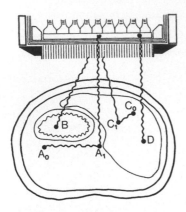

Figure 3-15   Side view showing arrangement of collimator, crystal, and photomultiplier tubes in an Anger camera. Photon A_0 scatters in the patient, producing photon A_1, which is detected in the crystal but has less energy and may be rejected by the pulse height analyzer; photon B is absorbed by collimator; photon C_0 scatters in the patient, resulting in photon C_1, which is absorbed by collimator; photon D does not scatter and is detected in the crystal. Collimators discriminate based on direction of flight, not on scattered versus nonscattered photons.

Collimators

A *collimator* is typically a 1/2- to 2-in thick piece of lead with a geometrical array of holes in it, and it has dimensions that are slightly larger than the scintillation crystal. The pinhole collimator is an exception to this general description. The lead between each hole is called a *septum;* collectively the lead represents *septa.* The collimator provides an interface between the patient and scintillation crystal by only allowing those photons traveling in an appropriate direction (i.e., those that can pass through the holes without being absorbed in the lead) to interact with the crystal. Collimators thus discriminate based on direction of flight, not on whether the photons are scattered or not. Several types of collimators are used with Anger cameras: parallel-hole, converging, diverging, and pinhole, as shown in Figure 3-16.

Types.   The most commonly used collimator is the *parallel-hole collimator,* which consists of an array of parallel holes essentially perpendicular to the crystal face and thus presents a real-size image to the detector. The resolution of a parallel-hole collimator is best at the collimator surface. The sensitivity is independent of the distance between the source and the collimator in most clinical applications. Although this seems to contradict the inverse square law, it really does not (Figure 3-17). The field of view of each hole increases

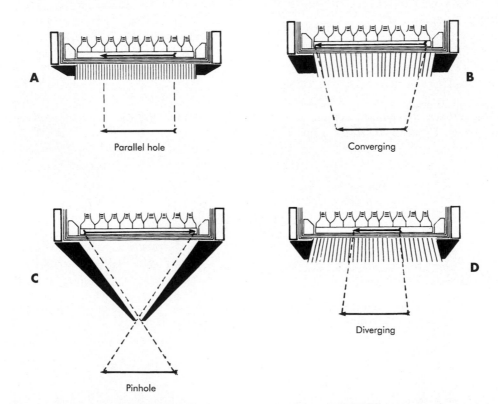

Figure 3-16   Four types of collimators for Anger cameras. Note how arrows are perceived by the crystal. **A,** Parallel hole; arrow is seen as actual size pointing to the left. **B,** Converging; arrow is magnified on crystal surface with point to the left. **C,** Pinhole; arrow is magnified on the crystal surface. Mirror image results with arrow pointing right. **D,** Diverging; arrow is minified on crystal surface with point to the left.

with increasing distance. This means that each hole "sees" a larger area at a greater distance from the collimator. Looking at it another way, more holes see the same source if it's farther away from the collimator. As a radioactive source is moved away from the face of the collimator, the count rate through each hole decreases because of the inverse square law. However, more and more holes see the source, and the total count rate remains constant. Because more holes see the source, its image is spread over a larger area of the crystal face (i.e., the image is progressively smeared out). Thus the resolution gets worse with increasing distance, as stated earlier.

Converging collimators have an array of tapered holes that aim at a point at some distance in front of the collimator; this point is called the *focal point*. The image that is presented to the crystal is a magnified version of the real object. Converging collimators have their best resolution at the surface of the collimator. The sensitivity of a converging collimator slowly increases as the source is moved from the collimator face back to the *focal plane* (the plane parallel to the collimator face that passes through the focal point) and then decreases.

Diverging collimators are essentially upside-down converging collimators. They have an array of tapered holes that diverge from a hypothetical focal point behind the crystal. The image presented to the crystal face is a minified image of the real object. This configuration is useful in patient studies when an organ or organs larger than the detector must be imaged. Because converging and diverging collimators are simply flipped versions of each other, some collimators may have an insert that can be flipped either way, in effect producing two collimators in one. This combination collimator is sometimes called a *div/con collimator*.

Pinhole collimators are thick conical collimators with a single 2- to 5-mm hole in the bottom center. As a source is moved away from the surface of a pinhole collimator, the camera image gets smaller. However, the camera image is magnified (i.e., larger than real size) from the collimator face to a distance equal to the length of the collimator. At larger distances it is then progressively minified.

Other types of collimators have more specialized functions. A *single-axis diverging collimator* is used for whole body scanning when the transverse field of view of the camera is smaller than the patient's width. This collimator has diverging holes in the transverse direction, but has parallel holes in the axial direction. A *fan-beam collimator* is a combination of a parallel-hole collimator (along one axis) and a converging collimator (along the other axis). It is used in some tomographic studies, such as brain scans.

Spatial Resolution and Sensitivity

As stated earlier, *spatial resolution* can be defined in terms of the amount by which a system smears out the image of a very small point source or a very thin line source of radioactivity. A profile of the counts along a line through the point source image (which is called the *point spread function*) or through the line source image (perpendicular to the line, which is called the *line spread function*) can be produced, usually with computer-aided analysis. Resolution is quantified as the FWHM of the point or line spread function and is generally expressed in millimeters. This measurement of spatial resolution is directly analogous to the measurement of energy resolution as the FWHM of the photopeak of a pulse height spectrum. In practice, the FWHM in millimeters will be nearly identical to the minimum distance by which two point or line sources must be separated in space to be distinguished as separate in an image. *Sensitivity,* on the other hand, is the overall ability of the system to detect the radioactive emissions from a source. The higher the sensitivity, the greater the fraction of the emissions that are detected. In practical terms, a higher sensitivity system detects more x rays or gamma rays when viewing the same radioactive source. In practice, there is always a trade-off between resolution and sensitivity. The simple relationship between spatial resolution and sensitivity for a pinhole collimator makes the point: the smaller the pinhole, the better the resolution and the worse the sensitivity, and vice versa for a larger pinhole.

Because of this trade-off, a collimator is not completely specified by its type. For multihole collimators sensitivity can be increased (at the expense of resolution) by increasing the size or shortening the length of each hole. This reduces the amount of lead in the path of the x rays or gamma rays so that a larger fraction can interact in the crystal. Resolution can be increased by using many more, smaller holes or by making the collimator longer (increasing the hole length). This reduces the sensitivity because of a net increase in the amount of lead in the collimator. *General all purpose* (GAP) collimators represent a compromise between high resolution and high sensitivity.

These relationships are illustrated in the following simplified equations for a parallel-hole collimator.

$$\text{Resolution} = \text{Diameter} \left(\frac{\text{Length} + \text{distance}}{\text{Length}} \right)$$

$$\text{Sensitivity} = \left(\frac{\text{Diameter}}{\text{Length}} \right)^2 \left(\frac{\text{Diameter}}{\text{Diameter} + \text{thickness}} \right)^2$$

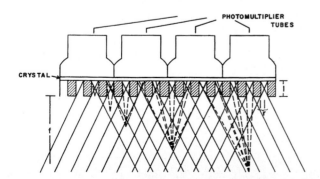

Figure 3-17 Relationship between each hole's field of view and distance from collimator face.

Resolution is the geometric resolution of the collimator (the smaller the number, the better); *diameter* is the diameter of each hole; *length* is the length of each hole; and *distance* is the distance between the face of the collimator and the patient or point in the organ of interest. Note that increasing the hole diameter or distance increases the resolution value (i.e., makes it worse), whereas increasing hole length decreases the resolution value (i.e., makes it better). *Sensitivity* is the geometric sensitivity of the collimator (the larger the number, the better), and *thickness* is septal thickness. Note that increasing the hole diameter increases the sensitivity value (i.e., makes it better), whereas increasing septal thickness decreases the sensitivity value.

It is important to note that the geometric spatial resolution of a collimator is only one of several factors that influence the actual spatial resolution in an image. In planar imaging, intrinsic camera resolution, collimator resolution, scatter, and "patient resolution" effects caused by patient or organ movement all influence the actual resolution in the image. A simple way to estimate total resolution from intrinsic, collimator, scatter, and patient resolution is

$$R_T = \sqrt{R_I^2 + R_C^2 + R_S^2 + R_P^2}$$

Note that the total resolution cannot be any better (i.e., a smaller value) than the largest term in the equation. Changes in intrinsic resolution of less than 1 mm rarely, if ever, influence image resolution.

In general, there is an inverse relationship between spatial resolution and sensitivity. However, when using a converging collimator, an additional parameter must be considered. The magnification provided by such a collimator provides increased spatial resolution and sensitivity compared with a parallel-hole collimator with equivalent holes. This is because the part of the patient within the field of view is spread over a larger area of the crystal. Of course the actual field of view with a converging collimator is proportionately smaller than that with a parallel-hole collimator because of the magnification. The possible increase in spatial resolution and sensitivity with magnification is sometimes exploited in single photon emission computed tomography (SPECT) with fan beam collimators.

Collimators are currently either cast or fabricated from corrugated lead strips (the latter are termed *foil* collimators). In general, it is harder to produce fabricated foil collimators with uniform septal thickness. This led some users to automatically consider cast collimators superior to foil collimators. At present, with improved manufacturing technology, excellent foil and cast collimators are available. Originally the collimator holes were circular in cross section. This meant that the lead septa were thicker in some areas than they needed to be to ensure that the thinnest areas were thick enough to absorb the x rays or gamma rays. Recent cast or corrugated collimators have square or hexagonal holes. With these collimators the septa are of uniform thickness around each hole. When compared with circular hole collimators, these newer collimator designs have better

sensitivity for a given resolution and better resolution for a given sensitivity.

Crystals

The properties of thallium-activated sodium iodide crystals as scintillation detectors were described earlier. As with crystals used in scintillation spectrometry, those used in Anger cameras are extremely sensitive to moisture and are sealed in an aluminum housing. In addition, they are sensitive to temperature, especially rapid changes in temperature, which can produce fractures. The crystals used in Anger cameras vary from 7 in to more than 25 in. In the past, virtually all crystals were circular in cross section. At present rectangular crystals are very popular because they typically provide an increased field of view. Crystals are typically 1/4 in to 1/2 in thick, with 3/8 in being the most common thickness. The thicker the crystal, the higher the probability that an incoming photon will interact, deposit its energy, and be detected. Thus the sensitivity of the camera is higher. However, the thicker the crystal, the poorer the spatial resolution because of the complex (geometric optics) interaction between the crystal, the photomultiplier tubes, and the light pipe that is generally used to optically couple the two. Crystals that are 1/4 in thick have about 1 mm better intrinsic resolution than crystals that are 1/2 in thick. When counting low-energy radionuclides such as ^{201}Tl, there is no difference in sensitivity. However, when counting ^{99m}Tc, crystals 1/4 in thick have 15% less sensitivity than crystals 1/2 in thick. At higher energies the difference in sensitivity is even more significant. Crystals with a thickness of 3/8 in to 1/2 in are required to efficiently detect gamma rays above 200 keV.

In recent times vendors have introduced cameras with thicker crystals ranging from 5/8 in to 1 in These crystals are primarily found in cameras that are used for coincidence imaging. Sensitivity is significantly increased for isotopes that emit high-energy photons such as I-131, In-111, and Ga-67, as well as positron emitters that produce annihilation photons. In crystals that are 1 in thick (Trade name "Starbright") the increase in sensitivity for medium- and high-energy photons is in the range of 50% to 100%. The challenge is to maintain satisfactory spatial resolution for routine clinical imaging with low-energy photons (e.g., Tc-99m and Tl-201). This challenge is met by cutting grooves into the crystal to reduce the spread of light, as shown in Figure 3-18. The grooves are 12.7 mm deep, 0.5 mm wide, and have a pitch of 6 mm. The boundaries of each "pixel" reflect light to the PMTs and produce a smaller light spot, which reduces interference between adjacent events (Figure 3-19). Pile-up is also decreased. Over 90% of the low-energy photons interact in the solid half of the crystal; high-energy photons interact evenly throughout the crystal. Clinical images of the same patient with 1 in and 3/8 in thick crystals are similar, but those from the 1 in crystals contain more counts or are acquired in less time.

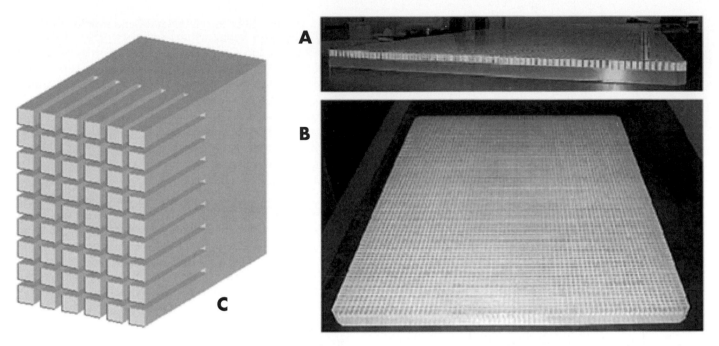

Figure 3-18   "Starbright" pixelated 1 in thick crystal. **A,** Side view of crystal. **B,** Oblique view of crystal. **C,** 3D diagram of section of crystal. (Courtesy of GE Medical Systems-Americas, Milwaukee, Wisconsin and Siemens Medical Solutions USA, Inc, Hoffman Estates, Illinois.)

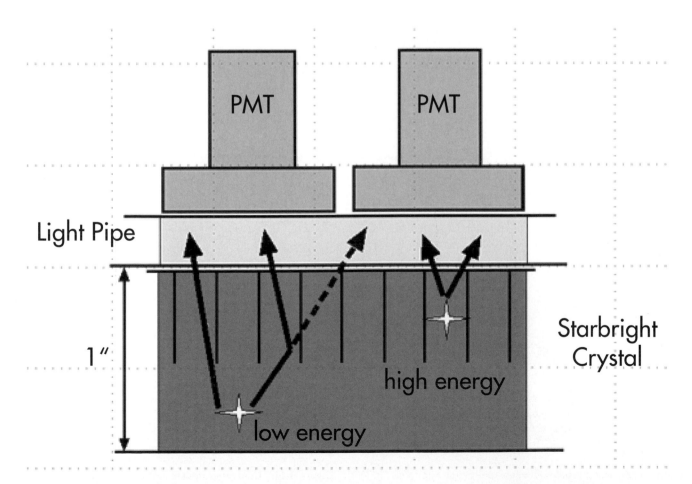

Figure 3-19   Reflection of light photons in second half of pixelated crystal.

Positioning Logic

Anger cameras have an array of photomultiplier tubes optically coupled to the back of the scintillation crystal (Figure 3-20). The actual number of tubes is determined by the size and shape of both the crystal and each individual photomultiplier tube. In circular-field cameras the tubes are typically arrayed in a hexagonal geometric configuration in which the number of tubes follows a "6n + 1" configuration (n is a whole number). For example, early cameras had 7 or 19 photomultiplier tubes. At present, it is common for cameras to have 37, 55, or 61 tubes. In general, the more photomultiplier tubes, the better the spatial resolution and linearity. Early photomultiplier tubes had a round cross section. Current tubes often have a hexagonal cross section to cover more of the crystal area for more efficient detection of scintillation photons.

When a scintillation event occurs, each photomultiplier tube produces an output pulse. The amplitude of the pulse from a given photomultiplier tube is directly proportional to the amount of light (number of scintillation photons) its photocathode has received. Those photomultiplier tubes closest to the scintillation event produce the largest output pulses. If only that tube with the largest pulse were used for positioning, the spatial resolution of the camera would be equivalent to the cross-sectional size of each tube. By combining the pulses from each photomultiplier tube, a higher resolution x, y coordinate of the gamma ray location can be generated, based on a centroid (center-of-mass) approach. The general equation for a centroid is

$$x = \frac{\Sigma x_i T_i}{\Sigma T_i}$$

where x is the centroid, x_i is the location of the ith tube, and T_i is the ith tube's output pulse size. Note that the centroid is the weighted average of the tube locations, with the weighting factors determined by pulse size. The y centroid is calculated with the same equation, except that y_i is used.

There are two ways in which the x and y centroids can be determined. In older, so-called analog cameras, an analog resistor network is used. A coordinate system is defined with the origin (0,0) at the center of the crystal (Figure 3-21).

The network creates four signals: x^+, x^-, y^+, and y^-. All photomultiplier tubes whose output is above a preset threshold contribute to all four signals. The contribution of any photomultiplier tube to the four signal lines (representing the four coordinate directions) is inversely proportional to the square of its distance from the respective coordinate and is controlled in a predetermined, fixed way by the resistor network. The sum of these four signals, called the z pulse, is proportional to the total energy deposited in the crystal by the photon interaction. The x coordinate of the interaction is given by

$$x = (x^+ - x^-)/z$$

Similarly, the y coordinate is given by

$$y = (y^+ - y^-)/z$$

Compare these equations to the general equation for a centroid given above. Note the similarities—remember that x^+, x^-, y^+, and y^- are already weighted sums of voltages (with the resistors providing the weighting factors), and that z is the sum of all tubes.

In newer, so-called digital cameras, each photomultiplier tube's output is digitized with an analog-to-digital converter. The resulting digital signals are then used with a software-based positioning algorithm. In many cases this algorithm is simply a "digital version" of Anger positioning logic with one significant difference. Many state-of-the-art cameras use a small cluster (also called zones or segments) of PMTs for calculating the position of an event. This scheme improves energy resolution and enables the camera to process events simultaneously, provided there is no spatial overlap of the clusters. The number of PMTs in the cluster varies between vendors. Some vendors use smaller PM tubes to increase the accuracy of positioning and increase the number of clusters that can be used.

In some cases more sophisticated algorithms are used. This highlights the theoretical advantage of a digital camera: the ability to more easily change and upgrade positioning algorithms. It should be noted, however, that the term digital camera does not have a universally accepted definition, and different vendors use the term to denote digitization of the signals at different stages. Although it is tempting to automatically consider a digital camera as superior to an analog camera, in practice, the functional performance, flexibility, and reliability of a camera determine its value. Excellent analog and digital cameras exist.

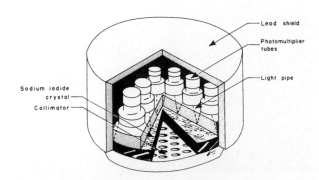

Figure 3-20 Arrangement of collimator, crystal, light pipe, photomultiplier tubes, and lead housing in an Anger camera.

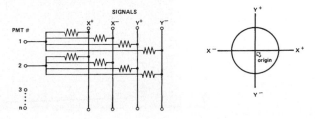

Figure 3-21 Coordinate system and resistor network for Anger positioning logic.

Energy Discrimination

The desired goal of the Anger camera is to create an image that portrays the distribution (i.e., sites and numbers of radioactive atoms) of radioactivity within the patient. Because the collimator only allows those photons traveling in predetermined directions to interact in the crystal, a line drawn from the scintillation event in the crystal through the nearest collimator hole is presumed to intersect the site of origin of the photon (i.e., the radioactive atom from which it originated) in the patient. If the photon has been scattered in the patient, a line drawn through its direction of flight will not intersect its site of origin, only the site of the Compton interaction. Thus photons scattered into the field of view could be falsely attributed to activity at the sites of Compton interactions in the patient. It is clearly not desirable to have these scattered photons contribute to the final image, because they may significantly degrade resolution and contrast. It is important to note that a large percentage of photons striking the crystal have been scattered in the patient.

The z pulse is used by the pulse height analyzer to discriminate against these scattered photons. The pulse height analyzer is used to set a window around the photopeak. Because the window has a finite width, some scattered photons may still be accepted (those that are scattered through a small angle and thus retain most of their energy). For example, 140 keV photons can scatter by as much as 55 degrees and still be accepted by the often-used 20% window.

In practice, proper window setting is vital because a window that is not centered on the photopeak (an offset window) can degrade field uniformity for many cameras (Figure 3-22). There is slightly better light collection efficiency directly under each photomultiplier tube. As a result events that occur under a tube tend to produce slightly

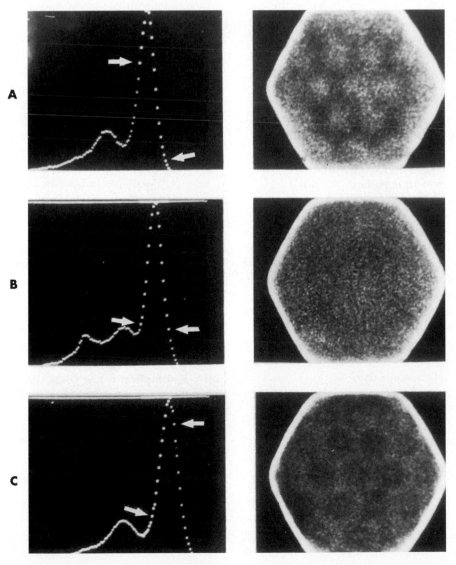

Figure 3-22 Effect of asymmetrically setting the pulse height window. **A**, Window set to high side of photopeak; **B**, window symmetrically positioned; **C**, window set to low side of photopeak.

larger z pulses, whereas those that occur between tubes tend to produce slightly smaller z pulses. If the manufacturer does not compensate for this effect, a pulse height window skewed to the "high side" of the photopeak will preferentially accept events occurring under tubes, producing a "hot-tube" pattern, whereas a window skewed to the "low side" will produce a "cold-tube" pattern. In practice, manufacturers of analog cameras frequently "tune" their cameras in a compensatory fashion to improve field uniformity. This has the effect of actually reversing the expected patterns with high-side and low-side peaking. Fortunately, newer cameras with microprocessor-based correction circuitry (described later), generally maintain fairly good uniformity even with slightly offset pulse height windows. Such cameras may be purposely peaked to the high side of the photopeak to further reduce scatter by eliminating any Compton scattered photons that show up in the lower half of the photopeak (because of every camera's less than perfect energy resolution). Some cameras have two or three separate pulse height windows to simultaneously image the multiple emissions of some radionuclides (e.g., those from ^{67}Ga). In this way counts are acquired in a shorter time as the multiple energy emissions are used.

The window can be set manually, or (in some cameras) automatically. Although *autopeaking* may be more accurate than manual peaking, automatic windows may be affected by the amount of Compton scatter that is present (which proportionately increases, for example, in larger patients) and generally perform poorly when multiple photopeaks are present.

Image Formation

An image can be formed in two ways. In analog cameras, particularly older cameras, photographic images are directly formed during acquisition. Virtually all current analog and digital cameras form images via digital acquisition. In older analog cameras, the scaler-timer controls the on/off cycle of the camera. The camera may be set up to acquire an image for a predetermined time interval (preset time mode) until a predetermined amount of radioactivity has been detected (preset count mode) or until a certain number of counts/cm^2 has been reached (preset information density mode). In current cameras, acquisition is under computer control, though typically the same criteria as above are used to define the end of acquisition.

Photographic image formation. For each z pulse that passes through the pulse height analyzer, its associated x and y pulses are used to position a finely focused dot of light on the CRT face. A collection of these light dots over time produces the image. Because it takes time for a complete picture to be obtained, some sort of integrating medium must be used to record the image. The most frequently used media are various types of photographic film. A photographic camera is mounted on the CRT, and the shutter is left open during the entire image acquisition period. The film is developed, and an image of the distribution of radioactivity is obtained.

An alternative camera recording system is a multiformatter. The heart of a multiformatter is a very high-quality CRT. The signals going to the multiformatter can be reduced and repositioned in such a way that the image only occupies a portion of the CRT. Thus it only exposes a corresponding portion of the photographic film. In this way up to 80 images can be produced on a single piece of film. The usual practice is to have four, nine, or sixteen images on one piece of 8×10 in film.

Digital image formation. The x, y signals from an Anger camera are frequently entered directly into the computer in real time during image acquisition. As scintillation events occur within the crystal of the camera, corresponding x, y signals stream into the computer and are digitized with the computer's analog-to-digital converters (which in the past had 8-bit resolution but at present have as much as 12- to 16-bit resolution). These x, y signals are stored in one of two ways, based on the mode selected by the operator before acquisition begins. These two acquisition modes are *frame mode* and *list mode* (also called *serial mode*).

In frame mode acquisition a digital image of the data is built in computer memory as the x, y signals are received. In frame mode the camera face is represented by a matrix of pixels, each of which corresponds to a certain area of the camera face and is designated by a specific range of x, y signal values. When the computer receives an x, y signal from the camera, the pixel associated with that particular x, y signal value is increased by one count. When data acquisition is complete, images are immediately available for display.

In list mode acquisition the x, y signals are transferred directly to computer memory in the form of a list of x, y coordinates. In addition to the x, y signals, other types of data can be inserted in the list. Typically, time markers are inserted every 1 to 10 msec. Physiologic trigger marks, such as the occurrence of the R wave from an ECG monitor of the patient's heart, can also be inserted. In list mode acquisition no matrices or images are formed within computer memory during acquisition. Although no images are produced immediately, list mode acquisition is useful because the x, y signals are permanently recorded in computer memory, allowing flexible control over subsequent formatting into digital matrices.

An extension of frame mode acquisition is *multiple-gated acquisition*. In this mode the data from the camera are distributed to a series of matrices in computer memory. A trigger signal (usually a physiologic trigger such as the R wave) controls the distribution of data among the matrices. Immediately after the trigger, data from the camera are placed in the first matrix for a fixed interval. When the interval has elapsed, data are then placed in the second matrix for the same interval. This process continues until the occurrence of a new trigger signal, at which time data distribution restarts at the first frame or until all the assigned matrices in computer memory are used, in which case no data are acquired until the occurrence of a new trigger signal. Multiple-gated acquisition is used to study a repetitive (cyclic) dynamic process. For example, in a cardiac-gated blood pool study, in which the circulating blood is labeled with radioactivity and the beating chambers of the heart examined, the data from the corresponding phases of many heartbeats are superimposed during acquisition, resulting in a series of images representing one "average" cardiac cycle. Typically, the cardiac cycle is divided into 16 to 64 frames, with each frame representing 1/16 to 1/64 of the cycle.

Three different types of data sets can be produced from an acquisition. A single, static image can be produced by acquiring a single frame mode image or by ignoring the time markers and formatting list mode data into a single matrix. A dynamic study can be produced by acquiring a series of frame mode images over time or by formatting list mode data into a series of matrices with reference to the embedded time markers in the list. These images may or may not represent equal intervals and may or may not be contiguous in time. A cyclic-gated study can be produced by multiple-gated frame mode acquisition or by formatting list mode data into a series of images representing a single average cycle with reference to the embedded trigger markers in the list.

The most common matrix sizes used in nuclear medicine are 64×64, 128×128, and 256×256. The larger the matrix size, the better the digital spatial resolution in the image. The digital sampling requirements necessary to preserve the "optical" or "geometric" spatial resolution that the camera is capable of producing are given by the Nyquist theorem. This theorem states that to accurately portray a signal, the spatial sampling frequency must be twice the highest spatial frequency present in the signal. Thus pixel dimensions should be smaller than half the system (collimator on) spatial resolution of the Anger camera. In practice, pixel dimensions range from 2 to 6 mm.

SOLID STATE CAMERAS

For some time several vendors have worked on developing a pixelated solid state camera. Early efforts centered on developing a detector that used an array of small cadmium zinc telluride crystals (CZT). Two of the vendors are continuing this effort, but a third has switched to a different material, cesium iodide. The scintillator is CsI(Tl), and the light signal is detected by a silicon photodiode. Its efficiency for collecting the light output from the CsI(Tl) is approximately 80%. CsI(Tl) has a higher atomic number than NaI(Tl), so its efficiency is higher. Because photodiode noise increases with temperature, a small thermoelectric cooler is used to maintain the temperature at a satisfactory level. The commercial system is pictured in Figure 3-23. The detector has a size of 21 cm × 21 cm and has 4096 CsI 3 mm × 3 mm sampling (64 × 64 pixels). The intrinsic spatial resolution of the output image is equal to a Gaussian profile with a FWHM of 2.0 mm.

Because the detector is quantized it has true digital event processing and the intrinsic spatial resolution is independent of energy. This is an important feature for imaging Tl-201. Furthermore, no distortion is present, and events are processed in parallel. Each pixel is an independent detector.

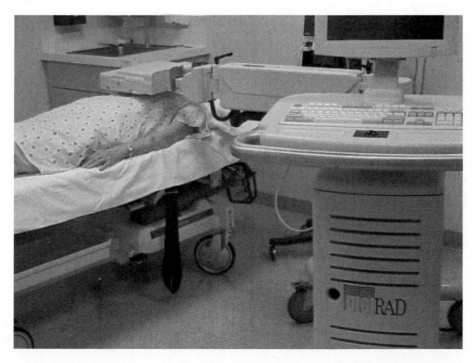

Figure 3-23   DigiRad 2020tc Imager solid state camera. (Courtesy of DigiRad Corporation, San Diego, California.)

In some clinical situations the small size of the detector is a problem. For cardiac SPECT there is no difficulty keeping the heart in the field of view (FOV). The small size also enables the technologist to acquire medial views of the breast and provides enhanced detectability of medial lesions. The lung and kidneys can be imaged, but a diverging collimator is required for large patients. The DigiRad camera can also be used for brain death studies. However, only limited bone scans can be done for adult patients.

EMISSION COMPUTED TOMOGRAPHY

Tomography is the process of producing a picture of a section or slice through an object. In medical imaging, tomography is performed either by transmitting x rays through an object (as in transmission computed tomography, CT scanning), by measuring proton density (as in magnetic resonance imaging, MRI), or by tomographically determining the distribution of radioactivity in a patient (as in emission computed tomography, ECT).

Emission computed tomography in its most general use refers to the process of producing a picture of the distribution of radioactivity in a slice through the patient. The slice can be oriented orthogonal to the patient's long axis (a transaxial slice), parallel with the patient's long axis (coronal or sagittal slices), or at any arbitrary oblique angle to the long axis of the body. In the past, ECT used either limited angle tomography systems or true transaxial tomographic acquisition and reconstruction (as in CT). At present, only transaxial approaches are in widespread use. These include single photon emission computed tomography (SPECT) and positron emission tomography (PET).

Single Photon Emission Computed Tomography

Single photon emission computed tomography is generally used today to refer to true transaxial tomography with standard nuclear medicine radiopharmaceuticals (i.e., those that emit a single photon on decay, as opposed to positron emitters, whose emissions ultimately result in two coincident annihilation photons). SPECT is performed with either specialized ring detector systems or rotating Anger cameras. The ring systems consist of an array of individual detectors (usually sodium iodide crystals) that surround the patient. These systems, which produce excellent tomograms, tend to be very expensive. By far the most popular method of doing SPECT is with a rotating Anger camera (usually with a large field of view detector) mounted on a special gantry that allows 360-degree rotation around the patient. The initial systems used a single Anger camera. At present, multidetector systems with two or three heads are common because they provide increased sensitivity.

The essence of emission transaxial tomography is similar to that of CT; an object is viewed at a number of angles between 0 and 180 or 360 degrees around it. Certain types of studies, such as myocardial perfusion studies, produce higher contrast when only 180 degrees of data (from RAO to LPO) are used for reconstruction. Images are acquired at many angles, each representing one *projection* of the object. In general, a parallel-hole collimator is used so that the projections have parallel beam geometry. In some cases it is useful to magnify the image in-plane. This is particularly true when the organ of interest encompasses only a small fraction of the system's field of view. In such a situation a fan-beam collimator may be used. This collimator has holes that converge in the plane of the slice but are parallel from slice to slice. Projections from such collimators have fan-beam geometry.

Reconstruction. To reconstruct a slice through an object, each projection need only be a one-dimensional linear scan of the object. The use of an Anger camera, which produces two-dimensional images, therefore allows simultaneous acquisition of data for a number of contiguous transaxial slices. Note, however, that the data used to reconstruct a given slice come from only that slice.

Tomographic reconstruction of transaxial slices by filtered back-projection is the most common computer algorithm for tomography. From the computer's point of view, it does not matter if the data are from a transmission CT scanner, a rotating Anger camera SPECT system, or a PET scanner. The essence of the reconstruction is the smearing back (*back-projection*) into the reconstruction space of each projection, maintaining the correct angular offset (Figure 3-24).

Filtering. Simple back-projection results in a blurred image, with streaks emanating from areas of high activity. This is called the "star" artifact. This artifact can be eliminated by understanding the underlying mathematics of reconstruction, as was first done by Radon in 1917. The mathematical function describing the reconstruction process contains a *filter* that is used to modify each projection before back-projection. Conceptually, this filter produces negative side regions around hot areas in each projection. The negative side regions cancel out the positive streaks from other projections during a reconstruction.

Mathematically a "perfect" filter exists called the *ramp filter.* This filter progressively boosts the power of higher and higher *spatial frequencies.* Spatial frequencies are analogous to audio (temporal) frequencies. Audio frequencies are expressed in cycles/time; spatial frequencies are expressed in cycles/distance. High spatial frequencies are generated by the edges of organs and other structures in the patient and by image noise. The ramp filter preserves spatial resolution, but also boosts noise significantly. In fact, the noise is no longer governed by Poisson statistics and is significantly worse. In practice, images are reconstructed with one of many different filters. These filters represent different tradeoffs between noise reduction and preservation of spatial resolution (Figure 3-25). In general, the filters used in practice are a combination of the ramp filter with a "low-pass" or "smoothing" filter, such as a Butterworth filter. The user

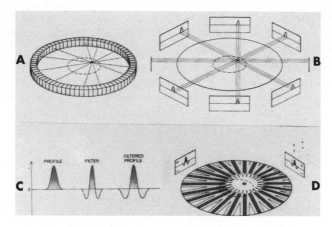

Figure 3-24   Reconstruction process. **A,** Arrangement of detection in positron tomography. **B,** So-called "parallel" detection geometry, from either reorganizing PET data or directly using Anger camera SPECT projections with parallel-hole collimation. **C,** Original single projection data profile, shape of filter used to modify data, and resulting filtered profile to back-project. **D,** Back-projection process to reconstruct image.

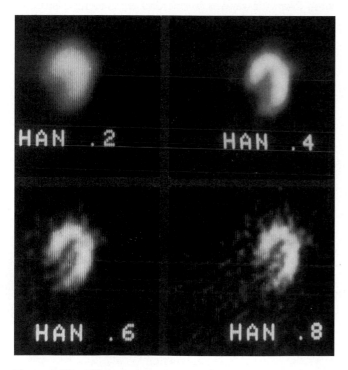

Figure 3-25   Effect of reconstruction of same raw projection data with four different filters. "Han" is an abbreviation for a Hann, sometimes called a Hanning, filter. The real number is the cutoff.

must specify certain characteristics of the low-pass filter, including the "cutoff frequency" or "critical frequency." The lower this frequency, the poorer the spatial resolution and the greater the noise reduction (i.e., the more the "smoothing" action of the filter).

Two-dimensional prefiltering followed by ramp filter reconstruction is preferable to one-dimensional filtering during reconstruction (provided a simple ramp filter is not used). With two-dimensional prefiltering, the spatial resolution in the data remains *isotropic* (uniform in all direc-

tions), whereas one-dimensional filtering produces a three-dimensional data set in which the transverse resolution is worse than the axial resolution. One-dimensional filtering thus produces coronal and sagittal images with horizontal smearing and oblique angle reorientations with nonuniform resolution. Contrast enhancing filters, such as the Wiener or Metz filter, are desirable in certain situations.

Sometimes, projection data from adjacent slices are combined to reconstruct transverse slices that are more than one pixel thick. In general, even if ultimately the slices will be displayed with greater than one pixel thickness, it is preferable to reconstruct one pixel thick transverse slices to use as the input for coronal and sagittal image formation and for oblique angle reorientation. After the slices are reoriented, they may be added together if necessary. The use of slices one pixel thick for reorientation is superior to starting with thicker transverse slices, because interpolation artifacts are significantly diminished. Automated reorientation approaches are frequently helpful, since these reduce analysis variability and particularly facilitate comparisons (both stress-to-rest and patient-to-database). In addition to reconstructing transaxial, coronal, sagittal, and oblique slices, it is often helpful to display the data in a "whole body" mode, particularly if the axial coverage is sufficient. This is often performed through a pseudo–three-dimensional volume rendering.

The availability of more powerful computers has made it possible to use iterative reconstruction for clinical studies. Filtered back-projection is ideal for computed tomography but cannot incorporate the physics of SPECT and PET that is needed. These elements are nonuniform attenuation correction, variation of resolution with depth, image noise, and scatter. However, the equations that include the physics for the projections require iteration, that is, multiple, repetitive steps. The ML-EM (Maximum Likelihood-Expectation Maximization) algorithm involves estimating a distribution of activity in the body that would have produced the measured projections. The EM algorithm iteratively estimates the distribution of radioactivity using estimates from previous iterations. The negative side is that this algorithm requires a large number of iterations (ten to hundreds) to produce the desired results. More recently a modification of the EM algorithm called OS-EM (Ordered-Subsets Expectation Maximization) has been developed that uses only some of the angles during each iteration (cycle). The sequence of iterations is "ordered" so that the final result includes all angles. By using only a subset of the angles the computation time is reduced to only a few minutes for each update and the number of iterations is reduced to less than ten. The results are better than with filtered back projection (FPB) because the correct physics is included in the reconstruction. Overall quality is improved, nonuniform attenuation is corrected, and streak artifacts and noise are reduced. An example of the difference in image quality is shown in Figure 3-26.

Multidetector SPECT. In an attempt to increase sensitivity, manufacturers are now producing SPECT systems that incorporate two or three detectors. The increase in sensitivity depends on the acquisition arc, as illustrated in Table 3-1.

Optimizing acquisition. In many SPECT acquisitions the organs or structures of interest are at a significant distance from the collimator face (as much as 25 to 30 cm or more in some views). In an attempt to increase resolution and, of greater importance, preserve good resolution with depth, the use of longer hole length collimation is desirable. Such collimators are typically labeled as "high-resolution" collimators. The corresponding loss in sensitivity is more than compensated for by the improved resolution at depth. The use of a multicamera system greatly facilitates the use of high-resolution collimation, because the loss of sensitivity with the use of high-resolution collimators can be (at least partially) compensated for by the increase in sensitivity with the use of multiple detectors. Frequently the increased sensitivity permits shorter imaging times, which reduces artifacts that might arise from patient motion or organ movement (e.g., so-called *upward creep* of the heart, a gradual upward movement of the heart during SPECT acquisition following a stress study). Shorter imaging times also reduce artifacts from tracer washout during acquisition.

Studies have shown that Anger cameras must have significantly better performance for adequate SPECT than for

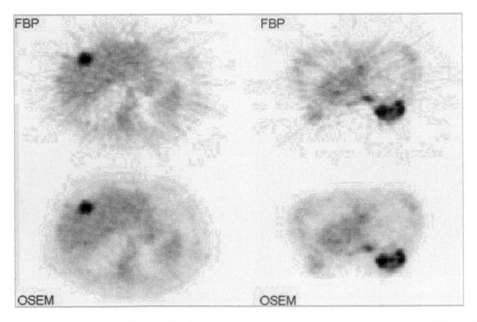

Figure 3-26   Comparison of transverse slice through the liver reconstructed with filtered back production (FBP) and Ordered-Subsets Expectation Maximization (OSEM). (www.osem.server-web.com/OSEM.html)

Table 3-1 Multidetector SPECT acquisition	360 degree acquisition		180 degree acquisition	
	Acq time	**Rel sens**	**Acq time**	**Rel sens**
Single	30	1	30	1
Double (heads at 180 degrees)	15	2	30	1
Double (heads at 90 degrees)	15	2	15	2
Triple	10	3	20	1.5

adequate planar imaging. For example, nonuniformity must be reduced to less than 1%. This requires acquisition of a 30 to 120 million count flood for subsequent computer correction of nonuniformities. In older cameras this correction had to be explicitly performed by the computer operator during the reconstruction process. In present systems, particularly those with microprocessor-based real-time correction circuits, the correction maps themselves contain sufficient counts to obviate the need for a separate SPECT uniformity correction procedure, provided collimator defects are not present. The camera image must also be mechanically aligned within the computer matrix, or a center-of-rotation correction must be made.

Positron Emission Tomography

One of the most exciting tomographic techniques is PET scanning. Positron-emitting radionuclides are used with this technique. A positron is an antimatter electron. Consider what happens when a positron-emitting radiopharmaceutical is distributed in a patient. After a positron is emitted, it travels a short distance (several millimeters in tissue) and deposits its kinetic energy. It then meets a free electron, and mutual annihilation occurs. By the law of conservation of energy two 511 keV annihilation photons appear; 511 keV is the energy equivalent to the rest mass of an electron or positron. By the law of conservation of momentum the annihilation photons are emitted 180 degrees back-to-back. We could use an Anger camera to individually detect these 511 keV annihilation photons. However, it makes more sense to surround the patient with a ring of detectors and electronically couple opposing detectors to simultaneously identify the pair of photons (Figure 3-27).

When two 511 keV annihilation photons are detected by opposing detectors in coincidence, we know that the annihilation event must have occurred along the line joining the two detectors. We thus know the direction of travel of the photons, without the need for a collimator. Conceptually the raw PET scan data consist of a number of these *coincidence lines*. Reconstruction could simply be the drawing of these lines They would cross and superimpose wherever there was activity in the patient. In practice, the data set is reorganized into projections, and filtered back-projection or OS-EM is used to reconstruct the images. PET differs from SPECT in that the "electronic collimation" of coincidence counting reduces the need for conventional lead collimation, thus increasing sensitivity.

The excitement about PET is due to both the chemistry and physics inherent in positron tomography. The most commonly used radionuclides—[11]C, ^{13}N, ^{15}O, and [18]F—are isotopes of elements that occur naturally in organic molecules. Fluorine usually does not, but is a bioisoteric substitute for a methane group. Thus radiopharmaceutical synthesis is simplified, and the tracer principle (which mandates as small a change in the molecule to be traced as possible) is better satisfied. Indeed, useful PET radiopharmaceuticals are now available for in vivo measurements of such important physiologic and biochemical processes as blood flow, oxygen, glucose, free fatty acid metabolism, amino acid transport: pH, and neuroreceptor densities. The short half-lives of the radionuclides (^{11}C, 20 min; ^{13}N, 10 min; ^{15}O, 2 min; and ^{18}F, 110 min) permit the acquisition of serial studies on the same day without background activity from prior injections interfering with the measurements. The physics of PET permits greater quantitative accuracy and precision. The use of small, high-density crystals improves spatial resolution (about 4 mm in the best commercial PET scanners). The lack of lead collimation to determine photon direction dramatically increases sensitivity. Finally, coincidence detection allows mathematically accurate attenuation correction.

Unfortunately, PET scanners generally cost between $700 thousand and $2 million. They require more space, more electricity, and more air-conditioning than Anger cameras. Although some generator systems exist (e.g., [68]Ge/^{68}Ga and [82]Sr/[82]Rb), a cyclotron is required to produce ^{18}F, 11C, ^{13}N, and [15]O. Because of the short half-lives of these radionuclides, the cyclotron is generally on site. Cyclotrons cost a minimum of $1 million and are quite expensive to install and operate. At the present time PET scanning is confined to about 400 centers around the world.

Positron Tomography With Scintillation Camera Systems

In theory, positron-emitting radionuclides could be used in SPECT in two ways: collimated detection of one or both of the two photons in noncoincidence mode (i.e., by one or more collimated heads in a conventional SPECT system), or uncollimated coincidence detection of both photons by opposing detectors (i.e., by a dual-head, uncollimated 180-degree SPECT system). Each approach has its advantages and disadvantages.

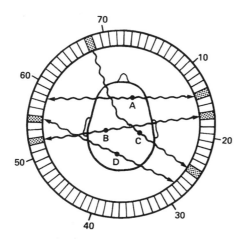

Figure 3-27 Geometry of PET detection system. Event **B** represents true coincidence detection; simultaneous detection of one annihilation photon from each of the events **A** and **D** produces accidental (random) coincidence detection; event **C** represents scatter coincidence detection.

must be measured A Geiger-Mueller counter is used for low-level surveys because of its higher sensitivity. They both require annual calibration and daily constancy testing with long-lived radionuclide standards. Calibration techniques are the same for both types of instruments.

Accuracy. Survey instruments are calibrated before their first use, annually, and following repair. Calibration is performed at two different operating points on the instrument's readout scale. The two points are approximately 1/3 and 2/3 of full scale. The standard that is used must be traceable within 5% accuracy to the National Institute of Standards and Technology (NIST, formerly known as the National Bureau of Standards). The same formula used to convert known exposure rate to activity can be rearranged to convert known activity to exposure rate:

$$E = AG/d^2$$

where E is the measured exposure rate, A is the activity of the source, d is the distance between the source and the detector, and G is the specific gamma ray constant. Readings are then made of the standard with the survey meter at those same distances. Each scale setting is calibrated over its entire range. Many departments send their instruments to qualified laboratories for calibration if they do not wish to keep a standard source on hand.

It is extremely important to remember the differences between ionization chambers and Geiger-Mueller counters. Ionization chambers respond in proportion to the total energy deposited in the detector. Thus the output of an ionization chamber can be directly related to exposure rate, no matter what the energy of each incoming photon. On the other hand, Geiger-Mueller detectors produce pulses with sizes that are independent of energy deposited. As a result, count rate may only be related to exposure rate if the energy of the radiation is known. Accordingly, the use of Geiger-Mueller counters to assess exposure is only possible if the photon energy used to calibrate the detector is the same as that of the source being measured.

Constancy. In addition to assessing accuracy, a reference source with a long half-life must be used to check the *constancy* of the survey meter's performance. The initial measurement of the source count rate (cpm) or exposure rate (mR/hr) is made at the time of calibration and should be conspicuously noted on the instrument. The source is then checked with the same geometry each day the instrument is used, after a battery change, and after any maintenance. If the exposure rate (or count rate) is not within 10% of the expected results, the instrument should be recalibrated.

Dose Calibrator Quality Control

The accuracy of the dose of radiopharmaceutical given to patients depends on the performance of the dose calibrator. An acceptable quality control program for radionuclide dose

calibrators consists of a series of procedures that measure its accuracy, linearity, geometry dependence, and constancy.

Accuracy. Instrument accuracy testing is performed at installation and annually thereafter. The accuracy of the dose calibrator is measured with at least two sealed reference standards whose activity is traceable to NIST. The instrument should be calibrated with standard sources of the radionuclide of interest whenever possible. Dose calibrators are normally calibrated by the vendor. When the use of short-lived nuclide standards is not possible, a long-lived standard of similar energy can be used, provided that the appropriate settings are employed. Several different radionuclides such as ^{57}Co, ^{137}Cs, and ^{133}Ba, may be used. The activity shall be at least $50\,\mu$Ci and preferably $200\,\mu$Ci or more. At least one of the sources must have a principal photon energy between 100 keV and 500 keV.

By correcting the standards for decay, the exact activity is known for comparison with the amount indicated by the dose calibrator. The average of several net-activity measurements should be compared with the activity calculated for that particular standard. According to the Nuclear Regulatory Commission (NRC), if the measured activity is within 10% of the standard, the dose calibrator is functioning with acceptable accuracy. So-called agreement states, such as Maryland and California, which regulate activities themselves under an agreement with the NRC, may have different limits.

Constancy. Constancy is checked each day the instrument is used. After the accuracy of the dose calibrator has been determined, the constancy of its performance is monitored by daily testing with a long-lived standard, preferably Cs-137, at each of the frequently used radionuclide settings. An activity control chart is established for each of the radionuclide settings (Figure 3-28). The average reading of the standard is obtained and plotted on semi-logarithmic graph paper. The activity level of the standard is calculated, with use of the appropriate decay schedule, and plotted. These

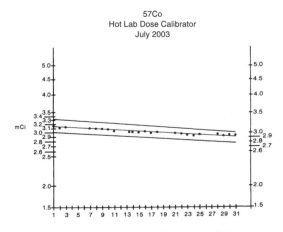

Figure 3-28 Typical activity control chart used for measurement of dose calibrator constancy.

points are connected with a straight line, which indicates the decay of the standard. Two straight lines are drawn, one above and one below the decay line, indicating the tolerance limits (±10% for NRC-regulated states). Daily readings of the standard are plotted and should fall within the tolerance limit lines. If a reading repeatedly falls outside the limits, the calibrator should be taken out of service until the problem is identified and corrected. Personal computer-based spreadsheets may easily be programmed to generate tables and graphs for this purpose.

Linearity. Instrument linearity is measured at installation and quarterly thereafter. The dose calibrator must function linearly over the range of its use between the highest dosage that will be administered to a patient and 30 µCi (for NRC-regulated states). Several methods may be used to determine the dose calibrator's response at different activity levels. A convenient method uses a vial of ^{99m}Tc that contains the desired amount of activity. The vial is assayed at frequent intervals, usually twice each day, over the appropriate range of activities. The observed activity versus time is plotted on semi-logarithmic paper, and a best-fit straight line is drawn through the points. A point is chosen on the line where the accuracy of the measurement has been established by a reference standard and a straight line constructed with a slope equivalent to the half-life of ^{99m}Tc (6 hours). Compare this straight line to the line generated by the data from the observed counts. Any difference greater than 10% (again, for NRC-regulated states) indicates the need for repair or adjustment. Note that the use of radionuclides with a longer half-life than that for ^{99m}Tc would require a correspondingly longer measurement period.

An alternative method uses a set of calibrated lead attenuation sleeves to assess changes in linearity once the system's linearity has been established. It offers the advantage of shortening the time required to perform the test from days to minutes.

Geometric calibration. Geometric calibration is performed at installation, whenever a change is made in the type of vial or syringe used in radiopharmaceutical processing, and after the chamber is repaired. Changing the radionuclide sample volume or configuration can significantly affect the measurement of the sample's activity. To measure the effect of changing the volume of liquid within a vial, a 30 ml vial containing 1 mCi of ^{99m}Tc in a volume of 1 ml is used. This is assayed, and the volume is increased with water in steps of 1, 4, 8, 10, 15, 20, and 25 ml, with assays being taken at each step. The net activity at each volume is determined by subtraction of the background. One of the volumes should be selected as the standard, and the correction factor for each of the other volumes can be calculated as the ratio of the measured activity for the standard reference volume divided by the measured activity for each of the other volumes. These volume-specific multiplicative correction factors should be plotted against the volume on linear graph paper. Alternatively, the data may be put in tabular form. One can

then calculate the true activity of a sample by taking the correction factor determined for that volume times the measured activity of the sample. This procedure should be used to determine the correction factors for various types and sizes of syringes, because significant changes in the measurement can occur when the radionuclide is assayed in different materials (plastic vs. glass) or the wall thickness of the container changes.

It is important to note that the sensitivity of a dose calibrator is affected by backscattering of photons by the shielding of the unit or other adjacent objects. An erroneous activity reading may be obtained if these variables are changed after calibration of the instrument.

The dose calibrator is a tool on which all nuclear medicine departments rely heavily. Assurance that the indicated activity on the dose calibrator is close to the true amount is important for the proper dispensing of radiopharmaceuticals to patients in the technologist's care.

Quality Control of Nonimaging Scintillation Detectors

Scintillation probes are employed for external organ counting, and well detectors are used for sample counting. Their reliable performance is essential for accurate results in a variety of in vivo and in vitro studies.

Calibration. Calibration initially involves energy calibration, in which the relationship between pulse height units and energy is determined (and set). First, the pulse height spectrum is obtained for a long-lived radionuclide, usually ^{137}Cs, by selection of a narrow window width (e.g., 10 pulse height units) and then by obtaining a series of counts at each 10 pulse height unit increment of the spectrum until the principal photopeak is passed or until the count rate approaches the background level. Plotting the resultant counts on linear graph paper will yield a pulse height spectrum. The pulse height position of the photopeak indicates the relationship between pulse height and energy. It is possible to adjust the amplifier gain or the high voltage across the photomultiplier tube to "move" the photopeak to a different pulse height position. It is frequently useful to move the photopeak to a pulse height position corresponding to the photopeak energy (e.g., 662 pulse height units for the 662 keV photon from ^{137}Cs).

By measuring the FWHM of the ^{137}Cs photopeak, one may determine the percent energy resolution for that radionuclide (see Figure 3-7). Typical values for percent energy resolution are less than 10%. Ordinarily this procedure is performed by the manufacturer, and the measured values are furnished with the instrument. It is prudent to repeat the procedure on installation and annually thereafter.

Daily calibration should include counting a long-lived reference source at specified window and base-line settings while either the fine gain or the high voltage is adjusted. This procedure is referred to as *peaking*. In other words, a series of counts at various voltages or gain settings are made until the maximum count rate is determined. The voltage or gain setting that yields the maximum or peak counts is recorded in the daily calibration log. Background counts accumulated for a statistically sufficient interval are recorded as well. The number of counts obtained at the peak is plotted on a control chart. This control chart is merely a graph of the number of source counts plotted on the ordinate, with time (usually 1 year) represented on the abscissa. A line is drawn representing the estimate of the source counts over time. Parallel lines representing ±1, 2, and 3 standard deviations are drawn as well. If daily counts fall outside the +/−3 standard deviation limits repeatedly, the instrument is not functioning properly. Quality control tests of probes require that the source be positioned in the center of the detector.

Reproducibility. The ability of the instrument to reproducibly and reliably record and display events detected can be assessed by performing standard statistical fits of repetitive sample counts obtained using a radioactive source. The most prevalent statistical models used are the chi-square test, Poisson standard deviation, and Gaussian standard deviation. These statistical goodness-of-fit formulas should be performed on a minimum of 10 repetitive counts (observations) and a statistically valid number of counts should be accumulated (greater than 10,000). It is sufficient to perform these tests initially when a program is begun or when a new instrument is placed in use. The data should be recorded and used for comparison at least twice per year and whenever the instrument is suspected of malfunctioning.

Reproducible sample geometry in multisample well counters is affected by the mechanical devices that position the sample in the well. There may be a combination of mechanical arms or elevators moving or lowering the sample into the well. Because of their mechanical design, the wearing of parts and belts or service adjustments may affect sample positioning and hence counting efficiency. This error may first appear as a decrease in the count rate of the long-lived standard used to monitor count rate stability and spectrometer calibration. As a result, it is not advisable to use the chi-square test for measurements made across samples that involve mechanical motion.

Calibration of Multicrystal Well Counters

The development of multicrystal gamma counters to increase the efficiency of counting large numbers of radioassay samples has introduced a special problem in assessing the balance or sensitivity of 10, 16, or 20 small sodium iodide crystals and their corresponding electronics. Discrepancies in the sensitivity of these multidetectors can drastically and insidiously affect the results of critically important tests. Most multicrystal systems employ a microprocessor-based program to assess the *balance* of detectors and usually match detector output by mathematically applying correction factors to counts from individual wells. The intrinsic balance of each well in these counters should be

evaluated daily using a single long-lived standard of appropriate energy and count rate, or a set of matched standards.

The actual measurement spread is determined by counting a source sequentially in all detectors for a minimum of 100,000 counts. The spread is defined by

$$\text{spread} = (\text{max} - \text{min})/\text{max} \times 100\%$$

where *max* and *min* are the maximum and minimum counts obtained from a set of detectors at any given count rate. The spread of absolute count rate should not exceed 3% at a counting rate not exceeding 10,000 counts/sec.

Scintillation Camera Quality Control

The performance of a scintillation camera system must be assessed each day of use to assure the acquisition of diagnostically reliable images. Performance can be affected by changes or failure of individual system components or subsystems and environmental conditions such as electrical power supply fluctuations, physical shock, temperature changes, humidity, dirt, and background radiation. Testing procedures that elucidate the presence of these performance-affecting variables must be used.

The most useful data to determine acceptability of camera performance reflect the parameters of field uniformity, spatial resolution, linearity, and sensitivity. These parameters must be measured at the time of installation to confirm specifications and provide the standard for all subsequent performance evaluations. These initial measurements are usually part of acceptance testing. It is also important to test the camera after service has been performed.

Uniformity. Perhaps the most basic measure of camera performance is *flood-field uniformity*. This is the ability of the camera to depict a uniform distribution of activity as uniform. It is assessed by "flooding" the camera with a uniform field of radiation and then assessing the uniformity of the resulting image. In the past, field nonuniformity was thought to arise primarily from differences in sensitivity across the crystal face. To correct the nonuniformity, a uniform flood or sheet source of radioactivity was imaged and recorded in an electronic memory in the camera. Clinical images were corrected during acquisition by either adding counts to the image in areas where the flood had too few counts relative to the other areas, or by subtracting (i.e., purposely not recording) counts in areas with too many counts. This process is usually done by *normalization,* that is, the counts in individual pixels are multiplied by a number greater than one (counts are added), less than one (counts are subtracted), or one (counts are not changed).

It is now well-known that most of the nonuniformity in a camera detector occurs as a result of *spatial distortion* (i.e., the mispositioning of events). To correct this distortion, references images are acquired and digital correction maps are generated and stored. Each map contains values that represent x, y correction shifts. Sophisticated microprocessor circuitry is used to reposition each count in real time during acquisition using these shifts. With many current cameras it is best to acquire correction maps with the same radionuclide as used for patient imaging. In some cameras several sets of corrections maps are stored on the computer, representing all the radionuclides used in the nuclear medicine department. The technologist must select the appropriate set for a given patient study.

Variation in the position of a pulse from different areas of the camera within the pulse height window can also produce nonuniformities. This spatially dependent energy variation may also be corrected by microprocessor circuitry. The combination of energy variation and spatial distortion is responsible for loss of spatial resolution and imperfect linearity and uniformity. In state-of-the-art cameras, explicit uniformity correction is typically carried out with multiplicative factors only after spatial distortion and spatially dependent energy response corrections have been applied. Some systems also include collimator-specific uniformity corrections.

Spatial resolution. Spatial resolution has been previously defined. A transmission phantom is commonly used to measure camera resolution. This type of phantom consists of some pattern in lead. The alternating patterns produce closely spaced areas of differing activity levels, which by definition allow for the analysis of resolution performance. The better the spatial resolution, the better the ability to detect small abnormalities manifested as different radionuclide concentrations in clinical images. In general a resolution pattern should be used without a collimator to measure intrinsic performance. In some multihead cameras it is difficult, or even impossible, and time consuming to measure intrinsic spatial resolution. It is also useful at times to assess resolution with a point or line source. The spread of the point or line is indicative of the degree of blurring (loss of resolution) of the camera.

Linearity. Linearity deals with the ability to reproduce a linear activity source as linear in the image. A phantom with a linear arrangement of bars or holes is usually used. The image produced should look exactly like the phantom (i.e., straight lines should be reproduced as straight).

Approaches to Camera Quality Control

When embarking on a scintillation camera quality control program, a department must make several decisions regarding methods and apparatus to be used. Three major decisions have to be made: which radionuclides to use, whether to use intrinsic or extrinsic testing or a combination, and which phantoms to use.

The radionuclide that is used should be of a similar energy to, if not the same as, the radionuclide used most frequently for actual patient imaging. Because of the widespread use of ^{99m}Tc-labeled radiopharmaceuticals, the two most commonly used radionuclides are ^{99m}Tc itself and ^{57}Co. There are advantages and disadvantages for both radionuclides. With a principal gamma-ray energy of 122 keV, ^{57}Co

meets the criterion of a similar energy. The half-life of 271 days allows for longer use before replenishment or replacement and also facilitates daily sensitivity checks. A disadvantage is the relatively high cost compared with ^{99m}Tc. Another consideration is that the microprocessor-based correction maps may be appropriate for the ^{57}Co setting (122 keV) but not for the ^{99m}Tc setting (140 keV). This is a possibility if ^{57}Co was used to acquire the maps. This could lead to a false sense of security when one sees acceptable ^{57}Co images, whereas the clinical images using ^{99m}Tc might be unacceptable. This would support the case for using ^{99m}Tc as a source, because it is the radionuclide used in the majority of nuclear medicine imaging procedures. Its availability makes cost an insignificant factor. The 6-hour half-life does necessitate daily replenishment.

Intrinsic testing (Figure 3-29, *A*) involves measuring the performance of the system without the collimator. A small volume or point source of the chosen radionuclide is positioned at a distance of five times the maximum dimension of the camera's useful field of view to give a uniform radiation flux across the crystal (Figure 3-30). Care must be taken to avoid contaminating or damaging the exposed crystal. The phenomenon known as *edge packing* is seen with some gamma cameras. This area of increased counts around the edge of the image must be masked off for those scintillation cameras that employ uniformity correction. The advantage of intrinsic testing is that a uniform radiation field is easily obtained using a small amount of radioactivity of the type used in clinical studies. The disadvantage is that the person who prepares the phantom receives some exposure to radiation and a source must be prepared each day.

Extrinsic testing (Figure 3-29, *B*) allows evaluation of the total system, including the collimator. When a collimator is used during assessment, a planar source having a uniform radionuclide distribution is placed on the collimator. Two types of planar sources are in use: a Lucite sheet impregnated with ^{57}Co and a liquid-filled, flat plastic phantom. The solid sheet consists of an epoxy type of material with ^{57}Co dispersed uniformly throughout the sheet, which ranges in size from 30 to 50 cm (Figure 3-31). New Co-57 floods

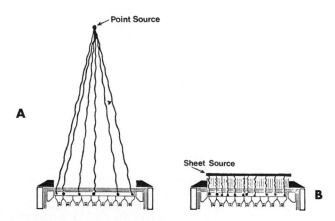

Figure 3-29 Schematic representation of intrinsic (**A**) and extrinsic (**B**) scintillation camera testing.

produce artifacts in the images acquired on some cameras because of the presence of relatively short-lived contaminates. In most cases this problem can be eliminated by placing the Co-57 flood on inverted foam cups.

A liquid-filled planar source (Figure 3-32), commonly called a *flood phantom,* is filled with water, and radioactivity must be added. The phantom is a sealable, flat, thin-walled container usually made of Lucite. It has a cavity that can be filled and then sealed. Thorough mixing of the radionuclide in the flood phantom is essential because any nonuniformity

in the distribution of radioactivity in the phantom could be interpreted as a camera malfunction. When this problem is suspected on a flood-field image, the phantom should be rotated 90 degrees and a second image should be obtained. A change in the pattern between images indicates a mixing problem in the phantom. Various examples are shown in Figure 3-33.

Analog cameras that are not interfaced to computers form photographic images in real time during acquisition. The use of exactly the same activity each day permits one to check the CRT intensity on such cameras. Figure 3-34 shows that a change in source strength greatly affects film density even though all imaging parameters, including total counts, were kept constant. This increased density at high count rates is due to two factors. When the electron gun in the CRT repeatedly strikes the same spot on the phosphor screen, the light output increases, or it experiences pulse buildup. Also, the high rate of light deposition on the film causes a failure of the reciprocal nature of producing the film density. The effects of film exposure on uniformity and resolution images are illustrated in subsequent figures. In addition, maintenance of a reproducible source strength produces a quality control check on the sensitivity or counting efficiency of the system.

Quality Control Phantoms

Many transmission phantoms have been developed for resolution and linearity testing, with several gaining the widest acceptance. An ideal phantom allows the accurate, simultaneous acquisition of an image that evaluates the parameters of spatial resolution, linearity, and spatial distortion. Some controversy exists regarding the ideal phantom to be used

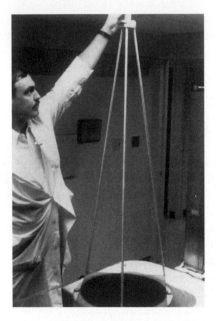

Figure 3-30   Tripod source receptacle used for intrinsic scintillation camera testing.

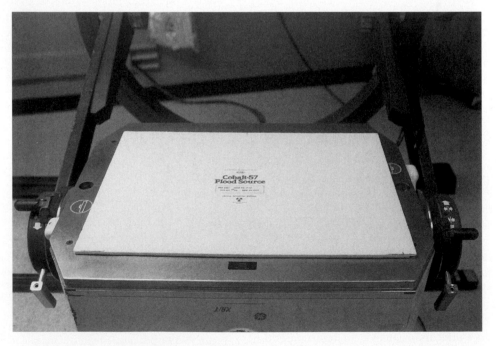

Figure 3-31   Planar disk source of ^{57}Co used for extrinsic scintillation camera testing.

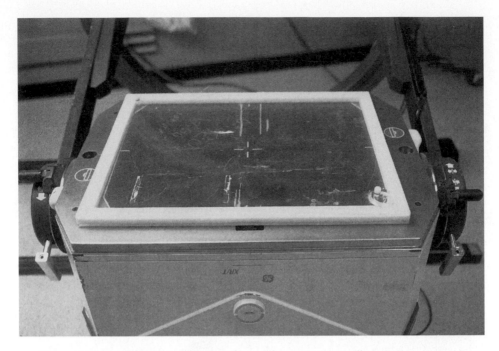

Figure 3-32 Liquid-filled planar source used for extrinsic scintillation camera testing.

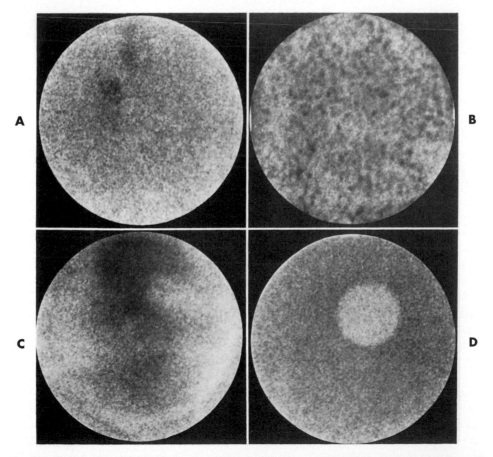

Figure 3-33 Complications arising from improper flood phantom preparation. **A,** Adherence of macroaggregated albumin particles to inner surface. **B,** Particulate formation within liquid. **C,** Incomplete mixing of radionuclide. **D,** Air bubble simulating a photomultiplier tube malfunction.

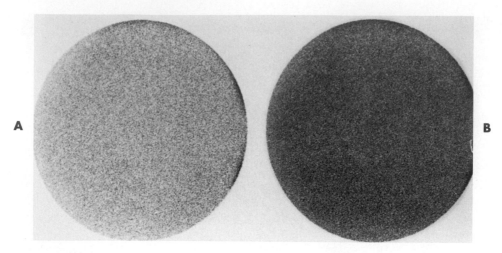

Figure 3-34 Effects of source activity on film density. Film density increases (**A** to **B**) when source activity is doubled. All other imaging parameters are kept constant.

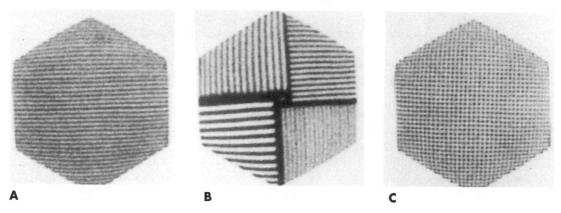

Figure 3-35 Transmission spatial resolution phantoms. **A,** Parallel-line equal-space (PLES) phantom. **B,** Four-quadrant bar phantom. **C,** Smith orthogonal-hole (OH) phantom.

in performing these checks. Two criteria must be met in selecting the phantom. First, the size and spacing of the holes or bars of the phantom selected should stress the maximum resolving capability of the instrument. Second, the same size pattern of holes or bars should be used to cover the entire camera field of view.

Three of the most widely used phantoms are pictured in Figure 3-35. The *parallel-line equal-space (PLES) phantom* consists of lead bars that have the same width and spacing and are embedded in Lucite. The bar width can be selected to match the lower limits of spatial resolution of the camera being evaluated. In departments that have more than one camera, optimal evaluation of spatial resolution and linearity may require that different patterns be purchased. Two transmission images acquired at an angle of 90 degrees relative to each other provide the assessment of spatial resolution, linearity, and spatial distortion for the entire detector area.

The *orthogonal-hole (OH) phantom* consists of a sheet of lead in which rows and columns of equal-diameter holes are arranged at right angles to one another. Phantoms are available with hole diameters 0.64 cm (1/4 in), 0.48 cm (3/16 in), and 0.32 cm (1/8 in) spaced at intervals of 1 cm (1/2 in), 0.96

cm (3/8 in), and 0.64 cm (1/4 in), respectively. A match of hole size to the lower limits of spatial resolution for the camera is important. A single image allows the assessment of spatial resolution, linearity, and spatial distortion for the entire detector area. The OH and PLES phantoms are considered comparable for all the parameters being assessed. As stated in the previous paragraph, optimal evaluation of spatial resolution and linearity may require more than one pattern if several different cameras must be tested.

Four different widths of bars and spaces are used in the *quadrant bar phantom.* The bars in the quadrants are arranged so that each set of bars is oriented 90 degrees from the set adjacent to it. The spaces and bars in each quadrant are equal. A higher resolution phantom going down to 2 mm bars is available for high-performance cameras. Measurement of the resolution of all detector regions requires imaging of the phantom in different positions, which is inconvenient. It should be noted that the effective resolution (FWHM) of the camera is about 1.7 times the smallest visible bars. The advantage of this phantom over the PLES and OH phantoms is that because of the presence of four different bar size/spacing combinations, the same phantom can be used to assess cameras with a range of intrinsic

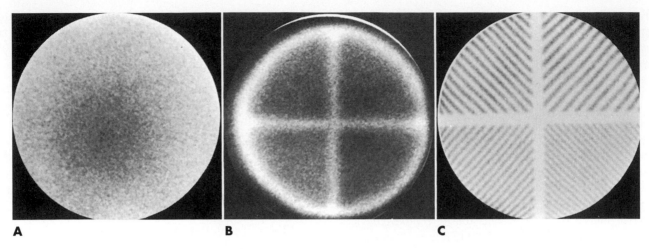

A   **B**   **C**

Figure 3-36   Source activity is important in assessing performance. Nonuniformity (**A**) and loss of resolution (**B**) occur when activity is too great. **C,** Resolution returns when activity is reduced to proper level. These effects are much less prominent in state-of-the-art cameras.

resolutions. Some facilities acquire one image and rotate the pattern by 90 degrees each successive week so that all quadrants are imaged with the most appropriate bar size every four weeks.

Whatever source is used, the count rate should not exceed 30,000 counts/sec. At excessive count rates, poor uniformity and spatial resolution arise because of counting losses and pulse pileup (Figure 3-36). However, it is important to note that state-of-the-art cameras show no significant loss of uniformity and spatial resolution at count rates as high as 75 Kcps. In general these transmission phantoms should only be used for intrinsic testing, without a collimator. However, system uniformity images can be acquired with Co-57 or Tc-99m floods provided certain conditions are met. First, a test of system (extrinsic) spatial resolution and linearity should only be done with a low-energy, preferably high-resolution, collimator. Use of the phantom with a collimator can produce a Moire type of artifact because of the interference patterns produced by the combination of the transmission phantom pattern with the "pattern" of holes in the collimator. This is particularly a problem with medium- and high-energy collimators (Figure 3-37). Second, it is also important to note that when acquiring transmission phantom images by computer, the digital acquisition matrix can act as a pattern. These types of images must be acquired with a large matrix (at least 256 × 256 and preferably 512 × 512).

Routine Camera Quality Control Procedures

Once the intrinsic-versus-extrinsic testing, source considerations, and phantoms have been discussed and decisions have been made, a daily quality control program for scintillation cameras can be established. One of the keys to a reliable quality control program is the standardized performance of the quality control procedures. A number of

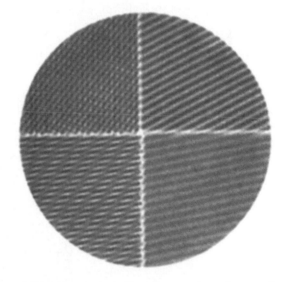

Figure 3-37   Extrinsic spatial resolution using a four-quadrant bar pattern, a medium energy collimator, and a Tc-99m flood source. (Courtesy of Ellinor Busemann-Sokole, Academic Medical Center, Amsterdam, The Netherlands.)

steps dealing with camera system setup must be taken prior to any quality control imaging.

Photopeak settings. The correct energy window for the radionuclide being used must be selected, and the photopeak must be centered in the window. If peaking is performed manually, the setting should be recorded. A correct photopeak setting is absolutely essential for optimum camera performance. All the parameters being assessed for quality control are adversely affected if the system is off-peak. The clinical ramifications of incorrect photopeaking are seen in Figure 3-22.

Orientation controls. Image orientation must remain constant for quality control images so that the same detector area is always recorded in the same position on the image. This is important in the evaluation of gradual performance degradation in a particular detector area.

Intensity. Daily use of the same CRT intensity settings and image size to produce field uniformity images should result in a comparable daily image density. This ensures that established CRT intensities used for clinical studies remain valid. When the same CRT intensity does not reproduce the same image density, the most common causes are electronic drift, aging of the CRT, and changes in the film processor (if transparency film is used). The same image-recording devices used for patient studies are also used to record all the quality control images.

Image size. The size of an image can have a significant impact on interpretation of the image. For this reason care must be taken to use the format and intensity each time.

Uniformity. Use one of the following methods daily.

Extrinsic method. If the system's extrinsic uniformity is to be evaluated, a collimator is installed and a planar source,

with a count rate that does not exceed 30,000 counts/sec, is centered over the detector. Covering the collimator surface with a plastic cover or enclosing the flood phantom in a plastic bag helps prevent contamination of the collimator.

1. Acquire a flood image that contains at least 3 million counts for a camera with a circular field of view and 5 million counts for a camera with a larger rectangular field of view.
2. If the camera has a microprocessor system for detector uniformity correction that can be turned off, daily flood-field images are acquired with and without microprocessor correction (Figure 3-38).
3. Evaluate and compare the image(s) with previous images of uniformity that were acquired.
4. Record the data, photopeak setting, CRT intensity setting, total counts, and elapsed imaging time.
5. Place the image in the appropriate file.

Intrinsic method. If an intrinsic protocol has been adopted, the collimator must be removed. Extreme care must be taken to avoid physical shock and radionuclide contamination of the crystal. A collimator can be removed if contaminated, but crystal contamination can shut the camera down for days.

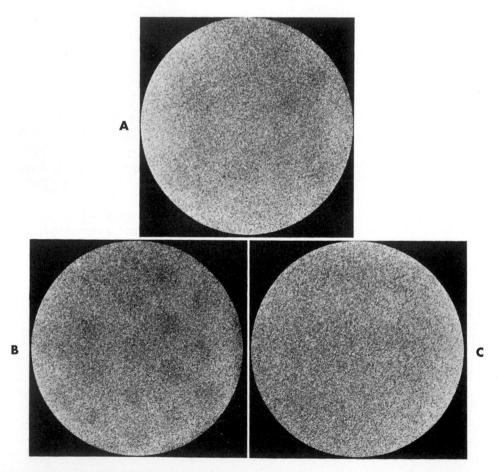

Figure 3-38 Detector performance without uniformity correction must also be assessed. **A,** Subtle nonuniformities. **B,** Increasing nonuniformity due to changes in energy and linearity correction maps with time. **C,** Uniformity corrected flood of detector in **B.** Uniformity correction should not replace good detector calibration.

1. Place an appropriate size lead mask ring on the face of the detector if the gamma camera's edge packing is not masked electronically or by the detector housing;
2. Position a point source, with a count rate not exceeding 30,000 counts/sec, at a distance of at least five times the maximum dimension of the camera's useful field of view. The source can be positioned above or below the detector, but keep in mind that a source that is positioned above the detector can fall and damage or contaminate the detector if is not covered with plastic. An alternative is to rotate the detector so it faces outward and tape the source to a wall or IV pole for acquisition of data.
3. Acquire a flood image that contains at least 3 million counts for a camera with a circular field of view and 5 million counts for a camera with a larger rectangular field of view.
4. If the camera has a microprocessor system for detector uniformity correction that can be turned off, daily flood-field images are acquired with and without microprocessor correction. Record the times taken to acquire both the corrected and uncorrected images and note the difference, if any.
5. Evaluate and compare the images with previous images for uniformity.
6. Record the date, photopeak setting, CRT intensity setting, total counts, and elapsed imaging time.
7. Place the images in the appropriate file.

Linearity and resolution. Spatial resolution and linearity should be checked weekly. An OH phantom can be used as long as the hole spacing is fine enough to "stress" present cameras. Other patterns may require multiple images of the phantom in different orientations for a complete evaluation of the system's performance, but as an alternative the test pattern can be rotated to a different orientation each week. Before the alternative is adopted the facility's radioactive materials license must be reviewed to verify that weekly rotation of the transmission phantom does not violate a license condition.

1. Remove the collimator from the camera and position the detector so it faces the source.
2. Place the appropriate size lead mask ring on the face of the crystal if the camera's edge packing is not masked.
3. Position the transmission phantom on the detector housing. Note: Some cameras have transmission phantoms that may be attached like a collimator. In such a case the camera may be positioned facing downward or in any other convenient direction.
4. A point source of appropriate activity is positioned at a distance of five times the maximum dimension of the camera's useful field of view. The count rate should not exceed 30,000 counts/sec.
5. Acquire an image that contains at least 3 million counts for a camera with a circular field of view and 5 million

counts for a camera with a larger rectangular field of view.
6. Remove the point source before removing the phantom, particularly if the source is attached to the ceiling.
7. Evaluate and compare the image with previous images for linearity and intrinsic resolution.
8. Record the findings in the camera log and place the image in the appropriate section of the logbook.

Collimators. The development of higher sensitivity and increased resolution low-energy collimators through the use of thinner septa and an increased number of holes has also produced the potential problem of physical damage or manufacturing defects, which can produce imaging artifacts (Figure 3-39). Checks for faulty or damaged collimators should be a part of a quality assurance program. These checks should include an initial check of all collimators plus subsequent checks at 12-month intervals. Each collimator should be evaluated by performing an extrinsic uniformity test in addition to a visual inspection for physical damage, dents, and separation of castings. The resultant images should be labeled with collimator name, date performed, total counts, time, and any pertinent comments. These images should be retained and used for comparison with quality control images obtained in the future.

Artifacts caused by the collimator can be confirmed by performing an extrinsic field uniformity image, then removing the collimator and rotating it 90 degrees or 180 degrees and reimaging (if possible). If the position of the artifact changes on the subsequent image, the collimator is the cause of the nonuniformity.

Photographic systems. Daily care and maintenance of the photographic system should be included as part of a quality assurance program. The CRT face and the lens and mirrors of the photographic camera system, including multiformatters, should be inspected and cleaned frequently. Dust and fingerprints on the mirrors and lens should be removed using professional lens paper. Do not use soap and water. The CRT face and protective cover can be cleaned with a lens cleaning solution. All surfaces should be checked for scratches and marks (Figure 3-40). It is not uncommon for the high resolution CRTs in multiformatters to gather dust and dirt and need to be cleaned by service personnel.

A suspected artifact in the photographic system can be confirmed or eliminated by the following procedure:

1. Obtain a flood-field image as described, noting the camera orientation, and observe where the suspected artifact is in the image.
2. Change the camera orientation by 90 degrees and obtain another flood-field image.
3. Compare the two images. If the artifact did not change locations with a change in camera orientation, the artifact is on the CRT or photographic system. If the artifact moves with a corresponding change in

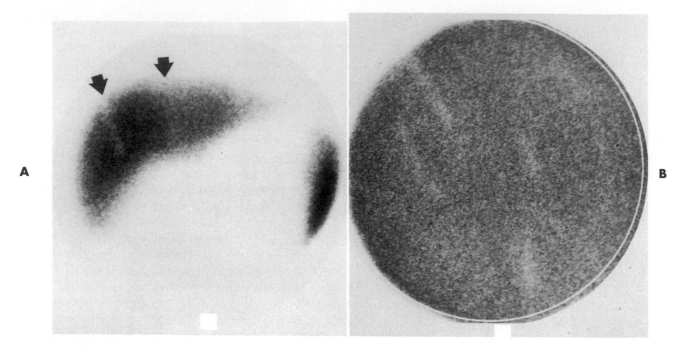

Figure 3-39   Anterior view **(A)** of liver with two photopenic areas suspected of being artifactual and planar flood image **(B)** demonstrating collimator damage as cause.

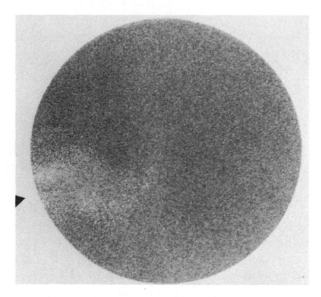

Figure 3-40   Cathode ray tube (CRT) artifact.

orientation, the display system can be eliminated as a cause.

Multiple window spatial registration. Cameras that are equipped with multiple pulse height windows must be evaluated for multiple window spatial registration. Unless positional information (x and y signals) from each window is the same, images will be distorted. This distortion typically manifests itself as decreased spatial resolution compared with single window acquisition. Consequently, a practical approach to assessment of multiple window spatial registra-

tion is to compare single window to multiple window ^{67}Ga images of a quadrant bar phantom. To use this approach, the bar phantom must be adequately thick to attenuate the higher energy photons from ^{67}Ga. In most cases it is.

Film Processor Quality Control

The processors used to develop nuclear medicine images require a program of maintenance and monitoring to assure that they function properly. A schedule should be established for cleaning, chemical change, temperature monitoring, and constancy of film development (density). This schedule should be strictly followed.

Computer Quality Control

The computer is an integral part of the imaging process for virtually all current scintillation cameras. Uniformity, linearity, resolution, dead time, and count rate response are important parameters that must be monitored on a timely basis. A number of these quality control procedures are very similar to those used for the scintillation camera and can be performed at the same time.

Uniformity. The same method chosen for the scintillation camera is employed each day of use for uniformity. At a minimum, a 128×128 matrix is used to collect the computer image; 256×256 is preferred. Evaluate and compare the image(s) with previous images for uniformity. A count profile across the field of view may be generated to aid in evaluation of uniformity. Many present computer systems have the National Electrical Manufacturer's Association

(NEMA) protocol for uniformity; this can be another useful aid in evaluation of uniformity. However, a word of caution is appropriate. Strictly speaking the NEMA protocol requires 20 to 30 M counts for acceptance testing. For quality control a smaller number of counts can be used. For example, 10 to 15 M counts are sufficient to provide a good estimate of the integral and differential uniformity. Quantification of uniformity should be done on a weekly basis; careful visual inspection of the images can be used the other days of the week. If uniformity is quantified, the initial value measured at the time the baseline tests are performed can generally be used to establish actions levels. A committee of camera manufacturers recommends three action levels. If the measured integral uniformity is less than XX%, the camera is satisfactory for clinical use. If greater than XX% but less than YY%, it can be used for clinical studies until service personnel arrive. If it is greater than YY%, the camera must not be used for clinical studies until the problem is corrected.

Linearity and resolution. For weekly monitoring the resolution test is used with the same technique described for scintillation camera resolution and linearity testing. The image is collected and displayed with the maximum digital resolution available (i.e., the largest matrix size). Linearity is evaluated by visually assessing the straightness of the rows and columns. Spatial resolution is checked by evaluating the definition of the bars or holes across the entire phantom image. Note that this test may produce erroneous results (Moire patterns) if too small a matrix (e.g., 64×64 or 128×128) is used.

Count rate performance. Follow one of the following procedures on a yearly basis.

Dead time determination

1. Prepare two sources of activity (approximately 300 to 500 μCi ^{99m}Tc); label one as source no. 1 and the other as no. 2. The activities of the sources must be within 10% of each other.
2. Remove the collimator and place the lead masking ring on the detector, if necessary.
3. Position the camera head to allow the sources to be placed approximately 1 meter from the center of the detector.
4. Collect 10 to 60 sec images in the camera (if analog) and the computer (64×64 matrix) of the individual sources and of the combined sources.
5. Calculate the dead time of the camera and the camera/computer system using the formula below

$$T = \frac{2R_{1,2}}{(R_1 + R_2)^2} \times \ln\left(\frac{R_1 + R_2}{R_{1,2}}\right)$$

where T is dead time in seconds, R_1 is counts/sec of source no. 1, R_2 is counts/sec of source no. 2, and $R_{1,2}$ is counts/sec of sources 1 and 2 combined.
6. Record these two values for comparison with subsequent monitoring measurements.

7. Identical counting conditions and nearly identical source activities must be employed each time the test is performed.

Maximum count rate

1. Prepare one source of activity (approximately 2 mCi of Tc-99m).
2. Remove the collimator, and place the lead masking ring on the detector, if necessary.
3. Tape the source to an IV pole at a position that is directly in line with the center of the detector and at a distance of 3 meters.
4. Set time to approximately 300 seconds, peak the camera using a 20% window, and start the camera.
5. Slowly move the IV pole toward the detector while observing the count rate.
6. Note the count rate when it stops increasing and begins to decrease.
7. Record the value for comparison with subsequent measurements.

Note: This setup may not be possible in some multihead cameras. In multihead cameras the results you obtain will probably depend on whether the detector(s) that are not being tested have collimators on them. The highest value of the maximum count rate will be obtained when the other detectors are covered. All these tests are used to detect changes in performance over time. The results are usually interpreted in a subjective manner, and a decision is then made to determine if the system can be used for clinical studies.

SPECT System Quality Assurance

Satisfactory SPECT demands stringent quality assurance procedures. Field uniformity tolerances of ±5% that are common for planar imaging may not be acceptable for SPECT imaging. Variations in uniformity of no greater than ±1% may be required. Additionally, alignment of the collimator crystal surface with the gantry axis of rotation, as well as alignment of the computer image matrix and axis of rotation, are critical.

Uniformity. Small changes in extrinsic camera uniformity may be misrepresented as different levels of activity or artifacts in reconstructed images (Figure 3-41). These artifacts typically take the form of alternating concentric hot and cold rings, which form a *bull's eye pattern*. Nonuniformities in multiple detector systems do not usually produce complete rings. SPECT imaging typically requires extrinsic uniformity variations that are less than 1%. This is particularly true for higher-count SPECT studies, and perhaps less true for lower-count (e.g., Tl-201 cardiac SPECT) studies. Extrinsic uniformity flood images (5 million counts, 64×64 matrix) should be acquired daily using clinical collimators. A uniform sheet source of ^{57}Co or ^{99m}Tc should be placed on the collimator, and the photopeak window should be prop-

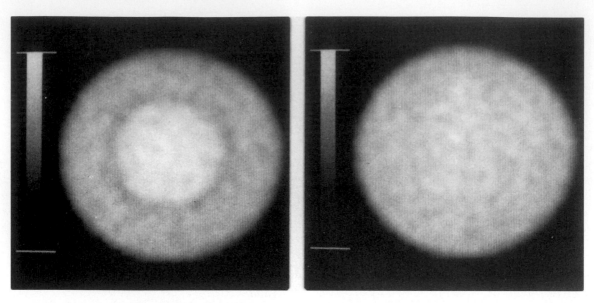

Figure 3-41 Slice through a water-filled cylinder containing a uniform distribution of ^{99m}Tc, reconstructed without *(left)* and with *(right)* compensation for nonuniformity in camera sensitivity.

erly set. Weekly, a 30 to 60 million count flood image using a 64 × 64 matrix should be acquired and analyzed for uniformity. (The matrix size that is required for analysis of integral and differential uniformity varies with vendor.) If a 128 × 128 matrix is to be used clinically, at least 120 million counts will be required for adequate statistical precision. Updated high-count flood images should be saved on the computer for performing uniformity correction. Different collimators and radionuclides may require that separate uniformity correction matrices be saved on the computer. Visual evaluation of high-count flood images is not adequate for quality assurance of SPECT equipment. Quantitative computer programs are required to evaluate the images to ensure that the extrinsic field variation is satisfactory.

^{57}Co sheet sources require no filling because the radionuclide is impregnated into the plastic. However, not all commercially available ^{57}Co disk sources have the required uniformity to evaluate SPECT imaging systems. Furthermore, these sources might need to be replaced every 6 to 12 months to maintain reasonable count rates. Fillable liquid sheet sources can be used for long periods and may be filled with different radionuclides. But care must be used in ensuring uniform mixing of the radionuclides with the liquid. Significant problems in filling or bulging with thin, fillable sheet sources may create artifacts in evaluating camera uniformity. A thick, water-filled phantom several centimeters thick can be used, but care must be taken that no contamination occurs when filling the sources and that no leaks occur in the phantom.

SPECT system alignment. Proper x, y centering and gain adjustments are extremely important in SPECT imaging. The x and y gains of the computer image matrix should be evaluated in both directions using two point source markers separated by a known distance. The number of pixels between

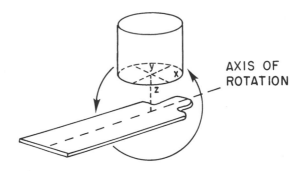

Figure 3-42 Camera x, y, and z coordinate system must be properly aligned with the axis of rotation of the SPECT gantry system. The camera y axis must be parallel to the axis of rotation for proper spatial registration on reconstructed images.

the two sources can be used to determine the dimension of a pixel. If the gains have drifted or are incorrectly set, they must be readjusted prior to any further SPECT imaging acquisitions.

The *axis of rotation* is an imaginary line that extends through the center of the camera gantry as a pencil would pass through a hole in a doughnut (Figure 3-42). As the camera moves in a circular orbit, the camera distance to this axis of rotation must not change. This requires that both the camera head and yoke rotation be carefully set to place the plane of the camera crystal parallel to the axis of rotation. Noncircular orbits may be implemented in several ways. In some approaches the camera head only moves in and out relative to the axis of rotation (i.e., the rotation radius changes). In this approach no additional alignment issues arise. In other approaches the gantry or bed may move in addition to the camera head. The effective axis-of-rotation changes from projection to projection and additional alignment relationships (e.g., between gantry and bed) must be proper.

The computer image matrix must also be correctly aligned with the axis of rotation (Figure 3-43). Any misalignment in the acquired images, independent of the source of error, will cause blurring and a loss of resolution in the reconstructed images. Reconstruction of an image with an incorrect axis of rotation can create or mask lesions. The initial calibration of camera gains and offsets, necessary for correct planar imaging, provides a starting point for more sophisticated center-of-rotation corrections.

Center of rotation. Most SPECT systems must be able to maintain center-of-rotation alignment (Figure 3-44). Center-of-rotation evaluation is done to ensure that alignment exists between the mechanical and observed reference point. Proper camera alignment with the mechanical center of rotation must be checked/calibrated at a frequency of 1 to 2 weeks (rotating collimators). Rotational image data are acquired with one or more point sources of ^{57}Co or ^{99m}Tc using a clinically used collimator and image matrix. A computer program is used to calculate the center-of-rotation error, and the pixel value is recorded. Reconstructed transaxial images (see Figure 3-44) may show enlarged point sources or even a cold center if the center of rotation is

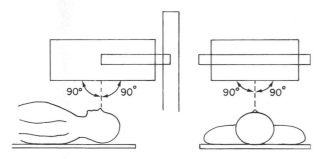

Figure 3-43 Camera head alignment must be perpendicular to the axis of rotation.

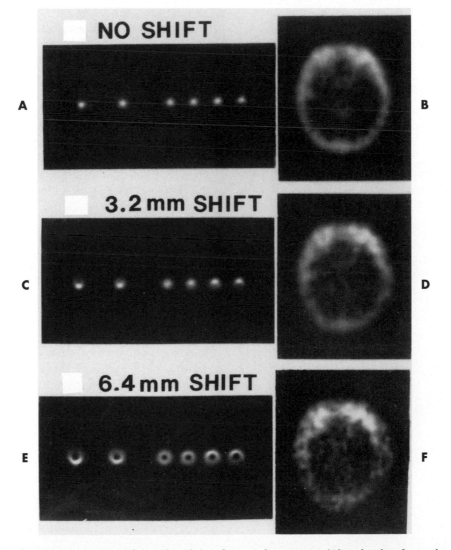

Figure 3-44 Top figures depict reconstructions for unaltered data from six line sources (**A**) and a slice from a brain scan (**D**). Centering error for **A** and **D** measured less than 1 mm. **B** and **E** show the effect of a 2 to 3 mm error in offset determination, accomplished by shifting the same projection data from **A** and **D** by one pixel (3.2 mm) prior to reconstruction. Note rapid deterioration of resolution and introduction of circular artifacts in **B** as compared to **A**. **C** and **F** show more dramatic changes than those seen in **B** and **E**, because the data were shifted 6.2 mm from the origin.

misaligned. Center-of-rotation shifts of 2 to 3mm can significantly alter the quality of reconstructed transaxial slices by producing a loss of resolution. Records of the center-of-rotation measurement (such as the correction shifts) should be kept to evaluate any slight shift that may require service.

Phantom evaluations. On a monthly to quarterly basis a full system test using a phantom (Figure 3-45) that can evaluate system uniformity and resolution simultaneously should be performed. These tests should always be performed with the same amount of radioactivity, collimator, and other acquisition and processing parameters. Phantom studies frequently require the use of high amounts of activity in the phantom and long acquisition times that exceed those that are used in clinical studies. A simple large plastic bottle filled with a uniform concentration of ^{99m}Tc can be used to evaluate reconstructed transaxial slices for uniformity.

Resolution phantoms should have a variety of sizes of cold defects. Some resolution elements should be fairly easy to resolve, and some should exceed the resolution capabilities of the system. Having this variety of resolution elements allows the overall system to be pushed to its limit. Data acquisition with clinical parameters and subsequent reconstruction with a variety of filters will allow the user to optimally evaluate parameter selection and provide the most information.

Sineogram display. An extremely useful way of displaying SPECT quality control data is the sineogram. This image consists of the projection data for a given slice. Each row in the sineogram represents the one row of pixels in the projection corresponding to the slice of interest. Thus the horizontal direction in the sineogram corresponds to the linear horizontal direction in the projection data, and the vertical direction in the sineogram corresponds to the projection angle.

Nonuniformities show up in the sineogram as straight vertical lines. Patient or organ motion or movement shows up as a "break" in the sineogram. Projections in which the organ moves out of the field of view produce sineograms with truncated activity.

National Electrical Manufacturers Association (NEMA) Standards

NEMA consists of approximately 550 electrical manufacturing companies in the United States. One of its eight product divisions is the Diagnostic Imaging and Therapy Systems Division, with a section devoted to nuclear imaging. This section is made up of manufacturers of nuclear medicine

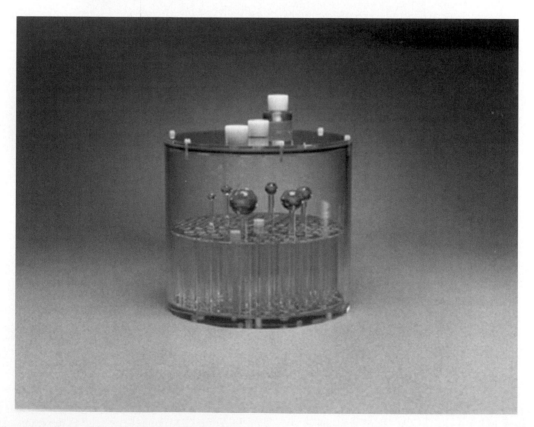

Figure 3-45 Commercially available SPECT phantom consisting of a cylinder with inserts to mimic hot or cold areas of activity. This type of phantom may be used to measure complete system performance. (Courtesy Data Spectrum, Inc., Hillsborough, North Carolina.)

equipment and includes all the major suppliers of scintillation cameras. This group has cooperatively formulated a set of standards that are used to measure the various performance characteristics of their products, including both planar imaging and SPECT performance.

After purchasing a scintillation camera it is prudent to perform some type of acceptance test and not rely on the word of the installer that the system is working correctly. The usual quality assurance checks of uniformity, spatial resolution, and linearity should certainly be done. However, most nuclear medicine departments lack the expertise or equipment to measure all the NEMA camera performance characteristics quoted by the manufacturer. For this reason, as well as the fact that there is a considerable dollar investment involved, it is wise to use the services of a consultant who has both the expertise and equipment to perform the NEMA measurements to ascertain that the system is performing as advertised.

MAXIMIZING IMAGE QUALITY

Image Quality and Signal-to-Noise Ratio

The goal of clinical nuclear medicine imaging is not to produce a "pretty picture" per se, but rather to aid diagnosis, prognosis, or treatment planning and monitoring. To do so, nuclear medicine images must be of high diagnostic and quantitative accuracy, depending on whether subjective visual interpretation or more objective quantitative analyses are used. In practice, the performance of a given instrument, technique, or study can only be judged in the light of rigorous assessment of diagnostic performance (by comparison with the results of "gold standard" tests or long-term follow-up) and quantitative accuracy (by comparison with the results of phantom studies and in vivo animal experiments). Subjective evaluation of "image quality," though frequently done in evaluations of new approaches, is of limited value in truly assessing the performance of an instrument or technique.

In general, the "quality" of an image can be described (quantitatively) by its *signal-to-noise* ratio (SNR). The SNR directly affects diagnostic and quantitative accuracy. In essence, then, a major goal of nuclear medicine imaging equipment is to maximize the SNR in an image.

The SNR describes the relative "strength" of the desired information and the noise (e.g., due to the statistics of radioactive decay) in the image. As a simple example, consider a bone scan with hot lesions. The signal in this example is the difference between the lesions and the surrounding bone activity. Note that the signal is not the bone itself, but rather the contrast (or difference in image counts) between the lesions and the rest of the bone. As another example, consider a liver scan with cold lesions. Again, the signal is the contrast or difference between the lesions and the normal liver. For either the bone or liver scan, the only way the lesions can be detected is if their activity is sufficiently

different than that of the surrounding areas. Contrast is often defined as

$$C = \frac{T - B}{T + B}$$

The greater the contrast between the lesions and the surrounding bone or liver, the greater the "signal" (Figure 3-46). In practice, this contrast is provided in the patient by the radiotracer's distribution. The goal of the imaging system is to preserve this contrast in the image. Contrast is maintained by avoiding blurring, which smears counts from higher activity regions into lower activity regions (and vice versa), thus reducing image contrast. Spatial resolution and contrast are closely linked. This relationship is quantitatively described by the imaging system's *modulation transfer function* (MTF). Although the MTF is obtained from the Fourier transform of the point or line spread function (a measure of spatial resolution), it is actually the ratio of the contrast in the image to that in the object as a function of spatial frequency.

When scattered photons are present, image contrast is reduced (see Figure 3-46). The imaging geometry of the system, along with its energy resolution, determines the amount of scatter that is present. It is important to note that the response of the imaging system to a point source of activity reflects both spatial resolution and scatter effects and can be used overall as an index of the ability of the system to preserve "signal."

The noise in the phantom shown in Figure 3-47 is the result of statistical fluctuation within the "lesions" and within the surrounding "tissue." This statistical fluctuation arises from the Poisson nature of radioactive decay. If there are few counts in the image, this fluctuation will be large, perhaps almost as large as the true contrast between the lesions and the rest of the bone. In such a case the viewer would not be able to recognize the lesions as being "different" from the rest of the tissue (see Figure 3-47).

For accurate quantification, many of the same factors that influence the image's SNR are involved. Accuracy refers to the degree to which the average value (e.g., of radioactivity concentration) corresponds with the truth. An average value implies the existence of multiple measurements. By strict definition the values of these individual measurements can vary. If the average value agrees with the truth, the overall measurement is *accurate*. Accuracy is influenced by the spatial resolution of the imaging system—by its ability to accurately portray the correct contrast present in the patient. Accuracy is also affected by other factors, such as photon attenuation.

Precision refers to the variation among the individual measurements. If all the values agree with one another, the overall measurement is *precise* or *reproducible*, even if it isn't accurate. Precision is influenced by the inherent statistical fluctuations due to the Poisson nature of radioactive decay and any further computer processing. For example, conventional 9-point weighted averaging (or "smoothing") improves the precision of each pixel's value.

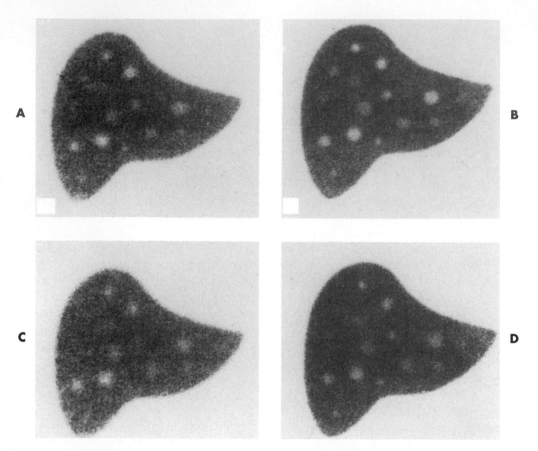

Figure 3-46 Effect of spatial resolution on image quality. Total counts are the same. **A,** High-resolution collimator with scattering material interposed. **B,** Same as **A** without scatter. **C,** Medium-energy collimator with scattering material interposed. **D,** Same as **C** without scatter. Note loss of contrast with scatter and lower resolution (medium-energy) collimator.

Instrumentation Factors Influencing SNR

To achieve a high SNR, high resolution and high sensitivity are required. Nuclear medicine imaging forces a compromise between resolution and sensitivity. In 1985 Dr. Gerd Muehllehner published an important study relating these two factors to perceived image quality. Observers viewed computer simulations of the Derenzo phantom and were asked to match images of similar image quality. "Image quality" in this context was based on the viewers' *perceived* ability to discriminate the hot spots from the background. Such a task would be influenced by the complicated interplay between image contrast and noise. Dr. Muehllehner found that an improvement in resolution of 2 mm (e.g., from 10 mm to 8 mm) resulted in comparable image quality with only about one fourth as many counts. In 1992 Dr. Fred Fahey and coworkers confirmed and extended Dr. Muehllehner's findings in a phantom study with a multi-camera SPECT system. These findings are consistent with the view that the image's SNR dominates perceived image quality and that the ratio may be increased by either increasing contrast (through improved spatial resolution) or decreasing noise (through increased sensitivity).

In practice, the technologist will find the concept of SNR very helpful in optimizing acquisition and processing pro-

tocols. By keeping in mind that the goal is to maximize an image's SNR, an optimum choice of collimator, for example, can be found that preserves contrast (through improved spatial resolution) while providing sufficient sensitivity to keep image noise to an acceptably low level. Similarly, an optimum reconstruction filter can be chosen. Usually the choice that maximizes SNR falls between the highest resolution choice and the highest sensitivity choice.

CONCLUSION

Nuclear medicine has always been a technology-intensive discipline in medicine. With the present emphasis on high-performance imaging devices and state-of-the-art computing, the technologist may be intimidated or overwhelmed with the knowledge and skills he or she is expected to possess. The basic principles of radiation physics, detection, digital computing, and image processing apply across the board to all clinical imaging. Thus the technologist is strongly encouraged to take the time and effort to fully learn these important principles and to become a fully participating member of the imaging team. A good technologist provides a unique and indispensable role and is valued accordingly.

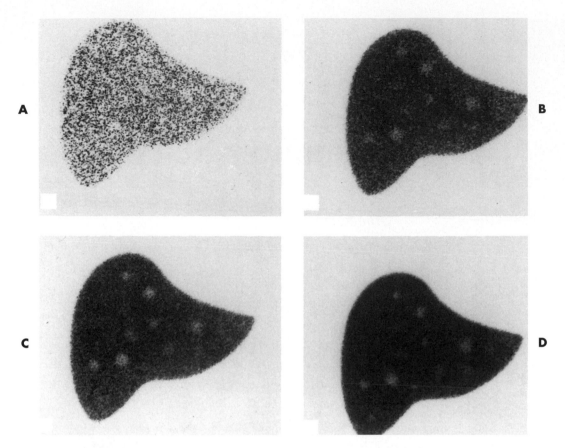

Figure 3-47 Effect of total counts on image quality. All other factors, including spatial resolution, are the same. **A,** 50,000 counts; **B,** 500,000 counts; **C,** 1,000,000 counts; **D,** 2,000,000 counts.

SUGGESTED READINGS

Chandra R: *Nuclear medicine physics: the basics,* ed 5, Baltimore, 1998, Lippincott Williams & Wilkins.

DePuey EG and Garcia EV, editors: Updated imaging guidelines for nuclear cardiology procedures, part 1, *J Nucl Cardiol* 8:G1–G58, 2001.

Henkin RE, Boles MA, Dillehay GL et al: *Nuclear medicine,* St. Louis, 1996, Mosby.

Hines H, Kayayan R, Colsher J et al: National Electrical Manufacturers Association recommendations for implementing SPECT instrumentation quality control, *J Nucl Med* 41:383–389, 2000.

Rollo FD: *Nuclear medicine physics, instrumentation, and agents,* St. Louis, 1977, Mosby.

Sandler MP, Coleman RE, Wackers FJTh et al: *Diagnostic nuclear medicine,* ed 4, Baltimore, 2002, Lippincott Williams & Wilkins.

Society of Nuclear Medicine procedure guidelines manual 1999, Reston, Va, 1999, Society of Nuclear Medicine, Inc.

Sorenson JA, Phelps ME: *Physics in nuclear medicine,* ed 2, Orlando, 1987, Grune & Stratton.

Wagner HN, Szabo Z, Buchanan JW: *Principles of nuclear medicine,* ed 2, Philadelphia, 1996, WB Saunders.

Paul E. Christian

Computer Science

Objectives

Describe the representation of data in decimal, binary, octal, and hexadecimal format.

Explain the function of the CPU.

Describe the operation and use of input/output devices.

Explain the principles and use of data storage media.

Describe the operation of disk drives.

Discuss the use, advantages, and limitations of data storage media.

Explain the operation of ADCs and the camera/computer interface.

List environmental factors for computers.

Define and discuss operating system.

Differentiate between high-level and machine code programs.

Discuss computer programming and programming languages.

Diagram and explain digital storage of images.

Discuss the advantages and disadvantages of different image size matrices.

Explain the acquisition of gated cardiac data.

Describe image processing operations.

Calculate a nine-point smooth for a 3 × 3 matrix.

Perform image region of interest placement and curve generation.

Explain the principles of normalization and calculate normalized background-corrected counts.

Describe frequency space representation of images.

Discuss the principles of SPECT and PET reconstruction.

Explain the use of frequency space filters to remove noise from SPECT and PET images.

Diagram computer network configurations.

Discuss uses for nonimaging computers.

Define the Internet, and discuss nuclear medicine applications.

---

*C*omputer: An electronic machine that stores instructions and information to perform rapid and complex calculations or to store, manipulate, and retrieve information.

By this definition the computer is distinguished from the calculator, a device used to make simple computations. In addition the computer is capable not only of storing information (numbers, data, images, or text) but also of following a set of instructions to make complex calculations and manipulate the information in some specific order. This can be as simple as adding two numbers or as complicated as calculating SPECT and PET 3D image volumes using advanced reconstruction algorithms. Not only are calculations performed, but also information can be evaluated, such as logical evaluations and sorting of information in a database.

Computers have become an integral part of the nuclear medicine department, with applications not only to imaging but also to less demanding but repetitive tasks such as billing, scheduling, patient reports, nuclear pharmacy records, and administrative and general office applications. However, this chapter concentrates primarily on the application of computers to acquire, store, and process images. Image processing is discussed in general, and specific applications are presented in later, clinical chapters.

HISTORY

Long ago, humankind realized the value of a device to help manipulate numbers. Around 1500 BC the Chinese invented the abacus, a device whose beads could be moved to add, subtract, multiply, and divide. For hundreds of years, few ways were found to improve number processing. By the mid-1600s Blaise Pascal and Baron von Leibniz had devised adding machines that, through a series of gears and dials, performed lengthy calculations. In 1804 Joseph Jacquard devised a technique of automating patterns to be woven into material. Jacquard's loom used a series of rods that "read" the perforations in a series of cards that dictated the pattern to be woven. This device was therefore the first encoding of instructions to a machine.

From 1822 to 1834 Charles Babbage constructed a device he called the *difference engine*. This mechanical instrument used a complex grouping of gears, rods, and wheels to perform a series of calculations according to a predefined instruction set. A more advanced design, the *analytical engine,* which was never completed, established the expression of all-purpose programming with the ability to follow a list of instructions with numbers as long as 50 digits. Babbage's assistant, Ada Lovelace, carefully documented the rules for encoding the instructions and wrote the first example of programs that could be used to control a computing machine.

In 1889 Herman Hollerith invented a machine that could sort, collate, and count information on punched cards. This machine was used to compile statistical information from the 1890 census. The company that Hollerith founded later became International Business Machines (IBM). Many types of mechanical calculating machines were developed in that era.

John Atanasoff and Clifford Berry in 1939 devised a prototype computer that used a binary numbering system. They had recognized that electronic circuits were well suited to handle binary (1 or 0 or on/off) representations of numbers.

Although several electromechanical computing devices were built in the mid-1940s, a fully electronic digital com-

puter was not operational until 1946. ENIAC (Electronic Numerical Integrator and Calculator) was the first electronic digital computer; it was used to calculate artillery-aiming tables for the U.S. Army and to solve problems for production of the hydrogen bomb. This room-sized computer used thousands of vacuum tubes and required programming by manual connection of hundreds of wires. In 1951 Remington-Rand became the world's first large-scale manufacturer of computers when it introduced the UNIVAC-I.

Although the transistor was invented in 1947, it was not fully developed nor was it generally available until the mid-1950s. Additional development of these semiconductor devices resulted in the placement of many components on a single circuit, or *chip*. These devices, called integrated circuits, created a revolution in computers over the next decade, with current technology being able to put millions of transistors on a single chip. Since the introduction of the integrated circuit, the transistor density on a chip has nearly doubled every 18 months.

In 1965 Digital Equipment Corporation introduced the PDP-8, the first successful minicomputer. Before this, computers had been room-sized machines requiring operation by many programmers and electronics technicians. The introduction of these minicomputers allowed thousands of small manufacturing plants, businesses, and scientific laboratories to purchase relatively low-cost systems with high reliability.

The first microprocessor, or computer on a single circuit board, was introduced in 1971. Around that time the performance of the computers was improving dramatically, while costs for these systems were dropping sharply. In 1973 IBM introduced the first low-cost high-speed magnetic storage device, the Winchester disk. This device allowed rapid storage and recall of large amounts of data, replacing the much slower tape drive. The Motorola 6800 microprocessor was released in 1975, representing the first low-cost computer on a chip. The foundation for the market of personal computers was established in 1977 when Steve Jobs and Steve Wozniak presented the first Apple Computer; that year the TRS-80 and Commodore personal computers also were released. IBM followed in 1981, manufacturing its first personal computer.

In the last 30 years, significant improvement has been seen in microprocessor technology. Very large-scale integration (VLSI) circuits have made possible the application of microprocessors in a variety of devices used in nuclear medicine. Devices internal to camera operation—such as energy, linearity, and uniformity correction circuits—are a product of microprocessor technology. The introduction of chips that have megabits of memory and operate at very high speeds with millions of switching operations per second has added significantly to imaging instrumentation performance.

The first introduction of computers into nuclear medicine imaging occurred in the late 1960s and early 1970s. Minicomputers were used to store the output from scintillation cameras and rectilinear scanners. At that time imaging was limited to static and dynamic studies; therefore the relatively unsophisticated and low-speed computers were able to manage all imaging requirements. These early computer systems were limited to single-function applications (i.e., only one acquisition or processing function could be performed at one time). In the mid-1970s, direct memory access and multitasking operations were implemented in minicomputers, which allowed image data to be processed while another study was being acquired. In 1977 the capability to perform multigated cardiac studies had been defined, which brought a tremendous new application for nuclear medicine imaging computers and started the proliferation of computers into the community hospital. During that time the performance and memory requirements of nuclear medicine computers were beginning to increase; however, outside of handling the pixel arrays of the images, the computing requirements of these systems were relatively modest.

The commercial availability of SPECT cameras in the early 1980s brought the first computationally intense applications to nuclear medicine in performing filtered backprojection reconstruction. It became immediately apparent that the time demands for reconstructing SPECT images were not feasible with minicomputers, and array processors were attached to perform SPECT reconstructions in a reasonable time. Within the last few years, memory and computing power have further increased, allowing use of Windows environments on image processing workstations. These powerful new systems allow the operator to interact with the computer using a mouse in each of several windows on the screen, each running different programs and all programs being executed simultaneously.

DATA REPRESENTATION

The most fundamental building block of all computers is the transistor; essentially the transistor is a switch that can be placed only in the on or off positions. Information stored by this switch is therefore *binary* and can be used to represent a 0 or 1. Also, the binary state can be used to signify a logical condition of true or false. All numbers and all logical conditions within the computer are represented in the binary form. The binary configuration, 0 or 1, is called a *binary digit* or *bit*.

Our customary decimal counting system of values 0 through 9 is not sufficient to represent all the numbers; therefore we use additional columns to represent powers of 10 (10, 100, 1000, etc.). In binary counting, each column is represented by powers of 2 (2^0, 2^1, 2^2, etc. or 1, 2, 4, 8, etc.).

The binary counting method is used for number representation in the computer, though other systems can also be employed by the computer within the system. Counting systems containing 8 bits (octal) or 16 bits (hexadecimal) can also be employed. The equivalent values to usual decimal counting follow.

Decimal	1024	512	256	128	64	32	16	8	4	2	0 or 1
Binary power	2^{10}	2^9	2^8	2^7	2^6	2^5	2^4	2^3	2^2	2^1	2^0
0	0	0	0	0	0	0	0	0	0	0	0
1	0	0	0	0	0	0	0	0	0	0	1
2	0	0	0	0	0	0	0	0	0	1	0
3	0	0	0	0	0	0	0	0	0	1	1
4	0	0	0	0	0	0	0	0	1	0	0
5	0	0	0	0	0	0	0	0	1	0	1
10	0	0	0	0	0	0	0	1	0	1	0
15	0	0	0	0	0	0	0	1	1	1	1
16	0	0	0	0	0	0	1	0	0	0	0
60	0	0	0	0	0	1	1	1	1	0	0
128	0	0	0	1	0	0	0	0	0	0	0
200	0	0	0	1	1	0	0	1	0	0	0
350	0	0	1	0	1	0	1	1	1	1	0

The decimal number 21 is represented as the sum of decimal numbers—$16 \times 4 + 1$:

$$\begin{aligned}
1 \times 2^4 &= 16 \\
0 \times 2^3 &= 0 \\
1 \times 2^2 &= 4 \\
0 \times 2^1 &= 0 \\
1 \times 2^0 &= \underline{1} \\
& \ 21
\end{aligned}$$

or all powers of 2 or in binary, resulting in 0 000 000 000 010 101. Note that 16 numbers are present in these examples, all zeros or ones. Most computers process numbers in groups of 16, 32, or 64 bits.

In hexadecimal counting (base 16) the usual decimal numbers 0 through 9 are supplemented with letters to obtain the full representation of numbers until the next column is needed. Sometimes computer users see numbers or need to enter certain codes that are in either octal or hexadecimal characterization.

Decimal	Octal	Hexadecimal
0	0	0
1	1	1
2	2	2
3	3	3
4	4	4
5	5	5
6	6	6
7	7	7
8	10	8
9	11	9
10	12	A
11	13	B
12	14	C
13	15	D
14	16	E
15	17	F
16	20	10
17	21	11
18	22	12
19	23	13
20	24	14

As mentioned, a bit represents a limited amount of information. A series of bits is needed to encode larger numbers. Eight bits form a *byte*. The maximum number that can be stored in a byte is 2^8, or 256 entries. Since the first number is 0, numbers from 0 to 255 can be stored in a single byte. Two bytes can be put together to form a word; a word is therefore 16 bits in length and is capable of storing a number as large as 2^{16}, or 65,536. Words are frequently used to represent the number of counts in a single image picture element, called a *pixel*. The range of counts that could be stored in a single word is 0 to 65,535. The most basic storage element of information on a magnetic tape or disk is to store the data in groups of bytes, called a *block*. For example, a disk sector might store a block of 256, 512, or 1024 bytes. Information, whether numbers, text, or executable programs, is called a *file*. The size of a file can be listed as the number of bytes needed to store the information.

Memory requirements are usually indicated as thousands of bytes, or kilobytes. When discussing the size of memory or the size of a file on disk, the prefix *kilo-* does not refer to the usual definition of 1000: it refers to 1024. Therefore 4 kilobytes of memory is 4×1024, or 4096.

To effectively communicate with the computer, humans need to exchange information not as zeros and ones or other numeric representation, but as standard written alphanumeric symbols. A set of numbers to represent alphanumeric characters has been established as the American Standard Code for Information Interchange (ASCII). Using this standard code, a byte can represent a letter of the alphabet, a number, punctuation character, or keyboard control character. Text files for word processing can be stored with one byte of information for each character of the document. In addition, ASCII code allows concise communication between the computer operator via the keyboard, computer, and display monitor, allowing the direct translation from alphanumeric characters into binary information. Text files, programs, and data all appear as binary information inside the computer. The confusion of data or text files for programs creates havoc within the computer and can halt operation of the system.

HARDWARE

Central Processing Unit

The nucleus of the computer is called the central processing unit, or CPU (Figure 4-1). Its three primary functions are to regulate the system operation and perform computations, to interact with memory to execute programs and store data, and to coordinate the control of input and output devices. The CPU as the central management area for program execution has two primary components: the control unit (CU) and the arithmetic logic unit (ALU).

Transistors execute instructions and other operations. Their switching from one state to another is controlled by a high-speed clock that "ticks" at rates now greater than 2 billion times per second (2 gigahertz). With each clock cycle

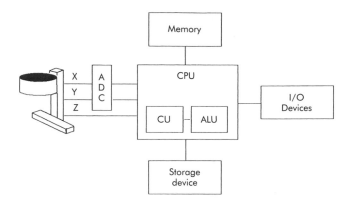

Figure 4-1 Nuclear medicine computer with the camera interfaced via an ADC to digitize x and y signals. The CPU controls the communication of information to the memory, input/output devices, and storage devices, disks, and tape.

the control unit coordinates the steps necessary to complete each instruction. Each instruction activates other areas within the CPU to perform operations, activates the ALU, and directs communication with memory and other devices. The ALU performs all arithmetic and executes all logic operations.

Memory

Because the CPU acts as the brain of the computer, it retains information by storing it in memory. Memory can be thought of as a group of mailboxes; each memory element has a specific address to store a single byte or word until it is needed. Memory consists of two types: read-only memory (ROM) and random access memory (RAM). The contents of ROM are permanent and remain in memory even when the machine is turned off. RAM is sometimes referred to as "read-and-write memory" and can be changed. When programs are loaded into the computer from an external storage device or when data are input into the computer, they reside in RAM. When the computer is turned off, information stored in RAM is lost.

ROM chips reside with the CPU and are used to store the instructions that "boot" the computer and read the first set of instructions from disk. They can also contain information that tests various internal components of the system, identifies and checks the amount of available memory, and identifies external devices.

When a computer is turned on, the electrical signal follows a permanently programmed path to the CPU and ROM chips that start the boot program. Additional ROM chips contain the basic input/output system (BIOS). The BIOS chips check the disk drive to locate the operating system, such as DOS or UNIX. The BIOS instructions then load and start the operating system program found on disk. The BIOS also communicates with other areas, such as the memory, keyboard, monitor, and disks.

RAM chips provide the computer with its tremendous flexibility in performing a wide variety of functions. Outside

devices. The instructions in a computer, called a *program,* can be executed only when they reside in memory. On early computer systems it was extremely laborious and time consuming to load the program or instructions into the computer before the program could be executed. After many years the idea of an operating system or master control program to load and run other programs was developed. The operating system is like a toolbox; it contains subprograms that interact with disks, the graphics display, modem, and camera interface and allows the user to list programs and files on disks in addition to loading and executing programs. Other programs in the operating system allow the user to create, copy, and delete files; to create, modify, and store data; and to run the editor to write programs, convert the instructions into an understandable format by the computer, and execute the new instructions.

When the computer is turned on, a set of instructions that reside in ROM chips is executed to pull up the system by its bootstraps, in other words, to boot the system. Operating systems are large programs and are stored on disk. A disk-operating system (DOS) has a monitor or executive program loaded from disk with the portions of the operating system not needed by memory retained on disk until they are needed. Examples of operating systems for personal computers are MS-DOS or Windows; System-10 for the Apple; and UNIX, NT or Linux for a variety of higher-level workstations.

The operating system is responsible principally for controlling the internal functions of the computer in running programs. Most personal computers and early nuclear medicine computers could run only one program at a time. Early nuclear medicine computers were limited either to image acquisition, image processing, or another applications program at one time. More advanced operating systems can provide foreground and background operations, apparently simultaneously. A foreground operation is a process that has priority for execution, such as an image acquisition program. When using DMA, an acquisition program should have minimal requirements of the CPU; therefore a background program can be running to perform some other type of operation such as image display. When the foreground program is not tying up the computer, the CPU works on the background program until it is interrupted again by foreground requirements.

The operating system manages the computer's activities, interfacing with the various devices and coordinating the systems. In addition, the operating system furnishes the user with a variety of programs needed for maintaining files on the computer. Disk and tape directories can be created, and programs and files can be listed, created, deleted, copied, moved, and typed. The operating system also loads programs into memory for execution.

A further enhancement of operating systems is a multitasking environment. Each of several tasks is allowed a portion of memory for the program and to store data required for each program operation. Tasks are assigned priorities, as with the foreground/background operating system. In some senses it is similar to a time-sharing system whereby jobs are swapped back and forth. Each user is given the impression of working alone on the system; however, increasing the number and complexity of tasks creates a slower response of the computer system.

Programming Languages

Machine-oriented language. The only instructions understood by the computer are represented by a series of zeros and ones, information that is virtually incomprehensible to humans. This form of instructions is machine language. Instructions at this level are extremely basic and perform only the most rudimentary tasks. Assembly language programs are written in short, very specific tasks. Simple instructions are followed one at a time to fetch instructions, decide on the operation to be performed, get values from memory, move these values to locations where operations can be performed, and so on. In assembly language even simple tasks such as adding two numbers and printing the result require many simple steps.

High-level programming languages. High-level languages are those in which instructions can be written in terms that more closely resemble English language communication. High-level languages allow programmers the ability to concentrate on writing the program without having to deal with the specifics of machine hardware and devices.

An editor is a program that allows keyboard entry of written material to create, modify, and save a written file that will become the program. The editor therefore is similar to a word processing program, allowing only entry of information, without any guarantee that the program will execute properly, or even execute at all.

The two general classifications of high-level languages are interpreted and compiled. Normally an interpreted program does not exist as a file of zeroes and ones that represent instructions the CPU can directly execute. An interpreted language is one in which the program is interpreted into machine code and one line of instructions is executed at a time. Any results are saved, and the next line of the program is then interpreted and executed, and so on. As one would expect, this language runs very slowly, because the instructions must be interpreted before they can be executed. Interpreted languages therefore do not lend themselves to large operations such as image processing. They do have an advantage; in working with small amounts of data the programs are effective and can be quickly changed without the need to recompile and link.

BASIC. A common example of an interpreted language is Beginners All-purpose Symbolic Instruction Code (BASIC). BASIC was readily available on some early personal computers, with the program available from programmable ROMs (PROMs). To write a program in BASIC, the lines of instructions within the program are numbered and executed according to the line number. BASIC and similar programs used for image processing usually have some assembly language subroutines available to perform elementary image processing functions quickly (such as image addition, smoothing, region of interest, curve generation, and SPECT reconstruction). This allows fairly rapid image manipulation with the flexibility of rapid programming changes.

A simple example program written in BASIC is shown below to use the decay equation to calculate the activity and volume of radioactivity needed for a clinical procedure at several time intervals. In the example, assume we are using ^{99m}Tc and that we enter the specific activity in mCi/ml at time zero into the computer. Then we have the computer print the specific activity and volume needed for a patient dose of 10 mCi at time intervals of 1 hr for a period of 4 hr. In BASIC this program could be written as:

```
10      REM Tc-99m DECAY EQUATION
            PROGRAM
20      T2 = 6
30      D = 10
40      INPUT "Enter the specific activity (mCi/ml)
            = ", A0
50      PRINT "Time(hr) Sp. Act.(mCi/ml)
            Vol.(ml)"
60      FOR T = 1 TO 4
70      A = A0 * EXP (−0.693 * T / T2)
80      V = D /A
90      PRINT, T, A, V
100     NEXT T
110     STOP
```

The program sets the half-life (*T2*) to 6, the dose (*D*) to 10, and prompts the user to enter the specific activity stored in a variable called *A0*. A control command, *FOR* and *NEXT,* sets up a loop to perform the calculation and printing of the results (*T, A* and *V*) for delay periods of 1, 2, 3, and 4 hr. When executed, the program output appears as:

Enter the specific activity (mCi/ml) = 13.7

Time (hr)	Sp.Act. (mCi/ml)	Vol. (ml)
1	12.205611	0.819295
2	10.874230	0.919605
3	9.688076	1.032197
4	8.631306	1.158573

In contrast to the interpreted language, compiled languages are used to create programs that execute directly and are therefore much faster. A compiler is a program that translates the written English file of instructions into an intermediate object code file. The compiler therefore translates the English version of the program into a form that is ready to accept subroutines to allow the program's instructions to interact with the CPU and peripheral devices. The linker is a program used to incorporate these library functions into the program, which then outputs an executable version of the program. This executable version now consists of zeros and ones, machine language instructions the computer can understand and perform.

FORTRAN. *Formula translation* (FORTRAN) is a scientific high-level language that is well established and available on a wide variety of systems from personal computers to mainframes. It has been widely used in nuclear medicine systems for commercial, research, and clinical applications. FORTRAN is a powerful language for performing computations dealing with large amounts of numeric data and for performing complex calculations. However, it is poor at dealing with data contained as text, with formal rules for the syntax that handles text. The example decay program shown in BASIC appears as follows when it is written in FORTRAN.

```
C    Tc-99m DECAY EQUATION PROGRAM
     REAL A, A0, T2, D, V
     INTEGER T
     T2 = 6
     D = 10
     PRINT*, 'Enter the specific activity (mCi/ml) = '
     READ*, A0
     PRINT*, 'Time(hr) Sp. Act.(mCi/ml) Vol.(ml)'
     DO 20 T = 1, 4
     A = A0 * EXP (−0.693 * T / T2)
     V = D / A
     PRINT*, T, A, V
20   CONTINUE
     END
```

The program is in many respects similar to the BASIC program. The lines that define and perform calculations are nearly identical. However, the lines that define variables and input and print data must deal with the strict syntax rules of FORTRAN to define, read, and write information.

COBOL. Many other high-level programming languages have been written for specific applications. Common Business Oriented Languages (COBOL) has been used for many years to permit easy handling of textual data with relatively modest requirements for complex numeric calculations.

Pascal. This is a language that provides a different approach to the logic of programming. Pascal uses a top-down approach in which the program's main objectives are defined as modules, and the details of the calculations are defined within each module.

C. This high-level language uses a wide variety of functions to perform many tasks that with other languages can be performed only with assembly code routines. The capability of C to interact more directly with the CPU and peripheral devices provides great power in performing complex applications such as graphics. Many Windows and workstation environments are written in C because of this power. An example of a decay program written in C follows.

```
#include <stdio.h>
#include <math.h>
main ()
{
```

requires 7,864,320 bytes (60 frames $\times$ 256 $\times$ 256 $\times$ 2 bytes per word).

Gated blood pool studies and SPECT image files are similar in size and storage format to dynamic studies. SPECT image files from a single detector camera can be acquired as 60 images of 64 $\times$ 64 pixels, or 245,760 words. Significant file space might be required when using multidetector SPECT cameras and acquiring 120 images in a high-resolution matrix of 128 $\times$ 128 pixels using 3,932,160 bytes.

On some computer systems dynamic, gated, or SPECT image files must be stored on sequential data blocks on the disk. When many image files have been acquired and deleted, there might not be enough sequential blocks of available storage, and data acquisition will not be allowed until appropriate space is available. In this case the disk must be "squeezed" to move data so there are no free data blocks between files. Most newer systems do not require contiguous blocks, and information from one file can be distributed into several groups of blocks spread over the disk. The file allocation table on the disk keeps track of the location of the various parts of the file and is totally transparent to the user. Disks that can distribute information in this way cannot be squeezed.

The acquisition of whole-body images into a digital form requires a very high-resolution matrix. The minimum matrix length should be at least a 512-pixel array; however, high-resolution cameras should use a 1024-2048 image matrix. Information acquired into an image matrix size smaller than these arrays has image resolution far below those acquired by spot film imaging.

Many types of imaging are applied to small organs, such as thyroid and heart, compared to the size of the detector. In acquiring computer images of these organs it is sometimes helpful to use hardware magnification, or zoom, to improve the resolution of the acquired image matrix in addition to presenting a larger image for viewing. When the hardware zoom mode is turned on, the x and y signals from the gamma camera are amplified by the zoom factor to fill the image matrix from the center point of the camera, and the outside perimeter of the image is lost. Although zooming increases resolution, there is a decrease in the number of counts per pixel, resulting in a noisier image.

Magnification of areas on digitized images can also be performed. Most commonly magnification is used to improve the visual display, though there is no increase in resolution. Software zoom is commonly applied to increase the size of the heart on SPECT myocardial perfusion imaging, because although the patient's whole chest fills the field of view, the only area of interest is the myocardium. Software zoom of areas on a digitized bone scan also can be useful in better appreciation of small detail, such as the vertebrae or hip joints.

Data acquisition of the gated radionuclide ventriculogram (RVG) requires synchronization of dynamic data acquisition with the cardiac cycle. More commonly known as multiple gated acquisition (MUGA), the RR interval of the ECG is divided equally into a series of images. From 16 to 32 images are used to acquire the data through the length of time for one cardiac cycle. An additional input to the computer to receive the R wave signal from an ECG is required. Data are acquired each time an R wave occurs. The time for each image frame is selected by dividing 60 seconds by the heart rate times the number of images in the sequence. For a 24-frame study, with a heart rate of 60, each frame represents only 42 milliseconds of data acquisition. With the detection of an R wave, acquisition begins with image data rapidly filling each frame in the sequence. If a new R wave is detected before the last frame is reached, acquisition into the first frame of the sequence begins again. Data from several hundred cardiac cycles are required to obtain a statistically accurate image. Images acquired in a 64 $\times$ 64 matrix with a hardware magnification are typically acquired for approximately 5 million counts. Usually this is accomplished in less than 10 minutes per view.

The technique just described acquires all data as R waves are detected. In patients with arrhythmias the quality of the data is compromised by premature ventricular contractions (PVCs) and the compensatory beats that follow PVCs. One technique to filter out bad beats is *dual buffering,* which allows information from a single cardiac cycle to be held in temporary image memory buffers. Before this information is added to the final set of data, the length of the cardiac cycle is determined to see if the RR interval is within a selected percentage of the patient's normal cardiac cycle. Heart rates outside the window indicate the buffer should be cleared, and no data from this cardiac cycle are saved. While the first beat is evaluated, images from the following beat are placed into the second buffer for RR interval evaluation. Data acquisition therefore alternates back and forth between the two buffers, evaluating RR intervals and placing only good cardiac intervals into the saved file of images.

Another mechanism for capturing gated cardiac data is list mode acquisition. In list mode the arrival of a z pulse indicates a gamma ray of proper energy has been detected. A timing mark is then stored along with the x and y locations of the scintillation event. In addition, when R waves are detected from the physiologic trigger, a physiologic marker is placed in the list of data. List mode acquisition requires a significant amount of disk space (several megabytes) to store a single study. The advantage of this technique is that after data have been acquired as a list of gamma ray events, the data can be evaluated, the desired RR interval can be selected from the acquired data, and images can be constructed only from those of desired heart rate. If the reformatted data are found unacceptable, a new RR interval can be selected and a new series of images can be formatted.

Data obtained from a gated cardiac study are most commonly evaluated by generating a time-activity curve of counts in the left ventricle. If the RR interval has been selected inappropriately, with too many R waves arriving early, image data do not fill the last images of the dynamic sequence equally; therefore counts in the last few frames can be artificially low, and the volume curve can tail off at the end. Also, if too many beats have been obtained from inadequately acquired data, the cardiac ejection fraction value may be wrong.

In recent years gated SPECT myocardial perfusion studies have proven to be helpful in evaluating myocardial perfusion, but this technique also displays the slice image as an ECG-gated cinematic study. Thus not only is perfusion evaluated by the radiopharmaceutical concentration but diminished perfusion also is correlated with corresponding decreased myocardial wall motion and thinning associated with myocardial infarction.

IMAGE DISPLAY AND PROCESSING

Gamma-ray scintillation events that occur at specific detector locations are stored as digital images by accumulating gamma-ray counts. As we have discussed, each pixel is stored as a byte or word, and an image is represented as an array or matrix of pixels. Once the information is stored, the image is displayed on a high-resolution CRT. Each pixel on the image is assigned a gray-scale value based on the number of counts. Images are typically displayed with the brightest pixel assigned to the maximum display intensity. Display screens and software usually allow images to be displayed as either black on white or white on black. Although the human eye can differentiate fewer than 100 shades of gray, most computer systems generate an 8-bit image, assigning display intensities from 0 to 255. The maximum pixel count is therefore assigned a display intensity of 255, and all other pixels are assigned scaled values from 255 down to 0. Some display systems may be assigned only 64 shades of gray, which is sufficient for viewing. Display artifacts can arise when too few shades of gray are assigned to the display. For example, an image displaying only 16 shades of gray shows the discrete count thresholds that will generate isocount lines where changes in count rate across the image jump from one count threshold to another.

The relationship between the number of counts and display intensity is usually linear (Figure 4-9), which provides a uniform shading between all count levels. Most computers also allow a logarithmic and an exponential relationship between pixel count and intensity. An exponential relationship suppresses the number of gray scales assigned to low-count values while expanding the number of shades of gray assigned to higher pixel counts (see Figure 4-9). This in effect reduces the low-count pixels, removing background. Conversely, the logarithmic relationship assigns more gray levels to low-count pixels and compresses the number of shades of gray assigned to high pixel values, enhancing differences in low-count densities.

Background subtraction is another enhancement technique to allow better appreciation of slight differences in count. Background enhancement selects a count threshold that is set to the lowest intensity and reassigns intensities between the threshold and the maximum pixel count.

The use of color is another technique to provide image enhancement. Typically a selected color table is used to

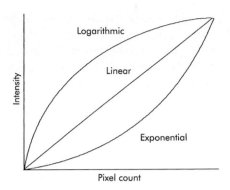

Figure 4-9 Gray-scale intensity can be assigned as a linear relationship relative to the pixel count. An exponential relationship suppresses low counts, providing background subtraction. A logarithmic relationship enhances low-count intensities.

enhance the differences between pixel count densities and to provide some visual background erase. The red, green, and blue guns of the CRT can be assigned intensity values from 0 to 255 and can be mixed to generate more than 16 million colors. A color table that has only ten different colors with discrete steps has the same effect of creating isocontour colors in the image as black-and-white images with limited shades of gray. The most effective color tables are those that have gradual and continuous shades of color. For example, the colors of the rainbow—from violet through red, representing low- to high-count values, respectively—provide some esthetically pleasing images. Another commonly used color table, the "hot iron" table, assigns gray scales from black to dark red through orange and white for the hottest pixel values. The result is an enhancement similar to an exponential scale to suppress low-count densities.

Image Algebra

The simplest image processing operations are those representing mathematical operations of add, subtract, multiply, and divide. Nuclear medicine computers allow images to be manipulated with these simple functions. For example, a dynamic flow study originally acquired at one frame per second can be reformatted through the addition of three images into one to create a dynamic set with each image representing 3 seconds. Image addition is usually performed to improve the count density of images or to compress a sequence of dynamic images into a smaller number of frames, which can be used more easily to identify time-activity changes within the images. Subtraction is commonly applied to an image matrix in one of two ways: subtraction of a numeric value from all pixels, and subtraction of one image from another. Subtraction of a number from the pixel count from each pixel of an image is used to perform background subtraction as an alternative to gray scale enhancement; this technique might be applied to an image where body background is to be eliminated from the image. Subtraction of one frame from another has many clinical uses, such as creation of a cardiac stroke volume image by subtracting the end-systolic image from the end-diastolic image, which leaves only the counts representing areas of myocardial contraction. Another example of frame subtraction is parathyroid imaging, where a technetium image of the thyroid is subtracted from a thallium image of the thyroid and parathyroids. The resultant image is a picture of only parathyroid tissue.

Other simple image manipulations are performed to shift an image a given number of pixels in the x or y direction or to rotate an image about its center point to correct alignment. Image manipulation is also necessary to move images from one position to another with any file of several images.

Image Smoothing

Image smoothing is performed to reduce noise from the random effects of radionuclide counting. The simplest technique is to average the counts of a given pixel with that of its eight surrounding neighbors and replace the center pixel count with the new value.

A most common type of simple image smoothing is a nine-point smooth, a filtering technique to modify a specific pixel value according to the values of its neighbors. The nine-point smooth uses a 3 × 3 matrix centered over each pixel in the image. The filter weighting values 4, 2, and 1 multiply the center and adjacent pixel values to allow the original value and closest pixels to have more influence on the result of filtering (Figure 4-10). The new computed value after filtering is placed into the pixel location of a new

filtered image. Nine-point smoothing blends pixel values with those of its neighbors, creating a smoother, more esthetic image (Figure 4-10). However, this smoothing results in a slight loss of resolution, and detail is slightly blurred. Filters can be based not only on a 3 × 3 matrix but also on a 5 × 5, 7 × 7, or larger filter matrix. In addition, filters with negative values around the edges can enhance or sharpen the edges of organs. These filters are sometimes used in applications for automatic edge detection programs.

Filtering of dynamic image sets can use a temporal filter, which performs weighted averaging of an image with those that occur just prior to and just following a dynamic image sequence. For example, Figure 4-11 shows an example of filtering frame B by multiplying the original frame B by a weighting value of 2 and adding one times the preceding frame A and one times the following image, frame C. Temporal filtering is applied most frequently to gated cardiac images with the filter applied in a closed loop. Temporal filtering removes noise without a loss of spatial resolution, as occurs with the nine-point smooth.

Cinematic Display

A dynamic sequence of images may be displayed as a continuous loop movie known as a cinematic display. The images to be displayed are formatted into an area of memory known as a buffer so that information can be retrieved quickly. Some systems may have insufficient memory, and a display buffer is created on disk. Dynamic studies, gated blood pool images, and SPECT images can all be displayed in a cinematic mode. The rate at which images are displayed can be changed; for example, the beating heart from a gated blood pool study can be displayed live time in a closed loop to provide an image of the beating heart. Longer dynamic studies, such as 30-minute kidney studies, can be displayed

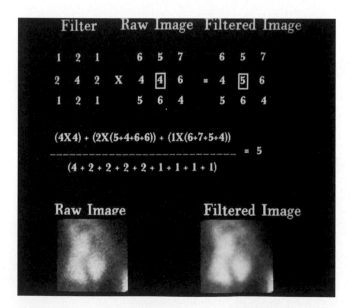

Figure 4-10 A nine-point smooth filter with values of 4, 2, and 1 is applied to the center pixel value (4) of a 3 × 3 pixel area of the raw image. Multiplying the raw image center point by 4, the side values by 2, and the corner pixel values by 1, and then dividing by the filter sum produces a new value (5), which is placed into the filtered image. Raw and nine-point smoothed gated cardiac images are shown at bottom.

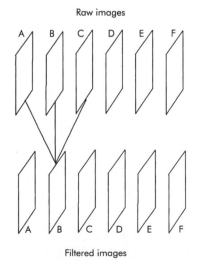

Figure 4-11 Dynamic series of images can be temporally smoothed by adding the previous and following images. Image B in the filtered image set is composed of an average of A, B, and C from the raw images.

to compress the set of images into a few seconds. The observer therefore has a better appreciation of physiologic changes that occur over a long time.

Image Quantitation

Digital nuclear medicine images are many times acquired to derive quantitative information. Counts in a particular area can be extracted from the image by defining a region of interest (ROI). An ROI is defined on the displayed image using a mouse, joystick, track ball, or light pen. ROIs can be defined as a rectangle or ellipse or manually drawn as an irregular shape. The ROI program usually allows an option to display or print the counts within the region, the number of pixels in the region, and the average count per pixel. Most computer systems allow 16 to 32 regions to be drawn on a single image. When defining ROIs, the area defined should be physiologically meaningful; for example, when drawing an ROI over the kidney, should the area include the whole kidney and renal pelvis, cortex, and collecting system, or simply the cortex? Different information can be extracted from the images, depending on how the ROI has been defined. Some clinical programs perform automated ROI definition. These programs can use a specific count threshold, maximum slope, isocount level, second derivative, or other criteria to identify the edge of an organ. A combination of techniques such as isocount level mixed with the profile maximum slope (second derivative) can be used in automatically defining the region of the left ventricle on a gated blood pool study.

Some nuclear medicine computer systems allow ROIs to be manipulated just as images can be manipulated. It might be desirable to add or subtract regions. For example, a region defining the renal pelvis could be subtracted from a region defining the whole kidney, leaving the area of the renal cortex. ROIs can be saved with the patient's study to allow reprocessing the information at a later time with the originally defined regions.

Curves

Quantitative information from a single image is derived by setting an ROI and obtaining the ROI counts. The ROI counts in sequential images from a dynamic study can be used to plot the radioactivity versus time change or time-activity curve. Physiologic information from dynamic studies might be appreciated more easily by generating time-activity curves. Curve displays are widely applied to a variety of clinical applications. Curves provide useful information in evaluating the accumulation and washout of radiopharmaceutical from the kidney, changes in left ventricular volume on gated studies (Figure 4-12), and changes in radionuclide distribution on gastrointestinal studies. Curves should be displayed to best demonstrate diagnostic information. When multiple curves are displayed on the same graph, such as the individual kidneys in a renal study, it is important that the curves be properly distinguished from one another and correctly labeled as to their region—left kidney, right kidney, and so on. Curve display software many times allows the user to select the options for the format of the display: a continuous line versus dots at each data point, the intensity or color of the curves, and display of axis labels. Curve information should also be scaled properly; that is, the extent of the data range along both the x and y axes

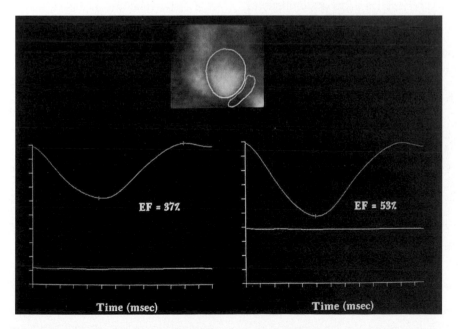

Figure 4-12   Regions of interest of the left ventricle and background can be drawn, and time activity curves generated. Curves on the left demonstrate the left ventricle curve *(upper)* and background curve *(lower)*. The background curve contains less activity and is smaller. Curves on the right show a higher background curve *(lower)* after area normalization. With normalization of the background counts, the ejection fraction is correctly computed at 53%.

changes the appreciation of changes in radioactivity. The appropriate scale of each axis should allow the observer to view most accurately changes of clinical significance in the study. For example, a renal scan with a y axis that is very short would display only a small change in radioactivity in a normal renal study.

The manipulation of curves is also valuable in data interpretation. Simple algebraic functions are useful for applications such as adding curves from two separate regions, performing subtraction of a background curve from an organ curve, or multiplying one curve to match the scaling of another curve.

Because of statistical limitations in counts, it is sometimes helpful to smooth curve data. Commonly a 1-2-1–weighted smooth is done for each curve point with its preceding and following neighbors. Another technique to reduce noise in curve data is to fit the curve points to a mathematical formula that allows additional quantitative information to be derived. Most commonly, a straight-line linear fit or an exponential function is fitted to the data. The fitted curve can then allow quantitative numbers to be measured, such as the slope of a linear function or the half-time of an exponential curve.

Normalization

Normalization is a concept in nuclear medicine that implies that a measurement has been brought to a standard. For instance, two images with different maximum counts may have their intensities normalized if the image with the lowest maximum count is multiplied so that the maximum count matches the second image. The two images, therefore, would be displayed with the same maximum intensity. Normalization is most commonly applied to two ROIs or curves. For example, the counts in ROI-1 are normalized to a second, larger ROI-2 by multiplying ROI-1 counts by a ratio of the number of pixels in ROI-2 divided by the number of ROI-1 pixels. Region normalization is performed most commonly to subtract background counts of one region from the counts from a different size region.

As an example, consider the subtraction of background in calculating left ventricular ejection fraction (EF) from a gated blood pool study (see Figure 4-12). Assume that the counts in an end-diastolic (ED) ROI are 89,485 and 56,375 in the end-systolic (ES) ROI. We can calculate the left ventricle ejection fraction using the equation

$$EF = (ED - ES)/ED \times 100$$

In our example and ignoring background, the ejection fraction would be

$$(89,485 - 56,375)/89,485 \times 100 = 37\%$$

This value is erroneously low because body background has not been subtracted. Let us assume the end-diastolic ROI contains 89,485 counts with an area of 586 pixels, that the end-systolic counts are 56,375 in 416 pixels, and that a background region contains 9134 counts in 89 pixels. To subtract the proper amount of background activity from the end-diastolic ROI, the area covered by the ROIs must be of the same size, thus the process of region count normalization. Since the background region is smaller than the left ventricle region, the background region counts are multiplied by a ratio of the region sizes (number of left ventricle pixels per number of background pixels).

$$\text{Normalized background counts} = \frac{\text{Background} \times \text{Number of heart pixels}}{\text{Number of background pixels}}$$

The background region contains 9134 counts in 89 pixels, and the end-diastolic heart region contains 586 pixels; the normalized end-diastolic background becomes 9134 × (586/89), or 60,140 counts. This can be subtracted from the end-diastolic count of 89,485, giving a background subtracted end-diastolic count of 29,345. The same normalization calculation can be made for the end-systolic region, which contains 56,375 counts in 416 pixels; the normalized background is 9134 × (416/89), or 42,693 counts. Subtracting this normalized background from the end-systolic left ventricle counts gives a net of 13,682 counts. With these normalized background-subtracted values, a background-corrected ejection fraction is calculated as

$$(29,345 - 13,682)/29,345 \times 100 = 53\%$$

With proper subtraction of background, the ejection fraction value has now been significantly changed.

These same principles of normalization can be applied to curve mathematics. Multiplying the background curve by the ratio of the organ region size divided by a smaller background region size properly increases the background curve for subtraction, significantly changing the ejection fraction value. Note that the background curve on the lower right of Figure 4-12 is increased after correct scaling by normalization and that the EF values have changed.

EMISSION COMPUTED TOMOGRAPHY (ECT) IMAGING

Emission computed tomography (ECT) is a general term describing the reconstruction of three-dimensional image volumes that are derived from one of two techniques: Single Photon Emission Computed Tomography (SPECT) or Positron Emission Tomography (PET). Both these techniques are similar in that they acquire information from different views, or projections, and this projection information from around the patient is used to determine mathematically the three-dimensional distribution within the body.

SPECT imaging is performed by obtaining planar images (projections) with the scintillation camera from many angles around the patient. Images are acquired from 360 degrees around the patient, except in myocardial perfusion studies, where 180-degree right anterior oblique to left posterior oblique images over the anterior chest are acquired. Images

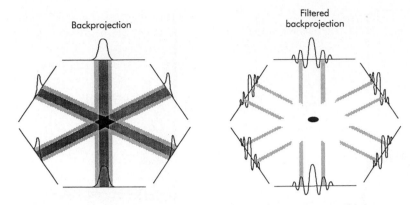

Backprojection

Filtered backprojection

Figure 4-13 Back-projection (*left*) in SPECT reconstruction creates a streak or star artifact. Filtered back-projection (*right*) creates negative values on the sides of high-count areas that cancel positive values and remove the star artifact.

are acquired in 64 × 64 resolution for most studies for single detector cameras or low-count images from multiple detector systems. Images of 128 × 128 resolution can be acquired on high-count studies. The planar projection SPECT images are first viewed cinematically to ensure no significant patient motion has occurred. Image data are then back-projected (Figure 4-13, *left*) to overlay areas of increased activity and create a transverse slice image. Back-projection produces a streak or star artifact that results from data being laid onto the slice image from various projections. A technique called filtered back-projection reduces the streak artifact. In the reconstruction process a frequency space filter is used to modify the projection data, in essence creating negative values on each side of areas of increased counts. These negative numbers, when combined with positive values, cancel each other out, eliminating streak artifacts (Figure 4-13, *right*). Streaks are also reduced by obtaining images from many angles, about 120 images in 360 degrees, essentially viewing objects from more angles.

PET information is created from lines drawn between two individual detectors, in a ring of detectors around the body, that simultaneously detect a pair of photons that result from a positron decay. All the lines measured from various directions provide information about the distribution of the radiotracer within the body. Using reconstruction techniques similar to SPECT, PET 3D images are then created.

Frequency Space and Filtering

SPECT reconstruction and filtering will be best understood after discussing the representation of images as a group of frequencies. The representation of objects as a frequency or a spectrum of frequencies is an unusual concept. A simple example is shown in Figure 4-14. This figure represents the count profile of an image with 0.5-cm bars and with spaces 0.5 cm wide. The counts in the profile of the bar appear as square blocks of activity, which can be approximated by the pattern of a wave with a specific wavelength and amplitude. The wavelength replicates the spacing of the bar pattern, and the amplitude replicates the height or in this case the

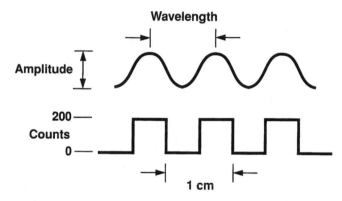

Figure 4-14 A simple application of frequencies would be to estimate the count profile of a parallel line bar phantom as represented at the bottom of the diagram, where 0.5-cm bars and spaces are shown in this count profile. A frequency space estimate of this pattern would be a sinusoidal pattern with wavelength of 1 cm and an amplitude that would correspond to 200 units. The total bar pattern image can now be roughly estimated by specifying a frequency of 1 cycle/cm with amplitude of 200.

number of counts. Therefore a simplistic representation of the bar pattern image would be frequency 1 cycle per centimeter with an amplitude of 200.

Image filtering to reduce noise depends on the information content of the image (e.g., counts, collimator, scatter, object distance, background activity). In frequency space filtering there will always be a trade-off or balance between reducing noise and degrading resolution, and vice versa.

Image information can be represented in frequency space by graphically plotting the frequency on the horizontal axis and the wave amplitude on the vertical axis. In Figure 4-15 a square count profile (*top*) of an object is roughly estimated by using a single wave with a specific wavelength and specific height or amplitude. To the right of the single wave in Figure 4-15 is the frequency space graph, showing a single frequency with a specific amplitude, thus representing a very rough estimate of the original square object. An improved representation is made by adding a second wave of higher

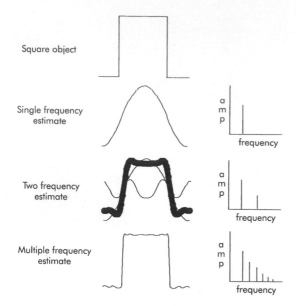

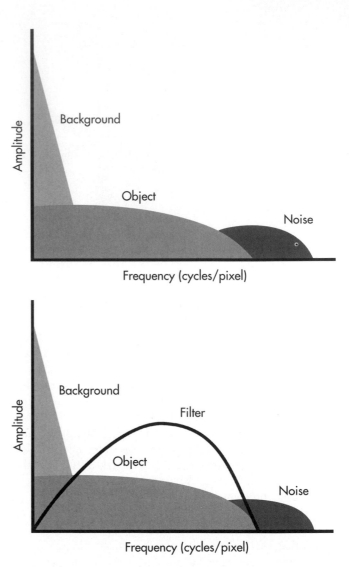

Figure 4-15 Count profile of a square object can be roughly estimated as a single frequency, or wave. The diagram on the right and top represents a single frequency with a specific amplitude to estimate the square object. Two frequencies can be added together (*dark curve*) to better estimate the profile of the original square object. Many frequencies (*bottom*) can be added to more accurately represent the original square profile. The group of frequencies in the lower right curve generate a frequency spectrum of the original object.

frequency, also with a specific amplitude. The dark line in Figure 4-15 shows two frequencies added, which better represents the original square object. When multiple waves are combined, they provide an accurate representation of the original object (*bottom*). The group of frequencies (*bottom right*) that now represent this object form a continuous curve—the frequency spectrum of the object. A mathematical process called the *Fourier transform* accomplishes the conversion of the image into its wave components. An inverse process called the inverse Fourier transform transfers the frequency group back into the x,y coordinate system, reconstructing the image. Images in the usual spatial domain are represented as counts in a pixel; in the frequency domain images are represented as amplitudes of various frequencies. The Fourier transform is computationally intense and is usually performed in an array processor to save time.

Frequency space can be thought of as analogous to a piano keyboard. The low keys create long frequency tones, and the upper keys create high frequencies. The combination of several frequencies, such as playing a chord, generates a certain sound. Changing a single frequency, such as changing one note in the chord, creates a sound with a different impression. Images are similarly characterized by properly mixing frequencies. Any object can be represented by a group of sine or cosine waves.

When images are converted to frequency space, objects or organs in the image are represented as a group of low and middle frequencies (Figure 4-16, *top*). The pixel-to-pixel

Figure 4-16 *Top,* Frequencies representing an image include high frequencies that are the noise in the image, and middle and low frequencies that represent the object and uniform body background. *Bottom,* The frequency space filter, when selected with the right cutoff frequency or point where it drops back down to zero amplitude, enhances the object while multiplying the noise frequency by zero to eliminate the noise.

count differences due to variations in counting statistics are represented as a group of high frequencies that we call noise. Figure 4-16 (*top*) shows body background activity as low frequencies, that is, constant activity (long wavelengths) in the body. The significant advantage of converting images to frequency space should now become clear; noise is represented by high frequencies, somewhat separate from the frequencies that represent the object organ of interest.

Filtering, or the reduction of noise, occurs in frequency space by reducing high-frequency information. Noise is reduced by multiplying the frequency space curve by a filter curve (Figure 4-16, *bottom*). The filter values at the low and middle frequencies multiply the object frequencies to retain the organs of interest in the image. The filter values at higher frequencies drop to zero, multiplying high frequencies by zero or very small values, thus eliminating noise.

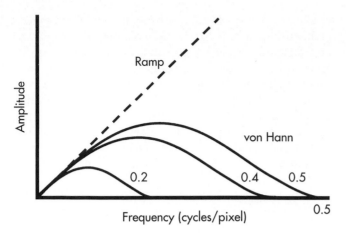

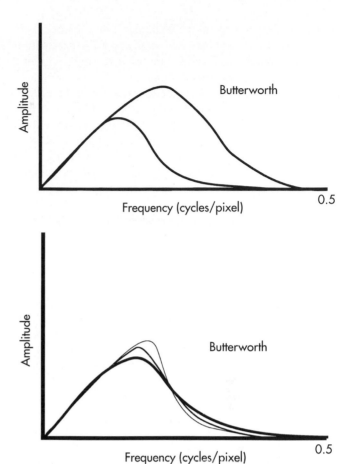

Figure 4-17 A ramp filter is the highest-resolution frequency space filter, but it also creates the largest amount of noise because of its high values due to its great amplitude at high frequencies. Von Hann filters with a cutoff frequency of 0.2, 0.4, and 0.5 cycles per pixel represent commonly used low-pass filters.

Filters are mathematical formulas that generate the curve shape, and cutoff values determine the dropoff point of the filter. Cutoff frequency is a common parameter used to generate and characterize filter shapes and may be measured in cycles/pixel, cycles/mm or just in millimeters. Commonly used are the ramp, von Hann (or Hanning), Butterworth, Parzen, Hamming, Wiener, and Metz filters. All these filters have the same basic purpose—to increase the amplitudes of the object frequencies and reduce the amplitude of the high frequencies. The ramp filter (Figure 4-17) is the highest resolution filter, but also significantly multiplies high frequencies, producing a noisy image. There is a group of filters classified as low pass, which includes von Hann, Hamming, Butterworth, Parzen, and others. Low-pass filters let low frequencies through. Each of these filters is actually a family of filters defined by various cutoff frequencies. For example, a low-pass filter with a higher cutoff frequency will produce a higher resolution but a noisier image. Using a von Hann filter with a cutoff frequency of 0.2 cycles per pixel produces a smooth image because image frequencies higher than 0.2 are multiplied by small filter values (or zero), therefore reducing noise. A von Hann filter with a cutoff frequency of 0.4 cycles per pixel (Figure 4-17) includes more high frequencies and produces a high-resolution image with little reduction in noise. Frequency space filtering must balance high resolution against noise reduction. Low-count images must remove many high frequencies and therefore must be smooth, low-resolution images. High-resolution filtered images can be obtained with high-count images.

Butterworth filters are in several aspects the best of the group of low-pass filters, because the mathematical formula contains not only a cutoff frequency parameter but also another parameter called the order that adjusts the downslope or roll off of the upper part of the filter. Figure 4-18 (*top*) shows two Butterworth filters, both with an order of 4 but with cutoff frequencies of 0.2 and 0.4 cycles/pixel. But-

Figure 4-18 The Butterworth filter has two parameters to define the shape of this low-pass filter. The order controls the downslope, and cutoff frequency defines the width or spread of the filter. The top curves represent Butterworth filters with order 4 and cutoff frequencies of 0.2 and 0.4. The bottom curves all have the same cutoff frequency (0.2) and orders of 3, 4, and 5.

terworth filters with a cutoff frequency of 0.2 and orders of 3, 4, and 5 (Figure 4-18, *bottom*) show steeper downslopes as the order increases. A steeper downslope will produce a higher resolution image.

Another group of filters is adaptive filters, sometimes called restorative filters. Adaptive filters (Metz and Wiener) are powerful filtering techniques in that they use some criteria about the resolution capabilities of the camera and collimator within the mathematical filter function. These filters differ from low-pass filters by not only suppressing noise but also preventing blurring and the smoothing of edges of objects. Metz and Wiener filters are both a family of curves with a multiplier value to create different curve shapes and control the point at which the downslope occurs (Figure 4-19).

Filtering and Tomographic Reconstruction

Many of the filters used for frequency space filtering can also be used in the filtered back-projection reconstruction algorithm. Finding proper filtering for each type of patient study to reduce noise and obtain high resolution remains a matter of personal preference in the final image appearance. There is a continual choice between obtaining a high-resolution image and obtaining a smooth image; increasing smoothing through filtering reduces resolution.

Image filtering is usually employed twice in SPECT reconstruction. On most computer systems filtering is performed first as a prefiltering function to remove noise from the planar projection images; then filtering is also incorporated into the reconstruction algorithm. The resultant image quality is influenced directly by image acquisition parameters (matrix size, number of stops, counts per image) and filtering. Although a ramp filter provides the highest resolution SPECT reconstruction, the slices contain a significant amount of noise; therefore optimum prefiltering or postfiltering of slices is an important factor in obtaining high-resolution SPECT. As an example of SPECT reconstruction, processing a ^{201}Tl myocardial study usually begins with a prefiltering of the images before reconstruction. Prefiltering is performed most commonly using a low-pass filter for noise reduction. A second filter is used in the filtered back-projection reconstruction. Studies such as thallium scans have very poor statistics in the planar images, and filtering is needed to provide an esthetic and interpretable set of slice images. SPECT imaging of the liver requires smooth slices, because abnormalities usually are seen as cold defects in a uniform area of radiopharmaceutical distribution. SPECT imaging of the lumbar spine on a bone scan has many counts and excellent resolution, whereas filters that retain the higher frequencies yield high-resolution slice images.

Prefiltering with low-pass filters using a small cutoff frequency (0.1 cycle per pixel) results in images slightly oversmoothed with some loss in resolution. When the image filter includes too many high frequencies, filtering and filtered back-projection algorithms create a mottled pattern in areas that should have uniform radionuclide distribution. Studies in which high counts are obtained with high-resolution collimators, such as bone imaging of the spine or brain imaging with ^{99m}Tc HMPAO, require the use of a low-pass filter with a fairly high cutoff frequency (0.35 to 0.5 cycles per pixel). With proper filter selection, these high-count studies yield images with high resolution and little noise. Multiple-detector scintillation cameras obviously have higher sensitivity than single-detector SPECT cameras and yield images with higher count statistics and higher resolution. In addition, the recent implementation of convergent collimators, such as fan beam, astigmatic, and cone-beam geometries also has improved sensitivity. Many more counts are obtained by these systems.

The speed of some new nuclear medicine computers will, in the near future, allow the use of reconstruction algorithms other than filtered back-projection techniques. These new computers have many megabytes of memory, and their ultrafast processors can execute computationally intense algorithms, such as maximum likelihood (ML), expectation maximization (EM), and conjugate gradient. These new algorithms give improved image quality with a reduction in streak artifacts.

Iterative Reconstruction Algorithms

More complex reconstruction algorithms, called *iterative reconstruction algorithms* have been introduced on some commercial systems in recent years. Iterative reconstruction techniques incorporate much more information about the physics of the imaging situation into the algorithm. Therefore these algorithms are computationally much more intense and may require several minutes to reconstruct. All iterative algorithms, as the name implies, consist of computing a series of improving images of the three-dimensional (3D) distribution of activity. Most algorithms provide clinically useful images after about 20 iterations. There are specific categories of iterative algorithms, such as maximum likelihood (ML), expectation maximization (EM), conjugate gradient, and maximum a priori (MAP). Each filter has its own distinct advantages. Most commonly used is the ordered subset expectation maximization (OS-EM) algorithm. This is an EM technique that evaluates subsets (subgroups) of the projections in order to calculate the 3D volume more quickly than calculating each point from all projections.

Reconstructions using iterative techniques do not have the streak artifacts that are produced by back-projection algorithms. Iterative reconstructed images have improved resolution compared to filtered back-projection, and the edges of organs look sharp with good image contrast. Therefore little postreconstruction filtering is required to produce clinical quality images.

Three-Dimensional Display

Although commercial SPECT systems have been available for more than 20 years, techniques to view the vast amount of data contained in a series of slice images have remained

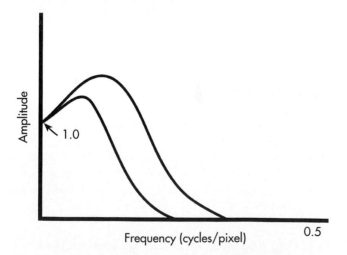

Figure 4-19 Adaptive filters, such as the Wiener, start with amplitude values of 1 and can be controlled by a parameter to enhance middle frequency to provide good smoothing and constant count areas. The rolloff portion of the curve provides excellent edge retention of objects with good contrast.

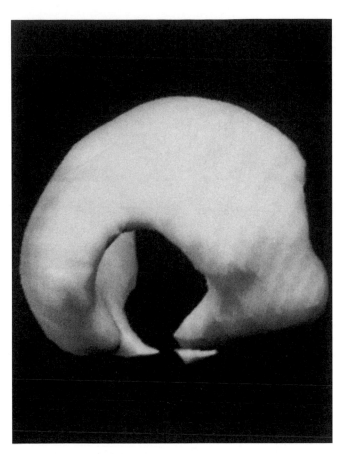

Figure 4-20 Three-dimensional surface renderings from SPECT data create an anatomic and pleasing display. This ^{201}Tl scan shows an inferoapical defect as seen from the 45 LAO projection.

limited. Surface display and volume rendering are two techniques for 3D viewing. Surface displays are created by selecting a count threshold for generating a 3D isocount surface. The problem, therefore, becomes to correctly set this threshold to include only clinically useful information; the proper threshold setting is critical for proper clinical interpretation of the 3D object. Because this display shows only a solid outer surface of the organ, information inside the organ is not seen; therefore the most suitable organs for surface displays are thin organs with cold abnormalities, such as the heart (Figure 4-20) and brain cortex. A very smooth set of slice images creates a smoother surface than the reconstructed slices for directed viewing. Volume rendering is a display technique that provides a translucent appearance to a 3D volume. A stack of reconstructed transverse slices (an image volume) are reprojected into planar images from multiple directions around the object volume like the original planar images (Figure 4-21, A). In this reprojection process the maximum pixel count along each projection line is selected as the maximum activity that would be seen for an individual pixel. This projection of the highest concentration of radioactivity provides the image a translucent appearance and also produces an image with very little noise. This technique is excellent for identifying hot abnormalities in SPECT image data and can be applied to a variety of studies, such as finding hot lesions on bone SPECT and identifying hepatic hemangiomas on labeled red-cell studies (Figure 4-21, B). The volume-rendered projections are viewed cinematically to produce a dramatic and esthetically pleasing display. Complex 3D volumes such as a whole body PET study may be quickly evaluated using volume rendering and displaying the images to see an image of the patient rotation in space. The human eye easily tracks moving objects, such

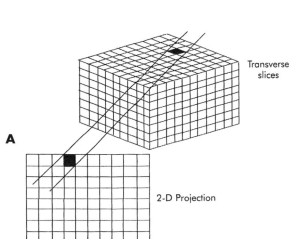

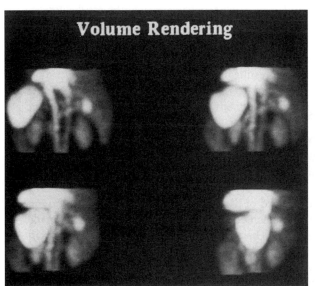

Figure 4-21 **A,** Volume rendering displays are generated from a stack of transverse slices by reprojecting the data into two-dimensional (2D) projections for cinematic viewing. The highest count pixel along the path for reprojection is placed into the 2D image. **B,** Volume-rendered translucent display of a hepatic hemangioma study shows the exact anatomic location of a hot lesion in the liver as seen from four different angles.

educational, and commercial computer centers. Although no one owns the Internet, there are organizations that promote the global exchange of information and provide technical direction and management.

The organization of computers on the Internet is controlled by an addressing system. Your own postal mailing address for your residence or business has information from the largest geographic area to a specific city, street, and number. Internet addresses have a set of names and numbers associated for both the computer and computer network. A location such as med.utah.edu indicates direction of the information to the education network domain, the University of Utah, and specifically to the Medical Center computer. Likewise, the information could have been directed to 155.100.78. An additional number would then specify a computer within this network. So IP addresses are actually four 8-bit numbers separated by a period. As we know, 8-bit numbers have a range of 0 to 255, so with four of these number composing the IP address we can connect 4,228,250,625 computer devices worldwide. Data files to be transferred on the Internet are broken up into small, manageably sized data packets that may actually be routed in different directions on the Internet but arrive and are reorganized into their original format at their destination. The transmission and reorganization of a file is transparent to the computer user and is part of the beauty of the software that uses the IP.

Computers within large institutions may be directly connected to the Internet, or their network may be connected to the Internet. Access to the Internet may also be provided using either standard telephone lines or special high-speed data lines that connect to another computer that resides on the Internet. Home service is most commonly provided through a commercial network provider for which you pay a nominal monthly fee and pay for your connection time. Often, nuclear medicine computers may not be connected to the Internet because of the concern over security issues. Any computer directly connected to the Internet should have appropriate security of user accounts and protection of data. Computer network system administrators may prevent unauthorized access to sensitive patient data and protect programs.

The Internet provides computer users with the ability to exchange and obtain information. Electronic mail (e-mail) uses a standard format of data called Simple Mail Transfer Protocol (SMTP) to allow various types of computers and software to send and receive mail. As previously mentioned, electronic mail must be addressed not only to a specific computer on a certain Internet domain but also to a specific individual account.

The transfer of information files can be done using ftp (File Transfer Protocol). This protocol uses a standard transfer method of data between Internet sites. Users may use ftp to enter computers where they have permission to look at a listing of files in different directories and *get* or *put* files. To use ftp, the user must have a fairly specific idea of the computer to be accessed and file directory to be reviewed to obtain the desired information. In the early 1990s a more friendly way of locating information was developed. One of these methods is the software called *Gopher.* Gopher was developed at the University of Minnesota to allow individuals to find specific documents without knowing the exact location of the information. Gopher uses a client-server mode, which connects to an institution's own Gopher server that provides menus of publicly available information. Gopher servers are linked together to provide a wide range of information to be searched and obtained. Other types of networking search programs such as Archie and Veronica allow users to access information that is indexed by keyword and title on a regular basis.

The most rapidly expanding part of the Internet is the World Wide Web (WWW or W3). The WWW is based on *hypertext* documents. Hypertext documents have "links" to other documents on the same computer or information at another location, which could be in another city or even country. Hypertext documents differ from other types of connectivity on the Internet in that they provide not only text but also image files, video files, and sound files, which are transferred at the click of a mouse button. A hypertext document is written in a special format language called hypertext markup language (html). Special formatting codes within these documents instruct the local computer to display a certain size font and text, where to position an image file on the page, and so forth. Links to other documents appear as colored text or small icons, which are activated by clicking on them with the mouse button. This may access a video file, an image or sound file, or may simply connect to another document.

Access to the World Wide Web is obtained using "browser" software that interprets hypertext documents. Browsers such as Mosaic, Netscape, and Internet Explorer are favorites and for personal computers are very reasonably priced. Browser software also contains access to search engines, which allow the user to type in words that describe any topic of interest, and then a list of sites using hypertext links is presented on the screen. The user may then move around or "surf" through documents at various sites to locate information.

The World Wide Web provides tremendous opportunities for locating or exchanging information between Web sites. For example, a Nuclear Medicine Department could create a Web server with documents relevant to its research, continuing education programs, or teaching files, all of which can be available online to anyone with access to the Internet. At this time many large teaching hospitals have Web sites with a variety of information.

SUGGESTED READINGS

English RJ: *SPECT: single photon emission computed tomography: a primer,* ed 3, New York, 1995, Society of Nuclear Medicine.

Erickson JJ: Nuclear medicine computer systems—
hardware, *J Nucl Med Technol* 13:97-102, 1985.

Erickson JJ: Nuclear medicine computer systems—
software, *J Nucl Med Technol* 13:140-149, 1985.

Erickson JJ, Rollo FD, eds: *Digital nuclear medicine,*
Philadelphia, 1983, Lippincott Williams & Wilkins.

Glowniak JV: An introduction to the Internet, part 1:
history, organization, and function, *J Nucl Med Technol*
23:56-64, 1995.

Glowniak JV: An introduction to the Internet, part 2:
obtaining access. *J Nucl Med Technol* 23:150-157, 1995.

Glowniak JV: An introduction to the Internet, part 3:
Internet services, *J Nucl Med Technol* 23:231-248,
1995.

Glowniak JV: An introduction to the Internet,
part 4: medical resources, *J Nucl Med Technol* 24:
1996.

Harkness B, Christian P, Rowell K: *Clinical computers in
nuclear medicine,* New York, 1992, Society of Nuclear
Medicine.

Lee K: *Computers in nuclear medicine: a practical approach,*
New York, 1991, Society of Nuclear Medicine.

Jay A. Spicer

chapter 5

Laboratory Science

Objectives

Use laboratory glassware appropriately, including beakers, flasks, graduated cylinders, pipets, and burets.

Use an analytical balance to perform mass measurements accurately.

Use and calibrate a centrifuge to separate solids from liquids.

Use a pH meter.

Describe the electronic structure of atoms.

Explain the structure of the periodic table of elements and discuss characteristics of various groups.

Explain ionic and covalent bonds.

Use the laws of constant composition and multiple proportions.

Describe the gram atomic weights, gram molecular weights, and the mole.

Describe molarity, molality, and normality.

Explain the characteristics and production of colloids.

Demonstrate and use chemical reaction equations.

Describe oxidation-reduction reactions and electrolytic reactions.

Define acids, bases, and neutralizing reactions.

Define and measure pH.

Explain the mechanisms of buffering solutions.

Describe the simple nomenclature of organic compounds.

*I*n the beginning humans were created as a fusion of two components, one spiritual and the other chemical. As has been and is now, the well-being of each component is vital to life. Although our spiritual involvement with patients is of utmost importance, knowledge of the chemical component of life is necessary to the successful practice of nuclear medicine.

Chemical principles are fundamental to an understanding of life and to the diagnostic processes used in the hope of maintaining a healthy life, but you should not consider this chapter as containing all there is to know. Space limitations make the following discussion of chemistry brief and often inadequate. Our hope and intention are that the individual instructors using this text will recognize the points that require further elucidation and will use their knowledge and talents to elaborate.

GLASSWARE AND INSTRUMENTATION

Glassware

The fundamental part of any scientific laboratory is the equipment, the most basic of which is the glassware. Figure 5-1 shows those items most commonly used in routine laboratory manipulations.

Beakers, flasks, and graduated cylinders. The most frequently used type of glassware is the beaker. Beakers range in capacity from a few milliliters to several liters and are used in the preparation of solutions and as weighing vessels when a high degree of accuracy is not required.

Erlenmeyer flasks are also used in these procedures and, because of their conic shape and small mouth, offer the advantage that solutions can be prepared by swirling the contents of the flask with little risk of spilling. This feature also makes the Erlenmeyer flask an ideal vessel for the substance in titrations. Neither the beaker nor the flask provides the accuracy (±5% to 10%) required for precise volume measurement.

Volume measurements requiring an accuracy of ±1% to 2% can be achieved by the use of the appropriate graduated cylinder (Figure 5-1). However, many laboratory procedures require the preparation of solutions accurate in concentration to ±0.001%. This precision can be attained by use of a volumetric flask. Flasks marked TC are calibrated "to contain" a specific volume, depending on the size of the flask, and allow volume measurement within the accuracy limits noted above.

Pipets and burets. In the normal course of laboratory work many occasions arise where a precise volume of a solution or solvents is required and an appropriate-sized volumetric flask is not available. In such cases a small (<5 ml) or nonintegral volume is usually required, and one must resort to the use of a pipet or buret.

Pipets (Figure 5-1) are transfer vessels used to measure and deliver a precise volume of solution or pure liquid. They are generally of two types: those that must be filled and drained manually, and automatic pipets, which measure and deliver a fixed volume when activated.

The ordinary pipets, which require manipulation, are of two styles: one is calibrated to deliver a fixed volume, whereas the other is graduated and may be used to deliver any increment of volume up to the full capacity of the pipet. Both styles are available in sizes ranging from microvolumes (a fraction of a milliliter) to a capacity of several hundred milliliters.

Care must be exercised in the use of pipets, because some are calibrated to deliver the stated volume by normal drainage (some solution remains in the tip of the pipet), and others are calibrated to deliver the entire volume drawn into the pipet, which requires "blowing out" the last traces of the solution. The blow-out pipets are identified by one or two bands placed near the top.

Automatic pipets are especially important to the radioimmunoassay laboratory, where knowing the accurate volumes of radioactive solutions is required.

Procedures such as titrations (p. 147), in which an accurately measured but unknown volume of solution must be determined, are conveniently performed by use of a buret. The buret, being graduated, allows a direct reading of the volume used in reaching the end point, the point at which the added titrant has reacted with the entire quantity of substance present in the sample.

Instrumentation

Just as certain types of glassware are important to the laboratory, so also are several instruments. All nuclear pharmacy or radioassay laboratories must be equipped with a minimum of three instruments: an analytic balance, a centrifuge, and a pH meter.

The analytic balance. The analytic balance (Figure 5-2) is vital to any laboratory where mass measurements of solids are routinely required, usually in small quantities (<1 g). The balance shown in Figure 5-2 allows mass measurements accurate to ±0.1 mg.

The balance is designed so that as the units on the weight dials are changed, the instrument automatically adds or removes weights from a knife-edge counterbalance inside the instrument. Newer, currently available analytic balances are automatic taring and provide a direct digital readout of weight. If handled with care, the balance will give dependable results with a minimum of service.

The centrifuge. Quite often it is necessary to separate solids from liquids, such as red blood cells from the plasma. When such separations are necessary, a centrifuge is used (Figure 5-3).

The centrifuge is composed of a balanced motor and shaft on which cups or holders are mounted. A container holding the mixture to be separated is placed in one cup, and a counterbalance container (having the same weight as the sample container) is placed in the cup opposite the sample.

The centrifuge exerts a strong centrifugal force on the sample by spinning the material at relatively high speeds (500 to 1500 rpm), and, as in the case of blood, the heavier red blood cells settle to the bottom of the container, leaving the lighter plasma on top. One can then draw off the plasma, thus effecting a separation of the two components.

The pH meter. The measurement of pH is generally accomplished by two methods, one of which provides reasonably accurate values, and the other, more precise values. The less sensitive method makes use of a paper containing a universal indicator. The universal indicator is a mixture of organic dyes, which themselves are acids and bases, and it undergoes changes in color on being converted from one form to the other, that is, acid to base or base to acid. These color changes occur at specific pH values.

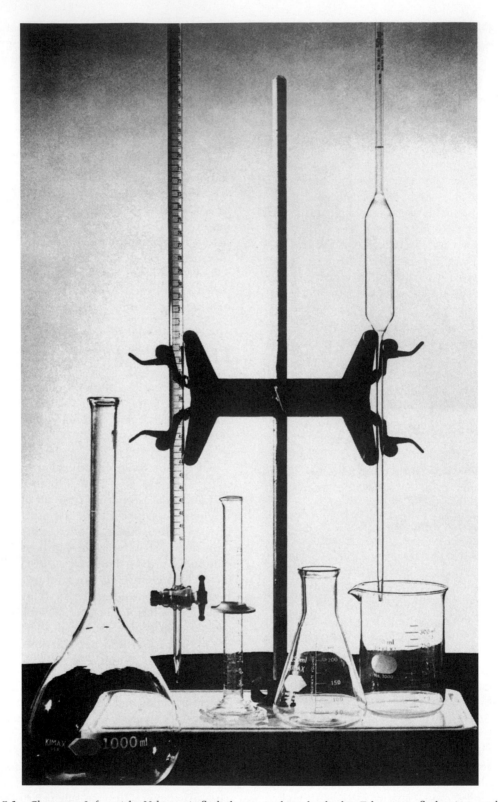

Figure 5-1 Glassware. *Left to right,* Volumetric flask, buret, graduated cylinder, Erlenmeyer flask, pipet, and beaker.

Accurate pH values, which are usually necessary in radioimmunoassay analysis or the preparation of radiopharmaceuticals, are determined by use of a pH meter (Figure 5-4).

A pH meter has two electrodes. Note that the one in Figure 5-4 contains both electrodes in a single probe. One electrode of known potential (a calomel electrode) serves as a reference and involves the following electrode reaction:

$$2Hg + 2Cl^- \leftrightarrows Hg_2Cl_2 + 2e^-$$

This reaction has a constant potential of $-0.27\,V$. The second electrode (a glass electrode) consists of a meter wire dipped

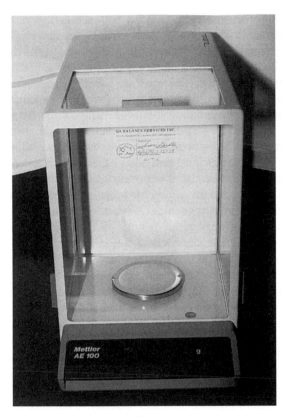

Figure 5-2 Analytic balance

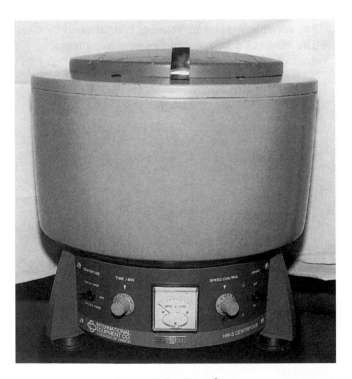

Figure 5-3 Centrifuge.

component of a pH meter is a voltmeter or potentiometer capable of measuring voltages accurate to at least ±0.01 V. The voltmeter or potentiometer is designed, based on the potential difference of the two electrodes, to give a reading in pH units.

ELEMENTS AND COMPOUNDS

In introducing the study of chemistry as it applies to nuclear medicine and nuclear pharmacy, it is desirable to define the word *chemistry*. Chemistry can best be defined as the study of matter and the changes that matter undergoes.

All matter exists in one of three physical states—solid, liquid, or gas. Each substance differs in physical and chemical properties from all other substances.

Physical properties are the attributes characteristic of a substance, such as odor, color, hardness, luster, density, and structure. These properties depend on the conditions imposed on the substance and may be affected by a change in temperature, pressure, or radiation. However, a substance, be it an element or a compound, that has undergone a change in physical properties because of a change in conditions will exhibit the initial properties when the substance is returned to the original condition. For example, sulfur, which is a yellow solid at room temperature, becomes a liquid when heated to 113°C and returns to the yellow solid when allowed to cool. Physical changes are readily reversible.

In contrast to a change in physical properties, chemical change results in a complex and deep-seated change. Chemical change always results in the formation of one or more "new" substances, each of which has chemical and physical properties unique to itself.

Most chemical changes are reversible only with great difficulty, and many—for example, the burning of wood or paper—are irreversible.

Electronic Structure

Because each element has unique chemical and physical properties, it is logical to ask why this is so. To answer this question, one must probe the very nature of the elements: their constitution and behavior.

Experimental evidence has shown that all elements are made up of minute particles called atoms and that an atom is the smallest unit of an element that can exist and still maintain the properties of the element. All atoms of a given element are identical in chemical properties, and the atoms of each element differ in properties from the atoms of all other elements. To understand why this is so requires knowledge of the structure of atoms and the components necessary to their formation.

Structurally, all atoms can be described as a sphere composed of two parts. One part is a small, compact nucleus located at the center of the sphere; the second part, a region of space surrounding the nucleus, is populated by small particles called electrons.

into a solution of known pH, and this solution is separated by a thin glass membrane from the solution whose pH is to be determined. The potential across the glass membrane, and thus the half-cell voltage of this electrode, is a function of the pH of the solution outside the membrane. A third

Table 5-1	Relationship of quantum numbers													
Shell (*n*)	1		2							3				
Subshell (*l*)	0	0	1			0	1			2				
m value	0	0	−1	0	+1	0	−1	0	+1	−2	−1	0	+1	+2
s value	±½	±½	±½	±½	±½	±½	±½	±½	±½	±½	±½	±½	±½	±½
Number of electrons*	↑↓	↑↓	↑↓	↑↓	↑↓	↑↓	↑↓	↑↓	↑↓	↑↓	↑↓	↑↓	↑↓	↑↓

*↑ denotes e⁻ with +½ spin; ↓ denotes e⁻ with −½ spin.

The next electron must now enter the second energy level, $n = 2$, and will occupy the 2s orbital; the same will be true for the next electron. The 2s orbital now containing two electrons, whose spins are paired, is filled, and the next electron must enter one of the three 2p orbitals. One might expect the next electron to enter the same p orbital to give paired electrons; however, spectroscopic evidence indicates that this electron enters one of the two remaining empty p orbitals and has the same spin number as the first p electron. This behavior is summarized by Hund's rule, which states that for an atom where orbitals of equal energies are being filled, the electrons will remain unpaired until each orbital is half filled, that is, one electron in each of the orbitals.

To facilitate the assignment of electrons to the lowest energy orbital available, the following sequence is helpful:

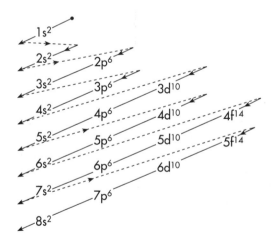

The arrows and broken lines indicate the proper order of filling. The symbols and their significance are as follows:

EXAMPLE: Given the term $4p^3$ indicate the *n*, *ℓ*, *m*, and *s* values.

1. $n = 4$, the fourth energy level.
2. Since p electrons are involved, $ℓ = 1$.
3. With $ℓ$ being 1, $m = −1, 0, +1$ (the three p orbitals), each of which can accommodate two electrons for a total of 6.
4. The superscript 3 denotes the presence of three electrons in the p orbitals. Following Hund's rule, each orbital (p_x, p_y, p_z) will contain one electron, all of which will have parallel spins ($s = +½$).

Had the electrons cited in the example been the electrons of highest energy in a neutral atom, the element to which they belong would be known. These being the highest energy electrons would indicate that all orbitals of lower energy had been filled. Thus, by counting the number of electrons (using the diagram above) and recalling that the number of electrons is equal to the atomic number of the element, we find that the element corresponding to the atom has an atomic mass of 33. The periodic table (Figure 5-8) shows element number 33 to be arsenic (As).

Periodic Table of the Elements

Early in the nineteenth century chemists noted a relationship between atomic weight and properties of the elements. Although many of the elements had not yet been discovered, chemists were able to recognize those elements having similar properties and to group them into families. Later in the century, around 1870, several chemists segregated the known elements into groups (families) and showed that properties were a function of atomic number rather than atomic weight and that the properties of a given element, both physical and chemical, were similar to those elements having an atomic number differing by 8, 18, 32, and so on. For example, lithium (atomic number 3), sodium (atomic number 11), potassium (atomic number 19), and rubidium (atomic number 37) exhibited similar physical properties in being shiny, ductile, malleable, and good conductors of electrical current. Chemically, these elements are similar in that they form compounds with other elements in the same proportions. Thus *one* atom of Li or Na reacts with *one* atom of fluorine, forming lithium fluoride (LiF) or sodium fluoride (NaF), but *two* atoms of Li or Na react with *one* atom of oxygen to form lithium oxide (Li_2O) or sodium oxide (Na_2O). Other families such as fluorine, chlorine, bromine, iodine, and astatine, or oxygen, sulfur, selenium, tellurium, and polonium are groups of elements exhibiting similar chemical and physical properties.

The periodic table contains the elements known at this time (Figure 5-8). Elements of similar properties, as discussed above, are grouped together in columns (placed vertically) to form a family having the same electron configuration in the outermost shell. For example, Li, Na, and so on, each contain *one* electron in the outer shell, whereas F, Cl, and so on, each contain *seven* electrons in the outer shell. However, the elements in a row (placed horizontally) differ from one another in chemical and most physical properties. From a consideration of the electron

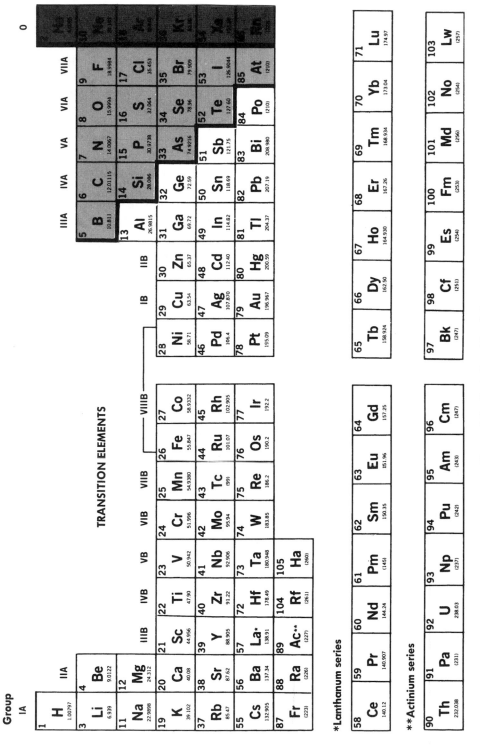

Figure 5-8   Periodic table of elements.

earth's atmosphere, exists as the molecule O_2. It is apparent that the electronegativity of each oxygen atom in the molecule is the same; therefore the electrons that bond these atoms cannot be attracted more strongly by one atom than by the other. This results in an equal sharing of electrons, *and the bond is completely covalent*. Other examples of non-polar covalent bonds are nitrogen (N_2, which is 80% of the earth's atmosphere), hydrogen (H_2), and the halogens (F_2, Cl_2, Br_2, I_2). As we shall find in a subsequent discussion, the carbon-hydrogen bond in organic molecules is essentially nonpolar covalent because both carbon and hydrogen have electronegativity values of approximately 2.5.

Coordinate Covalent Bonds

Those compounds containing coordinate covalent bonds are similar to those compounds containing covalent bonds in that the bonding electrons are shared by two atoms. However, the electrons used in forming these bonds are donated by *one atom only*. As an example, let us consider the reaction in which a molecule of sulfuric acid is formed from the following elements:

$$2H_\square + \; _{oo}^{oo}S_o + 4\,^{x}O^{x} \rightarrow H\,^{xx}_\square O\,^{oo}_{oo}S\,^{o}_{o}O_\square H$$

or

$$H—O—\underset{\downarrow}{\overset{\uparrow}{S}}—O—H$$
$$O$$

The symbol — represents a covalent bond, and ↑ represents a coordinate covalent bond in which the arrow points toward the atom that did not contribute any electrons to bond formation.

Considering each bond in the sulfuric acid molecule, and the electrons used in forming each bond, it is apparent that the hydrogen-oxygen bonds and two of the sulfur-oxygen bonds are polar covalent, whereas the remaining two sulfur-oxygen bonds are coordinate covalent bonds, in that the electrons used in forming these bonds are contributed by the sulfur atom only.

Complex Ions and Chelates

The formation of coordinate covalent bonds need not occur by reaction of neutral elements, as shown in the preceding section. In many reactions a coordinate covalent bond is formed by the interaction of a neutral molecule with an ion. In reactions of this type the driving force, or reason for reaction, is that an atom contained within the neutral molecule has not attained the electron configuration of a noble gas. In previous discussions the metals were assumed to react by transfer of their electrons to form ionic compounds.

However, elements such as aluminum (Al) have been found to form compounds in which the bonds are largely polar covalent. This being true, it is apparent that the aluminum atom needs three electrons to attain the noble gas configuration of argon (Ar). Consequently aluminum chloride ($AlCl_3$), in a nonpolar solvent, reacts with anhydrous chloride gas (Cl_2) according to the following equation:

$$_{xx}^{x}\text{CL}_{xx}^{x}{}^{-} + \text{Al}_{oo}^{oo}\text{Cl} \rightarrow \left[\text{Cl}_{x}^{x}\text{Al}_{oo}^{oo}\text{Cl} \right]^{-} + {}_{xx}^{x}\text{Cl}{}^{+}$$

The electrons used in forming the fourth chlorine-aluminum bond are donated by the chloride ion, resulting in the formation of a coordinate covalent bond. The ions that provide the bonding electrons are called *ligands*.

A second example of coordinate covalent bond formation is that in which a positive ion undergoes reaction with a neutral molecule, as illustrated in the following reaction:

$$H^{+} + {}_{o}^{o}N_{x}^{ox}H \rightarrow \left[H{}_{o}^{o}N_{x}^{ox}H \right]^{+}$$

The products resulting from reactions of neutral molecules with either a cation or an anion are called *complex ions*.

Although elements such as aluminum and nitrogen can share one pair of electrons with simple ions to form complex ions, other elements, especially the transition elements, must accept two or more pairs of electrons to attain a noble gas electron configuration. These complexes are especially important in nuclear medicine and in many cases involve the formation of chelates in which the electron pairs (two or more pairs) are donated by functional groups present in the ligand molecule. The term *chelate*, from the Greek word *chēlē* (claw), is reserved for these ligands. The complex ytterbium-pentetic acid (Yb-DTPA) (Figure 5-11), used as a cisternographic imaging agent, is an excellent example of a chelate. In this case the electrons used in forming the coordinate covalent bonds are donated by the functional groups present in the pentetic acid molecule.

Although the structures of many complex ions of technetium are still under investigation, it is reasonable to assume that their structures are similar to those formed by ytterbium.

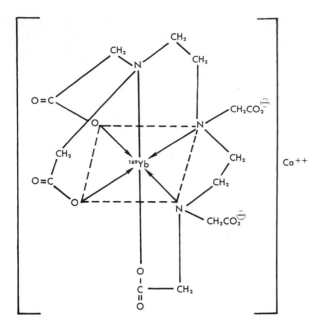

Figure 5-11 Ytterbium-pentetic acid (Yb-DTPA) complex. *Arrows,* Coordinate covalent bonds; *dotted line,* plane through these atoms.

LAWS OF CONSTANT COMPOSITION AND MULTIPLE PROPORTION

The fact that elements generally react with other elements to attain a noble gas electron configuration leads to the conclusion that any two elements that undergo reaction must do so in a definite ratio of atoms, that is, one Na to one F and one C to four Cl. It then follows that the elements must also react to definite ratios by weight. This is stated by the *law of constant composition:* A compound, regardless of its origin or method of preparation, always contains the same elements in the same proportions by weight.

In some cases, depending on reaction conditions, an element will combine with another to give products that differ in the ratio of atoms of the two elements. For example, sodium usually reacts with oxygen to form sodium oxide (Na_2O), but under other conditions they react to form sodium peroxide (Na_2O_2). However, in each case the ratio of sodium to oxygen is definite. This is stated by the *law of multiple proportions:* When two elements combine to form two or more different compounds, the ratio of the mass of one element that combines with a fixed mass of a second element is a simple ratio of whole numbers, for example, 2:1 or 3:2.

Sample Problems

EXAMPLE 1: When subjected to quantitative elemental analysis, two samples of a compound containing only carbon and oxygen give the following data:

	Weight of sample	Weight of C found	Weight of O found
Sample 1:	0.7335 g	0.2002 g	0.5333 g
Sample 2:	0.6162 g	0.1682 g	0.4480 g

Do these data uphold the law of constant composition? If the law is upheld, the percentage of carbon and oxygen must be the same in each sample. To determine this, the ratio of the weight of each element to the total weight of the sample must be equal to the ratio of the percent of the element to 100%.

Sample 1:

$$\text{Percent carbon} = \frac{0.2002}{0.7335} = \frac{\% C}{100\%} \quad \% C = 27.29$$

$$\text{Percent oxygen} = \frac{0.5333}{0.7335} = \frac{\% O}{100\%} \quad \% O = 72.71$$

Sample 2:

$$\text{Percent carbon} = \frac{0.1682}{0.6162} = \frac{x\% C}{100\%} \quad \% C = 27.29$$

$$\text{Percent oxygen} = \frac{0.4480}{0.6162} = \frac{x\% O}{100\%} \quad \% O = 72.71$$

The percentage of carbon and oxygen being the same for both samples indicates that they are of identical composition and thus support the law of constant composition.

EXAMPLE 2: A third sample, obtained from a different source, was also found to contain only carbon and oxygen and gave the following data upon analysis:

	Weight of sample	Weight of C found	Weight of O found
Sample 3:	0.3599 g	0.1543 g	0.2056 g

Show that these data illustrate the law of multiple proportions. Follow the procedure used in example 1.

Sample 3:

$$\text{Percent carbon} = \frac{0.1543}{0.3599} = \frac{\% C}{100\%} \quad \% C = 42.87$$

$$\text{Percent oxygen} = \frac{0.2056}{0.3599} = \frac{\% O}{100\%} \quad \% O = 57.13$$

Obviously this composition indicates that sample 3 was obtained from a compound different from that of samples 1 and 2. Although the samples differ in composition, the law of multiple proportions states that the ratios of the masses of the elements in each compound should be related as simple whole numbers. Thus:

$$\text{For sample 1:} \frac{\% O}{\% C} = \frac{72.71}{27.49} = 2.66$$

$$\text{For sample 3:} \frac{\% O}{\% C} = \frac{57.13}{42.87} = 1.33$$

Therefore the ratios of oxygen to carbon in sample 1 and sample 3 are related by the ratio of 2.66:1.33 or 2:1.

GRAM ATOMIC WEIGHTS, GRAM MOLECULAR WEIGHTS, AND THE MOLE CONCEPT

The chemistry discussed thus far has been based on the interactions of individual atoms. Although this description is a valid one, the isolation and use of single atoms in the laboratory is neither practical nor possible. The smallest sample that can be accurately measured in the laboratory will contain 10^{15} to 10^{17} atoms or molecules.

For a reaction to be accurately described by a chemical equation, it is necessary only that the number of atoms or molecules of the reactants be present in the *ratio* given by the coefficients for these substances. In the following reaction, the ratio of hydrogen (H_2) molecules to oxygen (O_2) molecules must be $2:1$.

$$2H_2 + 1O_2 \rightarrow 2H_2O$$

The chemist, being unable to count the number of atoms or molecules necessary for a given reaction, must resort to an indirect method to achieve this ratio. The fact that each element possesses a unique atomic mass (see Figure 5-8) indicates that even though equal weights of hydrogen and oxygen could be measured, the number of molecules of hydrogen present in the sample would be 16 times that of the oxygen molecules; that is, one hydrogen molecule has a weight of 2 relative to a weight of 32 for one oxygen molecule. A convenient method that allows the measurement of the required quantities of the reactants by accurate weighing of each substance is based directly on their gram atomic weight (gaw) or gram molecular weight (gmw). By definition, these are the weights in grams that are numerically equal to the atomic weights (amu) or molecular weights (the sum of the atomic weights of all atoms present in the molecule) of the elements or compounds involved. From this definition it is apparent that 1 gmw of any two substances will contain the same number of atoms or molecules. The number of atoms or molecules in 1 gaw or gmw has been shown by experiment to be 6.02×10^{23}. This number is called *Avogadro's number*, and 1 gaw or gmw of any substance is commonly referred to as 1 *mole*.

These concepts are illustrated in the following examples:

EXAMPLE 1: How many moles (gram atomic weights) of chromium (Cr) are contained in 28 g? From the periodic chart the atomic weight of chromium is found to be 52 amu; therefore the weight of Cr contained in 1 mole (gaw) is 52 g.

$$\frac{1\,mole}{52\,g} = \frac{x\,mole}{28\,g}$$

$$x = \frac{(28\,g)(1\,mole)}{52\,g}$$

$$x = \frac{28}{52}\,mole$$

$$x = 0.538\,mole$$

EXAMPLE 2: How many grams are contained in 0.59 moles (gram molecular weights) of sulfuric acid? Sulfuric acid, H_2SO_4, being a molecule, requires that we first determine its molecular weight.

$$2H \times 1\,amu = 2\,amu$$
$$1S \times 32\,amu = 32\,amu$$
$$4O \times 16\,amu = 64\,amu$$
$$\text{Molecular weight} = 98\,amu$$

Therefore 1 mole (gmw) would contain 98 g of sulfuric acid, and

$$\frac{98\,g}{1\,mole} = \frac{x\,g}{0.59\,mole}$$

$$x = \frac{(98\,g)(0.59\,mole)}{1\,mole}$$

$$x = (98\,g)(0.59)$$

$$x = 57.82\,g$$

EXAMPLE 3: How many molecules are contained in 0.50 mole of nitrogen (N_2)? One mole (gmw) of N_2 (28 g) would contain Avogadro's number of molecules (6.02×10^{23}), therefore

$$\frac{6.02 \times 10^{23}\,molecules}{1\,mole} = \frac{x\,molecules}{0.50\,mole}$$

$$x = \frac{(0.50\,mole)(6.02 \times 10^{23}\,molecules)}{1\,mole}$$

$$x = (0.50)(6.02 \times 10^{23})\,molecules$$

$$x = 3.01 \times 10^{23}\,molecules$$

EXAMPLE 4: How many moles of water (H_2O) are present in a sample containing 5×10^{12} molecules? One mole of H_2O contains 6.02×10^{23} molecules, therefore

$$\frac{1\,mole}{6.02 \times 10^{23}\,molecules} = \frac{x\,mole}{5.0 \times 10^{12}\,molecules}$$

$$x = \frac{(1\,mole)(5.0 \times 10^{12}\,molecules)}{6.02 \times 10^{23}\,molecules}$$

$$x = \frac{(5.0 \times 10^{12})\,mole}{6.02 \times 10^{23}}$$

$$x = 0.83 \times 10^{-11}\,mole$$

$$x = 8.3 \times 10^{-12}\,mole$$

EMPIRICAL AND MOLECULAR FORMULAS

All substances now known were initially obtained from natural resources or chemical reactions, and in many cases their elemental composition and structures were unknown. The elements present in such compounds must be determined by *qualitative chemical analysis,* and the relative amount of each element by *quantitative chemical analysis.* The information obtained in these analyses is useful in determining the empirical formula of a substance.

The ratio of the elements contained in a substance (the relative number of each kind of atom present) is indicated by the empirical formula. However, the empirical formula may not truly reflect the molecular formula of the substance, which may be a whole number multiple of the empirical formula. For instance, the organic substance oxalic acid, which is a constituent of some plants, has an empirical formula of CHO_2 but a molecular formula of $C_2H_2O_4$.

EXAMPLE: A compound, on analysis, was found to have the following composition by weight:

Carbon (C) = 50.7%
Hydrogen (H) = 4.25%
Oxygen (O) = 45.1%

What is the empirical example of the compound?

Because percentage is based on 100, it may be assumed that a 100 g sample of the compound would contain

$$50.7 \text{ g C}$$
$$4.25 \text{ g H}$$
$$45.1 \text{ g O}$$

Also knowing that a definite atomic weight (and gram atomic weight) is a unique property of each element, the relative abundance of each element is obtained by the following:

$$\text{Carbon:} \frac{50.7 \text{ g}}{12 \text{ g}} = \frac{x \text{ gaw}}{1 \text{ gaw}}$$

$$x = \frac{50.7 \text{ g}}{12 \text{ g}} (1 \text{ gaw})$$

$$x = 4.23 \text{ gaw}$$

$$\text{Hydrogen:} \frac{4.25 \text{ g}}{1 \text{ g}} = \frac{x \text{ gaw}}{1 \text{ gaw}}$$

$$x = \frac{(4.25 \text{ g})(1 \text{ gaw})}{1 \text{ g}}$$

$$x = 4.25 \text{ gaw}$$

$$\text{Oxygen:} \frac{45.1 \text{ g}}{16 \text{ g}} = \frac{x \text{ gaw}}{1 \text{ gaw}}$$

$$x = \frac{(45.1 \text{ g})(1 \text{ gaw})}{16 \text{ g}}$$

$$x = \frac{45.1}{16} \text{ gaw}$$

$$x = 2.82 \text{ gaw}$$

However, each element must be present in an integral value of its atomic weight, or gram atomic weight. To obtain integral values for each element, we must divide the above values of the gram atomic weight by the smallest value obtained. Thus:

$$\text{Oxygen:} \frac{2.82 \text{ gaw}}{2.82 \text{ gaw}} = 1$$

$$\text{Carbon:} \frac{4.23 \text{ gaw}}{2.82 \text{ gaw}} = 1.5$$

$$\text{Hydrogen:} \frac{4.25 \text{ gaw}}{2.82 \text{ gaw}} = 1.5$$

These values indicate that the empirical formula of the compound is $C_{1.5}H_{1.5}O_1$. Obviously, these values are not integral, and the actual number of atoms present in the molecule must be a multiple of these. Multiplying the value for each element by 2 results in an empirical formula of $C_3H_3O_2$, indicating an integral or whole number value for each element.

Further analysis of the above substance indicates its molecular weight to be 142. What is the molecular formula of the compound?

The molecular weight of the compound is derived from the following empirical formula:

Carbon	(3)(12) = 36	
Hydrogen	(3)(1) = 3	
Oxygen	(2)(16) = 32	
Empirical weight	= 71	

Inasmuch as the molecular formula must be a multiple of the empirical formula, that is, $142/71 = 2$, the molecular formula is $C_6H_6O_4$.

Empirical or molecular formulas may be characteristic of several different compounds and provide no information pertinent to the structure of the molecule.

SOLUTIONS AND COLLOIDS

Much of the chemistry encountered in nuclear medicine involves solutions. A solution is a homogeneous mixture of two substances: the *solute* can be a gas, liquid, or solid, and the *solvent* is generally a liquid. One must choose a solvent that will dissolve the solute and yet not undergo chemical reaction with the solute.

In working with solutions one must know the concentration of solute in a given volume of solution and therefore must be familiar with the methods and units used in defining concentrations.

Molarity

Molarity expresses the number of moles of solute contained in 1 L of solution.

$$\text{Molarity (M)} = \frac{\text{Number of moles of solute}}{\text{Number of liters of solution}}$$

Sample Problems

EXAMPLE 1: What is the molarity of a solution prepared by dissolving 16 g of barium chloride ($BaCl_2$) in sufficient water to give a total volume of 450 ml?

Step 1: How many moles of $BaCl_2$ are in the 16 g sample?

$$1 \text{ mole } (BaCl_2) = 137.5 \text{ g} + 2(35.5 \text{ g})$$
$$1 \text{ mole } (BaCl_2) = 208.5 \text{ g}$$

$$\frac{1 \text{ mole}}{208.5 \text{ g}} = \frac{x \text{ mole}}{16.0 \text{ g}}$$

$$x = \frac{(16.0 \text{ g})(1 \text{ mole})}{208.5 \text{ g}}$$

$$x = \frac{16.0 \text{ mole}}{208.5}$$

$$x = 0.077 \text{ mole}$$

Step 2: Molarity (M) $= \dfrac{\text{mole}}{\text{liter}}$

$$M = \frac{0.077 \text{ mole}}{0.450 \text{ L}}$$

$$M = \frac{0.171 \text{ mole}}{\text{L (molar)}}$$

EXAMPLE 2: How would 20 L of 6.0 M sodium hydroxide (NaOH) solution be prepared from solid NaOH?

Step 1: How many grams of NaOH are in 6.0 moles?

$$1 \text{ mole (NaOH)} = 23\,g + 16\,g + 1\,g$$
$$1 \text{ mole (NaOH)} = 40\,g$$
$$\frac{x\,g}{6.0 \text{ moles}} = \frac{40\,g}{1 \text{ mole}}$$
$$x = \frac{(40\,g)(6.0 \text{ moles})}{1 \text{ mole}}$$
$$x = (40)(6.0)\,g$$
$$x = 240\,g \text{ in } 6.0 \text{ moles of NaOH}$$

Step 2: One liter of 6.0 molar (M) solution requires 240 g of NaOH. Therefore for 20 L of 6.0 M solution, (20)(240 g) = 4800 g of NaOH dissolved in sufficient water to give a total volume of 20 L.

EXAMPLE 3: How could the solution prepared in example 2 be used to obtain 1.0 L of 0.50 M NaOH solution?

Step 1: The 6.0 M NaOH must be diluted with additional water. What volume of the 6.0 M solution contains 0.50 moles of NaOH?

$$\frac{1.0\,L}{\substack{6.0 \text{ mole} \\ (NaOH)}} = \frac{x\,L}{\substack{0.50 \text{ mole} \\ (NaOH)}}$$
$$x = \frac{(1.0\,L)(0.50\,M)}{(6.0\,M)}$$
$$x = \frac{0.50\,L}{6.0}$$
$$x = 0.083\,L$$

Step 2: If 0.083 L of 6.0 M NaOH contains 0.50 moles of NaOH, then to obtain a 0.50 M solution, one must add enough water to bring the volume to exactly 1.0 L.

Molality

A *molal* solution is defined as the number of moles of solute contained in 1 kilogram (kg) of solvent.

$$\text{Molality (m)} = \frac{\text{Number of moles of solute}}{\text{Number of kilograms of solvent}}$$

Whereas 1 L of a *molar* solution is prepared by the addition of sufficient solvent to the solute to give a total volume of 1 L, a *molal* solution is prepared when the solute is dissolved in 1 kg (in the case of water, 1 L) of solvent. The total volume of a 1 molal solution will generally be greater than that of a 1 molar solution.

EXAMPLE: Calculate the molality of a solute prepared by dissolving 20.4 g of sodium chloride (NaCl) in 192 g of H_2O.

Step 1: How many grams are contained in 1 mole of NaCl?

$$1 \text{ mole (NaCl)} = 23\,g + 35.5\,g$$
$$1 \text{ mole (NaCl)} = 58.5\,g$$

Step 2: How many moles are contained in 20.4 g of NaCl?

$$\frac{1 \text{ mole}}{58.5\,g} = \frac{x \text{ mole}}{20.4\,g}$$
$$x = \frac{(20.4\,g)(1 \text{ mole})}{58.5\,g}$$
$$x = \frac{(20.4)}{58.5} \text{ mole}$$
$$x = 0.349 \text{ mole}$$

Step 3: From the definition of molality:

$$m = \frac{0.349 \text{ mole}}{0.192 \text{ kg}}$$
$$m = 1.82 \text{ molal solution}$$

It should be noted that most solutions are usually expressed in terms of molarity rather than molality.

Normality

A third method of expressing concentration, and one that is in general more useful than that of molarity or molality, is normality (N). Normality is defined as the number of equivalents (Eq) of solute per liter of solution. The number of equivalents present in a solution, rather than being defined as the number of moles of solute per liter, is defined as the number of moles of reactant species contained in 1 mole of the solute. For example, as we have discussed earlier, in the reaction $H^+ + {}^-OH \rightarrow H_2O$ the reactants must arise from two different substances, one of which provides H^+ and another that provides ^-OH (conventionally OH^-, also ionically OH^-). Those compounds that give H^+ ions are called acids, as we shall discuss later. Two of the most common acids are hydrochloric acid (HCl) and sulfuric acid (H_2SO_4). Both these acids may be considered to be completely ionized in aqueous solution to give the H^+ ion and the corresponding anions. It should be apparent that ionization of 1 mole of HCl will give rise to 1 mole of H^+ ion, whereas the ionization of 1 mole of H_2SO_4 will give rise to 2 moles of H^+ ion. Thus in comparing HCl with H_2SO_4, we note that 0.5 mole of H_2SO_4 will provide the same number of H^+ ions that would be provided by 1 mole of HCl. Therefore the weight of H_2SO_4 that will provide 1 Eq of H^+ ion (1 mole) is half its molecular weight: 98 g/2 = 49 g, whereas the weight of HCl required to produce 1 Eq (1 mole) of H^+ is equal to its molecular weight (36.5 g). Similarly, the substances that provide OH^- ion (called bases) will have equivalent weights dictated by the number of moles of OH^- that will be provided by 1 mole of the base. Thus:

$$\text{Normality (N)} = \frac{\text{Number of equivalents}}{\text{Number of liters of solvent}}$$

and

$$\text{Normality (N)} =$$
$$\frac{(\text{Moles of solute})(\text{``Moles'' of reactant provided})}{1\,L \text{ of solution}} =$$

$$\frac{\text{Equivalents}}{\text{Liter}} = \frac{\text{Eq}}{L}$$

A second type of reaction to utilize *normal* solutions is that in which an oxidation-reduction is involved. This type is yet to be discussed, and suffice it to say at this point that the equivalent weight of a reagent in an oxidation-reduction reaction is determined by the number of electrons that it accepts or donates.

How are equivalent weights calculated? The equivalent weight, in grams, of an acid is calculated when the gram molecular weight of the acid is divided by the number of potential hydrogen ions contained in the molecule. For a base the gram molecular weight is divided by the number of hydroxide ions.

Problems

EXAMPLE 1: What is the equivalent weight of HCl?

$$\text{Equivalent weight} = \frac{\text{gmw}}{\text{Number of } H^+ \text{ ions}}$$

$$\text{Equivalent weight} = \frac{36.5\,g}{1} = 36.5\,g$$

EXAMPLE 2: What is the equivalent weight of H_2SO_4?

$$\text{Equivalent weight} = \frac{\text{gmw}}{\text{Number of } H^+ \text{ ions}}$$

$$\text{Equivalent weight} = \frac{98\,g}{2}$$

$$\text{Equivalent weight} = 49\,g$$

EXAMPLE 3: What is the equivalent weight of 1 mole of calcium hydroxide, $Ca(OH)_2$?

$$\text{Equivalent weight} = \frac{\text{gmw}}{\text{Number of } H^- \text{ ions}}$$

$$\text{Equivalent weight} = \frac{74\,g}{2}$$

$$\text{Equivalent weight} = 37\,g$$

From the foregoing discussion it is evident that the normality of a solution must be a whole number multiple of a corresponding molar solution.

EXAMPLE 4: What is the normality of a 90 ml sample of a solution that contains 10 g of NaOH?

Step 1:

$$1\text{ equivalent weight of NaOH} = \frac{1\text{ gmw of NaOH}}{1\,OH^- \text{ ion}}$$

$$1\text{ equivalent weight} = \frac{40\,g}{1} = 40\,g\text{ of NaOH}$$

Step 2: The number of equivalents of NaOH in solution:

$$\frac{1\,Eq}{40\,g} = \frac{x\,Eq}{10\,g}$$

$$x = \frac{(1\,Eq)(10\,g)}{40\,g}$$

$$x = \frac{10}{40}\,Eq = 0.25\,Eq\text{ of NaOH}$$

Step 3: Normality equals equivalents/liter, therefore

$$N = \frac{Eq}{L} = \frac{0.25}{0.09}$$

$$N = 2.78\text{ normal}$$

Note: Because normality equals molarity for NaOH, this solution is both 2.78 N and 2.78 M.

EXAMPLE 5: What are the normality and molarity of 100 ml of an aqueous solution containing 50.0 g of phosphoric acid (H_3PO_4)?

Step 1: How many grams of H_3PO_4 are contained in 1 gew (gram equivalent weight)?

$$1\text{ gew} = \frac{1\text{ gmw}}{\text{Number of } H^+ \text{ ions}}$$

$$1\text{ gew} = \frac{98.0\,g}{3} = 32.7\,g\text{ of }H_3PO_4$$

Step 2: What is the number of equivalents in 50 g of H_3PO_4?

$$\frac{1\,Eq}{32.7\,g} = \frac{x\,Eq}{50.0\,g}$$

$$x = \frac{(1\,Eq)(50.0\,g)}{32.7\,g}$$

$$x = \frac{50.0\,g}{32.7\,g} = 1.53\,Eq\text{ of }H_3PO_4$$

Step 3: Normality, by definition:

$$N = \frac{1.53\,Eq}{0.100\,L}$$

$$N = 1.53\text{ normal}$$

Step 4: Because H_3PO_4 is triprotic (3 H^+ ions), the molarity of this solution will be

$$m = \frac{N}{3} = \frac{15.3}{3}$$

$$m = 5.10\text{ molar }H_3PO_4$$

Colloids

A second type of mixture, one that is important in nuclear medicine, is the *colloid*. Unlike true solutions, colloids consist of minute particles that are suspended in a dispersing medium. Colloid particles vary in shape, and range in size from 10^{-9} to 10^{-7} m in diameter. Although several important types of colloids exist, we restrict our discussion to the colloid in which a solid is dispersed in a liquid—a *sol*.

Although one might expect the particles to settle out on standing, the dispersed colloid particles remain suspended in the dispersing medium indefinitely. This behavior is attributed to a constant bombardment of the dispersed particles by the molecules of the dispersing medium; thus the colloid particles are in constant motion. This phenomenon is called *Brownian movement* and may be observed with the proper type of microscope.

Unlike true solutions, colloids exhibit an optical effect characterized by the scattering of light when a narrow beam is passed through them. The scattering of light is attributa-

giving either a H_3O^+ ion or a OH^- ion. In reality, only *strong acids* such as HCl, HBr, HI, H_2SO_4, and HNO_3 may be considered to be completely ionized in aqueous solutions; thus:

$$H_2SO_4 + 2H_2O \rightarrow 2H_3O^+ + SO^-$$

The common bases NaOH and KOH are *strong bases* and dissociate completely when dissolved in water; thus:

$$NaOH + H_2O \rightarrow Na^+ + OH^- + H_2O$$

Many acids are defined as being *weak* in that they do not completely dissociate in water because the conjugate base of the acid is of nearly the same base strength as water. Some of the common weak acids are acetic acid, carbonic acid, phenol, water, and boric acid. For example, less than 0.5% of the acetic acid molecules in a 1 M solution undergo reaction with water to produce H_3O^+ ion: the remaining 99.5% of the molecules remain undissociated. Equations for such reactions are written as follows:

$$CH_3COOH + H_2O \rightleftharpoons CH_3COO^- + H_3O^+$$

The double arrow separating reactants and products indicates that a dynamic equilibrium is established in which the rate of the reverse reaction, thus:

$$H_3O^+ + CH_3COO^- \rightarrow CH_3COOH + H_2O$$

is equal to the rate of the forward reaction

$$CH_3COOH + H_2O \rightarrow CH_3COO^- + H_3O^+$$

Thus at equilibrium the concentration of each species in the solution remains constant. The disproportionate length of the arrows in the equation simply indicates that the acetic acid remains largely undissociated.

A similar situation exists for aqueous solutions of *weak bases*, for example, NH_3, Na_2CO_3, and H_2O. Thus a 0.1 M solution of NH_3 in water undergoes reaction to the extent of 0.5%.

$$NH_3 + H_2O \rightleftharpoons NH_4^+ + OH^-$$

EQUILIBRIUMS AND EQUILIBRIUM CONSTANT

The extent of dissociation of weak acids and bases and the resulting equilibriums have been studied exhaustively. These studies have resulted in a mathematic statement that allows calculation of the degree of dissociation. The mathematic expression describing the general equilibrium reaction

$$HY + H_2O \rightleftharpoons Y^- + H_3O^+$$

is expressed as follows:

$$K_{HY} = \frac{[Y^-][H_3O^+]}{[HY][H_2O]}$$

Note: The brackets [] indicate concentration of the species in moles per liter.

The equation states that the mathematic product of the concentrations of the reaction products divided by the mathematic product of the concentrations of the reactants is a constant (this is valid only at a given temperature). For example, the equilibrium expression for

$$NH_3 + H_2O \rightleftharpoons NH_4^+ + OH^-$$

is expressed as follows:

$$K_{NH_3} = \frac{[NH_4^+][OH^-]}{[NH_3][H_2O]}$$

Inasmuch as water is present in large excess in most solutions, its concentration remains essentially constant; therefore the term for the concentration of water is incorporated with the equilibrium constant, and the mathematic expression is normally

$$K_{NH_3} = \frac{[NH_4^3][OH^-]}{[NH_3]}$$

Experiments have shown that K_{NH_3} is equal to 1.8×10^{-5} m at 25 °C. In general, the larger the numeric value of K, the stronger the acid or base, depending on whether H_3O^+ or OH^- ion is one of the products.

A most important equilibrium reaction is that involving pure water, because reactions involving acids and bases are normally conducted in aqueous medium. Even though water is neutral, it was classified as both a weak acid and a weak base in the preceding section.

Experiments have shown that water undergoes autoionization, in which one molecule of water functions as an acid and a second molecule functions as a base, giving the following equation:

$$H_2O + H_2O \rightleftharpoons H_3O^+ + OH^-$$

It is apparent that even though autoionization is occurring, water is neutral, because the concentration of H_3O^+ ion is exactly equal to the concentration of OH^- ion. The equilibrium expression for water is

$$K = \frac{[OH^-][H_3O^+]}{[H_2O]}$$

or

$$K_W = [H_2O]K = [OH^-][H_3O^+]$$

The concentration of water being constant gives

$$K_W = [OH^-][H_3O^+]$$

K_W has been determined experimentally to be $1 \times 10^{-14} M^2$. For pure water

$$[H_3O^+] = [OH^-] + \sqrt{1 \times 10^{-14}} = 1 \times 10^{17} M$$

THE pH CONCEPT

Following the logic of the preceding discussion, an aqueous solution, no matter whether acidic, basic, or neutral, must have a concentration of H_3O^+ and OH^- ions, the product of which must equal 1×10^{-14}.

$$K_W = [H_3O^+][OH^-] = 1 \times 10^{-14} \ M^2$$

Any solution in which $[H_3O^+]$ is equal to $[OH^-]$ must be neutral, and any solution in which $[OH^-]$ and $[H_3O^+]$ are unequal must be either basic or acidic. However, at all times $[H_3O^+] \times [OH^-]$ equals $1 \times 10^{-14} M^2$. As with the solutions discussed previously, the concentration of H_3O^+ is expressed as moles/liter. This has been further simplified and is commonly expressed in terms of pH (from the French *puissance d'hydrogene*, meaning power of hydrogen) as a number between 0 and 14.

The pH of a solution is defined as being equal to the negative log of the $[H_3O^+]$; thus:

$$pH = -\log[H_3O^+]$$

and a neutral solution having a concentration of H_3O^+ equal to 10^{-7} has a pH of 7.

$$pH = -\log[H_3O^+] = -\log 10^{-7} = 7$$

For those solutions in which $[H_3O^+]$ is larger than 10^{-7}, the solution will contain a concentration of H_3O^+ ions greater than that of OH^- ions, and will therefore be acidic. Whenever the $[H_3O^+]$ is greater than $[OH^-]$, the pH will be less than 7, and for those solutions in which the $[H_3O^+]$ is less than $[OH^-]$, the pH will be greater than 7 and the solution will be basic.

Values of pH

1, 2, 3, 4, 5, 6   7   8, 9, 10, 11, 12, 13, 14
Acidic   *Neutral*   *Basic*

In an analogous manner, the pOH of a solution is the negative log of $[OH^-]$; therefore, knowing that pH is equal to $-\log[H_3O^+]$ and that K_w is equal to 1×10^{-14}, we find that pOH must equal $14 - pH$. For example, if a solution is found to have a $[H_3O^+]$ of $1 \times 10^{-3} M$, the pH of the solution will be $-\log (1 \times 10^{-3})$, or 3, and the pOH therefore must be $14 - 3$, or 11.

EXAMPLE 1: What is the pH of a solution that has a $[H_3O^+]$ of $2.3 \times 10^{-5} M$? Using the relationship $pH = -\log[H_3O^+]$, we proceed as follows:

$$pH = -\log (2.3 \times 10^{-5})$$
$$pH = -(\log 2.3 + \log 10^{-5})$$
$$pH = -(0.36 + [-5] \log 10)$$
$$pH = -(0.36 - 5)$$
$$pH = -(-4.64)$$
$$pH = 4.64 \text{ (The solution is acidic.)}$$

EXAMPLE 2: A solution is found to have a concentration of OH^- equaling $3.0 \times 10^{-8} M$. What is its pH?

a. Using $pOH = -\log[OH^-]$, find pOH.

$$pOH = -\log (3.0 \times 10^{-8})$$
$$pOH = -(\log 3.0 + [-8] \log 10)$$
$$pOH = -(0.477 + [-8])$$
$$pOH = -(-7.523)$$
$$pOH = 7.52$$

b. Using $pH + pOH = 14$, find pH.

$$pH + 7.52 = 14$$
$$pH = 14 - 7.52$$
$$pH = 6.48 \text{ (The solution is acidic.)}$$

EXAMPLE 3: Find the $[H_3O^+]$ of a solution that has a pH of 9.8 using $pH = -\log[H_3O^+]$.

$$9.8 = -\log[H_3O^+]$$
$$\log[H_3O^+] = -10 + 0.2$$

Using antilogs, find the $[H_3O^+]$.

$$[H_3O^+] = (\text{antilog } 0.2)(\text{antilog } -10)$$
$$[H_3O^+] = 1.58 \times 10^{-10} \text{ M}$$

EXAMPLE 4: Given the following information for a solution of acetic acid:

$$K_a = 1.8 \times 10^{-5}$$
$$[HOAc] = 0.5 \text{ M (HOAc is acetic acid.)}$$

Find the pH of the solution.

a. The equilibrium reaction is

$$HOAc \rightleftharpoons H^+ + OAc^-$$
$$0.5 \text{ M} \quad x \text{ M} + \quad x \text{ M}$$

We know that

$$K_a = \frac{[H^+][OAc^-]}{[HOAc]}$$

Assuming that x M of HOAC dissociates, the concentrations at equilibrium are

$$[HOAC] = 0.5 - x$$
$$[H^+] = x$$
$$[OAc] = x$$

Thus:

$$1.8 \times 10^{-5} = \frac{x^2}{5 \times 10^{-1} - x} = \frac{x^2}{5 \times 10^{-1}}$$

HOAc, being a weak acid, is largely undissociated, and x, compared to 5.0×10^{-1}, is very small and may be eliminated from the denominator without seriously affecting the value calculated for x.

$$x^2 = (1.8 \times 10^{-5})(5 \times 10^{-1})$$
$$x^2 = 9 \times 10^{-6}$$
$$x = 3 \times 10^{-3} \text{ M} = [H^+] = [OAc^-]$$

b. Using $pH = -\log[H_3O^+]$, proceed as follows:

$$pH = -\log (3 \times 10^{-3})$$
$$pH = -(\log 3 + [-3] \log 10)$$
$$pH = -(-2.52)$$
$$pH = 2.52 \text{ (The solution is acidic.)}$$

Table 5-6	Normal alkanes (C_nH_{2n+2})		
Number of carbons	**Name**	**Expanded formula**	**Condensed formula**
1	Methane	$H-\overset{\displaystyle H}{\underset{\displaystyle H}{C}}-H$	CH_4
2	Ethane	$H-\overset{\displaystyle H}{\underset{\displaystyle H}{C}}-\overset{\displaystyle H}{\underset{\displaystyle H}{C}}-H$	CH_3-CH_3
3	Propane	$H-\overset{H}{\underset{H}{C}}-\overset{H}{\underset{H}{C}}-\overset{H}{\underset{H}{C}}-H$	$CH_3-CH_2-CH_3$
4	Butane	$H-\overset{H}{\underset{H}{C}}-\overset{H}{\underset{H}{C}}-\overset{H}{\underset{H}{C}}-\overset{H}{\underset{H}{C}}-H$	$CH_3-(CH_2)_2-CH_3$
5	Pentane	$H-\overset{H}{\underset{H}{C}}-\overset{H}{\underset{H}{C}}-\overset{H}{\underset{H}{C}}-\overset{H}{\underset{H}{C}}-\overset{H}{\underset{H}{C}}-H$	$CH_3-(CH_2)_3-CH_3$
6	Hexane	$H-\overset{H}{\underset{H}{C}}-\overset{H}{\underset{H}{C}}-\overset{H}{\underset{H}{C}}-\overset{H}{\underset{H}{C}}-\overset{H}{\underset{H}{C}}-\overset{H}{\underset{H}{C}}-H$	$CH_3-(CH_2)_4-CH_3$

Starting with pentane, the alkanes are named systematically with a numeric prefix indicating the number of carbon atoms, that is, pent-, hex-, hept-, oct-, non-, dec-, undec-, dodec-, tridec-, tetradec-, pentadec-, hexadec-, heptadec-, octadec-, nonadec-, eicos- (20), heneicos- (21), docos-, tricos-, tetracos-, and so on.

The alkynes, having chemical properties similar to the alkenes, are also of interest as potential sources of radiopharmaceuticals.

Arenes and aromatic compounds. This family of compounds contains at least one aromatic ring, which is characterized by benzene, the simplest of the aromatic compounds.

The chemistry of these compounds differs greatly from that of the alkenes and alkynes in that rather than addition reactions, they undergo substitution reactions in which one or more hydrogens are replaced by another atom or group. For example, the iodination of benzene is

$$+ I_2^* + HNO_3 \rightarrow \text{(incomplete and unbalanced)}$$

This reaction is found to be especially useful in the preparation of *ortho*-iodohippuric acid, which has found use as a renal function agent.

Among other aromatic substances containing a radioactive halogen are the estrogens, which have been approved for experimental imaging procedures in humans.

An especially important radiolabeled aromatic compound used for determination of thyroid function is T_3.

facilitate substitution reactions in which radioactive halogens are introduced into the aromatic ring.

Halides. Radiopharmaceuticals that contain halogens, especially those containing radioactive bromine or iodine, again for example, rose bengal, T_3, and brominated estrogen, are of utmost importance and have great effectiveness in the practice of nuclear medicine, solely because of the presence of the radioactive halogen in these molecules. However, the functional molecules are of equal importance in that they determine the organ or site in which the total radioactive substance is localized.

Aldehydes and ketones. The carbonyl function

$$(-\overset{\overset{\displaystyle O}{\|}}{C}-)$$

is common to both aldehydes and ketones. The presence of this functional group is not especially important to the labeling of organic molecules, but, as noted in the preceding section, its presence is vital in determining the biodistribution of the radioactive substance.

Carboxylic acids. Several compounds containing the carboxyl function have been noted in previous sections. In addition, pentetic acid (DTPA) forms a complex with ^{169}ytterbium to give ^{169}Yb-pentetic acid (^{169}Yb-DTPA), a cisternographic imaging agent.

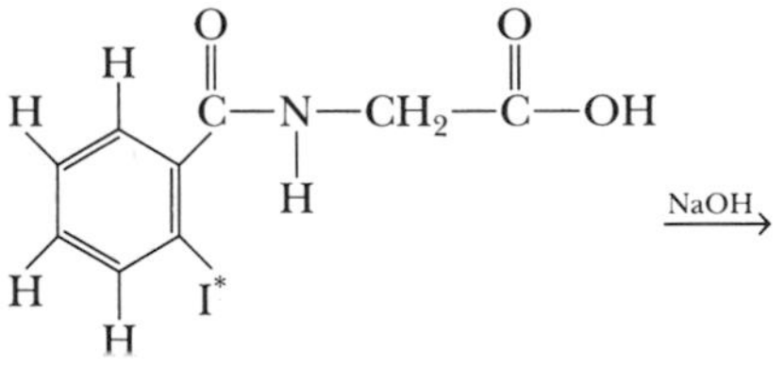

o-Iodohippuric acid

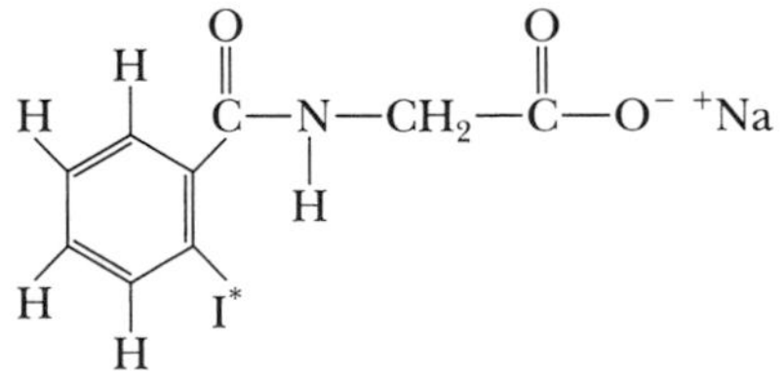

Hippuran

The sodium salt of *o*-iodohippuric acid, hippuran, in filtering through the glomeruli of the kidneys, provides an effective means of evaluating kidney function, especially important to patients who have received a kidney transplant.

Esters, functioning as derivatives of carboxylic acids, are formed by means of an acid-catalyzed condensation reaction between a carboxylic acid and an alcohol. These substances have not as yet been found to be useful as precursors to radiopharmaceuticals.

$$R-\overset{\overset{\displaystyle O}{\|}}{C}-OH + R'-OH \overset{H^+}{\rightarrow} R-\overset{\overset{\displaystyle O}{\|}}{C}-O-R' + H_2O$$

Table 5-7 Alkyl groups derived from the alkanes by removal of one hydrogen

	Common alkyl groups	Derived from
Methyl	CH_3-	Methane
Ethyl	CH_3-CH_2-	Ethane
Propyl	$CH_3-CH_2-CH_2-$	Propane
Isopropyl	$CH_3-CH-CH_3$	Propane
Butyl	$CH_3-CH_2-CH_2-CH_2-$	Butane
sec-Butyl	$CH_3-CH-CH_2-CH_3-$	Butane
Isobutyl	CH_3 / $HC-CH_2-$ / CH_3	Butane
tert-Butyl	CH_3 / CH_3-C- / CH_3	Butane

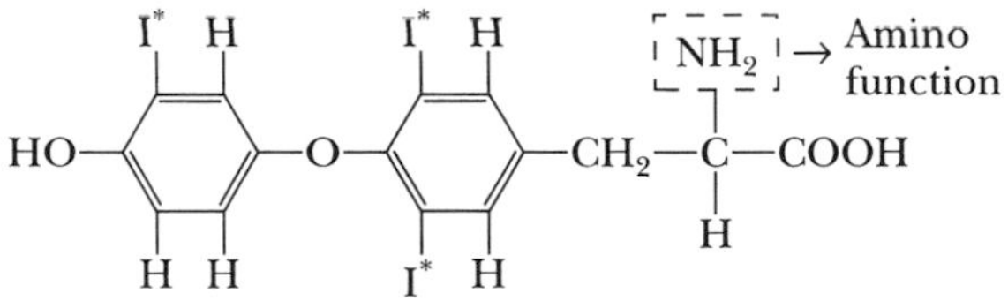

3,5,3′–Triiodothyronine (T₃)

Alcohols and phenols. Alcohols and phenols contain the functional group —OH. Inspection of the structures of rose bengal and T_3 shows that each contains a phenolic hydroxyl (—OH) function as a part of the molecule. Likewise, brominated estrone, mentioned in the preceding section, also contains this functional group.

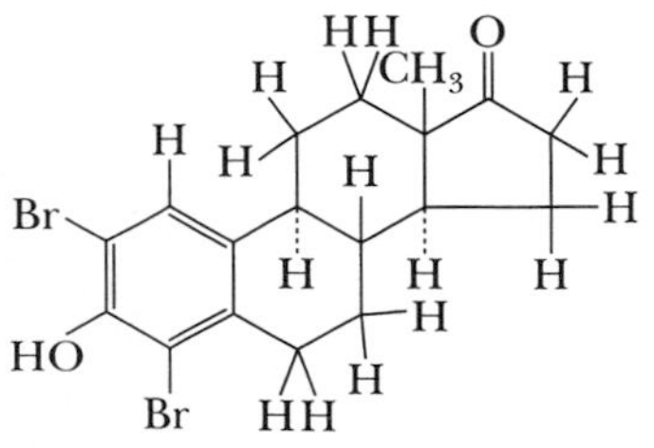

2,4–Dibromoestrone

Molecules containing this structural feature are highly important in preparation of radiopharmaceuticals.

Ethers. The ether linkage, R—O—R, also occurs in rose bengal and T_3, and its importance as a structural feature, as with the phenolic —OH function, lies in its ability to

Amides. Hippuran (previous section), in addition to the carboxylate group, also contains an amide function. Components of all biologic tissues have amide functions, which usually are referred to as peptide linkages. The protein human serum albumin (HSA), whose structure is not completely known, when labeled with ^{99m}Tc, is used as a blood pool imaging agent.

Amines and thiols. Amines and thiols are the nitrogen and sulfur analogs of the alcohols. Substances in which the amino groups ($—NH_2$) are an important structural component are the proteins and amino acids from which they are derived.

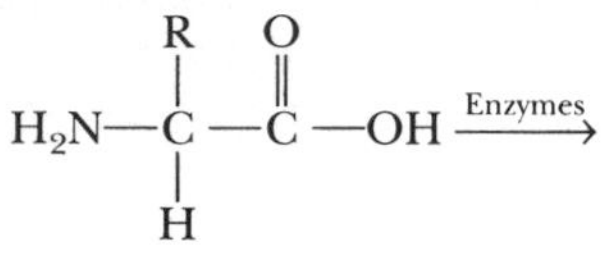

Amino acid

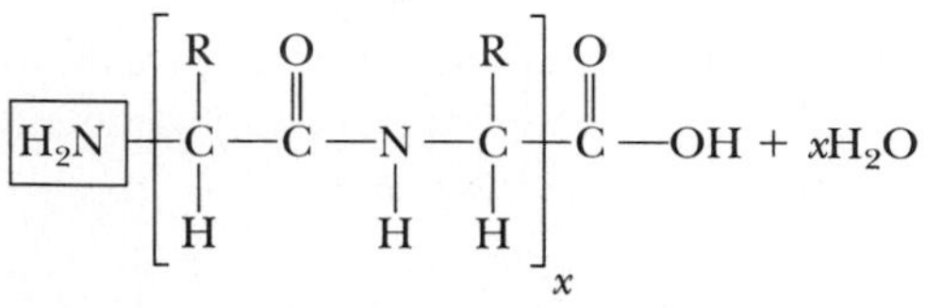

Protein

Of the compounds useful in nuclear medicine, one of the most important is pentetic acid (DTPA; see the previous carboxylic acids).

SUMMARY

The foregoing comments, in which the significance of the various organic functional groups to nuclear medicine have been noted, should not be considered by the student to be a complete description of the chemistry of these compounds. A thorough understanding of each of the radiopharmaceutical compounds requires knowledge of not only their structure and biologic fate but also ultimately of the chemical processes by which they are prepared. A discussion of the procedures used in preparing these substances is contained in Chapter 6. Of course, a thorough understanding of the theoretical and preparative techniques of organic chemistry as related to nuclear medicine and to an insight into the chemical basis of life is an unending quest.

SUGGESTED READINGS

Chang, R: *Chemistry,* ed 7, New York, 2002, McGraw-Hill.
Harris, DC: *Quantitative chemical analysis,* ed 6, New York, 2003, WH Freeman.
Wade LG Jr: *Organic chemistry,* ed 5, New York, 2003, Prentice Hall.

Sally W. Schwarz, Carolyn J. Anderson

chapter **6**

Radiochemistry and Radiopharmacology

Objectives

Discuss nuclear stability and its relationship to radioactive decay.

Describe the basic mechanisms for radionuclide production in a reactor.

Describe the fundamentals of particle accelerator operation and the production of radionuclides using particle accelerators.

Describe generator kinetics in the production of radionuclides, and detail the difference between transient and secular equilibrium.

Diagram a wet column and dry column molybdenum-technetium generator, and explain the elution process.

Describe the chemical properties of the pertechnetate ion.

Explain the technetium labeling processes used by reduction methods.

Discuss the chemical and labeling processes of gallium and indium radiopharmaceuticals.

Describe the pharmacokinetics of thallium as a myocardial perfusion imaging agent.

Explain iodination techniques.

List and describe the properties of PET radiopharmaceuticals and advantages of using these compounds.

Describe the differences between quality control relative to radionuclide purity, radiochemical purity, and chemical impurities.

Describe how particle sizes are measured.

Discuss the difference between sterile compounds and compounds containing pyrogens, and tests for ensuring these properties.

PRODUCTION OF RADIONUCLIDES

Nuclear Stability

Approximately 275 different nuclei have shown no evidence of radioactive decay and hence are considered stable with respect to this type of transformation. Figure 6-1 shows the relationship of the number of neutrons to the number of protons in the known stable nuclei. In the light elements, stability is achieved when the numbers of neutrons and protons are approximately equal. As the elements become heavier, the ratio of neutrons to protons (N/P ratio) for nuclear stability increases from 1 to about 1.5. If a nucleus has an N/P ratio too high for stability (neutron rich), it will undergo radioactive decay in a manner such that the N/P ratio decreases to approach the line of stability. The consequence is the production of a negative beta particle (β^-) as shown by the following example:

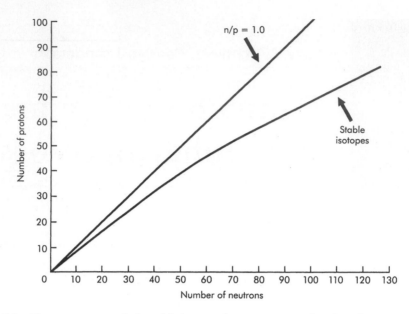

Figure 6-1   Neutron-proton ratio in stable isotopes becomes greater than 1 as the mass increases.

$$n \rightarrow p + e^- + \overline{\nu} \ (\beta^- \ \text{decay})$$

If the N/P ratio is too low for stability, radioactive decay occurs in a manner that will reduce the number of protons and increase the number of neutrons by the net conversion of a proton to a neutron. This is accomplished through either positron emission (β^+) or absorption by the nucleus of an orbital electron (electron capture, or EC). Examples are shown in the following reactions:

$$p \rightarrow n + e^+ + \nu \ (\beta^+ \ \text{decay})$$
$$p + e^- \rightarrow n + \nu \ (\text{electron capture})$$

Beta decay often leaves the daughter nucleus in an excited state. This excitation energy is removed either by gamma-ray emission or by a process called internal conversion. Generally, emission of a gamma ray occurs immediately after the beta decay (within 10^{-12} sec), but in some cases the nucleus may remain in the higher energy state for a measurable length of time. When this occurs, the excited nucleus is said to be in a metastable state, indicated by the letter *m*. An example is ^{99m}Tc, which decays with a half-life of 6 hr to ^{99}Tc. The transition of a radionuclide from an upper energy state to a lower energy state by the emission of gamma rays is referred to as an *isomeric transition*.

If a nucleus is capable of emitting a gamma ray, there is also a probability that the photon may eject an electron from an extranuclear shell. This process is an alternative to isomeric transition and is known as *internal conversion*. As an upper-level electron undergoes a transition to occupy the lower energy electron site, an x ray is emitted, characteristic of the electron shell that is being filled. In a process similar to internal conversion, these x rays may cause the ejection of an additional outer shell electron known as an *Auger electron*. The process continues until all inner shell

vacancies have been filled by "cascading" electrons from outer shells, with corresponding emissions of x rays or Auger electrons.

Positron decay leaves the daughter nuclide two electron mass units lower than the parent, requiring at least 1.022 MeV (2×0.511 MeV/electron) of transition energy. Once released from the nucleus, the β^+ reacts with an electron, resulting in the release of two 0.511 MeV photons, which are called annihilation radiation, emitted in opposite directions. Some positron-emitting radionuclides decay to excited states of the daughter nuclide. These excited daughter nuclides can further decay by isomeric transitions as discussed earlier.

Alpha decay occurs primarily for nuclei heavier than lead. In alpha decay the proton number is reduced by 2 and the mass by 4 units. It is represented by the following equation:

$$^A_Z X \rightarrow (^{A-4}_{Z-2})Y + \ ^4He$$

The probability of alpha decay is greater for nuclei with an even number of neutrons or protons than for nuclei with an odd number. Radionuclides that decay by alpha emission are not useful in nuclear medicine imaging, but may have future therapeutic applications.

Radionuclides used to label radiopharmaceuticals for nuclear medicine imaging should decay by either gamma or positron (β^+) emission. Gamma radiation emitted from radiopharmaceuticals readily penetrates tissues and escapes from the body, allowing external detection by gamma cameras. Positron-emitting radionuclides produce two 0.511 MeV gamma photons emitted in opposite directions from the positron-electron annihilation. The angle of nearly 180 degrees of the emitted 0.511 MeV photons is exploited in positron emission tomography (PET) to allow electronic collimation of the radiation and determination of the three-dimensional location of the decay event.

Reactor-Produced Radionuclides

The two major principles of a nuclear reactor are that neutrons induce fission in uranium and that the number of neutrons released by this fission is greater than one. Thus:

$$^{235}U + n \rightarrow \text{fission products} + \nu n$$

For each neutron consumed, an average of 2.5 new neutrons (νn) are released with an energy of 1.5 eV. These new neutrons can be used to fission other ^{235}U nuclei, leading to the release of more neutrons, self-propagating the reaction. These nuclear chain reactions are controlled by the use of moderators and neutron absorbers (materials used to reduce neutron energy [thermalize] to 0.025 eV) in a reactor so that an equilibrium state is reached. Radionuclides can be produced in a nuclear reactor by two methods: (1) irradiation of material within the neutron flux (neutrons $\times$ cm^{-2} $\times$ sec^{-1}) or (2) separation and collection of the fission products.

Thermal neutron reactions. The neutrons around the core of a nuclear reactor are low-energy (thermal) neutrons that typically induce the following types of nuclear reactions:

$$^A_Z X + n \rightarrow {}^{A+1}_Z X + \gamma \qquad (1)$$
$$^A_Z X + n \rightarrow {}^{A}_{Z-1} Y + p \qquad (2)$$

In a reaction of the first type the target atom X, with atomic number Z and atomic mass A, absorbs a neutron, and energy is emitted in the form of gamma rays. This is written as a (n,γ) reaction. The following are examples:

$$^{98}Mo(n,\gamma)^{99}Mo$$
$$^{112}Sn(n,\gamma)^{113}Sn$$

In the second type of reaction a proton is emitted after absorption of a neutron by the target atom. Since this changes the atomic number of the nucleus, an isotope of a different element (Y) is formed. Examples of this type of nuclear reaction (n,p) are as follows:

$$^{14}N(n,p)^{14}C$$
$$^{3}He(n,p)^{3}H$$

The (n,γ) reaction forms a radioisotope from a stable isotope of the same element, precluding production of high specific activity material. The specific activity is defined as the decay rate (dpm) of a radioactive isotope per gram of that same element. In a (n,p) reaction the product nuclide is an isotope of a different element, enabling the production of high specific activity, carrier-free (no stable isotope of the same element) radioisotopes.

The previously described reactions will produce neutron-rich products, decaying primarily by β$^-$ emission. Radionuclides that decay by β$^-$ emission are not generally used in imaging. However, products of (n,γ) reactions include parent isotopes used in nuclear generators. In a radionuclide generator the daughter radionuclide is the isotope of interest and is usually separated from the parent isotope by column chromatography. Examples of the parent-daughter system of radionuclide generators are as follows:

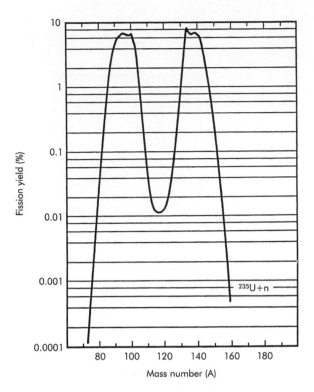

Figure 6-2 Relative yields of fission products of various mass formed after uranium fission.

$$^{98}Mo(n,\gamma)^{99}Mo \xrightarrow[t_{1/2} \; = \; 67 \text{ hours}]{} {}^{99m}Tc \; (t_{1/2} = 6 \text{ hours})$$
$$^{112}Sn(n,\gamma)^{113}Sn \xrightarrow[t_{1/2} \; = \; 115 \text{ days}]{} {}^{113m}In \; (t_{1/2} = 99.8 \text{ minutes})$$

Fission product separation. The fission process itself results in the formation of lighter radionuclides of unequal mass, some of which are used in nuclear medicine (^{99}Mo, ^{131}I, ^{133}Xe) (Figure 6-2). The neutron interacts with the ^{235}U nucleus to form unstable ^{236}U, which then undergoes fission. An example of a fission reaction occurring in a nuclear reactor is as follows:

$$n + {}^{235}_{92}U \rightarrow {}^{236}_{92}U \rightarrow {}^{89}_{36}Kr + {}^{144}_{56}Ba + 3n$$

Similar to products of (n,γ) reactions, fission products tend to decay by β$^-$ emission, and only a limited number have found use in nuclear medicine. However, unlike radionuclides formed from (n,γ) reactions, fission products can be produced carrier free. For example, fission-produced ^{99}Mo is formed from uranium, whereas thermal neutron-produced ^{99}Mo is made from bombarding a ^{98}Mo target. Unfortunately, a major problem associated with fission-produced radionuclides is the difficulty in chemically separating the product of interest from the others formed to obtain a radiochemically pure preparation.

Accelerator-Produced Radionuclides

Accelerators are devices that increase the energy of charged particles to enable a nuclear reaction on impact with a target.

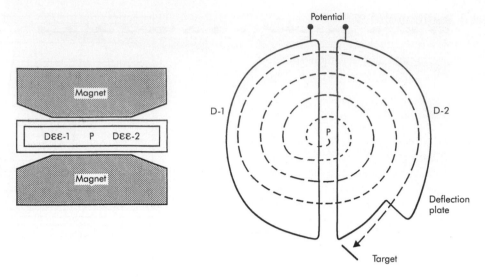

Figure 6-3 Schematic diagram of the operation of a positive ion cyclotron.

Either a cyclotron or a linear accelerator can be used to produce radionuclides, depending on the type of nuclear reaction and the yield desired. In linear accelerators, ions are repeatedly accelerated through small potential differences. The accelerator tube consists of a series of cylindrical electrodes called *drift tubes*. A high-frequency alternating voltage is applied between the two electrodes, resulting in acceleration of the ions at each gap between electrodes. Acceleration to high energies requires relatively long acceleration tubes, creating obvious size-related problems for general use of these machines.

The invention of the cyclotron in 1930 was a successful attempt to overcome the difficulties associated with the length of high-energy linear accelerators. The basic principles of the cyclotron are shown in Figure 6-3. In the simplest cyclotron design the particles are accelerated in spiral paths inside two semicircular flat evacuated metallic cylinders called dees. The dees are placed between the two poles of a magnet so that the magnetic field operates on the ion beam, constraining it to a circular path. At the gap between the dees the ions experience acceleration due to the imposition of an electrical potential difference. The beam particles originate from the ion source at the center of the cyclotron, acquiring energy for each passage across the gap. Eventually the high-energy particle beam reaches the periphery of the dees, where it is deflected onto an external target. Fixed-frequency cyclotrons can accelerate positively charged ions up to about 50 MeV for protons. Techniques have now been developed to use cyclotrons at much higher energies. Linear accelerators can accelerate particles up to energies of several hundred MeV.

The majority of cyclotrons built before 1980 accelerated positively charged particles such as protons ($^1_1H^+$) or deuterons ($^2_1H^+$), ^3H particles and α particles. The first negative-ion cyclotron designed specifically for PET was built by Computer Technology and Imaging, Inc. (CTI, Knoxville, Tennessee).

Medical cyclotrons currently being marketed accelerate negative ions, either hydrogen or deuterium ions. The negative ion design allows for a simple deflection system, in which the beam is extracted by interaction with a very thin carbon foil. The carbon foil strips electrons from H^-, resulting in the formation of positively charged proton, which changes direction without a final magnetic deflection due to the change in charge on the particle. The proton beam then bombards the target in a manner similar to that in a positively charged particle cyclotron. It is also possible to extract the beam at two points with the negative ion machines, allowing production of two radioisotopes simultaneously. CTI currently markets a proton only machine. GE Medical Systems (Uppsala, Sweden) (Figure 6-4), Ebco (Vancouver, British Columbia), and IBA (Louvain, Belgium) market machines that have both proton and deuteron capability.

The cost of radionuclide production depends on the method employed. In a reactor there are many positions for thermal neutron irradiation of samples, allowing several isotopes to be produced simultaneously. This allows the cost of operation to be divided among several reactor-produced radionuclides. The overall price of fission products produced in a nuclear reactor is largely associated with the extensive separation process. Alternatively, the cost of accelerator-produced isotopes is quite high. Because the machine is most frequently used to produce a single radionuclide, the entire cost of operating the accelerator must be charged for each production.

Generator Systems

Certain parent-daughter systems involve a long-lived parent radionuclide that decays to a short-lived daughter. Since the parent and daughter nuclides are not isotopes of the same element, chemical separation is possible. The long-lived parent produces a continuous supply of the relatively short-lived daughter radionuclide and is therefore called a gener-

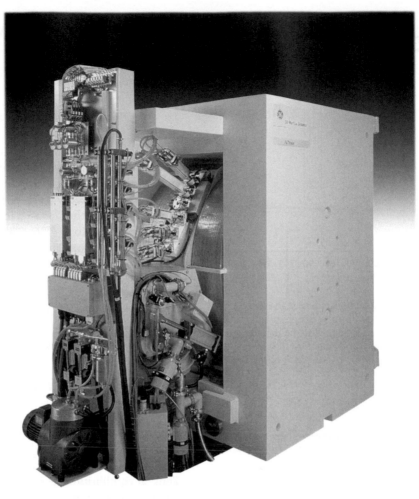

Figure 6-4 GE PETtrace® negative ion cyclotron.

Table 6-1	Decay properties for parent and daughter radionuclides of several generators		
Generator	**Parent $t_{1/2}$**	**Daughter $t_{1/2}$**	**Daughter E_γ (%)**
^{99}Mo-^{99m}Tc	2.78 d	6 hr	140 keV (90)
^{81}Rb-^{81m}Kr	4.7 hr	13 sec	190 keV (65)
^{113}Sn-^{113m}In	115 d	1.7 hr	393 keV (64)
^{68}Ge-^{68}Ga	280 d	68 min	511 keV (176)
^{62}Zn-^{62}Cu	9.3 hr	9.8 min	511 keV (196)
^{82}Sr-^{82}Rb	25 d	1.3 min	511 keV (192)

ator. The generator systems used in nuclear medicine are listed in Table 6-1.

The two types of parent-daughter relationships are transient and secular equilibrium. In a transient equilibrium system the half-life of the parent is a factor 10 to 100 times greater than that of the daughter, whereas in secular equilibrium the half-life of the parent is 100 to 1000 times greater than that of the daughter. The ^{99}Mo-^{99m}Tc generator, where ^{99}Mo has a 67-hr half-life and ^{99m}Tc has a 6-hr half-life, is an example of transient equilibrium (Figure 6-5). The

generator system ^{113}Sn($t_{1/2} = 115$ days) $- ^{113m}$In($t_{1/2} = 1.7$ hr), shown in Figure 6-6, is an example of secular equilibrium. The time required to reach equilibrium dictates how frequently each generator can be eluted and depends on the half-lives of the parent and daughter.

Equations governing generator systems. Assuming there is initially no daughter activity present in a generator, the daughter activity at any given time can be calculated from the following general equation:

^{68}Ge-^{68}Ga generator. Gallium-68 ($t_{1/2} = 68$ min) emits a 2.92 MeV positron in 89% abundance, making it very useful in PET imaging. The ^{68}Ge/^{68}Ga generator is not FDA approved, and only a few ^{68}Ga radiopharmaceuticals have been investigated clinically. These include ^{68}Ga macroaggregated albumin (MAA), ^{68}Ga citrate, and ^{68}Ga ethylenediaminetetraacetic acid (EDTA). Several generator systems have been developed to separate ^{68}Ga from ^{68}Ge. The early generators consisted of ^{68}Ge adsorbed onto an alumina column. The ^{68}Ga was eluted with a 0.005 M solution of EDTA at pH 7.[14] However, because ^{68}Ga forms such a strong complex with EDTA at neutral pH, it was difficult to dissociate ^{68}Ga from ^{68}Ga-EDTA to allow formation of other complexes. A solvent extraction ^{68}Ge-^{68}Ga generator was later developed that produces a ^{68}Ga-oxine chelate.[10] Although ^{68}Ga-oxine was a weaker chelate than ^{68}Ga-EDTA, problems with the operation of the generator system prevented it from becoming clinically useful. Most recently, a generator yielding ^{68}Ga in an ionic form has been developed.[20] In this generator ^{68}Ge is loaded onto a tin dioxide column and ^{68}Ga is eluted using 1 M HCl. The only problem incurred in this generator is the presence of trace metals, which sometimes reduces the amount of complexation with ^{68}Ga. This is the only ^{68}Ge-^{68}Ga generator produced commercially.

^{62}Zn-^{62}Cu generator. Copper-62, a positron-emitting radionuclide (98% abundance) with a 9.7 min half-life, is an attractive radionuclide for PET imaging. ^{62}Cu-labeled pyruvaldehyde bis (N^4-methylthiosemicarba-zone) (^{62}Cu-PTSM) has been used in clinical investigations for heart and brain blood flow measurement.[13] The parent isotope, ^{62}Zn, is cyclotron produced via the ^{63}Cu(p,2n)^{62}Zn reaction. Facilities for the production of ^{62}Zn exist at a number of commercial facilities as well as at several clinical PET centers. The major disadvantage is the short half-life of ^{62}Zn (9.3 hr), which requires generator replacement at 1- or 2-day intervals. Two different ^{62}Zn-^{62}Cu generator systems have been developed. In one design, ^{62}Zn is loaded onto a column containing Dowex 1 × 8 anion exchange resin, which retains Zn^{2+} and allows Cu^{2+} to be eluted using 0.2N HCl/1.8N NaCl or 2N HCl.[25] The other system employs a column containing a strong cation exchange resin adsorbent (CG-120, Amberlite), and ^{62}Cu is eluted in 0.2 M glycine.[12] The eluant in the latter generator is suitable for direct intravenous injection.

Clinical use of a ^{62}Cu-tracer requires a convenient method for routine, repetitive, high-yield radiopharmaceutical synthesis using the eluate of a ^{62}Zn/^{62}Cu generator. While previous work with ^{62}Cu-PTSM relied on a fairly simple remote system for radiopharmaceutical synthesis,[21] ^{62}Cu-radiopharmaceutical preparation has been further simplified by integration of reagent mixing operations into the 20 × 30 × 40-cm housing of a modular generator unit (Figure 6-8), available from Proportional Technologies, Inc. (Houston, Texas).[17,29] This modular generator can directly deliver the ^{62}Cu-PTSM in a sterile, pyrogen-free solution suitable for intravenous injection. The radiopharmaceutical synthesis time is the 40-second period required for generator elution. Such a modular ^{62}Zn/^{62}Cu generator system, nationally or regionally distributed from commercial medium-energy cyclotron facilities, may effectively support PET imaging centers as a source of short-lived radiopharmaceuticals for evaluation of tissue perfusion.

TECHNETIUM RADIOPHARMACEUTICALS

Technetium-99m was discovered in 1937 by Perrier and Segre in a sample of naturally occurring ^{98}Mo that had been irradiated by neutrons and deuterons. It was introduced into nuclear medicine in 1957 with the development of the ^{99}Mo/^{99m}Tc generator at the Brookhaven National Laboratory. The first clinical use of technetium, in 1961 at the University of Chicago, heralded a new era for nuclear medicine. The widespread use of ^{99m}Tc as the radionuclide of choice for a variety of nuclear medicine imaging procedures has been based mainly on its physical properties. These properties include a $t_{1/2}$ of 6 hr; a 140 keV photon (88% abundance), which provides good tissue penetration and imaging capabilities for use with gamma decay–providingcameras; and no beta decay—providing a low radiation absorbed dose. Another advantage is its ready availability from the ^{99}Mo/^{99m}Tc generator.

Oxidized Technetium Complexes

Technetium is obtained from a generator in normal saline (0.9% NaCl) as the pertechnetate ion, ^{99m}TcO$_4^-$. In this form Tc is in the +7 valence state as pertechnetate and has all seven of the outer electrons involved in covalent bonding. This is the most stable of all valence states of technetium in aqueous solution. The single negative charge of pertechnetate and the geometry of the compound–compound—oxygens in the four corners of a tetrahedron—give it a charge and size similar to the iodide ion (Figure 6-9). As a result the biodistribution of ^{99m}TcO$_4^-$ is similar to the iodide anion (I^-). It concentrates primarily in the thyroid, salivary glands, gastric mucosa, and choroid plexus. Pertechnetate crosses the placental barrier, so the fetal radiation dose must be considered when determining the suitability of a study employing pertechnetate for a pregnant woman. Pertechnetate is excreted primarily via the gastrointestinal tract and the kidneys. It is used for thyroid imaging and first-pass radionuclide angiocardiography. It has also been used in the past for brain imaging.

Pretreatment of a patient with potassium perchlorate, Lugol's solution (a solution of 5% iodine and 10% potassium iodide), or a saturated solution of potassium iodide (SSKI) influences the distribution of technetium. Perchlorate is approximately the same size as pertechnetate and competitively inhibits the uptake of ^{99m}TcO$_4^-$ into the thyroid and salivary glands, choroid plexus, and gastric mucosa. Stable iodine-127 is also taken up by these tissues and blocks the uptake of ^{99m}TcO$_4^-$. Activity in the choroid plexus presents a problem in interpreting brain images, so it is

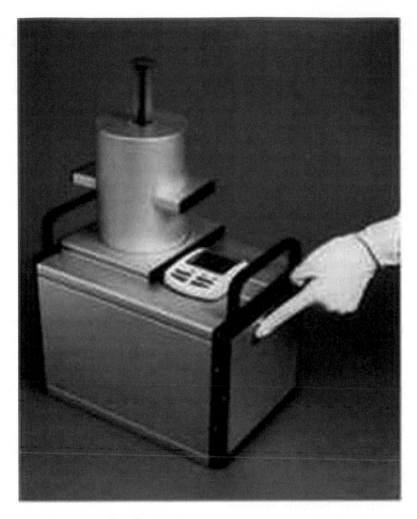

Figure 6-8 Commercially available ^{62}Zn-^{62}Cu generator. (Courtesy Proportional Technologies, Inc. Houston, Texas)

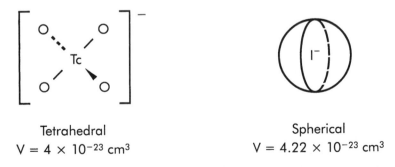

Tetrahedral
$V = 4 \times 10^{-23}$ cm^3

Spherical
$V = 4.22 \times 10^{-23}$ cm^3

Figure 6-9 Spatial comparison of TcO$_4^-$ and I$^-$ ions.

advantageous to block the uptake into this tissue using one of these pharmaceuticals.

Other than pertechnetate, the only radiopharmaceutical containing technetium possibly in a +7 valence state is technetium-sulfur colloid. ^{99m}Tc-sulfur colloid (^{99m}Tc-SC) is prepared from commercially available kits that contain sodium thiosulfate, phosphoric or hydrochloric acid, gelatin, and a buffer. Sodium thiosulfate and gelatin are added to an acid-

ified solution of ^{99m}Tc-pertechnetate. The mixture is heated in a boiling water bath for 5 to 10 min. Following heating, the vial is vented and a buffer is added. ^{99m}Tc-SC exists as ^{99m}Tc-heptasulfide coprecipitated with colloidal sulfur particles, which are generated from acid decomposition of the sodium thiosulfate. The final suspension is maintained at a pH of 5.5 to 6.0 to avoid conversion of the heptasulfide back to pertechnetate. The particle size range is 10 nm to 2.0 μ.

to ^{131}I-Hippuran.[27] The preferential nuclear properties of ^{99m}Tc make ^{99m}Tc-mertiatide superior to ^{131}I-Hippuran as a renal agent. The kit method of preparing ^{99m}Tc-mertiatide requires boiling for 10 min. The quality control method for the kit formulation employs Sep-Pak chromatography, which is discussed later under quality control.

Cardiac imaging agents. One of the goals of nuclear medicine has been to develop a ^{99m}Tc complex that has a biodistribution similar to [201]Tl. Recently several technetium agents taken up by the myocardium in relation to blood flow have been developed (Figure 6-12).

One of these cardiac agents is ^{99m}Tc-methoxyisobutyl isonitrile (MIBI), also known as ^{99m}Tc-sestamibi (Cardiolite®) (Figure 6-12). The kit method of production is a 10-min boiled preparation involving a ligand exchange labeling reaction. This results in the formation of a ^{99m}Tc-hexakis-isonitrile complex with ^{99m}Tc in an oxidation state of +1. The method of myocardial localization is not known, though it has been determined that it does not occur via the Na⁺/K⁺ pump, which is the mechanism of uptake for [201]Tl.[26] ^{99m}Tc-sestamibi has approximately a 65% cardiac extraction efficiency; minimal or no redistribution occurs. The amount of liver uptake that occurs has presented some problems in reading the resulting cardiac images.[9]

The second commercially available technetium cardiac agent is a neutral boronic acid adduct of a technetium dioxime complex (BATO). This agent, ^{99m}Tc-teboroxime (Cardiotec®), is a neutral complex with ^{99m}Tc in a +3 oxidation state (Figure 6-12). The kit formulation is a 15-min boiled preparation employing a template synthesis, which indicates that the complex is formed around the ^{99m}Tc once it is added to the reaction. The method of uptake into the myocardium has not yet been determined. ^{99m}Tc-teboroxime exhibits 95% extraction efficiency but shows rapid washout from the myocardium.[7] This allows imaging to be initiated

as early as 3 to 4 min after injection but necessitates completion of imaging within to 15 to 20 min because of the rapid clearance.

The most recently available cardiac agent is ^{99m}Tc-tetrofosmin (Myoview®), a cationic ^{99m}Tc-complex of an ether-substituted phosphine ligand. The kit formulation of ^{99m}Tc-tetrofosmin involves an exchange reaction during the 15-min, room-temperature incubation. The unreconstituted kit should be stored in the refrigerator, protected from light. The method of quality control is detailed in the section on radiopharmaceutical quality assurance. Uptake into the myocardium reaches a maximum of 1.3% of the injected dose (ID) at 5 min postinjection, falling to 1% ID by 2 hr. The mechanism of uptake into the myocardium has not been established. Imaging may be initiated 15 min postinjection.

Hepatobiliary imaging agents. A group of N-substituted iminodiacetic acid ligands that contain hydrophilic groups for ^{99m}Tc complexation and possess the necessary hepatocellular specificity have been developed. The first of this group of radiopharmaceuticals was ^{99m}Tc-lidofenin (HIDA). A variety of ^{99m}Tc-iminodiacetic acid analogues that have different groups substituted on the aromatic ring have also been developed (Figure 6-13). Generally, the newer agents offer improved hepatocellular specificity, more rapid blood clearance, and reduced renal clearance. These agents provide information regarding hepatocyte function, outline the biliary tract, and provide evidence of bile flow or obstruction. The hepatobiliary imaging agents are removed from the blood by carrier-mediated processes that also transport and excrete bilirubin. The uptake and clearance are therefore affected by increasing levels of bilirubin. The newer agents, ^{99m}Tc-disofenin (Hepatolite®) and ^{99m}Tc-mebrofenin (Choletec®), show an improvement in competitive uptake of the radiopharmaceutical even in cases of significantly elevated bilirubin levels.

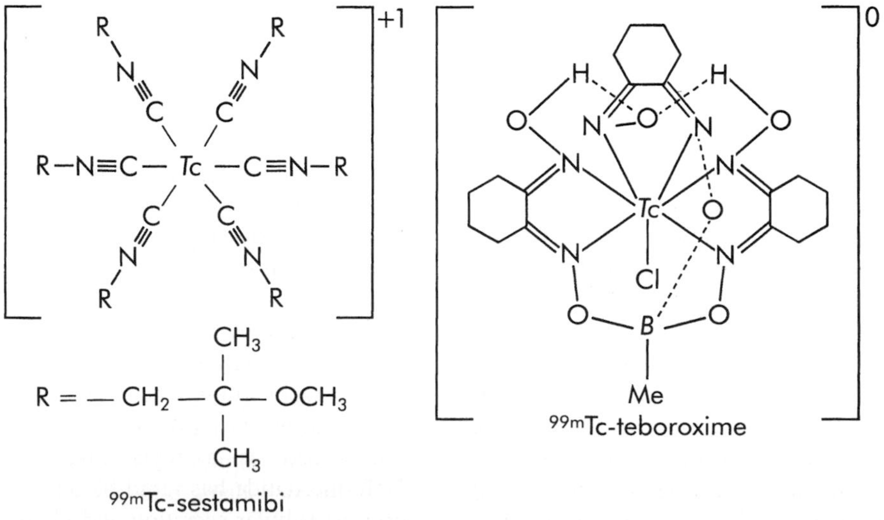

Figure 6-12 Two technetium cardiac agents developed as replacements for [201]TlCl.

Hepatobiliary excretion of a compound has been found to be related to several physicochemical characteristics: (1) a molecular weight of 300 to 1000; (2) the presence of a strong anionic polar group ionized at plasma pH; (3) the presence of a nonpolar group to decrease renal excretion; (4) lipophilic character; and (5) binding to plasma proteins, which can promote transfer into the hepatocyte. The original work done on ^{99m}Tc-HIDA determined the structural configuration to exist as a dimer (Figure 6-14).[19] The ^{99m}Tc atom serves as a bridge between two ligand molecules. Dimerization is one of the major factors determining the hepatobiliary route of excretion for this radiopharmaceutical.

Brain imaging agents. With the advent of single photon emission computed tomography (SPECT) came renewed interest in brain imaging. One of the new lipophilic brain agents is ^{99m}Tc-hexamethyl propylamineoxime (HMPAO), also known as exametazime. ^{99m}Tc-exametazime (Cerutec®) is rapidly extracted into the brain (about 6% ID at 1 min after injection), then immediately decomposes in vivo to a more polar metabolite that does not diffuse out of the brain. Evidence has been presented to indicate that the conversion to the nondiffusible form can be accomplished by an intra-

cellular reaction with glutathione.[23] The main problem with the original commercial kit formulation is instability; it must be used within 30 min of preparation, and quality control must be done before injection. A recent modification of the kit formulation of HMPAO is the immediate addition of methylene blue to the kit preparation after the addition of ^{99m}TcO$_4^-$ to stabilize the ^{99m}Tc-exametazime. After preparation of ^{99m}Tc-exametazime, the kit can be used for 4 hr. Since the final injectant is a dark blue color and therefore cannot be checked for the presence of particulate matter, it must be injected through a 0.22 μ filter, which is provided by the manufacturer.

Additionally, white blood cells (WBCs) have been labeled with technetium using ^{99m}Tc-exametazime. The original kit formulation, not the stabilized kit formulation, must be used for ^{99m}Tc-WBC labeling. Radiolabeling is accomplished in the presence of plasma, in vitro. Unlike the labeling of WBCs using ^{111}In-oxine, transferrin does not adversely affect the ^{99m}Tc-labeling process. Although diagnostic equivalent images can be obtained with ^{99m}Tc-labeled WBCs, the 6 hr half-life of technetium can make imaging 24 hr after injection difficult, when abscess-background ratios typically are maximized.

A second commercial technetium brain agent is ^{99m}Tc-L,L-ethylcysteinate dimer (ECD®). ^{99m}Tc-ECD (Neurolite®) has approximately 5% of the injected dose extracted into the brain within 2 min postinjection. This agent shows more rapid brain clearance and a higher brain/soft tissue ratio than ^{99m}Tc-HMPAO.[18] The commercial kit formulation is also stable for 6 hr.

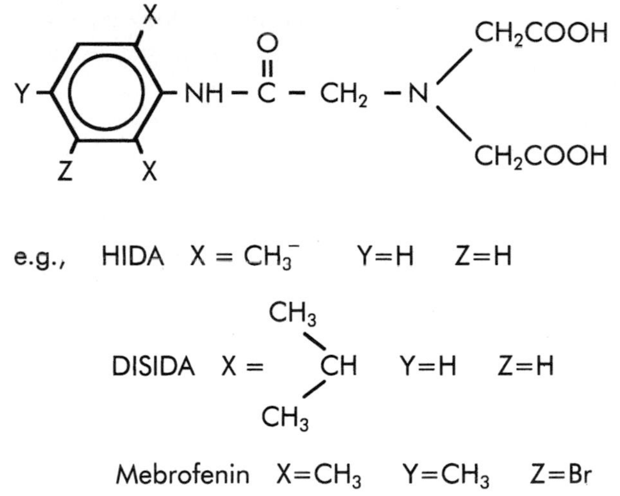

GALLIUM AND INDIUM RADIOPHARMACEUTICALS

The four radionuclides of indium and gallium that have been used in nuclear medicine applications are ^{67}Ga, ^{68}Ga, ^{111}In, and ^{113m}In. As discussed previously, ^{68}Ga and ^{113m}In are generator produced. Cyclotron production of ^{67}Ga (t$_{1/2}$ = 78 hr) and ^{111}In (t$_{1/2}$ = 67 hr) can be accomplished by several different nuclear reactions:

$$^{67}Zn(p,n)^{67}Ga$$
$$^{68}Zn(p,2n)^{67}Ga$$
$$^{111}Cd(p,n)^{111}In$$
$$^{109}Ag(\alpha,2n)^{111}In$$

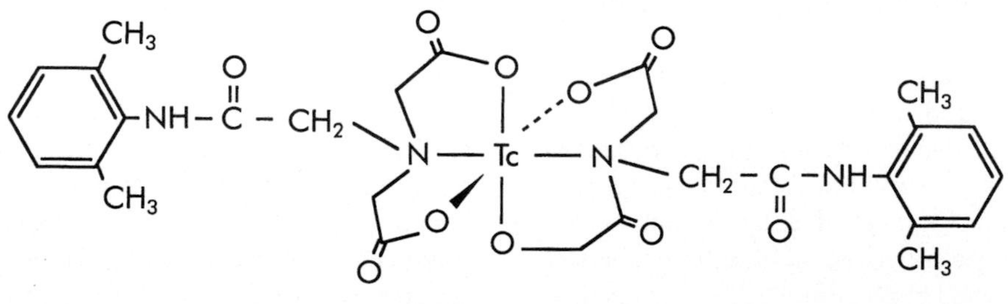

Figure 6-13 ^{99m}Tc-hepatobiliary analogs developed with different groups substituted on the aromatic ring of the iminodiacetic acid structure.

Figure 6-14 Dimeric configuration of Tc-HIDA.

Analysis of the decay schemes for ^{67}Ga and ^{111}In indicates the following gamma photon energies and abundances: ^{67}Ga, 93 keV (40%), 184 keV (24%), 296 keV (22%), and 388 keV (7%); ^{111}In, 173 keV (89%) and 247 keV (94%). The physical half-lives and decay characteristics of ^{67}Ga and ^{111}In make them well-suited for nuclear medicine. The gamma energies of ^{111}In are in the optimum range of detectability for the commercially available gamma cameras, and the abundance of gamma emissions provides 183 photons for every 100 disintegrations. Although the gamma energies of ^{67}Ga are in a range suitable for detection, their abundances are low. Therefore more than twice as much ^{67}Ga as ^{111}In would have to be injected to obtain a comparable image.

In aqueous solution, gallium and indium exist only as Ga^{3+} and In^{3+}, making radiopharmaceutical production simpler than with ^{99m}Tc, because a reduction does not have to be performed. The solution chemistry of both indium and gallium is similar to that of iron, with In^{3+} and Ga^{3+} forming very strong complexes with the plasma protein transferrin. To see the desired biodistribution using an indium or gallium radiopharmaceutical, a complex must be formed that is stronger than that of the metal with transferrin.

The solubility of indium hydroxides varies with the pH. At values higher than 4.5 indium hydroxide becomes very insoluble. In aqueous solution the free hydrated Ga (III) ion is stable only under acidic conditions. Hydrolysis occurs as the pH is raised, leading to the formation of insoluble gallium hydroxide. Unlike indium hydroxide, gallium hydroxide is amphoteric, dissolving in alkaline as well as acidic solutions. Thus, as pH is raised to ~3, $Ga(OH)_3$ precipitates but then redissolves as $Ga(OH)_4^-$ at pH greater than 7.4.[15]

The most widely used ^{67}Ga radiopharmaceutical is ^{67}Ga-citrate, an agent used for imaging tumors and sites of inflammation. On injection of the ^{67}Ga-citrate, more than 90% of the gallium becomes bound to plasma proteins, particularly transferrin, resulting in slow clearance from the plasma. However, when transferrin is saturated with stable gallium or iron prior to injection of radioactivity, the plasma and urinary clearance are improved. Under these conditions gallium distribution shifts from soft tissue to bone, though uptake by tumors does not seem to be affected. Alternatively, increasing ^{67}Ga protein transferrin binding causes an increase in soft tissue activity and decreased tumor activity. The mechanisms of ^{67}Ga localization in tumors and sites of inflammation are not completely understood, but the uptake of gallium into intracellular components by one or more mechanisms, possibly involving transferrin binding, is strongly indicated.

^{68}Ga is used to prepare radiopharmaceuticals for PET imaging. ^{68}Ga-citrate is used in studies of regional plasma volume. ^{68}Ga-EDTA forms an ionic chelate complex that is excluded from the brain by the blood-brain barrier following intravenous injection in normal subjects, and it has been used to assess the size and extent of blood-brain barrier disruption in patients with brain tumors. The commercial

MAA kits designed for preparation of ^{99m}Tc-MAA have also been used to prepare ^{68}Ga-MAA.[3] The major use for ^{68}Ga-MAA has been as a reference flow marker in PET imaging studies.

Because of the great stability of indium and gallium with transferrin, only very strong chelates can be used in vivo to direct the localization of the radionuclides to other sites. Strong chelators such as EDTA or DTPA can be easily labeled with gallium or indium using citrate or acetate as a transfer ligand. ^{111}In-DTPA has been used for renal and brain imaging and is currently used for cisternography.

Gallium and indium colloids can be prepared easily and conveniently as the insoluble hydroxides. By adding a small amount of ferric chloride to the radionuclide to act as a carrier, increasing the pH, and adding gelatin as a stabilizer, colloids that can be used as liver/spleen-imaging agents are formed. Larger particles prepared in a similar manner can be used for lung imaging.

Platelets and WBCs can be labeled with ^{111}In to provide agents for imaging inflammatory processes and thrombi. A weak complex is formed between the ^{111}In radiometal and 8-hydroxyquinoline (oxine). Because the ^{111}In-oxine complex is weak, the metal rapidly exchanges with transferrin in the plasma. In the absence of plasma, the complex diffuses across the cell membrane and the metal binds to intracellular sites. Isolation of the desired blood component from plasma permits easy labeling of either platelets or WBCs. This is routinely accomplished using centrifugation or sedimentation.

Procedures to label WBCs and platelets with ^{111}In-oxine vary, but the overall process can be summarized as follows:

1. Draw the patient's blood into an anticoagulated syringe and sediment the WBCs or platelets by centrifugation. Remove and save the leukocyte-poor (LPP) or platelet-poor plasma (PPP).
2. Wash the cells with 0.9% NaCl (saline) to remove plasma transferrin. Remove the saline wash, and resuspend the cells in saline.
3. Add ^{111}In-oxine to the cell suspension and incubate 15 min at room temperature.
4. Add a portion of the LPP or PPP to the ^{111}In-labeled WBCs or ^{111}In-labeled platelet preparation. Centrifuge the cells.
5. Resuspend the labeled cells in the remaining LPP or PPP for reinjection.

Overall labeling efficiencies (percentage of ^{111}In bound to cells) for WBCs is 70% to 90% and for platelets is 50% to 70%. Care must be taken to avoid damaging the cells during the labeling procedure.

^{111}In has also been conjugated to octreotide as an agent for the scintigraphic localization of primary and metastatic somatostatin receptor positive neuroendocrine tumors.[1] Somatostatin is a naturally occurring 14 amino acid peptide responsible for hormonal regulation of a number of organ systems. However, octreotide (Sandostatin®), an eight-amino acid analogue of somatostatin, has a much longer biologic half-life and even greater regulatory properties than the native peptide.[18] For these reasons it is a much better target for labeling than somatostatin. A labeled form of octreotide is commercially available as the DTPA chelated compound ^{111}In-DTPA-octreotide (^{111}In-pentetreotide, Octreoscan®). The most commonly diagnosed tumors have been carcinoids and gastrinomas, with a lower success rate noted for insulinomas and neuroblastomas. In the kit formulation, ^{111}In is complexed using sodium citrate, added to the pentetreotide, and incubated for 30 min at room temperature. Quality control must be performed before patient administration using C_{18} Sep-Pak chromatography.

Monoclonal antibodies (MAb) have been labeled with ^{111}In using bifunctional chelates. The chelating agent is first conjugated to the antibody, and then ^{111}In binds to the conjugated MAb via the chelating agent. The MAb B72.3 (satumomab) is an intact MAb that is directed to a high molecular weight, tumor-associated glycoprotein. The expression of this glycoprotein has been demonstrated in a variety of adenocarcinomas. This MAb has been conjugated using a derivatized DTPA ligand, then radiolabeled with [111]In. The kit formulation contains 1 mg of satumomab pendetide (Oncoscint®). ^{111}In-acetate is prepared by addition of ^{111}In chloride to a vial of sodium acetate buffer. The ^{111}In-acetate is then transferred to the MAb reaction vial. The vial is incubated for 30 min at room temperature and filtered through a low protein-binding $0.22\,\mu$ filter. The preparation should be stored at room temperature and used within 8 hr of preparation. The indication for ^{111}In-satumomab pendetide is determination of the extent and location of extrahepatic malignant disease in cases of colorectal or ovarian carcinoma.

THALLIUM CHLORIDE

[201]Tl is a monovalent cationic metal used in cardiac imaging. It is ultimately obtained from a [201]Pb-^{201}Tl generator. [201]Pb is produced by bombarding natural thallium metal with protons, according to the following nuclear reaction:

$$^{203}\text{Tl}(p,3n)^{201}\text{Pb} \xrightarrow[\text{(EC)}]{T_{1/2}\ =\ 9.4\ h}\ ^{201}\text{Tl}$$

The [201]Pb is then complexed, and undesirable target material is removed by ion exchange chromatography. The purified lead radioisotopes are affixed to another column. [201]Pb decays by electron capture with a $t_{1/2}$ of 9.4 hr to give [201]Tl. A second purification by column chromatography is required to remove the [203]Pb radiocontaminant, which is present at the end of purification at a level less than 0.5% per mCi ^{201}Tl at calibration. The ^{201}Tl is isolated carrier-free, has a $t_{1/2}$ of 74 hr, and decays by electron capture with gamma emissions between 140 and 170 keV.

Thallium clears rapidly from the blood, with maximum concentration in the heart approximately 10 to 30 min after injection in the resting state and 5 min after stress induced either by exercise or pharmacologic intervention at the time of administration. Uptake of ^{201}Tl into the myocardium occurs intracellularly in proportion to blood flow. Additionally, adequate tissue oxygenation is required to support ^{201}Tl uptake in myocardial cells, because oxygen supports the Na-K-ATPase concentrating mechanism. Similarities between [201]Tl^{+} and K^{+} include monovalent charges, comparable ionic radii, and involvement in the membrane Na-K-ATPase pump.

A number of pharmacologic stress inducers are available for use with [201]Tl. Dipyridamole (Persantin®) is a coronary vasodilator that has been employed in ^{201}Tl cardiac imaging to simulate exercise stress testing in patients who cannot exercise adequately. The dose employed is 0.142 to 0.570 mg/kg/min and is infused over 4 min. The most frequent adverse reaction reported was chest pain/angina pectoria. Parenteral aminophylline (50 to 250 mg over 30 to 60 sec by slow intravenous injection) should be available during dipyridamole stress testing for relieving adverse reactions such as bronchospasm or chest pain.

Adenosine (Adenocord®) is another coronary vasodilator for use in perfusion imaging. The initial dose of 6 mg is infused as a rapid intravenous bolus. It has a much shorter $t_{1/2}$ in plasma than dipyridamole (<10 sec versus <30 min), which allows more rapid reversal of the pharmacologic effect. The most common adverse effects are facial flushing and shortness of breath.

IODINATED RADIOPHARMACEUTICALS

Sodium iodide, either [123]I- or ^{131}I-labeled, is used for thyroid imaging, uptake measurements, and therapy (in the case of ^{131}I) as a capsule or a solution for oral administration. [123]I ($t_{1/2}$ of 13.2 hr) decays by electron capture with emission of a 159 keV gamma (83%), whereas [131]I ($t_{1/2}$ of 8 days) decays by β^{-} emission with subsequent gamma emission of 364 keV (82%). [131]I has also been used to label monoclonal antibodies for in vivo tumor imaging and therapy. HSA labeled with [125]I ($t_{1/2}$ of 60 days decays by electron capture with a 35 keV gamma) is used to measure plasma volume, and ^{125}I-labeled antibodies are used for radioimmunoassay.

To label proteins, particularly antibodies, with iodine the use of mild iodination agents that do not denature the protein is important. Iodination of proteins involves the formation of positively charged iodine species that react with various groups of the protein. Under general conditions used for iodination, the tyrosine residues in the protein are iodinated to the greatest extent, giving monoiodotyrosine and diodotyrosine.

The method of iodination chosen depends on the application. Retention of biologic activity of the protein is probably the most important consideration in the choice of the labeling technique. However, the overall labeling yield is also a key factor in determining the ultimate utility of a method. A variety of methods have been used to oxidize iodide to a positively charged species to effect protein iodination. Some of the most commonly used methods for iodination of proteins are outlined below.

1. I_2 iodination (δ indicates partial charge)

2. Iodine monochloride iodination.

$$ICl + {}^*I^- \xrightarrow{pH\,4} {}^*ICl \xrightarrow{pH\,8}$$

3. Chloramine-T iodination. Chloramine-T is a strong oxidizing agent that converts iodide ion to an iodinating species (possibly HOI). The exact mechanism of chloramine-T iodination is unknown.
4. Enzymatic iodination. Various peroxidases have been found to catalyze the iodination of proteins. Lactoperoxidase is most commonly used. In a typical iodination reaction the protein, enzyme, radioiodine, and a small amount of hydrogen peroxide are mixed to effect the labeling.
5. Indirect iodination. Most methods of direct iodination involve the addition of an oxidizing agent to the protein. This can be avoided by first iodinating a molecule with a structure similar to tyrosine, which can then be attached to the protein. N-succinimidyl-3-(4-hydroxyphenyl) propionate (SHPP) is a molecule that has been used for this application. SHPP is initially iodinated, usually by the chloramine-T technique, separated from the iodinating solution, and then added to the protein at pH 5.
6. Iodogen iodination. Iodogen, chloroglycoluril, is a mild iodinating agent that is quite popular. The iodogen is coated on the reaction vessel or bound to insoluble beads. The protein and radioiodine are added in an aqueous solution. Because the iodogen is not water soluble, it remains bound to the reaction vessel or beads, allowing easy separation of the labeled protein.

Other iodinated compounds used in nuclear medicine are ${}^{131}I$-orthoiodohippuran for renal imaging, ${}^{131}I$-metaiodobenzylguanidine (MIBG) for adrenal tumor imaging, ${}^{123}I$-iodoamphetamine for brain imaging, and ${}^{123}I$-labeled fatty acids for myocardial imaging.

Cyclotron production of ${}^{123}I$ can be accomplished by several methods. Enriched ${}^{124}Te$ can be bombarded with

protons, resulting in the ${}^{124}Te(p,2n){}^{123}I$ reaction. The most likely contaminant of this reaction is ${}^{124}I$, which emits a high-energy photon that can affect image resolution. Alternatively, this can be produced by the ${}^{127}I(p,5n){}^{123}I$, where the main contaminant is ${}^{125}I$. This contaminant does not pose a problem in imaging but will deliver a higher radiation dose to the patient because of the $t_{1/2}$ of 65 days. ${}^{131}I$ is obtained predominantly as a chemically separated fission product.

PET RADIOPHARMACEUTICALS

The most frequently used positron-emitting radionuclides for PET imaging are ${}^{15}O$ ($t_{1/2} = 2\,min$), ${}^{13}N$ ($t_{1/2} = 10\,min$), ${}^{11}C$ ($t_{1/2} = 20\,min$), and ${}^{18}F$ ($t_{1/2} = 110\,min$). Their decay characteristics are described in Table 6-2. Unlike the larger radionuclides used in conventional nuclear medicine, most PET radionuclides are identical to those found in naturally occurring biomolecules, and therefore the biochemical and physiologic processes in the body can be studied directly. Although fluorine is not usually native, labeling with ${}^{18}F$ only minimally changes the structure of a biomolecule, because its size is similar to the hydrogen it replaces. The short half-lives of these isotopes require production and radiopharmaceutical synthesis close to where the PET imaging takes place. This often requires an on-site cyclotron; however, for ${}^{18}F$-labeled radiopharmaceuticals, centralized radiopharmacies that supply regional hospitals and PET centers are becoming more common.

Oxygen-15

Oxygen-15 is cyclotron produced, generally by the ${}^{14}N(d,n){}^{15}O$ nuclear reaction. With a half-life of 2.04 min, PET radiopharmaceuticals labeled with ${}^{15}O$ are limited to a few simple molecules such as ${}^{15}O$-labeled water ($H_2{}^{15}O$), ${}^{15}O$-labeled oxygen gas (${}^{15}OO$), ${}^{15}O$-labeled carbon dioxide ($CO{}^{15}O$), and ${}^{15}O$-labeled carbon monoxide ($C{}^{15}O$). The short half-life and the low radiation absorbed dose allow amounts of activity up to 100 mCi to be administered in imaging procedures, which can be repeated at 8- to 10-min intervals.

Table 6-2 Decay properties of several short-lived positron-emitting radionuclides used in nuclear medicine

Nuclide	$t_{1/2}$ (min)	E_β^+ max (MeV)	Preferred Method of Production
${}^{15}O$	2	1.72	${}^{14}N\ (d,n)\ {}^{15}O$
${}^{13}N$	10	1.19	${}^{16}O\ (p,\alpha)\ {}^{13}N$
${}^{11}C$	20	0.96	${}^{14}N\ (p,\alpha)\ {}^{11}C$
${}^{18}F$	110	0.64	${}^{18}O\ (p,n)\ {}^{18}F$

^{15}O-labeled gas can be used directly to study O_2 metabolism, or the ^{15}O oxygen can be converted to ^{15}O-labeled CO, CO_2, or H_2O. Labeled carbon oxides are produced by passing the ^{15}O oxygen through an activated carbon furnace. The furnace temperature determines whether $C^{15}O$ or $CO^{15}O$ is produced. High specific activity ^{15}O can be produced that allows ^{15}O-labeled CO to be safely administered to patients by inhalation. Carbon monoxide labeled with ^{15}O binds to hemoglobin found in the RBC, allowing the study of red blood cell volume.

^{15}O-labeled water is usually produced from $CO^{15}O$ via the carbonic acid mediated exchange reaction by bubbling $CO^{15}O$ through saline. The ^{15}O-labeled water is produced in a form suitable for immediate intravenous injection. This tracer can also be produced by passing labeled oxygen gas and hydrogen gas over a suitable catalyst. The most common use for ^{15}O-labeled water is as a tracer for cerebral and myocardial perfusion.

Nitrogen-13

Currently ^{13}N is cyclotron produced by the $^{16}O(p,\alpha)^{13}N$ nuclear reaction. This nuclear reaction is performed in-target using a 5-mM solution of ethanol in water to yield ^{13}N in the form of ammonia.[5] Ethanol is used as a scavenger to reduce the amount of ^{13}N-nitrates formed. The ^{13}N-ammonia is delivered from the target through an anion exchange resin and a Millipore 0.22 μm sterile filter. N-N-13 labeled ammonia has been used as a tracer for cerebral and myocardial blood flow because it undergoes relatively high extraction into these organs and exhibits prolonged retention. A major fraction of the extracted ^{13}N-ammonia is metabolically incorporated into amino acids.

Carbon-11

Carbon-11 is generally produced by the $^{10}B(d,n)^{11}C$ or $^{14}N(p,\alpha)^{11}C$ nuclear reactions. C-11 labeled carbon monoxide (^{11}CO), carbon dioxide ($^{11}CO_2$), and cyanide ($^{11}CN^-$) are the most commonly used synthetic precursors. The number of different ^{11}C-labeled compounds that have been synthesized as radiopharmaceuticals for PET studies is extensive. This chapter briefly discusses a few of the more clinically useful ones.

One compound routinely prepared is ^{11}C-acetate, a tracer used in the study of myocardial metabolism. C-11 CO_2 is bubbled through the grignard, methylmagnesium bromide, and the intermediate formed is hydrolyzed with acid, and final sterile filtered.[24] C-11 acetate is converted to acetyl coenzyme A by the enzyme acetyl CoA synthetase after myocardial uptake. Acetyl coenzyme A enters the tricarboxylic acid cycle (TCA or Kreb's cycle) and is predominately metabolized to the end product $^{11}CO_2$. Because the TCA cycle is closely linked to oxidative phosphorylation ^{11}C-acetate metabolism can provide an index of oxidative metabolism.

C-11 glucose is also used to study metabolism. Early methods to prepare ^{11}C-glucose were lengthy compared to the 20 min half-life of ^{11}C; however, modifications have corrected this. The glucose analogue 2-deoxy-D-glucose labeled with ^{11}C in the C-1 position has been synthesized rapidly from the $H^{11}CN$ precursor. This analog of glucose has similar characteristics except that it fails to undergo intracellular enzymatic glycolysis beyond initial phosphorylation. It is metabolically trapped in brain and myocardial cells and has been used for measurement of cerebral and myocardial glucose metabolism.

Fluorine-18

Fluorine-18 fluoride is produced either by the $^{18}O(p,n)^{18}F$ or the $^{20}Ne(d,\alpha)^{18}F$ nuclear reaction. The proton irradiation of ^{18}O-labeled water is the preferred method of producing ^{18}F. The target body is constructed of metals such as silver, copper, titanium, nickel, or stainless steel. The target has small cavities for the target water, which are 0.1- to 3-mL in volume and covered by thin metal foils. The production of ^{18}F in most ^{18}O-labeled water targets is excellent, with yields of greater than 1.0 Ci at end of bombardment (EOB). The major problem in producing ^{18}F using ^{18}O-labeled water is the limited availability and high cost of the enriched isotopic target material. To aid in the conservation of the ^{18}O-labeled water, the recovery of unused target material by ion exchange chromatography is frequently practiced.

The most frequently used ^{18}F-labeled radiopharmaceutical is 2-deoxy-2-[^{18}F]fluoro-D-glucose (FDG). The FDA-approved indications for FDG are lung, esophageal, colorectal, head and neck, thyroid, and esophageal cancers; lymphomas; melanoma; refractory seizures; and myocardial viability. The indication for breast cancer at this time is still under consideration.

The mechanism of ^{18}F-FDG trapping follows the glucose biochemical pathway. ^{18}F-FDG is transported into the cell and metabolized by phosphorylation with hexokinase to ^{18}F-FDG-6 phosphate. However, unlike glucose, ^{18}F-FDG-6-phosphate is then trapped in the cell because of the stereochemical and structural demands of the enzyme responsible for further catabolism (Figure 6-15).

The most commonly used method for production of ^{18}F-FDG involves the method developed by Hamacher, et al.[13] The method utilizes a nucleophilic displacement reaction with mannose triflate. After displacement of the triflate with ^{18}F, acid hydrolysis of the acetylated intermediate, tetra acetyl-^{18}F-glucose (TA-^{18}F-FDG), gives ^{18}F-FDG (Figure 6-16). The Hamacher synthesis uses Kyrptofix®Kryptofix® 2.2.2 as a phase transfer catalyst to increase the reactivity of the $^{18}F^-$ anion.[16]

FDG synthesis modules available on the market employ several chemistry methods to prepare the ^{18}F-FDG. The original CTI FDG synthesizer uses Kryptofix® chemistry with acid hydrolysis. Nuclear Interface (Figure 6-17) modules use a nucleophilic reaction with either Kryptofix®[16] or tetra-

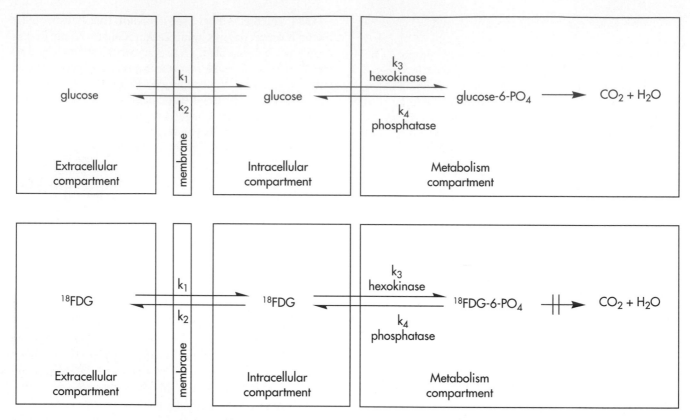

Figure 6-15 FDG undergoes metabolism similar to glucose, by hexokinase, but is metabolically trapped, because phosphorylization cannot proceed.

butylammonium hydrogen carbonate, then hydrolysis with HCl.[2]

The Coincidence Technologies FDG synthesizer also uses the nucleophilic substitution method.[13] The resulting tetra acetyl-^{18}F-glucose is trapped on a standard reverse phase extraction cartridge, and the acetyl groups are removed using base hydrolysis.[11] The CTI Quadrax® synthesizer employs Kryptofix® nucleophilic radiofluorination with acid or base hydrolysis.

The use of a neon gas target containing 1% F_2 provides labeled fluorine gas, [18]F[19]F. The production of ^{18}F involving F_2 gas using this nuclear reaction is inherently carrier added, and there are practical limits on the specific activity that can be obtained. Using [18]O gas via the [18]O(p,n)[18]F produces [18]F_2 using a no carrier added reaction, allowing higher specific activities for production of ^{18}F-FDOPA. The positron-emitting fluorinated L-dopa analog, 6-^{18}F-fluoro-L-3,4-dihydroxyphenylalanine, ^{18}F-FDOPA, (Figure 6-18), has been used as an imaging agent for brain dopamine neurons. The chemical structure of fluorodopa differs from L-dopa only at the 6 position of the catechol moiety where a fluorine atom replaces a hydrogen atom. Fluorodopa F-18 Injection was added to the USP in 1991. Because dopamine cannot cross the blood-brain barrier, its precursor, ^{18}F-FDOPA, the analog of L-dopa that crosses the blood-brain barrier, is administered. Once ^{18}F-FDOPA crosses into the brain, it is converted to 6-^{18}F-flurodopamine (^{18}F-FDA) by decarboxylation (Figure 6-18), is actively stored in sympa-

thetic synaptic vesicles in the brain, and can be released by sympathetic nerve stimulation. ^{18}F-FDOPA has been used to study parkinsonism and other neurologic disorders.

A commercial synthesis module manufactured by Nuclear Interface has been modified to produce FDOPA using the one-pot synthesis of deVries.[8] The method uses a fluorodestannylation reaction followed by acidic removal of the protecting groups.

THERAPEUTIC RADIOPHARMACEUTICALS

Sodium ^{32}P-phosphate is an FDA-approved radiopharmaceutical indicated for treatment of polycythemia vera, chronic myelocytic leukemia, and chronic lymphocytic leukemia, and for palliation of metastatic bone pain. It is prepared as a solution for intravenous administration. Chromic ^{32}P-phosphate is a suspension of ^{32}P used for intracavity installation for treatment of peritoneal or pleural effusions caused by metastatic disease. Phosphorus-32 decays by β^- emission with a $t_{1/2}$ of 14.3 days. The major toxicity noted is significant marrow suppression in approximately one third of patients receiving this radiopharmaceutical. The duration of response is 1.5 to 11 months.

Recently ^{89}Sr-chloride (Metastron®) has been approved by the FDA for relief of bone pain in cases of painful skeletal metastases. The compound behaves biologically as calcium does and localizes in hydroxyapatite crystal by ion exchange. Strontium uptake occurs preferentially at sites of

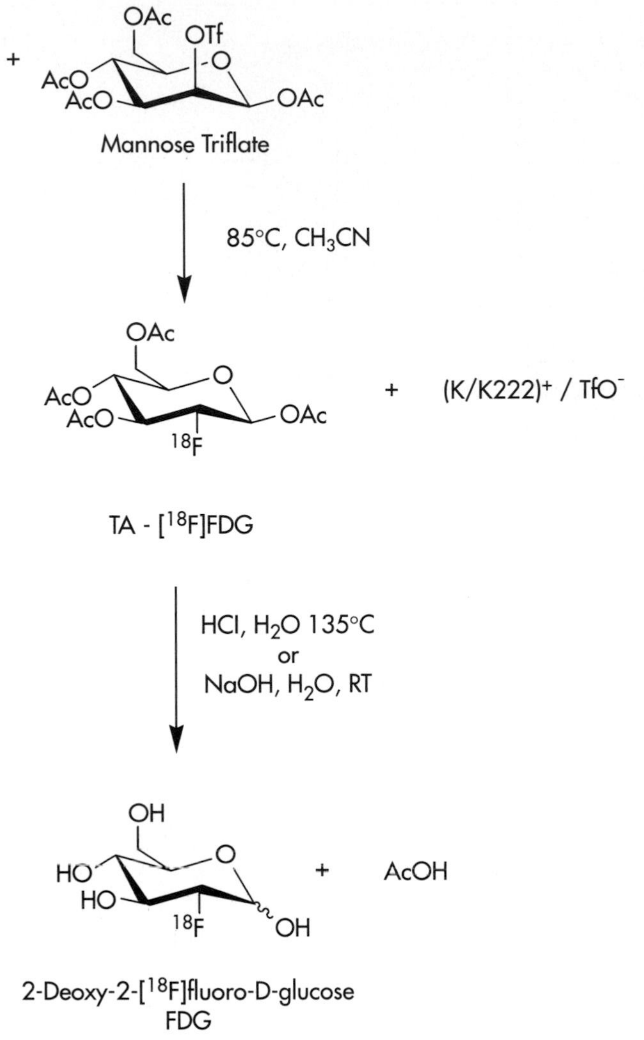

Figure 6-16 FDG synthetic scheme using Kryptofix® chemistry with acid or base hydrolysis.

active osteogenesis. This allows primary bone tumors and areas of metastatic involvement to accumulate significantly higher concentrations of strontium than surrounding normal bone. ^{89}Sr decays by β^- emission with a $t_{1/2}$ of 50.6 days.

In 1997, ^{153}Sm-EDTMP (Quadramet®) was approved by the FDA for relief of bone pain for similar indications as ^{89}Sr-chloride. Samarium-153 decays only by β^- emission and has a $t_{1/2}$ of 46.3 hr. Samarium-153 is complexed with a bone-seeking ligand, EDTMP, which localizes in bone metastases by chemisorption. The duration of response is 1 to 12 months. The main toxicity of this radiotherapeutic is mild transient bone marrow suppression.

In February 2002 the first radiolabeled monoclonal antibody (mAb) received FDA approval for radioimmunotherapy. Yttrium-90-labeled MX-DTPA-anti-CD20 antibody (^{90}Y-ibritumomab tiuxetan [Zevalin®]) is used to treat patients with non-Hodgkin's lymphoma (NHL). The unlabeled mAb, Rituximab®, targets the CD20 antigen present in most B-cell NHL's, and also has FDA approval for treating

patients with NHL. In a Phase III clinical trial carried out by IDEC Pharmaceuticals (San Diego, Calif.), Zevalin® was compared to Rituximab® in 143 patients. Preliminary data on 90 of these patients showed an overall response rate of 80% with Zevalin® vs. 44% for Rituximab®. The complete response rate for Zevalin® of 21% was also higher than that of Rituximab® (7%). Toxicity of Zevalin® was hematologic and reversible. For a review on the Phase I-III clinical trials of Zevalin®, see Witzig.[30]

RADIOPHARMACEUTICAL QUALITY ASSURANCE

Radionuclidic Purity

Radionuclidic purity is defined as the proportion of the total radioactivity present as the stated radionuclide. As such, measurement of radionuclidic purity requires determination of the identity and amounts of all radionuclides that are present. Radionuclidic impurities can have significant effects on the overall radiation dose to the patient and the quality of the images obtained. The identities and amounts of radionuclidic impurities found in a radiopharmaceutical depend on the method of radionuclide production used. As an example, ^{99m}Tc obtained from a generator prepared using neutron bombardment-produced ^{99}Mo has different impurities than ^{99m}Tc obtained from a generator containing fission-produced ^{99}Mo. The requirements for radionuclidic purity as listed by the *United States Pharmacopoeia XXV (USP)* for sodium ^{99m}Tc-pertechnetate solution are listed in Table 6-3.

An assay using a multichannel analyzer for detection and identification of all gamma-emitting radiocontaminants present in a sample is usually performed by the manufacturer. In the case of ^{99m}Tc, one expected radionuclidic impurity is parent ^{99}Mo. It is possible for the user to assay routinely for ^{99}Mo breakthrough using a gamma-ionization dose calibrator and a lead vial holder thick enough to absorb the 140 keV gamma of ^{99m}Tc but to allow penetration of the 720 and 740 keV gammas of ^{99}Mo (Figure 6-19). The Nuclear Regulatory Commission (NRC)-allowable ^{99}Mo contamination is less than 0.15 μCi/mCi of ^{99m}Tc. NRC regulations require that the first elution from a ^{99}Mo-^{99m}Tc generator be tested for ^{99}Mo breakthrough and that the records be maintained for 3 years.

Radiochemical Purity

Radiochemical purity is defined as the proportion of the stated radionuclide that is present in the stated chemical form. The radiation absorbed dose, the biologic distribution, and thus the quality of the image are directly related to the radiochemical purity. Several chromatographic methods can be used to determine radiochemical purity, including gel-permeation chromatography, gas-liquid chromatography, and paper chromatography. The method applicable to routine in-house quality control of technetium radiopharmaceuticals is paper or instant thin-layer chromatography (ITLC).

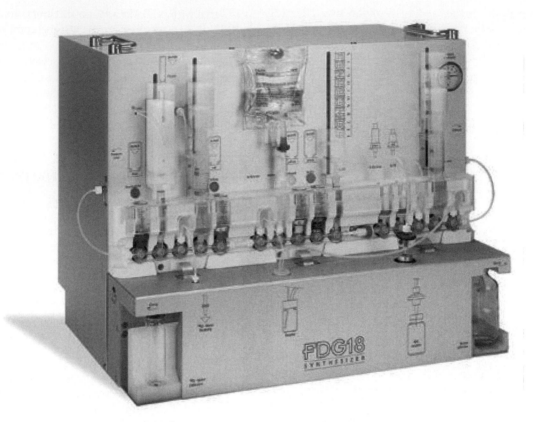

Figure 6-17   GE Medical Systems TRACERlab MX$_{FDG}$.

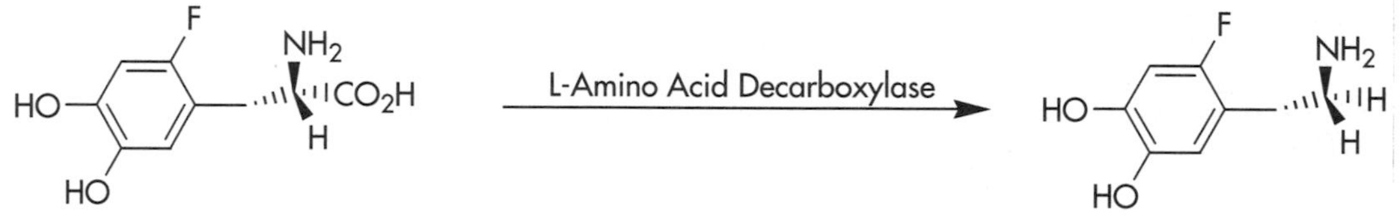

Figure 6-18   FDOPA decarboxylation to FDA.

6-FDOPA

L-Amino Acid Decarboxylase

6-Fluorodopamine

Table 6-3	NRC allowable radionuclidic impurities in ^{99m}Tc-pertechnetate

Neutron bombardment ^{98}Mo (n,γ) ^{99}Mo	Fission-separation ^{99}Mo

^{98}Mo (n,γ) ^{99}Mo
^{99}Mo < 0.15 μCi/mCi ^{99m}Tc
 	
Other gamma-emitting radionuclides:
   0.5 μCi/mCi ^{99m}Tc
   <2.5 μCi/administered dose
	^{99}Mo < 0.15 μCi/mCi ^{99m}Tc
	
	Other gamma-emitting radionuclides:
	   ^{131}I < 0.05 μCi/mCi ^{99m}Tc
	   ^{103}Ru < 0.05 μCi/mCi ^{99m}Tc
	   ^{89}Sr < 0.0006 μCi/mCi ^{99m}Tc
	   ^{90}Sr < 0.00006 μCi/mCi ^{99m}Tc
	Remaining β + γ < 0.1 μCi/mCi ^{99m}Tc
	   α < 0.001 μCi/mCi ^{99m}Tc

Chromatography involves the separation of a chemical mixture into its components along a stationary phase (adsorbent) as a result of different velocities in the mobile phase (migrating solvent). Radiochromatography differs from regular chromatography only in that the presence of the component is determined by the location of its radioactivity rather than by some other physical or chemical property. The R_f of a compound is defined as the measure of its migration distance, where

$$R_f = \frac{\text{Distance of center of spot from origin}}{\text{Distance of solvent front origin}}$$

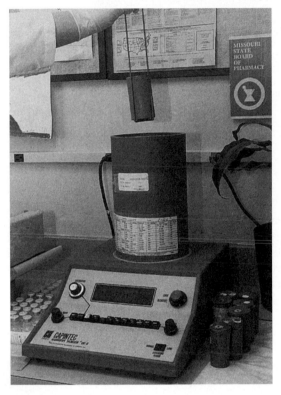

Figure 6-19   Molybdenum-99 assay chamber being placed in a dose calibrator.

When the $R_f = 1$, the component migrates with the solvent front; whereas when the $R_f = 0$, the component remains at the point of application (origin).

The ideal separation of a component in a solvent system gives an R_f value greater than 0 but less than 1. A component that migrates at the solvent front ($R_f = 1$) or remains at the origin ($R_f = 0$) is not truly separated. However, for routine rapid quality control of technetium radiopharmaceuticals and the separation of known impurities, free pertechnetate ($^{99m}TcO_4^-$) and free reduced technetium ($^{99m}TcO_2$) from the labeled radiopharmaceuticals, R_f values of 1 and 0 are considered acceptable.

A typical thin-layer radiochromatogram of ^{99m}Tc-sulfur colloid with $^{99m}TcO_4^-$ contaminant is shown in Figure 6-20. The radioactivity associated with the peaks may be measured in several ways. The simplest method, which was used to obtain the data, involves the use of a radiochromatogram scanner (Figure 6-21). In this system the paper chromatography strip is moved across a detector, a ratemeter indicates the count rate, and the counts are graphically printed out by a strip chart recorder. A manual counting system can also be employed, in which the chromatogram is cut into strips, and each strip is counted using a well counter or an ionization dose calibrator.

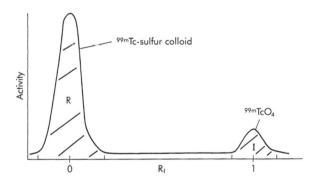

Figure 6-20   Radiochromatogram scan of ^{99m}Tc-sulfur colloid (R) indicating radiochemical purity. The only radiocontaminant present is $^{99m}TcO_4^-$ (I).

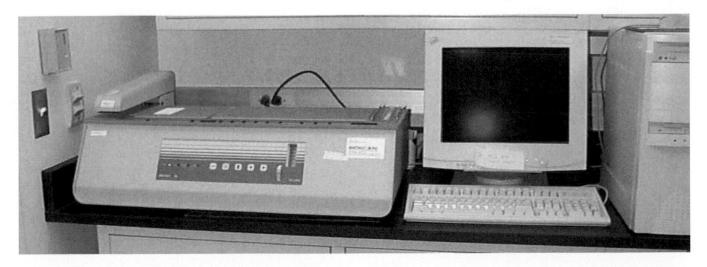

Figure 6-21   Radiochromatogram scanner used for radiochemical purity analysis and calculation of percent radiochemical purity.

Table 6-4 Chromatographic systems used for quality control of ^{99m}Tc radiopharmaceuticals

Radiopharmaceutical	Solvent	Solid Support	R_f		
			Free ^{99m}TcO$_4^-$	Free ^{99m}TcO$_2$	^{99m}Tc-labeled Radiopharmaceutical
Sulfur colloid	Acetone or saline	ITLC-SG	1.0	—	0
MAA	Acetone or saline	ITLC-SG	1.0	—	0
PYP	Acetone and	ITLC-SG	1.0	0	0
MDP/HDP/	Saline	ITLC-SG	1.0	0	1.0
DTPA					
GHP					
DMSA					
Disofenin/	20% NaCl	ITLC-SA	1.0	0	0
Mebrofenin	H$_2$O	ITLC-SG	1.0	0	1.0
Sestamibi	100% EtOH	Aluminum oxide TLC	0	0	1.0
Teboroxime	Saline	Whatman 31ET	1.0	0	0
	Saline-acetone (1:1)	Whatman 31ET	1.0	0	1.0

The radiochemical purity of a radiopharmaceutical preparation can be calculated using the following expression:

Percentage of radiochemical purity
= Area R (Area R + Area I)
= Counts in strip R (counts in strip R + Counts in strip I [total counts])

where R refers to the radiopharmaceutical and I refers to the impurity.

Routine rapid radiochromatography can be performed to evaluate the percentage of radiochemical purity of ^{99m}Tc radiopharmaceuticals. The most commonly employed procedure involves the use of instant thin-layer chromatography silica gel-impregnated (ITLC-SG) glass-fiber sheets as the solid support. These strips are developed in solvents such as saline, acetone, and methyl ethyl ketone (MEK). ^{99m}Tc radiopharmaceuticals can be divided into three groups based on their chromatographic behavior.

1. Oxidized, particulate: This group contains ^{99m}Tc-sulfur colloid. Because the technetium is present in the +7 oxidation state, it is not necessary to analyze for free reduced ^{99m}Tc in these preparations. The chromatographic system used involves a single solvent (saline, acetone, or MEK) to determine the amount of free pertechnetate.
2. Reduced, particulate: This group includes the ^{99m}Tc-labeled lung perfusion imaging agent MAA. The rapid chromatographic procedures described for sulfur colloid can be used only to determine free pertechnetate. It is not possible to separate free reduced ^{99m}Tc (which is colloidal at physiologic pH) and the

^{99m}Tc MAA using this rapid system. It is possible, however, to use an indirect method to detect ^{99m}TcO$_2$ impurity levels. The radiopharmaceutical is first filtered through a Millipore® filter with a $1\,\mu$ pore diameter, which retains the ^{99m}Tc MAA but allows the colloidal free reduced ^{99m}Tc to pass through. Once the macroparticles have been removed, rapid chromatography on the filtrate (using either saline, acetone, or MEK) enables the determination of free ^{99m}TcO$_4^-$ and ^{99m}TcO$_2$.
3. Reduced, soluble: This group contains the soluble, reduced ^{99m}Tc-radiopharmaceuticals, including DTPA, glucoheptonate, methylene diphosphonate, pyrophosphate, DMSA, and albumin. The chromatographic procedure for this group involves two solvents (saline and an organic solvent, such as acetone or MEK) to determine the percentages of free pertechnetate, free reduced technetium, and labeled radiopharmaceutical.

The R_f values of the technetium radiopharmaceutical and the relevant impurities are outlined in Table 6-4 for each of these groups. The steps in a typical chromatographic procedure for a reduced, soluble ^{99m}Tc-radiopharmaceutical are as follows:

1. Place 1 mL of saline in a small glass vial; repeat this procedure with the organic solvent.
2. Mark two 1-cm by 6-cm ITLC chromatography strips at 2 cm and 5 cm with a pencil.
3. Place a small spot of the radiopharmaceutical in the center of each strip (near the mark located 2 cm from the bottom of the strip) using a tuberculin syringe.

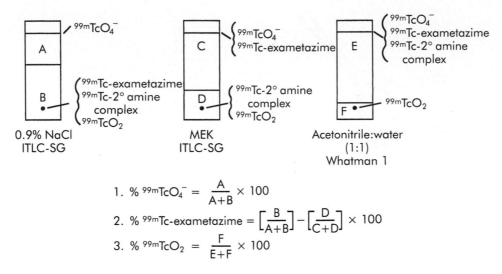

1. $\% \ {}^{99m}TcO_4^- = \dfrac{A}{A+B} \times 100$

2. $\% \ {}^{99m}Tc\text{-exametazime} = \left[\dfrac{B}{A+B}\right] - \left[\dfrac{D}{C+D}\right] \times 100$

3. $\% \ {}^{99m}TcO_2 = \dfrac{F}{E+F} \times 100$

Figure 6-22 Chromatographic system used for radiochemical purity determination for ^{99m}Tc-exametazime and calculation of percentage of radiochemical purity.

4. Place one strip into each solvent before the spot has air-dried to prevent air oxidation of the radiopharmaceutical. Allow the solvent front to move up each strip until it has reached the line at 5 cm.
5. Cut the strips in the middle between the pencil markings and count each portion of the strips for activity, or use a radiochromatogram scanner (Figure 6-21) to measure the amount of activity along the intact strips.
6. In the dual solvent system, the percentage of free ^{99m}TcO$_4^-$ is calculated from the strip developed in the organic solvent, and the percentage of free ^{99m}TcO$_2$ is determined using the strip developed in saline. Subtraction of the percentages of these two impurities from 100% yields the overall radiochemical purity of the ^{99m}Tc radiopharmaceutical.

Radiochemical testing using ITLC is easily performed in any nuclear medicine laboratory. Testing each lot of a radiopharmaceutical kit on a weekly basis is a reasonable approach for routine radiochemical testing. Additional testing should be performed if there are questions concerning purity of a given preparation. Several of the newer technetium radiopharmaceuticals require more specific types of quality control methods. In the preparation of the lipophilic ^{99m}Tc-exametazime, three radiochemical impurities can be present: a secondary ^{99m}Tc-amine complex, ^{99m}TcO$_4^-$, and reduced hydrolyzed ^{99m}Tc. A combination of three chromatographic systems is necessary for radiochemical purity determination: 0.9% NaCl (ITLC-SG); MEK (ITLC-SG); and acetonitrile-water (1:1). In the 0.9% NaCl (saline) solvent the ^{99m}TcO$_4^-$ migrates at the solvent front, whereas the ^{99m}Tc-exametazime, secondary ^{99m}Tc-amine complex, and free reduced ^{99m}Tc remain at the origin. In the MEK solvent, ^{99m}TcO$_4^-$ and ^{99m}Tc-exametazime migrate at the solvent front, whereas the secondary ^{99m}Tc-amine complex and the free

reduced ^{99m}Tc remain at the origin. Use of the acetonitrile-water (1:1) solvent causes ^{99m}TcO$_4^-$, ^{99m}Tc-exametazime, and the secondary ^{99m}Tc-amine complex to migrate with the solvent front, whereas the free reduced ^{99m}Tc remains at the origin. The calculations used for determining the percentage of ^{99m}Tc-exametazime are shown in Figure 6-22.

The radiochemical purity of ^{99m}Tc-mertiatide is determined using Sep-Pak® chromatography. The Sep-Pak® is made of C$_{18}$ hydrocarbon chains that retain nonpolar compounds. Initially the Sep-Pak® is prepared by washing with 100% ethanol to remove nonpolar impurities, then with 0.001N HCl to remove polar impurities. A sample of the ^{99m}Tc-mertiatide is then placed on the Sep-Pak® and eluted with a 0.001N HCl solution, which elutes any polar impurities present in the preparation. This fraction is retained and labeled fraction 1. Then the Sep-Pak® is eluted with an ethanol-saline (1:1) solution, which solubilizes and elutes the ^{99m}Tc-mertiatide. This fraction is labeled 2, and the Sep-Pak® is labeled 3. Fractions 1, 2, and 3 are counted in the dose calibrator. Figure 6-23 shows the calculation for ^{99m}Tc-mertiatide purity determination.

A single solid support, aluminum oxide, and a single solvent, 100% ethanol, are used for quality control of ^{99m}Tc-sestamibi. The ^{99m}Tc-sestamibi migrates at the solvent front. Pertechnetate is thought to form a complex with the aluminum and remains at the origin. The ^{99m}TcO$_2$ also remains at the origin.

Quality control for ^{99m}Tc-teboroxime involves use of a two-solvent system. Solvents and solid supports for this analysis are outlined in Table 6-4.

^{99m}Tc-tetrofosmin quality control requires the ITLC-SG as the solid support and a 35/65 (v/v) mixture of acetone and dichloromethane. After spotting the ITLC-SG, the solvent is allowed to migrate 15 cm. The strip is removed from the solvent and cut into three pieces, each approximately 5 cm long. The percent ^{99m}Tc-tetrofosmin will be equal to the

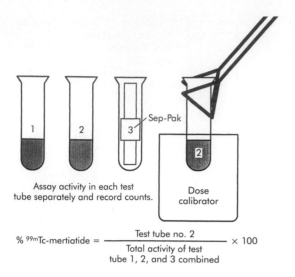

$$\% \ ^{99m}\text{Tc-mertiatide} = \frac{\text{Test tube no. 2}}{\text{Total activity of test}} \times 100$$
$$\text{tube 1, 2, and 3 combined}$$

Figure 6-23 Calculation of percent radiochemical purity of ^{99m}Tc-mertiatide.

activity of the center piece of the strip, divided by the total activity of the three pieces, multiplied by 100.

Completion of quality control, involving C_{18} Sep-Pak chromatography, is recommended before patient administration for ^{111}In-pentetreotide. The Sep-Pak is prepared for use by initially flushing with 10 mL of methanol, followed by 10 mL of water. A sample of ^{111}In-pentetreotide is placed on the Sep-Pak and eluted with 5 mL of water. The fraction is labeled fraction 1. The Sep-Pak is then eluted with 5 mL of methanol, which solubilizes ^{111}In-pentetreotide. This is labeled fraction 2, and the Sep-Pak® is labeled fraction 3. Each fraction is assayed in the dose calibrator, and the percent purity of the ^{111}In-pentetreotide is determined (Figure 6-24).

Chemical Impurities

Chemical impurities are all the nonradioactive substances present in a radiopharmaceutical preparation that either affect labeling or directly cause adverse biologic effects. In microgram concentrations aluminum can affect the formation of ^{99m}Tc-labeled radiopharmaceuticals. The NRC states the concentration of aluminum should not exceed 10 μg/mL. The presence of excess Al^{3+} can cause formation of colloidal ^{99m}Tc-Al particles, resulting in liver uptake, aggregation of sulfur colloid to larger particles with resultant capillary blockade and lung visualization, and ^{99m}Tc-RBC aggregation, which results in uptake of the damaged cells in lungs and spleen.

Aluminum can be detected using a spectrophotometric method. Aluminum solutions of known concentrations are reacted with aluminon reagent (the ammonium salt of aurin tricarboxylic acid), and the absorbance in the visible region of the spectrum is measured. A standard curve is then prepared by plotting the absorbance versus the aluminum concentration; this curve can be used to determine aluminum concentrations of unknown samples. A more convenient

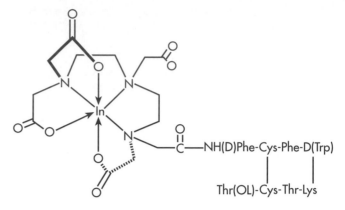

Figure 6-24 Spatial configuration of ^{111}In-pentetreotide (OctreoScan®).

method for aluminum determination is the use of a commercially available indicator paper impregnated with aluminon reagent that turns pink when Al^{3+} is present in a spot of the eluant solution. A standard solution of Al^{3+} (10 μg/mL) is used as a color comparison.

Most of the commercially available technetium kits contain stannous ion as the reducing agent. In most cases more stannous ion is contained in each kit than is actually required to reduce and bind the technetium that is added; this excess of stannous ion has been found to cause some problems. For example, liver uptake has been noted on an otherwise normal bone scan, which may be attributable to the formation of ^{99m}Tc-tin colloids. Another problem that can occur with excess stannous ion is inadvertent RBC labeling. As mentioned previously, excess stannous ion injected into a patient receiving a reduced ^{99m}Tc radiopharmaceutical remains in the circulation. This can cause RBC labeling on subsequent administration of ^{99m}Tc-pertechnetate for brain or thyroid imaging.

Microbiologic Testing

Sterility testing. The objective of sterility testing is to provide assurance that the sterilization process was conducted properly. The sterility test required by the *USP XXV* involves inoculation of the product in both fluid thioglycollate and soybean-casein digest media. Fluid thioglycollate provides conditions for growth of aerobic and anaerobic bacteria. Soybean-casein digest medium supports growth of fungi and molds. The official sterility test requires 14 days, but because of the short half-life of ^{99m}Tc, the *USP XXV* allows for the release of these radiopharmaceuticals before the completion of the tests. The cold kits used to prepare the ^{99m}Tc radiopharmaceuticals are tested for sterility and pyrogen content.

Pyrogen testing. The *USP XXV* also requires pyrogen testing. Pyrogens are any agents that cause a rise in temperature and are generally considered to be heat-stable byproducts of the growth of bacteria, yeasts, and molds. The word *pyrogen* is often used to mean bacterial endotoxin. Previously, to test for the presence of pyrogens the *USP XXV* required the monitoring of three healthy rabbits for 3 hr after intravenous injection of the test sample. The test was positive if any rabbit showed an increase of 0.6 °C or more above the baseline temperature or if the sum of the three temperature increases exceeded 1.4 °C.

The *USP XXV* now uses bacterial endotoxin testing (BET) as the approved method of pyrogen testing. The BET test involves the use of the limulus amebocyte lysate (LAL), which is isolated from the horseshoe crab (Limulus). LAL reacts with gram-negative bacterial endotoxins in nanogram or greater concentrations to form an opaque gel. Gram-negative endotoxins are recognized as the most important source of pyrogen contamination. The BET test is both a rapid and a very sensitive in vitro method.

Manufacturers are required to perform sterility and apyrogenicity testing on all their products before release into the marketplace. The short half-life of ^{99m}Tc, however, prohibits testing of ^{99m}Tc-labeled radiopharmaceuticals for sterility and apyrogenicity before patient administration. Because this is the case, it is imperative that the user emphasize aseptic technique. The use of laminar airflow enclosures improves the environment for radiopharmaceutical formulation, because these enclosures contain high-efficiency particulate air (HEPA) filters to remove particles of 0.3 μ and larger with an efficiency of 99.97%. Vertical laminar airflow hoods are preferred in a radiopharmacy, because horizontal flow presents a potentially serious contamination hazard to personnel by forcing radioactivity out into the room. If the laminar airflow cabinet is reinforced, it can support a leaded glass shield to provide radiation protection for the technologist during preparation of the radiopharmaceuticals.

USP quality control requirements for ^{18}F-FDG. ^{18}F-FDG is currently being dispensed and distributed according to the *USP XXV* monograph requirements for ^{18}F-FDG because the FDA has not finalized yet the regulatory status of PET.[28]

Pre-release USP quality control (QC) testing for PET radiopharmaceuticals includes identity testing, pH, visual appearance, radiochemical and chemical testing, including residual solvent analysis and BET (<175 EU/mL) at end of synthesis (EOS). Each of these tests must include adequate standards testing as part of the analysis. Final product should be filtered through a 0.22 μm filter to assure sterility.

Sterility testing is required postrelease for every batch of PET radiopharmaceutical prepared for human use. An aliquot of the batch must be inoculated for sterility within 24 hours EOS. Radionuclidic purity testing, commonly involving gamma analysis with a multichannel analyzer (MCA) must be performed on a regularly defined interval.

For radiopharmaceuticals having a $T_{1/2} < 20.0$ minutes, the *USP XXV* allows preparation of a separate batch, called a "sub-batch" for QC testing before preparation of the patient batch. The QC batch must be tested for all pre- and postrelease tests as noted above.[28]

The following tests should be performed prerelease for each batch of ^{18}F-FDG:[28]

1. Identity testing for ^{18}F-FDG involves decay analysis over a defined period of time. This test is performed using a dose calibrator. The half-life is determined mathematically using linear regression. The acceptable $t_{1/2} = 109.7$ (with an allowable range of 105–155 min).

2. The pH must be between 4.5 and 7.5. An aliquot of each batch ^{18}F-FDG is tested with pH paper.

3. The batch is checked visually (using adequate shielding) to ensure a clear colorless solution that is free of particulate matter.

4. The radiochemical purity of ^{18}F-FDG can be determined by using silica gel 60 TLC plates developed in acetonitrile/water (95:5). A nonradioactive FDG standard should be chromatographed with the ^{18}F-FDG. This system allows separation of ^{18}F-FDG ($R_f = 0.4$), ^{18}F-fluoride ($R_f = 0.1$) and TA-^{18}F-FDG, the nonhydrolyzed intermediate ($R_f = 0.6$). Acceptable radiochemical purity is ≥90%.

5. The chemical purity of each batch of ^{18}F-FDG must be checked pre-release. If the synthetic method of ^{18}F-FDG production involves the use of Kryptofix®, which is a toxic substance, *USP XXV* requires determination of the concentration of Kryptofix® in the final product. The *USP XXV*-approved method to test for the presence of Kryptofix®, developed by Chaly and Dahl,[4] involves a rapid, simple, TLC quality control procedure using a silica gel thin-layer chromatographic plate developed in a mixture of methanol/ammonium hydroxide (9:1). The developed plate is dried, and an iodine vapor chamber is used for visualization. A yellow spot ($R_f = 0.4$) indicates the presence of Kryptofix® 2.2.2. The *USP XXV* test takes about 30 minutes to complete. Mock et al[22] have also developed a color spot test for FDG that can determine the presence of Kryptofix® to as low as 2.0 μg/mL in about 5 minutes. The test uses pretreated strips of plastic-backed silica gel TLC (Eastman Kodak), saturated with iodoplatinate reagents that are over-spotted with drops of ^{18}F-FDG and Kryptofix® standard solutions. The test requires less than 10 minutes to perform, but must be validated against the USP method. The Kryptofix® concentration must be <50 μg/mL. Residual solvent concentrations such as acetonitrile, ethanol, and ether must be tested if they are used in the synthesis before release of ^{18}F-FDG. Gas chromatographic methods have been developed for the measurement of residual solvents that allow precision and linearity over the range of concentration levels suggested by the FDA,[6] and required by the USP. The concentration of acetonitrile must be 0.04% w/v (0.4 mg/mL), ethanol 0.5% w/v (5 mg/mL), and ether 0.5% w/v (5 mg/mL).

6. Every batch should be tested using BET. The acceptable endotoxin limit is <175 EU/mL EOS.

Postrelease sterility testing must be performed for each batch of ^{18}F-FDG. The product should be inoculated in both fluid thioglycollate and soybean-casein digest media within 24 hours EOS. Radionuclidic purity should be determined on a defined interval by γ-ray spectroscopy using a suitable gamma counting device. An MCA is often used to determine the presence of any gamma photon energy other than that characteristic of ^{18}F, including 511 keV, 1.02 MeV or Compton scatter. The radionuclidic purity must be >99.5%.

REFERENCES

1. Bauer W, Briner U, Doepfner W, et al: SMS 201-995: a very potent and selective octapeptide analogue of somatostatin with prolonged action, *Life Sci* 31:1133, 1982.

2. Brodak JW, Dence CS, Kilbourn MR, Welch MJ: Robotic production of 2-deoxy-2[^{18}F]fluoro-D-glucose: a routine method of synthesis using tetrabutylammonium [^{18}F]fluoride, *Int J Rad Appl Instrum [A]* 39:699-703, 1988.

3. Brodack JW, Kaiser SL, Welch MJ: Laboratory robotics for the remote synthesis of generator-based positron-emitting radiopharmaceuticals, *LRA* 1:285, 1989.

4. Chaly T, Dahl JR: Thin layer chromatographic detection of Kryptofix 2.2.2. in the routine synthesis of [^{18}F]-2-fluoro-deoxyglucose, *Nuc Med Biol* 16:385, 1989.

5. Channing MA, Dunn BB, Kiesewetter DO, et al: The quality of [13N]ammonia produced by using ethanol as a scavenger, *J Labelled Comp Radiopharm* 35:334, 1994.

6. Channing MA, Huang BX, Eckelman WC: Analysis of residual solvents in 2-[^{18}F]FDG by GC, *Nuc Med Biol* 28:469, 2001.

7. Coleman RE, Maturi M, Nunn AD, et al: Imaging of myocardial perfusion with Tc-99m SQ 3Q217: dog and human studies, *J Nucl Med* 27:893, 1986.

8. deVries, EFJ, Luurtsema G, Brussermann M, et al: Fully automated synthesis module for the high yield one-pot preparation of 6-[18F]fluoro-L-DOPA, *Appl Rad Isot* 51:389, 1999.

9. Dudczak R, Leitha T, Kletter K, et al: Comparison of Tc-99m-methoxyisobutyl-isonitrile (MIBI) for myocardial imaging in man, *J Nucl Med* 29:794, 1988.

10. Ehrhardt GJ, Welch MJ: A new germanium-68/gallium-68 generator, *J Nucl Med* 19:925, 1978.

11. Füchtner F, Steinbach J, Mading, P Johannsen B: Basic hydrolysis of 2-[18F]fluoro-1,3,4,6-tetra-O-acetyl-C-glucose in the preparation of 2-[18F]fluoro-2-deoxy-D-glucose, *Appl Radiat Isot* 47:61, 1966.

12. Fujibayashi Y, Matsumoto K, Yonekura Y, et al: A new zinc-62/copper-62 generator as a copper-62 source for PET radiopharmaceuticals, *J Nucl Med* 30:1938, 1989.

13. Green MA, Mathias CJ, Welch MJ, et al: Copper-62-labeled pyruvaldehyde bis (N^4-methylthiosemicarbazonato) copper (II): synthesis and evaluation as a positron emission tomography tracer for cerebral and myocardial perfusion, *J Nucl Med* 31:1989, 1990.

14. Green MW, Tucker WD: An improved gallium-68 cow, *Int J Appl Radiat Isot* 12:62, 1961.

15. Green MA, Welch MJ: Gallium radiopharmaceutical chemistry, *Nucl Med Biol* 16:435, 1989.

16. Hamacher K, Coenen HH, Stocklin G: Efficient stereospecific synthesis of NCA 2-[^{18}F]fluoro-2-deoxy-D-glucose using aminopolyether supported nucleophilic substitution, *J Nucl Med* 27:235, 1986.

17. Haynes NG, Lacy JL, Nayak N, et al: Performance of a ^{62}Zn/^{62}Cu generator in clinical trials of PET perfusion agent ^{62}Cu-PTSM, *J Nucl Med* 41:309, 2000.

18. Leveille J, Demonceau G, DeRoo M, et al: Characterization of technetium-99m-L,L-ECD for brain perfusion imaging. Part 2. Biodistribution and brain imaging in humans, *J Nucl Med* 30:1902, 1989.

19. Loberg MD, Fields AT: Chemical structure of technetium-99m-labeled N-(216-dimethylphenyl-carbamoylmethyl)-iminodiacetic acid (Tc-HIDA), *Int J Appl Radiat Isot* 29:167, 1978.

20. Loc'h C, Maziere B, Comar D: A new generator for ionic gallium-68, *J Nucl Med* 21:171, 1980.

21. Mathias CJ, Margenau WH, Brodack JW, et al: A remote system for the synthesis of copper-62-labeled Cu(PTSM), *Appl Radiat Isot* 42:317, 1991.

22. Mock BH, Winkle W, Vavrek MT: A color spot test for the detection of Kryptofix 2.2.2 in [^{18}F]FDG preparations, *Nuc Med Biol* 24:193, 1997.

23. Neirinckx RD, Burke JF, Harrison RG, et al: The retention mechanism of technetium-99m-HMPAO: intracellular reaction with glutathione, *J Cereb Blood Flow Metab* 8:54, 1988.

24. Pike VW, Eakins MN, Allan RM, Selwyn AP: Preparation of [1-11C]acetate—an agent for the study of myocardial metabolism by positron emission tomography, *Appl Radiat Isot* 33:505, 1982.

25. Robinson GD, Zielinski FW, Lee AW: Zn-62/Cu-62 generator: a convenient source of copper-62 radiopharmaceuticals, *Int J Appl Radiat Isot* 31:111, 1980.

26. Sands H, Delano ML, Gallagher BM: Uptake of hexakis (t-butylisonitrile) technetium (I) and hexakis (isopropylisonitrile) technetium (I) by neonatal rat myocytes and human erythrocytes, *J Nucl Med* 27:404, 1986.

27. Taylor Jr A, Eshima D, Fritzberg AR, et al: Comparison of iodine-131 OIH and technetium-99m MAG$_3$ renal imaging in volunteers, *J Nucl Med* 27:795, 1986.

28. USP/NF. *United States Pharmacopoeia XXV*, Rockville, MD, 2002, United States Pharmacopoeial Convention, 754-755, 2068-2071.

29. Walhaus TR, Lacy J, Whang J, et al: Human biodistribution and dosimetry of the PET perfusion agent ^{62}Cu-PTSM from a compact modular ^{62}Zn/^{62}Cu generator, *J Nucl Med* 39:1958, 1998.

30. Witzig TE: Radioimmunotherapy for patients with relapsed B-cell non-Hodgkin's lymphoma, *Cancer Chemother Pharmacol* 48(suppl 1):S91, 2001.

SUGGESTED READINGS

Fowler JS, Wolf AP: The synthesis of carbon-11, fluorine-18 and nitrogen-13 labeled radiotracers for biomedical applications. In *Nuclear Science Series, Nuclear Medicine,* Washington, DC, 1982, Technical Information Center, U.S. Department of Energy.

Kilbourn MR: Fluorine-18 labeling of radiopharmaceuticals. In *Nuclear Science Series, Nuclear Medicine,* Washington, DC, 1990, National Academy Press.

Kowalsky RJ, Perry JR: *Radiopharmaceuticals in nuclear medicine practice,* Norwalk, CT, 1987, Appleton & Lange.

Krenning EP, Bakker WH, Kooij PPM, et al: Somatostatin receptor scintigraphy with Indium-111-DTPA-D-Phe[1]-octreotide in man: metabolism, dosimetry and comparison with Iodine-123-Tyr-Octreotide. *J Nucl Med* 33:652, 1992.

Rydberg J, Liljenzin JO, Choppin G: *Radiochemistry and nuclear chemistry,* ed 3, Oxford, England, 2001, Butterworth-Heinemann.

Steigman J, Eckelman WC: Chemistry of technetium in medicine. In *Nuclear Science Series, Nuclear Medicine,* Washington, DC, 1992, National Academy Press.

Swanson DP, Chilton HM, Thrall JH: *Pharmaceuticals in medical imaging,* New York, 1990, Macmillan.

Verbruggen AM: Radiopharmaceuticals: state of the art, *Eur J Nucl Med* 17:346, 1990.

Welch MJ, Kilbourn MR: Positron emitters for imaging. In Freeman L, ed: *Freeman and Johnson's clinical radionuclide imaging,* ed 3, vol 1, Orlando, FL, 1984, Grune & Stratton.

Marleen M. Moore

chapter **7**

Radiation Safety in Nuclear Medicine

Objectives

List and define units of radiation, absorbed dose, and dose equivalent.

Discuss sources of radiation exposure to the general population.

List the regulatory limits for radiation exposure.

Define ALARA and detail a comprehensive ALARA program for nuclear medicine.

Discuss patient radiation exposure and describe exposure to critical organs (with examples).

Explain the appropriate use of ionization chambers.

Use Geiger counters and scintillation detectors for laboratory surveys and decontamination procedures.

Describe the appropriate clinical use of the dose calibrator to be in compliance with federal and state regulations.

Discuss the use of personnel monitoring devices.

List the criteria for posting warning signs for exposure to radiation.

Discuss the receipt, disposition, and disposal of radioactive materials and radioactivity.

Discuss the methods of testing for and controlling radioactive contamination.

Define the criteria that constitute a misadministration.

Discuss the necessary precautions when using therapeutic radionuclides.

Describe the effects of ionizing radiation.

---

*T*he practice of nuclear medicine includes handling radioactive materials and exposure to radiation. To do this safely requires precautions to ensure minimum radiation exposure to personnel and the general population and only appropriate exposure to patients. In addition, procedures must be used to prevent contamination from unsealed sources. Federal and state regulations mandate many of these policies and procedures. The medical use of radioactive materials is regulated by the Nuclear Regulatory Commission, either directly or in agreement with states. The practices discussed in this chapter comply with these regulations, which provide for safe use of radioactive materials.

UNITS

A system of measurement is required to determine the amount of radioactivity used and to quantify the resulting radiation. Nuclear medicine now officially uses the system of units known as the Systeme International d' Unités (SI), which was introduced in Chapter 1. The commonly used traditional system of units and appropriate conversion factors are listed in Table 7-1.

Table 7-1	SI-derived units adopted for specifying ionizing radiation levels		
Quantity	**Name**	**Symbol**	**Relationship to replaced unit**
Radiation exposure	X unit	C per kg 3881	Roentgens per X unit
Absorbed dose	Gray	Gy	100 rad per gray
Dose equivalent	Sievert	Sv	100 rem per sievert

Three important concepts of determining radiation levels are exposure, absorbed dose, and dose equivalent.

Radiation Exposure

X-ray and gamma radiations have the property of producing ions, that is, liberating electrical charge when interacting with matter. A common method of determining the intensity of x-ray or gamma radiation is to measure the magnitude of the electrical charge (of either sign) liberated in air. The quantity that denotes the amount of electrical charge per unit mass of air is termed the exposure. The definition of exposure (X) is the quotient Q/m, where Q is the sum of the electrical charges of all the ions of one sign produced in a volume of air whose mass is m, that is:

$$X = Q/m$$

There are several important aspects to the concept of exposure:

1. The concept applies only to ionizing electromagnetic radiation, such as x rays and gamma rays, and not to particle radiations, such as beta particles and neutrons.
2. Air is the interacting medium.
3. The measured endpoint is the amount of ionization per unit mass of air.
4. It becomes operationally difficult to fulfill the requirements for measuring exposure for photon energies less than several keV and more than several MeV. Accordingly, the use of this concept is limited to photons with energies of 3 MeV or less.
5. Devices expressly designed to measure exposure are referred to as air ionization chamber instruments.

The concept of exposure is expressed in fundamental units of coulomb/kg of air in SI units. In traditional units, radiation exposure is measured in roentgens. A roentgen (R) is defined as 2.58×10^{-4} coulomb/kg of air. This is also equivalent to the older definition of 1 electrostatic unit of charge (ESU)/cm^3 of air at standard temperature and pressure.

Absorbed Dose

Radiation damage often depends on the amount of energy absorbed per unit mass of the irradiated material. The quantity that specifies the energy imparted to a material by any type of ionizing radiation per unit mass at the point of interest is termed the absorbed dose. Absorbed dose (D) is defined as the quotient of E/m, where E is the energy absorbed by material of mass m:

$$D = E/m$$

The SI unit for this quantity is the gray (Gy), which is defined as the energy deposition of 1 joule/kg of material. The concept of absorbed dose applies to all categories of ionizing radiation dosimetry, to all materials, and to all forms of ionizing radiation. The traditional unit is the rad, which is defined as energy deposition of 0.01 joule/kg. Thus, 1 Gy = 100 rad.

Dose Equivalent

The dose equivalent concept originated from the observation that different biologic effects can be produced for the same absorbed dose by different types of radiation. The dose equivalent is a computed quantity that expresses a measure of the biologic harm imparted to tissue. The dose equivalent (H) at a point of interest in tissue is defined by the following equation:

$$H = DQN$$

where D is absorbed dose, Q is a modifying quantity called the quality factor, and N is the product of all other appropriate modifying factors that apply to a given situation. The quality factor concept is based on research studies that have shown that the biologic effects of ionizing radiation are not solely determined by the absorbed dose but also by the density of ionization produced along the path of the ionizing particles. A measure of the ion density along the path of an energetic particle is the particle's linear energy transfer (LET), which expresses the energy transfer per unit path length. The LET of an ionizing particle is often expressed in the units of keV/mm or keV/μ. The quality factors used for radiation safety purposes have been obtained from measurements of the relative biologic effect (RBE) of specific types of radiation as a function of the LET of the ionizing radiation. The ratio of the absorbed doses of a reference type of radiation and the type of radiation in question that produces the same biologic effect is the RBE. For example, if 20 cGy (20 rad) of x rays (250 kVp lightly filtered x radiation is generally used as the reference radiation for RBE determinations) produce the same biologic endpoint as 1 cGy (1 rad) due to neutron irradiation, the RBE of the neutron radiation is 20. Table 7-2 shows the QF dependence on LET; Table 7-3 lists QF values for several types of ionizing radiation. Although several modifying factors have been proposed, the only one commonly employed is the quality factor.

Table 7-2 Relationship between quality factor and linear energy transfer

LET (keV/μ in water)	QF
3.5 or less	1
3.5–7.0	1-2
7.0–23	2-5
23–53	5-20
53–175	10-20

Table 7-3 Quality factor values for selected types of ionizing radiation

Type of radiation	QF
X rays, gamma rays, beta particles, and electrons	1
Thermal neutrons	5
Neutrons	20
Protons	20
Alpha particles	20

From U.S. Nuclear Regulatory Commission Title 10, Code of Federal Regulations. Part 20: Standards for protection against radiation, *Fed Reg* 56(98):23390, 1991.

The special unit of dose equivalent is the sievert (Sv). The dose equivalent in Sv is numerically equal to the absorbed dose in Gy multiplied by the appropriate modifying factors. The use of this concept is illustrated by the following example:

EXAMPLE: A radiation worker employed at a cyclotron facility incurs whole body absorbed doses of 2 cGys due to gamma radiation and 0.1 cGy due to fast neutrons. Compute the worker's whole body dose equivalent H.

$$H (cSv) = \Sigma \text{ (absorbed dose in cGy for each type of}$$
$$\text{radiation multiplied by the corresponding QF)}$$
$$= (2 \times 1) \text{ gamma radiation} + (0.1 \times 20) \text{ fast}$$
$$= 4 \text{ cSv}$$

where the symbol Σ denotes the sum of the terms described in parentheses, and the QF values are taken from Table 7-3. In traditional units the dose equivalent is the rem. This is numerically equal to the absorbed dose in rad multiplied by the quality factor. Thus, 1 Sv = 100 rem.

The example above goes beyond the medical situation. For the radiations used in a medical setting, the quality factor equals one, so the absorbed dose and dose equivalent will be equal. Further, when using traditional units, the exposure in roentgens will be approximately equal to the dose in rad to tissue at that location.

Table 7-4 Organs and weighting factors used for computing effective whole-body dose equivalent*

Organ/tissue	Weighting factor
Gonads	0.25
Breast	0.15
Red bone marrow	0.12
Lungs	0.12
Thyroid	0.03
Bone surfaces	0.03
Whole body	1.0
Remaining tissues◆	0.30

*Average for a large population consisting of persons of both sexes and all ages.
◆The factor for the remaining tissues is equally (0.06) divided among the remaining five organs or tissues having the highest doses.

EFFECTIVE DOSE EQUIVALENT

The radiation doses imparted to the various organs of the body because of either external irradiation or the presence of internal radioactivity can vary markedly depending on the type of radiation and, in the case of internal radioactivity, on the biologic characteristics of the material. The International Commission on Radiation Protection (ICRP) has introduced a quantity, the effective dose equivalent, which reflects not only specific organ doses but also the relative radiosensitivity of the organs.[9] The effective dose equivalent (H_E), is defined as

$$H_E = \Sigma w_i H_i$$

where H_i is the dose equivalent of a specified organ and w_i is the corresponding weighting factor. The weighting factor (w_i) represents the ratio of the radiation detriment resulting from a given dose equivalent to a specific organ to the detriment due to a uniform whole body dose equivalent of the same magnitude. The tissue weighting factors are based on the assumption that the health detriment associated with a given dose to a specific organ can be expressed as the product of the probability of harm and the severity of the resultant illness.

The numeric values of the weighting factors recommended by the ICRP are shown in Table 7-4. As an example of the significance of the values, it is assumed that the radiation detriment or risk of a given dose to the red bone marrow is about 12% of the corresponding risk of receiving a uniform dose of the same amount to the whole body. The attraction of the effective whole body dose equivalent is that it provides, in a single computed quantity, a measure or index of the biologic harm of radiation exposure even in those cases in which the body is not uniformly irradiated. Use of the weighting factors shown in Table 7-4 results in indices of both somatic (cancer induction) and genetic risks

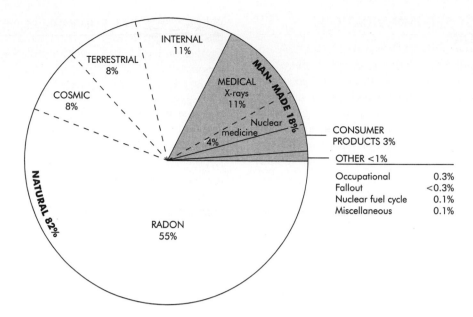

Figure 7-1   Percentage contribution of various radiation sources to the total average effective dose equivalent in the U.S. population.

associated with radiation doses. The weighting factor for the gonads can be omitted, and the resultant recalculated weighting factors can be used to compute cancer-induced risks alone. This approach yields a computed effective dose equivalent that is generally called the *somatic dose index*. For example, the somatic dose index for a diagnostic nuclear medicine procedure requiring the administration of 3 mCi of ^{99m}Tc colloid has been computed to be 1.7 mSv (170 mrem).[4] This means that the somatic radiation risk of the examination is approximately the same as that associated with a uniform whole body dose equivalent of 1.7 mSv (170 mrem).

SOURCES OF RADIATION EXPOSURE

The primary source of exposure for much of the population is what is called background radiation. Humans have always been exposed to background levels caused by the following:

1. Terrestrial radiation from the presence of naturally occurring radioactivity in the soil, primarily due to uranium and its by-products. The levels of radiation may vary significantly, depending on the location. For example, the Colorado plateau in the Rocky Mountains has higher levels of terrestrial radiation because of greater amounts of uranium.
2. Cosmic radiation that results from the interaction of particles from outer space with the atmosphere and high-energy photons from outer space. Cosmic radiation levels will be higher at a higher altitude because of less shielding from the atmosphere.
3. Internal radioactivity due to naturally occurring radioactivity deposited in the body. An example is ^{40}K, a naturally occurring isotope of potassium.

The average annual whole body radiation dose equivalent in the United States is approximately 0.82 mSv (82 mrem)/yr, varying from about 0.65 mSv (65 mrem)/yr in the Atlantic and Gulf Coast regions to about 1.4 mSv (140 mrem)/yr in the Colorado plateau. Recent estimates of the annual radiation dose to the population have also included the contribution due to radon gas. The estimated whole body dose equivalent due to radon is approximately 2 mSv (200 mrem)/yr, though the only tissue of concern is the lung.[7] Thus, the average total estimated whole body dose equivalent is 3 mSv (300 mrem)/yr, of which 1 mSv (100 mrem)/yr is due to penetrating radiations (Figure 7-1).

The only other significant source of radiation to the general population in the United States is medical radiation exposure, presumably for beneficial reasons. As shown in Table 7-5, the average per capita radiation dose equivalent due to medical radiation is approximately 0.53 mSv (53 mrem)/yr.[12] This estimate includes 0.39 mSv (39 mrem)/yr due to diagnostic x rays and 0.14 mSv (14 mrem)/yr due to use of radiopharmaceuticals.

The remaining contributors to the average per capita radiation dose equivalent are consumer products, nuclear industry, weapons testing, and perhaps of most interest, occupational exposure.[6] Although the average whole body dose equivalent for nuclear medicine personnel is estimated to be 3 mSv (300 mrem)/yr, the number of personnel is small (approximately 10,000) compared with the total population. Thus, the dose averaged over the population results in about 0.001 mSv (0.1 mrem) of the occupational exposure contribution. The total annual effective dose equivalent due to both natural and man-made sources in the United States is estimated to be 3.6 mSv (360 mrem)/yr.[12]

RADIATION DOSE RECOMMENDATIONS AND REGULATIONS

The benefits of radiation have been recognized for more than a century. The potential for harm was also recognized shortly after radiation was first used for medical and therapeutic uses. Various advisory groups exist to review the use of radiation, evaluate the risk, and make recommendations on safe use, including exposure levels for personnel and the general population. The most prominent international organization is the International Commission on Radiological Protection (ICRP). In the United States, the National Council on Radiation Protection and Measurements (NCRP), a private organization, provides radiation dose recommendations that often serve as the basis for adoption by regulatory agencies.

Regulations for use of radioactive materials and radiation exposure are enforced by a number of federal and state agencies, primarily the Nuclear Regulatory Commission (NRC). This agency is charged by Congress to regulate the use of by-product radioactive materials. This is accomplished either directly or, in many states, indirectly. In "agreement states" the NRC delegates the authority for regulation to the state with the proviso that state regulations may not conflict with federal regulations. In agreement states the regulations extend to use of all radioactive materials, because these states are not restricted to use of by-product materials.

Other agencies that regulate various portions of the medical use of radioactive materials are the Food and Drug Administration (FDA), Department of Transportation (DOT), Environmental Protection Agency (EPA), and Occupational Safety and Health Administration (OSHA). However, it is the regulations of the NRC with which the worker in nuclear medicine must be familiar.

The NCRP provides recommendations for radiation workers and for areas with sources of radiation that result in exposure to the general population.[16] The current recommendations are shown in Table 7-6. The current federal regulations for radiation workers due to occupational exposure are shown in Table 7-7. These reflect the regulations that were implemented by the NRC in January of 1994.[22] These regulatory and recommended limits are just for external and internal occupational exposure and exclude background level radiation and personal medical exposure.

Table 7-5	Annual effective dose equivalent in the United States population

Source	Dose (mSv)	% of total
Natural sources		
Radon	2.0	55
Other	1.0	27
Medical		
Diagnostic x rays	0.39	11
Radiopharmaceuticals	0.14	4
Occupational	**0.009**	**0.3**
Consumer products	**0.05-0.13**	**2.0**
Nuclear industry		
weapons testing research, etc.	0.0011	1.0
ROUNDED TOTALS	3.6	100

From Ionizing radiation exposure of the population of the United States, *National Council of Radiation Protection Report No. 93,* Washington, DC, 1987, The Council.

Table 7-6	Dose-limiting recommendations of the National Council on Radiation Protection

Category of recommendation	Recommended effective dose equivalent
Occupation exposure	
Whole body (prospective)	50 mSv (5 rem) in any 1 year
Skin	500 mSv (50 rem) in any 1 year
Hands	750 mSv (75 rem) in any 1 year
Forearms	300 mSv (30 rem) in any 1 year
Other organs, tissues, and organ systems	150 mSv (15 rem) in any 1 year
Fetus of radiation worker	5 mSv (0.5 rem) in gestation period
General public or occasionally exposed individuals	
Individual (whole body)	Up to 5 mSv (0.5 rem) in any 1 year
Average to population (genetic and somatic)	1.7 mSv (0.17 rem) in any 1 year
Students (whole body)	1 mSv (0.1 rem) in any 1 year

Modified from National Council of Radiation Protection: Recommendations on limits for exposure to ionizing radiation. In *National Council of Radiation Protection report no. 91,* Washington, DC, 1987, The Council.

ALARA

The NRC requires that licensees, including those in agreement states, make every reasonable effort to keep radiation exposures and regulated releases of radioactive materials as low as reasonably achievable. This philosophy of "as low as reasonably achievable" is the basis of the acronym ALARA. A statement signed by the institution administrator who has authority to commit funds must be submitted as part of a license. This commitment is meant to ensure that resources will be allocated to implement policies and procedures that minimize occupational exposure. It is the belief of the NRC that medical occupational exposures can be maintained at values of 10% or less of the limits given in the federal regulations.[5,11,19]

PATIENT DOSIMETRY

The amount of activity used for patient studies also results in an absorbed dose. The consideration of what constitutes an acceptable dose for clinical studies is different in that patients receive a benefit from the study via the information provided to the referring physician.

The absorbed dose received depends on the type of radioactivity, the amount of activity administered, the distribution, amount of time in each organ, and the physical relationship to other organs. A straightforward method for calculating the dose has been developed called the Medical Internal Radiation Dose Committee (MIRD) system. However, in day-to-day operations it is rare that such a dose calculation is needed. In most cases a quick estimate of the dose to one or more organs will suffice. The radiopharmaceutical package insert contains a table that gives doses for the "average" patient as a function of administered activity. A simple calculation using this table and the activity administered provides the approximate dose, which may have been requested by the clinician or patient. In cases where a more accurate dose calculation is required, a medical physicist is often consulted.

RADIATION SAFETY AND LABORATORY INSTRUMENTATION

Instruments used in the Radiation Safety Program are designed to allow detection ranging from extremely small amounts of activity associated with wipe tests to the much higher levels of exposure rates around generators or patients containing therapeutic amounts of radioactivity. To meet these requirements a variety of instruments are required.

Survey Instruments

Geiger-Mueller (GM) instruments. A portable survey meter using a GM tube is used for area surveys for contamination. The GM tube (see Chapter 3) provides high gas amplification, resulting in an ability to detect individual ionizing events. The GM meter is operated to display the rate at which the individual events are detected, usually using a ratemeter, which is calibrated in counts per minute (cpm). This simplicity of design results in an instrument that is inexpensive and reliable.

The GM probe consists of a gas-filled tube with a metal housing. Usually, one section of the housing is replaced with a thin window, such as mica, which is covered with a removable cap, often plastic. With the cap removed, all except the lowest energy beta particles (e.g., ^{3}H) are able to penetrate the thin window and are readily detected. With the cap in place, only higher-energy beta particles and x rays and gamma rays penetrate. A typical commercial meter is shown in Figure 7-2, *A*.

A GM meter is not the best instrument for measuring exposure rates. GM meters are often energy dependent and also have a large dead time, resulting in significant loss at high count rates. However, it is possible to calibrate a GM meter in mR/hr with a calibration source of an energy comparable to the energy of radiations that will be monitored. The unit must be calibrated at least annually and in accordance with license requirements. At calibration the count rate or exposure reading from a check source, usually attached to the side of the meter, is recorded on a label attached to the meter. Before each use of the meter, a reading of the check source must be obtained to ensure proper operation.

Ionization chamber instruments. Survey instruments operated in the ionization region of the gas amplification curve are designed to measure radiation exposure or exposure rate. These instruments operate in the current mode rather than pulse mode, and so require the detection of a large number of events. Survey meters are unable to detect very small amounts of activity, such as with contamination. Adequate sensitivity for low exposure levels is obtained by using a rather large air-filled chamber (Figure 7-2, *B*). Ionization survey meters may be used to measure high expo-

Table 7-7	Federal dose limits for occupational exposure of radiation workers

Dose category	Dose equivalent limit per calendar quarter (13 weeks), except for fetus
Whole body, head and trunk, active blood forming organs, lenses of the eyes, gonads	12.5 mSv (1.25 rem)
Hands, forearms, feet, and ankles	187.5 mSv (18.75 rem)
Skin of whole body	75 mSv (7.50 rem)
Fetus of radiation worker	5 mSv (0.5 rem) during entire gestation period

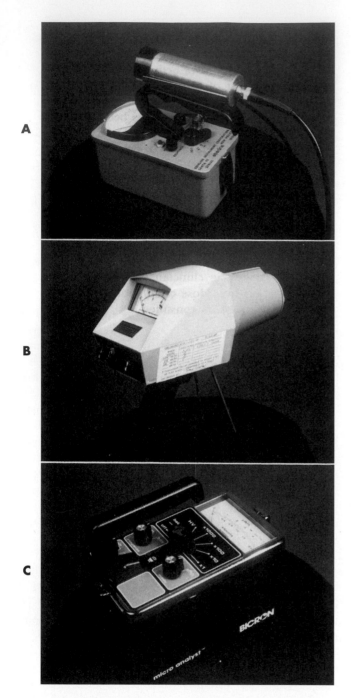

Figure 7-2 Variety of portable radiation survey instruments. **A,** Geiger-Muller (GM) device with an end window probe. **B,** Ionization chamber-based instrument of the "cutie pie" design. **C,** Scintillation detector (NaI) survey instrument.

sure rates accurately and should be used when surveying a large source of radioactivity, such as a generator, or a patient treated with a therapeutic amount of radioactive iodine.

Portable ionization chamber instruments must also be calibrated annually and must have a check source reading obtained at calibration. The check source often is sent separately and mounted in a convenient location in the radiopharmacy when returned. As with GM meters, a reading of the check source is made before each use.

A portable ionization chamber may have a removable cap. This allows detection of the presence of higher-energy beta particles, such as those from ^{32}P or ^{89}Sr. The concept of exposure is defined only for x rays and gamma rays, however, so a measurement of beta-particle intensity is not possible.

Scintillation instruments. Scintillation detectors using a sodium iodide crystal are found as portable devices and also as fixed devices, such as well counters. As portable devices, a probe consisting of a crystal and photomultiplier tube is connected to electronics similar to that found with a GM tube. The high sensitivity of the scintillation detector makes it particularly useful for detecting very low levels of activity (Figure 7-2, *C*). For quantitative measurements, however, it is necessary to calibrate the detector with the radionuclide of interest and also to use the same geometry. A system such as this may be used, for example, in checking the thyroid of personnel who have cared for ^{131}I-therapy patients.

MEASUREMENT OF RADIOACTIVITY

Well Counter

A sodium iodide well counter is used for determination of radioactivity, usually in dpm, from wipe tests and leak tests. As described in Chapter 3, the well counter may be used to accurately quantitate very small amounts of radioactivity. With a well counter it is necessary to determine the minimum radioactivity that may be detected (MDA) for any radionuclide that will be used. The MDA will depend on the background counting statistics, counting time, and detector efficiency

$$MDA = 4.66\,\sigma_b + 3/Kt$$

where σ_b is the standard deviation of the background, K is the detector efficiency (with conversion to µCi), and t is the counting time. The conditions of the radioactive materials license require that instruments used for wipe tests be able to detect contamination of less than 0.005 µCi.

Routine quality control of the well counter should also include daily calibration with a standard, usually ^{137}Cs. The gain or high voltage at which proper calibration occurs should be recorded. A 1-minute count at a fixed window width should also be recorded. This allows monitoring for any drift in the system. Monthly, a check of the FWHM of the ^{137}Cs photopeak should be obtained. Spread in the photopeak may be, among other possibilities, indicative of degradation of the crystal. See Chapter 3 for additional discussion of testing.

Radionuclide dose calibrator. The radionuclide dose calibrator is an ionization chamber that allows assay of gamma emitters. The operation and quality control testing for a dose calibrator are described in Chapter 3 and discussed later in this chapter under Operational Radiation Safety.

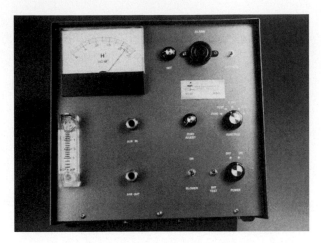

Figure 7-3 Ion chamber air sampler that provides instantaneous readings of airborne activity.

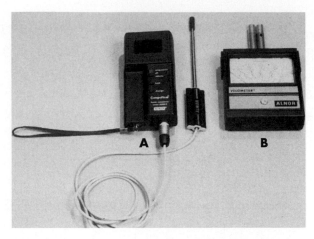

Figure 7-4 Two types of anemometers. **A,** Thermal (hot-wire) anemometer. **B,** Gravitational anemometer.

Airborne Activity Samplers

The concentration of radioactivity in air can be determined with the aid of a variety of equipment in operation; this is termed air sampling. Such methods as filtration, precipitation, and continuous measurement are used. The devices most commonly used to evaluate airborne activity levels associated with nuclear medicine procedures involving ^{133}Xe gas, labeled aerosols, ^{131}I sodium iodide, and so forth are ion chamber and filtration samplers.

Ion chamber samplers. The method most generally applicable to radioactive gases (e.g., ^{133}Xe) is to continuously draw the air to be sampled through a sensitive ion chamber. The resultant ion current produced because of the radioactivity in the air can be converted directly into the air concentration of the radionuclide. Such monitors continuously draw air through the ion chamber at a known rate, detect the radioactivity, and display the computed concentration, typically in μCi/m^3. Most radioactive gases may be monitored with this type of instrument (Figure 7-3).

Filtration samplers. The presence of either radioiodine or labeled aerosols in air can be monitored by assaying the activity deposited by air in appropriate filtering media when the air is drawn through the filters at a known rate. For example, airborne radioiodine activity is evaluated by drawing a measured quantity of air through activated charcoal filters to trap the radioiodine efficiently. The trapped activity is then assayed by counting the filter contents in a scintillation well counter of known sensitivity for the sampled radionuclide. The quotient of trapped activity to sampled air volume yields the average airborne concentration, provided the trapping efficiency is 100%. The airborne concentration of ^{99m}Tc aerosols can be evaluated by a similar method, except that laminated glass filters are used rather than activated charcoal filters.

Small, compact personal air samplers that allow the wearer to perform work without interference are commercially available. These devices consist of a pump unit in series with a filter—typically, an activated charcoal filter to trap radioiodine or a paper filter to trap radioactive particles.

Air Flow Measuring Devices

A variety of ventilation measurements must be made periodically to demonstrate that certain nuclear medicine procedures involving radioactive gases or volatiles are being performed in a safe environment. For example, the performance of fume hoods is tested by measuring the average face velocity of the air being drawn through the hood opening. Similarly, the negative pressure required of rooms in which ^{133}Xe gas is used can be established by measuring the rates of ventilation input and output. A variety of instruments are available for making such measurements. These devices, often termed *anemometers,* use either gravitational or thermal methods to measure the linear flow rate (e.g., in feet per minute) of the air movement at the point of measurement. Figure 7-4 shows a variety of anemometers. Airflow measurements are often made by the engineering or safety services staff in the institution.

PERSONNEL DOSIMETERS

Personnel exposed to ionizing radiation are monitored to determine their occupational exposure. Although this primarily consists of monitoring external exposure, it is also necessary to assess the need to monitor internal exposure and, if necessary, incorporate it into a worker's total exposure history. External monitoring can be accomplished by using a photographic film, thermoluminescent, or pocket dosimeter (Figure 7-5).

Photographic Film Dosimeters

Photographic film is sensitive to ionizing radiation, and when it is used as a monitor, the amount of film darkening is a measurement of the radiation exposure. For use as a monitor, a filmstrip in a light-tight cover is placed in a special holder. The combination of the filmstrip and the holder constitutes the film monitor, and is referred to as a film badge. This film badge has a small, open window that allows the film to be exposed with most x- ray and gamma radiations and high-energy beta radiations. The film badge also contains a set of plastic and metal filters. Because these filters will attenuate different types and energies of radiation differently, the pattern on the processed film may be used to determine the type, approximate energy, and intensity of the exposure. Because film response is energy dependent, this approximate energy determination allows use of a film energy response calibration curve. Such monitors can be used to measure exposures as low as 0.01 mSv (10 mrem) and as high as several Sv. Although limited by the large size of the film badge, the shape may be adapted so that film badges may be used to monitor the whole body, hands, wrist, and so on, depending on where the film badge is worn. Some advantages of film badges include the following:

1. *Permanent record.* The manufacturer of the film badge retains the film. If a suspicious reading is noted, the film may be reread. This is particularly useful when an employee receives an exposure that is of an energy or type of radiation that should not have been encountered, where a review of the film may indicate that the film was worn incorrectly or handled improperly.
2. *Energy and nature of exposure.* The pattern on the film may indicate the angle of exposure, whether the exposure was a series or single event, and the energy, which may be correlated with the employee's working environment.
3. *Cost.* Film badges remain the least expensive way of monitoring personnel. They are inexpensive enough

that it is possible to monitor employees who may receive little if any exposure, thus providing both reassurance and an assessment of the working environment.

There are, however, disadvantages to the use of film dosimetry, including:

1. *Energy dependence.* Because of the energy dependence, the film must be properly placed between the filters in the badge holder, or erroneously high readings will be observed. A rereading of the film will identify this if it is noted that no filter pattern is present.
2. *Fading.* Film also fades with time, so it may not be used for extended monitoring. Typically, film cannot be accurately evaluated if returned beyond 3 months.
3. *Size.* The size of film limits the ability to monitor fingers or eye level.

Thermoluminescent Dosimeters

A small semiconductor material called a thermoluminescent dosimeter (TLD) may also be used to monitor radiation exposure. When radiation interacts with a TLD, the energy is stored in the material. When heated, the energy is released as light, and the amount of light is proportional to the amount of energy stored. The TLD most commonly used for monitoring is lithium fluoride, usually found as chips that are 1/8 inch square. This size is readily incorporated into rings for finger monitoring and into plastic-encased clips or elastic bands for attachment to eyeglasses.

The advantages of a TLD are primarily its size and limited energy dependence. In addition, it is relatively insensitive to temperature and humidity and does not fade with time. Where the circumstance warrants, as in low exposure areas, TLD monitors may be used for more extensive periods, typically 3 months.

One disadvantage of TLD is that once it is heated and the reading is recorded, the only permanent record is the reading. It is not possible to reread the TLD should there be a questionable result. The signed, written record maintained by the supplier is, however, a legal document. Another disadvantage is the cost. In situations where dosimeters are exchanged monthly, the TLD is more expensive.

Pocket Dosimeters

When it is necessary to evaluate possible radiation exposure quickly, a pocket dosimeter may be used. It may be used as a second monitor in high-dose rate operations, to provide immediate information to other personnel, such as nurses, caring for therapy patients, or to evaluate possible exposure in new operations. Two general types of pocket dosimeters may be used: small ionization chambers with direct or indirect read and compact GM-based digital dosimeters.

Pocket ionization chambers are designed to measure the ionization events within an air-filled chamber. Both direct and indirect read chambers are constructed of a cylinder of

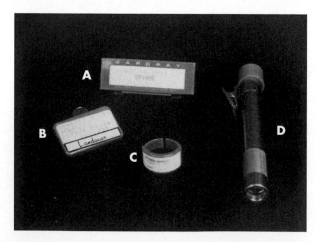

Figure 7-5 Variety of personnel monitoring devices. **A,** Photographic film badge. **B,** Thermoluminescent dosimeter body monitor. **C,** Thermoluminescent dosimeter ring monitor. **D,** Pocket ionization chamber dosimeter.

metal (Figure 7-5, *D*). Direct read chambers operate on the principle of an electroscope. Exposure to radiation results in discharge of the chamber, which may be seen by looking through the chamber and viewing the position of a hairline on a scale. With indirect read chambers, it is necessary to use a special reader to determine the exposure. This type of dosimeter is subject to erroneous readings due to electrical leakage and being hit or dropped. They are also not accurate for extended exposures.

Digital dosimeters that use a GM tube have features that make them particularly useful (Figure 7-6). The exposure and/or exposure rate may be provided on a digital display, allowing simple evaluation of the radiation field. Many have audible signals, emitting chirps at a frequency proportional to the intensity of the radiation. The units are small, easily fitting into a pocket or clipped onto a belt. They are not subject to erroneous readings due to physical conditions or rough handling by personnel.

PERSONNEL MONITORING

Personnel who are working in areas where there is a reasonable likelihood of receiving a measurable exposure to radiation should be issued personnel dosimeters. The conditions of the radioactive materials license require that dosimeters be issued to personnel who could receive in excess of 10% of the occupational limit (i.e., 500 mrem/yr).[22]

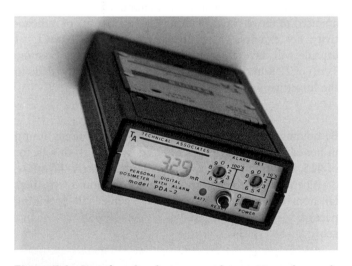

Figure 7-6 Digital pocket dosimeter with numeric readout and adjustments for audio alarm.

Many workers are unlikely to receive such a radiation exposure but should be monitored to demonstrate compliance with institutional ALARA goals, to provide useful information to employees regarding their working environment, and to provide data for the Radiation Safety Officer (RSO) to assess any changes in the working environment.

The primary monitor that is issued should be worn between the neck and waist to monitor the whole body exposure. A film badge is often used for personnel monitoring. The whole body badge monitors exposure to the trunk. Film badges are usually exchanged monthly, though a more frequent cycle is possible. In addition to the whole body badge, monitors for the hands are issued to workers handling radioactive materials. Ring badges containing a TLD chip are often used for this. The ring badge is worn with the sensitive material facing toward the palm of the hand, on the hand that is likely to receive the highest exposure. Furthermore, the ring badge is worn under protective gloves to prevent accidental contamination of the ring that does not reflect exposure to the skin and hand.

The reports that provide the results of personnel monitoring should be reviewed and initialed when received by the RSO. Any unusual exposures should be promptly investigated (Table 7-8). If the exposure exceeds ALARA Level I, it is necessary to evaluate the cause. If the exposure exceeds ALARA Level II, the employee must be notified in writing and an explanation must be generated and corrective action proposed. A summary report of personnel monitoring, giving any Level I or II exposures, should be included in the quarterly Radiation Safety Committee (RSC) meeting. Depending on the size of the institution, either the original or a duplicate report should be posted for personnel to review and initial. Records of personnel monitoring must be maintained as permanent records.

For the pregnant worker, other conditions may exist. As soon as a worker learns she is pregnant, she should notify her supervisor and the RSO. The pregnant employee should read the information on the risks of radiation in pregnancy as contained in USNRC Regulatory Guide 8.13 *Instruction Concerning Prenatal Radiation Exposure, Rev. 3, 1999*. As a "declared pregnant worker" she will be asked to sign a statement that she is pregnant and has been informed of the risks. The exposure limits are 500 mrem to the fetus during gestation. This is monitored by a separate badge, which should be worn at the abdomen. To provide quicker feedback on exposure, this badge may be exchanged more frequently

Table 7-8	ALARA investigation levels example reporting levels and timelines		
	Immediately	**24 hours**	**30 days**
Eye	75 rem/event	15 rem/event	15 rem/year
Skin or extremity	250 rem/event	50 rem/event	50 rem/year
Single organ	No criteria	No criteria	50 rem/year
Total body	25 rem/event	5 rem/event	5 rem/year

- Do not eat, drink, smoke, or apply cosmetics where radioactive material is stored or used.
- Do not store food or drink where radioactive material is stored or used.
- Wear personnel monitoring devices correctly.
- Dispose of radioactive waste in designated receptacles.
- Never pipette by mouth.
- Conduct surveys and wipe tests as required.
- Keep flood sources and other radioactive materials in shielded, labeled containers.
- Assay each patient dose before administration.
- Use a cart or wheelchair to move large sources.

Other aspects of initial and annual training should include a review of the license conditions, rights of radiation workers as given in *Form NRC-3 Notice to Employees* (Figure 7-8), emergency procedures, personnel monitoring reports, and radiation safety procedures specific to the institution. A written record of training, including the date of the training and a legible list of attendees, must be maintained.

Control of Radioactive Materials

Ordering and receiving. All radioactive materials that are ordered must be listed on the radioactive materials license and must not exceed any limits given on the license. To meet this requirement the RSO must review radioactive materials orders. Generally, standing orders for general use must be reviewed annually, whereas "special" orders should be reviewed on a case-by-case basis. In addition, manufacturers or commercial radiopharmacies must keep a copy of the license on file and should check that materials ordered are approved on the license.

Procedures for receiving radioactive materials should detail how the delivery will reach the nuclear medicine pharmacy. If packages are received at a loading dock, personnel working in that area must be trained on safe handling techniques, including the need for visual checks of packages and procedures to follow if a package is damaged. Packages received after hours must be delivered to a designated location. Typically that location will have a locked, possibly shielded storage space, or a protocol will be in place for security personnel to deliver the package to the radiopharmacy. Again, it is necessary for security personnel to be

trained in radiation safety techniques. The most straightforward situation exists where a commercial radiopharmacy delivers radioactive material directly to the nuclear medicine department. Often this eliminates transport by security or distribution personnel.

Opening packages. Radioactive materials received in the nuclear medicine department must be checked in within 3 hours during normal working hours and, if any are received at other times, as soon as the department reopens. This check should consist of donning disposable gloves to conduct a visual inspection of the package. If there is any evidence of damage or wetness, indicating leakage, the package should be immediately secured and the RSO should be notified. Next, all packages requiring White I, Yellow II, or Yellow III Department of Transportation labels must be wipe tested when received. The wipe should cover 300 cm^2 of the package surface area. The amount of radioactivity measured should not exceed 22 dpm/cm^2 for beta and gamma radiations and 2.2 dpm/cm^2 for alpha material. The package should then be opened, and a second visual check should be made to ensure that the contents are what was indicated on the packing slip and that there is no damage. Indications of damage would be breakage, less liquid than expected, or discoloration of the packing material. If indications of damage are observed, the package should be secured and the RSO should be contacted. Finally, the contents should be removed and the empty shipping package should be surveyed for contamination with a low-range GM meter. Before disposal, all radioactive symbols must be defaced. During all these steps, good radiation safety practices should be used, such as wearing disposable gloves and using tongs to move the source. Records of receipt of the material and the findings of the wipe test must be maintained.

Dose calibrator testing. The dose calibrator, used to assay doses of prepared radiopharmaceuticals, must be tested to verify proper function. The required tests and frequency are listed in Table 7-10.

These tests (see Chapter 3) will ensure that an assay is accurate and reproducible. On installation and then annually, certified standards should be assayed to test for accuracy of the unit. The recorded radioactivity must be within 10% of the limits of the National Institute of Standards and

Table 7-10	Dose calibrator tests	
Test	**Test frequency**
Accuracy test using two or more standards of certified radioactivity.	At installation, at least annually thereafter.
Linearity tests through the range of radioactivities assayed.	At installation, at least quarterly thereafter.
Geometric or volume-of-source dependence evaluation for each of the source configurations used.	At installation, before implementation of new source configurations.
Constancy-of-response tests using a long-lived reference source.	Once each day of use before use.

UNITED STATES NUCLEAR REGULATORY COMMISSION
Washington, D.C. 20555

NOTICE TO EMPLOYEES

STANDARDS FOR PROTECTION AGAINST RADIATION (PART 20); NOTICES, INSTRUCTIONS AND REPORTS TO WORKERS; INSPECTIONS (PART 19); EMPLOYEE PROTECTION

WHAT IS THE NUCLEAR REGULATORY COMMISSION?

The Nuclear Regulatory Commission is an independent Federal regulatory agency responsible for licensing and inspecting nuclear power plants and other commercial uses of radioactive materials.

WHAT DOES THE NRC DO?

The NRC's primary responsibility is to ensure that workers and the public are protected from unnecessary or excessive exposure to radiation and that nuclear facilities including power plants are constructed to high quality standards and operated in a safe manner. The NRC does this by establishing requirements in Title 10 of the Code of Federal Regulations (10 CFR) and in licenses issued to nuclear users.

WHAT RESPONSIBILITY DOES MY EMPLOYER HAVE?

Any company that conducts activities licensed by the NRC must comply with the NRC's requirements. If a company violates NRC requirements, it can be fined or have its license modified, suspended or revoked.

Your employer must tell you which NRC radiation requirements apply to your work and must post NRC Notices of Violation involving radiological working conditions.

WHAT IS MY RESPONSIBILITY?

For your own protection and the protection of your co-workers, you should know how NRC requirements relate to your work and should obey them. If you observe violations of the requirements, you should report them.

HOW DO I REPORT VIOLATIONS?

If you believe that violations of NRC rules or of the terms of the license have occurred, you should report them immediately to your supervisor. If you believe that adequate corrective action is not being taken, you may report this to an NRC inspector or the nearest NRC Regional Office.

WHAT IF I WORK IN A RADIATION AREA?

If you work with radioactive materials or in a radiation (controlled) area, the amount of radiation exposure that you may legally receive is limited by NRC Regulations. The limits on your exposure are contained in sections 20.101, 20.103, and 20.104 of Title 10 of the Code of Federal Regulations (10 CFR 20). While those are the maximum allowable limits, your employer should also keep your radiation exposure as far below those limits as is "reasonably achievable."

MAY I GET A RECORD OF MY RADIATION EXPOSURE?

Yes. Your employer is required to tell you, in writing, if you receive any radiation exposure above the limits set in the NRC regulations or your employer's license. In addition, if your job involves radiation, you may request from your employer a record of your annual radiation exposures and a written report of your total exposure when you leave your job.

HOW ARE VIOLATIONS OF NRC REQUIREMENTS IDENTIFIED?

NRC conducts regular inspections at licensed facilities to assure compliance with NRC requirements. In addition, your employer and site contractors conduct their own inspections to assure compliance. All inspectors are protected by Federal law. Interference with them may result in criminal prosecution for a Federal offense.

MAY I TALK WITH AN NRC INSPECTOR?

Yes. Your employer may not prevent you from talking with an NRC inspector and you may talk privately with an inspector and request that your identity remain confidential.

UNITED STATES NUCLEAR REGULATORY
COMMISSION REGIONAL OFFICE LOCATIONS

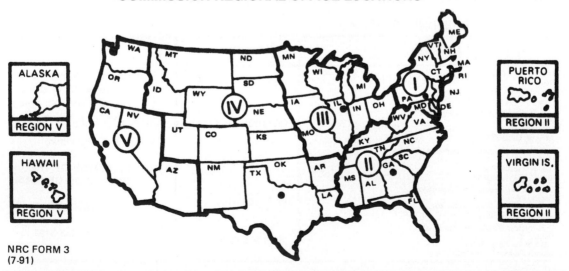

NRC FORM 3
(7-91)

Figure 7-8 U.S. Nuclear Regulatory Commission radiation protection standards *Notice to Employees.*

MAY I REQUEST AN INSPECTION?

If you believe that your employer has not corrected violations involving radiological working conditions, you may request an inspection. Your request should be addressed to the nearest NRC Regional Office and must describe the alleged violation in detail. It must be signed by you or your representative.

HOW DO I CONTACT THE NRC?

Notify an NRC inspector on-site or call the nearest NRC Regional office collect. NRC inspectors want to talk to you if you are worried about radiation safety or other aspects of licensed activities, such as the quality of construction or operations at your plant.

CAN I BE FIRED FOR TALKING TO THE NRC?

No. Federal law prohibits an employer from firing or otherwise discriminating against a worker for bringing safety concerns to the attention of the NRC. You may not be fired or discriminated against because you:

- ask the NRC to enforce its rules against your employer;
- testify in an NRC proceeding;

- provide information or are about to provide information to the NRC about violations of requirements;
- are about to ask for or testify, help, or take part in an NRC proceeding.

WHAT FORMS OF DISCRIMINATION ARE PROHIBITED?

No employer may fire you or discriminate against you with respect to pay, benefits, or working conditions because you help the NRC.

HOW AM I PROTECTED FROM DISCRIMINATION?

If you believe that you have been discriminated against for bringing safety concerns to the NRC, you may file a complaint with the U.S. Department of Labor. Your complaint must describe the firing or discrimination and must be filed within 30 days of the occurrence.

Send complaints to:

Office of the Administrator
Wage and Hour Division
Employment Standards Administration
Room S3502
U.S. Department of Labor
200 Constitution Avenue, NW
Washington, DC 20210

or any local office of the Department of Labor, Wage and Hour Division. Check your telephone directory under U.S. Government listings.

WHAT CAN THE LABOR DEPARTMENT DO?

The Department of Labor will notify the employer that a complaint has been filed and will investigate the case.

If the Department of Labor finds that your employer has unlawfully discriminated against you, it may order you to be reinstated, receive back pay, or be compensated for any injury suffered as a result of the discrimination.

WHAT WILL THE NRC DO?

The NRC may assist the Department of Labor in its investigation. NRC may conduct its own investigation where necessary to determine whether unlawful discrimination has prevented the free flow of information to the Commission. Also, if the NRC or Department of Labor finds that unlawful discrimination has occurred, the NRC may issue a Notice of Violation to your employer, impose a fine, or suspend, modify, or revoke your employer's NRC license.

A representative of the Nuclear Regulatory Commission can be contacted at the following addresses and telephone numbers. The Regional Office will accept collect telephone calls from employees who wish to register complaints or concerns about radiological working conditions or other matters regarding compliance with Commission rules and regulations.

Regional Offices

REGION	ADDRESS	TELEPHONE
I	U.S. Nuclear Regulatory Commission Region I 475 Allendale Road King of Prussia, PA 19406-1415	(215) 337-5000
II	U.S. Nuclear Regulatory Commission Region II 101 Marietta St., N.W., Suite 2900 Atlanta, GA 30323	(404) 331-4503
III	U.S. Nuclear Regulatory Commission Region III 799 Roosevelt Road Glen Ellyn, IL 60137	(708) 790-5500
IV	U.S. Nuclear Regulatory Commission Region IV 611 Ryan Plaza Drive, Suite 400 Arlington, TX 76011-8064	(817) 860-8100
V	U.S. Nuclear Regulatory Commission Region V 1450 Maria Lane, Suite 210 Walnut Creek, CA 94596-5368	(510) 975-0200

To report incidents involving fraud, waste or abuse by an NRC employee or NRC contractor,

telephone:

OFFICE OF THE INSPECTOR GENERAL

HOTLINE

1-800-233-3497

Figure 7-8   U.S. Nuclear Regulatory Commission radiation protection standards *Notice to Employees.*—cont'd

Technology (NIST) for traceable certified radioactivity. Also on installation, the variation in recorded radioactivity with geometry should be evaluated. Keeping the radioactivity constant, the volume in a vial and also in a syringe will be varied, and the reading should be noted. The variation between the standard vial reading and a syringe reading should also be determined. The linearity should be tested quarterly to ensure that readings are accurate for the range of radioactivities that are assayed. Finally, before patient doses are assayed each day, the constancy of response should be checked using a long-lived source, such as ^{137}Cs. For this test the most commonly used setting, usually ^{99m}Tc, should be checked daily, and other commonly used settings should be checked weekly. A schedule of the required times for the other tests should be placed in a conspicuous place on the calibrator. The results of testing should be reviewed and signed by the RSO.

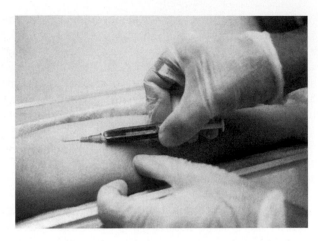

Figure 7-9 Proper technique for administration of radiopharmaceutical.

Radionuclide generator testing. Each eluate of a ^{99}Mo/^{99m}Tc generator must be tested to determine the contamination levels of the parent radionuclide, ^{99}Mo. The maximum contamination level that is acceptable for human administration is 0.15 μCi of ^{99}Mo per mCi of ^{99m}Tc. This level must not be exceeded during the shelf life of a prepared radiopharmaceutical (e.g., 6 hours after preparation). The molybdenum radioactivity is usually determined by placing the eluate vial in a specially designed lead holder that attenuates effectively all the lower-energy ^{99m}Tc photons, while allowing transmission of some percentage of the higher energy ^{99}Mo photons. The total radioactivity of molybdenum should then be determined; the method used depends on the calibrator used. The concentration must be calculated, and the acceptability of the eluate must be verified. A record of the radioactivity of ^{99m}Tc and of ^{99}Mo; the ratio, time, and date of measurement; and the name of the person conducting the test must be maintained. The procedure manual should contain a description of the method used for molybdenum contamination. A list of authorized personnel trained in the procedure should be maintained.

Measurement and records of radiopharmaceutical use. Before administration, each patient dose must be assayed. For beta emitters, such as ^{89}Sr, this may be done by measurements and calculations or by obtaining the dose in unit form from an approved manufacturer or preparer. Records must be maintained that include identification of the radiopharmaceutical, identification of the patient, the results of the assay, the date and time of the assay, and identification of the individual preparing the dose. In addition, the syringe must be labeled to identify its contents and either its use (i.e., the clinical procedure) or the patient. This labeling is an important way of preventing administration of the wrong radiopharmaceutical, particularly in departments where more than one technologist may handle the dose.

Administration of patient dose. Syringe shields in sizes to fit the syringes used must be available in the department for use in the preparation and administration of radiopharmaceuticals. If possible, each technologist should have a syringe shield in the most commonly used size. Use of syringe shields significantly reduces exposure to the hands and eyes and should be used at all times. Disposable gloves must also be worn. These serve two purposes: protecting the hands from radioactive contamination and serving as a barrier to infectious diseases (Figure 7-9).

Infection control procedures, as required by the OSHA Laboratory Standards Act, also require methods to prevent infectious diseases from needle sticks. Needles used for patient injections must not be recapped by hand. Many departments use needle boxes for immediate, safe disposal.

Daily and weekly surveys for exposure and contamination. Area surveys for external radiation exposure levels and removable contamination must be performed regularly in all areas of the nuclear medicine department.

At the end of each day that radioactive materials are used, a survey of external exposure levels must be performed. This includes weekends or holidays when a procedure is performed on call. All areas where radioactive materials have been prepared or used, radiopharmacy lab, injection room, and applicable imaging rooms, must be surveyed, and the results must be recorded. A portable survey instrument, either an ionization chamber or a wide-range GM meter or both, with a range of 0.1 mR/hr to 1 R/hr, should be used. The readings should be recorded in mR/hr. A background level reading in an area known to be free of radiation should also be recorded. Action levels, which are typically two or three times the average levels for that area, should be established. If a reading exceeds the action level, corrective action, such as checking that all sources are in lead storage or removing a flood source from a room, must be taken, and the action taken should be recorded on the survey form. A survey of all wastebaskets may prevent contaminated materials from being disposed of via this route.

Surveys to detect removable contamination must be performed weekly. A wipe should be made with a filter paper disk or cotton swab over an area 10 cm × 10 cm on designated areas. These areas should be where it is more likely that contamination will be found, such as the floor near the camera or treadmill, work surfaces, and telephones. Wipes should be performed in each area of use. The wipes should then be counted in a well counter. Wipe test results in counts per minute should then be converted to disintegrations per minute, using the counting efficiency that has been determined for the counter. Results should be recorded in dpm/100 cm². Action levels must also be established for wipe test results. If an area exceeds 200 dpm/100 cm², decontamination must be performed[21] and the area must be wipe tested again. Action levels for intervention by the RSO are often established so that the source of the contamination may be investigated.

Posting of Signs and Notices

Certain signs should be posted near the entrance to each room where radioactive material is used or stored to inform individuals entering the area of the presence of a potential hazard and to denote radiologic safety evaluation and control of the area. Signs commonly employed include the following:

Sign	Intended use
CAUTION RADIOACTIVE MATERIALS	To signify areas in which radioactive material is used or stored in amounts exceeding quantities specified by state and federal regulatory agencies, typically when the quantities exceed 10 times the quantity specified in Appendix C of Part 20 of the NRC regulations.[17]
CAUTION RADIATION AREA	To signify areas accessible to personnel in which a major portion of the body of a person could receive more than 5 mrem in 1 hour.
CAUTION HIGH RADIATION AREA	To denote areas accessible to personnel in which a major portion of the body of a person could receive a dose in excess of 100 mrem in any 1 hour.
CAUTION AIRBORNE RADIOACTIVITY AREA	To signify that the airborne activity level in the area may transiently exceed the restricted area limit or may exceed 0.6% of the Annual Limit of Intake (ALI) or 12 DAC hours.

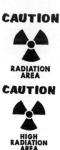

Each of these signs must bear the three-bladed symbol, which is the international warning symbol for ionizing radiation. Generally the trefoil is magenta against a yellow background.

Various other signs and notices are often posted near the entrance of or in areas where radioactive material is used or stored. These include notices to radiation workers that provide information as required by federal or state regulatory agencies, for example, the NRC *Form NRC-3 Notice to Employees* (see Figure 7-8); signs that provide instructions for the actions necessary in the case of an accident or emergency; and signs that provide the evacuation time necessary for a room in which an accidental release of gaseous activity has occurred.

CONTAMINATION CONTROL

Sealed Source Leak Tests and Inventory

Sealed sources used for dose calibrator testing and for camera quality control must be inventoried and leak tested for removable contamination. A written inventory and exposure survey of the source storage area must be performed quarterly. The inventory should be taken and the leak test should be performed every 6 months. The inventory and leak test must include all photon-emitting sources of greater than 100 µCi. A general procedure for the test is as follows:

1. Wipe the source with a dampened cotton swab or paper wipe held with forceps. Place wipe material in a marked test tube. Obtain a background level sample with the same wipe material.
2. Using a wide window, count in a well counter that is capable of detecting a minimum of .005 µCi of radioactivity.
3. Record the results. Calculate the removable radioactivity.
4. Any sealed source with more than 0.005 µCi removable radioactivity of the source material must be removed and stored. The appropriate regulatory agency must be notified.

Note that if radioactivity is detected, external contamination rather than leakage must be ruled out. If counting is done in a multichannel analyzer, there must be confirmation that the observed counts are at the photopeak of the sealed source and not a clinical nuclide.

Sources no longer in use, such as ⁵⁷Co sources too weak for the intended use, may be placed in long-term storage until disposed of. If the source is taped shut with the date recorded and a note indicating that it is not in use, a leak test is not required.

Control and Evaluation of Airborne Activity

Special efforts are required to evaluate and document that radioactive materials, which are either volatile or potentially volatile, are safely controlled. Considerations should include safety precautions that are practiced while the materials are used or stored, evaluations of concentrations of the materials breathed by workers in restricted areas, and evaluations of the airborne concentrations in applicable nonrestricted areas including points of release to the atmosphere. Such efforts are indicated not only for radioactive gases, such as ¹³³Xe, but also for dispersible materials, such as ⁹⁹ᵐTc DTPA aerosols and for materials with a volatile component, the best example of which is ^{131}I sodium iodide. The evaluations or surveys are often calculations based on certain physical measurements, that is, ventilation or discharge rates and knowledge of the quantities of materials periodically used by the nuclear medicine facility.

Storing and Using Radioactive Gases and Other Dispersible or Volatile Materials

Rooms in which gaseous radioactive material is used and the nuclear pharmacy should be maintained at a negative pressure with respect to the surrounding areas. Maintaining such an area at negative pressure means that the direction of airflow at the boundaries of the room is into the room. Thus, airborne activities generated within the room are removed by the exhaust system that maintains the negative pressure, and the activity should not, to any appreciable extent, passively diffuse into the surrounding nonrestricted areas such as corridors or waiting areas. The exhaust system serving areas in which volatile radioactive materials are used or stored should serve only those areas (a dedicated system), should provide enough ventilation to sufficiently dilute radioactivity released within the room, and should exhaust the radioactivity at release points properly located away from the general population, for example, on the rooftop of the building and away from any air intakes. Measurements should be made to demonstrate that the airflow at the boundaries of such rooms is toward the room, and measurements should be periodically made thereafter, about every 6 months, to show that the situation is unchanged.

It is important to properly store radioactive gases and volatiles. Containers of ^{133}Xe are generally stored in a fume hood so that any inadvertent leakage of activity is routed away from the immediate work area. Optimum storage of ^{131}I sodium iodide solution intended for oral administration involves several considerations. Although the fraction of the vial activity that is gaseous is kept at a low value (about 0.0001 to 0.001) by maintaining it at a basic pH, the volatile fraction can be further reduced by keeping the stored vials refrigerated and in the dark. According to manufacturers of ^{131}I sodium iodide, the basic pH minimizes the labeled I_2 species, whereas reduced temperature assists in controlling the volatile HI component. Also, when preparing the radioactivity for patient administration, it is important to minimize agitation or handling of the vial and to avoid exposure of the contents to bright light.

It is generally recommended that information be posted in imaging rooms in which ^{133}Xe is used that specifies the period of time that the room should be evacuated by personnel following an accidental release of gas within the room. A common criterion used to calculate the evacuation time is to delay reentry until the average concentration of ^{133}Xe in the room has decreased to the occupational limits specified for restricted areas. (This criterion is very conservative, because the airborne activity to which radiation workers are exposed in restricted areas may be averaged over the 520 working hours of a calendar quarter to demonstrate

compliance with the specified limit of airborne activity concentration.) Such a calculation employs the volume of room air into which the activity was released and the net ventilation rate of the room. In equation form the time of evacuation can be expressed as

$$T = (V/Q) \ln (A/CV)$$

where T is the time of evacuation in minutes, A is the released activity of ^{133}Xe in mCi, V is the room air volume in ml (1 ft^3 = 28,300 ml), Q is the net ventilation rate of the room in ml/min, and C is the airborne activity concentration limit of ^{133}Xe in the air of a restricted area (3 × 10^{-5} μCi/ml).

EXAMPLE: Compute the evacuation time that should be posted in a ^{133}Xe imaging room if the greatest radioactivity used is 30 mCi, the dimensions of the room are 10 ft × 12 ft × 8 ft, and the net ventilation rate of the room is 250 ft^3/min.

$$T = V/Q \ln (A/CV)$$

where $V = 960 \, \text{ft}^3 = 2.7 \times 10^7 \, \text{ml}$

$Q = 250 \, \text{ft}^3/\text{min} = 7.1 \times 10^6 \, \text{ml/min}$

$C = 3 \times 10^{-5} \, \mu\text{Ci/ml}$

$A = 30 \, \text{mCi} = 3 \times 10^4 \, \mu\text{Ci}$

$$T = \frac{2.7 \times 10^7 \, \text{ml}}{7.1 \times 10^6 \, \text{ml/min}}$$

$$\frac{3 \times 10^4 \, \mu\text{Ci}}{(3 \times 10^{-5} \, \mu\text{Ci/ml})(2.7 \times 10^7 \, \text{ml})}$$

$T = 3.8 \ln 37 \, \text{min}$

$T = 13.7 \, \text{min}$

Evaluation of the average concentrations of airborne activity in nonrestricted areas should also be performed and documented. The practice of maintaining rooms in which gaseous activities are used at a negative pressure with respect to the surrounding nonrestricted areas helps to ensure that the airborne levels in those areas are at acceptably low values. However, it is prudent to periodically document the low levels by conducting airborne activity surveys to measure the levels (refer to the RADIATION SAFETY and LABORATORY INSTRUMENTATION sections of this chapter for descriptions of various airborne sampling devices). Such surveys, usually conducted during representative use of the gaseous or volatile radionuclide, permit the evaluation of the peak or worst-case airborne concentration levels. If the measured peak levels are less than the nonrestricted area concentration limit for a specific radionuclide, there is compliance. If the transient peak levels are significantly higher than the nonrestricted area limit, however, a calculation should be made over an extended time—from a month to a year—to demonstrate that the time-averaged concentration is less than the applicable limit.

A special case is the evaluation of the average concentration at the site where a ventilation system serving a gaseous activity use area, such as a ^{133}Xe imaging room, releases the air to the atmosphere. For the release site to be a nonrestricted area the average airborne activity of the exhaust must be less than the nonrestricted area limit for the radionuclide under consideration. Calculation of the average concentration requires knowledge of the discharge rate of the exhaust and the activity released from the site in a given period. The following example illustrates such a calculation.

A room used for ^{133}Xe examinations has a continuously operating ventilation system whose measured discharge rate is 2000 ft^3/min, and it is assumed that all the administered activity for an average patient workload of 12 examinations per week is released from the ventilation exhaust. If the average administered activity is 10 mCi per patient, show that the average concentration at the release point, based on a representative week, is less than the USNRC limit for ^{133}Xe in the air of a nonrestricted area, 3×10^{-7} µCi/ml (a useful conversion factor is 28,300 ml/ft^3).

The total estimated release of activity per week is

$$(12 \text{ patients/wk})(10 \text{ mCi/patient}) =$$
$$120 \text{ mCi/wk} = 1.2 \times 10^5 \text{ µCi/wk}$$

The total volume of air released per week is

$$(2000 \text{ ft}^3/\text{min})(10,080 \text{ min/wk})(28,300 \text{ ml/ft}^3) =$$
$$5.7 \times 10^{11} \text{ ml/wk}$$

The average concentration for the week is then

$$c = \frac{1.2 \times 10^5 \text{ µCi / wk}}{5.7 \times 10^{11} \text{ ml / wk}} = 2.1 \times 10^{-7} \text{ µCi / ml}$$

The computed average in this example represents 70% of the NRC limit. Thus, although such a situation satisfies the commission's regulation, it provides a small margin of safety and does not fulfill the ALARA goal of licensees' voluntarily reducing environmental releases to 10% or less of the legal requirements. When results indicate that air concentrations are in excess of the desired level, several corrective actions can be taken. These include increasing the discharge rate, decreasing the released activity by using activated charcoal filters to trap most of the radioactive xenon, and considering the location of the exhaust (e.g., on a rooftop) as a restricted area. However, the last approach is often operationally burdensome—the boundary of the restricted area must be clearly established and posted—and access to the location must be restricted.

When charcoal filters are used to reduce the concentration released to the atmosphere, the user must be able to demonstrate that the filters are effective and are performing as assumed. Measurements to determine the trapping efficiency and whether a filter has become saturated should be periodically performed.

Spills and Accidents

With even the most careful attention to radiation safety procedures, it is possible for an accident to occur, usually a spill. Because this may also include personnel contamination, procedures for handling personnel and area control and decontamination must be posted in any area where unsealed radioactive material is routinely handled. If there is a possibility that a spill could occur resulting in an immediate room shutdown, the procedure should be posted in more than one location.

A procedure to handle a radioactive spill should include the following:

1. *Clear the area.* Have anyone else in the immediate area move to a more distant location and remain there until checked for contamination. If there is any chance of shoe contamination of these people, have them remove their shoes at a boundary quickly defined as the clean area. If there are noncontaminated personnel present, ask one of them to assist.
2. *Notify* a supervisor or the RSO. The posted form must clearly list current notification numbers.
3. *Contain the spill* with absorbent paper. If the radioactive material is high activity, attempt to shield the source, if this can be done quickly.
4. *Evaluate the severity* to determine the best way to decontaminate and whether assistance from the Radiation Safety Office should be obtained.
5. *Decontaminate personnel.* Removing and bagging outer clothing, including shoes, will remove most contamination. Skin contamination is removed by gentle washing with tepid water and soap or a commercial decontaminating agent. Do not irritate or abrade the skin, which may cause absorption of the contaminant. Check the effectiveness with a low-range GM survey meter, and continue until the radiation level is at or near background. Residual radioactivity on the hands may be removed by using powder-lined gloves taped at the wrist, causing the radioactivity to be released with sweat.
6. *Decontaminate the spill area,* using personnel and radiation safety precautions appropriate for the radioactivity and type of radionuclide. For low-activity spills, immediately start using absorbent paper. Work from the outside to the center of the spill. If necessary, wash with small amounts of decontaminant, making sure that the liquid does not spread the contamination. Place all contaminated materials in a plastic bag, label it, and place it in radioactive waste. For high-activity spills with greater possibility for high exposure to personnel, it is reasonable to plan the decontamination procedure before starting, including an assessment of the exposure rate. Depending on the findings, it may be necessary to use more than one person or to allow some time for decay.
7. *Survey* using a low-range GM tube. Record the findings, noting the location and reading. When no additional contamination is removable, take wipe tests to confirm successful decontamination. Record these results.
8. *Write up a report,* describing the accident and steps taken to clean up the spill.

An all too common spill may occur when injecting a patient who is being stressed on a treadmill. The radioactive material often lands on the treadmill and may also land on the patient. In this case, stop the treadmill, have the patient step off (if possible onto a towel or absorbent paper), and contain the radioactivity. Have the patient step out of his or her shoes to a clean area, and decontaminate the skin if necessary. Decontaminate the treadmill as much as possible. If any radioactivity remains, as often happens, have patients wear booties until no radioactivity is detectable on the treadmill.

Radioactive Waste Disposal

The objective of radioactive waste management is to prevent human contact with concentrations of material or radiation levels significantly above background level. Most of the waste material generated in nuclear medicine may be disposed of by holding the material in storage for extensive decay, diluting and dispersing the material to the atmosphere or sanitary sewer system, or returning the spent material to the manufacturer or supplier. Rarely, these techniques are not appropriate, and materials are concentrated and shipped for land burial. Recommended techniques for safe disposal follow. As with all aspects of nuclear medicine, records of the disposal must be maintained by the department.

Return to manufacturer or supplier. This method is very useful for long-lived materials found in nuclear medicine. Departments using molybdenum generators may be able to return the old, partially decayed generator to the manufacturer. As part of the purchase of new long-lived sealed ^{57}Co flood source or dose calibrator constancy checks, the old source may be exchanged if it was purchased from the same manufacturer. Programs may exist where the contaminated materials used with long-lived materials, such as for ^{89}Sr therapy, may be returned. The specific requirements for such returns must be arranged in advance with the manufacturer or supplier, who will also usually supply the appropriate paperwork, copies of which are maintained by the department.

Dry waste. Most of the dry waste generated in nuclear medicine consists of items contaminated with radionuclides with relatively short physical half-lives. Radioactive waste with half-lives of 60 days or less may be stored for extensive decay before disposing of the material. State and federal regulatory authorities permit the disposal of short-lived radionuclides by decay-in-storage programs. The material is held in storage a minimum of 10 half-lives and then is carefully monitored with an appropriate survey instrument of good sensitivity. If the survey indicates that the material has decayed to less than two times background levels, it may then be transferred to the appropriate regular trash for disposal (e.g., needle containers to biohazard waste). Before disposing of the material, all radiation signs and symbols must be obliterated or defaced. This is most easily and safely accomplished as the item is placed in waste, so that it is not necessary to later go through a waste bag. The radionuclides

for which decay is used are usually separated by half-lives to minimize the time shorter half-lived material must be stored and therefore the space required for decay in storage.

Long-lived materials, usually found only in research programs, may require the material to be shipped to a federally approved low-level radioactive material land burial site. Waste materials shipped for disposal must be properly packaged and labeled according to U.S. Department of Transportation requirements. A number of commercial companies act as brokers in the handling of radioactive waste material destined for either burial or incineration.

Liquid waste. Small quantities of liquid waste that are either soluble or dispersible in water can be discharged in a designated sink to a sanitary sewer system provided the collective amounts disposed of by this method do not exceed concentrations and annual amounts specified in 10CFR20 Appendix B. The maximum permitted concentrations specified by regulatory authorities are based on the total water discharge rates of the licensee (water discharge rate can generally be assumed to be equal to the water consumption rate; hence water bills provide a record of the licensee's water discharge rates) and the released radioactivity. To demonstrate compliance with the concentration limits, the released concentrations can be averaged over extended periods, such as a month. Records of the date of disposal and the type and amount of radioactivity must be maintained by the department.

Gaseous wastes. Certain gases, principally ^{133}Xe, are often disposed of after their use by discharging them to the atmosphere. This does not apply to unused xenon, which is held for decay. This method of waste disposal is discussed in the Control and Evaluation of Airborne Activity section. An important alternative method of disposing of ^{133}Xe is to use activated charcoal to trap the gas after its use. The activated charcoal traps containing the ^{133}Xe are periodically placed in storage for an extended period to permit most of the radioactivity to decay before reuse of the filter. Several precautions are important with this method. Other gases, such as CO_2 and water vapor, compete with the xenon for trapping by the charcoal. Thus, the traps can become saturated and ineffective in trapping ^{133}Xe and should be periodically replenished with fresh charcoal.

Part 20 of Title 10 of the Code of Federal Regulations[17] defines a category of waste that can be disposed of without regard to its radioactivity, ^{3}H and ^{14}C in liquid scintillation cocktails or animals that have a concentration less than 185 Bq/g ($0.05\,\mu$Ci/g). This category of waste can be found in many hospitals and universities involved with clinical and biomedical research. It only has to be treated as hazardous waste and can be incinerated as nonradioactive.

Radiation safety audit. A review of the Radiation Safety Program should be conducted quarterly to ensure that procedures are followed. The review, which is conducted by a medical physicist or other appropriate personnel, should include a visual check of personnel safety practices and camera quality control records. The department policy and procedures and related records must be reviewed annually by a medical physicist. The results should be presented to the RSC.

PATIENT PRECAUTIONS

The radiation dose that the patient receives is considered acceptable in that the study provides needed medical information, which is a benefit. To ensure that the use of radioactivity is beneficial, procedures must be in place so that the correct patient receives the correct amount of radioactivity for an appropriate study. All studies must be properly requisitioned. When the patient arrives, his or her identity must be clearly ascertained. This may be done in a number of ways, such as by checking an in-patient wristband or asking for date of birth, which may be checked against the requisition. The radiopharmaceutical to be used must be checked, and the proper material must be selected. For example, if kits are prepared in the department, color-coding may be used so that a bone agent is not confused with pertechnetate. Before administration, the radionuclide must be assayed, the radioactivity must be compared with the recommended amount, and the syringe must be properly labeled. Last, the correct route of administration must be used, and care must be taken to prevent administration of a useless radiation dose to the patient, such as extravasation.

Additional precautions, using a written directive, must be taken for medical procedures that have a higher risk to the patient, for example, using any ^{131}I or ^{125}I procedures greater than $30\,\mu$Ci, or any other unsealed source therapy procedures such as ^{32}P or ^{89}Sr. For these procedures, a written directive must be completed by the authorized user (i.e., the nuclear medicine physician authorized for unsealed source therapy procedures). The written directive must identify the patient, the procedure, radiopharmaceutical form, and route of administration. The directive must be signed and dated. Before administration, the patient must be identified in two ways. Prior to administration by the authorized user, the material must be assayed and documentation must be provided that the radioactivity is within 10% of the prescribed amount. There must also be documentation that the administration is in accordance with the written directive, for example, by having the physician who administers the material sign the dose slip. The written documentation must be kept on file. The description of how these additional precautions will be addressed and the mechanism for review should be contained in the institution's Quality Management Program (QMP). It is a requirement of the materials license that a QMP be in place. At specified intervals (e.g., quarterly) the paperwork should be reviewed to further evaluate whether problems have occurred. The files of patients who fall into the above categories should be reviewed for accuracy and completeness during inspections by federal or state regulators.

If an error is made in dosing a patient, the incident should be documented. It must then be determined if the event is one that should be reported to the appropriate regulatory agency. Incidents that must be reported are *misadministrations*. A misadministration occurs when (1) a radiopharmaceutical other than ^{131}I or ^{125}I is administered to the wrong patient; the prescribed dose differs by more than 20% from the administered dose; or the wrong radiopharmaceutical is administered, AND the dose to the patient is greater than 5 rems effective dose equivalent or 50 rems dose equivalent to any organ, or (2) a dose of greater than $30\,\mu$Ci of ^{131}I or ^{125}I or another therapeutic dose is administered to the wrong patient; a dose is administered by the wrong route of administration; the wrong radiopharmaceutical is used; or there is more than a 20% difference between the prescribed and administered dose. In the case of a misadministration, it is necessary to notify the appropriate regulatory agency immediately. Because it is highly unlikely that a diagnostic study would meet the whole body or organ dose requirement, most misadministrations result from errors in the Quality Management Program (QMP). Another category of reporting is the *recordable event,* which is of lower severity and involves errors in the QMP. A recordable event occurs when there is no written directive for any ^{131}I or ^{125}I or therapeutic administration or when the measured dose differs from the prescribed dose by more than 10%. For these circumstances, a written record describing the event and the steps taken to prevent a reoccurrence must be maintained. Although generally not required, it is good practice to document also any incorrect administration, investigate the cause, and determine possible methods to prevent reoccurrence.

Studies of women of childbearing age also require additional precautions. Before beginning the study, the last menstrual period (LMP) must be ascertained and documented, such as on the requisition. If a woman is pregnant or late in her menstrual cycle, the nuclear medicine physician and the referring physician must decide if the study should be performed. If the study is performed, documentation of the administered radioactivity and type of study should be recorded so that the probable dose to the fetus may be calculated. If the woman is nursing, she should discontinue for a designated time following the study.

Therapeutic Procedures

Specific authorization for therapeutic procedures must be given in the radioactive materials license. Often, smaller institutions are not licensed for therapy administrations, and patients are treated at larger facilities.

Treatments with radioactive iodine typically comprise the greatest percentage of therapeutic use. Treatments under 30 mCi are usually done on an outpatient basis. This would include ^{131}I hyperthyroid treatment and some thyroid carcinoma ablations. For these procedures, few special precautions need to be taken. Because only nuclear medicine personnel are involved, the annual training is adequate. The

Table 7-11	^{131}I Patient discharge instructions

A time interval (usually 3–7 days) should be specified for each instruction depending on the patient's household

	Days
Try to keep the time you spend in close contact with others to a minimum.	_____
Minimize the time spent with young children or pregnant women.	_____
Sleep alone if possible.	_____
Practice good hygiene habits; wash your hands after each toilet use.	_____
Drink plenty of liquids.	_____
Use separate bath linens; wash these linens and your underclothing separately from other laundry.	_____
Use separate (or disposable) eating utensils.	_____
Discuss with your physician how long after treatment you should wait to try to become pregnant.	_____

documentation required for the QMP must be accurate and complete. The iodine is often given as a capsule, minimizing the possibility of volatilization or a spill. The patient may leave immediately with discharge instructions as shown in Table 7-11. In the event that a patient is treated while hospitalized, the precautions described below should be followed, providing a consistent Radiation Safety Policy.

For treatments of greater than 30 mCi, hospitalization is required for regulatory purposes. Because these treatments often exceed 150 mCi of ^{131}I, precautions must be in place to protect personnel and members of the public from exposure during the treatment and contamination following the treatment. A room that is identified on the license must be used. The room must be designed so that any patient in adjacent areas will not receive greater than 10 mrem/yr. A large room on an outside corner often works best, particularly if a roof is above or the floor-to-floor heights are large. The room must also have a private bathroom. Before the patient is admitted, the room should be prepared so that any contamination can easily be removed. Areas that the patient is likely to touch, such as chairs, the floor, and doorknobs, should be covered with plastic or plastic-backed paper. If a phone is present in the room, it should either be covered or replaced with a phone that may be removed for decay. Disposable service should be ordered for meals so that all

contaminated materials may be surveyed and disposed of properly.

Instruction of the nursing staff is critical. These instructions must cover radiation safety principles, techniques for reduction of exposure, methods for caring for the patient, and the requirements of the QMP. For example, emphasis should be placed on the use of time and distance to reduce exposure; lead shielding at the energy of ^{131}I is only effective if it is approximately 1 in thick. Most iodine patients who must be hospitalized are self-care patients, so use of distance when talking with the patient is very effective. This instruction must be documented. Personnel caring for the patient must also be issued radiation dosimeters.

Before the patient receives the iodine, it is useful to review the precautions that he or she must take, such as staying in the room and flushing twice after using the toilet. The choice of whether the patient may have visitors is one that must be decided by the institution. It is possible, particularly with larger rooms, to mark the line behind which the exposure rate is 2 mR/hr. If the patient remains at the location for the measurement, visitors may stay behind the marked line without regard to time. Staff and visitors must not use the patient's bathroom or sink.

The iodine may be administered as a capsule(s) or liquid. It is possible to obtain the liquid in a sealed vial, which may be punctured by a long needle with a straw attached. In this way the convenience of drinking the material rather than taking many capsules is possible, and the potential for spills is almost eliminated. Any staff in the room at the time of the administration must have a thyroid bioassay. Following administration of the material, an exposure rate measurement is taken 1 meter from the patient. This serves as the baseline measurement for determination of when the radioactivity remaining is below 30 mCi. For example, if the patient receives 100 mCi and has an initial exposure rate of 25 mR/hr, the patient may be discharged when the exposure rate is below 7.5 mR/hr.

$$\frac{30\,\text{mCi}}{100\,\text{mCi}} = \frac{X\,\text{mR/hr}}{25\,\text{mR/hr}}$$

Measurements are made once or twice a day to determine when the patient is below the calculated level. The patient may then be discharged, with instructions such as given in Table 7-11.

Following discharge, it is necessary to decontaminate the room. All contaminated items are removed to waste storage. The room is then surveyed with a low-range GM meter. Any area above background level must have a wipe test and must be further decontaminated until wipes result in less than 200 dpm. All patient measurements and room surveys must be documented.

Other therapeutic procedures that may be performed are injection of ^{32}P and ^{89}Sr. These procedures are usually performed on an outpatient basis. The primary precaution during the administration of these injections is to use a thick plastic syringe shield to attenuate the beta particles. Following injection, all personnel and the room used should be surveyed with a GM meter with the end cap off, which makes the meter extremely efficient for detecting beta particles. Because some of the material will end up in the urine, the patient should be instructed to use care when urinating and flush twice. If it is necessary to treat an inpatient, any bandages that are removed following injection should be retained to determine if they are contaminated. In the case of ^{89}Sr for treatment of metastatic bone pain, many institutions only treat on an outpatient basis and further recommend that the patient be continent. For this material, the exposure rate around the patient is minimal and requires no special precautions.

BIOLOGIC EFFECTS OF IONIZING RADIATION

The radiation safety practices that have been described are intended to minimize the dose received (i.e., energy deposited) to the body due to ionizing radiation. This is necessary because biologic effects due to radiation have been observed, either directly as in the case of high, single exposures, or in some percentage of a population as in the case of somewhat lower exposures. A knowledge of these biologic effects helps to assess the risks associated with exposure to radiation.

Acute Effects

A high, single radiation exposure to all or most of the body results in acute effects (i.e., those showing rapid onset, severe symptoms, and a short course). At a minimum whole body dose of 2 Sv (200 rem), radiation sickness will be observed. Note that this results from a dose to the whole body delivered in a short time, a situation that would occur only because of a severe radiation accident. Within an hour or two of exposure, nausea, vomiting, and, at higher doses, diarrhea will be observed. Neurologic symptoms such as headache, decreased blood pressure, and fatigue are also observed. This is called the *prodromal stage*. Except with the highest doses, a *latent period* follows, during which the victim shows no visible signs and symptoms of radiation injury.

The radiation syndrome (the signs and symptoms) exhibited, depends on the whole body dose received. The dose levels given are approximate in that there is fortunately little human data. At doses of 100 Gy (10,000 rad) *cerebrovascular* damage results in death in a matter of hours. Although the exact cause of death is unknown, it appears that vascular damage results in rapid accumulation of cerebral fluid, resulting in disorientation, diarrhea, convulsions, coma, and death. At doses of a 10 Gy (1000 rad) and higher, the damage that results in death is due to damage of the *gastrointestinal* system. Following a short latent period, the victim will exhibit severe diarrhea, dehydration, loss of weight, and exhaustion. Death occurs in approximately 3 to 10 days. Death of the immature cells of the epithelial lining of the intestine, which are normally sloughed off and replaced, results in inability to absorb necessary nutrients and main-

tain body fluid balance. At doses of approximately 0.2 to 0.8 Gy (200 to 800 rads), the dose is not high enough to seriously affect the gastrointestinal tract. It is high enough to kill mitotically active precursor blood cells. It will be the *hematopoietic* system, then, that will be affected. In humans, a rather long latent period lasts a few weeks. During this time, as mature blood cells die off naturally, the supply of immature cells is inadequate for replacement. At about 3 weeks, fatigue, petechial hemorrhages, ulceration of the mouth, and bleeding may occur. More seriously, infections and fever from white blood cell depression may occur. If other symptoms are not too severe, infection may be controlled by antibiotics.

One way of expressing the lethality of a dose is the LD_{50}. This means the dose that will result in a specified endpoint, in this case death, to 50% of the population. For humans, the LD_{50} is thought to be about 3 to 3.5 Gy (300 to 350 rads) for healthy adults irradiated but with no medical intervention. With medical intervention, particularly prevention and treatment of infection, it may be possible to raise this by a factor of two.[8]

Cataract Induction

The lens of the eye differs from other organs in that dead and injured cells are not removed. Damage to the lens caused by a single dose of approximately 5 Sv (500 rem) will induce opacities that interfere with vision within a year. When the dose occurs over a protracted time, a total dose of 8 Sv (800 rem) or larger is required, and the cataract appears several years after the last exposure.[10] The 1980 BEIR report[2] concludes that cataract induction should not be a concern for the doses currently permitted radiation workers. For example, even if a worker received 0.05 Sv/yr to the eyes for a working lifetime of 40 years, (both high estimates), the lifetime dose would be 2 Sv, which is still well below the threshold.

Fertility Effects

Doses of a few Sv to the human testes can lead to permanent sterility; smaller doses cause only a temporary reduction in the number of sperm cells. A single dose of 4 Sv (400 rem) to the ovaries is required to produce permanent sterility; at 0.5 Sv (50 rem) temporary amenorrhea (SP) can occur. Occupational exposure levels will not result in fertility effects.[6]

Late Effects

Radiation has also been shown to produce effects that may occur long after the dose is received because of damage to cells that is expressed much later. If this cell is a germ cell (oocyte or sperm), damage may result as a genetic mutation. Damage to all other cells of the body, *somatic cells,* may result in leukemia or cancer in the exposed individual. These are *stochastic* effects, meaning there is a probability of occurrence that has no threshold, increases with increasing doses to the individual, but does not increase with severity as a function of the dose. For example, both a dose of 0.1 Sv (10 rem) and 1 Sv (100 rem) may cause leukemia to develop later in life, but in both cases the leukemia is the same in severity. The difference is that the probability of occurrence will be greater with the higher dose.

Knowledge of somatic late effects of radiation is based on studies of groups of people who were exposed to ionizing radiation. There have been a number of such groups, the largest of which are the survivors of the bombing of Hiroshima and Nagasaki, who have been carefully followed. Many other examples exist, often with irradiation to specific areas of the body, such as children irradiated for an enlarged thymus who developed subsequent thyroid cancer and women irradiated for pneumothorax who developed subsequent breast cancer. In all cases the dose received and the time to acquire the dose are estimated and the data plotted (Figure 7-10). Animal studies will expand the data. The data points in Figure 7-10 demonstrate the difficulty that arises in estimating the risk at low doses. Most of the data available are for high total doses and often high dose rates, defined as greater than 0.1 Gy/min. The doses of concern are at much lower doses and dose rates. It is necessary to attempt to interpret the data to develop a mathematical model that may be used to predict the response at low doses. Groups such as the National Academy of Sciences Committee on the Biological Effects of Ionizing Radiation (BEIR V) have done extensive reviews and analysis of the data. The two most common models, as shown in Figure 7-11, are the linear model (*curve 1*) and linear-quadratic model (*curve 2*). There is disagreement, however, about which model should be used for estimating risk. The most current recommendation is to use the linear model, but with the proviso that the risk at low dose rates, as found in most diagnostic situations, is a factor of two or more lower than predicted by that model.

Two additional difficulties are present in estimating late effects. A *natural incidence,* often rather large, of the cancers

and leukemia is observed,. Also, a *latent period* follows exposure before the effect is observed. Beyond the latent period, there will be an increase in the incidence of the cancer or leukemia, the *radiogenic increment* (Figure 7-10). This may increase at a constant rate with time or extend for a given number of years beyond exposure, depending on the cancer.

Organs and tissues differ greatly in their susceptibility to cancer induced by radiation. The organs most sensitive to radiation-induced carcinogenesis are the active bone marrow, thyroid, female breasts, and lungs.[13] Risk coefficients of radiation-induced malignancies are listed in Table 7-12. Because of the relatively high susceptibility of female breast and thyroid tissues, women have an overall greater somatic risk than men. Radiation-induced leukemia is better understood than other types of radiocarcinogenesis because of the natural rarity of the disease, the relative ease of its induction, and its short latent period. However, the combined risk of induced solid tumors (such as thyroid, lung, and female breast) exceeds that of leukemia. The fatal risk from all malignancies is likely to be on the order of 10^{-2}/Sv, that is, the probability of death due to a radiation-induced

Table 7-12   Risk coefficients for selected organs

Tissue	Risk coefficient (probability of biologic change per Sv)
Gonads	$40 \times 10^{-4}\,Sv^{-1}$ ($40 \times 10^{-6}\,rem^{-1}$)
Breast	$25 \times 10^{-4}\,Sv^{-1}$ ($25 \times 10^{-6}\,rem^{-1}$)
Red bone marrow	$20 \times 10^{-4}\,Sv^{-1}$ ($20 \times 10^{-6}\,rem^{-1}$)
Lung	$20 \times 10^{-4}\,Sv^{-1}$ ($20 \times 10^{-6}\,rem^{-1}$)
Thyroid	$5 \times 10^{-4}\,Sv^{-1}$ ($5 \times 10^{-6}\,rem^{-1}$)
Bone surfaces	$5 \times 10^{-4}\,Sv^{-1}$ ($5 \times 10^{-6}\,rem^{-1}$)
Remainder	$50 \times 10^{-4}\,Sv^{-1}$ ($50 \times 10^{-6}\,rem^{-1}$)
TOTAL	$165 \times 10^{-4}\,Sv^{-1}$ ($165 \times 10^{-6}\,rem^{-1}$)

From National Council of Radiation Protection: Recommendations on limits for exposure to ionizing radiation. In *National Council of Radiation Protection report no. 91,* Washington, DC, 1987, The Council.

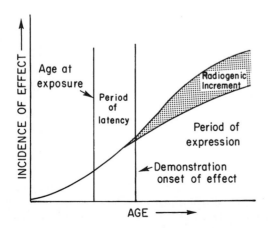

Figure 7-10   Graph illustrating the periods of latency and expression.

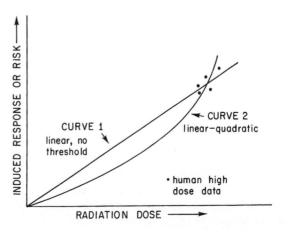

Figure 7-11   Dose response relationships.

Table 7-13 Risk coefficients for selected organs

Tissue or site	Age of exposure (years)	Years at risk*	Absolute risk coefficient[♦]	
			Male	**Female**
Leukemia	0-9	5-26	1.7	1.1
	10-19	5-26	0.85	0.54
	20–34	5-26	1.1	0.67
	50+	5-26	1.6	0.99
Lungs	10-19	10-33	0.30	0.3
	20-34	10-33	0.56	0.56
	35-49	10-33	0.86	0.86
	50+	10-33	1.2	1.2
Breast	0-9	10-35	—	3.8
	10-19	10-35	—	7.6
	20-29	10-35	—	4.9
	30-39	10-35	—	4.9
	40-49	10-35	—	1.3
	50+	10-35	—	0.8
Thyroid	0-9	10-34	1.5	5.0
	10-19	10-34	1.5	5.0
	20-34	10-34	0.5	1.5
	35-49	10-34	0.5	1.5
	50+	10-34	0.5	1.5

From Rall JE et al: *Report of the National Institutes of Health working group to develop epidemiological tables,* NIH publication no. 85-2748, Washington, DC, 1985, U.S. Government Printing Office.
*Number of excess cases of cancer per million persons per year per rem of organ dose (low-level, low-LET radiation) averaged over the specified period of expression.
♦Following the radiation exposure.

malignancy is approximately one chance in a hundred per Sv of whole body radiation dose. The ranges of fatal risk estimates are listed in Table 7-13. The risk factors shown in Table 7-13 were derived to apply to acute doses of about 10 rem or more and should not be used for doses comparable to natural background levels or even many occupational exposures. In fact, the 1980 BEIR report refuses to discuss the effects of exposures below 0.1 Sv (10 rem) and states, "Below these doses, the uncertainties of extrapolation of risk were believed by some members of the committee to be too great to justify the calculation." Accordingly, the use of the risk factors for lower doses will yield upper-limit estimates of the fatal cancer risk of radiation exposure. Incidentally, the malignancy will result in death roughly half the time. Thus the risk of cancer induced by radiation is of the order of 2×10^{-2}/Sv.

The risks due to radiation may be compared with other occupational or overall risks. The American Cancer Society[3] has reported that approximately 25% of adults in the 20- to 65-year age bracket will develop cancer at some time from all possible causes including cigarettes, food, drugs, air pollutants, and naturally occurring background level radiation. Thus, in any group of 10,000 workers not exposed to radiation on the job, about 2500 will develop cancer. If each of this entire group of 10,000 workers were to receive an occupational exposure of 10^{-2} (1 rem), the risk factor of 2×10^{-2}/Sv (2×10^{-4}/rem) would predict an additional two cases of cancer.

An interesting measure of risk is the life expectancy lost on the average because of radiation-induced cancer. It is estimated that the average loss of life expectancy due to radiation exposure is about 1 day/rem of whole body dose equivalent. Table 7-14 lists comparative loss of life expectancy attributed to selected health risks.

Another useful comparison is the relative fatal risk of certain everyday endeavors. For example, an NCRP publication[15] states that a one in a million risk of death has been attributed to each of the following:

400 miles by air
60 miles by car
3/4 of a cigarette
20 minutes of being a man of age 60
0.1 mSv (10 mrem) of whole body radiation

In conclusion, the only somatic effect thought to occur at occupationally permitted levels is cancer induction. The probability of death due to radiation-induced cancer is conservatively believed to be less than 10^{-2}/Sv (10^{-4}/rem) when applied to the situation of a few Sv received over several

Table 7-14	Estimated loss of life expectancy from selected health risks

Health risk	Estimated days of life expectancy lost, average
Smoking 20 cigarettes per day	2370
Overweight (by 20%)	985
All accidents	435
Auto accidents	200
Alcohol consumption (U.S. average)	130
Home accidents	95
Drowning	41
10 mSv (1 rem)/year for 30 years	30
Natural background radiation	8
All catastrophes (earthquakes, floods, etc.)	3.5
10 mSv (1 rem)/year occupational radiation DE	1

From U.S. Nuclear Regulatory Commission: Instruction concerning risk from occupational radiation exposure. In *Draft regulatory guide,* Washington, DC, 1980, The Commission.

years. This risk, approximately one chance in 100/Sv of whole body dose, is low when compared with the risks of fatality associated with smoking, driving, being overweight, and so on.

Genetic Effects

Radiation may also result in a genetic mutation. A mutation is an inherited change in a *gene,* a finite segment of DNA within a chromosome. Mutations are, generally speaking, *dominant* or *recessive.* Dominant genes are expressed in the first generation. Recessive genes are expressed only when matched with similar recessive genes, and so may not be expressed for a number of generations. The genetic mutations that occur are not unique. Rather, there may be an increase in the occurrence of mutations that occur naturally or spontaneously in the population.

Radiation genetic risk estimates have been derived primarily from mouse data. Large-scale human genetic studies that have been carried out to date show no significant increase in genetic endpoints with increasing dose. In particular, ongoing studies of Japanese bomb survivors have shown no statistically significant increase in five different genetic endpoints. However, based on the mouse data, there is reason to believe that humans receive radiation-induced genetic effects in a somewhat similar fashion. The current estimate of radiation-induced genetic effects is that the risk of serious genetic disorders is 6 to 35 first generation cases per 10^6 live births per 10 mSv.

The *doubling dose* is the dose of radiation that will double the spontaneous mutation rate in a biologic system. Data

from mouse studies and Japanese survivors have been used by groups such as BEIR V to estimate the doubling dose in humans. The current estimate as given in BEIR V is 1 Sv (100 rem).

Developmental Effects

At high doses of in utero exposure (single exposures greater than approximately 0.25 Sv), effects on the fetus have been observed. These effects include growth and developmental retardation, congenital abnormalities, and prenatal or neonatal death. Below this level, these effects are not observed or are at levels low enough to be indiscernible above the normal incidence of abnormalities, which is approximately 6% of live births. The effects are dose related and are also related to the time in pregnancy. The three periods of concern are *preimplantation,* which extends to roughly 10 days after conception; *organogenesis,* which extends to 7 weeks after conception; and *fetal development* through birth.

During preimplantation, radiation damage results in either death of the fertilized egg or survival with no measurable effect.[1] Outwardly, no effect would be noticed other than a failure to conceive.

Irradiation during organogenesis is the period of most concern. For this reason, it is often noted that radiation should be particularly limited "during the first trimester." The implanted egg multiplies rapidly, and differentiation occurs, with development of organ systems. The effect of radiation is to produce congenital abnormalities. In early organogenesis these may be skeletal effects, whereas in late organogenesis neurologic effects are noted. In addition, there may be some form of growth retardation due to loss of cells. Much of the information available, however, is based on studies of mice and rats, which develop at a rate that varies from humans in extent and timing. This makes it difficult to extrapolate to the expected human effect. These effects have not been observed at less than a 0.1 Sv (10 rem) dose delivered to the embryo.

After organogenesis, the fetus continues to grow and develop. Irradiation during this stage at higher doses may result in growth retardation or damage to organs. There is contradictory evidence that lower doses result in an increased incidence of leukemia.[8]

In nuclear medicine the possibility for exposure to the embryo or fetus is very small. Of particular concern is that there not be accidental exposure of the fetal thyroid due to administration of radioactive iodine. The fetal thyroid takes up iodine after the tenth week of pregnancy. Because pregnancy may be easily ascertained, any woman of childbearing age who receives radioactive sodium iodide should have pregnancy status confirmed.

REFERENCES

1. AAMP Report, College Park, MD, American Association of Physicists in Medicine.

2. Advisory Committee on the Biological Effects of Ionizing Radiations: *The effects on populations of exposure to low levels of ionizing radiation,* Washington, DC, 1980, Division of Medical Science, National Academy of Sciences, National Research Council.
3. American Cancer Society: *Cancer facts and figures,* New York, 1978, The Society.
4. Brill A, Adelstein A, Johnston R, et al, editors: *Low-level radiation effects: a fact book,* New York, 1985, Society of Nuclear Medicine.
5. Brodsky A: *Principles and practices for keeping occupational radiation exposures of medical institutions as low as reasonably achievable,* Washington, DC, 1977, U.S. Nuclear Regulatory Commission Office of Standards Development.
6. Environmental Protection Agency: *Proposed federal radiation protection guidance for occupational exposure,* Washington, DC, 1981, U.S. Environmental Protection Agency Office of Radiation Programs.
7. National Council of Radiation Protection: Exposure of the population of the United States and Canada from natural background radiation. In *National Council of Radiation Protection report no. 94,* Washington, DC, 1987, The Council.
8. Hall EJ: *Radiobiology for the radiologist,* ed 3, Philadelphia, 1978, JB Lippincott.
9. International Council of Radiation Protection report no. 26: *Ann Intern Comm Radiol Protect* 1 (3), 1977.
10. International Council of Radiation Protection report no. 41: nonstochastic effects of ionizing radiation, *Ann Intern Comm Radiol Protect* 1 (3), 1977.
11. National Council of Radiation Protection: Implementation of the principles of ALARA for medical and dental personnel. In *National Council of Radiation Protection report no. 107,* Washington, DC, 1990, The Council.
12. National Council of Radiation Protection: Ionizing radiation exposure of the population of the United States. In *National Council of Radiation Protection report no. 93,* Washington, DC, 1987, The Council.
13. Laws P: Evaluation of health detriment from delayed effects of ionizing radiation. In *Proceedings of a symposium on biological effects, imaging techniques and dosimetry of ionizing radiations,* HHS Publication FDA 80–8126, Rockville, MD, 1980, Bureau of Radiological Health.
14. Nishiyama H: Administration of radiopharmaceuticals to patients, In Sodd V, editor: *Radiation safety in nuclear medicine: a practical guide,* HHS Publication FDA 82–8180, Rockville, MD, 1981, Bureau of Radiological Health.
15. Pochin EE: Why be quantitative about radiation risk estimates? *Lauriston S. Taylor lecture no. 3,* Washington, DC, 1978, National Council of Radiation Protection.
16. National Council of Radiation Protection: Recommendations on limits for exposure to ionizing radiation. In *National Council of Radiation Protection report no. 91,* Washington, DC, 1987, The Council.
17. U.S. Nuclear Regulatory Commission: Title 10, Code of Federal Regulations, Part 20: *Standards for protection against radiation,* Washington, DC, 1987, The Commission.
18. U.S. Nuclear Regulatory Commission: Title 10, Code of Federal Regulations, Part 35: *Human uses of byproduct material,* Washington, DC, 1987, The Commission.
19. U.S. Nuclear Regulatory Commission: Information relevant to insuring that occupational radiation exposures at medical institutions will be as low as reasonably achievable. In *Regulatory Guide 8.18,* Washington, DC, 1977, The Commission.
20. U.S. Nuclear Regulatory Commission: Applications of bioassay for I-125 and I-131. In *Regulatory Guide 8.20,* Washington, DC, 1978, The Commission.
21. U.S. Nuclear Regulatory Commission: Guide for the preparation of applications for medical programs. In *Regulatory Guide 10.8,* Washington, DC, 1980, The Commission.
22. U.S. Nuclear Regulatory Commission: Title 10, Code of Federal Regulations, Part 20: Standards for protection against radiation, *Fed Reg* 56(98): 23390-23470, 1991.

Marcia Boyd, Kathy E. Thompson, Donna Mars

chapter 8

Patient Care and Quality Improvement

Objectives

List the positive attributes of patient encounters.

Demonstrate the proper techniques for transferring patients from wheelchairs and stretchers.

Demonstrate the proper method of moving patients to obtain imaging positions.

Discuss medications commonly prescribed for patients and medications used in nuclear medicine.

Demonstrate precautions for using and disposing of sharps.

Perform the proper technique in venipuncture and intravenous administration.

Discuss monitoring and care of intravenous lines.

List and discuss sources of infection and methods to prevent disease transfer.

Discuss techniques used in universal precautions.

Demonstrate good hand-washing technique.

Obtain accurate respiration rate, pulse rate, and blood pressure measurements.

Describe actions to be taken in various medical emergencies and how to activate emergency teams in your institution.

Discuss quality improvement programs and their relationship to nuclear medicine services.

Describe methods to provide quality improvement in custom service.

Discuss techniques to obtain and analyze data relative to patient care, including problem solving.

*I*t is the responsibility of the nuclear medicine technologist to provide quality care to the patient during all procedures. The nuclear medicine technologist is often the only person available to provide basic care to the patient while performing the nuclear medicine procedure. In competitive markets it is also the responsibility of the nuclear medicine technologist to provide excellent customer-oriented, quality services. This chapter discusses the various responsibilities associated with the first encounter with the patient, including patient care and patient assessment. This chapter also provides a framework for continuous performance improvement in nuclear medicine.

PATIENT PREPARATION

The patient's first encounter with nuclear medicine personnel may be the most important in establishing trust and cooperation. This encounter may be with the clerical support employee, transportation employee, or the technologist.

However, the technologist may be the primary contact for patient encounters from scheduling to completion of the procedure.

There are multiple settings for nuclear medicine, such as outpatient diagnostic centers, physicians' offices, mobile units, and hospitals. Patient encounters are modified based on the setting, but basic quality service must be maintained, and efforts to continuously improve the process must be investigated.

The first step is usually to review the referring physician's order to correlate the procedure with the history and to determine if there are any contraindications. The format used by physicians when ordering a procedure will vary with the setting. A hospitalized patient will have orders written in the medical chart or entered electronically in the information system. Orders for an outpatient may be electronically transmitted, verbally ordered, or presented on arrival in written format. Restrictions may be placed on the method of ordering procedures based on institutional policy or legal requirements. An example would be Medicare regulations related to written orders.

Some nuclear medicine procedures require special standardized patient preparation. Standardized protocols should be established with the scheduling source, for example, nursing units, physician offices, or clinics. A reminder by nuclear medicine personnel regarding patient preparation at the time of scheduling can help prevent delays in performing the procedure. The scheduling source should also be aware of any conflicting exams, such as barium radiographs, nuclear medicine procedures, or interfering medications.

Basic information included on the request should be the patient's name, identification number, referring physician's name, and clinical indications for the procedure. Hospitalized patients will have additional information, such as room number and mode of transportation.

Arrangements must be made for the availability of the radiopharmaceutical required for the procedure. Orders must be placed for radiopharmaceuticals not routinely stocked. When ordering radiopharmaceuticals, the timing from preparation to injection must be a consideration. Ample time must be allocated when ordering from a nuclear pharmacy so that arrival of the patient and the radiopharmaceutical dose are synchronized.

A simplified flow chart of the process of scheduling a patient is presented in Figure 8-1. Several preparations must be made before the patient's arrival:

- Quality control measurements must be performed on all equipment, for example, dose calibrator and gamma camera.
- Personnel must be trained in the technical aspects of procedures and in customer service.
- Necessary supplies must be assembled.
- Radiopharmaceutical doses must be assayed.
- Interventional agents must be ordered, if applicable.
- Emergency equipment and supplies must be available.

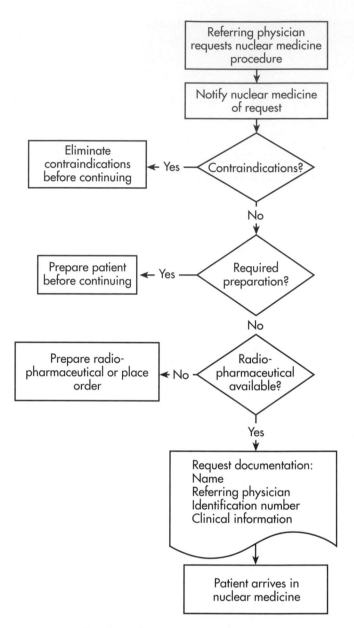

Figure 8-1   Flowchart of scheduling process in nuclear medicine department.

PATIENT ENCOUNTER

A person's perception concerning the quality of his or her care is formed during the first 30 seconds of the encounter. The person greeting the patient, whether the transporter, technologist, or clerical personnel, must do so in a friendly, professional manner. It is important to remember that most patients have limited knowledge of nuclear medicine procedures and the term *nuclear* alone may initiate unrealistic fears.

The patient must be clearly identified on arrival. The wristband serves as an identifying tool for the hospitalized patient. In order to properly identify an outpatient, the patient may be asked to repeat his or her name, spell the name, or recite the address and social security number. Demographic information may be obtained at the time of arrival by reviewing the outpatient's billing information.

When the patient arrives in the nuclear medicine department, further investigation must be made to ensure that the correct procedure is scheduled and that there are no contraindications. Before beginning the procedure, the technologist must obtain a complete medical history. The medical history will give the technologist information concerning any contraindications, such as medications or disease states that may interfere with the procedure. These situations may call for special precautions or an alternative protocol. For outpatients, a thorough medical history may not be available; therefore it is the technologist's responsibility to obtain the history from the patient. Hospitalized patients normally arrive with their medical charts, and the current medical status can be determined by reviewing the chart. If preparation for the procedure is required, a determination must be made that orders were clearly followed.

Patients expect the courtesy of receiving an explanation of what is expected of them, how the procedure will be performed, any discomfort they will experience, the required length of time for the procedure, and how and when they will hear about the results. Effective communication at this point will help ensure cooperation throughout the procedure. It is important to use terminology appropriate to the patient's understanding.

The technologist must determine the extent of the patient's physical ability. Patients who are physically challenged may have special care needs. Assistance must be provided for those patients unable to move on and off imaging tables. The geriatric patient may have a hearing loss, making it difficult to follow instructions. Pediatric cases require special handling techniques, and the psychiatric patient may have special needs.

Information is presented in the next few pages on body mechanics, medications and their administration, infection control, using specialized equipment, and basic patient care skills such as obtaining vital signs and responding to the patient during emergency procedures. Establishing a quality or performance improvement process, which involves strategic planning, process management, customer satisfaction, analysis and management of data, and specific problem-solving tools and techniques for the individual technologist and nuclear medicine teams, is also discussed.

BODY MECHANICS

The principles of proper body alignment, movement, and balance are referred to as body mechanics. Practicing the concepts of body mechanics is important in terms of the health and wellness of the technologist as well as the safety of the patient.

Concepts of Body Mechanics (Figure 8-2)

Base of support—Provide wide and stable base of support by standing with feet shoulder width apart and one foot slightly advanced.

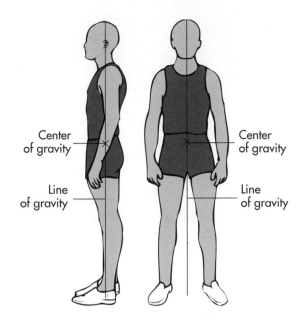

Figure 8-2   Correct body alignment.

Center of gravity—Keep objects close to the body. The weight of an object is multiplied by a factor of 10 for every inch it is held away from the body.

Body alignment—When lifting objects off the floor, bend the knees and keep the back straight and avoid twisting the trunk.

Lifting Tips

- Avoid lifting heavy objects above shoulder or below the waist level.
- Keep stomach muscles tight, using legs for lifting and abdominal muscles for support.
- Bend the knees when lifting below the waist level.
- Avoid using back muscles to lift.

Pushing/Pulling Tips

- When moving heavy objects or equipment, push rather than pull while using leg and abdominal muscles.
- If pulling is necessary, do so by walking forward.

Carrying Tips

- Hold loads with arms and legs working together.
- Avoid bending neck to the side when carrying a load on the shoulder.
- Vary carrying techniques and pause for rest when carrying for long distances.

Patient Transfers

The first step is to determine that the technologist has the correct patient. The next step is to assess the patient's ability to move and explain to the patient his or her role in the transfer.

Wheelchair Transfers

To transfer a patient from the bed to a wheelchair, start by lowering the bed to the level of the wheelchair seat and elevating the head of the bed. Position the wheelchair at a 45-degree angle to the bed with wheels locked, and remove footrests. Position patient on the edge of the bed by placing one arm under the patient's shoulders and the other arm under the knees to raise the patient to a sitting position. Allow time for the patient to adjust to the upright position. Take precautions to ensure patient safety by supporting the patient. Many patients suffer from orthostatic hypotension after long periods of rest and feel light-headed or faint when changing to an upright position suddenly. After this adjustment period, most patients will be able to move to the wheelchair with only minimal assistance.

Orthopedic or neurologically impaired patients require more assistance. Always position the patient's strongest side toward the area he or she is being transferred to. Stand facing the patient. Reaching under the patient's shoulders, place hands over scapulae. The patient's hand may rest on your shoulders. While using proper body mechanics, lift upward. If the patient has an injured leg or foot, place your feet on either side of the affected foot. Using your knees, block the patient's knee to provide additional support. Pivot the patient toward his or her strong side and into the wheelchair.

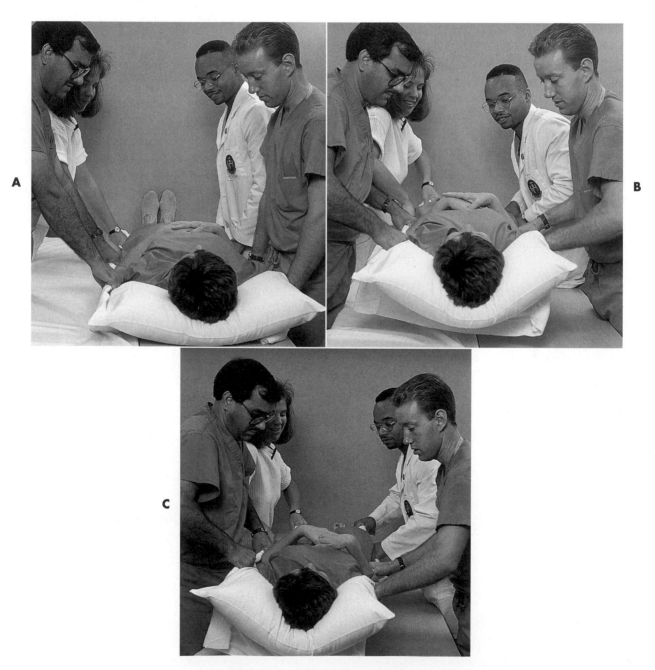

Figure 8-3 Patient transfer using a sheet.

To move a patient from the wheelchair to a locked imaging table, place the wheelchair at a 45-degree angle to the table with the patient's strongest side toward the table. Lock the wheels, remove footrests, and help the patient stand, using face-to-face assist as described. Have the patient place one hand on the footstool handle and one arm on your shoulder and step onto the footstool, with strong side first, pivoting with the patient's back to the table. Ease the patient into a sitting position. Place one arm around the patient and the other arm under the patient's knees. With a single motion, place the legs on the table while lowering the head and shoulders into the supine position.

If a patient is unable to stand, a stretcher should be used. Start with the patient in the supine position with knees flexed and feet flat. Position the stretcher parallel to the imaging table toward the patient's strongest side and lock the stretcher wheels and imaging table. Place one arm under the patient's shoulders and the other arm under the pelvis. Instruct the patient to push with feet and elbows as you assist in the transfer to the imaging table. The maneuver should be repeated until the patient is secure on the imaging table.

Use "draw sheet" lifts or a slide board when a patient is unable to assist in the transfer. A draw sheet is a sheet folded in half that is placed under the patient. Align the patient's head and torso in order to move the patient as one unit, while supporting the patient's head. When transferring the patient, the sheet is rolled up close to the patient to provide a handhold for lifting and pulling the patient onto the imaging table. A slide board can be used in conjunction with the draw sheet. Roll the patient onto his or her side and insert the board under the draw sheet, being sure to include the patient's head and torso. The slide board provides a hard surface to make the transfer easier. The use of antistatic spray will prevent the buildup of static electricity on the board. Note: these techniques require two or more persons (Figures 8-3 and 8-4).

Safety straps must be used on all patients being transferred by a wheelchair or stretcher. Safety straps should also be used on imaging tables if possible. Stretcher side rails should be in place during transport of the patient. The use of restraints requires a physician's order. For more information on the use of immobilizers, see Chapter 18.

MEDICATIONS AND THEIR ADMINISTRATION

Technologists are required to be proficient in the administration of radioactive and nonradioactive medications. It is the responsibility of the technologist to be familiar with the routes of administration, pharmacology, and the adverse effects. No medication is given without the order of a physician. The order may be written or verbal. Verify the order by checking patient's written records. The medication may be ordered by its generic or trade name. The generic name of a medication identifies its chemical family. Different pharmaceutical companies may manufacture the same generic substance under a different proprietary or trade name. A useful resource that lists medications alphabetically according to their generic classes, trade names, or indications is the Physician's Desk Reference (PDR) (Tables 8-1 and 8-2).

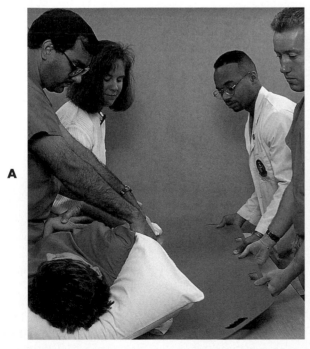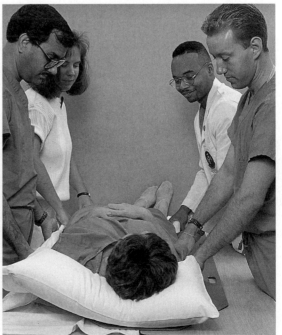

Figure 8-4   Patient transfer using a slide board. **A,** Logroll the patient to one side and position the slide board. **B,** Slide the patient onto the slide board.

Table 8-1 Overview of clinical pharmacology

Class	Why used	Examples (brand names) other uses
Antihistamines		
Allergies	Prevent allergic reactions	diphenhydramine (*Benadryl*) astemizole (*Hismanal*)
Anti-infectives		
Antibiotics	Treat/prevent Bacterial infections	Aminoglycosides (IV) gentamicin, tobramycin—nephrotoxic Penicillins, cephalosporins amoxicillin (*Amoxil*), *Unasyn, Timentin*, cefazolin, cefuroxime, ceftriaxone (*Rocephin*) Quinolones ciprofloxacin (*Cipro*), ofloxacin (*Floxin*) Other miscellaneous clindamycin, erythromycin, metronidazole, trimethoprim/sulfamethoxazole (*Bactrim*), vancomycin, doxycycline fluconazole (*Diflucan*)
Antifungals	Treat/prevent Fungal infections	amphotericin B—nephrotoxic cyclophosphamide, ifosfamide—nephrotoxic
Antineoplastics	Treat cancer	doxorubicin, fluorouracil, methotrexate, cisplatin, carboplatin, vincristine, vinblastine
Autonomic		
Anticholinergics	Inhibit effects of parasympathetic nervous system activity	atropine, preop for salivation; causes dry mouth, constipation Ipratropium (*Atrovent*)—inhaled for COPD
Adrenergics	Bronchodilation Increase HR, BP	albuterol (*Ventolin*)—inhaled for asthma See cardiac drugs
Coagulation		
Anticoagulants	Treat/prevent blood clots: for DVT/PE, AMI, Afib	heparin (IV) Warfarin (*Coumadin*)
Thrombolytics	Break up clots for AMI	TPA, streptokinase
Cardiovascular		
Cardiac drugs	Increase heart's contraction	digoxin (*Lanoxin*)—also for Afib dobutamine (*Dobutrex*) Dopamine Low dose increases urine output High dose increases heart contractility
	Treat arrythmias	lidocaine, bretylium
Antilipemic	Treat elevated cholesterol	lovastatin (*Mevacor*) cholestyramine (*Questran*)
Hypotensives	Reduce blood pressure	ACE-inhibitors—also CHF, diabetes, captopril (*Capoten*), enalapril (*Vasotec*) Beta-Blockers—also post MI, atenolol (*Tenormin*), metoprolol (*Lopressor*) Calcium channel blockers diltiazem (*Cardizem*), verapamil (*Calan*), Nifedipine (*Adalat, Procardia*) Central a_2 agonists clonidine, methyldopa (*Aldomet*) Peripheral a_1 antagonists prazosin (*Minipress*), terazosin (*Hytrin*)

Table 8-1	Overview of clinical pharmacology—cont'd

Class	Why used	Examples (brand names) other uses
Vasodilators	Angina, acute MI	Nitrates nitroglycerin, isosorbide dinitrate (*Isordil*)
CNS-agents		
Analgesics and antipyretics	Pain and fever	Aspirin—also antiplatelet (stroke, MI, angina) acetaminophen (*Tylenol*) NSAIDs—Can be nephrotoxic esp w/ACE inhibitor, ibuprofen (*Motrin*), indomethacin (*Indocin*)—also for gout
Analgesics	Pain Reverse opiate-induced sedation and respiratory depression	Opiates morphine, meperidine (*Demerol*) Opiate antagonist naloxone (*Narcan*) (IV) phenytoin (*Dilantin*)
Anticonvulsants	Prevent seizures	carbamazepine (*Tegretol*) valproic acid (*Depakene*)
Psychotherapeutics	Depression Psychosis, agitation	amitriptyline (*Elavil*) fluoxetine (*Prozac*) haloperidol (*Haldol*)
Anxiolytics	Anxiety, insomnia	Benzodiazepines midazolam (*Versed*), lorazepam (*Ativan*)
Water/electrolytes		
Diuretics	Remove fluid	Loop—also in CHF, furosemide (*Lasix*) Thiazide—also in HTN, hydrochlorothiazide
Gastrointestinals		
Miscellaneous	Prevent acid secretion	H₂ blockers ranitidine (*Zantac*), cimetidine (*Tagamet*) Proton pump inhibitors Omeprazole (*Prilosec*)
Prokinetics	Speed passage of food out of stomach	metoclopramide (*Reglan*) cisapride (*Propulsid*)
Antiemetics	Prevent/treat nausea/vomiting	promethazine (*Phenergan*) ondansetron (*Zofran*)
Hormonal		
Adrenals	Supplement, anti-inflammatory	prednisone (PO) methylprednisolone (IV) triamcinolone (*Azmacort*)—inhaled-asthma
Antidiabetics	Replace insulin Stimulate insulin release Increase glucose uptake	insulin (many kinds) Sulfonylureals glipizide (*Glucotrol*), glyburide (*DiaBeta, Micronase*) metformin (*Glucophage*) Contraindication: Must not give within 2 days of radiological procedures, and then hold metformin until renal function returns
Thyroid	Replace Suppress	levothyroxine (*Synthroid*) propylthiouracil
Miscellaneous		
Asthma/COPD	Relax bronchial muscle	theophylline (*Theo-Dur*), aminophylline
Gout	Acute Chronic	colchicine, allopurinol Benztropine (*Cogentin*)
Parkinson's disease	Restore dopamine/ACh balance	Carbidopa-levodopa (*Sinemet*)

From McEvoy GK, editor: *American hospital formulary service—drug information,* Bethesda, MD, 1996, American Society of Health-System Pharmacists. Modified by Ted Morton, PharmD, Baptist Memorial Hospital, Memphis, TN.

Table 8-2	Nonradioactive pharmaceuticals used in nuclear medicine		
Pharmaceutical	**Indication**	**Dosage**	**Adverse effects**
Acetazolamide (*Diamox*)	Brain perfusion	1 g in 10 ml sterile water, IV over 2 min	Tingling sensations in extremities and mouth, flushing, lightheadedness, blurred vision, headache
Adenosine (*Adenocard*)	Cardiac stress imaging	140 μg/kg/min for 6 min, or 50 μg/kg/min increased to 75, 100, and 140 μg/kg/min each min to 7 min	Chest, throat, jaw, or arm pain, headache, flushing, dyspnea, ECG changes
Bethanechol (*Urecholine*)	Gastric emptying	2.5 to 5 mg subcutaneously	Abdominal discomfort, salivation, flushing, sweating, nausea, fall in blood pressure
Captopril (*Capoten*)	Renovascular hypertension evaluation	25 to 50 mg orally 1 hr before study	Orthostatic hypotension, rash, dizziness, chest pain, tachycardia, loss of taste
Cholecystokinin (*Kinevac*)	Hepatobiliary imaging	0.02 μg/kg in 10 ml saline, IV over 5 min	Abdominal pain, urge to defecate, nausea, dizziness, and flushing
Cimetidine (*Tagamet*)	Meckel's diverticulum imaging	Adult: 300 mg/kg Pediatric: 20 mg/kg in 20 ml saline, IV over 2 min with imaging 1 hr later	Diarrhea, headache, dizziness, confusion, and bradycardia
Dipyridamole (*Persantine*)	Cardiac stress imaging	0.57 mg/kg IV over 4 min (0.142 mg/kg/min)	Chest pain, nausea, headache, dizziness, flushing, tachycardia, shortness of breath, and hypotension
Dobutamine (*Dobutrex*)	Cardiac function reserve	Incremental dose rate of 15 μg/kg/min up to 15 (child); up to 40 μg/kg/min every 3 min (adult)	Angina, tachyarrhythmia, headache, nausea, and vomiting
Enalaprilat (*Vasotec IV*)	Renovascular hypertension evaluation	0.04 mg/kg in 10 ml saline, IV over 5 min	Orthostatic hypotension, dizziness, chest pain, headache, vomiting, and diarrhea
Furosemide (*Lasix*)	Renal imaging	Adult: 20 to 40 mg Pediatric: 0.5 to 1 mg/kg, IV over 1 to 2 min	Nausea, vomiting, diarrhea, headache, dizziness, and hypotension
Glucagon	Meckel's diverticulum imaging	Adult: 0.5 mg (range 0.25 to 2 mg) Pediatric: 5 μg/kg, IV or IM	Nausea, vomiting
Morphine (*Astramorph, Duramorph*)	Hepatobiliary imaging	0.04 mg/kg, diluted in 10 ml saline, IV over 2 min (range 2 to 4.5 mg)	Respiratory depression, nausea, sedation, light-headedness, dizziness, and sweating
Pentagastrin (*Peptavlon*)	Meckel's diverticulum imaging	6 μg/kg subcutaneously	Abdominal discomfort, urge to defecate, nausea, flushing, headache, dizziness, tachycardia, and drowsiness
Phenobarbital (*Luminal*)	Hepatobiliary imaging	5 mg/kg/day orally for 5 days	Respiratory depression, nausea, vomiting, dizziness, drowsiness, headache, and paradoxical excitement in children
Vitamin B_{12} (*Cyanoject, Cyomin*)	Schilling test	1 mg IM 2 hr after radioactive B_{12} dose	None

Modified from Park HM, Duncan K: Non-radioactive pharmaceuticals in nuclear medicine, *J Nucl Med Technol,* 22 (4): 1994.

Medication Administration

The correct administration of pharmaceuticals include the five rights system as follows:

1. Right dose
2. Right medication
3. Right patient
4. Right time
5. Right route

Medications may be administered by topical, sublingual, oral, or parenteral routes.

Topical Route—Medication is applied to a limited area for a local effect. The medication is absorbed through the skin and into the bloodstream. Examples are solutions, creams, or transdermal patches applied directly to the skin.

Sublingual Route—Medication is placed beneath the tongue and is absorbed into the bloodstream. An example of a sublingual medication is nitroglycerin. Administration of nitroglycerin results in a dilation of the coronary arteries. This produces a systemic effect to counteract angina pectoris.

Oral Route—Oral medications are supplied in a variety of forms, such as tablets, capsules, granules, and liquids. Sodium iodine I-123 or I-131 is administered by mouth, usually in capsule or liquid form, for thyroid uptakes, scans, and therapy. Radioactive vitamin B_{12} is administered in capsule form by mouth.

Oral medications are administered as follows:

- Wash hands.
- Read the label and prepare for administration.
- If physician is administering the medication, show him or her the label.
- If the physician requests the technologist to administer the medication, check the patient's identification and read the label again before administering. Stay with the patient while the medication is swallowed, and offer water if permitted.

Parenteral route—These are medications injected directly into the body and are classified according to the depth of the injection (Figure 8-5).

- *Subcutaneous* (under the skin) medications are injected at a 45-degree angle using a 5/8-inch needle with a 23

to 25 gauge. The most common injection sites are the upper arm or outer aspect of the thigh. Injection volume is usually 2 ml or less. Example: allergy injections.
- *Intramuscular* (into the muscle) medications are injected into the deltoid muscle of the upper arm, the upper quadrant of the gluteus maximus muscle in the hip, or the vastus lateralis muscle of the lateral thigh at a 90-degree angle. The injection volume may be up to 5 ml, and the needle size can range from 22 to 25 gauge. Example: vitamin B_{12} injections.
- *Intradermal* (between the layers of skin) medications are administered using a tuberculin syringe with a very small needle (26 or 27 gauge). Example: tuberculin skin test and injections for lymphoscintigraphy.
- *Intravenous* administration is the parenteral route most often used in nuclear medicine and will be discussed in more depth later.

Withdrawal of Nonradioactive Materials

Assemble the syringe and needle. Read the label to verify the correct medication, concentration, and expiration date. If the drug is supplied in a single dose ampule, a small file is needed to score the neck of ampule. Snap off the top by using a 2 inch × 2 inch gauze to protect fingers (Figure 8-6). A filter needle may be used to draw up the medication and eliminate possible glass particles. If the drug is supplied in a vial, a metal or plastic cap will need to be removed. If the vial is used for multiple doses, clean the rubber septum with alcohol after the first puncture. When withdrawing nonradioactive substances, a volume of air equal to the dose may be inserted into the vial before withdrawing the dose. Remove the needle cover, taking care not to contaminate the needle. Insert the needle into the rubber septum at a 45-degree angle, straighten the needle when puncturing the septum, and withdraw the desired amount while checking for any air bubbles. Air bubbles may be removed by tapping the sides of the syringe.

Withdrawal of Radioactive Materials

Gloves should always be worn when handling radioactivity. Required lead glass syringe shields are available in several

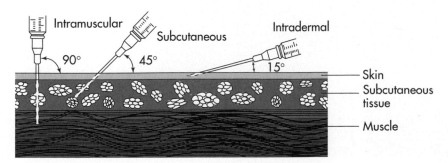

Figure 8-5 Comparison of the angles of needle insertion.

syringe sizes to decrease the exposure when withdrawing and injecting radioactivity. Assemble the syringe and needle, and lock them securely into the syringe shield. Remove the needle cover, taking care not to contaminate the needle. Clean the rubber septum of the shielded vial with alcohol and insert needle at a 45-degree angle, straightening the needle when puncturing the septum. This will prevent breaking off pieces of the rubber septum and introducing them into the vial. Turn the vial upside down and withdraw the desired volume while checking for air bubbles. Do not inject air into vial when withdrawing radiopharmaceuticals (Figure 8-7).

Preparation for Venipuncture

The antecubital or median cubital vein on the anterior surface of the elbow is usually used. Other sites that may be used include the medial basilic veins, cephalic veins, veins of the anterior wrist, or veins of the posterior hand. Dilate the vein by applying the tourniquet 4 to 6 inches above the

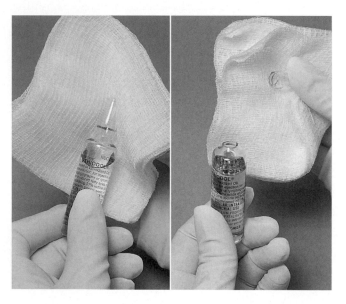

Figure 8-6 Preparing medication from an ampule.

venipuncture site. Ask the patient to hold a tight fist. Apply gloves. Palpate the area, using the first or second finger to locate a vein. Appropriate veins for venipuncture will demonstrate a rebound sensation on palpation. Avoid superficial veins or veins that feel hard or knotty with palpation. Prepare the site using an alcohol swab, working outward from the center of the site in a circular motion (Figure 8-8).

Intravenous Equipment

Venipuncture may be accomplished with a butterfly set, a hypodermic needle, or an intravenous catheter. A butterfly set is often used for direct injections with a syringe. Before the butterfly needle is inserted into the vein, the tubing may be filled with saline or sterile water to avoid injecting air. To insert a winged steel needle of a butterfly set, remove the cover and turn the bevel of the needle up, grasping the wings of the device between the thumb and index finger. The wings of the device may be taped to the patient's skin after the needle is in place. This prevents movement of the needle in the vein (Figure 8-9).

The use of hypodermic needles is generally restricted to withdrawing blood samples or for single injections. Hypodermic needles are supplied in various diameters and lengths. The gauge of a needle indicates the diameter. As the gauge increases, the diameter of the bore decreases. The length of the needle is measured in inches, and may vary from 1/2 inch for intradermal use to 4 1/2 inches for intrathecal (spinal cord) injections. To insert a hypodermic needle, remove the needle cover and turn the bevel upward.

Venipuncture technique is the same whether using a butterfly set, hypodermic needle, or intravenous catheter. Anchor the vein by stretching the vein firmly in the opposite direction of the course of the needle. Hold needle at a 30-degree angle, and penetrate the skin just below the point where the vein is to be entered. Avoid touching the insertion site after cleaning it with alcohol. Advance the needle quickly but cautiously, penetrating the vein with the needle point. As the vein is entered, usually there is a sensation of resistance followed by an ease of penetration and a flashback

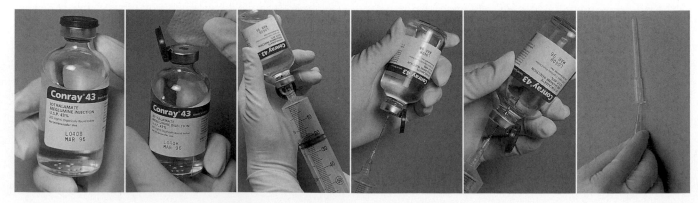

Figure 8-7 Drawing up medication from a vial.

of blood into the tubing with the butterfly set, or into the needle hub in the case of the hypodermic needle. While continuing to hold the skin taunt, carefully advance the needle in a direct line with the vein to prevent puncture of the vein's posterior wall.

To confirm that the needle is in the vein, withdraw a small amount of blood into the hypodermic needle and syringe before injecting the radiopharmaceutical. To confirm placement of needle using a butterfly set, inject sterile water or saline before injecting the radiopharmaceutical. Observe for signs of possible infiltration such as puffiness in the area of injection. If signs are present, discontinue the injection immediately. Release the tourniquet and withdraw the needle. Apply pressure immediately with a dry gauze or cotton ball and maintain pressure for approximately 1 minute or until bleeding stops.

Intravenous catheters frequently are used when repeated intravenous injections, infusions, or bolus injections will be administered. An over-the-needle catheter is composed of a silicon catheter with a stylet/needle inside the catheter lumen. To insert an over-the-needle catheter, remove the needle cover and turn the bevel of the stylet/needle up. Anchor the vein and insert the needle at a 20- to 30-degree angle. Lower the needle unit until it is almost flush with the skin, and enter the vein. This is to prevent piercing of the posterior wall of the vein. Check for vein entry by observing a flashback of blood, and advance the needle 1/4 inch farther into the vein to establish the catheter tip. Holding the stylet/needle hub with one hand, use the thumb and forefinger of the other hand to gently advance the catheter off the stylet/needle and into the vein. Do not reinsert the stylet/needle into the catheter. Release the tourniquet and relax the tension on the skin. Remove the stylet/needle from the catheter and attach the adapter or syringe. To prevent excessive flashback of blood, use the index finger to apply digital pressure on the vein above catheter. A 2 inch × 2 inch sterile gauze pad may be placed under the catheter hub to prevent leakage of blood onto the patient's skin (Figure 8-10).

Needleless Systems

Blunt cannulae can be used to draw up medications and to access established intravenous lines for blood draws and medication administration. (Figures 8-11, 8-12, and 8-13).

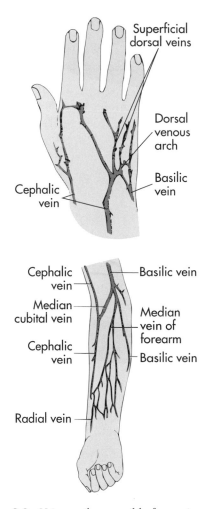

Figure 8-8 Veins easily accessible for venipuncture.

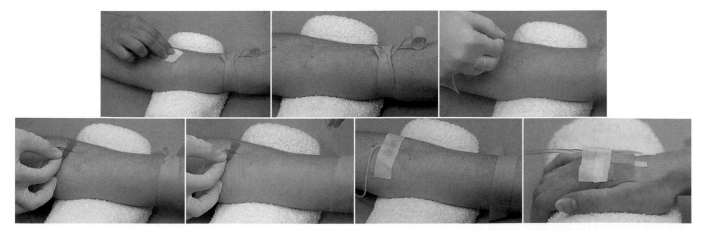

Figure 8-9 Venipuncture.

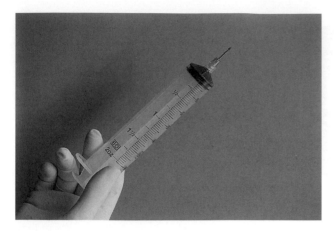

Figure 8-11 Interlink vial access cannula. (Courtesy Baxter Health Care.), (Syringe courtesy BD) BD and BD logo are trademarks of Becton, Dickinson and Company, copyright 2003 BD.

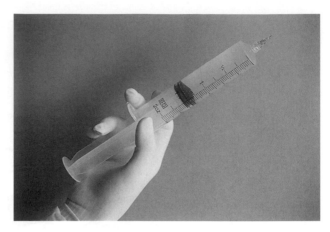

Figure 8-13 Interlink syringe cannula. (Courtesy Baxter Health Care.), (Syringe courtesy BD) BD and BD logo are trademarks of Becton, Dickinson and Company, copyright 2003 BD.

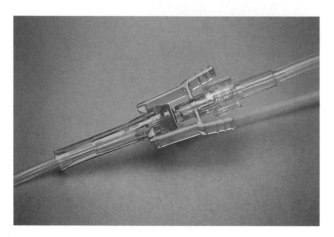

Figure 8-12 Needleless system interlink level lock for intravenous piggyback medication administration. (Courtesy Baxter Health Care.), (Syringe courtesy BD) BD and BD logo are trademarks of Becton, Dickinson and Company, copyright 2003 BD.

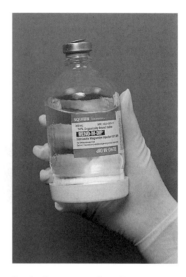

Figure 8-14 Check the name of medication, its strength, and the expiration date.

avoid a painful hematoma. Document that the infiltration occurred.

Needle Disposal

Dispose of all syringes and needles directly into a puncture-proof container without recapping. Containers are labeled according to the type of contamination: biohazard and/or radioactive.

Radioactive syringes sometimes will require recapping before disposal to avoid radioactive contamination. If it is necessary to recap a used needle, use a needle cap holder or place the needle cover on a firm surface and insert the needle using one-handed technique.

Several additional points must be remembered when administering medications:

1. Know the indications and side effects of the medication before administration.
2. Follow the established rules of the aseptic technique.

3. Read the label three times: before and after withdrawal of the medication and before administration. The technologist is responsible for medication that he or she administers, regardless of who has prepared it.
4. Check medication for proper concentration and expiration date (Figure 8-14).
5. Check patient identification before administration.
6. Monitor the patient for side effects. Be familiar with any medication that may require an antidote and where the emergency cart is located.
7. A medication error must be reported according to institutional policy. The patient's physician must also be notified.

Monitoring Intravenous Lines

The drip or flow rate of an intravenous (IV) line can be determined by reviewing the patient's medical chart. An infusion rate of 15 to 20 drops/min or approximately 60 ml/hr is common. The infusion rate can be controlled by a clamp or medication pump.

Several precautions should be taken when monitoring an IV. Always keep the IV solution 18 to 20 inches above the level of the vein. If the solution is inadvertently placed lower than the vein, blood will flow back into the needle or tubing and may clot. An IV solution that is too high may cause fluid to infiltrate into surrounding tissues because of the increased hydrostatic pressure.

Precautions in caring for patients with IV lines include the following:

- Call in advance and inform the nurse if the procedure will be lengthy.
- Whenever possible, plug the IV pump into an electrical outlet rather than relying on battery power.
- Watch IV fluid levels and allow enough time for fluid replacement before the IV fluid is exhausted.
- If an IV set does run out or if an alarm sounds despite appropriate troubleshooting, call the nursing service immediately rather than waiting until the patient is returned to the nursing unit.
- When performing IV injections through appropriate IV lines, flush with a minimum of 10 cc saline or sterile water.
- Have a good understanding of the pumps used in the facility.

Charting Medications

Notation that the study was completed and any medications given should be recorded in the patient's records. The notation should include the time of day, the name of the drug, the dosage, and the route of administration. The entry must include the identification of the person who charted it. For legal purposes the technologist who charts medications must use the procedure established by the institution.

Infection Control

Medical asepsis is the technique used to prevent the spread of infection or disease by reducing the number of infectious microorganisms or pathogens. Microorganisms include bacteria, viruses, protozoans, and fungi.

The cycle of infection involves a pathogenic organism, reservoir of infection, means of transmission, and a susceptible host (Figure 8-15).

The reservoir of infection can be any place that microorganisms can find nutrients, moisture, and warmth. The human body provides this type of medium. Some microorganisms live on or within the body as part of normal flora and aid in digestion and skin preservation. These organisms are nonpathogenic as long as they are confined to their usual environment, but can assume a pathogenic role outside their environment. Pathogens can also live in the bodies of healthy individuals without causing apparent disease. These persons are called carriers and may be a reservoir for infection without realizing it.

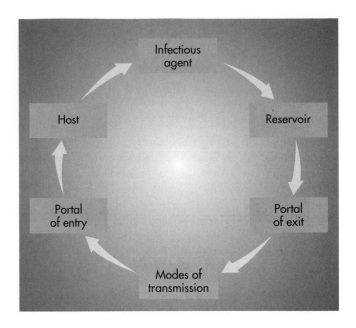

Figure 8-15   The cycle of infection.

Although the human body is the most common reservoir of infection, any environment that will support growth of the microorganisms has the potential to be a secondary source. Such sources may include contaminated food or water or any damp, warm place that is not cleaned regularly.

Compromised immune systems of patients make them susceptible hosts. They may develop a secondary problem or nosocomial (hospital-acquired) infection. The incidence rate of nosocomial infections is approximately 5% of patients admitted to hospitals yearly. Most of these infections are not life threatening. The most common nosocomial infection is a urinary tract infection. However, statistics indicate that 20,000 patients a year die of hospital-acquired infections and that more than half of these are preventable.

The most direct way to intervene in the cycle of infection is to prevent transmission of the pathogen from the reservoir to susceptible host. The most effective system to prevent transmission of disease is by practicing "Standard Precautions," which are aimed at reducing risk of transmission of microorganisms from both recognized and unrecognized sources. "Universal Precautions" were designed to reduce the risk of transmission of bloodborne pathogens. "Body Substance Isolation" was designed to reduce the risk of transmission of pathogens from moist body substances. The new term "Standard Precautions" combines the major features of "Universal Precautions" and "Body Substance Isolation" into one standard. This standard applies to all patients, regardless of their diagnosis or presumed infection status, and is based on the use of protective barriers for contact with all body substances rather than focusing on the isolation of a patient with a particular diagnosis. All patients are treated as potential reservoirs of infection. The Center for Disease Control (CDC) recommends a two-tiered system for health care workers that implements "Standard Precautions" and

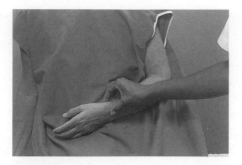

Figure 8-18 Measuring the radial pulse.

count the beats of the pulse for at least 30 seconds and multiply by two to obtain beats per minute. For irregular rhythms, a complete cycle of 1 minute is required. (Figure 8-18).

The normal respiratory rate is 12 to 16 breaths/min. Notify the physician of any change in the patient's breathing pattern. Difficult or labored respiration is called dyspnea. Rapid breathing is tachypnea or hyperventilation. Oxygen is a prescribed drug and may only be administered to the patient with a physician's order. It may be difficult for the patient with lung disease to lie flat for even a short period. Many times, a change in position will alleviate the dyspnea.

Count the respirations without the patient being aware and count the breathing sequence (in and out) as one respiration. Count for 30 seconds and multiply by two to obtain respirations per minute.

Blood pressure is the lateral pressure exerted on the walls of the arteries by blood flowing through the arteries. It reflects the rhythm of the heartbeat and is a measure of the volume of blood pushed into the vessels by the heart. The pressure of blood within the arteries is highest whenever the heart contracts and is called systolic pressure. Between beats, when the ventricles are at rest, arterial pressure is at its lowest and is called diastolic pressure.

Blood pressure is measured in millimeters of mercury (mm Hg). Normal blood pressure varies, depending on age, weight, and physical status, but blood pressures of 100/60 to 140/90 are considered to be within the acceptable range. The top number, systolic (s for squeezing of the heart muscle) is a measure of the pumping action of the heart muscle itself. The diastolic pressure (d for down or dilation of the heart muscle) indicates the ability of the arterial system to accept the pulse of blood that is forced into the system by the contraction of the left ventricle. Elevated blood pressure is hypertension; low blood pressure is hypotension and may indicate shock. In a changing or emergency situation, the physician will need accurate readings to be able to make a valid evaluation of the patient's status.

The most common site for taking blood pressure is the brachial artery of the upper arm, but arteries of the lower arm, thigh, and calf may also be used. When the arm is used, the patient should either sit or lie down with the arm and blood pressure cuff at the level of the heart.

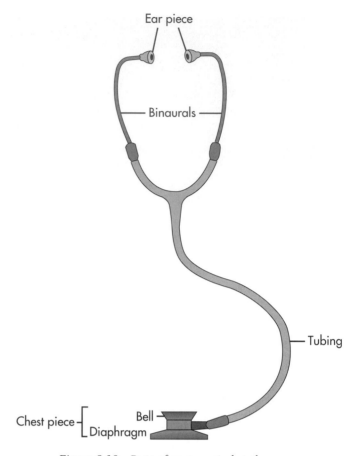

Figure 8-19 Parts of an acoustical stethoscope.

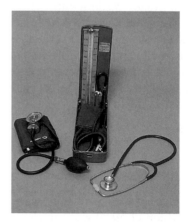

Figure 8-20 Aneroid (*left*) and mercury (*right*) manometers.

Equipment used to measure blood pressure includes a sphygmomanometer, a cuff, and a stethoscope. The procedure is begun by inflating the cuff to 180 to 200 mm Hg. The cuff contains an inflatable rubber bladder that should be centered over the brachial artery, 1 to 2 inches above the elbow. Cuffs should be wrapped snugly but not tightly. If the cuff is too loose, systolic and diastolic readings will both be falsely elevated (Figures 8-19 and 8-20).

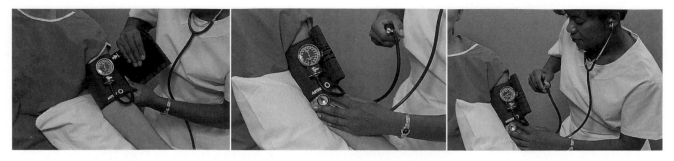

Figure 8-21 Assessing blood pressure.

A stethoscope with a flat diaphragm is best for taking blood pressures. After locating the brachial artery by palpation, place the diaphragm of the stethoscope over the artery without touching the cuff or patient's clothing. Gentle application of the stethoscope should be used, because too much pressure can cause abnormally low diastolic sound (Figure 8-21).

Blood Pressure Procedure

1. Explain the procedure to the patient and make him or her comfortable in a sitting or recumbent position.
2. The patient should be resting for 5 minutes before the blood pressure is taken.
3. Select the site and use the same site consistently because of variations in blood pressure taken in different locations. Blood pressure should also be taken with the patient in the same position each time.
4. Expose the site and position the patient's arm on a supporting structure at heart level.
5. Place the cuff so that its lower edge is 1 to 2 inches above the elbow, leaving space over the brachial artery free.
6. Using the middle and index fingers, palpate the brachial artery, which is located on the medial aspect of the arm at the level of the elbow.
7. Place the diaphragm of the stethoscope directly over the point of strongest pulsation.
8. Holding the rubber bulb in the palm of one hand, close the valve on the bulb with your thumb and finger, then rapidly inflate the cuff by pumping the bulb.
9. Inflate the cuff to about 20 to 30 mm Hg above the expected systolic reading, or approximately 180 mm Hg. Inflation of the cuff should take 7 seconds or less.
10. Slowly open the valve on the bulb, releasing the pressure on the cuff steadily. Listen carefully for sounds of the first heartbeat, and note the reading on the sphygmomanometer. This reading represents the systolic pressure.
11. After the first sound, the pulsing will get louder as the pressure is released slowly from the cuff (approximately 2 to 3 mm Hg per heartbeat). Continue

deflation until all sound stops or the intensity of the sound suddenly decreases and seems muffled. This reading represents the diastolic pressure.
12. Open the valve to deflate cuff rapidly.
13. Remove the cuff and record values as systolic/diastolic (e.g., 120/80).
14. If you need to repeat a reading, let all the air out of the cuff and wait 15 seconds before inflating the cuff again. Do not reinflate the cuff during the reading.
15. Wipe the eartips and diaphragm of the stethoscope with alcohol before storing.

If there is difficulty hearing the diastolic sounds, completely deflate the cuff. Wait 15 seconds, have the patient raise his or her arm for a few seconds, and then retake the blood pressure. The diastolic sounds may become muffled before stopping or may remain muffled down to zero. In this case, record the diastolic pressure at the point the change is distinguished from clear to muffled, as well as when the sound ends completely (e.g., 120/80/62).

EMERGENCY CARE

Patient assessment is critical in determining the action to be taken when a patient experiences difficulty in breathing. Obstructed airways, heart attacks, strokes, seizures, and syncope are common causes of medical emergencies. The universal sign of a choking person is the hand placed around the throat area. If the patient can cough and/or talk, the technologist should observe the patient and take no action. If the patient's coughing reflex does not remove the object, and the patient loses the ability to cough and/or talk, this represents an obstructed airway.

Obstructed Airway—Conscious Victim (Figure 8-22)

Abdominal thrusts can be performed with the person standing, sitting, or lying down as follows:

1. Ask the victim, "Are you choking?"
2. Give quick upward thrusts to the abdomen slightly above the navel, applying pressure upward against the diaphragm just below the ribs.

Diabetes

The diabetic patient cannot metabolize glucose because of the lack of insulin production by the pancreas. These patients are usually on some form of insulin, which has the potential to cause problems when they have taken their insulin and can have nothing by mouth (NPO). These patients may develop hypoglycemia (low blood sugar). The onset of symptoms may be sudden and include the following:

- General weakness
- Sweating, clammy, cold skin
- Tremors, nervousness, and irritability
- Hunger
- Blurred vision
- Loss of consciousness

The condition can be quickly remedied by the administration of sugar (candy or fruit juice). Report the occurrence of such symptoms to a physician. Protect the patient from falling by laying the patient down until the sugar takes effect. People can have hypoglycemia without diabetes; the treatment is the same.

Asthma

Bronchospasms cause difficulty in breathing or dyspnea in asthmatic patients. Stress or anxiety, such as having a nuclear medicine procedure, can precipitate this condition. The treatment of choice is to relieve the bronchospasm without the administration of oxygen. If the patient has a nebulizer that contains bronchodilating medication, this usually relieves the symptoms. An injection of epinephrine will relieve the symptoms of an acute episode and must be ordered and administered by a physician.

Emergency Carts

Emergency carts contain essential items that could be needed during an emergency. The carts are located throughout the hospital and should be easily accessible to all areas. The items may vary slightly, but most carts contain artificial ventilation equipment, emergency medications, bags of intravenous solutions, a defibrillator, blood pressure cuff, and stethoscope. These carts are inventoried and locked to keep them ready for use. To be able to assist if needed, the technologist should become familiar with the location of the cart and its components (Figure 8-26).

SPECIALIZED EQUIPMENT

Intravenous Equipment

Computerized infusion pumps are used in most institutions to regulate the drip rate of the prescribed fluids. Unless authorized, the technologist should not change the rate of flow. The technologist should know how to troubleshoot, as in the case of an occluded line in the system.

Nasogastric (NG) Tubes

This tube is inserted through a nostril and terminates in the stomach. It is used for feeding, to obtain specimens, or to drain fluids. Nasoenteric tubes go farther into the intestinal tract to remove fluid and gas that may cause distention. Precautions should be taken to make sure the tubes are not pulled or tugged on when moving or positioning patients. The technologist needs to report any leakage in the tube or suction system. Suction or feeding can be discontinued if the patient needs to be transferred to the department.

Oxygen Administration

In caring for a patient receiving oxygen, always note the flow rate in the medical chart or doctor's orders. Oxygen can be administered by high-flow—rate or low-flow—rate devices. The low-flow—rate devices most often used are the nasal cannula or simple oxygen masks. The nasal cannula is inserted into the patient's nostrils, providing a direct source of oxygen at a minimum flow rate of 0.5 and a maximum rate of 6 L/min. Simple masks must be set at an oxygen flow rate of no less than 6 L/min to prevent the buildup of exhaled carbon dioxide. Masks with reservoir bags should be set with a liter flow rate high enough to ensure that the bag never completely deflates during patient breathing. The mask fits over the mouth, nose, and chin of the patient (Figures 8-27 and 8-28).

During transport, portable oxygen is contained in cylinders. These cylinders may be made of steel or aluminum. For the safety of the patient and the practitioner, steel cylinders must not be used in the presence of a magnetic field. The stem valve on the top of the cylinder must be opened

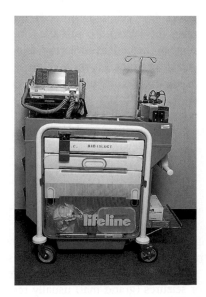

Figure 8-26 Emergency cart with defibrillator.

at least one to two turns to allow oxygen to flow into the regulator. The regulator has a pressure gauge that will give an indication of how much oxygen is in the cylinder. A knob on the regulator allows for flow adjustment to the patient in liters per minute. Both valves must be turned on for the patient to receive oxygen. A common oxygen rate is 3 to 5 L/min. Trauma (in shock) patients may require a higher rate of oxygen administration. Patients with chronic obstructive pulmonary disease (COPD) receive oxygen at a lower rate, usually less than 3 L/min. The carbon dioxide level controls the respiratory rate in these patients, and if too much oxygen is delivered, the respiratory rate may slow down to the extent that ventilation is insufficient (Figure 8-29).

Currently most health care facilities use bulk liquid oxygen systems rather than oxygen supplied in gaseous form because of two factors: (1) gases shipped in bulk are less expensive than gases shipped in cylinders, and (2) liquid oxygen takes up less space than gaseous oxygen. Portable liquid oxygen systems are available for patient transport. The portable device is filled from the bulk liquid oxygen system and provides an 8- to 12-hour supply of oxygen. Care must be taken to avoid spillage when filling the portable unit. Because of the extremely low temperature of liquid oxygen, direct contact will cause frostbite to the skin or eye injury. Avoid placing the portable unit in direct contact with the patient.

Precautions when using oxygen cylinders or liquid oxygen units include the following:

- Cylinders should be secured at all times and never allowed to stand free. Always use liquid oxygen units in the upright position.
- Care must be taken to prevent fire when oxygen is in use. Never place cylinders or liquid units near a heat source.
- Always determine the amount of oxygen in the cylinder or liquid unit before transporting the patient. Liquid oxygen units will vent gas when not in use.
- When transporting, secure cylinders in the cylinder cart and liquid oxygen units by straps. Never use the patient's stretcher to transport oxygen.

Catheters

The most common type of catheter is the urinary catheter. Plastic tubing is inserted through the patient's urethra and into the bladder. Urine is drained from the bladder and flows through the tubing into the urine bag. To prevent backflow of urine, the bag must be kept below the level of the bladder. Catheterization is a sterile technique and needs to remain a closed system to prevent urinary infections. The catheter bag can be attached to the bed, stretcher, or wheelchair, but should never be placed directly on the floor.

Surgical Drains

Colostomies (surgical opening into the colon) and ileostomies (surgical opening into the ileum) allow for drainage of feces. The opening (stoma) is covered by plastic disposable bags or pouches (appliances), which must be changed frequently. Clean rather than sterile technique is needed when changing these appliances.

Dressings should be maintained, and any signs of fresh bleeding should be reported immediately. If hemorrhaging

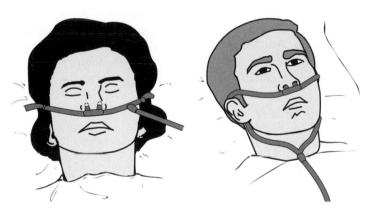

Figure 8-27 Nasal cannula.

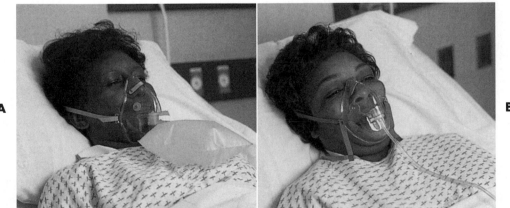

Figure 8-28 Oxygen face masks. **A,** Plastic face mask with reservoir bag. **B,** Simple face mask.

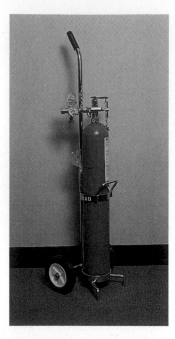

Figure 8-29   Oxygen tank.

occurs, apply direct pressure to the site while calling for assistance.

QUALITY IMPROVEMENT

In the present health care arena, the nuclear medicine facility must maintain reliable quality outcomes, a cost-efficient operation, easy access, and superior customer service to remain competitive in the marketplace.

The words *quality management, quality improvement, continuous improvement, performance improvement,* and *total quality management (TQM)* are often used interchangeably in present health care. These words describe designs to improve the processes of the work performed. In nuclear medicine many different processes are started and completed within the service (internal), and others involve outside parties (therefore are external). An example of an internal process is completing the quality control studies on a camera. Obtaining a radiopharmaceutical and its ultimate disposal may involve personnel outside the nuclear medicine department (external). Sets of tasks in a continuum are referred to as a process. For example, nuclear medicine procedures are a part of the continuum of care of a patient. *Case management, care paths, critical paths,* and other similar terms are used to describe a process or continuum of care for a patient. Care paths often list nuclear medicine procedures to be obtained at critical times during the patient's care. The Joint Commission on Healthcare Organizations (JCAHO) no longer looks at nuclear medicine as a separate entity to be evaluated but rather considers how nuclear medicine relates to other functions within the total care of a patient.

To function in a continuous improvement mode, the nuclear medicine technologist, physician, support person-

nel, and other interactive groups should focus on planning, customer requirements, process management, analysis and management of data, and problem-solving models.

PLANNING

Any quality or performance improvement plan must relate to the overall strategic plan of the nuclear medicine facility. This is a continuation of the institutional plan if nuclear medicine is part of a larger organization. Short-term plans are usually developed for 1 year or less, and long-term planning normally extends to 3 years. Planning should take into account customers' needs and expectations, fiscal restraints, and the environmental influences.

There are a number of environmental factors to consider in planning. The type of market will have a direct effect on the nuclear medicine facility. In a capitated market with heavy managed care contracts there will be more restrictions on the types of nuclear medicine procedures performed and the amount of reimbursement. A good understanding of the actual case mix is important in any planning. The competition must be considered. This includes other nuclear medicine facilities as well as other modalities. As algorithms are developed for patient care, nuclear medicine may or may not play a role in the diagnostic care of a patient or group of patients.

Fiscal restraints must be considered, especially in the area of human resources and facilities. The most efficient use of staff may mean addressing issues of cross training, productivity, threats of downsizing, and staff recruitment and retention. Equipment must be operationally sound, and replacement plans must be developed. Routine suppliers should be evaluated, and partnerships must be established, when feasible.

CUSTOMER SERVICE

It is imperative for a nuclear medicine facility to identify its customers and assess their needs and expectations. A customer is anyone to whom a service, product, or information is provided. Nuclear medicine facilities normally identify the referring physician as an important customer. The referring physician's staff may be direct contacts in scheduling and providing important information about the patient. In many instances nuclear medicine must depend on a unique customer/supplier relationship for patients. As more regions operate in a managed care market, third-party payers, such as insurance companies and health maintenance organizations (HMOs), may actually be the primary customers because they dictate to the patient where he or she will go for services. Clinical outcomes become an important factor in assessing the quality of ancillary services. Third-party payers are interested in clinical outcomes, accessibility, and overall satisfaction of their clients when they select nuclear medicine suppliers.

The patient's needs and expectations must be considered in developing quality and performance improvement plans.

The primary type of patient will influence perceptions of good customer service. For example, a geriatric population and a pediatric population will not view exceptional service in exactly the same manner.

Not to be forgotten is the internal customer, both within the department and the institution. Many of the deficiencies within a process occur when accountability moves from one party to the next. Many times the nuclear medicine technologist's contact with other customers or suppliers can affect the success or failure of the total process, as in, for example, scheduling the patient, ordering or preparing the radiopharmaceutical, performing the procedure, generating the report, and correlating with other modalities.

Understanding the customer's needs and expectations will involve asking the right questions. This is normally done in survey format and focus group settings. Only by asking these questions and addressing the issues can the nuclear medicine department provide viable services.

PROCESS MANAGEMENT

The greatest improvements can be seen in a nuclear medicine facility through efficient process management. One of the most effective ways of evaluating a process is to develop a flowchart. By using a flowchart, the technologist can identify those "bottlenecks" that cause delays or confusion. Time becomes an important factor in customer satisfaction, as well as cost-effectiveness. When turnaround time is decreased, quality, productivity, and cost-effectiveness improve. Once the time deficiencies have been identified, various problem-solving techniques can be used to address the root cause of the problem.

It may be of value to identify "best practices" through benchmarking. Once a process has been determined and fully understood, it may be necessary to network with other nuclear medicine facilities to determine which facility has the most efficient process management, for example, who has the shortest turnaround time, lowest expense, and most accurate results. Studying another type of business may also be of value when looking at processes. For example, bank billing practices may be related to nuclear medicine billing practices; delivering a package on time may be related to transporting a patient on time; and the patient check-in process may be related to the hotel check-in process.

ANALYSIS AND MANAGEMENT OF DATA

It has been said that we can only manage that which we can measure. Within any system, measurements must be reliable and accurate. The decisions as to what data to collect should be based on relative importance. Often in nuclear medicine, measurements have been done for accreditation without affecting overall improvement. Measuring must be selective and meaningful and should support process management, planning, and customer satisfaction. Measurement outcomes can benefit patient care.

PROBLEM-SOLVING MODELS

Understanding and properly using problem-solving tools and techniques can help the nuclear medicine technologist to improve a process.

Plan, Do, Check, Act (PDCA)

The Shewhart Cycle, or a similar model, is commonly considered the format for problem solving. It begins with the "Plan" phase, determining the problem or what needs to be changed or improved. The "Do" phase involves data collection and analysis; the root cause of the problem is determined. Based on the data, possible solutions are determined, and controls are established. A change is initiated in the "Check" phase. In the "Act" phase, results of the change are reviewed and modified as necessary, and continuous monitoring is established. Modifications of the Shewhart Cycle include the Ten-Step JCAHO Model and other methods that use a number of steps but follow the same principle.

PROBLEM-SOLVING TECHNIQUES

Many problem-solving techniques or tools may be used in combination or alone to improve a process.

Brainstorming is a technique used to generate ideas from several people. Specific rules to obtain the most positive outcomes may include the following:

- Select a topic.
- Record *all* ideas.
- Record one idea at a time in the sequence given.
- Pass over participants who have no spontaneous ideas.
- Do not criticize any of the ideas listed.
- Continue brainstorming until all ideas are listed or the time limit is reached.
- Clarify all ideas listed.

The *affinity diagram* is another brainstorming method that is effective with large groups. It is most often used with groups who do not work together, when full participation is required, in political environments, or when "group think" should be avoided. It is also an effective method when the topic under consideration is sensitive, there is a need to break from traditional ideas, thinking is chaotic, or many creative ideas are needed. The procedure includes the following steps:

- Select a broad topic.
- Write each idea on a separate adhesive note or card.
- Be clear and concise.
- Mix responses together randomly.
- Group similar cards together without discussing the ideas.
- Select a heading (main topic) for each group of ideas.

Fish bone (also referred to as the "cause and effect" diagram) is a method that is used to determine the causes of a problem. Causes are most commonly grouped under the following categories:

- Methods
- Machines
- People
- Materials
- Measurements

Force-field analysis is used to identify the forces that drive a situation and those that restrain it. The procedure for using the method is as follows:

- Identify the current situation.
- Identify the desired (ideal) situation.
- Identify the driving forces (those that make the desired situation achievable).
- Identify the retraining forces (those that prevent the current situation from becoming the desired situation).
- Determine which factors can be altered to achieve the desired situation.

The *flowchart* is one of the most useful tools to identify and improve a process. By listing process steps in a symbolic format, areas that are "bottlenecks" can be more easily identified and removed or changed. Typical symbols are used in Figure 8-1 (the rectangle indicates a step in the process; the diamond indicates a decision point; the curved rectangle indicates a document; and arrows indicate a connector to the next step).

The *contingency diagram* is an effective method for looking at the negative parts of a problem and then reversing them to take positive action steps. The usual format to complete a contingency diagram is as follows:

- Identify the problem.
- Brainstorm for ideas to ensure that the problem will continue and possibly worsen.
- Review each idea to determine if the opposite can occur.
- Develop an action plan.

An *interrelationship digraph* is a method of linking related ideas. It involves the following procedure:

- Randomly space the ideas/issues.
- Select the first idea and relate it to the nearest idea/issue.
- Ask the question: Does this idea/issue cause or influence the idea/issue it is being related to?
- If the answer is yes, draw an arrow from the first idea to this idea.
- Return to the original idea/issue and relate it to the next idea/issue.
- Continue to ask the question and draw arrows.
- When the first idea/issue has been related to all the other ideas/issues, follow the same sequence for each of the other ideas/issues.
- Identify the idea/issue that has the greatest influence on the others (the one with the most arrows pointing away from it).
- Identify the idea/issue that is most influenced by the others (the one with the most arrows pointing to it).

This method will help determine which ideas/issues to work on for the greatest possibility of altering a situation.

Measurements

Most problem solving involves measurement, which may be in any phase of the PDCA cycle but is most important during the analysis (check) phase. The more common types of measurement include the following:

A *Pareto chart* consists of a bar graph from the highest frequency to the lowest and is used to help determine which area to work on first.

The *check sheet* is used to collect data to identify patterns.

The *run chart* is used to measure trends.

A *control chart* is a run chart with upper and lower acceptable limits.

The *histogram* is a bar graph of the distribution of data, which demonstrates variation.

A *scatter diagram* is used to correlate two variables to look for cause and effect.

Practical Application of Problem-Solving Techniques

The following example illustrates how a team could use several of the problem-solving tools and measurements discussed above to improve a process.

PROBLEM: Patient wait time has been identified as the greatest source of dissatisfaction for patients scheduled for nuclear medicine procedures.

A team is formed to develop a solution that will ensure the best outcome. During the planning phase, the team analyzes data already available (Figures 8-30 and 8-31). Of the patients studied in nuclear medicine, 65% are outpatients, and 35% inpatients. The team develops a flowchart of the process of scheduling patients through the department and discovers that the "bottleneck" causing longer waiting times for outpatients is during the check-in phase; for inpatients it is waiting for transportation to return to the nursing units after the procedure has been completed. Based on the data, the team determines that improving the process of checking in outpatients will have the greatest impact on outpatient satisfaction because they make up the greatest number of patients and are most dissatisfied with patient waiting time.

The team can use a number of tools to find solutions to the problem. The fish bone diagram can be used to brainstorm for root causes (Figure 8-32). Once causes have been identified, the team can develop measures to determine which causes can be changed to bring about the greatest impact on outpatient satisfaction. The contingency diagram can be used to identify those factors that will cause the problem to continue or worsen (Box 8-1). The force-field analysis can be used to identify the desired situation, (i.e., that outpatient waiting time for nuclear medicine procedures be decreased) and then identify the forces that would drive the desired outcome and those that are currently preventing it (Table 8-3).

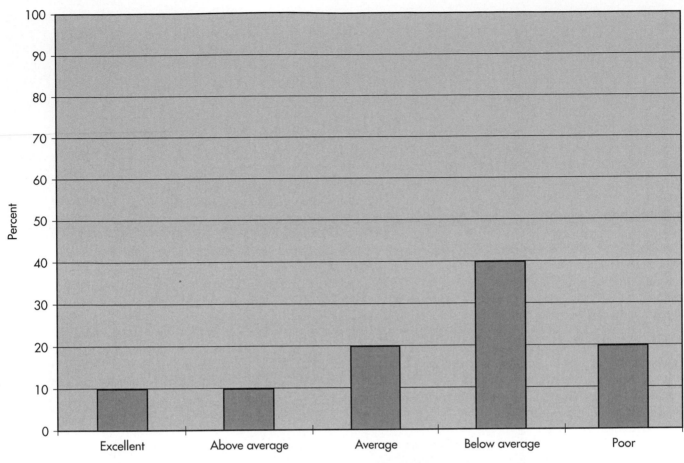

Figure 8-30 Outpatient satisfaction—timeliness of staff.

Box 8-1 Contingency diagram

QUESTION: How can we ensure that outpatient satisfaction for timeliness of staff continues to be low?

Do not change the current process.

Wait until patients arrive to tell them what information is needed.

Schedule all patients for same arrival time.

Eliminate the job position of nuclear medicine clerk.

Keep the old, unreliable copier.

Do not service the copier.

Increase the information required of patients.

Do not communicate with HMOs and insurance companies.

Do not provide information to referring physicians' offices.

Box 8-2 Force-field analysis

CURRENT SITUATION: Wait time for outpatients is too long during check-in.

DESIRED SITUATION: Decrease waiting time for outpatient check-in to improve patient satisfaction.

Driving forces

Require less information on patients.

Get information before patient's arrival.

Electronically communicate with referring physicians' offices.

Electronically communicate with HMOs and insurance companies.

Cross train others to help obtain information.

Restraining forces

Billing department requires too much information.

Patient is not told of information needed before arrival.

Lack of communication with referring sources.

Only one person in the nuclear medicine department is trained to obtain information.

Patient's perception that waiting time is too long.

Process has too many steps.

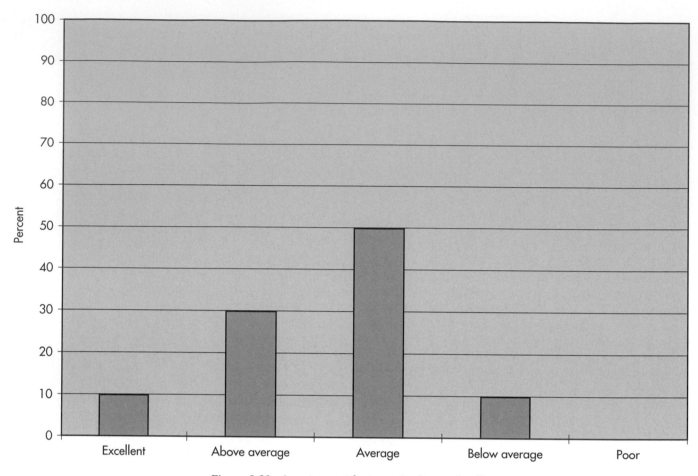

Figure 8-31 Inpatient satisfaction—timeliness of staff.

Once the team has determined what they believe to be the major causes of the problem, measurements must be taken to prove the hypothesis. The checklist is commonly used to measure multiple variables. It may be necessary to divide the measurements, such as for different days, times of the day, and source of the patient referral. It is important to determine all the parameters that may be important when solving the problem before measurements begin in order to prevent having to take additional measurements later. Examples of possible checklists for this particular problem are presented in Tables 8-4 and 8-5.

To analyze the data, the information is usually plotted on a Pareto chart, which identifies the cause having the greatest impact on the problem. This is sometimes referred to as the 80:20 rule, which means that 20% of the factors cause 80% of the problem, and if the 20% are fixed, 80% of the "headaches" will disappear. Unfortunately, those 20% are usually the hardest factors to fix.

Another chart that is helpful is the run chart, which is used to identify trends over time. If the team analyzed the data charted in Figure 8-33, they would conclude that something was causing greater delays on Wednesday and would look for causes such as the clerk not working and more patients being scheduled from a particular referring physician.

Based on the data analysis, the team might develop the following action plan:

- Work with the billing department to evaluate the amount of information required of outpatients and eliminate what is unnecessary.
- Develop a checklist of patient demographics and insurance requirements, and distribute this to referring physicians' offices to give to patients before their arrival in the nuclear medicine department.
- Determine what information can be provided by the referring physicians' offices before the patient's arrival.
- Work more closely with referring physicians' offices whose patients were least informed to better educate their staff regarding the information that will be required from patients.
- Reschedule the clerk's off time to better cover Wednesday mornings.

When the action plans are in place, the team must continue to monitor for improvements and alter the actions accordingly. Once the outpatient satisfaction starts improving, the team should begin to tackle causes of the "bottleneck" identified for inpatients, using similar techniques.

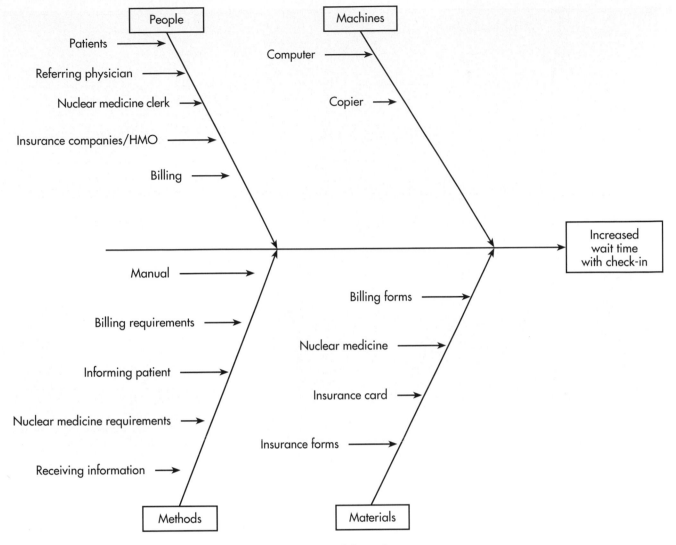

Figure 8-32   Fish bone diagram.

Table 8-3	Checklist					
Reason for wait	**Mon**	**Tue**	**Wed**	**Thur**	**Fri**	
Copier broken.						
Clerk not available.						
Patient arrives with no information.						
Patient arrives late.						
Patient arrives early.						
Patient unable to fill out form.						
Other						

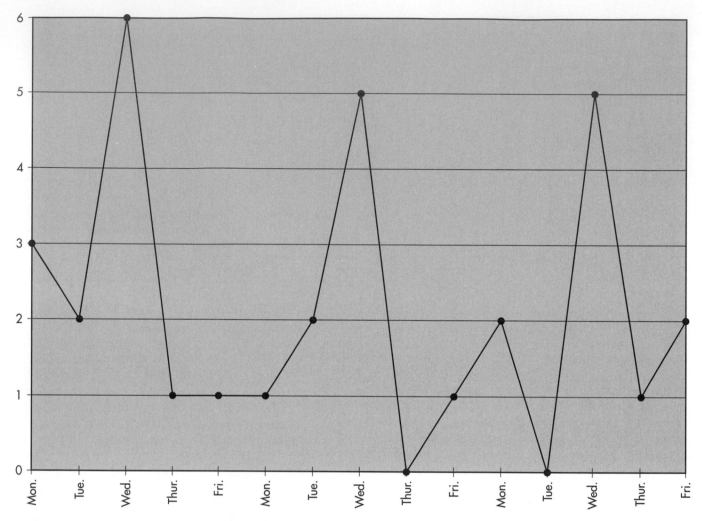

Figure 8-33 Number of patient delays at check-in.

| Table 8-4 | Checklist |

Patients arriving without billing information

Referral source	Week 1	Week 2	Week 3
HMO A			
HMO B			
HMO C			
Dr. Jones			
Dr. Smith			
Dr. Johns			
Neurology group			
Cardiology group			
Pulmonary group			

SUGGESTED READINGS

Brassard M: *The memory jogger plus*[+], Methuen, MA, 1989, GOAL/QPC.

Craig C: *Introduction to ultrasonography and patient care,* ed 1, Philadelphia, 1993, WB Saunders.

Ehrlich RA, Daly JA, McCloskey ED: *Patient care in radiography with an introduction to medical imaging,* ed 5, St. Louis, 1999, Mosby.

Hibbard W: *Laboratory manual for nuclear medicine technology,* New York, 1984, Society of Nuclear Medicine.

Keefer BS: Back to basics: the ABCs of back injury prevention, *RT Image* October 1991.

Leathers D: Oh, my aching back! *RT Image* December 1993.

Scholtes PR: *The team handbook,* Madison, WI, 1988, Joiner Associates.

James R. Galt, Tracy Faber

chapter **9**

Principles of Single Photon Emission Computed Tomography (SPECT) Imaging

Objectives

Discuss advantages of SPECT compared with planar imaging.

Describe characteristics of the SPECT gantry.

Discuss issues relative to multiple detector SPECT systems.

Describe collimators used in SPECT.

List SPECT acquisition modes.

Compare circular and body contour orbits.

Describe principles of tomographic reconstruction.

Discuss reconstruction algorithms, including their respective advantages and computational requirements.

Describe frequency space filtering.

List types of low-pass filters.

Discuss the use and effect of cutoff frequency and its effect on image smoothness and noise.

Define Nyquist frequency.

List units in which frequency may be defined.

Describe reorientation planes used in cardiac SPECT.

Discuss volume rendering techniques and their advantages for display presentation.

Describe surface rendering of SPECT data sets.

Discuss the physics of SPECT relative to attenuation, scatter, and detector response.

Describe attenuation correction performed by transmission imaging.

Discuss scatter correction methods.

Describe the general techniques used in automatic reorientation.

Discuss gray scale versus color display.

Describe techniques used to acquire gated cardiac SPECT studies.

List quality control tests performed specifically for SPECT.

SINGLE PHOTON EMISSION COMPUTED TOMOGRAPHY

Clinicians use planar images in the diagnosis of many types of disease. X-ray images show the distribution of materials of different densities in the body by imaging the attenuation of photons passing through the body. Scintigrams, produced by a scintillation camera, are planar images of the distribution of a photon-emitting radioactive tracer administered to a patient. An inherent difficulty in the interpretation of planar images is the fact that they represent a projection through the body. Each point, or pixel, in the image represents the superimposition of all the material (in the case of an x-ray) or activity (in the case of a scintigram) in front of and behind it. In addition, the two-dimensional aspect of projection images means that objects perpendicular to the imaging plane appear to be shortened or are difficult to view at all. Determining the shape of the distribution requires that the physician assimilate the information in several views. Computed tomography helps overcome this problem by using several planar images to reconstruct tomographic images in which each pixel represents a single point within the subject (Figure 9-1). The pixels actually represent a small volume, often called a *voxel,* for volume element. Unlike planar images, tomographic images do not suffer from the overlap of structures in front of or behind the organ of interest.

In medical terminology, emission computed tomography (ECT) is distinguished from x-ray computed tomography (CT) in that the photons used in ECT originate within the subject instead of from an external source. Consequently, emission computed tomography is a process-oriented measurement that records where the tracer is located within the patient. Single photon emission computed tomography (SPECT) produces images of gamma rays (or sometimes x-rays) emitted by a radioactive tracer. Positron emission tomography (PET) images the two 511 keV photons produced when a positron comes into contact with an electron.

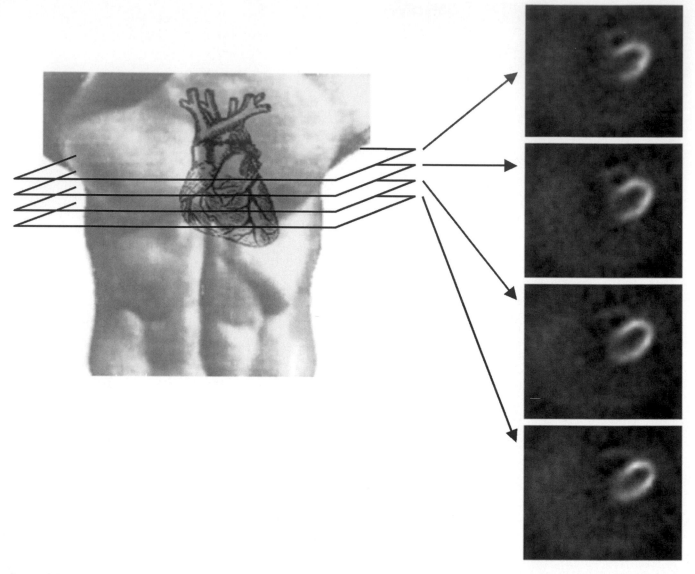

Figure 9-1   Tomography creates a stack of slices through the axis of the body; the slices show the distribution of radionuclide at each point. Here, myocardial perfusion images that slice through the chest are displayed.

CT, however, measures the attenuation of photons as they pass through the patient and thus provides a measurement of anatomy in the form of attenuation coefficients.

Image Properties

The most common measurements of image quality are resolution, contrast, and noise. No matter which kind of image is produced, resolution refers to how well objects can be separated in space (as opposed to blurring them together); contrast to how well different levels of brightness can be seen (brightness representing density for x-rays and radionuclide concentration in scintigrams); and noise to random additions to the image that interfere with the viewer's perception. In a scintigraphic image, resolution allows us to separate two objects that are close together. Contrast allows us to determine if two objects have different activity concentrations.

Noise is primarily due to counting statistics, giving planar images a speckled appearance and producing more complex problems in tomographic images.

Contrast in scintigraphic images can be defined as the measure of counts (or intensity) in the target (the object we are trying to image) compared with the intensity in a background region. It is measured as

$$\text{Contrast} = (C_0 - C_b)/C_b$$

where C_o is the organ count and C_b is the background count. The higher the contrast, the more visible the target. Low contrast can make the target fade into the background. Contrast is most easily measured by graphing a *count profile* (the counts encountered along a line drawn through a region of interest in the image). The peak counts in the graph are taken to be C_o, and the minimum count level is taken to be C_b. Figure 9-2 shows profiles taken through the left

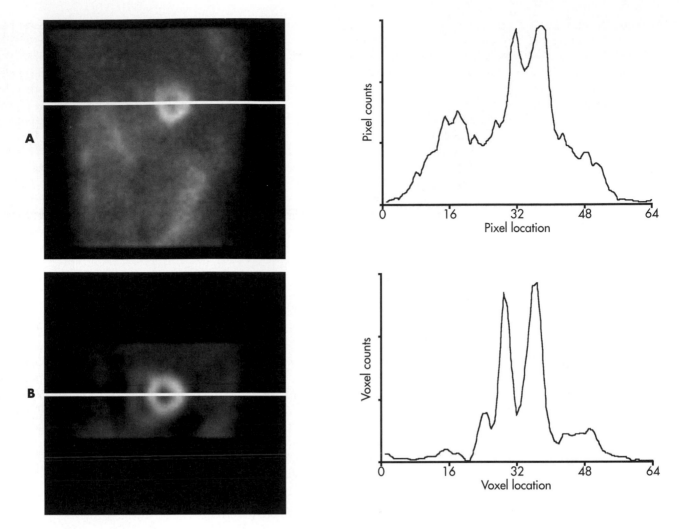

Figure 9-2 Profiles taken through the myocardium in a planar image (**A**) and a tomographic image (**B**) from a myocardial perfusion study show properties related to image quality. The lower background count level of the tomographic image results in improved image contrast. A profile of an image is a graph of counts versus location.

ventricle in both planar and tomographic images from a myocardial perfusion study. The decreased background count level in the tomographic image causes increased contrast compared with the planar image.

Resolution in scintigraphic images is the measure of how close two point sources of activity can get and still be distinguished as separate. Because no medical imaging modality is perfect, a point source never appears as a single bright pixel but rather always as a blurred distribution. Two blurry points eventually smear together into a single spot when they are moved close enough to each other. Resolution is measured by taking a profile though a point source and analyzing the resulting curve. A profile through a perfect point source would look like a sharp single spike rising above the flat background. A profile through a real point source appears as a gaussian-shaped curve. Resolution is the width of the gaussian curve at a level of one half of its maximum, or the full-width half-maximum (FWHM).

Noise in scintigraphic images is primarily the result of the random nature of counting statistics. Each pixel in a planar

scintigram is assigned a number (or pixel value) that represents the number of photons detected in a small area of the camera's crystal. The random nature of nuclear decay produces random fluctuations in the number of counts detected in adjacent pixels. Noise can be thought of as a measure of irrelevant information in the image. Noise appears as a speckle in nuclear medicine planar images and is particularly noticeable in background regions. Noise is measured relative to the useful image information, called the *signal*. In planar scintigrams, the signal is proportional to the counts (N), and the noise is proportional to the square root of N. Because the signal (N) increases faster than its square root, noise is a more serious problem for low-count images. As image counts increase, noise becomes less evident. Therefore, in low-count images, image quality can be improved greatly by even a small increase in the number of acquired counts. If count rates are high, the images will not be improved even by acquiring twice as many counts.

The effect of noise on tomographic images can be difficult to predict because each voxel is the product of the projection of that point in space from several different angles. In that sense, each voxel represents the summation of several projections and has better noise characteristics than individual projections. Tomographic reconstruction techniques, however, tend to increase noise.

SPECT images are superior to planar images in contrast but at some cost to resolution. Because each image represents a slice through the patient, much of the background activity is eliminated, increasing the contrast. Resolution decreases with distance from a scintillation camera. Because the camera must view the patient from all angles, it cannot be close to the organ of interest in all views. Practically, however, occlusion and superimposition of structures tend to reduce apparent resolution in planar images. For example, two point sources can be feet apart but still be seen as only one point in a planar image if one is in front of the other. Tomography, which eliminates these effects, often appears to provide higher resolution than planar imaging. This apparent increase in resolution can be seen in Figure 9-2. If the widths of the profiles taken through the myocardium are compared, the steeper slope of the profiles in the tomographic image implies a higher resolution.

INSTRUMENTATION

The main components of SPECT systems are the scintillation camera, the gantry (the frame that supports and moves the heads), and the computer systems (hardware and software). These components work together to acquire and reconstruct the tomographic images.

Scintillation Cameras

The basic components of a scintillation camera are a collimator, a sodium iodide (NaI) crystal, photomultiplier tubes (PMTs), pulse height analyzers (PHAs), and spatial positioning circuitry. Gamma rays (photons) pass through the collimator and cause a scintillation event (a short burst of visible light) in the crystal. The glow of the scintillation is converted into electrical signals by the PMTs. The location of the scintillation event is determined by the positioning circuitry based on the relative signals from the different PMTs. The brightness of the scintillation is proportional to the energy of the photon, which is measured by the PHAs. Scintillation cameras as described here were developed by Hal Anger of the University of California at Berkley in the late 1950s and early 1960s and are still the most widely used cameras.[1] Early cameras were completely analog devices in which the output was sent to an oscilloscope, creating a flash on the screen. A lens focused the screen on a piece of x-ray film that was exposed one flash at a time. This allowed for planar imaging, but for SPECT the images must be made available to the computer digitally.

A *digital scintillation camera* may be defined as a camera system in which the computer is an integral part of system and is used for processing the scintillation event. Digital cameras provide a digital output, or images in the form of a computer matrix, rather than strictly analog signals sent to an oscilloscope. In reality, no commercial system is totally analog or totally digital. Most camera systems convert the position and pulse height signals generated from analog circuitry in the camera to digital signals, which may then be further corrected for energy and position through digital processing. Camera designs that allow the output of each PMT to be converted to a digital signal have become common. Separation of the processing for each PMT leads to the ability to image at higher count rates. Digitization of each PMT's signal allows computer software to replace the complicated analog circuitry for positioning and pulse height analysis. This allows greater processing flexibility, resulting in improved energy and spatial resolution. The evolution of scintillation cameras from analog to digital devices is shown in Figure 9-3.

Gantry

The frame that supports the scintillation camera used for SPECT must be able to rotate and position the camera precisely, making size and stability important factors. Size is a practical issue because the gantry is the largest part of the SPECT system, and its size determines the amount of room space needed. The gantry must be able to rotate the scintillation camera with its heavy collimator and lead shielding. This makes the gantry/camera combination very heavy (floor loading must be considered when positioning a camera within a department).

SPECT Systems

SPECT cameras consisting of a single scintillation camera mounted on a ring gantry formed the backbone of tomographic nuclear medicine for years, and their utility and flexibility maintain their importance today. Circular cameras are more easily manufactured and dominated through the 1980s. Most scintillation cameras manufactured today have a rectangular head shape because a rectangular *field of view* (the usable imaging area of the camera) is more efficient for SPECT and whole body imaging. Rectangular heads do not give a significant advantage in cardiac imaging, however, and the patient's arms may interfere with the corners of the camera during SPECT.

Multiple detector SPECT systems are systems with more than one scintillation camera (Figure 9-4). They are more commonly sold today than single detector systems. The most obvious benefit of adding more detectors to a scintillation camera system is the increase in sensitivity. It seems obvious that doubling the number of heads doubles the number of photons that may be acquired in the same amount of time. The user may take advantage of the increase in sensitivity by acquiring more counts, by adding higher-resolution collimation, or by increasing throughput.

When two large field-of-view rectangular cameras are mounted opposite each other (180 degrees), they may speed whole body bone imaging by allowing simultaneous

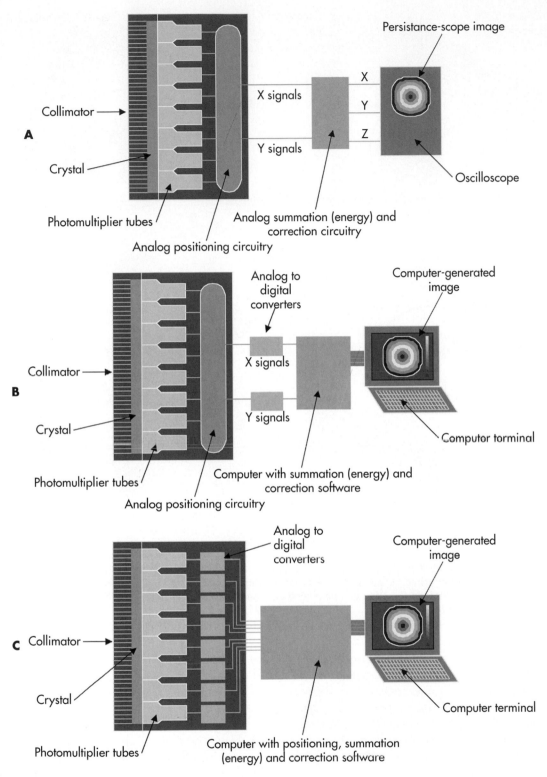

Figure 9-3   Scintillation cameras have evolved over the years from strictly analog devices in the early 1960s (**A**) to devices that produce computerized images (**B**). Many cameras today digitize the output of the PMTs (**C**), which allows most of the signal processing to be done in software.

acquisition of anterior and posterior images. A dual detector SPECT system capability can also increase throughput for 360-degree SPECT imaging by halving imaging time while collecting the same number of counts. A full 360 degrees of projections can be acquired by rotating the gantry

180 degrees. The gain in sensitivity may be traded off to achieve more precise images by allowing the use of higher resolution collimators.

However, these improvements may mean very little for cardiac SPECT, in which a 180-degree orbit is

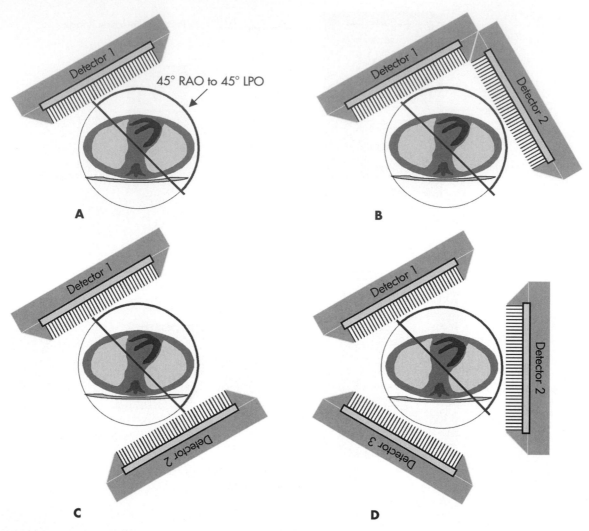

Figure 9-4   SPECT cameras may be configured with one, two, or three detectors. **A,** Single detector camera. An important consideration is that for ^{201}Tl myocardial SPECT, more than 66% of the counts are collected in the 180 degrees between 45 degrees RAO (right anterior oblique) and 45 degrees LPO (left posterior oblique). **B,** Addition of a second detector at 90 degrees doubles the sensitivity for both 180-degree and 360-degree orbits and is preferred for cardiac imaging. Flexibility may be lost, however, where simultaneous anterior and posterior images are desired. **C,** Addition of a second detector at 180 degrees doubles the sensitivity for 360-degree SPECT, but no increase in sensitivity is seen if a 180-degree orbit is recommended. **D,** A three detector system, with detectors mounted at 120-degree intervals, increases the sensitivity for 180-degree SPECT by only 50% but triples the sensitivity for 360-degree orbits.

recommended. The addition of a second head does not result in doubled sensitivity for cardiac imaging because counts in posterior planar images are much more severely attenuated than those of the anterior projections. In systems designed for cardiac SPECT, the two detectors are mounted next to each other (at 90 degrees) on the gantry. This allows a full 180-degree orbit to be acquired while rotating the gantry only through 90 degrees.

The drawbacks of double-headed cameras include the increase in quality control required by the addition of the second head and some loss of flexibility. Double detector systems do not allow the same flexibility of movement that is enjoyed with many single-headed systems. This may prevent them from being easily used for some types of planar imaging (e.g., gated blood pool) in which it is often difficult to position the camera correctly. There is a great deal of variation between manufacturers in the camera movement

allowed for planar imaging. Most manufacturers market dual detector systems that allow the cameras to be rotated to 180 degrees for general SPECT or 90 degrees for cardiac SPECT.

Triple detector cameras are usually dedicated to SPECT imaging. The three heads, as discussed for double-headed systems, result in increased sensitivity that may be used to increase throughput, counts, or resolution. However, if the three detectors are mounted rigidly at 120 degrees from one another, the system cannot perform simultaneous anterior/posterior imaging, which greatly reduces its utility for planar imaging. These systems also do not have a great impact on cardiac imaging with 180-degree orbits, for the reasons discussed above. Triple-headed SPECT systems are best suited for clinics that do a great deal of 360-degree SPECT imaging and can afford to have a camera dedicated solely to that task.

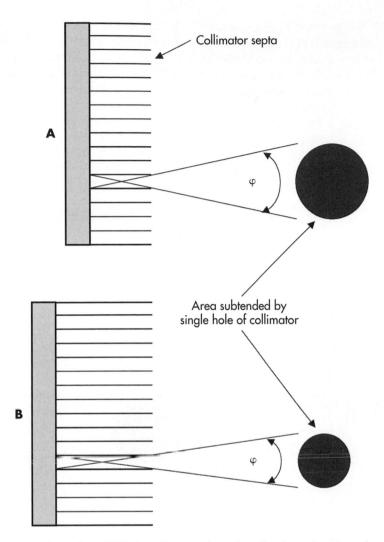

Figure 9-5   The resolution and sensitivity of parallel hole collimators depend on the shape, length, and size of the holes. **A,** Each hole in the collimator restricts the photons that may strike the crystal to those that originate within the arc φ. **B,** Lengthening the holes of the collimator reduces φ and the area exposed through each hole at a given distance. The longer the holes, the greater the resolution and the lower the sensitivity. It should also be noted that regardless of the length of the hole, the resolution degrades with the distance from the collimator.

Collimators

The collimator is the focusing device of a SPECT camera. Gamma rays have too much energy to be focused by a lens in the same way that visible light photons are in a film or digital camera. Instead, collimators are made up of an array of long, narrow (usually) parallel holes that exclude all photons except those traveling parallel to the direction of the hole (Figure 9-5). Collimators are rated by their sensitivity and resolution. In general, the sensitivity and resolution of a collimator are inversely related: a very high sensitivity collimator has low resolution, and a very high resolution collimator has low sensitivity. These properties are determined by the area, length, and shape of the collimator's holes.

Low-energy all-purpose (LEAP) and general purpose (GAP) collimators have relatively short, wide holes that accept more photons than high resolution (HRES) collimators with long, narrow holes. This can be seen in the example in Figure 9-5. Increasing the length of the hole increases resolution by decreasing the angle subtended by the hole. This increase in resolution comes at the expense of sensitivity. In general, images with better resolution do not need as many counts to achieve the same image quality. Unless the images are very count poor or must be acquired very quickly, HRES collimation is generally preferred to LEAP collimation, particularly when multiple detector SPECT systems are used.

Collimators must be made of material that cannot be easily penetrated by photons of the range used in nuclear medicine (70 to 300 keV). This limits the selection to dense metals such as lead, silver, gold, and tungsten. Most collimators are made of lead, but some tungsten collimators are available at great expense. LEAP, GAP, and HRES collimators are all low-energy collimators and are suitable for imaging thallium-201 (^{201}Tl) (~72 keV), technetium-99m (^{99m}Tc)

(140 keV), and iodine-123 (^{123}I) (159 keV). If higher energy radionuclides are used, the collimator septa (the walls that form the holes) must be thicker for the collimator to be effective. Thickening the septa reduces sensitivity for the simple reason that more of the crystal is covered by lead. Collimators designed for indium-111 (^{111}In) (171 and 245 keV) and gallium-67 (^{67}Ga) (93, 185, and 300 keV) are medium-energy collimators. Collimators designed for iodine-131 (^{131}I) (364 keV) are high-energy collimators. Ultra-high-energy collimators have been designed for SPECT imaging of the 511 keV annihilation photons of positron-emitting radionuclides, but their use has been accepted only for myocardial imaging with fluorodeoxyglucose ^{18}FDG. These collimators are extremely heavy, and their weight may put a strain on the SPECT gantry. To recapture some of the sensitivity lost by thicker septa, most medium- and high-energy collimators are designed for lower resolution than low-energy collimators.

Parallel hole collimators are most commonly used for SPECT, but increased sensitivity can be obtained with converging collimators in which the holes converge on a line (fan beam) or a point (cone beam). Converging collimators require more complex setup procedures than do parallel hole collimators if used for SPECT, and once the images have been acquired, they require special image reconstruction software that may result in much longer reconstruction times. Converging collimators allow more of the crystal to be used, which increases sensitivity, as shown in Figure 9-6. This increase in sensitivity is realized with a decrease in the size of the field of view. In practice this usually limits the clinical use of converging collimation to brain imaging.

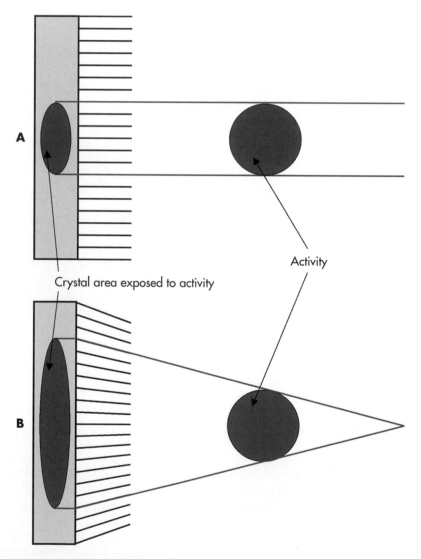

Figure 9-6 Converging collimators improve sensitivity at the expense of field of view. **A,** Parallel hole collimators expose the crystal only to photons that originate directly in front of the collimator. The image formed is a projection of the radionuclide distribution the same size as the distribution. **B,** Fan beam collimators have holes that are directed toward a line at a fixed distance in front of the collimator (parallel to the imaging table). The projection is magnified, more of the crystal is used, and sensitivity is increased. Objects at differing distances from the collimator are magnified by different amounts, resulting in a distorted image. Cone beam collimators are similar but converge to a point instead of a line.

Converging collimators pose a problem for cardiac SPECT because the field of view does not necessarily cover the entire thorax. This truncation of data can lead to artifacts in the reconstruction. Currently, the best compromises have been either to use fan beam collimators with a very slight angle to improve resolution slightly with no truncation or to create a collimator with holes that change the pitch of their angles according to their location in the field of view. The latter type of collimator has holes that get closer to parallel toward their sides, which means that objects in the center of the field of view are imaged with higher resolution than those at the edges, but there is no truncation.

TOMOGRAPHIC ACQUISITIONS

SPECT images are created by mathematically combining many planar scintigrams (called *projections*) that have been collected at many angles around the body. The theory of SPECT requires that the scintillation camera acquire enough images of the patient at different angles to obtain a complete description of the distribution of the radioactive tracer. Several projections over a 180-degree orbit would be satisfactory if there were no scatter or attenuation. Because this is not often the case, 360-degree orbits are used for most SPECT studies (the exception is cardiac SPECT). Numerous parameters define exactly how the rotating gamma camera travels around the patient in the process of collecting these images. These acquisition parameters help determine the quality of the final tomographic image.

SPECT Data Acquisition Modes

Most SPECT systems move in a fashion called *step-and-shoot* as they orbit the patient. The camera moves, stops, acquires an image, moves again, stops, and acquires another image. The optimum number of stops is determined by the system resolution and the pixel size (the better the resolution and the smaller the pixels, the more stops are required). The time

during which the camera is moving and turned off is called *dead time*; it typically is 3 to 5 seconds per projection but may be as high as 8 seconds per projection. Long dead times increase acquisition time, reducing patient comfort, without benefit to image quality.

Continuous orbit cameras try to resolve this problem by acquiring counts at all times, even while the camera moves. Traditionally, continuous motion cameras move slowly and smoothly while counts from designated arcs are collected to form the planar projections. The smaller the arc used for each projection, the less the blurring from the camera's motion.

A final acquisition mode combines step-and-shoot with continuous acquisition; it therefore is termed *continuous step-and-shoot*. The camera is stopped at discrete projection angles but is not turned off during rotation. This minimizes the blur seen with continuous-rotation acquisition but maximizes the number of collected counts in a given time.

Table 9-1 shows the lost time resulting from step-and-shoot motion for both long acquisition (16 minutes, typical of most cardiac SPECT) and short acquisition (3 to 5 minutes), assuming that the lost time per frame is 3 seconds. Most cardiac SPECT studies use 32 or 64 total frames, whereas most general SPECT studies use 64 or 128 total frames. The 16-frame entry in the table assumes a 90-degree dual detector SPECT system and an acquisition with 32 total projections (16 per detector).

180-Degree versus 360-Degree Data Acquisition

As noted above, the exception to the rule that 360-degree orbits are preferred is cardiac SPECT. The heart is located forward and to one side of the center of the thorax, resulting in a great deal of attenuation when the camera is behind the patient. The angles chosen for the 180 degrees are those closest to the heart, from 45 degrees right anterior oblique

Table 9-1 Time to complete a SPECT study using step-and-shoot and continuous acquisitions

Number of frames	Seconds/frame	Acquisition time in minutes		
		Continuous	Step-and-shoot	Lost time*
Long acquisition				
16	60	16.0	16.8	5%
32	30	16.0	17.6	9%
64	15	16.0	19.2	17%
Short acquisition				
16	12	3.2	4.0	20%
32	6	3.2	4.8	33%
64	3	3.2	6.4	50%

*Assuming lost time per frame due to camera motion: 3 seconds.

(RAO) to 45 degrees left posterior oblique (LPO). These projections are affected least by attenuation, scatter, and detector response because they are the closest to the heart. Reconstructions from 180-degree acquisitions have higher resolution and contrast than those from 360-degree acquisitions, particularly with ^{201}Tl images.[2,3] However, because 180-degree reconstructions are not truly complete (i.e., additional information is available from the other 180 degrees of projection), occasional artifacts are seen with 180-degree reconstructions that can be avoided with 360-degree reconstructions.[4-6]

Circular versus Body Contour Orbits

Most SPECT systems offer a choice of circular or body contour orbits. In the simple motion of circular orbits, the gamma camera is limited to rotating in a circle. The position of the detector is fixed at a given radius with respect to the center of rotation. A minimal radius is chosen that allows the camera to clear the body at every angle. However, forcing the camera to stay at a fixed radius at one angle may result in it being very far from the body at another angle (after all, most people are not circular in cross section).

Body contour orbits seek to keep the camera as close to the body as possible throughout the tomographic acquisition, thereby maximizing resolution.[7] The radius is changed angle by angle to minimize the distance while maintaining the same angles used in a circular orbit. The simplest body contour orbits assume the shape of an ellipse, although some manufactures offer sophisticated sensors that minimize the

camera-body distance in real time at each angle. Body contour orbits are illustrated in Figure 9-7.

For general SPECT images, the results of body contour orbits are superior to those of circular orbits. Some manufacturers' complicated setup procedures have made the body contour technique prohibitively complex for use in the clinical setting. Use of body contour orbits for cardiac SPECT is not as widely accepted. Because the resolution varies from angle to angle, the resulting reconstruction may be different from one created with a circular orbit. In cardiac SPECT, the heart is often put at or near the center of rotation when a circular orbit is used, which ensures that the heart is imaged with approximately the same resolution for all angles. Use of a noncircular orbit changes the distance from the detector to the center of rotation, or the heart, at each angle. This has been reported to cause apical defects,[8] or the base and septum of the heart to appear as having slightly decreased counts, because these regions are relatively farther from the detector during a body contour orbit.[9] These "artifacts" may be related to exactly how the noncircular orbit is effected; that is, how the gantry, camera heads, and patient table are moved during the acquisition. Others have found no significant difference in perfusion quantification applied to acquisitions performed with circular and noncircular orbits.[10,11]

Other Factors

Three important variables are the size of the image pixels, the average number of counts collected for each pixel, and

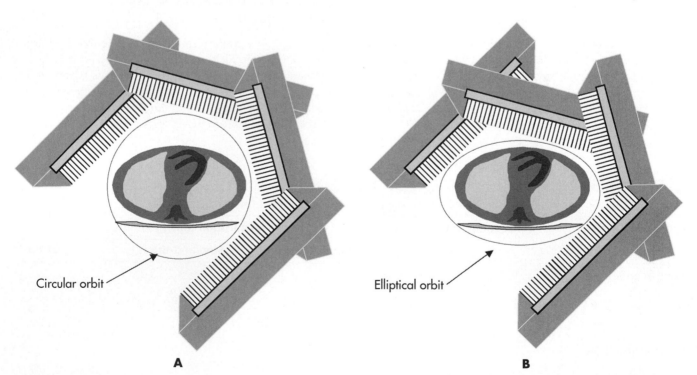

A   **B**

Figure 9-7   Elliptical and body contour orbits keep the camera close to the patient during the entire SPECT acquisition. **A,** When a circular orbit is used, the camera is close to the body in some projections but far away in others. **B,** Elliptical and body contour orbits try to maximize resolution by keeping the camera as close to the body as possible during the entire orbit. In cardiac imaging the asymmetric position of the heart in the body may lead to a widely varying heart-to-camera distance (and thus widely varying resolution) during the orbit, resulting in reconstruction artifacts.

the number of views obtained. In general, the pixel size should be less than one third the system resolution (measured as FWHM). The number of counts in each pixel is also related to the system resolution; the higher the resolution, the lower the number of counts obtained per pixel. In most cases the number of counts should be maximized without exceeding radiation dose limits or the patient's ability to remain immobile. The number of views depends on the resolution and the pixel size. If too few views are taken, resolution is lost and artifacts may be introduced.

SPECT imaging of the thorax, abdomen, or pelvis usually uses the camera's full field of view. A 128 × 128 pixel matrix is preferred for most low-energy studies because this gives a pixel size of about 4 mm for a typical 51 cm wide large-field-of-view camera. For the study, 128 views should be acquired over 360 degrees. In some cases using medium- or high-energy collimation in which the pixel counts are low, a 64 × 64 matrix may be satisfactory.

Pixels 6 to 6.5 mm in size have proved to be adequate for cardiac SPECT. This size is obtained by using a 64 × 64 pixel matrix for systems with a field of view of 38 to 40 cm. In these studies, 64 projections over 180 degrees are preferred, but 32 projections are often used with satisfactory results. To achieve a field of view of this size in a large-field-of-view camera, some of the scintillation crystal area can be discarded through a process know as *zoom*. When a zoom factor is used, the field of view is reduced and the pixels of the image are used more efficiently (more of the image is occupied by the organ of interest, in this case the heart). A zoom factor of 1.3 reduces the field of view of a 51 cm camera to 38 cm. Camera zooms are described in Figure 9-8.

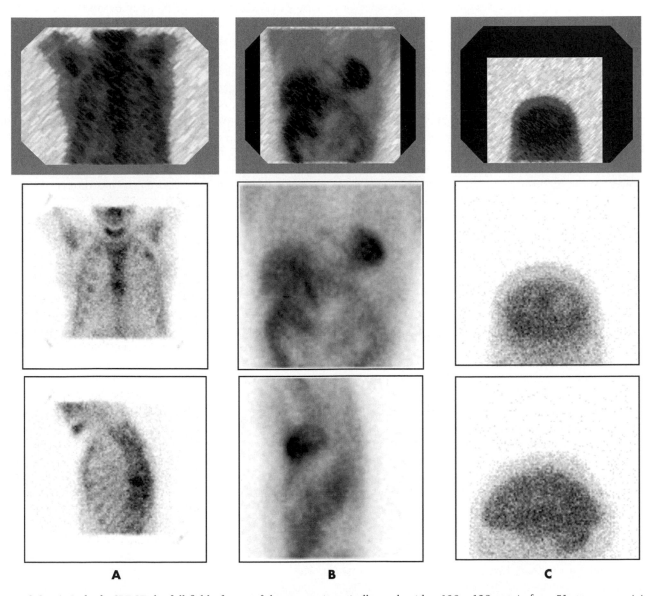

A   **B**   **C**

Figure 9-8   A, In body SPECT the full field of view of the camera is typically used, with a 128 × 128 matrix for a 51 cm camera giving 4 mm/pixel. **B,** Myocardial SPECT does not require the full field of view, which may be reduced by zooming the image. A zoom factor of 1.3 reduces the field of view to 38 cm and gives a pixel size of 6 mm for a 64 × 64 matrix. **C,** The brain is relatively small compared to the camera, and a zoom factor of 1.6 reduces the field of view to 32 cm, with a 2.5 mm/pixel for a 128 × 128 matrix. Note that the zoomed area is shifted to the bottom of the camera, reducing the distance from the edge of the image to the edge of the camera. This helps the operator bring the camera closer than the patient's shoulder during setup.

The scintillation camera should remain as close to the head as possible for brain SPECT. This allows for excellent resolution compared with body SPECT (remember that resolution decreases as the distance from the collimator increases). A zoom factor of 1.5 reduces the pixel size to less than 3 mm with a 128×128 matrix. For the study, 128 views should be acquired over 360 degrees. An important consideration in choosing a camera for brain SPECT is the *brain reach*, or the distance from the edge of the camera to the usable field of view. If this distance is too great, it becomes difficult to position the camera close to the head (over the shoulder) without cutting the lower portion of the cerebellum out of the field of view.

Specific guidelines for the setup of different SPECT procedures can be found in *Procedure Guidelines Manual*, published by the Society of Nuclear Medicine.[12] The American Society of Nuclear Cardiology has published *Guidelines for Nuclear Cardiology Procedures*,[13] which has the recommended procedures for nuclear cardiology.

SPECT RECONSTRUCTION

Methods of reconstructing the radionuclide distribution from planar projections have been the subject of investigation since the possibility was proven by L. Radon in 1917. The advent of computers accelerated research into different methods of image reconstruction, and many have been proposed. These reconstruction algorithms fall into two categories: iterative methods and analytic methods. Analytic methods are based on exact mathematical solutions to the image reconstruction problem, whereas iterative methods estimate the distribution through successive approximations. Accurate corrections for attenuation and other degradations require more complex iterative reconstruction techniques.

Filtered Back-Projection Reconstruction

Filtered back-projection, the most frequently used method of image reconstruction,[14] is an analytic reconstruction algorithm. As its name implies, filtered back-projection is a combination of filtering and back-projection. When a projection image is acquired, each row of the projection contains counts that emanate from the entire transverse plane. When projection images are obtained from many angles about the body, enough information is available in each row of the set of angular projections to reconstruct the original corresponding transverse slice. Figure 9-9 shows projections acquired from a phantom over many angles. The projections can be reordered such that single lines from each of the projection angles are stacked on top of each other. This type of image is called a *sinogram*, because a point source in this image traces out a sine wave (Figure 9-9, *C*). A sinogram has all the projection data necessary to reconstruct a single slice of the original activity distribution.

Back-projection assigns the values in the projection to all points along the line of acquisition through the image plane from which they were acquired. This is shown in Figure 9-10. This operation is repeated for all pixels and all angles; the new values are added to the previous ones in what is known as a *superposition operation*. As the number of angles increases, the back-projection improves.

Although simple back-projection is useful for illustrative purposes, it is never used in practice without the step of filtering. Note that the back-projection in Figure 9-10, *D* is quite blurred compared with the original distribution from which it was created. Also, Figure 9-10, *B* and *C* both show instances of the *star artifact*, which consists of radial lines near the edges of the object. This artifact is a natural result of back-projection applied without filtering. In clinical practice, a ramp filter is applied to each projection before back-projection (ramp filters are discussed in more detail later in the chapter). The ramp-filtered projections are characterized by enhancement of edge information and the introduction of negative values (or *lobes*) into the filtered projections. During superposition in the back-projection process, these negative values cancel portions of the other angular contributions and in effect help eliminate the star artifact (Figure 9-11). However, enough projections must be acquired to ensure that proper cancellation is obtained. Radial blurring or streaking toward the periphery of the image often indicates that too few projections were acquired. Finally, a noise-reducing filter, such as a Butterworth or Hanning filter, usually is applied before, during, or after the back-projection operation. These filters are discussed in more detail in following sections.

Iterative Reconstruction

Iterative reconstruction techniques require many more calculations and thus much more computer time to create a transaxial image than does filtered back-projection. As computers have progressed in speed and memory, they have made the transition from a research tool to routine clinical use. Their primary importance is their ability to incorporate corrections for the factors that degrade SPECT images. Iterative techniques use the original projections and models of the acquisition process to predict a reconstruction. The predicted reconstruction is then used again with the models to create new predicted projections. If the predicted projections are different from the actual projections, these differences are used to modify the reconstruction. This process is continued until the reconstruction is such that the predicted projections match the actual projections. The primary differences between various iterative methods are the ways the predicted reconstructions and projections are created and the ways they are modified at each step. Practically speaking, the more theoretically accurate the iterative technique, the more time-consuming the process. Maximum likelihood methods allow noise to be modeled, whereas least squares techniques, such as the conjugate gradient method, generally ignore noise.[15-17] Iterative filtered back-projection (IFBP) methods create the new reconstruction at every iteration by using filtered back-projection.[18,19]

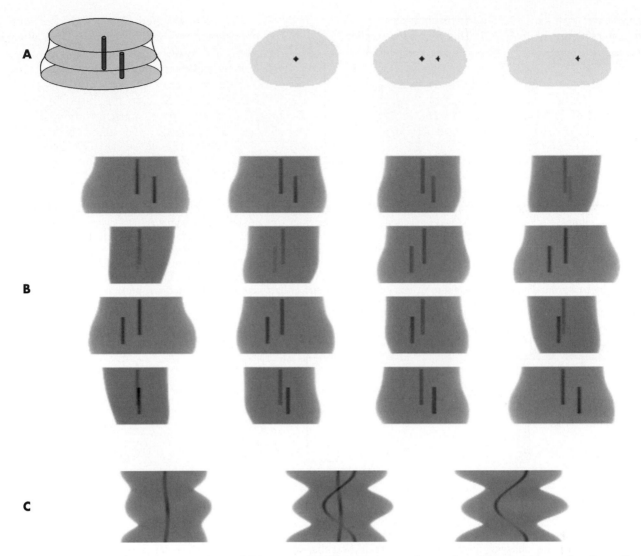

Figure 9-9   Projections and sinograms. **A**, Original 3D activity distribution is a tapered part of an ellipsoid, with two hot lines offset in two directions. Three slices through the original distribution are shown. **B**, Sixteen original projections created from the activity distribution. From top left to bottom right, these projections were acquired from the rear of the object, rotating around to the left, to the front, to the right, and then returning to the rear. **C**, Three sinograms created from the projections. Each sinogram contains a single horizontal line taken from each of the 16 projections, so that a single sinogram contains all of the information necessary to reconstruct a single slice of the original image. The left-most sinogram was taken from near the top of the projections shown in **B**, so that the outer background of the object is relatively small and the single hot spot is near the center. The right-most sinogram was created using a line taken from near the bottom of the projection set. Note that in this sinogram, the outer boundary of the background of the object is larger and the hot spot, which is offset from the center, traces a sine wave within the sinogram. The center sinogram was created using a line taken from near the center of the projection.

Based on the maximum likelihood criteria commonly used in statistical analysis, the most widely used iterative reconstruction method is maximum likelihood expectation maximization (MLEM).[15,20] The MLEM algorithm attempts to determine the tracer distribution that would "most likely" yield the measured projections given the imaging model and a map of attenuation coefficients if available. The MLEM algorithm converges slowly, requiring many more iterations than IFBP algorithms. The slowly converging characteristics of this algorithm yield greater control over image noise.[20,21] An example of the reconstruction of the myocardium with the MLEM algorithm is shown in Figure 9-12. The point of convergence of this algorithm and the related number of

iterations for clinical use are a source of debate.[22] In practice, there is no common rule for stopping the algorithms after a number of iterations on clinical data, and protocols describing the optimum number of iterations are largely empirically based.

Another approach to the MLEM algorithm for iterative reconstruction is the ordered subsets expectation maximization (OSEM) method,[23] in which the projection data are ordered into subsets, which are used in the iterative steps of the reconstruction to greatly speed up the process. The advantage of OSEM is that an order of magnitude increase in computational speed can be obtained.

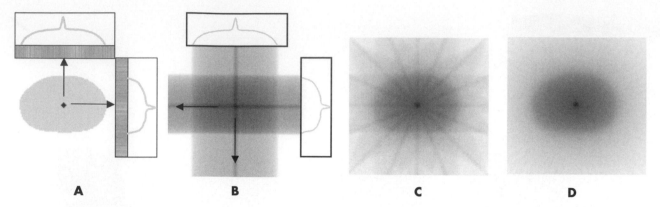

Figure 9-10 Simple back-projection. **A,** Two projections are acquired from a single slice. The original activity distribution is shown in the center, with the two projections to the top and right. Profiles through the projections are shown within each. **B,** Counts from the two projections are spread back out over the reconstruction, with counts from each projection being added to, or superposed on, the previous one. **C,** More projections added to the back-projection process start to make the reconstruction recognizable as the original transverse slice. **D,** Use of many projections gives a blurry representation of the original object. Note the rays from the back-projection process in the background of this image and in **C,** demonstrating the star artifact inherent in simple back-projection.

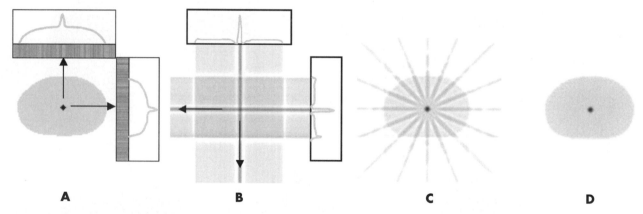

Figure 9-11 Filtered back-projection. **A,** Two projections are acquired from a single slice. The original activity distribution is shown in the center, with the two projections to the top and right. Profiles through the projections are shown within each. **B,** A ramp filter is applied to the projections, changing the profiles through each. Note that now the background of the object is reduced, and the point source has higher contrast. These two effects are the direct result of ramp filtering. Counts from the two filtered projections are spread back out over the reconstruction, with counts from each projection being added to, or superposed on, the previous one. **C,** More projections added to the filtered back-projection process start to make the reconstruction recognizable as the original transverse slice. **D,** Use of many projections gives a sharp, accurate reconstruction of the original object. Note that the star artifact is also reduced in both this reconstruction and the one shown in **C.**

FILTERING OF SPECT IMAGES

In SPECT, filters are used either to enhance or to remove the high-frequency components of the image.[24] High-frequency components are sharp changes in image intensity, such as those seen at edges between the heart and the background or in noise points. Low frequencies contain information about slowly changing or constant intensities of the image, such as uniform regions of perfusion. Filters that remove high frequencies are called low-pass filters because they preserve (pass) only the low frequencies. This reduces noise but blurs edges. Filters that enhance high frequencies are called high-pass filters. They operate in the opposite manner; they pass only the high frequencies while attenuating low frequencies. This sharpens organ boundaries but increases noise.

A Fourier transform (implemented on the computer as a fast Fourier transform, or FFT) decomposes an image into its various frequency components. The frequency components are the spatial frequencies that make up the image. These frequencies are expressed in terms of cycles per distance (usually cycles/centimeter or cycles/pixel).

Low frequencies reflect the overall shapes of an image. High frequencies are the result of areas with sharp changes in pixel counts, such as edges (and image noise). The highest frequency in a digital image is 0.5 cycles/pixel, representing alternating bright and dark pixels. This frequency is called the *Nyquist frequency.* Because filters are defined in terms of spatial frequencies, it is important that careful attention be given to the units of the frequency. Some manufacturers define filters in terms of cycles/pixel, others use cycles/cm, and still others use a percentage of the Nyquist frequency; the difference is as important as the difference between inches, centimeters, and miles.

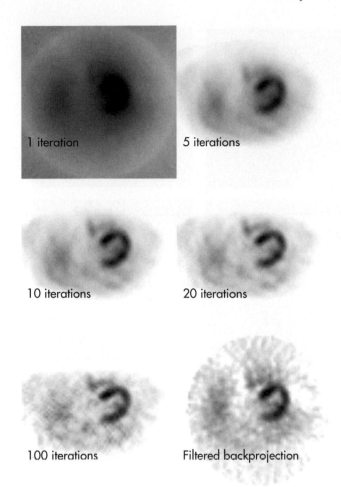

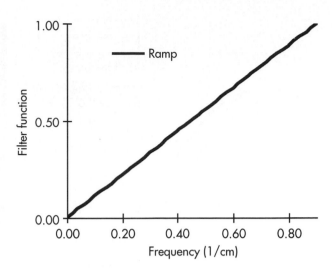

Figure 9-13   The ramp filter, the filter referred to in filtered back-projection, is used to remove the blurring given by simple back-projection. Note that the filter ends at a little greater than 0.8 1/cm, or the Nyquist frequency for 0.6 cm pixels. Also note that the ramp filter allows more high frequencies than low frequencies and is considered to be a high-pass filter.

Figure 9-12   Iterative reconstruction of a ^{99m}Tc sestamibi patient study (transaxial slices). The quality of images reconstructed with the maximum likelihood algorithm (beginning with a uniform image) improves with successive iterations. After a point, however, image noise begins to degrade the image, as can be seen in image produced by 100 iterations.

Ramp Filter

A *ramp filter,* which is a high-pass filter, is the most important filter for SPECT because the ramp filter erases the blurring of simple back-projection. When we speak of filtered back-projection, we are speaking of the ramp filter. It is important to note that the ramp filter is applied only in the transaxial plane because this is the only plane that experiences blurring in simple back-projection. The formula for the ramp filter is given by

$$w(f) = |f|$$

where $w(f)$ is the filter function, and f represents the spatial frequencies of the image. When graphed, the filter has the shape of a ramp (Figure 9-13).

Hanning Filters

Hann (or *Hanning*) *filters* (Figure 9-14) are among the most commonly used smoothing (or noise reduction) filters for SPECT. The formula for a Hann filter is given by

if $|f| < f_m$,

$$w(f) = 0.5 + 0.5 \cos\left(\frac{\pi f}{f_m}\right)$$

or if $|f| > f_m$,

$$w(f) = 0$$

where $w(f)$ is the filter function, f represents the spatial frequencies of the image, and f_m is the maximum frequency, or *cutoff frequency,* of the filter. The Hann filter has a value of 1 at zero frequency ($\cos(0) = 1$) and decreases to zero at the cutoff frequency. Thus the cutoff frequency is the parameter used to define the Hann filter. The lower the cutoff frequency, the more high frequencies are removed from the image and the smoother the filtered image.

Butterworth Filters

Another common filter is the *Butterworth filter* (Figures 9-15 and 9-16), which is more versatile (and more complicated) than the Hann filter. The Butterworth filter is given by the equation

$$w(f) = \frac{1}{\sqrt{1 + \left(\frac{f}{f_c}\right)p}}$$

where $w(f)$ is the filter function; f represents the spatial frequencies of the image; f_c is the maximum frequency, or *critical frequency,* of the filter; and p is the *power factor* of the filter. The Butterworth filter has a value of 1 at zero frequency and decreases to (but never quite reaches) zero. The Butterworth filter is characterized by a level plateau and a drop-off defined by the critical frequency. The power factor defines the steepness of this drop-off. It is important to note

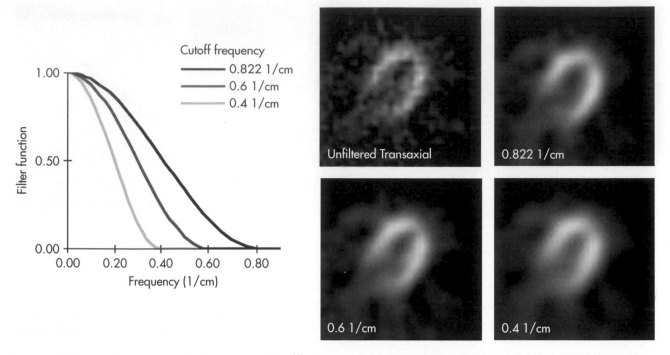

Figure 9-14 Results with three Hanning filters, applied to ^{201}Tl myocardial perfusion SPECT and using different cutoff frequencies, are plotted. The lower the cutoff frequency, the smoother the image after the filter is applied. When no smoothing filter is applied, the image might be considered too noisy for clinical use. A cutoff frequency of 0.4 cm^{-1} smoothes most of the details out of the image.

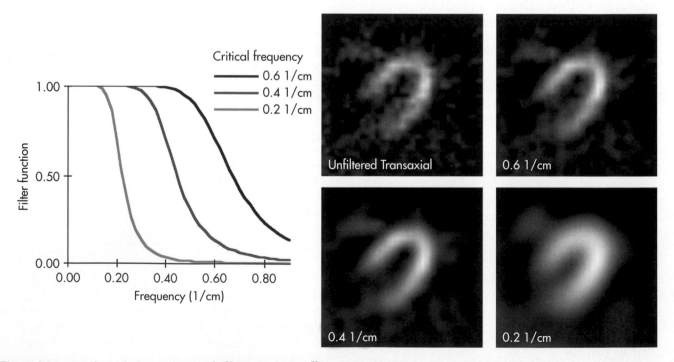

Figure 9-15 Results with three Butterworth filters, applied to ^{99m}Tc sestamibi SPECT and using different critical frequencies, are plotted. The lower the critical frequency, the smoother the image after the filter is applied. The same power factor (10) is used for each of the filters. The higher the critical frequency, the more high frequencies are retained in the filtered image and the less smooth it appears.

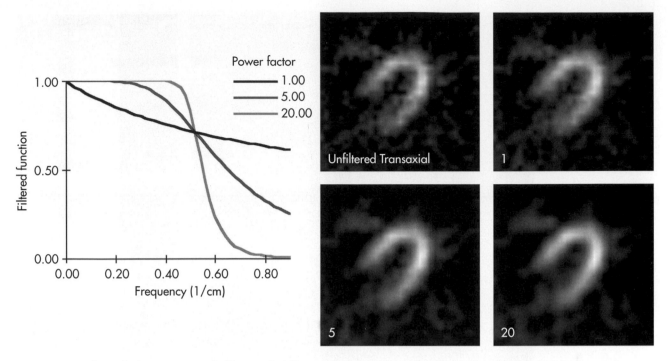

Figure 9-16   Results with three Butterworth filters with different power factors are plotted. The lower the critical frequency, the smoother the image after the filter is applied. The same critical frequency (0.52 1/cm) is used for each of the filters. The effect of changing the power factor is less apparent than that of the critical frequency. Lower power factors retain more high frequencies but at the expense of middle and low frequencies.

that the critical frequency of the Butterworth filter differs from the cutoff frequency of the Hanning filter. At $f = f_c$ the Butterworth filter equals $1/\sqrt{2}$, not zero. Some manufacturers refer to the critical frequency as a cutoff frequency in an attempt to avoid confusion.

Alternate definitions of the Butterworth filter are:

$$w(f) = \frac{1}{\sqrt{1 + \left(\frac{f}{f_c}\right)2n}} \quad \text{and} \quad w(f) = \frac{1}{1 + \left(\frac{f}{f_c}\right)2n}$$

In the first example n is the *order* of the filter. The only difference is that the order is one half the power factor. The second example removes the square root and at $f = f_c$, the Butterworth filter equals one half.

When to Filter

Smoothing filters can be applied before, after, or during back-projection. There are advantages and disadvantages to each method, but filtering in three dimensions is generally preferred to filtering in two dimensions (Figure 9-17).

Prior to back-projection. A two-dimensional filter applied to each of the planar projections before back-projection actually filters in all three dimensions. After image reconstruction the image will have the same resolution in all three dimensions. This offers an advantage if sagittal, coronal, or oblique images are needed. This is sometimes called a *pre-*

filter because it precedes the ramp filter, which is applied only in the transverse direction (perpendicular to the axis of the table). A two-dimensional pre-filter is the preferred method of soothing and noise reduction for SPECT images.

During back-projection. A one-dimensional smoothing filter is sometimes combined with the ramp filter and applied during the back-projection process. The advantage is that only one filter must the applied (i.e., a ramp-Butterworth, the combination of a ramp and a Butterworth filter), and computations are reduced. The disadvantage is that no smoothing has been done in the axial dimension. If sagittal, coronal, or oblique images are cut from the resulting image set, they will not have been equally smoothed in all directions and will appear to have horizontal streaks.

After back-projection. Filters may also be applied after image reconstruction, but they should be applied in all three dimensions. If a two-dimensional filter is applied to the transaxial images, however, the same problems will occur as with filtering during back-projection: the images will not have been smoothed in the axial dimension. Another filter must then be applied (sometimes called a *y filter*) to compensate before images at other orientations are extracted. This leads to more computations (and longer processing times) than are required when filtering is performed before back-projection. Three-dimensional post-reconstruction filtering is preferred for iterative reconstruction techniques.

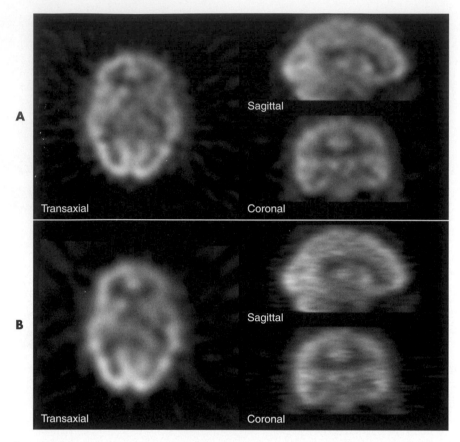

Figure 9-17 Filtering during back-projection leads to uneven resolution or smoothness in different directions. **A,** These SPECT brain images have been smoothed in three dimensions, either by pre-filtering or by using a 3D filter after reconstruction. **B,** These images were smoothed with a ramp-Butterworth filter during reconstruction. The smoothing filter was applied only in the transaxial plane (as is the ramp filter). Horizontal streaks are evident in the sagittal and coronal images.

Table 9-2 Conversion of units of frequency (multiply by column to get row)

	From Nyquist	From cycles/cm	From cycles/pixel
To get Nyquist	1	2 * pixel size	2
To get cycles/cm	1/(2 * pixel size)	1	1/pixel size
To get cycles/pixel	1/2	pixel size	1

Pixel sizes are assumed to be centimeters (cm).

Units of Frequency

The implementation of filters varies widely among manufacturers of nuclear medicine computers. In addition to the alternate definitions of the Butterworth filters and the choices of when to apply smoothing filters mentioned above, manufacturers specify cutoff and critical frequency values using different units, including cycles/cm, cycles/pixel, and Nyquist, which is equivalent to cycles/2 pixels. Table 9-2 is presented as an aid to conversion of the various units.

SPECT IMAGE DISPLAY

Color Versus Gray Scale

Different color scales may be used to highlight different features in SPECT images. Certain color scales may help distinguish normal from abnormal regions in some studies. Conversely, gray scale is actually better for highlighting very dim objects. Because color scales can be used to enhance or diminish various features, the same image can be made to look very different simply by changing the color table. SPECT images, therefore, should always be scaled and displayed in a reproducible and standardized manner to ensure reproducibility in qualitative analysis. In the past few years some automatic techniques for performing this task have been described.

Image Reorientation

Transaxial images. The natural products of rotational tomography are images that represent cross-sectional slices of the body perpendicular to the imaging table (or long axis

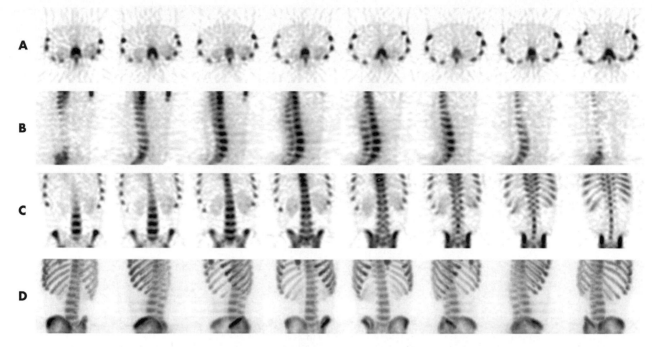

Figure 9-18   A, Original transaxial slices taken from a normal bone SPECT study. Transaxial slices are oriented such that the patient's right side is on the left side of the image. The patient's anterior is to the top of the image. Consecutive slices are displayed from the patient's superior to his inferior. **B,** Consecutive sagittal slices of the same study. Sagittal slices are oriented such that posterior structures are on the left and anterior structures are on the right. Consecutive slices are displayed from the patient's right to his left. **C,** Coronal slices taken from the same study. Coronal images are oriented such that the left side of the patient is shown on the right side of the image. Consecutive slices are displayed from the patient's anterior to his posterior. **D,** Volume-rendered maximum activity projection images displayed from different angles. Note that the whole "hot" skeleton can be seen, with bones closer to the viewing point more intense than those farther away.

of the body). These images are called *transverse* or *transaxial slices* (Figure 9-18, *A*).

Longitudinal images. SPECT images can be reconstructed so that the image slices are contiguous and the slice thickness is equal to the pixel size (defined as the length of one side of the square pixels). Once we recognize that the pixels have depth as well as width, the terminology must be altered, and the pixels are more aptly called voxels (volume elements; pixel stands for picture element). The images may then be thought of as a three-dimensional matrix of information about the patient. Using the computer, this three-dimensional matrix can be resliced to give images at different orientations. Coronal slices are parallel to the surface of the imaging table. Sagittal slices are perpendicular to both transaxial and coronal slices. Sagittal and coronal slices are shown in Figure 9-18, *B* and *C*, respectively.

Oblique images. We are not restricted to the natural *x, y,* and *z* directions, however, for the extraction of images. The computer may be used to extract images at any orientation, and these images are called *oblique images*. The short and long axis images commonly used in myocardial tomography are examples of oblique images. Oblique images may also be used to retrospectively obtain a desired image orientation for brain imaging. The important oblique sections used for

viewing cardiac images are described in the section on cardiac quantification.

Three-Dimensional Displays

Interest in three-dimensional (3D) displays for SPECT data has increased over the past several years. Currently, the most common display mode is a two-dimensional (2D) interactive slicing program that allows a user to view a 3D data set one slice at a time. Such displays are limited when the examiner is trying to gain an accurate idea of the size and shape of an organ or tumor or the extent and severity of disease. For these reasons, efforts have been underway to generate true 3D displays.[25-27] These displays generally fall into two categories, volume rendering and surface rendering.

Volume rendering. Volume rendering offers the advantage of visualizing an object in 3D without having to explicitly identify the surface. The most common type of volume rendering in SPECT is the technique of maximum intensity projection (MIP) developed by Wallis and Miller.[28] In this approach, the reconstructed transaxial slices are first stacked to form a 3D tomographic volume. Maximum intensity projection involves rotating this 3D tomographic volume into a desired viewing angle and extracting the maximum pixel along each row and column of the rotated volume onto a

2D image plane. To enhance the 3D effect of the image, the volume can be depth-weighted to emphasize structures in the front of the volume and deemphasize structures in the rear of the volume before the maximum pixel is extracted. Because the maximum pixel is always extracted, this type of volume rendering emphasizes hot spots and is very useful in blood pool and tumor imaging procedures. Maximum intensity projections of the normal bone scan shown in Figure 9-18 can be viewed in the final row. A similar example of both longitudinal slices and a MIP rendering of an abnormal bone scan is shown in Figure 9-19.

Wallis and Miller[27,28] and Miller, Wallis, and Sampathkumaran[29] have noted several advantages of volume-rendered gated cardiac blood pool studies using MIP. The most noticeable advantage of MIP is the enhanced contrast over standard planar imaging. Also, a volume-rendered display can be generated for any desirable viewing angle, allowing a clinician to view each structure of the myocardium from the best possible angle, even those views that cannot be routinely acquired during a planar study. The disadvantage of MIP is that it is essentially a modified planar technique with improved contrast but increased processing time. As such, it is well suited for hot spot imaging procedures but has limited application in demonstrating cold lesions.

Surface rendering. Surface rendering refers to methods that display an organ or region based on explicitly detected boundaries. Generation of a surface-rendered display, therefore, requires segmentation. *Segmentation* is the process of separating the organ from the background or nearby structures. It can be accomplished using various methods, such as hand tracing the volume of interest, using a thresholding technique in which pixels with values greater than the threshold are assumed to be part of the organ and all other pixels are assumed to be background, or complicated boundary detection algorithms. Usually, a thresholding segmentation process produces a binary data set in which myocardial voxels have a value of 1 and background voxels have a value of zero. A boundary tracking algorithm is then used to identify the surface of the myocardium as the boundary between 1s and 0s and convert it into geometric primitives, such as squares or triangles. In contrast, hand tracing and boundary detection methods usually result in a set of discrete surface points, which are then connected into geometric primitives, usually triangles.

Surface-rendered models are generally displayed using standard computer graphics packages, which allows rotation and translation of the "model," positioning of one or more light sources, and adjustment of the model's *opacity* (the amount of light shining through the model) or *reflectance* (the amount of light reflecting off the model). The speed of a three-dimensional surface rendering depends greatly on the type and number of individual elements from which the model is composed. In general, however, surface-rendered displays are quite fast and often can be rotated and translated interactively. The accuracy of such displays depends primarily on the surface detection and the mapping of func-

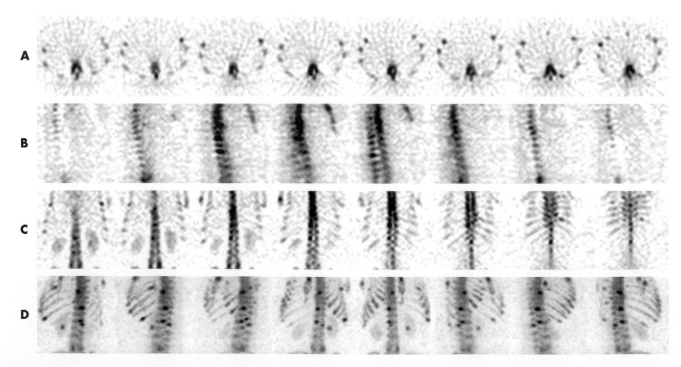

Figure 9-19 **A,** Original transaxial slices taken from an abnormal bone SPECT study. This patient has hot metastases at numerous locations in the spine and rib cage. **B,** Consecutive sagittal slices of the same study. **C,** Coronal slices taken from the same study. **D,** Volume-rendered maximum intensity projection images displayed from different angles. Note that the whole skeleton can be seen, but the hotter metastases are also obvious, and their locations are more effectively visualized than with serial slices.

tion onto the surface, when this is performed. Figure 9-20 shows the surface renderings of two SPECT brain studies of the same patient, a baseline study and a Diamox challenge. The surfaces of these two brains were defined using a single threshold for segmentation.

The advantage of this kind of display is that it is often fast and easy to implement and with the proper segmentation can give useful results. The disadvantage of this technique is that many SPECT studies contain both physiologic and anatomic information. Segmentation of a SPECT study into a binary data set using thresholding techniques often ignores some of the important physiologic information present in the scan. In fact, improper segmentation from use of an incorrect threshold can give erroneous results. Unfortunately, because single thresholds are used for segmentation in most commercial packages, improper segmentation is a common finding. However, when this technique is applied with appropriate boundary detection algorithms, it is the most realistic way to view the results of quantitation.

SPECT PHYSICS AND IMAGE ARTIFACTS

Artifacts in SPECT images arise from the combined effects of photon absorption, Compton scatter, and the degradation in resolution with distance from the collimator. Each of these interrelated factors produces inconsistent information in the planar projections, in violation of the assumptions behind filtered back-projection (FBP), the most widely used tomographic reconstruction algorithm. The effect of these factors on SPECT images is quite complex, and each is discussed separately.

Attenuation

An example of the attenuation process in myocardial SPECT is shown in Figure 9-21, *A*. Photons emitted from the heart and picked up by the detector in an anterior view have traversed a relatively small amount of tissue (soft tissue and bone). In a lateral view, photons must traverse a greater distance but through different materials (including lung) to

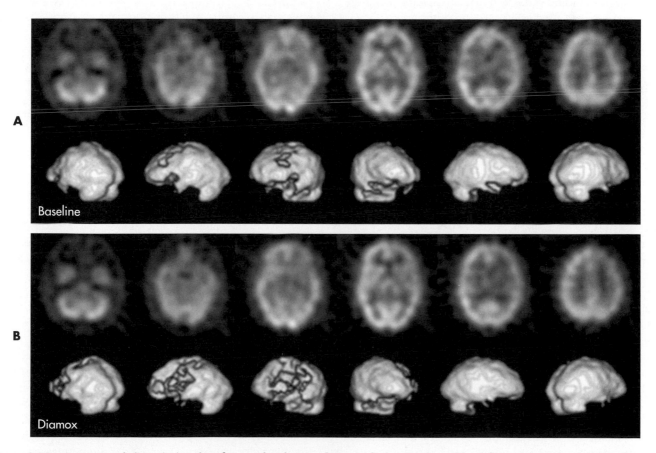

Figure 9-20 **A,** Transaxial slices (*top*) and surface-rendered views (*bottom*) of a baseline brain blood flow study. A threshold has been applied to the original images, and the resulting pixels have been connected into a single polygonal object that is then displayed from different angles using surface rendering. Note the "hole" in the left superior part of the brain, an effect created because of the pixels that did not survive the chosen threshold. The part of the brain corresponding to this "hole" may have decreased blood flow. **B,** The same serial slices and 3D views as seen in **A** from the same patient after a Diamox challenge. Diamox should increase brain blood flow in regions where the arterial blood supply is normal and thereby show relative decreases in blood flow distal to constricted or otherwise abnormal vessels. In this case, a relative decrease is seen in the same left superior region as in **A**, but with this pharmaceutical challenge, the abnormality is more profound. This can also be seen on the 3D image, because the "hole" in the brain surface is much larger in these views.

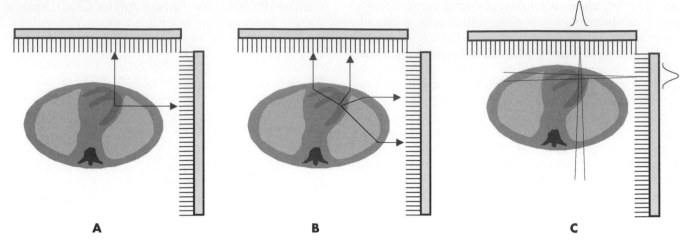

A   **B**   **C**

Figure 9-21   Physical factors that compromise SPECT include nonuniform attenuation (photons emitted from a single point in the heart pass through different materials in different planar projections) (**A**); Compton scatter (photons emitted from that point no longer appear to originate there) (**B**); and varying resolution (the farther the distance from the point to the camera in each projection, the poorer the resolution) (**C**).

reach the detector. As the detector moves about the patient, the projection profile varies with the attenuation along the projection ray and the distance to the collimator.

Attenuation is described quantitatively by the linear attenuation coefficient (commonly depicted by the Greek letter mu [μ]). For example, the value of μ for ^{99m}Tc in soft tissue is approximately equal to that of water: 0.154 l/cm^{-1}. The process of attenuation is described by

$$A_x = A_0 e^{-\mu x}$$

where A_x is the activity measured after attenuation through a thickness of tissue x and A_0 is the true activity at a point in the body.[30] Thus the term $e^{-\mu x}$ represents the fraction of photons that are attenuated over a distance x.

The probability of absorption increases as photon energy decreases; thus attenuation artifacts are reported to be more severe with ^{201}Tl agents than with ^{99m}Tc.[8,31] The most frequently noted effects of attenuation in myocardial SPECT are artifacts associated with breast attenuation in women and diaphragmatic attenuation in men.[8,31,32] Breast attenuation artifacts are commonly identified as a region of decreased count density over the anterior myocardial wall. If the breast position is the same between scans, the appearance of a "fixed" perfusion defect may result and may be interpreted as scar or partial reversibility (ischemia). A breast that is not in the same position between rest and stress scans may masquerade as a reversible defect. Similar changes in apparent perfusion patterns in the inferior myocardial wall can result from differences in diaphragmatic attenuation between resting and stress scans.

Compton Scatter

When a photon undergoes Compton scattering though interactions with an electron, it changes direction and loses energy (Figure 9-21, *B*). If detected in the photopeak energy window, Compton-scattered photons are likely to be miss-

positioned in the transverse image, leading to reduced image contrast and reduced lesion detection. Just as with attenuation, scatter can be a more severe problem with ^{201}Tl than with ^{99m}Tc, particularly in myocardial SPECT.

In myocardial SPECT, scatter affects the apparent extent and severity of the hypoperfused regions detected with ^{201}Tl or ^{99m}Tc. In some patients the scatter from high concentrations of activity in abdominal organs (primarily liver and bowel) may artifactually increase the counts in the inferior wall of the myocardium.[33-35]

Detector Response

The most important factors in the spatial resolution of images made with a conventional scintillation camera are the geometry of the collimator and the distance from the camera face. The resolution of both fan beam and parallel hole collimators degrades with distance. This effect is shown with a parallel hole collimator in Figure 9-21, *C*. As the camera orbits the patient for a circular acquisition, the only point in the patient that maintains the same distance from the collimator in all the views is at the center of rotation. Because the spatial resolution at any given point in a SPECT image is a result of the resolution in each of the planar projections, the center of rotation is the only point in the reconstructed image with symmetric resolution. This spatially varying resolution can lead to significant distortion in the reconstructed images, particularly for 180-degree acquisitions.[4,6] Although combining the two opposing views of a 360-degree acquisition degrades spatial resolution, it also minimizes its variation across the transverse plane.[16]

ATTENUATION CORRECTION, SCATTER CORRECTION, AND RESOLUTION RECOVERY

Methods exist to correct for attenuation, scatter, and variable resolution effects in SPECT. Some are straightforward and easily implemented; however, the trend is toward applying physical models of each of the effects within an iterative reconstruction technique.

The American Society of Nuclear Cardiology and the Society of Nuclear Medicine have issued a position statement on "the value and practice of attenuation correction for myocardial perfusion SPECT imaging."[36] This statement concludes that "attenuation correction should be regarded as a rapidly evolving standard for SPECT myocardial perfusion imaging" and that "the adjunctive technique of attenuation correction has become a method for which the weight of evidence and opinion is in favor of its usefulness."

Attenuation Correction

Although artifacts caused by attenuation, Compton scatter, and varying resolution present a problem for all SPECT imaging, the most commonly cited complications (and the most difficult to correct because of the variable media of the thorax) are attenuation artifacts in myocardial perfusion SPECT. These artifacts are often cited as the most significant factors limiting interpretative accuracy.[8,31,32] They reduce the specificity of cardiac SPECT by causing variations in normal tracer patterns that may overlap known coronary territories and resemble patterns associated with coronary artery disease.

Procedures for minimizing the clinical impact of attenuation. One method of handling attenuation artifacts is simply to reduce their clinical impact through scanning techniques and knowledge of their location and severity when they occur. For example, the effect of attenuation can often be detected in the rotating planar projection images where a "shadow" moves laterally across the body profile relative to the cardiac uptake. Compared with true hypoperfusion, attenuation artifacts can move "independent" of the heart and attenuate background activity in some of the projection images. The existence of such artifacts, when supplied to a physician, can reduce false positives. In addition, SPECT imaging in the prone position has been reported to minimize attenuation artifacts in myocardial perfusion studies in which the inferior wall may be involved.[37] When the patient is positioned this way, the heart, diaphragm, and subphrenic structures shift to reduce inferior wall attenuation while potentially increasing anterior wall attenuation.

Conventional correction methods. The most common correction methods used in commercial systems until recently have been a pre-reconstruction method based on work by Sorenson[38] and a post-reconstruction method developed by Chang.[39] Both of these methods assume that the attenuation within the body is homogeneous, and both have been used effectively for SPECT applications in which the attenuation is approximately homogeneous, such as liver imaging. These methods have been shown to

be inadequate for myocardial perfusion SPECT imaging because the attenuating material in a patient's thorax is too varied for a constant attenuation coefficient approximation to be effective.[20]

Transmission scan–based correction methods. The concept of using transmission scanning with radionuclide imaging was suggested early in the days of nuclear medicine.[40] After acquisition, the transmission projections are reconstructed using either FBP or statistical-based reconstruction algorithms.[41] Once a map of the attenuation values has been reconstructed, a physical model of the attenuation process can be incorporated into an iterative reconstruction technique to correct the degradation of attenuation.

Currently, the most widely disseminated configuration for transmission imaging is the scanning line source approach with gadolinium-153 (^{153}Gd) as the external source.[42] It was initially commercialized on triple and dual 90-degree detector systems but can also be used on single detector systems. Scanning line source systems (Figure 9-22) use an electronic window that moves simultaneously and opposite the external source to separate transmission and emission data. Other methods of acquiring transmission scans are shown in Figure 9-23.[41,43-45]

The use of conventional x-ray sources and detectors to acquire transmission scans has potential to yield much higher quality maps that can also be used for anatomic reference.[46] This approach has recently been introduced commercially[45] and produces attenuation maps that exceed the quality obtainable by the sealed-source systems described above. The transmission scanning apparatus is mounted on the SPECT gantry, and the transmission scan is performed with rapid rotation of the gantry as the table moves through the x-ray beam.

Many transmission-based SPECT systems use simultaneous acquisition of emission and transmission data. This provides efficient acquisition and essential alignment of transmission and emission scans. However, it is very important that the technologist recognize that artifacts in the transmission scan can have a detrimental effect on the attenuation-corrected images. Careful and thorough quality control procedures, therefore, must be used with the transmission scan. The transmission projections and tomograms should be reviewed by the technologist to identify technical problems such as motion, missing frames or counts, truncation of the body, and gating artifacts. In addition, many of the quality control concepts used for conventional SPECT imaging extend to systems that perform transmission imaging. For example, center of rotation alignment, which limits reconstruction accuracy in SPECT, can also affect transmission projection data alignment.

Scatter Correction

Scatter correction methods for SPECT require estimation of the number of scattered photons in each pixel of the image. This is a complex matter because the scatter component of

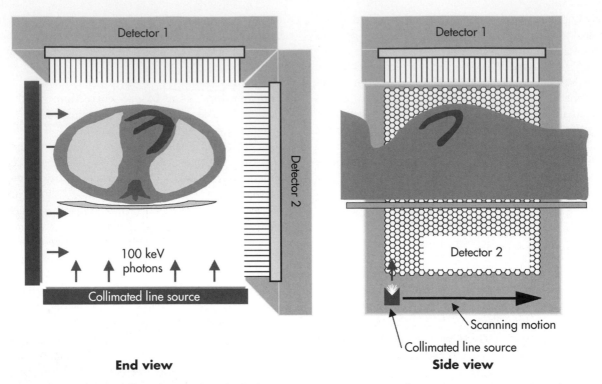

Figure 9-22   The most commonly implemented method of acquiring transmission scans for attenuation correction uses line source scanning. During each projection of a step-and-shoot acquisition, a line source (usually filled with ^{153}Gd) scans across the camera's field of view. An electronic window opposite the line source acquires only counts with an energy that matches the line source.

the image depends on the energy of the photon, the energy window used, and the composition and location of the source and the scattering medium.[47,48]

Energy window–based methods. One of the most widely used scatter correction methods is the dual window scatter subtraction method suggested by Jaszczak et al[49] for ^{99m}Tc. This method requires a second energy window at a lower energy (127 to 153 keV) than the photopeak window (89-123 keV). A fraction of this window is subtracted from the photopeak window. The dual window technique makes the assumption that the scattered photons in the scatter window are linearly proportional to the scattered photons in the photopeak window. The triple energy window (TEW) technique uses scatter windows on either side of the photopeak window. The contribution of scattered photons to the photopeak window is estimated as the average counts in the two scatter windows normalized to the photopeak window.[50] At best, energy window–based methods can provide only approximate scatter correction, and they may increase image noise.[51]

Iterative correction techniques. Reconstruction-based methods incorporate compensation for Compton scatter directly into the iterative reconstruction.[52-54] The physics of photon interactions provides a relationship between image scatter and the attenuation distribution in patients, suggesting that a measured attenuation map (from a transmission

scan) can be used in conjunction with the source distribution provided by the emission scan to provide a study-specific correction.[55] Reconstruction-based techniques use this information to incorporate a physical model of the scattering process into the iterative reconstruction algorithm information.[56-59]

Resolution Recovery

Several approaches have been proposed to compensate for the loss of resolution with distance from the collimator and the resulting distortions produced in SPECT images. Analytic approaches to the problem of distance varying resolution model the shape of the collimator response to remove the effects from the image.[60,61] Another approach is to use the *frequency distance principle*,[62,63] which states that points at a specific source-to-detector distance correspond to specific regions in the frequency space of the sinogram's Fourier transform. Applying a spatially variant inverse filter to the sinograms performs the resolution recovery. This inverse filtering is relatively fast but may also amplify noise in the image.

Resolution recovery can also be included in iterative reconstruction methods. It is possible to include resolution recovery in both iterative filtered back-projection[64,65] and maximum likelihood reconstruction techniques.[66,67] These methods take considerably more computations to implement than the frequency distance principle (FDP) but have

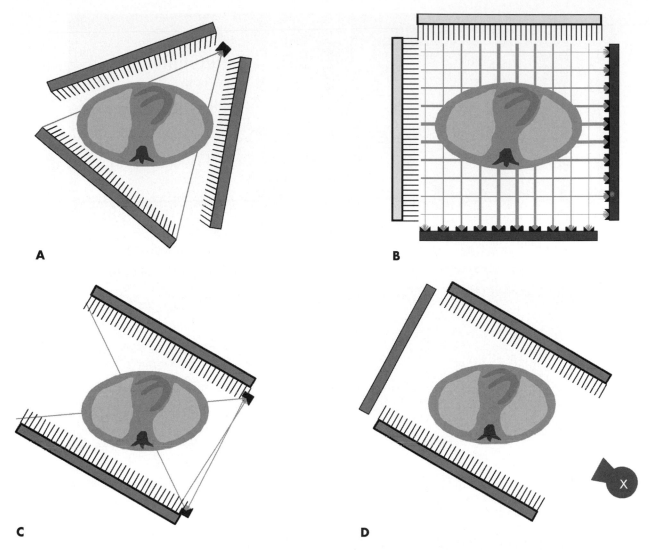

Figure 9-23   Other SPECT-based transmission hardware configurations include line source and fan beam collimation for fan beam systems (**A**), arrays of line sources mounted opposite both cameras of a dual 90-degree camera system (**B**), asymmetric fan beam geometry using high-energy photons that penetrate the septa of a low-energy collimator (**C**), a conventional x-ray source and detector mounted on the SPECT gantry (**D**). Note that the systems in **C** and **D** can also be used with a 90-degree camera configuration.

the potential to compensate more accurately for the resolution response.[68]

Combining Attenuation Correction, Scatter Correction, and Resolution Recovery

As described in the literature, optimum accuracy of SPECT image reconstruction requires correction for Compton scatter, attenuation, distance-dependent spatial resolution, and image noise.[68-70] For example, it has been demonstrated that attenuation compensation without scatter compensation can result in an artificial increase in inferior wall counts.[35,71] Other reports demonstrate that scatter compensation is essential for accurate attenuation compensation.[18,70] An example of the application of both attenuation correction and scatter compensation to a myocardial perfusion scan is shown in Figure 9-24. In this example, the original emission and transmission projections are shown for a myocardial perfusion study. Transaxial slices of the emission and transmission studies after reconstruction with filtered back-projection are shown in Figure 9-24, *B*. Figure 9-24, *C* shows short axis slices reconstructed with filtered back-projection and an iterative technique that corrects for both attenuation and scatter. Corresponding vertical long axis slices are shown in Figure 9-24, *D*. In the FBP reconstruction, breast attenuation artifactually decreases the counts in the anterior wall of the heart, but the attenuation and scatter corrections resolve this problem.

Iterative reconstruction algorithms provide the opportunity to investigate complete compensation of cardiac SPECT images for the effects of the patient's anatomy as described by the attenuation map and the limited, spatially varying resolution of SPECT. It is anticipated that further improvements in the accuracy of cardiac SPECT reconstruction and diagnostic accuracy will result as these methods evolve.

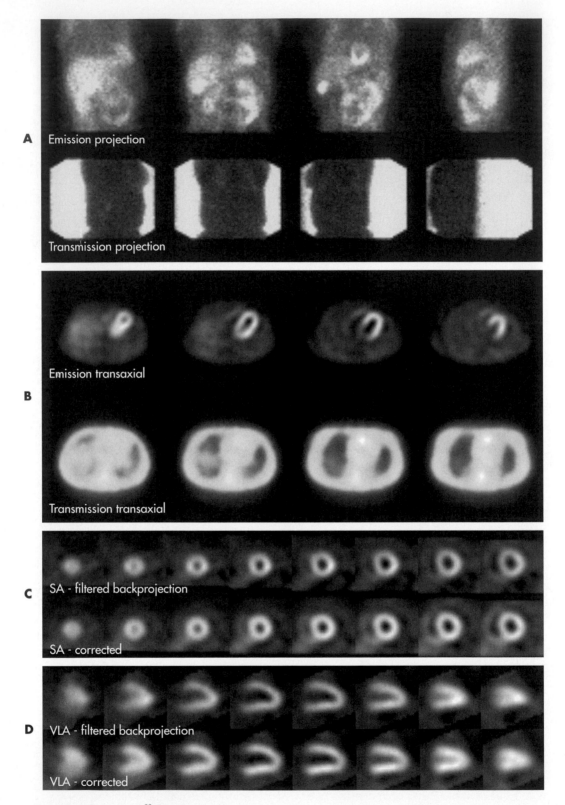

Figure 9-24   Attenuation correction of ^{99m}Tc SPECT of a normal female. **A,** Emission and transmission projections from a SPECT system equipped with scanning line sources. **B,** Emission and transmission transaxial slices through the heart. **C,** Short axis slices reconstructed with filtered back-projection, which may be compared with those produced with corrections for attenuation and Compton scatter. **D,** Corresponding vertical long axis images. Breast attenuation artifactually decreases the counts in the anterior wall of the heart, a problem that is resolved when the corrections are applied.

CARDIAC SPECT QUANTIFICATION

Cardiac Reorientation

Most cardiac images are viewed in a standard format consisting of short axis, horizontal long axis, and vertical long axis slices. Short axis slices are also necessary for some automatic perfusion quantification algorithms. Generation of these standard sections from the original transaxial images has been performed interactively, requiring the user to mark the location of the left ventricular axis. The following sections describe the process of interactively creating these standard sections, along with their definitions.

Vertical long axis slices. Using a display of a transaxial slice through the middle of the left ventricle, the position of the long axis is denoted with a line drawn by the user. The three-dimensional set of transaxial sections (some of which are shown in Figure 9-25, *A*) is resliced parallel to the long axis and perpendicular to the transaxial slices. Each of the resulting oblique images is called a *vertical long axis slice* (Figure 9-25, *B*). The slices are displayed with the base of the left ventricle toward the left side of the image and the apex toward the right. Serial slices are displayed from medial to lateral, left to right.

Horizontal long axis slices. Using a display of a midventricular vertical long axis image, the user once again denotes the left ventricular long axis. The three-dimensional block of vertical long axis slices is recut parallel to the denoted long axis and perpendicular to the stack. The resulting oblique cuts are called *horizontal long axis slices* (Figure 9-25, *C*). They contain the left ventricle with its base toward the bottom of the image and its apex toward the top. The right ventricle appears on the left side of the image. Serial horizontal long axis slices are displayed from inferior to anterior, left to right.

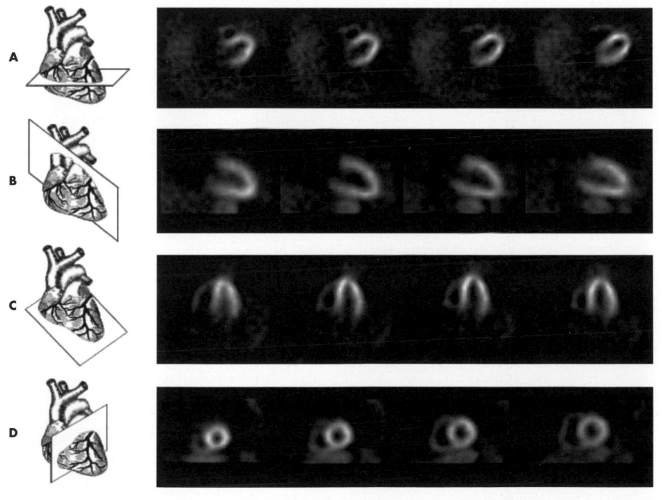

Figure 9-25   Standard oblique sections for viewing cardiac data. **A,** Original transaxial slices. The left side of the body is to the right in each slice, with the anterior side at the top. Slices are displayed from inferior to superior, left to right. **B,** Vertical long axis slices. The base of the left ventricle is toward the left side of the image, and the apex is toward the right. Slices are displayed from medial to lateral, left to right. **C,** Horizontal long axis slices. The base of the left ventricle is toward the bottom of the image, and its apex is toward the top. The right ventricle appears on the left side of the image. Serial slices are displayed from inferior to anterior, left to right. **D,** Short axis slices. The anterior wall of the left ventricle is toward the top, the inferior wall is toward the bottom, and the septal wall is toward the left. Slices are displayed from apex to base, left to right.

Short axis slices. Slices perpendicular to the denoted long axis and perpendicular to the vertical long axis slices are also cut from the stack. These are called *short axis slices* (Figure 9-25, *D*); they contain the left ventricle with its anterior wall toward the top, its inferior wall toward the bottom, and its septal wall toward the left. Serial short axis slices are displayed from apex to base, left to right.

Automatic reorientation. Two approaches[72,73] start by identifying the left ventricular region in the transaxial images, using a threshold-based approach that includes knowledge of the expected position, size, and shape of the left ventricle (LV). Once this region has been isolated, the approach described by Germano et al[72] uses the original data to refine the estimate of the myocardial surface. Lines at 90 degrees (vectors) to an ellipsoid fit to the LV region are used to resample the myocardium; a gaussian function is fitted to the profiles obtained at each sample. The best-fit gaussian function is used to estimate the myocardial center for each profile, and after further refinement based on image intensities and myocardial smoothness, the resulting mid-myocardial points are fitted to an ellipsoid, the long axis of which is used as the final LV long axis. This method was tested on 400 patient images and the results compared with interactively denoted long axes. Failure of the method was described as either not localizing the LV, presence of significant hepatic or intestinal activity in the "LV" region of the image, or greater than 45 degrees' difference between automatically and interactively determined axes. Using these criteria, the method was successful in 394 of the 400 cases.

Mullick and Ezquerra[73] use a more complex heuristic technique to determine the optimal LV threshold and isolate it from other structures. After this has been accomplished, they use the segmented data directly to determine the long axis. The binary image is tessellated into triangular plates, and the normal of each plate on the endocardial surface is used to "point to" the LV long axis. The intersection of these normal vectors (or near-intersections) are collected and fitted to a three-dimensional straight line, which is then returned as the LV long axis. This method was tested on 124 patient data sets, and the automated long axis orientation was compared with interactively determined angles. Failure was described as a failure to isolate the left ventricle; this method succeeded in 116 of 124 cases.

Slomka et al[74] take a different approach entirely to automated reorientation. Their method registers the original image data to a "template" image in which the orientation of the LV is known and standardized. The template is created by averaging a large number of registered, normal patient data sets, and separate templates are created for males and females. The registration is done by first translating and scaling the image based on principal axes; the match is refined by minimizing the sum of the absolute differences between the template and the image being registered. This method was not compared with interactively reoriented images but was evaluated visually for 38 normal and 10 abnormal subjects and found to be successful for all.

Perfusion Quantification

All commercially available quantification methods for myocardial perfusion in SPECT are based on the idea that sampled counts in the myocardium of a patient's image can be compared with similar counts sampled from a set of normal subjects. In its basic form, the quantitation algorithm samples the left ventricular myocardium in short axis slices to determine the maximum count values within the myocardium at evenly spaced angles about the left ventricular long axis. For each short axis slice, the resulting maximum count values are graphed against the angle at which they were encountered; such a graph is called a *circumferential profile.*

Circumferential profiles are amassed for a large number of normal subjects. The profiles are generally normalized for each person so that the maximum count value in each study is rescaled to a standard value, such as 100. This accounts for variations in uptake, dose, and overall perfusion rates. For each angle on each slice, both a mean normal value and its standard deviation are computed over the set of normal subjects. Normal boundaries or normal limits for each point in each profile are created based on these statistical values; for example, they may be set at 2 or 2.5 standard deviations below the mean normal value. By comparing a patient's circumferential profile angle by angle and slice by slice to the normal limits, perfusion defects can be pointed out automatically. Figure 9-26 shows the creation and use of circumferential profiles.

Generally, analysis is performed and normal limits are created for the stress study and for a normalized difference between the stress and rest studies. (If ^{201}Tl washout images are being quantitated, the percentage change between the stress and the washout images is analyzed instead of the normalized difference between the two.) Separate normal limits must be created for males and females because normal differences in body shape cause different normal attenuation and scatter artifacts in the reconstructions. Abnormal areas or defects seen in the stress images that persist on the rest study are considered fixed. Abnormal regions in the stress study that improve or normalize in the rest study are considered reversible.

Methods vary primarily in the way in which the myocardium is sampled, For example, the previous description of short axis circumferential profiles has been extended to a hybrid cylindric/spheric coordinate system[8] and to ellipsoid sampling.[75] Another difference is the way in which the normal limits are generated; one approach uses receiver-operator curves to generate an optimum threshold for each myocardial region.[76] All the methods are similar, however, in that they sample the counts at discrete points in the myocardium and compare those values to some known "normal" values to localize perfusion defects.

Because few studies have compared these various approaches to perfusion quantification, it is not a simple matter to choose one based on its comparative accuracy. More practical issues, therefore, may be the most useful

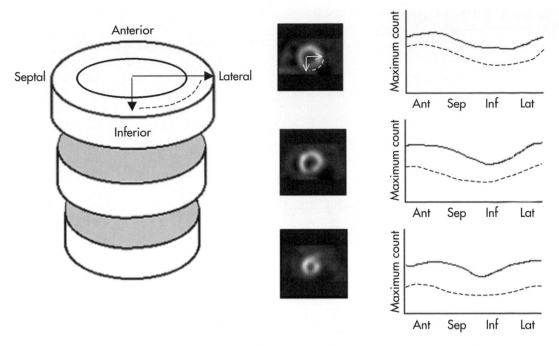

Figure 9-26 Creation of circumferential profiles for perfusion quantification. Short axis slices are sampled at numerous angles about the center of the left ventricle; the maximum count in the myocardium at each angle is graphed against the angle. The result is a circumferential profile for each short axis slice, seen as the solid line in the graphs at the right. Normal limits are created for each profile by studying normal subjects; these normal limits are shown as dotted lines in the graphs. Whenever a part of the circumferential profile falls below the normal limit, that portion of the patient's myocardium is considered to have a perfusion defect. The subject shown here is normal.

guide to choosing which of the methods may be best for clinical use. Certainly it is important to make sure that the approach has been validated and the results published. The manufacturer should have U.S. Food and Drug Administration (FDA) approval to market it for clinical use. It is also important that the methodologies be kept up-to-date. New normal files are often required for new protocols, and a program that is no longer in active development will not be applicable to the latest technologies. For instance, some programs may not have normal files for dual isotope perfusion analysis. Others that were developed for use with all-purpose collimators may never provide normal limits for use with high-resolution collimators. In any case, the most important thing to keep in mind when using quantitative programs is to follow the acquisition and processing protocols developed for the technique exactly. Even small changes in reconstruction filtering or acquisition time can compromise the accuracy of the quantitation.

CARDIAC DISPLAY

Polar Maps

Polar maps, or bull's-eye displays, are another way to view circumferential profiles. They give a quick, comprehensive overview of the circumferential samples from all slices by combining them into a color-coded image. The points of each circumferential profile are assigned a color based on normalized count values, and the colored profiles are shaped

into concentric rings. The most apical slice processed with circumferential profiles forms the center of the polar map, and each successive profile from each successive short axis slice is displayed as a new ring surrounding the previous. The most basal slice of the left ventricle makes up the outermost ring of the polar map. Figure 9-27, *A* shows polar maps created by applying the CEqual quantification method to a ^{99m}Tc sestamibi study. This kind of display allows immediate and comprehensive viewing of the quantitative results of the entire myocardium.

The use of color also can aid the identification of abnormal areas at a glance. Abnormal regions from the stress study are often assigned a black color, thus creating a blackout map. Blacked-out areas that normalize at rest are color-coded white, thus creating a whiteout reversibility map.[77] This can be seen in Figure 9-27, *A* (it is also shown in the color plate section). Additional maps, such as a standard deviation map that shows the number of standard deviations below normal of each point in each circumferential profile, can aid in evaluation of the study by indicating the severity of any abnormality.

Although they offer a comprehensive view of the quantitation results, polar maps distort the size and shape of the myocardium and any defects. Numerous improvements in the basic polar map display have helped to overcome some of these problems.[8] For instance, "distance-weighted" maps are created so that each ring is the same thickness. These maps have been shown to be useful for accurate localization of abnormalities. "Volume-weighted" maps are constructed

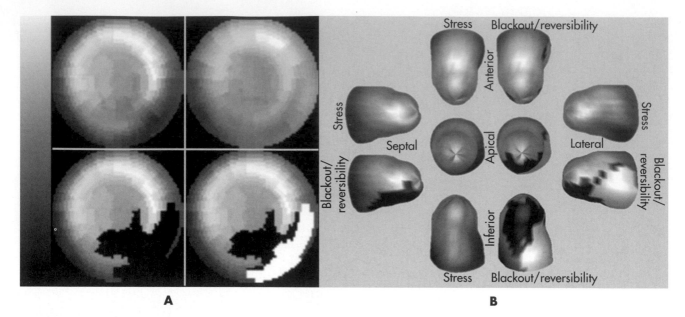

Figure 9-27 Polar (bull's-eye) maps and three-dimensional displays of perfusion, quantified from a stress ^{99m}Tc sestamibi/rest ^{201}Tl study. **A,** Polar plots of stress perfusion *(top left),* rest perfusion *(top right),* stress blackout *(bottom left),* and reversibility whiteout *(bottom right).* In polar plots, the anterior wall is toward the top, the septal side is toward the left, the lateral wall is toward the right, and the inferior wall is toward the bottom. For each plot, colors are scaled from 0 to 100% of the maximum myocardial counts. The blackout plot shows in black all abnormal regions in the stress image, determined from comparison with normal limits. The regions that normalize at rest are shown in white in the whiteout map. **B,** Three-dimensional displays of the same data as in **A.** Here, only stress and blackout/reversibility whiteout data are shown. Five different views of the left ventricle are provided; clockwise from top, they are anterior, lateral, inferior, and septal, with an apical view in the center. Note that the size and shape of the left ventricle can be better appreciated in this three-dimensional display. Also, the size, shape, and location of the defects are immediately obvious.

such that the area of each ring is proportional to the volume of the corresponding slice. This type of map has been shown to be best for estimating defect size. However, more realistic displays have been introduced that do not have the distortions of polar maps.

Three-Dimensional Cardiac Displays

Three-dimensional graphics techniques can be used to overlay results of perfusion quantification onto a representation of a specific patient's left ventricle.[78,79] In the most basic form of such techniques, the pixel locations of the maximum-count myocardial points sampled during quantitation are used to estimate the myocardial surface. These points can be connected into triangles, which are then color-coded in a way similar to a polar map. Figure 9-27, *B* displays the same information seen in the polar maps of Figure 9-27, *A* using a three-dimensional representation. Such displays routinely can be rotated in real time and viewed from any angle with current computer power. They have the advantage of showing the actual size and shape of the left ventricle and the extent and location of any defect in a very realistic manner. Some studies have shown that the 3D models are more accurate for evaluating the size and location of perfusion defects than polar maps[79] or slice-by-slice displays.[80,81]

The biggest disadvantage of 3D displays is that they require more computer screen space (and therefore more film or paper for hard copies) than polar maps. The entire left ventricle can be visualized in a single circular polar map but only one side of the left ventricle can be seen when it is displayed using 3D graphics.

CARDIAC GATING

Standard cardiac SPECT images suffer from motion blur, because the heart is always in motion. These images can show only a picture of the average position of the heart. It is well known that because the heart is moving, contracting and relaxing, perfusion defects can be missed or underestimated; they are, in a sense, "averaged" with normal myocardium that may move into the location previously occupied by the defect earlier in the cardiac cycle. In addition, it is well understood that the intensity of the myocardium in nuclear medicine images is related not only to radiotracer uptake but also to relative myocardial thickness.[82] As the heart contracts, the myocardium appears brighter in the reconstructed image. This effect also is "averaged" into a standard static (ungated) acquisition and may result in impaired diagnostic accuracy.[83]

Cardiac gating allows heart motion and contraction to be resolved by dividing the projections into discrete time parts coupled with the cardiac cycle. The electrocardiogram (ECG) is used to determine the heart rate and the onset of contraction at the QRS complex. The cardiac cycle is divided into a set number of predetermined time intervals, called *frames,* and counts collected during each frame are directed to a different projection set. Counts are directed into the first frame during the initial T/N seconds after the QRS complex is detected, where *N* is the number of frames and *T* is the length in seconds of the cardiac cycle. Then, counts are directed into the second frame for the second T/N seconds, and so on. This is repeated for each heartbeat during the acquisition, at every angle. At the end of the acquisition, there are N sets of complete projection images. When these are reconstructed, the result is N three-dimensional sets of slices showing the heart at N points during the cardiac cycle. These four-dimensional data allow three-dimensional analysis of motion and myocardial thickening,[26,84,85] as well as perhaps enabling better discrimination of the extent and location of perfusion abnormalities.[86] It has even been proposed that exercise ejection fraction can be measured using gated tomographic perfusion imaging by acquiring gated projections rapidly (in about 6 minutes) during stress. Although the resulting images are of poor quality and probably not useful for perfusion analysis, the endocardial surfaces may be detected with enough accuracy to compute end-diastolic and end-systolic volumes for ejection fraction calculation.[87]

There are a number of practical considerations for cardiac gating. First, each projection set and reconstruction will be reduced in counts by a factor equal to the number of collected frames. This precludes gating studies, which are normally low count, because image quality becomes too poor. Also, gating software should be able to deal with abnormal heartbeats and "reject" or ignore counts from these contractions. Similarly, the acquisition should be able to adjust to changing heart rates and direct counts to the projection frames accordingly. One commonly seen result of a change in heart rate is late frame drop-off. If the heart rate speeds up but the software fails to adjust, the heartbeat ends before counts have been directed into the last few frames. When the next contraction begins, counts are directed back into the first frames. Therefore relatively fewer counts are seen in the late end-diastolic frame. Motion blur is also reintroduced, because for some early projections, the cardiac cycle is divided into 8 frames, but for late projections, it is divided into 6 frames. Finally, the size of a gated data set increases proportionally to the number of frames collected. This raises both processing time and storage space for gated studies.

Quantifying Function

It is possible to obtain quantitative functional information from gated perfusion SPECT images. Global variables such as left ventricular volumes, mass, and ejection fraction can be calculated. Local properties of wall motion and myocardial thickening are also obtainable; these can then be displayed using either polar maps or three-dimensional graphics. Most commercially available programs for quantifying cardiac function are fully three-dimensional approaches, which start by detecting endocardial and epicardial surface points through the cardiac cycle. For instance, the QGS program determines the locations of the surface points through fitting of count activity profiles across the myocardium to asymmetric gaussian curves.[84] Other methods seek definition of the same points by analysis of percent systolic count increases resulting from partial

volume effect[88] analysis of count gradients followed by iterative relaxation labeling[26,89] or analysis of moments of the count distribution.[90]

Global variables. Once the left ventricular endocardial (inner wall) and epicardial (outer wall) boundaries have been determined, the number of pixels within the chamber or left ventricular wall can be determined. Because the pixel sizes are known, the total volume in the chamber or myocardium can be computed. Myocardial mass is calculated by multiplying the myocardial volume by an assumed density, usually 1.05 g/cc. The end-diastolic volume is determined to be the largest chamber volume found in the gated set of images; the end-systolic volume is the smallest. The ejection fraction is computed using these values.

Endocardial wall motion. If the endocardial surface is detected at each point in the cardiac cycle, regional endocardial wall motion can be assessed by computing how each surface point moves. Wall motion is difficult to compute with much accuracy because it is impossible to say with certainty that a particular point in one time frame moves to a particular location in the next. In addition, there is a global translational component to left ventricular motion, which is difficult to assess and/or remove. In fact, most analyses of left ventricular wall motion rely heavily on simplified models of motion originally developed for two-dimensional contrast ventriculograms or radionuclide ventriculograms. These models may assume, for example, that every point moves radially toward the left ventricular center of mass; regional motion is therefore forced to be "radial." Two approaches[88,91] use a three-dimensional extension of the centerline method originally developed for contrast ventriculograms.[92] In this method, each left ventricular surface point is assumed to move in a direction perpendicular to the surface at that point. Note that no method for modeling endocardial motion is completely accurate in every case, therefore quantitated left ventricular wall motion should be considered in conjunction with perfusion information.

Myocardial thickening. Myocardial thickening is known to be a better indicator of myocardial viability than endocardial wall motion; therefore the ability to quantify this variable accurately from perfusion tomograms would be very valuable. The most promising methods use the fact that, as a result of detector response, myocardial thickness is linearly related to image intensity in perfusion images when the myocardial thickness is less than two times the resolution of the reconstructed images.[82] Because current SPECT systems provide resolution on the order of 1 cm, this thickness/intensity relationship should hold true for the vast majority of cases, in which the range of myocardial thickness is 0.5 to 2 cm. Note that there is no way to tell absolute thickness with this method; instead, only the change in thickness over the cardiac cycle can be assessed. For example, if the peak counts at one point of the myocardium double from end-diastole to end-systole, it can be postulated that the wall has doubled in thickness during contraction at that point.

One approach to quantification of wall thickening using this theory samples the myocardial counts at numerous locations (more than 4,000) for every gated frame.[85] Then a time/intensity curve is created for each of the myocardial points. The curve is "smoothed" by fitting a cosine function to its values. The amplitude of the fitted cosine wave is used as a measure of the change in thickness from end-diastole to end-systole at the point in question. Thickening polar plots or three-dimensional displays can be created to show the resulting "percent thickening" computed around the left ventricle. This method has proved to be very robust with respect to noise in simulation studies. However, quantification of myocardial thickening from perfusion SPECT images has not at this writing been truly tested in the clinic.

QUALITY CONTROL

Quality assurance is the approach taken to ensure that a quality product is provided. Suboptimal images can make diagnosis difficult or even lead to misdiagnosis. *Quality control* encompasses the specific tests needed to achieve quality assurance. Several tests must be performed on scintillation cameras to verify that they meet performance specifications.[93] Although at one time these tests were performed using similar methods on almost any manufacturer's camera, today methods of testing and calibrating cameras vary widely from manufacturer to manufacturer.

Although the methods for performing quality control procedures for multiple detector systems vary widely among manufacturers, the same procedures required of single detector systems apply. The additional quality control calibrations and procedures required of multiple detector SPECT systems primarily deal with the registration of images between the two heads. All of the detectors may have excellent spatial resolution independently, but if images produced by the different detectors do not fall precisely on top of one another, this resolution will be lost.

Planar Gamma Camera Quality Control

Quality control for SPECT cameras must include the quality control procedures common to all scintillation cameras. On a daily basis the camera energy peaks should be checked, and a uniformity test should be done. On a weekly basis the camera's resolution and linearity should be checked.[13,94] It is important to note that not only do these tests need to be done, the results also need to be analyzed with a critical eye. It does no good to perform the tests if action is not taken when warranted.

SPECT Quality Control

SPECT reconstruction techniques depend on the consistency of the images from different views. Imperfections that go unnoticed in planar imaging can be amplified in the reconstruction process, resulting in severe artifacts in the transaxial images. Two calibrations uniquely important to

SPECT are uniformity corrections and center of rotation calibrations. These must be part of any clinic's routine quality control procedures and must be performed weekly or monthly, depending on the manufacturer's recommendations and the user's experience with the equipment. Multiple-camera systems require additional tests to ensure that the two systems are adequately aligned.[94] Patient motion is a concern and should be monitored during the acquisition and checked after the acquisition. After acquisition, it is also important to maintain consistency in the processing of SPECT images. Standard protocols should be developed for reconstruction, filtering, and display.

Uniformity correction. All scintillation cameras must correct for differences in energy responses from different photomultiplier tubes. Although these corrections are important for reducing uniformity errors in planar projections, uniformity requirements for SPECT are more stringent and require further correction. Next to photomultiplier tubes, the greatest sources of image nonuniformities are imperfect collimators. A local nonuniformity is propagated in the reconstructed transaxial slice in the form of a circular, or *ring,* artifact because the same nonuniformity is back-projected at each of the angles of acquisition (Figure 9-28). The higher the acquired counts for that slice, the more prominent the artifact, because it rides above the random noise error. Also, the closer the local nonuniformity to the axis of rotation, the higher the amplitude of the artifact, because the back-projected lines are closer together (more overlapping of count values).

Uniformity defects are most easily seen in flood tests and in phantom acquisitions in which a large area of uniform activity is present (Figure 9-29). Artifacts can be much more difficult to detect in multihead SPECT because the uniformity defect does not usually complete the ring artifact. Clinical radiotracer distributions usually have low count rates in most of the image, making uniformity defects difficult to detect (Figure 9-30).

Figure 9-29 A SPECT phantom should be imaged quarterly as part of a clinic's routine quality control procedure. The resulting images should be compared with previous images to ensure that image quality has not degraded. Each camera of a multiple detector SPECT system should undergo quality control independently, and the system should be tested as a whole. In this example, camera 2 of a dual detector system has a uniformity defect (created by a clay mask approximately the size of a photomultiplier tube). **A,** Anterior and posterior projections from a 360-degree acquisition. Low count rates in SPECT acquisition with camera 1 are shown, along with a transaxial slice. The slice is uniform, except for the effects of attenuation, and defects (*solid plastic spheres*) are clearly seen. **B,** An identical acquisition using only camera 2 clearly shows the uniformity defect and the resulting ring artifact in the transaxial image. **C,** When the two cameras are used as a unit, the 360-degree acquisition is accomplished by rotating each camera through 180 degrees. The uniformity artifact in the transaxial slice is still significant but more difficult to diagnose.

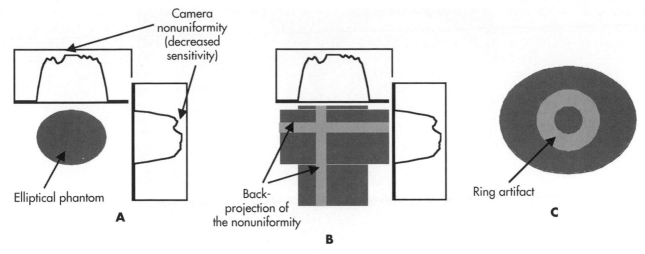

Figure 9-28   Uniformity artifacts are formed when there is an area of decreased sensitivity on the camera face. **A,** A quality control phantom is filled with uniform tracer solution. An area of decreased sensitivity resulted in a uniformity defect in the activity profiles of the two planar projections shown. **B,** When back-projected, these areas originate from the same pixels in each projection. **C,** The intersections of the uniformity defects from each of the projections scribes a circular defect in the transaxial image.

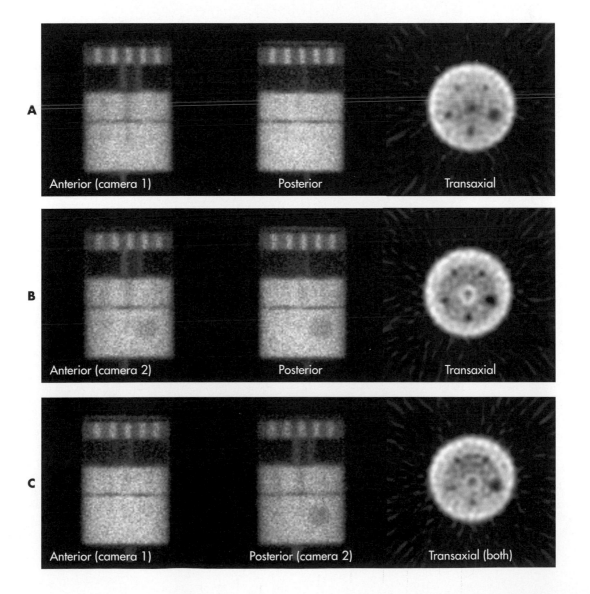

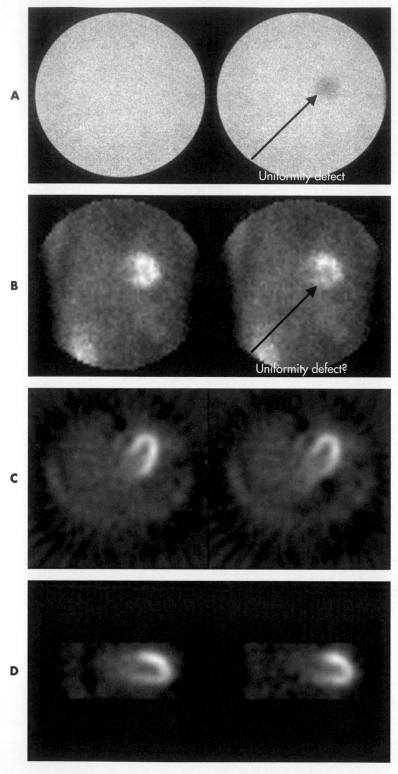

Figure 9-30　Uniformity artifacts are more difficult to detect in clinical images. **A,** Daily flood images from a system working correctly on the left and with a simulated uniformity defect on the right (similar to that of a faulty photomultiplier tube). **B,** This same uniformity was applied to clinical ^{201}Tl SPECT. Although it was easy to identify the defect in the flood image, it was very difficult to identify the defect in the clinical image, even when rotating the projections in cine mode. **C,** No ring artifact is evident in the transaxial images. The ring is incompletely formed because of the 180-degree camera orbit and the low background counts. **D,** Note the decreased counts in the inferior wall of the left ventricle resulting from the uniformity artifact. This could easily be mistaken for a perfusion abnormality. Clinical diagnoses could be further complicated if the patient is positioned differently between the stress and rest acquisitions and the defect appears in different areas of the body in the two scans, giving the appearance of a reversing defect.

Center of rotation. Artifacts caused by errors in the center of rotation (COR) are unique to SPECT. The center of rotation is the axis about which the camera rotates (Figure 9-31). The COR measurement determines the offset between the center of the camera matrix and projection of the center of rotation of the camera face (they do not automatically correspond). If this offset is very large (more than 2 pixels), the reconstruction of a point source looks like a bright ring (Figure 9-32). COR errors too small to create a ring (as small as 0.5 pixel) can blur the image by spreading out the counts and possibly creating artifacts. Also, 180-degree reconstruc-

tions of a point source do not produce a full ring, but rather a shape similar to a tuning fork (Figure 9-33). This can be much easier to detect than the simple blurring of 360-degree orbits.

Patient motion. Patient motion is one of the more significant causes of artifacts in SPECT images, because motion as small as 0.5 pixel can yield significant artifacts.[95,96] The technologist should warn the patient not to move, should make sure the patient is comfortable so that movement is less likely, and should monitor the patient during acquisition.

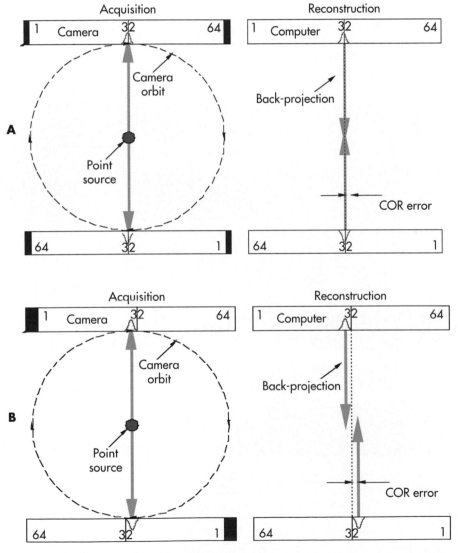

Figure 9-31 When properly calibrated, the digital image matrix is perfectly centered on the camera face and the central pixels always align with the imaginary line around which the camera rotates (center of rotation). **A,** When properly calibrated, a point source placed at the center of rotation projects to the center of the pixel matrix (pixel 32 in this example). Upon reconstruction the back-projection of opposing views overlay exactly. **B,** When improperly calibrated (illustrated by shifting the pixel matrix to one side of the camera), the point source projects to one side of the center of the matrix. Upon reconstruction the projections do not meet in the center but are shifted to either side of the center of the matrix. The center of rotation calibration measures and corrects for this shift (COR error).

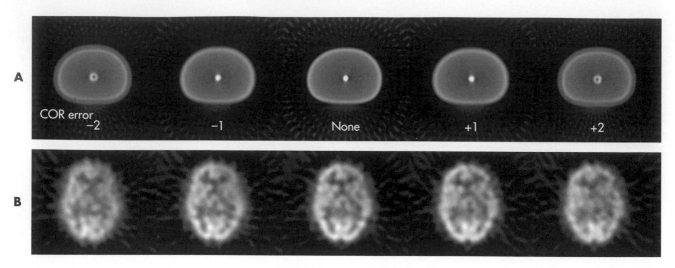

Figure 9-32   Center of rotation errors are most easily identified using a line or point source; they can be difficult to detect in clinical images. **A,** A simulated quality control phantom containing a line source is imaged using a 360-degree acquisition with center of rotation errors of −2, −1, 0, +1, +2 pixels. Extreme errors convert the single point of the line to a ring, but typical clinical errors (on the order of 1 pixel or less) severely degrade resolution. **B,** The same errors in brain SPECT produce loss of resolution and distortions that can be difficult to identify as center of rotation problems.

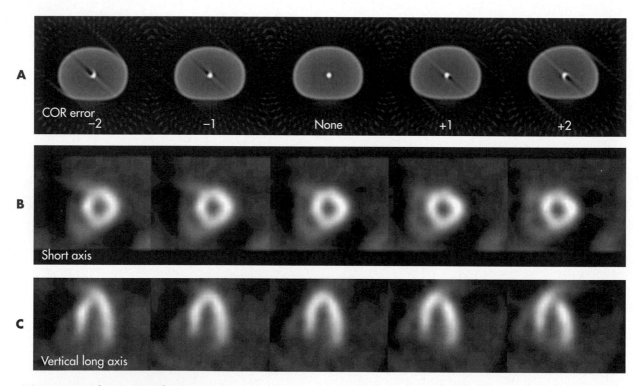

Figure 9-33   Center of rotation artifacts in 180-degree acquisitions have a different appearance from those in 360-degree acquisitions. **A,** The simulated quality control phantom from Figure 9-32 is imaged using a 180-degree acquisition with center of rotation errors of −2, −1, 0, +1, +2 pixels. Even small center of rotation errors produce an artifact typically described as the shape of a tuning fork. **B,** The same errors in cardiac SPECT produce an apparent mismatch between the septal and lateral walls of the heart. **C,** The mismatch is most easily seen in the horizontal long axis images, as is a characteristic defect near the apex of the heart.

Images should be viewed after the procedure to check for patient motion, attenuation, or other factors that may reduce the accuracy of the reconstructed images. Patient motion can be detected by summed projections, sinograms, or cine displays (Figure 9-34).

Summed projections are formed by adding all the planar projections for the SPECT acquisition. The heart can be seen as a blurry horizontal line across the center of the summed images of Figure 9-34. To evaluate motion, the technologist should look for a change in the height of the heart (in this

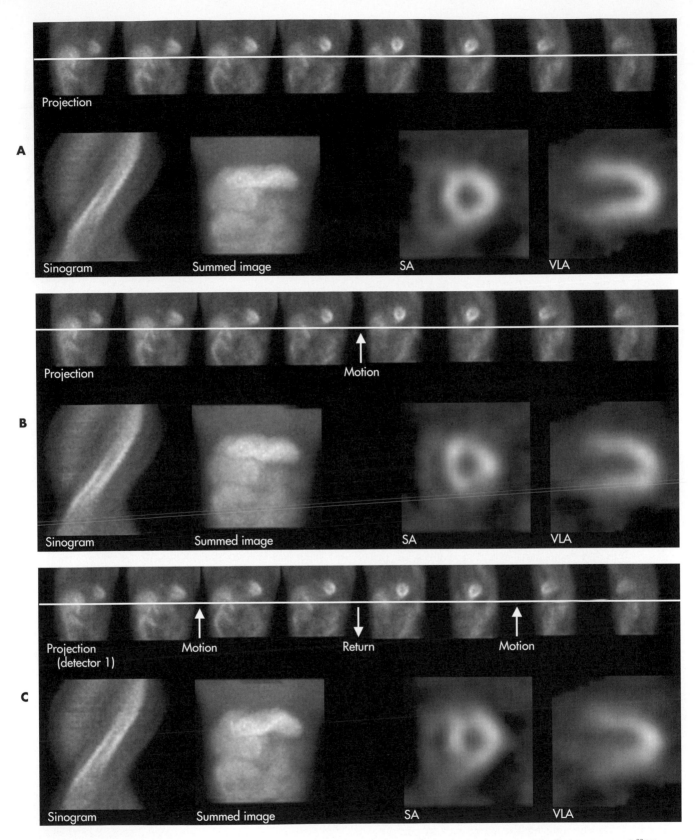

Figure 9-34 The projections in these diagrams illustrate how patient motion might be detected in a cine display in a normal ^{99m}Tc sestamibi cardiac SPECT scan. If the distance between the heart and the horizontal line is compared in each panel, a 2 pixel vertical movement can be detected in the second two panels. This motion, easily detectable in the cine display, is difficult to detect using the sinogram and summed images. **A,** The heart maintains a uniform height above the line, and the resulting short axis (SA) and vertical long axis (VLA) images are fairly uniform. **B,** Shifting the projection up 2 pixels in the second half of the study simulates motion in a single detector system. Significant artifacts are evident in the SA and VLA images. **C,** Shifting the projection up 2 pixels in the second half of the study simulates motion in a 90-degree dual detector system. The motion appears one fourth of the way through the study because each detector simultaneously acquires one half of the projections. The heart appears to return to the original position at the midpoint of the cine (the first projection for detector 2). Significant artifacts are again evident in the SA and VLA images but do not appear to be as great as in the example above.

example) that would indicate movement during acquisition. This works best for vertical motion (i.e., along the table).

The heart can be seen as a bright stripe from the top right to the lower left in the sinograms in Figure 9-34. The technologist should look for a break in this stripe that would represent the patient moving left to right. Sinograms, therefore, are best for detecting horizontal motion (i.e., across the table). Sinograms also show vertical motion but not as well as horizontal motion.

Cine displays of the planar projections are the simplest and most effective way of detecting patient motion. The playback of the acquisition can be watched as a movie to detect all types of motion, and this should be a routine part of the reconstruction process. The technologist should watch the movie of the planar projections at a fairly rapid rate and observe the images for up and down motion. It should be noted that the best way to detect and correct motion is for the technologist to observe the patient and repeat the scan if motion occurs. Immediately repeating the scan might prevent the patient from having to return to the clinic on another day for a repeat scan if the motion renders the scan uninterpretable.

Motion is much more easily detected with multihead systems (Figure 9-34, C) because of the transition between detectors seen during cine of the projections. Sudden motion will be seen twice for each detector in cines: once when the motion occurs and once when the cine makes the transition from one camera to the next. The observer should remember that, unlike a cine produced on a single-head camera, the sequence in projections does not correspond directly to time. For example, if a dual-headed camera is used to acquire 64 projections over 180 degrees, 32 projections will be acquired by each camera head. If patient motion occurs halfway through a scan, the motion will be visible in frame 16 (acquired by camera 1) and in frame 48 (acquired by camera 2). In addition, if the patient does not return to the original position, apparent motion will be visible between frame 32 (acquired by camera 1 at the end of the scan) and frame 33 (acquired by camera 2 at the beginning of the scan). The fact that motion is more easily detected by multihead systems does not mean that it will more severely affect the reconstructed images. Overall, the effects of the motion should be reduced when compared with a single-head system because the patient has less time to move. If significant motion is detected, however, the scan should be repeated.

Most manufacturers offer some sort of motion correction software. Manual corrections require the operator to shift projections (either by dragging the image with the computer mouse or by specifying the motion by pixels) based on visual analysis. Automated methods perform the operation based on a number of different algorithms. Regardless of the implementation, these methods should be used with great care and the results of the correction should be evaluated by observing rotating cines of the corrected and uncorrected projections, as well as the reconstructed images.

Standards and Procedures

The National Electrical Manufacturers Association (NEMA) is a trade association for manufacturers of electrical products. The Nuclear Section of the Diagnostic Imaging and Therapy Systems Division developed the *NEMA Standards Publication for Performance Measurements of Scintillation Cameras.*[97] This document defines standards by which scintillation cameras may be measured. No performance standards have been set by NEMA; rather, the intent of the published standards is to define methods by which scintillation camera performance can be measured so that a comparison can be made between performance claims by different manufacturers. The American Association of Physicists in Medicine has published several pamphlets on scintillation camera quality control and acceptance testing that can provide additional guidance in designing quality control procedures.[98-100] The American Society of Nuclear Cardiology has released guidelines for instrumentation quality assurance and performance and quality control procedures for transmission-emission tomographic systems to be used for attenuation correction.[13]

REFERENCES

1. Anger HO: Scintillation camera with multichannel collimators, *J Nucl Med* 5:515-531, 1964.
2. Maublant JC, Peycelon P, Kwiatkowski F et al: Comparison between 180° and 360° data collection in technetium-99m MIBI SPECT of the myocardium, *J Nucl Med* 30:295-300, 1989.
3. Hoffman EJ: 180° compared to 360° sampling in SPECT, *J Nucl Med* 23:745-746, 1982.
4. Eisner RL, Nowak DJ, Pettigrew RI et al: Fundamentals of 180° reconstruction in SPECT imaging, *J Nucl Med* 27:1717-1728, 1986.
5. Go RT, MacIntyre WJ, Houser TS et al: Clinical evaluation of 360° and 180° data sampling techniques for transaxial SPECT thallium-201 myocardial perfusion imaging, *J Nucl Med* 26:695-706, 1985.
6. Knesaurek K, King MA, Glick SJ et al: Investigation of causes of geometric distortion in 180° and 360° angular sampling in SPECT, *J Nucl Med* 30:1666-1675, 1989.
7. Gottschalk SC, Salem D, Lim CB et al: SPECT resolution and uniformity improvements by noncircular orbit, *J Nucl Med* 24:822-828, 1983.
8. Garcia EV, Cooke CD, Van Train KF et al: Technical aspects of myocardial perfusion SPECT imaging with Tc-99m sestamibi, *Am J Cardiol* 66:23-31E, 1990.
9. Maniawski PJ, Morgan HT, Wackers FJT: Orbit-related variation in spatial resolution as a source of artifactual defects in thallium-201 SPECT, *J Nucl Med* 32:871-875, 1991.

10. Van Train KF, Silagan G, Germano G et al: Noncircular versus circular orbits in quantitative analysis of myocardial perfusion SPECT, *J Nucl Med* 36:46P, 1995 (abstract).

11. Keyes JW: SPECT and artifacts: in search of the imaginary lesion, *J Nucl Med* 32:875-877, 1991.

12. *Society of Nuclear Medicine procedure guidelines manual 2001*, Reston, Va, 2001, Society of Nuclear Medicine.

13. DePuey EG, Garcia EV, editors: Updated guidelines for nuclear cardiology procedures, part 1, *J Nucl Cardiol* 8:G1-G58, 2001.

14. Brooks RA, DiChiro G: Principles of computer assisted tomography (CAT) in radiographic and radioisotopic imaging, *Phys Med Biol* 21:689-732, 1976.

15. Shepp LA, Vardi Y: Maximum likelihood reconstruction for emission tomography, *IEEE Trans Med Imag* 1:113-122, 1982.

16. Budinger TF, Gullberg GT: Three-dimensional reconstruction in nuclear medicine emission imaging, *IEEE Trans Nucl Sci* 21:2-20, 1974.

17. Tsui BMW, Zhao X, Frey E et al: Comparison between ML-EM and WLS-CG algorithms for SPECT image reconstruction, *IEEE Trans Med Imag* 38(6):1766-1772, 1991.

18. Galt JR, Cullom SJ, Garcia EV: SPECT quantification: a simplified method for attenuation correction for cardiac imaging, *J Nucl Med* 33:2232-2237, 1992.

19. Ye J, Cullom SJ, Kearfott KK et al: Simultaneous attenuation and depth-dependent resolution compensation for 180° myocardial perfusion SPECT. Proceedings of the Medical Imaging Conference, *IEEE Trans Nucl Sci* 39:1056-1058, 1992.

20. Tsui BMW, Gullberg GT, Edgerton ER et al: Correction of nonuniform attenuation in cardiac SPECT imaging, *J Nucl Med* 30:497-507, 1989.

21. Lalush DS, Tsui BMW: Improving the convergence of iterative filtered backprojection algorithms, *Med Phys* 21:1283-1285, 1994.

22. Snyder DL, Miller MI, Thomas LJ Jr et al: Noise and edge artifacts in maximum-likelihood reconstructions for emission tomography, *IEEE Trans Med Imag* MI-6(3):228-238, 1987.

23. Hudson HM, Larkin RS: Accelerated image reconstruction using ordered subsets of projection data, *IEEE Trans Med Imag* MI-13:601-609, 1994.

24. Galt JR, Hise LH, Garcia EF et al: Filtering in frequency space, *J Nucl Med Technol* 14:152-162, 1986.

25. Cooke CD, Garcia EV, Folks RD et al: Visualization of cardiovascular nuclear medicine tomographic perfusion studies. In *Proceedings of the first conference on visualization in biomedical computing*, Atlanta, 1990, IEEE Press.

26. Faber TL, Akers MS, Peshock RM et al: Three-dimensional motion and perfusion quantification in gated single-photon emission computed tomograms, *J Nucl Med* 32(12):2311-2317, 1991.

27. Wallis JW, Miller TR: Three-dimensional display in nuclear medicine and radiology, *J Nucl Med* 32:534-546, 1991.

28. Wallis JW, Miller TR: Volume rendering in three-dimensional display of SPECT images, *J Nucl Med* 31:1421-1430, 1990.

29. Miller TR, Wallis JW, Sampathkumaran KS: Three-dimensional display of gated cardiac blood-pool studies, *J Nucl Med* 30:2036-2041, 1989.

30. Sorenson SA, Phelps ME: *Physics in nuclear medicine,* ed 3, Philadelphia, 1987, WB Saunders.

31. DePuey EG: How to detect and avoid myocardial perfusion SPECT artifacts, *J Nucl Med* 35(4):699-702, 1994.

32. DePuey EG, Garcia EV: Optimal specificity of thallium-201 SPECT through recognition of imaging artifacts, *J Nucl Med* 30:441-449, 1989.

33. Germano G, Chua T, Kiat H et al: A quantitative phantom analysis of artifacts due to hepatic activity in technetium-99m myocardial perfusion SPECT studies, *J Nucl Med* 35(2):356-359, 1994.

34. Nuyts J, DuPont P, Van den Maegdenbergh V et al: A study of the liver-heart artifact in emission tomography, *J Nucl Med* 36(1):133-139, 1995.

35. King MA, Xia W, DeVries DJ et al: A Monte Carlo investigation of artifacts caused by liver uptake in single-photon emission computed tomography perfusion imaging with Tc-99m–labeled agents, *J Nucl Cardiol* 3:18-29, 1996.

36. Hendel RC, Corbett JR, Cullom SJ et al: The value and practice of attenuation correction for myocardial SPECT imaging: a joint position statement for the American Society of Nuclear Cardiology and the Society of Nuclear Medicine, *J Nucl Cardiol* 9:135-143, 2002.

37. Esquerre JP, Coca FJ, Martinez SJ et al: Prone decubitus: a solution to inferior wall attenuation in thallium-201 myocardial tomography, *J Nucl Med* 30(3):398-401, 1989.

38. Sorenson JA: Quantitative measurement of radioactivity in vivo by whole body counting. In Hine JH, Sorenson JA, editors: *Instrumentation in nuclear medicine,* ed 2, New York, 1974, Academic Press.

39. Chang LT: A method for attenuation correction in radionuclide computed tomography, *IEEE Trans Nucl Sci* 1:638-643, 1978.

40. Kuhl DE, Hale J, Eaton WL: Transmission scanning: a useful adjunct to conventional emission scanning for accurately keying isotope deposition to radiographic anatomy, *Radiology* 7:278, 1966.

41. Ficaro EP, Fessler JA, Ackermann RJ et al: Simultaneous transmission-emission thallium-201 cardiac SPECT: effect of attenuation correction on

myocardial tracer distribution, *J Nucl Med* 36(6):921-931, 1995.

42. Tan P, Bailey DL, Meikle SR et al: A scanning line source for simultaneous emission and transmission measurements in SPECT, *J Nucl Med* 34:1752-1760, 1993.

43. Tung CH, Gullberg GT, Zeng GL et al: Nonuniform attenuation correction using simultaneous transmission and emission converging tomography, *IEEE Trans Nucl Sci* 39:1134-1143, 1992.

44. Cellar A, Sitek A, Stoub E et al: Multiple line source array for SPECT transmission scans: simulation, phantom, and patient studies, *J Nucl Med* 39:2183-2189, 1998.

45. Patton JA, Delbeke D, Sandler MP: Image fusion using an integrated, dual-head coincidence camera with x-ray tube–based attenuation maps, *J Nucl Med* 41:1364-1368, 2000.

46. Lang TF, Hasagawa BH, Liew SC et al: Description of a prototype emission-transmission computer tomography imaging system, *J Nucl Med* 33(10):1881-1887, 1992.

47. Floyd CE, Jaszczak RJ, Coleman RE: Scatter detection in SPECT imaging: dependence on source depth, energy, and energy window, *Phys Med Biol* 33:1075-1081, 1988.

48. Frey EC, Tsui BMW: Modeling the scatter response function in inhomogeneous scattering media for SPECT, *IEEE Trans Nucl Sci* 41:1585-1593, 1994.

49. Jaszczak RJ, Greer KL, Floyd CE Jr et al: Improved SPECT quantification using compensation for scattered photons, *J Nucl Med* 25:893-900, 1984.

50. Ichihara T, Ogawa K, Motomura N et al: Compton scatter compensation using the triple energy window method for single- and dual-isotope SPECT, *J Nucl Med* 34(12):2216-2221, 1993.

51. Buvat I, Rodriguez-Villafuerte M, Todd-Pokropek A et al: Comparative assessment of nine scatter correction methods based on spectral analysis using Monte Carlo simulations, *J Nucl Med* 36:1476-1488, 1995.

52. Frey EC, Tsui BMW: A practical method for incorporating scatter in a projector/backprojector for accurate scatter compensation in SPECT, *IEEE Trans Nucl Sci* NS-40:1007-1016, 1993.

53. Frey EC, Ju ZW, Tsui BMW: A fast projector/backprojector pair modeling the asymmetric, spatially varying scatter response function in SPECT imaging, *IEEE Trans Nucl Sci* NS-40:1192-1197, 1993.

54. Beekman F, Eijkman E, Viergever M et al: Object shape–dependent PSF model for SPECT imaging, *IEEE Trans Nucl Sci* NS-40:31-39, 1993.

55. Mukai T, Links JM, Douglass KH et al: Scatter correction in SPECT using nonuniform attenuation data, *Phys Med Biol* 33:1129-1140, 1988.

56. Meikle SR, Hutton BF, Bailey DL: A transmission-dependent method for scatter correction in SPECT, *J Nucl Med* 35:360-367, 1994.

57. Welch A, Gullberg GT, Christian PE et al: A transmission map–based scatter correction technique for SPECT in inhomogeneous media, *Med Phys* 22(10):1627-1635, 1995.

58. Beekman FJ, den Harder JM, Viergever MA et al: SPECT modeling in nonuniform attenuating objects, *Phys Med Biol* 42:1133-1142, 1997.

59. Kadrmas DJ, Frey EC, Karimi SS et al: Fast implementations of reconstruction-based scatter compensation in fully 3D SPECT image reconstruction, *Phys Med Biol* 43(4):857-873, 1998.

60. Soares EJ, Byrne CL, Glick SJ et al: Implementation and evaluation of an analytical solution to the photon attenuation and nonstationary resolution reconstruction problem in SPECT, *IEEE Trans Nucl Sci* NS-40:1231-1237, 1993.

61. Pan X, Metz CE, Chen CT: Noniterative methods and their noise characteristics in 2D SPECT image reconstruction, *IEEE Trans Nucl Sci* 44:1388-1397, 1997.

62. Lewitt RM, Edholm PR, Xia W: Fourier method for correction of depth-dependent collimator blurring, SPIE vol 1092, Medical Imaging III: Image processing, pp 232-243, 1989.

63. Glick SJ, Penney BC, King MA et al: Noniterative compensation for the distance-dependent detector response and photon attenuation in SPECT imaging, *IEEE Trans Med Imag* 7:135-148, 1988.

64. Rigo P, Van Boxem PH, Safi JF et al: Quantitative evaluation of a comprehensive motion, resolution, and attenuation correction program: initial experience, *J Nucl Cardiol* 5:458-468, 1998.

65. Younes RB, Mas J, Pousse A et al: Introducing simultaneous spatial resolution and attenuation correction after scatter removal in SPECT imaging, *Nucl Med Commun* 12:1031-1043, 1991.

66. Tsui BMW, Hu GB, Gilland DR: Implementation of simultaneous attenuation and detector response correction in SPECT, *IEEE Trans Nucl Sci* 35:778-783, 1988.

67. Zeng GL, Gullberg GT, Tsui BMW et al: Three-dimensional iterative reconstruction with attenuation and geometric point response correction, *IEEE Trans Nucl Sci* 38:693-702, 1991.

68. Tsui BMW, Frey EC, Zhao X et al: The importance and implementation of accurate 3D methods for quantitative SPECT, *Phys Med Biol* 39:509-530, 1994.

69. Ye J, Liang Z, Harrington DP: Quantitative reconstruction for myocardial perfusion SPECT: an efficient approach by depth-dependent deconvolution and matrix rotation, *Phys Med Biol* 39(8):1263-1279, 1994.

70. Tsui BMW, Frey EC, LaCroix KJ et al: Quantitative myocardial perfusion SPECT, *J Nucl Cardiol* 5:507-522, 1998.

71. Matsunari I, Boning G, Ziegler SI et al: Effects of misalignment between transmission and emission scans on attenuation-corrected cardiac SPECT, *J Nucl Med* 39:411-416, 1998.

72. Germano G, Kavanagh PB, Su HT et al: Automatic reorientation of three-dimensional transaxial myocardial perfusion SPECT images, *J Nucl Med* 36:1107-1114, 1995.

73. Mullick R, Ezquerra NF: Automatic determination of left ventricular orientation from SPECT data, *IEEE Trans Med Imag* 14:88-99, 1995.

74. Slomka PJ, Hurwitz GA, Stephenson J et al: Automated alignment and sizing of myocardial stress and rest scans to three-dimensional normal templates using an image registration algorithm, *J Nucl Med* 36:1115-1122, 1995.

75. Germano G, Kavanaugh PB, Waechter P et al: A new algorithm for the quantitation of myocardial perfusion SPECT. I. Technical principles and reproducibility, *J Nucl Med* 41:712-719, 2000.

76. Van Train KF, Areeda J, Garcia EV et al: Quantitative same-day rest-stress technetium-99m sestamibi SPECT: definition and validation of stress normal limits and criteria for abnormality, *J Nucl Med* 34:1494-1502, 1993.

77. Klein JL, Garcia EV, DePuey EG et al: Reversibility bull's-eye: a new polar bull's-eye map to quantify reversibility of stress-induced SPECT Tl-201 myocardial perfusion defects, *J Nucl Med* 31:1240-1246, 1990.

78. Faber TL, Cooke CD, Pettigrew RI et al: Three-dimensional displays of left ventricular epicardial surface from standard cardiac SPECT perfusion quantification techniques, *J Nucl Med* 36:697-703, 1995.

79. Cooke CD, Garcia EV, Folks RD: Three-dimensional visualization of cardiac single photon emission computed tomography studies. In Robb RA, editor: *Visualization in biomedical computing 1992*, SPIE 1808:671-675, 1992.

80. Quaife RA, Faber TL, Corbett JR: Visual assessment of quantitative three-dimensional displays of stress thallium-201 tomograms: comparison with visual multislice analysis, *J Nucl Med* 32:1006, 1991.

81. Santana CA, Garcia EV, Vansant JP et al: Three-dimensional color-modulated display of myocardial SPECT perfusion distributions accurately assesses coronary artery disease, *J Nucl Med* 41:1941-1946, 2000.

82. Galt JR, Garcia EV, Robbins WL: Effects of myocardial wall thickness on SPECT quantification, *IEEE Trans Med Imag* 9:144-150, 1990.

83. Eisner RL, Schmarkey S, Martin SE et al: Defects on SPECT "perfusion" images can occur due to abnormal segmental contraction, *J Nucl Med* 35:638-643, 1994.

84. Germano G, Kiat H, Kavanagh PB et al: Automatic quantification of ejection fraction from gated myocardial perfusion SPECT, *J Nucl Med* 36(11):2138-2147, 1995.

85. Cooke CD, Garcia EV, Cullom SJ et al: Determining the accuracy of calculating systolic wall thickening using a fast Fourier transform approximation: a simulation study based on canine and patient data, *J Nucl Med* 35:1185-1192, 1994.

86. Corbett JR, McGhie AI, Faber TL: Perfusion defect size and severity using gated SPECT sestamibi: comparison to ungated imaging, *J Nucl Med* 35:115P, 1994 (abstract).

87. Germano G, Kiat H, Mazzant M et al: Stress perfusion/stress wall motion with fast (6.7 min) Tc sestamibi myocardial SPECT, *J Nucl Med* 35:81P, 1994 (abstract).

88. Faber T, Cooke C, Folks R et al: Left ventricular function and perfusion from gated SPECT perfusion images: an integrated method, *J Nucl Med* 40(4):650-659, 1999.

89. Faber TL, Stokely EM, Peshock RM et al: A model-based four-dimensional left ventricular surface detector, *IEEE Trans Med Imag* 10(3):321-329, 1991.

90. Goris ML, Thompson C, Malone LJ et al: Modeling the integration of myocardial regional perfusion and function, *Nucl Med Commun* 15(1):9-20, 1994.

91. Germano G, Kavanagh PB, Kiat H et al: Automatic analysis of gated myocardial SPECT: development and initial validation of a method, *J Nucl Med* 35:116P, 1994 (abstract).

92. Sheehan FH, Bolson EL, Dodge HT et al: Advantages and applications of the centerline method for characterizing region ventricular function, *Circulation* 74:293-305, 1986.

93. Graham LS: Quality control for SPECT systems, *Radiographics* 15:1471-1481, 1995.

94. Nichols KJ, Galt JR: Quality control for SPECT imaging. In DePuey EG, Garcia EV, Berman DS, editors: *Cardiac SPECT imaging*, Philadelphia, 2001, Lippincott Williams & Wilkins.

95. Eisner R, Churchwell A, Noever T et al: Quantitative analysis of the thallium-201 myocardial bull's-eye display: critical role of correcting for patient motion, *J Nucl Med* 29:91-97, 1988.

96. Botvinick EH, Zhu YY, O'Connell WJ et al: A quantitative assessment of patient motion and its effect on myocardial perfusion SPECT images, *J Nucl Med* 34:303-310, 1993.

97. *Performance measurements of scintillation cameras*, NEMA Standards Publication NU1-1994, Washington, DC, 2001, National Electrical Manufacturers Association.

98. *Scintillation camera acceptance testing and performance evaluation*, AAPM Report No. 6, New York, 1980,

American Association of Physicists in Medicine, American Institute of Physics.

99. *Computer-aided scintillation camera acceptance testing,* AAPM Report No. 9, New York, 1981, American Association of Physicists in Medicine, American Institute of Physics.

100. *Rotating scintillation camera SPECT acceptance testing and quality control,* AAPM Report No. 22, New York, 1987, American Association of Physicists in Medicine, American Institute of Physics.

Paul E. Christian

chapter *10*

Fundamentals of Molecular Imaging with PET

Objectives

Describe positron decay and the production of annihilation photons.

List positron-emitting radionuclides and their properties.

List detector crystals that can be used for PET imaging and describe their properties.

Explain the fundamental operation of dedicated PET scanners and their design.

Describe the detection of true, scatter, and random events.

Describe transmission imaging and its need and use in attenuation correcting PET images.

Characterize the visual presentation of nonattenuated and attenuation-corrected images.

Define SUV and explain how it is calculated and used; discuss critical elements in generating quantitative measurements.

Describe the process of storing reconstructed data in sinograms and reconstruction methods.

List calibrations required of dedicated PET scanners.

Discuss 2D and 3D imaging and the advantages and disadvantages of each.

Describe how PET scanners acquire and store data.

Discuss reconstruction of PET images.

Describe attenuation correction techniques in PET.

Discuss the implications of image fusion and describe the PET/CT scanner.

Discuss the safe handling of PET radiotracers to maintain ALARA principles.

*P*ositron emission tomography (PET) is a powerful technique to image simple chemical or physiological processes within the body. The metabolic and biologic activity of disease always precedes any anatomic evidence of the illness. PET as a biologic imaging technique does not replace anatomic imaging, but adds the characterization of simple molecular processes that are taking place in normal or diseased tissues within the body. X ray, CT, or MRI may see the anatomic defect, but PET as a molecular analysis adds information about the chemical activity of normal and abnormal tissue. Nature has provided very short-lived positron-emitting forms of the some of the simple elements (^{11}C, ^{13}N, and ^{15}O) used in the most basic and fundamental biochemical reactions. These radionuclides, along with fluorine-18, represent the core of PET tracers that can be used to study the interaction of elementary chemical processes of all life, such as $^{15}O_2$, $H_2{}^{15}O$, $C^{15}O_2$, and ^{18}F-glucose (sugar) (Table 10-1). More than 3000 different chemical compounds have been radiolabeled with PET tracers and have been used to image molecular processes.

Table 10-1	Positron radionuclides for PET		
Radionuclide	Half-life	Maximum range (mm)	Mean range (mm)
^{11}C	20 min	5.0	0.3
^{13}N	9 min	5.4	1.4
^{15}O	2.1 min	8.2	1.5
^{18}F	110 min	2.4	0.2
^{82}Rb	75 sec	15.6	2.6

In recent years, PET has moved rapidly from a well-established research tool into routine clinical practice. Payment approval by Medicare and private insurance companies for PET imaging in some diseases relating to oncology, cardiology, and brain imaging has opened the way for the expanded use of this powerful modality and its availability to physicians and patients. The availability of PET radiotracers through commercial distribution networks has also allowed hospitals and clinics to add PET as a new service and has promoted the expansion of independent outpatient imaging centers and mobile PET imaging services.

The basic science principles of PET (i.e., physics, radiochemistry, scintillation detectors) are discussed in earlier chapters. This chapter focuses on how these science fundamentals are brought together specifically for imaging positron-emitting radionuclides. Clinical applications of PET to brain and heart imaging are discussed in the respective organ system chapters. The application of PET in oncology is discussed in a separate chapter in this book.

PHYSICS OF POSITRONS

In 1927, P.A.M. Dirac theorized the existence of the positron (positively charged electron) as an antiparticle of the negatron (negatively charged electron). The existence of the positron was later confirmed experimentally by C. Anderson in 1932. Proton-rich nuclei decay by either electron capture or by positron emission. These alternative decay pathways may exist in the same nuclei and be alternate forms of decay in some atoms, such as in naturally occurring potassium-40. In many of the radionuclides used for PET imaging, most decay pathways are predominantly positron emission alone.

When a positron is expelled from the nucleus of an atom, it travels within a range of only a short distance. During this travel across several millimeters, adjacent atoms are ionized and the positron loses energy and slows down. The positron then pairs up with an electron, and these two particles spiral in toward each other for a tiny fraction of a second, forming a two-particle atom call positronium (Figure 10-1). When the antiparticle positron/electron pair interact, they annihilate each other, and the mass of each particle is completely converted into energy through Einstein's equation, $E = mc^2$. Since the masses of the positron and electron are exactly the same, the annihilation process converts the mass of each particle into pure electromagnetic energy (511 keV from each particle). Therefore a pair of 511 keV gamma rays is produced, with the gamma rays being emitted in nearly opposite directions, 180+/– ~0.5 degrees apart. The minor variation from exactly 180 degrees apart is due to the motion of the particles at the time when the annihilation event occurs.

Each PET radionuclide emits its positron with a different energy, higher energy particles having greater path lengths and greater mean ranges for the travel of the positron. Table 10-1 lists the maximum and the mean ranges of some of the most useful PET radionuclides, along with the half-life of each. In those PET radionuclides that have very large mean ranges, the positron may travel a substantial distance (a few millimeters) before the annihilation event occurs. This large particle range results in a slight mispositioning of the annihilation event from the actual location of the positron-emitting atom. Therefore a scan performed with ^{18}F (2.4 mm maximum and 0.2 mm average range) will produce a higher resolution image than ^{82}Rb, which has a 15.6 mm maximum and 2.6 mm mean range.

PRODUCTION OF PET RADIOTRACERS

Physics teaches us that positrons are produced by proton-rich nuclei. Therefore to manufacture positron-emitting radiopharmaceuticals requires a device that can add protons to the nucleus. Small linear accelerators or cyclotrons provide a source of positively charged protons or deuterons of an appropriate energy to create these nuclei. Small medical cyclotrons are typically used for producing PET radiopharmaceuticals. The chapter on radiochemistry and

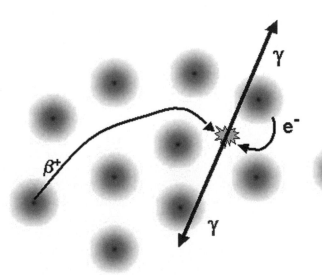

Figure 10-1   Once the positron is emitted from the nucleus, it travels a few millimeters and ionizes many atoms before pairing with an electron and undergoing an annihilation interaction, which produces a pair of 511 keV gamma rays that travel in opposite directions.

radiopharmacology discusses both cyclotrons and the production of PET radiopharmaceuticals. (See Figures 6-3 and 6-4 for a diagram and photograph of a cyclotron.) A cyclotron costs about $2 million and must be accompanied by a radiochemistry laboratory that can manufacture the short-lived radiotracers of ^{18}F, ^{11}C, ^{13}N, and ^{15}O. ^{18}F is the only radiopharmaceutical that has a half-life long enough (110 min) to be transported any substantial distance from the cyclotron. Therefore radiotracers ^{11}C, ^{13}N, and ^{15}O must be imaged on a scanner that is in the same facility where the cyclotron is located. At this time ^{18}F-flurodeoxyglucose is the only ^{18}F label compound currently approved by the FDA for general distribution. ^{18}F-FDG can be shipped by ground or air transportation within a distance of a few hundred miles. Most oncology studies are performed using FDG.

Generator-produced rubidium-82 is FDA approved, but it is used at only about a dozen sites in the United States. Rubidium is an analog of potassium and is therefore a myocardial perfusion imaging agent, which has a half-life of 75 seconds. These generators are rather expensive and can only be afforded by those sites that can guarantee several myocardial perfusion studies every day. PET scanners produce much higher resolution images with significantly more counts than single photon emission computed tomography (SPECT) and therefore provide substantially better quality.

PET radiotracers that are produced on-site and those obtained from commercial PET radiopharmaceutical companies must be produced according to pharmaceutical current Good Manufacturing Practices and according to FDA and USP standards. Quality control of the radiotracers must be performed as with any radiopharmaceutical. The production of a single PET radiopharmaceutical will require very expensive equipment, including the cyclotron, target, automated synthesis module, hot cell (to contain the synthesis module), and any additional radiopharmaceutical quality control and precursor preparation equipment.

PET RADIATION DETECTORS

Detecting 511 keV coincidence photons in PET would be most ideal if the scintillation material had a high density to stop the high-energy photons. Ideally, the material should also be a very efficient scintillator and create a large amount of light that would be released from the crystal very quickly. Most scintillation crystals are lacking in at least one of these ideal attributes at 511 keV. However, many materials are efficient at high gamma-ray energy, some of which are listed in Table 10-2. The critical issue is to stop the annihilation gamma rays and thus detect the radiation. Therefore most PET scanners use bismuth germanate ($Bi_4Ge_3O_{12}$) or BGO. Bismuth has a high atomic number and is therefore very good at stopping the 511 keV photons. BGO is unfortunately a relatively slow scintillator and yields a relatively small amount of light compared with NaI(Tl). In addition, BGO has poor energy resolution that requires energy windows that span from about 300 to 600 keV. The stopping power

| Table 10-2 | PET scintillation detector properties |

	NaI(Tl)	BGO	LSO	GSO
Density (gm/cm^3)	3.7	7.1	7.4	6.7
Effective atomic #	51	75	71	59
Emission intensity	100	15	75	25
Decay time (nsec)	230	300	40	30–45
Hygroscopic	Yes	No	No	No

of BGO compensates for its other deficiencies, and BGO is currently the most commonly used scintillator in dedicated PET scanners.

Some dedicated PET scanners use other scintillation crystal materials. Leutetium orthosilicate ($Lu_2SiO_5[Ce]$ or LSO) and gadolinium orthosilicate ($Gd_2SiO_5[Ce]$ or GSO) are now available in some commercial PET systems. Both these crystals have slightly lower stopping power than BGO, but produce much more light per keV of detected gamma ray energy than BGO. However, the main reason that these materials are used is that they are fast scintillators. Because the positron is identified by the coincidence detection of the gamma rays on opposite detectors, faster materials are desired. Scanners using the fast scintillators, LSO or GSO, have been designed to operate only in 3D acquisition mode to provide higher detection sensitivity.

A 511 keV gamma ray travels across the detector ring in about one nanosecond. Slow scintillator materials will not allow an exacting measurement of simultaneous event detection. Thus very fast light-emitting crystals provide more exact time measurements of simultaneous event detection. Very fast scintillators, such as BaF_2 (0.5 nsec light decay time) can allow the measurement of estimated spatial location along the coincidence line of detection by measuring the difference in the gamma ray arrival times at opposing detectors. This type of scanner is referred to as a "time of flight" scanner and has been limited in use to research systems.

PET SCANNER DESIGN

PET imaging requires the placement of detectors on opposite sides of the patient in order to simultaneously detect the coincidence photons produced by the annihilation process. PET systems have most often been referred to either as dedicated PET scanners or as gamma camera-based hybrid systems. Gamma camera hybrid PET scanners have two or three gamma camera detectors that can be used in coincidence mode to identify an annihilation gamma pair and to determine a line of response (LOR) path representing the path of the photon pair. They detect fewer photon pairs and therefore produce poorer images than machines dedicated solely to image PET radiotracers. The lack of adequate imaging statistics—and subsequently, lower lesion detectability—has limited the reimbursement from health care payers for PET imaging on gamma camera-based PET systems.

BGO is the most commonly used detector material in dedicated ring systems. BGO, LSO, and GSO systems have rectangular crystals about 3 to 4 mm in size and 10 to 30 mm in length. Dedicated PET scanners have 8,000 to 20,000 of these crystals laid out to form several rings of detectors. Each crystal is too small to have its own photomultiplier tube; therefore a group of crystals is put together in a detector block. Most commonly, four photomultiplier tubes are used on a block to collect the light from all the crystals, measure the gamma-ray energy, and identify which crystal in the block was struck by the gamma ray. These multicrystal blocks are typically constructed in one of two ways: as a "cut block" or as a reflective block of crystals. A cut block design is created from one larger crystal as shown in Figure 10-2, *A*, where cuts are made at different depths through the crystal that allow the reflected scintillation photons to be distributed in a specified pattern over the four PMTs. The PMTs signal output can then determine which of the crystal elements in the block detected the radiation. The alternative reflective block approach is to create a block from a group of small individual crystals (Figure 10-2, *B*); each crystal is surrounded by a carefully designed amount of reflective material that spreads the light in a designated pattern onto the PMTs. Therefore both the cut block and reflective block designs do the same thing, namely, use reflective surfaces on the sides of individual crystals to distribute the scintillation photons to the PMTs. The four PMTs are used to detect the scintillation light, and the output signals identify which crystal has detected the event using pulse strength information, similar to the Anger camera positioning circuitry. The output from the array of four PMTs—A, B, C, and D (Figure 10-3)—is used to calculate the transverse location X and Z-axis location of the event within the detector block by $X = (B + D)/(A + B + C + D)$ and $Z = (C + D)/(A + B + C + D)$. The output from a 6×6 crystal detector block is shown in Figure 10-4. PMT centers are shown by the curved contour lines for 36 crystals in this example of a reflective design detector block, and straight lines show the edges of the regions that define the effective crystal boundaries. Software can be used to adjust these boundaries that define each crystal. Several detector blocks

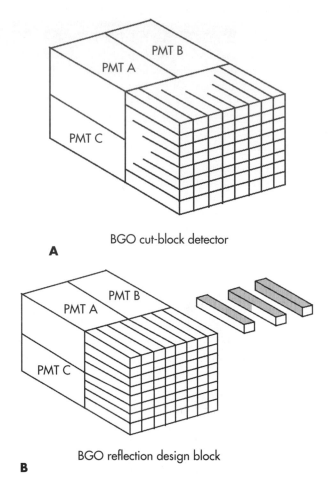

BGO cut-block detector

A

BGO reflection design block

B

Figure 10-2 **A,** A cut-block detector formed from one crystal with partial cuts to create the effect of many small crystals. The cuts form reflective surfaces to reflect light to four PMTs. A reflection design block **(B)** is made from small individual crystals, each wrapped with a certain amount of light reflector to distribute the light to the four PMTs. Both block designs accomplish the same reflective distribution of light to four PMTs that can then determine which crystal element within the block detected the scintillation event.

are combined to form detector "buckets" or "modules." Dozens of these modules or buckets form rings of detectors around the patient (Figure 10-5). Each block of crystal/PMT assemblies forms this series of rings of detectors, and each ring acquires one image slice from the patient. Dedicated PET scanners, as shown in Figure 10-6, typically have 18 to

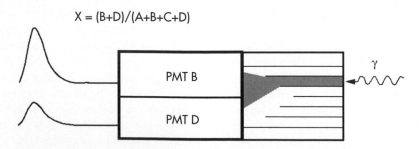

$$X = (B+D)/(A+B+C+D)$$

PMT B

PMT D

γ

Figure 10-3 Light from a scintillation event in a single crystal element is distributed by the reflective surfaces onto the PMTs in a specific pattern. Analysis of the pulse strength from each PMT is used to determine the X or Y location of the gamma ray.

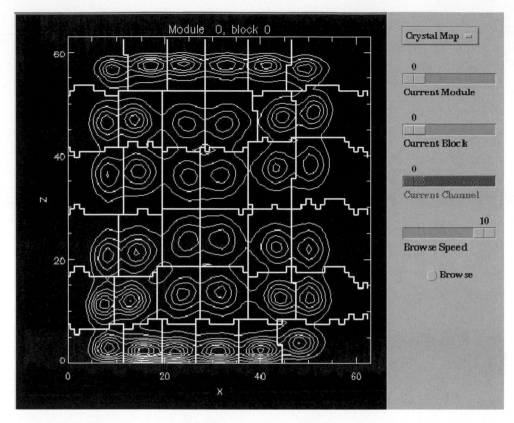

Figure 10-4   The output map from each crystal in a block is shown on the computer display as circular patterns of light intensity from each crystal in the detector block. Automated computer software shows the overlying linear pattern that defines the effective location of each crystal and balances the sensitivity of each crystal element.

30 consecutive rings of crystals and create a field of view along the patient of about 15 cm. Images of small organs, such as the heart or brain, may be acquired with a single bed position of the patient within the scanner. However, the possibility of distant metastases in cancer patients requires

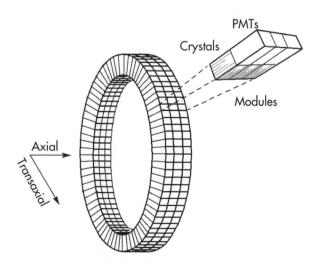

Figure 10-5   Detector blocks, or modules, are used to construct a ring of detectors around the patient. Hundreds of blocks are used to create 18 to 30 consecutive rings of detectors that form a cylindrical field of view about 6 inches long and that can acquire many slices of coincidence data at one time.

that a large area of the body be imaged. "Whole body" PET scans are used in most oncology studies, which actually only cover from the hips up through the base of the brain (approximately 90 cm) or about six bed positions. Total body (nearly head to toe) scans are required with certain types of cancer where malignant tissue may grow in any area of the body, as with melanoma. In this case the number of bed positions will be increased to cover the total body area, ≥10 bed positions. Scans of the whole body or total body are obtained by moving the imaging table many times to cover the desired length over the body, and the total time for data acquisition is 40 to 90 minutes.

One drawback with BGO systems is the relatively poor energy resolution of this crystal, as compared with NaI(Tl), LSO, or GSO. With poorer energy resolution, the energy window when using BGO must be set somewhat wide. With most scintillation materials, a narrow energy window is effective at rejecting scattered photons, which will have a lower energy. The wide window employed with BGO is thereby not very efficient at rejecting scattered photons, and a method for scatter correction will be used during reconstruction.

One manufacturer of dedicated PET scanners uses six large curved single NaI(Tl) crystals, each with 48 PMTs. Each of these six detector/PMT assemblies operates much like a single photon scintillation camera, but the assemblies operate only in coincidence mode, forming a dedicated large

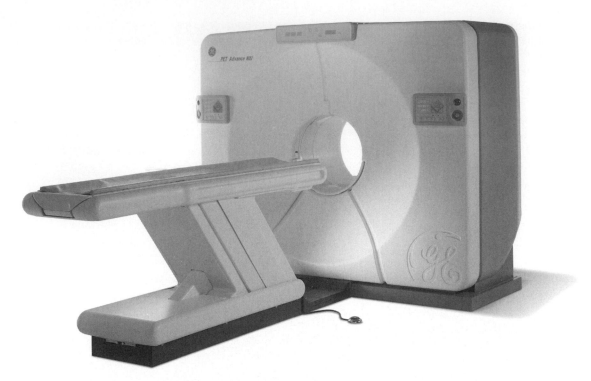

Figure 10-6   Dedicated BGO ring scanner containing 12,096 crystals that obtains 35 slices simultaneously. (Courtesy of General Electric Medical Systems, Waukesha, Wisconsin.)

area of view (~30 cm FOV) PET scanner. This NaI(Tl) based scanner is much less expensive, though the NaI(Tl) crystals stop fewer high-energy photons than BGO. It also has limited count rate capabilities. Therefore there are fewer counts in the images, which gives slightly lower performance than BGO systems in detecting either small or low-contrast lesions.

COINCIDENCE DETECTION: TRUE, SCATTER, AND RANDOM EVENTS

PET imaging is based on the detection of the annihilation pair of 511 keV gamma rays. In theory these gamma rays are detected simultaneously from scintillation detectors that are positioned on opposing sides of the patient. The arrival of the 511 keV photons should take place within a short time of one another, which in theory should ensure that the photons are from the same annihilation event. A coincidence timing window measures the arrival time interval of the electrical pulses. The interval is very short, about 6 to 12 nanoseconds (electromagnetic radiation travels 30 cm/nanosecond).

A pair of annihilation gamma rays striking two detectors at the same time is termed a "true" coincidence annihilation event (Figure 10-7, *A* and *D*). When two atoms decay at nearly the same time, photons from two different annihilation events may be detected within the timing window. When this happens, a false event, referred to as a "random" event, is recorded (Figure 10-7, *C* and *F*), and its false line of response is shown as a dotted line on the diagram.

Because many atoms are decaying at nearly the same time, random events cannot be avoided. However, techniques exist for estimating corrections of these false events. Random count rates are also higher when there is more activity present or when the scanner is in 3D mode. In certain clinical situations, such as where there is a hot source of radioactivity just outside the scanner field of view (brain, bladder, tumor, injection site), the random events may be 50 percent of all coincidence events detected. Without correction the image will have very low contrast of true hot lesions, and some tumors may be missed. A common way to estimate the random events' contribution is to collect and subtract data from a "delayed event" timing window (>12 nanoseconds) and to use this information as a measure for randoms correction. Using data from the long timing window ensures that all events with this delay are randoms, and a fairly accurate correction may be made. Additional techniques may also be available on some systems.

Another mispositioning error of PET data comes from the scatter of gamma rays between their origin and the detectors (Figure 10-7, *B* and *E*). Normally, nuclear medicine imaging reduces scatter in the image by selecting a relatively narrow energy window, which eliminates the detection of the scattered photons. However, BGO has relatively poor energy resolution, and the energy window is rather wide, and therefore a narrow energy window technique is not practical. Scatter is always present in clinical imaging, representing about 15 percent of data in 2D mode, and reconstructed images will require correction. The original 2D scanner design using septa between detector rings was to aid in reducing both scatter and randoms. Scanner manufacturers provide various techniques that are employed in factory set reconstruction macros to either estimate or mathematically model scatter and make a correction during image reconstruction. Scatter correction is very important in 3D imaging, particularly when hot organs are nearby or just outside the FOV of the detectors. Approximately 50 percent of photons scatter within the body. Therefore scatter correction and accurate attenuation correction are imperative when quantitative information is needed.

Scatter is affected by the distribution of radioactivity, size, and density of the object or objects and their locations relative to the detectors. Scatter cannot be measured directly, but various estimates and mathematical models may be used for estimated corrections, with various techniques for 2D or 3D mode acquisition. The most accurate techniques may look at the pair of emission and transmission slices and adjust the model to the size and activity distribution within the patient. Complex scatter corrections are based on estimating the scattering physics within the emission and transmission images but may be computationally intense

and require a longer time to reconstruct slices. However, reasonable estimates for scatter correction are provided in the manufacturer's reconstruction software.

Correction techniques may also be employed for the deadtime loss, particularly in 3D mode where accurate compensation for count rate losses is important because count rates are very high, and deadtime losses become a measurable and significant fraction of all counts. It is important to remember that scatter and randoms are a 3D effect as demonstrated in the lower diagrams of Figure 10-7, *D-F*. Randoms, scatter, and deadtime corrections should be a routine part of the image correction and reconstruction process.

DATA ACQUISITION

The detection of an annihilation photon pair by opposing crystals creates one event or line of response (LOR) between two detectors. Millions of these LORs will be acquired and stored for use in the reconstruction of the 3D distribution of radiotracer. If two photons are from

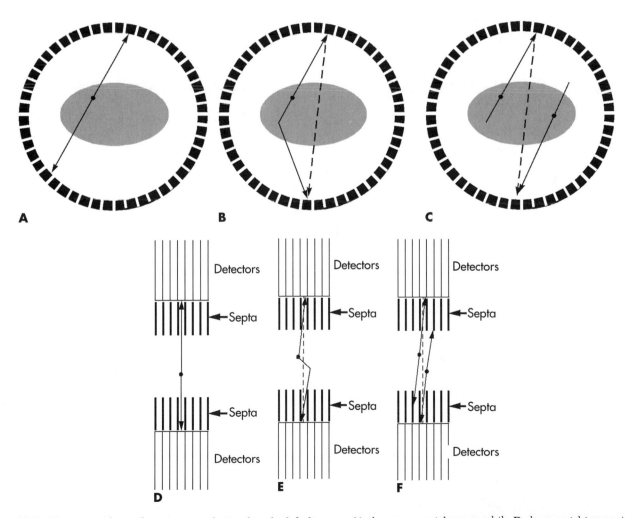

Figure 10-7   True coincidence detections are depicted in the left diagrams (**A** shows transaxial event, while **D** shows axial interactions). Scattered gamma rays (**B, E**) also create a false location of the coincidence (*dotted line*) by misdirecting gamma rays to a false location. Random events (**C, F**) occur when two disintegrations happen within the timing window and one gamma from each creates a false coincidence shown as a dotted line.

the same annihilation interaction, they should be detected by opposing crystals at about the same instant. As mentioned above, the coincidence circuit sets a narrow timing window to ensure that the pulses are detected within about 6 to 12 nanoseconds or less. Data acquisition may also include acquisition of delayed events (those that are definitely random events), using the delayed timing window.

Spatial resolution of PET scanners is determined primarily by the size of the crystals and their separation. The spatial resolution of PET images will therefore be very close to the size of the crystal, typically 3 to 5 mm. Thus the full width at half-maximum (FWHM) will be about the same resolution over the diameter of the ring (Figure 10-8, *A*), and therefore the resolution of dedicated PET is significantly better than SPECT (about 4 mm reconstructed resolution for PET and >12 mm for SPECT). With a large number of crystals and hundreds of independently operating PMTs, the count rate capability of the PET scanner is significantly higher than scintillation cameras. On gamma cameras, collimators have an efficiency that is a small fraction of 1 percent, or only a very few photons are detected for a thousand decaying atoms in the patient. Ring PET systems are not limited by multihole collimators, and about 1.5 to 2 percent of all photons produced in the patient are detected by the PET scanner. The

PET scanner is therefore about 50 to 100 times more sensitive than the gamma camera, which is why PET images are of higher quality than SPECT. Also the higher sensitivity for detecting events, much higher count-rate capability, better resolution (independent of depth), and many more counts in the study give PET the highest resolution and highest count density images in all of tracer imaging. PET scans are produced from many dozens of millions of events. The higher spatial resolution images will only be possible when very high data density is obtained.

As mentioned, PET information is acquired by recording a LOR between two individual crystals as coincidence photons are detected. As shown in Figure 10-8, *A*, the spatial resolution measured in FWHM will be about the same size as an individual pixel and will have similar resolution all the way across the detector ring. However, as shown in Figure 10-8, *B*, the resolution near the edge of the ring will be slightly worse because of the thickness of the crystal and the possibility for the event to be detected at different depths within that crystal. This is a well-known issue with ring detector systems, that small sources of radioactivity near the edge of the ring will have slightly reduced resolution because of the length of the crystals and the variation in the depth in the crystal in which the scintillation event may take place.

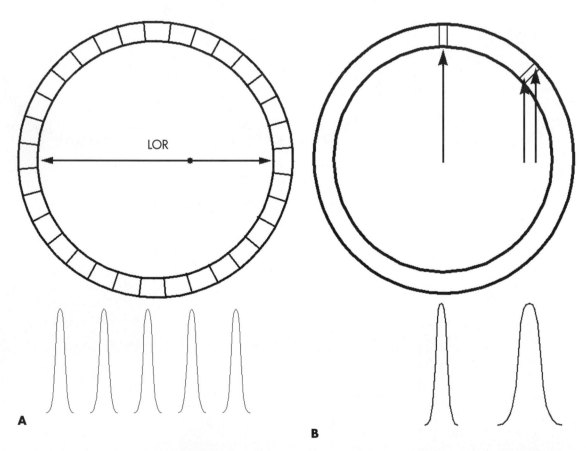

Figure 10-8 **A,** Pair of gamma rays creates a coincidence detection that represents a line of response *(LOR)*. Resolution is only limited by the size of the detectors, as shown by the equal full width at half-maximum (FWHM) curves below. Axial resolution degrades at the edges of the field of view **(B)** because of variations in the depth of interactions that can occur. Therefore, sources of radioactivity near the edge of the gantry ring have poorer resolution (wider FWHM) than sources at the center.

The crystals in a ring scanner detect coincidence LORs over a wide angle of almost 90 degrees, so meaningful information is obtained over a fan-shaped region of the ring (Figure 10-9, *A*). The top crystal of the ring therefore has a 90-degree angle of sensitivity for radiation detection. Each crystal around the ring creates a different fan-shaped sensitivity pattern of LORs (Figure 10-9, *B, C*). Therefore angular sampling around the gantry takes data from the patient from many very small angles to produce high resolution and high data density images. LOR data acquired from the thousands of crystals are sorted into lines of response that are parallel

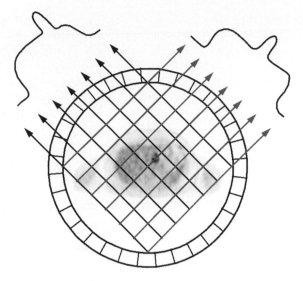

Figure 10-10　Parallel LORs provide the equivalent of projection information from all angles around the patient.

and thus form projection information as shown in Figure 10-10. Once the raw LOR data are reformatted to form projection data from each angle, the result can be thought of as being similar to SPECT raw projection count profiles.

For each slice, the count profiles may be taken from each projection angle and laid out to form a sinogram (Figure 10-11). Each horizontal row in the sinogram represents the

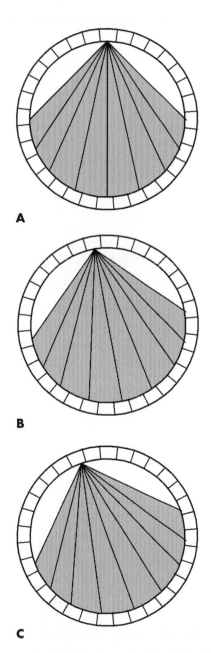

A

B

C

Figure 10-9　Each detector is limited to having coincidence detection over about 90 degrees, which creates a fan pattern of possible coincidence detection LORs. Each crystal (**A, B, C**) has a different orientation of its sensitivity pattern so that all crystals are used to provide a complete set of LORs from around the patient.

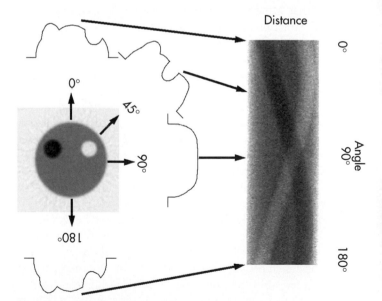

Figure 10-11　For each slice, the projections from each angle are placed in a horizontal row of a matrix called a sinogram. The sinogram plot is represented as the distance across the field of view of the scanner plotted against the angle from which the projection is taken. Each projection through 180 degrees is used to form a complete set of projection information. Hot and cold objects within a cylinder filled with radioactivity each create a sine wave pattern on the sinogram (*right*). Only 180 degrees of data are needed to form a complete set of projection information, as the next 180 degrees would be a repeat. One sinogram represents the data from which only one slice in the data will be formed; therefore one sinogram must be acquired per slice.

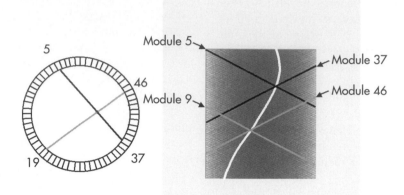

Figure 10-12 Sinogram information is also represented by the intersection of two detectors. Each detector module creates a line of possible detection with opposing detectors as represented by an angular dark line. Module 5 on one side of the ring detects a photon at the same time as module 37. The intersection of these two detector lines represents the LOR at which this event was detected. The intersection by another detector pair, 19 and 46, also demonstrates this. As these two LORs were obtained from the same point in space, a sinusoidal pattern (*right*) that represents the pattern is seen on the sinogram from that point in space.

count profile (or projection) across the distance of the gantry as seen from each angle. The vertical axis of the sinogram is the angle from which the projection is taken over 180 degrees. Projection information from the next 180 degrees around the object is not needed, because it is a repeat of the first 180 degrees. The sinogram will therefore contain all the data that will be needed to reconstruct one transaxial slice. Reconstruction of a transaxial slice will therefore be somewhat similar to reconstructing SPECT; both are projections at various angles. Viewing sinogram data is sometimes helpful in identifying that data were adequately received from all detectors.

Let's look at Figure 10-12 to see how a sinogram may be formed during 2D data acquisition. A point source in the scanner emits an annihilation pair, and one module, 5 for instance, may have coincidence detection with any of the modules on the opposite side of the ring. On the sinogram, module 5 interactions occur along a downward angle toward the right. Module 37 on the opposite side of the ring uses a downward left angle to represent the possible LORs for this module. When a coincidence event occurs between modules 5 and 37, the pixel value at the intersection of those detectors is incremented by one event. If another annihilation pair is emitted from the same point, but on a different angle, a different pair of detectors, 19 and 46 for example, will have the LOR data stored as a pixel count at the intersection of those modules. As you can observe in Figure 10-12, *right*, all counts from this fixed point source will create a sine curve-shaped pattern down the sinogram as shown by the white curve. All possible detector pairs that may observe this interaction will have LOR data stored on this curve. The reconstruction process will calculate the activity represented at each projection (the horizontal line of the sinogram matrix) as observed from all angles, represented by the vertical sinogram axis.

Acquisition software allows a wide variety of operational modes. Scans may be simple one-bed position static images; dynamic; gated; 2D or 3D; or whole body, multiple bed position studies. They may also include the acquisition of emission data alone, transmission data alone, or a combination of emission and transmission images acquired in various orders (acquisition of all emission data, then all transmission data, all transmission data then all emission data, or interlacing a transmission/emission study at each bed position). Images are most commonly terminated by a specified amount of time for the acquisition. A standard patient dose will produce good-quality images, as standard protocols are used that use predefined times for emission and transmission data. Deviations from the department standard protocol will therefore require the technologist to modify the acquisition times or processing parameters to provide optimal quality images.

An acquisition interface program is available on all systems and allows the technologist to use predefined acquisition protocols. The program also allows changes to any parameters necessary. The time of acquisition, orientation of the patient on the table, and mode of acquisition may all be changed as needed to accommodate tailoring the study to the requirements for the individual patient. Likewise, processing protocols with override options are available on all commercial systems to facilitate easy and standardized operation.

2D AND 3D DETECTOR CONFIGURATION

Most ring-design dedicated PET scanners have tungsten or lead septa that sit inside the ring of crystal detectors and are positioned between detector rings (Figure 10-13). The septa are 1 to 3 mm thick and project about 8 to 10 cm into the axis of the gantry. These septa serve two purposes: (1) to limit the field of view of events to those within the same detector ring, or events with contiguous planes, and (2) to reduce the number of scatter and random events from outside the plane. With the septa in place, the scanner operates in what is termed 2D mode–that is–coincidence photon detection events are for the most part, limited by the septa to a single ring. Thus single slice or information from one 2D plane is acquired. The detector electronics and septa also allow the detection of an additional slice between the crystal rings (see the dotted lines in Figure 10-13). These virtual planes are termed interplane slices and create nearly twice the number of image slices as there are rings of crystals. For example, a scanner with 18 rings of crystals will generate an additional 17 interplane slices for a total of 35 slices. An interplane slice is created by the coincidence events of ring 1 with ring 2, and also those events between ring 2 with ring 1; therefore the interplane slices may have a different sensitivity than the direct (same ring) slices. As a point of interest, the resolution of the scanner may not be the same in all directions. The resolution along the z-axis (axis along the center of the rings) may have slightly different resolution than the resolution in the x or y axis across a slice.

On more recently manufactured scanners, retracting the septa creates the ability to place the scanner in 3D detection mode, where annihilation photon pairs can now be detected through a wide angle across the detector rings, thereby significantly increasing the sensitivity of the scanner (Figure 10-14). The retraction of the septa increases the sensitivity by a factor of 4 to 10 times, depending on the individual scanner design and on the organ and distribution of radiotracer being imaged. Without the septa, the number of possible LORs between a given crystal, and opposing crystals, increases significantly, thus dramatically increasing the number of LOR events detected, and thus increasing the data density in the image. Although 3D imaging demonstrates a theoretical improvement in imaging, the lack of septa results in a significant increase in both scattered photons and random coincidence events. Good correction techniques for both those factors must be made to exclude image artifacts when performing 3D imaging. The comparative 2D and 3D brain images shown at the bottom of Figure 10-14 demonstrate the advantages of using 3D mode for brain imaging. There is a significant improvement in the resolution and contrast because noise is reduced as the number of detected events is dramatically increased. In 3D mode, high amounts of activity just outside the detector FOV will create a significant increase in random events. Inadequate correction for randoms will reduce image contrast, which may mask subtle lesions adjacent to these sites of high activity, such as around the brain, bladder, or myocardium. Some dedicated PET scanners, those with NaI(Tl), LSO or GSO crystals, and some PET/CT scanners have no septa and therefore only operate in 3D mode.

Although 3D mode acquires significantly more events (4 to 10 times more), reconstruction algorithms may require more complex 3D randoms and scatter correction than 2D imaging. With much more data and added complexity of corrections, there is a significant increase in the reconstruction time of 3D data. 3D data sets will be 8 to 12 times larger than 2D data, and they typically require 6 to 8 times longer to reconstruct than do 2D. The disk space and archival storage space for 3D data sets also slow down processing, transferring, and archiving of 3D data.

Whole-body imaging with the scanner in 3D mode improves patient throughput because it provides an increase in scanner sensitivity and may allow a decrease in the time required for emission imaging. One consideration when applying the 3D mode to whole-body imaging is the reduced sensitivity at the ends of the FOV as compared with the sensitivity at the center of the scanner. To compensate for this sensitivity variation, a significant overlap of scanned area with two adjacent bed positions is performed. An overlap of several centimeters is done to provide adequate data acquisition over the entire scanned area.

Whole-body imaging in 3D mode provides very high count rates, and some data are lost because of deadtime limitations of the system. Technologists must carefully adjust the injected dose of activity, delay time before imaging, and count rate measured by the scanner to ensure that there is no compromised imaging due to the high count rate performance of the scanner. In addition, deadtime correction techniques must be employed for 3D data.

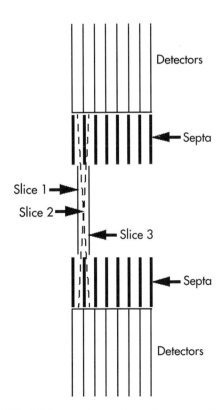

Figure 10-13   With septa in position, photons are limited to striking mostly one ring. However, one photon may strike one ring, and another photon may strike an adjacent second ring, creating a virtual slice in between that is called an interplane slice. The interplane slices provide improved resolution and nearly double the number of image slices beyond the actual number of detector rings.

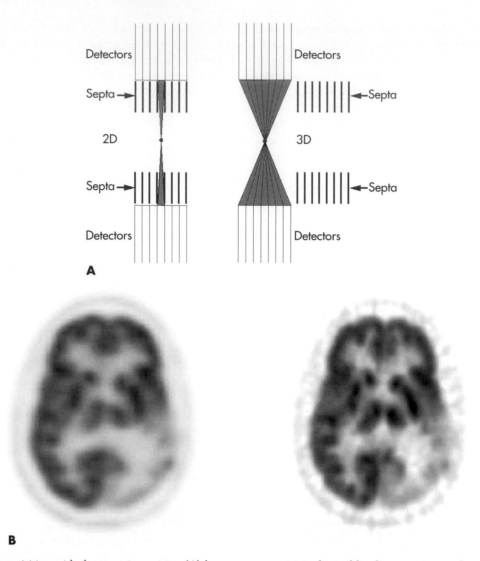

Figure 10-14 2D acquisition with the septa in position (**A**) has scanner sensitivity limited by the septa. 3D mode with the septa retracted from the gantry significantly increases the sensitivity. Brain images (**B**) demonstrate 2D *(left)* and a higher quality 3D image *(right)*.

PET is by the nature of its physics a 3D imaging technique. The use of septa for 2D imaging in the past was necessary to reduce scatter and randoms and limit the count rate. Recent improvements in detector materials, electronics, correction techniques, and algorithms have facilitated the application of 3D imaging to routine clinical use. Such 3D techniques are principally desired to increase the sensitivity of the scanner, but they create additional challenges or problems, resulting in count rate limitations, and may therefore limit the quantity of radioactivity that may be injected into the patient. The increase in sensitivity may allow for more accurate data and result in a more precise observation of the true distribution of radiotracer. New designs of PET scanners that operate only in 3D mode rely solely on electronic collimation. The elimination of the septa may also enlarge the gantry opening and thus reduce claustrophobia, accommodate larger patients, and allow some positioning variation so that the patient position is more similar to radiation treatment planning positions.

Whole-body imaging in 3D mode presents some challenges and has disadvantages. The advantage of higher sensitivity creates problems with deadtime and countrate limitations, requiring the use of smaller amounts of radiotracer. There is a significant increase in the size of 3D data sets that must be stored, accessed, reconstructed, and archived. These steps take a much longer time because of the increased volume of data. In particular, the reconstruction of complex 3D data must be rebinned correctly before more advanced algorithms produce the slices. The 3D mode also creates a significant increase in the number of random events that are detected, which then requires the application of accurate correction techniques during reconstruction.

RECONSTRUCTION ALGORITHMS

The LORs are stored during data acquisition, and this raw data must first be reformatted into sinograms, each sinogram representing one image slice. Filtered back-projection (FBP) techniques are the simplest and quickest way to create the image slice from the projection information stored in a sinogram. However, FBP creates severe streak or star artifacts, increasing image noise and thus reducing contrast, which may mask lesions (Figure 10-15, *left*). Faster computers and computational capacity now allow more sophisticated algorithms to be routinely used. Iterative reconstruction algorithms are techniques that sequentially refine estimated pixel values and provide a more accurate reconstruction of the actual radiotracer distribution in the body. Iterative algorithms significantly reduce streak artifacts compared with FBP reconstruction techniques and provide images with a lower signal to noise ratio (Figure 10-15, *right*). Maximum Likelihood Expectation Maximization (MLEM) or a faster and more efficient version, Ordered Subset Expectation Maximization (OSEM) algorithms are used for iterative reconstruction. OSEM selects subsets of the projection data instead of all the data, which can then be used with fewer iterations than MLEM to rapidly reconstruct slices.

As mentioned, 3D imaging significantly increases scanner sensitivity and the volume of acquired data. The 3D LOR information must first be rebinned into projection sinograms using algorithms such as Single Slice Rebinning (SSRB) or Fourier Rebinning (FORE). Iterative reconstruction of a large number of these 3D projection sinograms takes significantly longer than 2D reconstruction. More advanced 3D reconstruction algorithms, with more accurate corrections, will become available and decrease reconstruction time as larger computer memory, faster data transfer technology, and more advanced computers become available.

ATTENUATION CORRECTION BY TRANSMISSION IMAGING

The accurate distribution of radiotracer can only be represented in the images when accurately measured attenuation correction values have been applied during image reconstruction. Why is attenuation correction so important in the high gamma-ray imaging in PET? PET imaging is based on detecting the coincidence gamma-ray pair that must travel the full width of the body, which becomes a significant amount of attenuation (Figure 10-16). In addition, the body has a complex mixture of tissues, each with a different effect on gamma-ray attenuation. In the chest, for example, lung tissue is filled mostly with air; both muscle and fat have similar attenuation; and bone tissue has higher gamma-ray absorption. The only way to accurately compensate for attenuation is to pass a beam of radiation through the body and measure the attenuation. The measured attenuation data for each slice are obtained by rotating a line source of radioactivity, as shown in Figure 10-17, around the patient at each bed position. These radioactive line sources are usually 5 to 20 mCi of Ge-68 or Cs-137. The radioactive line source is held in a shielded housing within the gantry, and a robotic system loads the source into a rotating ring that moves around the patient during transmission scanning mode. The transmission scan usually takes 1 to 3 minutes per bed position and may be performed before or after the emission data are acquired, or preferably acquired at each bed position. Most scanners use an interlaced acquisition of emission-transmission-transmission-emission (ETTE) mode during whole-body imaging. Transmission scan data are reconstructed into attenuation correction maps for each slice. Figure 10-18, *A*, shows the transaxial, coronal, and sagittal reconstructed images without attenuation correction. Note that the lungs (low-attenuation areas) appear falsely filled with radiotracer, while areas deep in the body show up falsely void of tracer. The reconstructed attenuation map (Figure 10-18, *B*) from the transmission scan shows dramatic attenuation differences between lung, soft tissues, and bone. Attenuation-corrected images (Figure 10-18, *C*) show the correct amounts of radioactivity in lungs, which have no uptake of tracer, while deep structures such

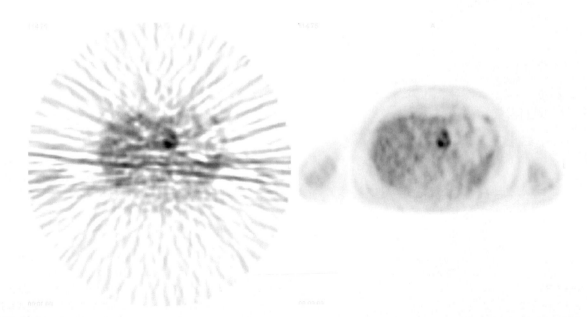

Figure 10-15   The filtered back-projection reconstruction algorithm (*left*) leaves significant streak artifacts on reconstructed slices, and lesion contrast may lower because of a higher background in the image. More advanced iterative reconstruction algorithms (*right*), such as Ordered Subset Expectation Maximization (OSEM) improves the overall quality of this image of a tumor within the liver.

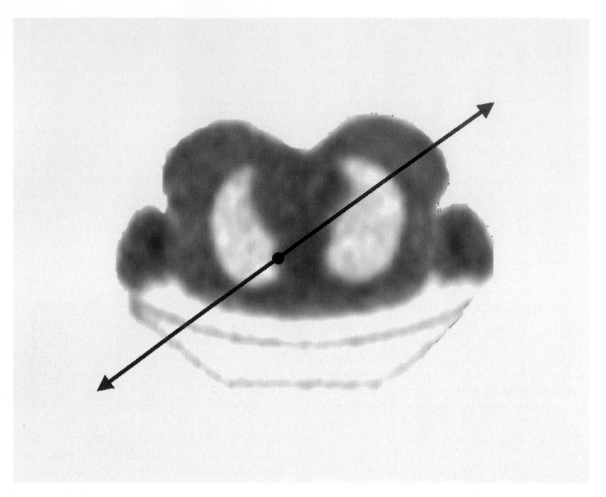

Figure 10-16 The pair of annihilation photons must traverse the entire width of the body. Although the photons are of high energy, the attenuation across the full width of the body is significant. Because of the complexity of tissues along this path (muscle, fat, lung, bone, and the imaging table), a measurement of radiation attenuation must be obtained.

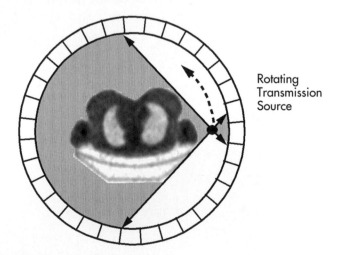

Rotating
Transmission
Source

Figure 10-17 A transmission image is obtained by acquiring data from a rotating transmission rod source of a long-lived positron-emitting radionuclide, usually Ge-68. The transmission data may be acquired before, after, or interleaved into the emission PET scan.

as the spine and internal organs are now appropriately brighter. Note that without attenuation correction the body appears to have radiotracer uptake in the skin, demonstrated as a bright outline, which disappears with attenuation correction. This artifact is due to a lack of any attenuation for annihilation photon pairs that travel transaxially to the detectors without passing through the patient, and is thereby misrepresented as a high-activity area.

Figure 10-19, *A*, shows the transaxial, coronal, sagittal, and maximum intensity projection anterior image on a patient study when no attenuation correction has been applied. Again the body appears to have increased tracer uptake in the skin; the lungs appear to take up the radiotracer; and deep organs are falsely faintly seen. The transaxial, coronal, and sagittal slices are all positioned through small lesions in the right lobe of the liver that are only very faintly seen and easily could be overlooked. It is not apparent that there is more than one lesion in this location. With the application of measured transmission attenuation correction (Figure 10-19, *B*), there is a dramatic change in the appearance of all images. The lesions in the right lobe of the liver are now much more evident, and the definition of at least two lesions becomes clear.

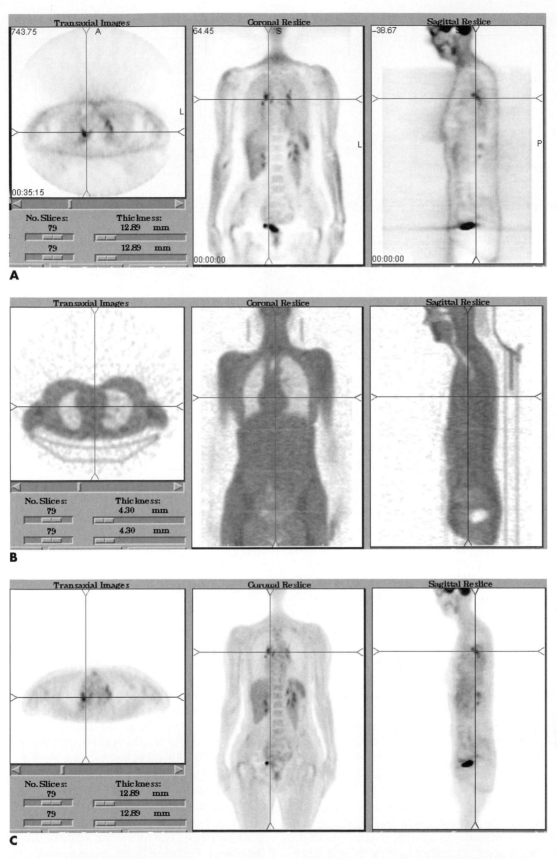

Figure 10-18 Without attenuation correction (**A**), transaxial, coronal, and sagittal images demonstrate falsely hot activity on the body surface and falsely low activity within deep structures. The lungs, an area of low attenuation, appear falsely hot. **B** shows transmission images at the same planes as **A** in all three projections. Areas of the lungs, nasopharangeal area, trachea, and other sites where attenuation is low are seen in white. **C** shows the same planes with attenuation correction. The hot skin artifact has been removed, and the lungs now appear appropriately void of radioactivity. Deep structures within the body are more easily seen as the images now demonstrate a correct relationship of activity.

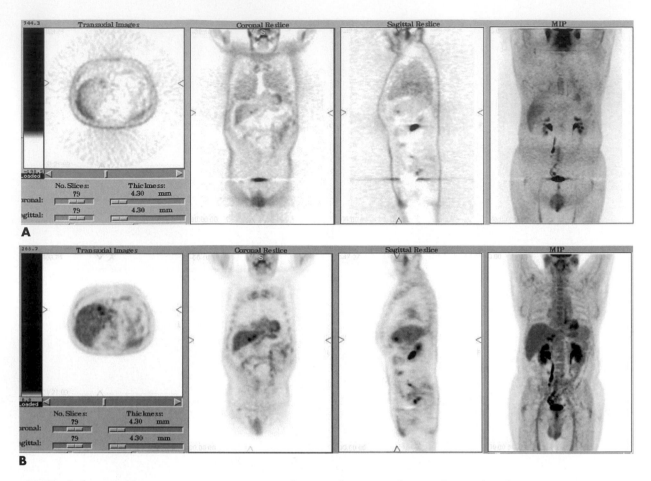

Figure 10-19 **A,** Images without attenuation correction are shown in the transaxial, coronal, sagittal, and MIP projections. **B,** Attenuation correction allows two lesions in the liver that may have been missed without attenuation correction to be seen easily.

SCANNER CALIBRATION AND QUALITY CONTROL

PET scanners differ significantly from nuclear medicine gamma cameras in image quality control issues. In general, PET scanners require more in the way of updating and refining calibration values rather than in viewing test images, as is done with gamma cameras. Therefore PET requires a meticulous program of calibrations and verification of image quality. This program should be built around the manufacturer's recommendations as a minimum set of calibrations and tests, then expanded or modified to the specific needs of the institution as experience is increased and instrument performance has been monitored. The terminology of the calibrations and tests discussed in this chapter may differ from terminology used by various vendors and the way in which the calibrations and tests are performed; however, all these calibrations are used with every type of scanner.

Calibrations may be separated into two general types: characterization (or operation) calibrations and correction calibrations. Characterization calibrations are those that are fundamental to the operation of the PET scanner, such as energy, position, PMT gain, and coincidence timing window. Correction calibrations are those that compensate for inherent variations in the scanner and perform meaningful scaling of the image, such as normalization, blank scan, and absolute activity (well counter) calibrations.

Characterization and Correction Calibrations

Energy window calibration. Energy window calibration is typically only performed after repair, during quarterly preventive maintenance (PM) service, or just before a normalization calibration is done. The energy resolution of BGO is relatively poor, and the energy window may be set as wide as 300 to 650 keV; because the PET scanner operates at only one radionuclide energy (511 keV), a check of the energy window is not required frequently. Scanners using other types of detector materials may require additional checks and calibrations for the energy setting. Energy calibration usually is performed by a service engineer, but on some systems, calibration may be performed by the technologist.

Gain settings. The calibration and adjustment of amplifier gains from PMTs are fundamental to ensure that a uniform sensitivity response from the individual detectors and modules is maintained. Frequent sensitivity drift may occur if gains are not updated at recommended intervals, or even more frequently. Gain settings should be adjusted to

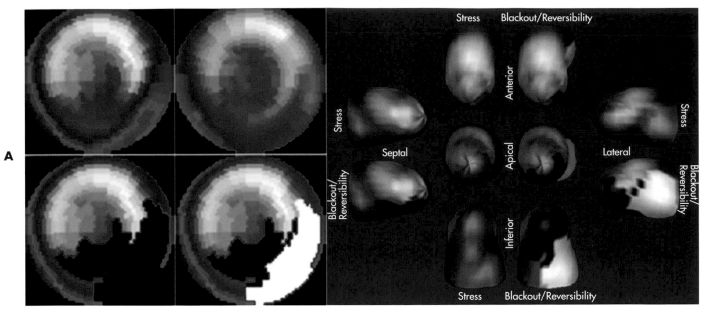

Plate 1 Polar (bull's-eye) maps and three-dimensional displays of perfusion, quantified from a stress ^{99m}Tc sestamibi/rest ^{201}Tl study. **A,** Polar plots of stress perfusion *(top left),* rest perfusion *(top right),* stress blackout *(bottom left),* and reversibility whiteout *(bottom right).* In polar plots, the anterior wall is toward the top, the septal side is toward the left, the lateral wall is toward the right, and the inferior wall is toward the bottom. For each plot, colors are scaled from 0 to 100% of the maximum myocardial counts. The blackout plot shows in black all abnormal regions in the stress image, determined from comparison with normal limits. The regions that normalize at rest are shown in white in the whiteout map. **B,** Three-dimensional displays of the same data as in **A.** Here, only stress and blackout/reversibility whiteout data are shown. Five different views of the left ventricle are provided; clockwise from top, they are anterior, lateral, inferior, and septal, with an apical view in the center. Note that the size and shape of the left ventricle can be better appreciated in this three-dimensional display. Also, the size, shape, and location of the defects are immediately obvious.

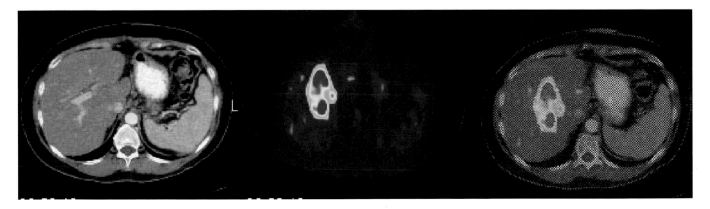

Plate 2 Software may be used to align a normal CT scan over the liver *(left)* with a PET scan with large hepatic tumor *(middle)* and create an overlay image of the two scans *(right).* However, the software does not completely align the outer body area in this case. Normally the overlay image is shown on a computer monitor with the CT (or MRI) as an anatomic reference image with the PET scan overlaid in color.

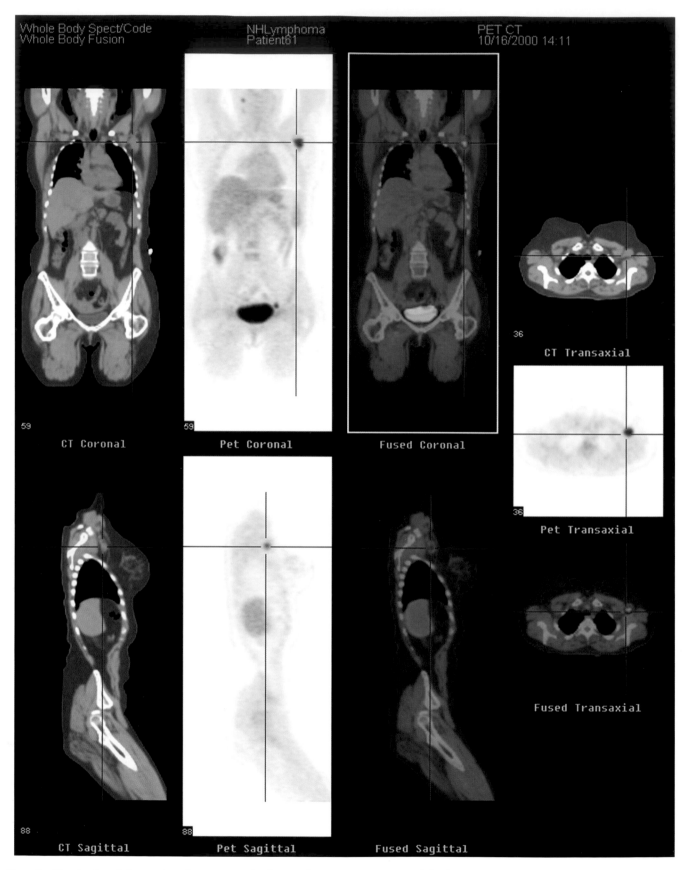

Plate 3 The display of the combined PET/CT study shows reference cursors on CT (*left column*) and PET images (*middle left*) at the same time, in addition to the overlay image (*middle right*). The transaxial images are shown in the right column. The advantage of the combined PET/CT is to have exact location correlation between the two modalities; CT, showing high-resolution anatomy, and PET, demonstrating molecular function of the tissue at that site. (Courtesy of GE Medical Systems, Waukesha, Wisconsin.)

compensate for temperature changes that affect the electronics performance and stability. This calibration is typically performed using the radioactive rod sources used for transmission imaging. Calibrations require a high number of events for fine tuning gain adjustments; therefore the procedure usually takes many minutes to acquire sufficient data. Depending on the manufacturer, these data may also be used to update crystal maps (See Figure 10-4), PMT gain, and energy window definition (The crystal maps may be adjusted by service engineers to match the sensitivity of individual detectors to the other detectors in a module). Gain updating compensates for variation in the changes in detector module gain over time. Gain update calibration procedures should be run at least weekly, or even daily, to keep systems in top performance and prevent sensitivity drift. The more frequently they are run, the more uniform the performance of the scanner.

Crystal map calibration and photomultiplier tube gains may be strongly linked on some systems. Therefore significant changes in the crystal maps will affect the PMT gain. If a map is distorted, attempts at further calibration may fail. The update gains program balances the gain characteristics of the four PMT channels on a specific block by aligning the photopeak to a specific histogram channel. PMT gain will drift with temperature changes and age. An increase in temperature is likely to affect the whole system, resulting in a change in system sensitivity but usually little change in spatial resolution. This results in quantitative image value errors, so quantitative information requires stable performance and frequent system calibration. A temperature shift of as little as 2 degrees Celsius may change the overall sensitivity of the scanner.

Coincidence timing calibration. Timing windows are significantly longer than the time it takes for photons to traverse the distance across the detector ring. The coincidence timing calibration adjusts for the timing differences in the event detection circuitry. Timing information is histogrammed (a histogram is a plot of time versus the number of events at each time) and analyzed to determine timing differences from various detector circuits.

Blank scan. Blank scans are performed daily to provide accurate transmission scan data for attenuation correction of images. Radioactive decay of the transmission sources, deadtime corrections, and detector sensitivity may vary frequently; therefore a blank scan must be obtained each morning before clinical use of the scanner. Blank scans are used as a reference uniformity measure for the transmission scan used in attenuation correction. It is very important to acquire and evaluate blank scans daily, because attenuation correction made with poor or outdated blank scans will have artifacts that will show up in the emission patient images. Patient data that are archived should have the results of that day's blank scan stored for reference if future image reconstruction is required. Blank scans are typically viewed by reconstructing the sinogram for each slice (Figure 10-20, *A*).

Sinogram information plots projection angle versus distance across the detector of the source location. Each point on the sinogram represents a specific location between two detectors operating in coincidence. Blank scans should be evaluated visually for any abnormal streaks (Figure 10-20, *B*) that show specific crystal or module variations and changes in regional sensitivity. Broad diagonal bands will be seen on the sinogram when PMT problems arise or signal is lost from a module. Some systems may use an algorithm to analyze the blank scan to evaluate daily variations statistically and report a quantitative parameter of detector uniformity performance.

In some respects, the blank scan may be thought of as viewing a daily uniformity flood image on a scintillation camera, providing an overall indicator of scanner performance. The blank scan, however, is data that represent the sensitivity response to the transmission source without any attenuating material (or patient) in the gantry ring. Any significant artifacts in the daily blank scan are an indication that there are problems with the system that should be investigated and resolved before injecting and imaging any patients.

Normalization calibration. The 2D normalization calibrations are done to measure the efficiency for all LOR. Normalization calibration is performed by rotating radioactive rod sources, which contain a low activity source of radioactivity, and acquiring data that will be used to balance the efficiency of all detectors in the scanner. The normalization calibration is used much like a high-count uniformity correction in the scintillation gamma camera. Very high statistics are therefore required, and the normalization scan takes at least 6 to 24 hours, depending on the strength of the radioactive source. It is done at low count rates to simulate the count rate of patient data and approximate the level of deadtime losses seen during patient acquisition. A normalization scan for 3D mode may need to be acquired separately. The normalization calibration table is used to correct for sensitivity from all detectors; therefore it is essentially a uniformity correction used in the reconstruction. Normalization calibrations are performed quarterly or after major service.

Absolute activity calibration (well counter calibration). Well counter calibration is a historical term for a calibration more appropriately referred to as absolute activity calibration. Absolute activity calibration factors are used to convert pixel values into a measure of absolute activity per voxel. This calibration is performed by taking a precisely known amount of activity and loading a water-filled phantom of accurately known volume. The phantom is imaged, reconstructed, and processed into a set of correction factors that allows the conversion of a patient scan into a representation of percent of injected dose per volume or gram of tissue. This conversion creates an image that represents a quantitative image for the measurement of Standard Uptake Values (SUV) of tissue or tumors. Separate acquisition and processing of data are required for 2D and 3D well counter

Box 10-1	PET scanner failures

Detector malfunction
High voltage drift
Energy drift
Gain drift
Cable breakage
Power supply drift or failure
Temperature drift or cooling system failure
Coincidence timing malfunction
Transmission source or robotics malfunction
Septa mispositioning or misalignment
Imaging table failure

calibration factors. Absolute activity calibrations are performed only after all other calibrations have been performed, and should be done quarterly or after major service.

Quality control

Quality control of any imaging device, including PET scanners, is a test or series of tests that verify proper operation of the scanner and allow checks that the calibrations are appropriate and working properly. The quality control tests must be sensitive enough to detect changes in the scanner performance and ensure that clinical images will be an accurate representation of the radiotracer distribution and that no artifacts are present. A list of problems that may occur with PET scanners is listed in Box 10-1. Daily tests must be performed and images reviewed to attempt to identify any variation in the operation of the scanner.

Daily quality control must be done to measure the performance of each detector and ensure that calibrations are properly applied. A blank scan that may be applied to attenuation correct patient studies for that day may be reconstructed as sinograms prior to being reformatted into a calibration table. The blank scan (Figure 10-20) will show artifacts if there are any problems with detector modules, signal cables, high voltage drift, gain changes, and so on. An alternative daily test may be to image a uniform cylinder of radioactivity, which can have a transmission scan applied to verify that the attenuation correction components are all working. A regular schedule of calibrations will optimize image quality by ensuring that the instrument is working correctly for all studies.

Detailed PET scanner acceptance testing and performance testing procedures are described by the National Electrical Manufacturers Association (NEMA), in its publication NU-2. In addition there should be a budget, plan, and schedule for replacing the calibration and transmission radioactive sources in the gantry. As radioactive sources decay, the transmission beam through the patient will become more limited in statistical accuracy, particularly in larger patients. Because months can go by before a source is replaced, it is helpful to slightly extend the transmission acquisition time to ensure that a sufficient data density is being achieved. Otherwise image noise and horizontal line artifacts on coronal and sagittal images may appear, caused by high noise in the transmission data that will limit the accuracy of attenuation correction in the reconstruction algorithms.

A quality control program must be established for PET scanners and should include daily, weekly, and quarterly tests in addition to a regular schedule of preventive maintenance service. An aggressive quality control program is needed to reduce artifacts, increase uptime, produce higher quality images, and thus ensure diagnostic accuracy.

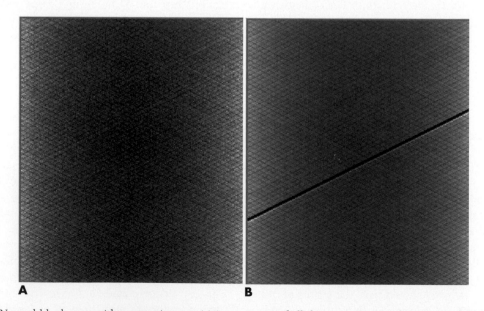

A   **B**

Figure 10-20   **A,** Normal blank scan with appropriate sensitivity response of all detectors. **B,** One detector module is displaying an inappropriate sensitivity as demonstrated by the dark diagonal line. Dark or white diagonal lines may been seen when one or more detector modules is malfunctioning or out of calibration.

QUANTITATIVE IMAGE INFORMATION

The absolute quantitative uptake of the radiotracer in tumors can be measured in an effort to differentiate between malignant and benign tissue. The standard uptake value (SUV) can be useful in measuring tumor metabolic function. PET scanner calibration of absolute activity (well counter calibration) allows the conversion of image data into an activity measure of radiotracer uptake per pixel or voxel in the image. SUV measurements are based on either the injected activity per patient weight in kilograms or per body surface area in meters squared. The injected activity (minus residual in the syringe) must be accurately known and the time of injection recorded. Activity measurements may be in microcuries or MBq. Body surface area is usually calculated:

$$BSA \ (m^2) = (weight \ in \ kg)^{0.425} \times (height \ in \ cm)^{0.725} \times 0.007184$$

Tumor SUV is determined by placing a region of interest (ROI) over the tumor and using computer programs to automatically calculate the value. The computer operator can select if the calculation is to be done per weight or per BSA. Calculations are based on the formula:

$$SUV_{BW} = (ROI \ activity, \ mCi/ml)/(injected \ activity,$$
$$mCi/patient \ weight, \ g) \ or$$
$$SUV_{BSA} = (ROI \ activity \ units)/(injected \ activity/BSA)$$

Accurate information is needed for the exact time of dose measurement, activity administered, injection time, patient height and weight, and the time at which the images were acquired at each bed position. SUV values change with time, so it is critical to specify the time at which the SUV image was obtained. If follow-up quantitative measurements are obtained, the precise time between injection and imaging must be repeated.

SUV values of 2.5 or greater have been used in differentiating benign from malignant lung lesions as reported by Lowe et al.[1] Figure 10-21 shows a solitary pulmonary nodule with a SUV of 3.0, indicating a likelihood of malignancy. The typical false positive in lung imaging is caused by an inflammatory process. Some benign lesions may take up FDG preferentially. These include tuberculosis, histoplasmosis, and rheumatoid nodules. It is also difficult to compare SUV values from different scanners or institutions because of factors such as glucose concentration, ROI size, resolution capabilities, and calibrations.

The usefulness of the SUV remains controversial. It is widely recognized that accuracy in calculating these values is difficult and that rigorous quality control and calibration are required. The technologist must also pay particular attention to the details of administering the radioactivity and to recording the time of injection and the time of imaging. Image reconstruction and filtering techniques may also affect the result of the SUV value. Moreover, small lesions are affected by the partial volume effect, where small sources of radioactivity have their activity distributed artificially among too many voxels, resulting in false resolution, contrast, and an underestimation of radioactivity. Accurate SUVs can only be obtained when the size of the lesion is two to four times the pixel size.

Investigations have shown value in measuring lesion uptake at two different points in time, for example, at 1 hour and 3 hours postinjection. Malignant tumors continue to accumulate FDG with time, whereas inflammatory processes

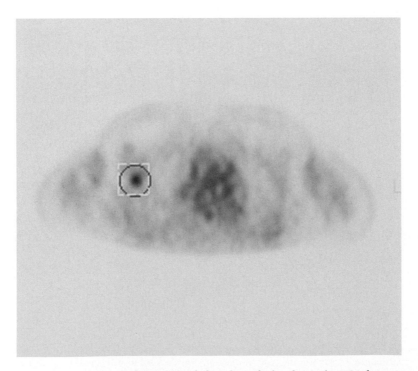

Figure 10-21   A lesion in the right lung is seen on this transaxial slice through the chest. The ROI demonstrates the area where a standard uptake value (SUV) of 3.0 indicates abnormally high activity, indicating a high likelihood of lung cancer.

decrease in activity with time. Therefore false positive studies with PET are avoided by characterizing the FDG kinetics by this dual point measuring technique. The sensitivity and specificity of PET in lung cancer and identification of solitary pulmonary nodules are each increased by about 10 percent.[1]

DISPLAYING PET DATA

The PET computer system creates image data of a volume within the patient that is represented by a series of adjacent slices. The small crystal size creates 3- to 5-mm slices along the long axis of the body. The challenge facing the physician and technologist is how to organize or reformat this large volume of information into the most meaningful display that (1) aids in rapidly identifying abnormalities and (2) provides the best spatial relationship to normal landmarks (organs) within the patient to provide an accurate location of any abnormalities. It is difficult to look through 200 to 300 transaxial slices of a whole-body PET study and be able to identify abnormalities and relate their location to structures that may be outside the axial plane that is being viewed. Even observing more than a dozen axial slices on the computer screen at one time does not allow the best relationship of a source of radiotracer to structures in other slices. Therefore the 3D volume should be reformatted to create planes through the volume that provide the most information about

normal and abnormal structures. Whole-body transaxial slices are reformatted to create a series of coronal and sagittal slices. The coronal slices are the most commonly viewed set of images because the symmetric view of the body allows the best comparison of right and left structures in addition to providing the view of the largest axis along the body. Coronal slices represent the way the we most commonly think of the distribution of organs within the body and also produce a convenient display to view the body in the fewest number of images.

Viewing all projections, transaxial, coronal, and sagittal slices at one time has significant advantages to provide the spatial relationship of lesions or questionable areas into the different projections. This is most convenient when reference lines appear on the images to identify the location of each plane through the volume (see Figure 10-18, *C*).

3D studies may be most dramatically displayed using the reprojection of the volume information back into a series of projections from around the body. This display technique is called the maximum intensity projection (MIP). The reconstructed volume of the body is projected back into 2D projection images at equally spaced angles around the body. A ray passing through each plane is used to project the maximum pixel value along that ray onto the 2D projection image (Figure 10-22). Therefore the pixel with the most counts, or brightest intensity, is placed into the image. In Figure 10-22 the tumor pixel intensity is highest and is

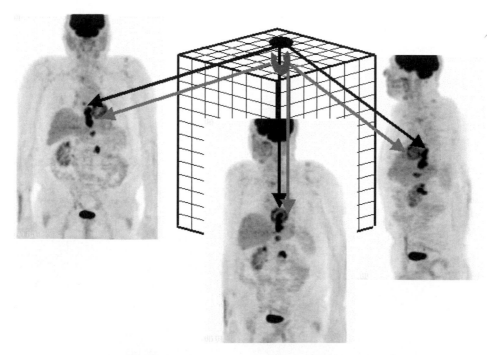

Maximum intensity projection

Figure 10-22 Once the volume of the scan has been reconstructed as shown by the 3D voxels, data may be reprojected along rays through the volume to show the volume projected at various angles around the patient. Each ray through the volume projects the maximum count onto images called the maximum intensity projection (MIP). A set of MIP images created at equal angles from around the patient volume may be displayed in a closed loop cinematic display to create a movie of the entire patient volume. The MIP images are a convenient media to quickly observe the whole patient.

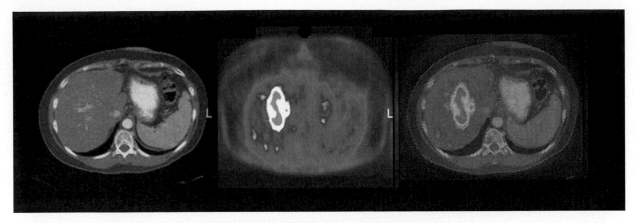

Figure 10-23 Software may be used to align a normal CT scan over the liver (*left*) with a PET scan with large hepatic tumor (*middle*) and create an overlay image of the two scans (*right*). However, the software does not completely align the outer body area in this case. Normally the overlay image is shown on a computer monitor with the CT (or MRI) as an anatomic reference image with the PET scan overlaid in color (refer to the color plate section).

therefore projected on each image. The 2D projection images are then displayed on the computer in a continuous loop cinematic mode to present the whole volume on one projection. Our eyes and brain sort out the 3D relationship of various structures as the images change in the movie display.

IMAGE FUSION

In the early 1990s, the fusion of SPECT brain scans with MRI or CT was shown to be very useful in the correlation of the exact site of anatomic (CT or MRI) and physiologic (PET or SPECT) information. Although radiology's anatomic images have high resolution, the anatomic images demonstrate disease only when it has progressed to create a change in tissue density (as seen on CT) or has changed in its proton density (as shown with MRI). Disease is therefore seen only when tissue has degraded in its structure by the illness. PET, as a biologic chemistry image, commonly shows disease changes at the molecular level, where problems may show up with PET before they are evident on CT or MRI. The PET 3D radiotracer information can be aligned or fused with a high-resolution image of anatomy. Tumor uptake of FDG or other PET radiotracers is often very high compared with surrounding normal tissues, but the exact location of the increased uptake may be difficult to determine.

Image fusion software is widely available that can import DICOM slice information from CT, MRI, SPECT, or PET and allow two image sets to be aligned by identifying anatomic points on each modality that should be aligned between two different modalities. The problem with using anatomic points is that the radiotracer modalities do not have sufficient spatial resolution to be precise (within a very few millimeters) in location. This problem can be somewhat resolved by placing external skin-surface markers on the patient that can be seen on both imaging modalities. These markers can contain a small amount of F-18 in addition to a material that will show up on CT or MRI. These points can then be aligned, which in theory should align the organs

within the body. However, this technique has a few logistical problems. CT or MRI is usually performed before the PET scan is ordered, and the images therefore do not have the external markers present. Insurance companies are unlikely to pay for another CT or MRI. CT scans also usually exclude the outer edge of the body, which may exclude the anatomic markers as well. In addition, patients are instructed to inhale and hold their breath during a CT of the chest. The chest or body is therefore a different size between the CT and PET scans, as seen in Figure 10-23 (refer to the color plate section), which may require stretching or morphing one of the image sets. Patients may also be positioned slightly differently between the two modalities, causing additional alignment problems. However, when the two imaging modalities are successfully aligned and fused, there is tremendous power in the resulting display. The ability to view the PET physiologic image and accurately place the exact anatomical site of that location is very valuable. PET images are usually displayed in color on the computer and are overlaid on a grayscale CT or MRI image. PET thus highlights in color those areas of increased metabolic activity, which are placed in the exact location on the grayscale anatomic image to improve the accuracy for both detecting and localizing disease.

PET/CT SCANNERS

The best device for image fusion is one that contains both the PET and CT scanner in one gantry. The PET/CT scanner was designed with a high performance dedicated ring PET scanner along with a high performance CT scanner in the same gantry. The PET/CT scanner (Figure 10-24) therefore solves many of the problems that may cause misalignment when software alone is used to fuse two separately acquired studies. When the patient is positioned on the scanner, a CT scan of the desired body area is rapidly acquired (usually in less than 1 minute for a whole-body scan). Afterward, the PET emission scan data are acquired. The CT scan

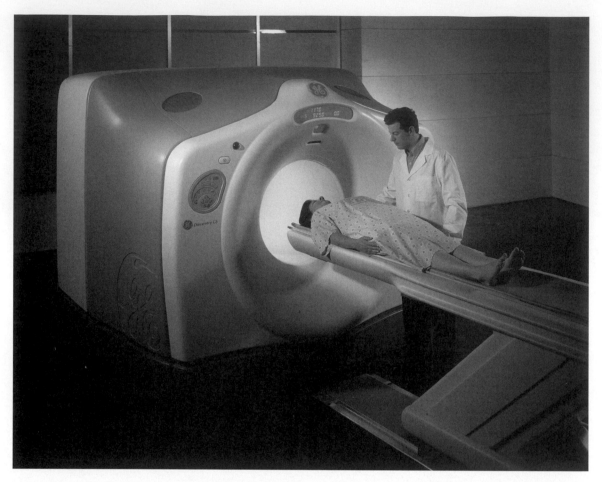

Figure 10-24 Combined PET and CT scanners in one gantry allow exact anatomic alignment of the two modalities in one patient study. The CT scan not only allows exact anatomic correlation with the PET scan, but the CT images can also be used for attenuation correction of the PET scan. (Courtesy of GE Medical Systems, Waukesha, Wisconsin.)

serves two purposes: (1) it iprovides a perfectly aligned anatomic image that matches the exact location of the functional image of the PET scan and (2) the CT scan may be transformed into an attenuation map for correcting the PET images. Viewing software allows the display of the PET, CT, and color overlaid PET on the CT scan (Figure 10-25). See the color plates for the color overlaid PET on the CT scan.

Cursor lines help identify the slice locations on 3D projections from the transaxial, coronal, and sagittal views simultaneously displayed at the same time on the computer screen. PET scans are most commonly viewed directly on the computer instead of on film so that the physician may essentially move around within the body and correlate lesion location in other projections.

An excellent example of the clinical utility of PET/CT is when cancer invades lymph nodes. On CT, lymph nodes are considered normal as long as they are less than 10 mm in size, and abnormal once they are 10 mm or larger. PET, on the other hand, shows the metabolic function of the tissue within the lymph node and can detect disease earlier than the anatomic manifestation occurs.

As previously discussed, the axial CT slices from the PET/CT scanner may be converted into a transmission map to be used for attenuation correction of the corresponding PET emission slices. Cancer patients referred for PET or PET/CT scans often have other imaging studies, which sometimes include the use of x-ray contrast material. If contrast is present, the CT Hounsfield values where the contrast is located will be very high, and when converted into 511 keV attenuation values, cause an overestimation of activity in the corrected emission image. Figure 10-26 (*top*) demonstrates increased FDG activity in the bowel on attenuation-corrected coronal slices. However, the coronal CT images generated from the PET/CT study demonstrate a significant amount of barium in the large intestine, creating overcorrection for attenuation correction (Figure 10-26, *middle row*). The nonattenuation-corrected images show no increased FDG uptake; therefore the barium caused falsely high attenuation values that overcorrected bowel activity that may have been erroneously interpreted as colitis.

A promising application of PET/CT fused images is in radiation therapy treatment planning. This is particularly useful in 3D conformal beam radiation therapy. Intensity modulated radiation therapy (IMRT) uses a multileaf collimator system to conform the shape of the therapy beam to the tumor. CT scans are normally used in IMRT treatment planning; however, the PET scan fused with the anatomic CT scan may allow the IMRT beam to be further refined to deliver more radiation to the most metabolically active areas of the tumor. Precise IMRT delivers more radiation to exactly where it is needed and less radiation to surrounding areas, thus reducing side effects and complications.

RADIATION SAFETY IN PET

Chapter 7 discusses some of the issues relative to the use and handling of PET radionuclides. Several comments are worth reviewing here as we discuss the specifics of PET fun-damentals. Technologists performing PET procedures commonly have higher radiation exposure than when working in nuclear medicine. This increased exposure is principally from two sources: handling millicurie quantities of high-energy gamma emitters and being in proximity to patients that have been injected with high-energy gamma radiation. The energy spectrum from the patient is not as high as might be expected. There are many Compton scattered gamma rays that the patient emits, and the mean energy is in the 200 to 300 keV range.

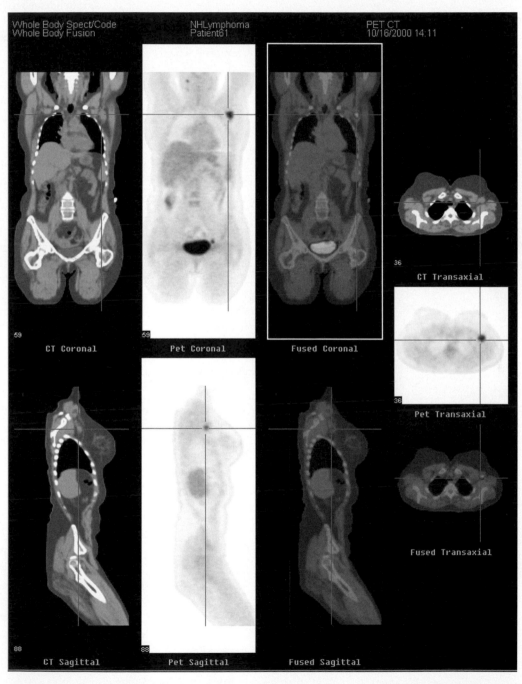

Figure 10-25   The display of the combined PET/CT study shows reference cursors on CT (*left column*) and PET images (*middle left*) at the same time, in addition to the overlay image (*middle right*). The transaxial images are shown in the right column. The advantage of the combined PET/CT is to have exact location correlation between the two modalities, CT showing high resolution anatomy and PET demonstrating molecular function of the tissue at that site. This figure is also seen in the color plate section. (Courtesy of GE Medical Systems, Waukesha, Wisconsin.)

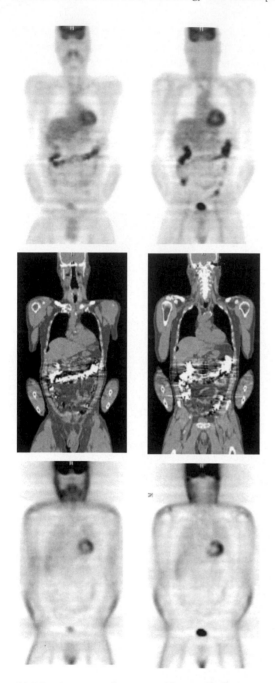

An additional small source of radiation exposure for patients and staff comes from the long-lived radioactive sources in the gantry that are used for transmission imaging and for scanner calibration. As with all nuclear medicine, PET uses the application of time, distance, and shielding to maintain ALARA radiation safety practices.

The 511 keV annihilation photons have a half-value layer of 4 mm of lead. This requires special syringe shields, typically made from tungsten, which has about 1.4 times the effectiveness as the same thickness of lead. Waste containers should also be of thicker shielding material, and the lab bench for handling PET radionuclides should have a 1- to 2-inch thick L-block of lead with a 4-inch thick lead glass viewing window. Tongs and remote manipulators should be employed whenever possible when handling vials, syringes, and sources. Reducing the time of handling radioactive materials has significant advantages when working with high-energy radionuclides. Time reduction and increased distance are particularly helpful during injection and uptake periods and when positioning the patient for imaging.

The exposure rate from a patient receiving 10 mCi of FDG will exceed 1 mR/hr at 1 meter. It would therefore be unwise to allow injected patients to immediately return to public waiting areas during the FDG uptake period before scanning. A dedicated injection/uptake room is most suitable; it may require one-eighth to one-quarter inch of lead in the walls of the room if this space is adjacent to unrestricted and heavily occupied areas. It may also be a beneficial to have the wall between the PET scanner and control room contain lead shielding in particularly busy laboratories. These details should be worked out with the radiation safety officer of the institution.

REFERENCE

1. Lowe VJ, Fletcher JW, Gobar L, et al: Prospective investigation of positron emission tomography in lung nodules, *J Clin Oncol* 16:1075-1084, 1998.

SUGGESTED READINGS

Fahey, FH: Data acquisition in PET imaging, *J Nucl Med Technol* 30:39-49, 2002.

Ruhlmann, J, Oehr, P, Biersack HJ, editors: *PET in oncology,* Berlin, 1999, Springer-Verlag.

Turkington TG: Introduction to PET instrumentation, *J Nucl Med Technol* 29:4-11, 2001.

von Schultess, GK, editor: *Clinical positron emission tomography,* Philadelphia, 2000, Lippincott Williams & Wilkins.

Wahl RL, editor: *Principles and practice of positron emission tomography,* Philadelphia, 2002, Lippincott Williams & Wilkins.

Figure 10-26   A patient who received barium before a PET/CT scan shows falsely increased uptake in the colon due to overcompensation of attenuation correction due to the barium in that location (*top row*). The CT portion of the study demonstrates the location of the barium (*middle row*). The nonattenuation correction images show no FDG uptake in the colon. Careful patient screening is needed to avoid false positive studies. (Courtesy of Henry Yeung, M.D., Memorial Sloan Kettering Cancer Center, New York.)

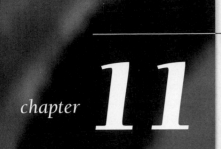

chapter **11**

Clinical PET Oncology

Objectives

Discuss the principles of PET FDG oncology imaging.

State the principal reasons for the recent rapid growth of PET oncology imaging.

Recognize the normal biodistribution of FDG and list those organs with intense, moderate, or mild FDG activity.

Describe the various patterns of normal FDG myocardial activity.

Discuss the normal patterns of head and neck FDG activity.

Discuss benign causes of increased FDG activity.

Describe the variations in FDG biodistribution caused by improper patient preparation.

Explain the steps in properly preparing a patient for an FDG PET scan.

Discuss the significance of peripheral blood glucose levels in FDG imaging.

List the necessary historical information that should be obtained from each patient.

List the various modes of PET acquisition and their uses.

Describe patient positioning and comfort issues that can hinder the acquisition of high-quality scans.

Discuss the value of future PET oncology radiotracers.

Discuss potential future directions of PET oncology.

*E*ach year approximately 1.2 million new cases of cancer are discovered in the United States, in addition to another 1 million cases of basal cell cancer and melanoma. Currently, 5 million to 10 million people have cancer and are undergoing treatment. Significant advances continue to occur in the development of both more powerful diagnostic techniques and more effective cancer treatments. Despite these advances, key questions persist regarding cancer staging, monitoring of therapy effectiveness, and identification of possible cancer recurrence. Although positron emission tomography (PET) cancer imaging is a relatively new tool, its availability is expanding. It is emerging as a widely used and accepted imaging modality. PET represents the best of nuclear medicine. Among nuclear medicine imaging devices, PET scanners have the best resolution, and among the different nuclear medicine radiotracers, positron-emitting radionuclides can be labeled to the most appropriate molecules for study of fundamental biochemical processes. PET offers an extremely powerful method to gather information about molecular processes in the human body.

PET instrumentation and PET radiopharmaceuticals developed rapidly during the 1970s and 1980s. Scanners went through several successive generations, medical cyclotrons specifically for positron-emitting radionuclides were refined, and the radiosynthesis of new PET pharmaceuticals proceeded from the research laboratory to highly automated modules that could reliably produce large amounts of common PET radiotracers.

During the initial PET development, the principal clinical investigations involved the heart and brain. However, in the late 1980s, investigators began to show the value of PET technology in cancer detection. During the early 1990s, scholarly investigations continued to support this early experience, clearly demonstrating that the sensitivity and specificity of PET in cancer detection exceeded those of most routine medical tests and radiologic imaging techniques. The continued proliferation of clinical investigations and scientific publications provided the necessary clinical validation of PET for certain types of cancer, and cost analyses demonstrated huge potential savings through avoidance of unnecessary tests and needless surgery.

In 1998 Medicare announced that fluorodeoxyglucose (FDG) PET scans would be reimbursed for patients with solitary pulmonary nodules or non-small cell lung cancer. This breakthrough in reimbursement opened the door for Medicare payments for other cancers in which experience had shown that PET was the most accurate imaging technique for identifying and staging the disease. Medicare coverage followed for melanoma, lymphoma, colorectal cancer, head and neck cancer, esophageal cancer, and recurrent breast cancer. Most third-party insurance companies now also cover FDG PET scans for a variety of cancer patients.

Payor reimbursement has been the driving force behind the rapid expansion in the number of PET facilities available to patients and referring physicians. However, to expand the number of locations offering PET services, it has also been necessary to simultaneously increase the number of cyclotron facilities that provide FDG. PET has expanded not only among academic institutions and large hospitals, but also among private business interests, which have brought free-standing imaging centers and shared mobile scanners to community hospitals and rural areas. Similar worldwide growth is occurring as PET begins to establish its position as a powerful and valuable oncologic imaging tool.

INTRACELLULAR F-18-FDG METABOLISM

In PET cancer imaging, the most widely used radiopharmaceutical is 2-[F-18]-fluoro-2-deoxy-D-glucose (F-18-FDG). Biochemically, F-18-FDG is a nonphysiologic compound with a chemical structure very similar to that of naturally occurring glucose; it serves as an external marker of cellular glucose metabolism.

The ability to externally image cellular glucose metabolism is important in oncologic applications because many cancer cells use glucose at higher rates than normal cells. Current research also demonstrates that numerous malignant tumors express higher numbers of specific membrane transport proteins, with greater affinity for glucose than normal cells. This permits increased glucose flow into cancerous cells. Additionally, once glucose has entered the tumor cells, hexokinase (the first intracellular enzyme involved in glucose breakdown) is usually much more active than in normal cells. These factors increase the probability of noninvasive visualization of malignant tumors in the body.

Both glucose and FDG are absorbed by facilitated diffusion into cells with the assistance of certain specific membrane transport proteins. Once in the cell cytosol, glucose is broken down in a series of enzymatic steps called *glycolysis*. The first step in this pathway occurs when hexokinase enzymatically adds a phosphate group to glucose, creating a new compound, glucose-6-phosphate (G-6-P). FDG follows the same process in its transformation to FDG-6-phosphate (FDG-6-P).

The cell membrane is impermeable to both of these intermediate phosphorylated compounds, and neither can re-cross the cell membrane. G-6-P continues through the next glycolytic step with its transformation into fructose-6-phosphate by the action of phosphoglucoisomerase. However, FDG cannot be enzymatically transformed into fructose-6-phosphate (Figure 11-1). Because FDG-6-P cannot be broken down or re-cross the cell membrane, it remains "trapped" within the cell. As more FDG molecules enter the cell and are transformed into FDG-6-P, they continue to accumulate within the cellular cytosol.

Intracellular FDG activity varies with different types of cancer. Increased intracellular localization usually correlates with more aggressive tumors and greater numbers of viable tumor cells. However, this correlation is not prefect. FDG PET provides a marvelous noninvasive imaging tool in a wide variety of cancers because these cancer cells demonstrate increased rates of facilitated glucose diffusion across the cell membranes, they have higher rates of glucose phosphorylation, and they demonstrate greater FDG-6-P accumulation within the cytosol than most normal cells.

Because FDG acts as visual marker of cellular glucose metabolism, it creates both advantages and problems. Because many different types of cancer demonstrate increased FDG utilization, FDG PET can serve as a powerful screening tool in a wide variety of cancers. However, this power comes at a price. Many normal and noncancerous conditions, such as infection, inflammation, atelectasis, healing tissues, and muscular activity, also can increase intracellular FDG utilization. Thus normal tissues or benign processes can masquerade as malignancies. Essentially, FDG PET cancer screening is a broad-based or "shotgun" approach. Cancers are detectable, but so are other occasionally confounding and potentially misleading benign processes.

Of greater concern are those cancers that utilize FDG at the same rate as normal surrounding tissues. In these cases tumors remain hidden within the normal imaging background and go unnoticed and possibly untreated. The fact that FDG PET fails at times to distinguish the presence of cancer has stimulated many attempts to develop new methods of PET cancer detection. Several additional PET

Normal cell FDG metabolism

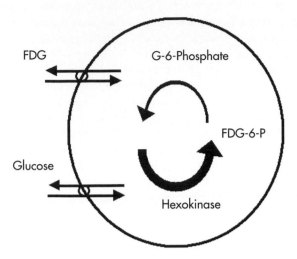

Cancer cell FDG metabolism

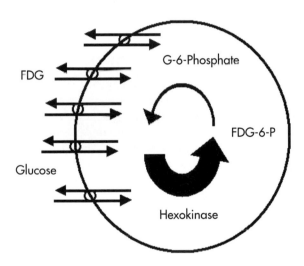

Figure 11-1 FDG avidly accumulates in cancerous cells for three main reasons: (1) cancer cells express more numerous specific membrane transport proteins with greater affinity for glucose than do normal cells (allowing for increased rates of facilitated diffusion into the cytosol); (2) the hexokinase enzymes in cancer cells transform FDG into FDG-6-P at higher rates than do normal cells; and (3) FDG-6-P cannot be further metabolized, therefore it remains "trapped" in the cytosol.

radiotracers are mentioned at the end of the chapter, but most of the chapter focuses on FDG as the predominant PET cancer imaging agent, with all its inherent advantages and problems.

PATIENT PREPARATION AND INJECTION

PET radiotracers provide images of fundamental metabolic processes within the body. These radiotracers, such as FDG, are extremely sensitive to small changes in tissue metabo-

lism. It is critical, therefore, to ensure that the patient's baseline metabolic activity starts at appropriately low levels and that the patient remains at rest prior to, during, and after injection of the radiotracer. Patients should not participate in strenuous exercise for 24 hours before the study, to reduce muscle uptake.

Before any FDG injection, the technologist should obtain a brief history to ensure that a PET scan is appropriate and should confirm the patient's identification. The history should include, at least, information about height, weight, fasting state, diabetes, pregnancy, breastfeeding, surgeries, prior chemotherapy or radiation therapy, and the results of any recent imaging procedures. The examination should be completely explained to the patient and any questions answered. After the intravenous line is started, the patient should be placed on a bed or in a reclining chair for 10 minutes and asked to relax and refrain from talking. If the brain is to be imaged, the patient should also close the eyes, and the room should be quiet and dark. At this point, the technologist should administer the FDG, followed by a 20 to 30 ml saline flush, and the patient should continue to rest for 45 to 90 more minutes. The IV line should then be removed and the patient imaged or escorted to an appropriate waiting area.

To reduce the peripheral blood glucose level, patients arriving for an FDG PET scan should be fasting for 4 to 6 hours before the appointment. The peripheral blood glucose level can be measured with a glucometer. Ideally, the value should be less than 120 mg/dl. Increased blood glucose levels can compete with FDG, resulting in little difference between tumor and normal soft tissue uptake and in very low contrast images. Some laboratories inject patients with glucose levels up to 180 mg/dl and have reported no degradation in image quality. However, there are no published, controlled scientific studies to adequately establish an upper limit for the measured peripheral blood glucose level.

Some laboratories contend that the peripheral blood glucose level should be measured in every patient. Other laboratories do not measure the glucose level, assuming that it will be sufficiently low as long as the patient has been fasting and has no history of diabetes or of blood relatives with diabetes. Patients with elevated peripheral blood glucose levels may sometimes be studied after the glucose level has been reduced, either by an additional time delay or after injection of fast-acting insulin formulations, as directed by a knowledgeable physician. However, insulin administration within 2 hours of FDG injections can also result in reduced tumor uptake of FDG, resulting in lower-contrast images.

FDG usually displays normally faint activity within the body, providing a general anatomic distribution of the solid organs. However, patients with diabetes and high peripheral blood glucose levels (>150 mg/dl) may demonstrate inhomogeneous or inadequate tissue activity because of the lack of insulin, insulin resistance, or competition from the increased nonradioactive extracellular glucose. Patients with diabetes mellitus must continue their standard snacks between meals and have their insulin injections before FDG PET scans. Such patients may present serious difficulties in the acquisition of diagnostic FDG PET studies, and the close involvement of knowledgeable referring physicians or endocrinologists before the scan date is prudent to avoid problems and potential havoc to the daily schedule.

FDG should be administered while the patient is in a resting state, therefore it is less disruptive to place an angio-cath in a peripheral vein of the upper extremities 10 minutes or more before the time of administration. This IV line may be used to access a small amount of blood for peripheral glucose testing. It is essential to use fastidious technique and to ensure proper placement of the angiocath before the FDG injection. Infiltration must be avoided. A 20 to 30 ml saline flush after the FDG injection helps to reduce venous FDG uptake in the upper extremity. Port-a-caths or indwelling central catheters should not be used to inject FDG unless absolutely necessary. Retention in the reservoirs and the tips of the catheter lines can cause errors in evaluation of the chest wall and, more important, the mediastinum.

The normal injected FDG dose ranges from 10 to 20 mCi. The most common adult dose, 10 mCi, is at the lower end of this range so as to reduce radiation exposure to the bladder. The pediatric dose is determined by body weight 150 μCi/kg. The injection is performed using a three-way stopcock attached to the IV line and to the dose syringe. Again, after injection, the IV should be flushed with 20 to 30 ml of saline to help eliminate any activity in nearby veins. The patient should rest completely during the injection and for approximately 45 to 90 minutes after the injection. Tumor concentration of FDG continues to increase with time, whereas soft tissue activity diminishes; therefore longer waiting times increase tumor to soft tissue contrast and improve lesion detection. Before imaging, the IV may be removed, and the patient should void.

PET SCAN ACQUISITION

Selecting the Scan Type and Body Area

PET oncology imaging can be performed in several ways: limited area scanning, dynamic imaging, whole body imaging, or total body imaging. Limited area imaging is used when the patient's history indicates the need to evaluate only a very specific area of the body, such as in patients who have a solitary pulmonary nodule discovered on a screening CT examination and no known cancer. Scanning protocols with a limited number of bed positions (approximately three or four) over the chest can cover both lungs entirely. Dynamic imaging requires continuous imaging in a single bed position; it would be done only if the exact position of the lesion is known and the study is tailored especially to evaluate the possibility of a benign or malignant process in a single well-defined lesion.

Patients most commonly receive whole body PET scans. Whole body oncology PET scans cover the area from the base of the brain through the pelvis (about 90 cm) and require five to seven bed positions, depending on the scanner's field of view. Normally these scans are obtained just after the patient has voided. They start from the pelvis and continue toward the head so that the bladder can be imaged while it is nearly empty.

Total body imaging is performed if there is a question that a cancer might include the head or legs. These scans cover from the top of the head through the feet and require more than 10 bed positions. Total body scans are most commonly used for patients with malignant melanomas. On some scanners the scanning protocol may be set up to start just above (or below) the bladder, scan the empty bladder first and continue in one direction along the body, then to return to the starting point and scan the remaining portions of the body in the opposite direction.

If cancer is suspected in the pelvis, it occasionally may be necessary to place a urinary catheter to reduce normal bladder activity. Some facilities use diuretics to promote enhanced excretion of FDG, whereas others add a continuous saline flow through the urinary catheter to further reduce bladder activity. However, in most cases these interventions are highly irritating to the patient and may actually end up being counterproductive.

Patient Positioning and Comfort

Before the imaging procedure, the patient should remove any metallic object that can cause attenuation artifacts. The patient should be placed in a comfortable recumbent position with a support sponge or pillow under the knees and a support to help hold the arms still. The PET physician should establish the preferred patient arm position. If the PET scan is to be compared to a chest CT, the physician may want the patient's arms to be positioned above the head. Some large patients may need arms-up imaging or may place their arms on their abdomen to fit into the scanner. Most commonly, however, the average patient can place the arms at the sides, and the selected scanning protocol can be performed. The technologist may use a strap to support the patient's arms, cover the patient with a blanket, and encourage the patient to relax and hold still during the scanning procedure.

Because PET scanners have much higher resolution than routine nuclear medicine imaging devices, the patient's cooperation and proper positioning are critical. Whole body imaging may require up to an hour, and total body imaging may extend well over 1 hour. Listening to music may help patients relax during the scan.

The imaging tables on scanners have a weight limit, and some tables sag significantly under the weight of a heavy patient even before the allowable weight limit is reached. The internal diameter of the scanner opening also limits the size of patients that can be imaged. Additionally, larger patients typically have greater attenuation and reduced image quality. For these reasons, acquisition times for both emission and transmission scans should be appropriately increased in such patients.

If there is a question of cancer involvement of the head or neck, it may be helpful to place the patient in a head holder fitted with a chin restraint to reduce possible motion. The patient should always be checked before the scanning protocol begins to ensure that the person is safe and that no body parts will be pinched as the table moves through the scanner. It also should be verified that the acquisition program is set for the desired orientation. Again, most PET scanners have significantly higher resolution than planar or SPECT cameras. The patient rotation and symmetry may be very important when the interpreting physician views the finished study.

The acquisition parameters should be properly set to acquire high-quality images. The acquisition mode, two dimensional (2D) or three dimensional (3D), depends on the technical capabilities of the individual scanner and its ability to appropriately correct for high random counts and an increased scatter fraction when in the 3D mode. The imaging matrix should be 128×128 or higher. Most scanners can overlap bed positions by at least one acquisition slice (or more) to help prevent sensitivity changes of the outer slices of each bed position, which may cause a "hot" or "cold" slice at the ends of each bed position. This can occur in either the 2D or 3D mode. In large patients, overlapping by three to seven slices further aids in the reduction of these artifacts. Although 3D mode yields more total counts, the number of random and scatter events increases dramatically. The manufacturer's recommendations may be a useful guide in establishing acquisition protocols at individual institutions.

Scanners that use radioactive rod sources for transmission attenuation correction may allow different acquisition ordering to acquire the transmission-emission images. Each technique should be selected so as to reduce the likelihood of patient motion, which can create misalignments between the acquired transmission and emission scans. The transmission and emission scans, therefore, should be interlaced so that both of these acquisitions are completed at each position before the table is shifted to the next position. The most time-effective protocol performs transmission scans at two different positions while the radioactive rods are exposed in the gantry. Thus the emission scan (E) and transmission scan (T), are interlaced as ETTE acquisitions; that is, emission, transmission, move the table, transmission, emission for adjacent bed positions.

NORMAL WHOLE BODY FDG DISTRIBUTION

In PET oncology, a thorough knowledge of normal anatomy and normal FDG distribution in the body is required before any evaluation of pathologic accumulations can be attempted.

Many organs and body structures accumulate FDG. The most common and constant sites of intense activity are:

- Brain
- Liver (moderate)

- Kidneys (especially the calyces and pelves)
- Bladder

Sites with variable activity include:

- Salivary glands
- Thyroid
- Heart and vascular structures
- Thymus (in children)
- Spleen
- Esophageal ampulla
- Stomach
- Bowel (especially the colon)
- Endometrium (during menses)
- Bone marrow
- Muscles
- Testicles

Although a completely normal whole body FDG PET scan (Figure 11-2) can be easily recognized, it is necessary to evaluate several hundred whole body FDG PET studies to feel comfortable with the many intriguing and sometimes quite disturbing normal variations in FDG localization.

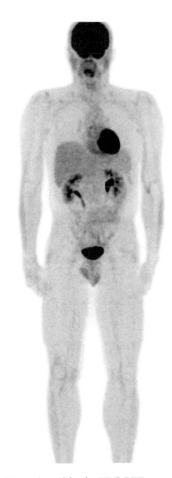

Figure 11-2 Normal total body FDG PET scan. Intense activity accumulates in the brain, pharyngeal constrictors, salivary glands, left ventricular myocardium (variable), urinary collecting system, and bladder. Moderate activity appears in the liver, spleen, and testicles.

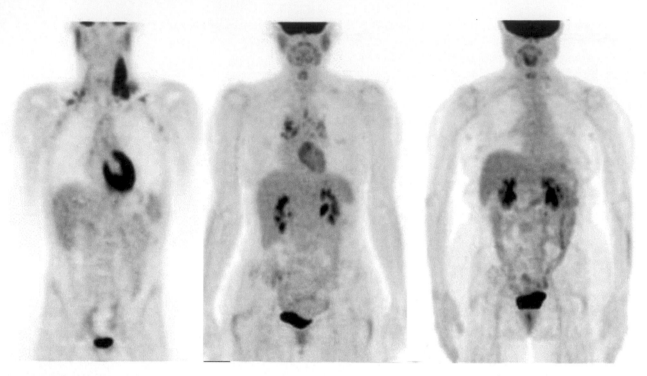

Figure 11-3   Normal left ventricular activity variations in patients with normal fasting peripheral blood glucose levels (<120 mg/dl) showing intense *(left)*, patchy *(middle)*, and absent activity *(right)*.

NORMAL VARIATIONS IN FDG LOCALIZATION

The purpose of this section is not to delineate all the possible variations in normal whole body FDG PET studies but to demonstrate some common differences in normal subjects. Occasionally, only hard-earned experience, focused histories, physical examinations, additional imaging studies, biopsies, or surgery can accurately determine what is (or is not) a normal variation. The value of a pertinent and accurate history of pathology results (usually obtained by the PET technologist) and of correlative imaging studies (e.g., ultrasound [US], computed tomography [CT], magnetic resonance imaging [MRI]) cannot be overemphasized.

Myocardial activity ranks as the most noticeable normal variation (Figure 11-3). Most fasting patients demonstrate little or no left ventricular activity, which is an advantage in the search for tumors, especially in the left lung base. However, intense left ventricular activity can occur normally in fasting patients. Also, heterogeneous activity frequently appears in diabetic patients even with blood glucose levels less than 120 mg/dl. Glucose "clamping" protocols, therefore, are used when myocardial PET imaging is performed in these patients.

Evaluation of the thyroid can be difficult because normal activity varies from a complete absence to a faint nodular pattern to an intense diffuse uptake (Figure 11-4). However, an intense nodule in the thyroid bed usually requires further investigation.

Many different normal patterns occur around the mouth. FDG accumulates in the salivary glands (including the parotid, submandibular, and sublingual glands), the labial

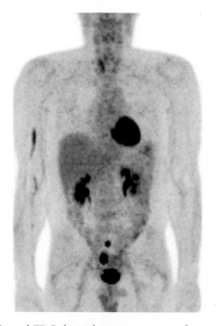

Figure 11-4   Normal FDG thyroid activity can vary from diffusely increased uniform activity to patchy activity (as in this example) or completely absent activity.

or buccal muscles, the laryngeal and anterior spinal muscles and, frequently, the pharyngeal constrictors (Figure 11-5). If a patient grinds the teeth or chews, the muscles of mastication may appear very prominent (Figure 11-6).

Extraocular muscles frequently demonstrate diffusely increased activity. Occasionally only certain complementary

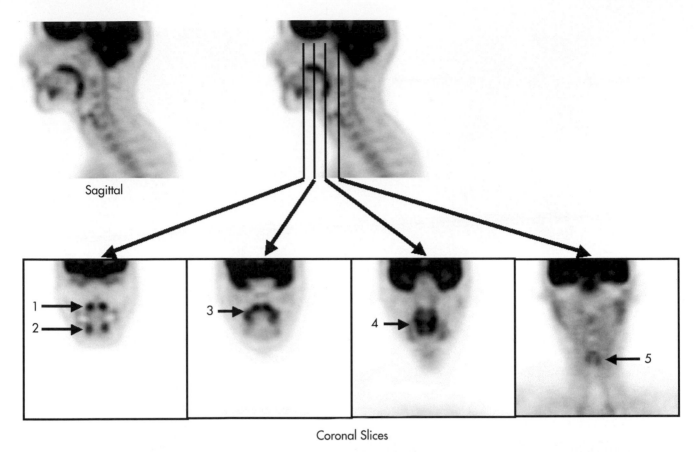

Figure 11-5   Normal physiologic activity around the nasopharyngeal area. Various coronal images demonstrate (1) bilateral symmetric nasopharyngeal activity, (2) salivary gland activity, (3) oropharyngeal activity, (4) hypopharyngeal activity, and (5) laryngeal activity.

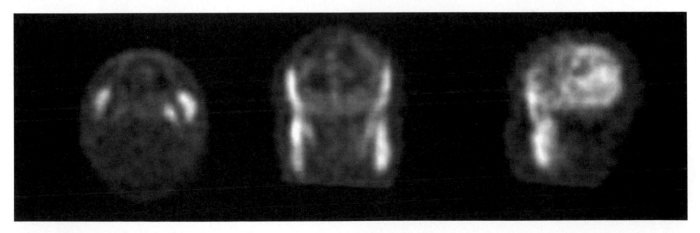

Figure 11-6   Normal activity in the muscles of mastication. This patient was chewing gum immediately after injection of FDG. Bilaterally increased muscle activity can be seen on the transaxial, coronal, and sagittal views.

muscle pairs or the muscles of a single eye appear (Figure 11-7).

Two sets of normal variations frequently cause diagnostic frustration and potentially important misdiagnoses: muscular or fat activity in the neck and shoulders (especially near the trapezius, sternocleidomastoid, and subclavius muscle groups) and gastrointestinal (GI) tract activity (especially in the colon).

Exercise, shivering, and muscular tension can lead to increased FDG utilization from the metabolic demands of the muscles and possibly the fat in the neck (Figure 11-8). Most of the time, the diffuse activity throughout the stressed muscles presents little diagnostic difficulty. However, activity in the neck and supraclavicular regions can be quite nodular, mimicking metastatic disease in the lymph nodes in these areas. Occasionally, unilateral neck activity causes

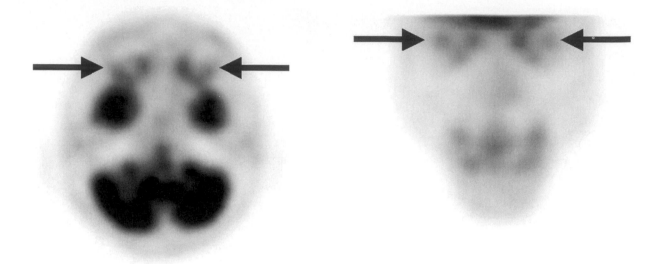

Figure 11-7   Normal extraocular muscle FDG activity present on transaxial *(left)* and coronal *(right)* slices. Activity normally occurs in the extraocular muscles *(arrows)* but can be variable. In this case, activity predominates in the medial rectus muscles. A relaxed patient with the eyes closed may demonstrate less activity.

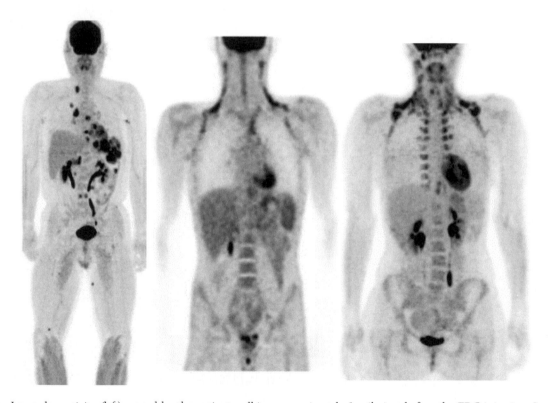

Figure 11-8   Lower leg activity *(left)* caused by the patient walking approximately 1 mile just before the FDG injection. In the middle image, the neck muscle activity is fairly smooth and symmetric. However, in another patient *(right image),* the neck muscle activity occurs in a much more nodular and somewhat asymmetric pattern, mimicking cancerous involvement of supraclavicular nodes. Neither patient had any adenopathy. Also, note the normal, fairly symmetric activity along both sides of the spine at the costovertebral joints.

even more anxiety. Physical examination or additional imaging (US, CT, or MRI) may help, but sometimes only a biopsy can answer the question of possible tumor involvement.

Variable amounts of normal, increased activity frequently occur within the small and especially the large bowel. FDG can present as a diffuse, focal or, commonly, scattered regional tubular pattern (e.g., ascending colon plus sigmoid colon) (Figure 11-9). The causes of these patterns are obscure but may be related to peristalsis or gas. The problem lies in the occasional difficulty of determining normal from inflammatory processes or even tumors. Again, more invasive measures (colonoscopy or barium enema) may be necessary to further evaluate the possibility of pathology.

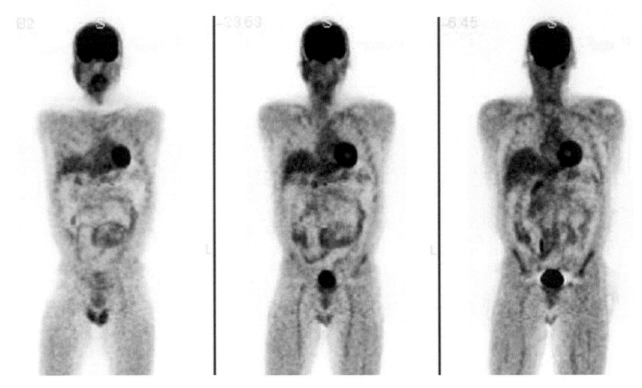

Figure 11-9   Normal gastrointestinal tract activity. These coronal slices demonstrate increased but normal tubular activity throughout large portions of both the small and large bowel.

Although not strictly normal variations, whole body PET oncology examinations show FDG accumulations in a variety of commonly encountered locations. Activity may occur in recent surgical incisions, ostomy sites, recovering hematopoietic bone marrow, arthritic joints (especially the acromioclavicular joints), infections, focal or diffuse inflammation (particularly after recent radiation therapy), pleural effusions, biopsies, or injection sites (Figs. 11-10 and 11-11).

PET ONCOLOGY APPLICATIONS

Although FDG PET imaging has been documented in the scientific literature to be effective in a wide variety of cancers, at this time the government and private insurance companies limit coverage to a select number of cancer groups. The following discussion focuses on these select primary indications for FDG PET oncology studies. In addition, examples of some other cancers for which patients might be referred for PET scans are also presented.

Solitary pulmonary nodules (SPNs) and non-small cell lung cancers (NSCLCs) were the first FDG PET oncology studies covered by Medicare. Reimbursement coverage has now been extended to melanoma, lymphoma, colorectal, head/neck, esophageal, and recurrent breast cancers. Private insurance companies may cover FDG PET studies in other types of cancer, usually after a thorough review of individual patient needs and circumstances. However, insurance carriers usually require preauthorization for any PET examination.

In the following discussion, the individual comparative statistical values (e.g., sensitivity, specificity) of FDG PET and complementary imaging modalities are not enumerated, because these values are very well presented in other sources.*

SOLITARY PULMONARY NODULE (SPN)

In the United States, lung cancer is the leading cause of cancer death, having a high prevalence and a poor prognosis. The chances of survival depend on many factors but generally are related to the particular type of cancer and its spread (stage) in the body. Usually, the smaller the original tumor and the less it has spread, the better the chance of survival. In patients with a high risk of developing lung cancer (e.g., cigarette smokers), screening protocols (chest radiographs and chest CT) increasingly are used in the hope of discovering lung cancer in its earlier and potentially more curative stages. With these screening examinations, many new single pulmonary nodules are discovered. However, both benign and malignant conditions can result in lung nodules. Biopsies of all these nodules in search of cancer would be extremely expensive and invasive and frequently would result in nondiagnostic findings.

Increased FDG utilization in an SPN suggests malignancy. However, benign processes (e.g., tuberculosis, fungal infection, pneumonia) also can demonstrate increased FDG

---

*See Gambhir SS et al: A tabulated summary of the FDG PET literature, *J Nucl Med* 42(suppl 5):1S–79S 2001.

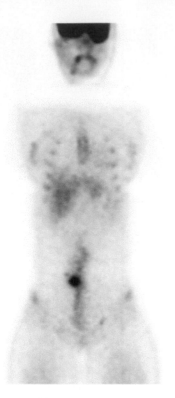

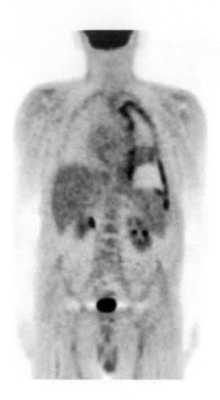

Figure 11-10   Mild to intense FDG activity commonly localizes in surgical wounds (*left*) and inflammatory conditions (*right*). In the latter case, the FDG accumulates in a diffuse inflammation of the left pleura.

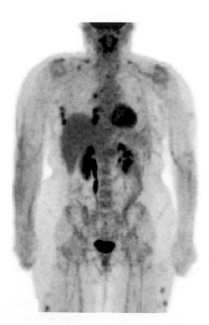

Figure 11-11   FDG localization at injection sites. The three areas of moderate activity in the thighs represent recent injection sites. Metastases are present in the thorax.

metabolism, and biopsies are often still needed to determine the true nature of the nodule. On the other hand, lesions with no FDG activity are almost always benign. Occasionally, low-grade lung cancers can show little or no FDG uptake (Figure 11-12).

PET outperforms CT in determining whether an SPN is benign or malignant. Even though PET is an expensive tool, cost analysis demonstrates that including FDG PET studies in the evaluation of solitary pulmonary nodules saves millions of dollars a year in the United States alone.

NON-SMALL CELL LUNG CANCER (NSCLC)

In evaluating newly diagnosed NSCLC, FDG PET is superior to CT and MRI in finding lymph node involvement and distant metastases, especially in the adrenal glands. This allows more accurate assessment of the tumor stage and better determination of whether a patient should undergo an invasive biopsy, would benefit from a potentially curative surgery, or should receive only noninvasive therapies (radiation, chemotherapy, or both).

Many pulmonary lesions identified by CT or MRI cannot be definitely classified as either benign or malignant, because anatomic imaging cannot provide all the information necessary to evaluate the functional status of individual lesions. FDG PET provides complementary metabolic information that helps direct the proper clinical management of each patient. However, because FDG PET identifies any process that utilizes FDG to a greater extent than normal surrounding tissues, FDG imaging also demonstrates many infections (especially fungal infections) and inflammatory processes. Furthermore, low-grade malignancies, bronchoalveolar cell carcinoma (BAC) in particular, may utilize

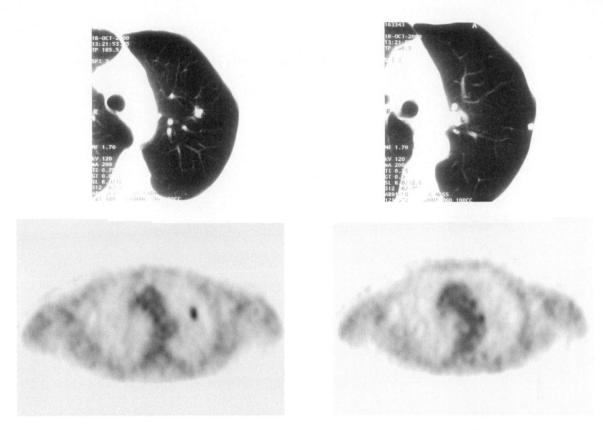

Figure 11-12   The top row demonstrates CT images of two pulmonary modules in the same patient. The bottom row shows FDG PET images corresponding to the CT images. On the left, noticeable activity occurs on the PET image corresponding to the nodule present on the CT image, suggesting cancer. On the right, there is no PET activity along the pleural surface where the second nodule resides on the CT image, strongly suggesting a benign process.

FDG at essentially the same levels as normal surrounding tissues and may be hidden within this background.

Standard uptake values (SUVs) cannot distinguish between benign and malignant diseases with any helpful degree of accuracy because, as mentioned previously, common fungal and infectious processes can utilize FDG at very high rates, and BAC or other low-grade tumors can utilize FDG at background levels.

Clinical investigations offer some hope that a more accurate differentiation between cancer and benign processes can be made by obtaining FDG utilization rates within a single region of interest (ROI) at various intervals, starting immediately after injection and extending up to 4 hours later. If the values continuously rise, cancer appears to be much more likely. If the values plateau or decline after the initial rise, benign processes seem much more likely. It remains to be clearly established whether these time-activity curves can be used clinically, which would help avoid many invasive procedures.

Physicians interpreting PET studies may prefer to image patients with their arms above their heads to correspond to patient positioning during CT scans. PET to CT imaging fusion may then be performed. However, CT examinations generally are acquired with breath-holding maneuvers, whereas PET studies are obtained while the patient breathes

normally. The images, therefore, may differ in size, resulting in possible image mismatches.

MELANOMA

The incidence of malignant melanoma has risen steadily over the past century. Currently, approximately 7000 people die each year from melanoma in the United States alone. Several factors help determine the chances of survival in patients with melanoma, including tumor thickness (Breslow index), depth of invasion (Clark index), tumor location, and metastases, among others. The presence of metastases dramatically lowers the chance of survival.

Melanoma avidly utilizes FDG, allowing whole body PET to assess the presence of metastases much more accurately than conventional techniques (US, CT, bone scintigraphy). PET stands out as the single best screening examination for high-risk melanoma patients and for patients in whom recurrence is suspected (Figure 11-13).

The search for possible metastases in the brain can be very difficult because the neurons also avidly utilize FDG. The normally intense neuronal activity can obscure metastases, which commonly occur at the gray-white junction. Also, with attenuation correction algorithms, small surface skin metastases may be difficult to visualize because of slight

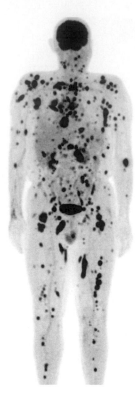

Figure 11-13 Very extensive metastases from malignant melanoma. Note the normal, intense brain activity that may hide metastases.

misalignments of the transmission and emission images. Some institutions use both attenuated and nonattenuated whole body PET images to help evaluate for the possibility of faint skin lesions (Figure 11-14).

Again, it is important for the technologist to obtain a history, including previous surgery, on all patients. Any patient with a history of melanoma, even if referred for another indication, should have a total (head to toe) body scan. Care should be taken to ensure that the site of the original melanoma is clearly included in the scan. Over the legs, the acquisition times for both the emission and transmission scans may be slightly reduced from the times used for the rest of the body.

LYMPHOMA

Lymphomas cover a wide variety of tumors of the immune system that are divided into two broad categories: Hodgkin's disease (HD), and non-Hodgkin's lymphoma (NHL). The presentations and therapies of these two groups differ. Hodgkin's disease occurs less often than NHL, usually involves the upper mediastinum, and tends to spread from one lymph node station to contiguous nodes (Figure 11-15). The type of therapy (radiation, chemotherapy, or both) depends mostly on the stage of the disease.

NHL covers a broader range of subtypes than HD and usually spreads more widely throughout the lymph nodes

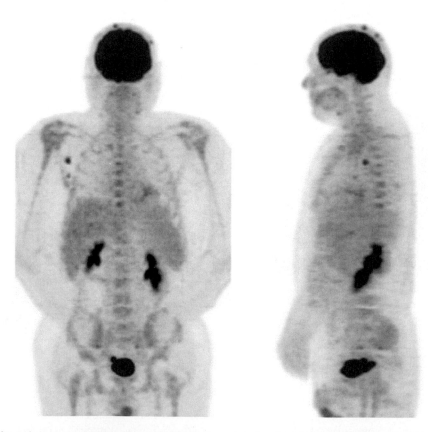

Figure 11-14 Faint scalp melanoma metastases present on both the coronal and sagittal views. There are also right axillary and posterior mediastinal metastases. Faint skin surface metastases may sometimes be missed with attenuation correction protocols if there are slight misalignments between transmission and emission scans.

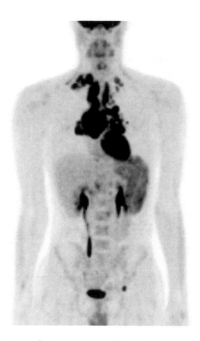
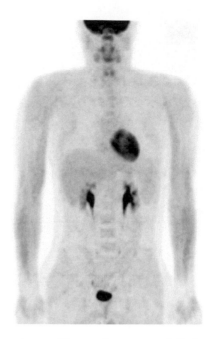

Figure 11-15   FDG evaluation of the response of lymphoma to chemotherapy. The pre-therapy scan *(left)* shows intense activity in multiple mediastinal, supraclavicular, splenic, periportal, and left inguinal metastases. After 5 months of therapy *(right),* the lymphoma is in complete remission.

and other organs of the body. Therapy for NHL depends more on the histologic subtype than the tumor stage.

Lymphomas (with the occasional exceptions of low-grade NHL and maltomas) tend to avidly accumulate FDG, which makes these tumors visible in almost all cases. FDG PET, therefore, is a valuable tool for accurately staging lymphomas and evaluating tumor response to therapy (see Figure 11-15). Pre-therapy whole body PET scans should be obtained to document the original state of FDG utilization (some low-grade tumors fail to accumulate FDG) and to allow accurate assessment of the response to therapy.

PET outshines all other anatomic imaging modalities in the evaluation of lymphomas (especially evaluation of the therapeutic response) because neither CT nor MRI can distinguish between scar tissue and residual tumor after therapy. Persistent FDG tumor activity after therapy strongly suggests residual or recurrent tumor. Lack of FDG activity essentially excludes persistent tumor, especially if FDG activity was present on the pre-therapy examination.

Gallium-67 (^{67}Ga) scintigraphy has provided the standard for assessing the response of lymphomas to treatment, with good results seen in the neck and thorax and poor results in the abdomen and pelvis. FDG PET detects significantly more disease (and smaller tumors) than ^{67}Ga scintigraphy because more lymphomas accumulate FDG than ^{67}Ga and because gallium scintigraphy has a lower resolution.

If the patient's history includes lymphoma of the head or neck, the patient should be placed in a head holder, and the head, neck, and shoulders should be carefully positioned to ensure anatomic symmetry in the coronal plane. The head holder also helps reduce patient motion.

COLORECTAL CANCER

Colorectal cancer ranks third behind lung and prostate cancers in men, and breast and lung cancers in women, in the number of newly diagnosed cases each year. These cancers frequently metastasize, particularly to the liver. Before potentially curative surgery is attempted, an intensive search for metastases should be undertaken, so that inappropriate surgery and exposure to possible surgical morbidity can be avoided.

CT is relatively good at evaluating for the presence of liver metastases but relatively poor at detecting extrahepatic sites of involvement. Whole body FDG PET more accurately assesses liver and, especially, extrahepatic tumor involvement, improving candidate selection for surgery (Figure 11-16). Although expensive, whole body PET is a superb, cost-effective screening tool for colorectal cancers, mainly because it identifies more sites of tumor involvement and more accurately determines nonresectable disease, thereby avoiding unnecessary and more costly surgical procedures.

When necessary, whole body FDG PET can be used to search for cancer when the patient's tumor markers are rising and conventional anatomic imaging techniques have failed to detect any disease or to differentiate scar tissue from recurrent tumor.

Figure 10-23 (p. 305) presents a dramatic example of a very large liver tumor that was invisible on a CT examination but completely obvious on the whole body FDG PET images. This case dramatizes the very important point that different imaging parameters (e.g., Hounsfield units for CT; FDG utilization for PET) may be needed to evaluate differ-

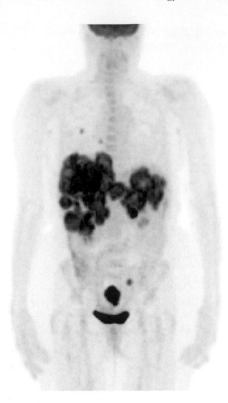

Figure 11-16 Extensive colorectal metastases, with disease occurring in the pre-sacral, left iliac, hepatic, splenic, and right pulmonary locations.

ent types of tumors or the same tumor type in different individuals. However, in the case of colorectal cancers, a critical analysis must be undertaken to determine whether FDG PET should replace all anatomic imaging modalities as the first-line screening method because of the very serious problems inherent in these conventional tools.

HEAD, NECK, AND ESOPHAGEAL CANCERS

Head and neck cancers are almost exclusively squamous cell carcinomas (95%). Fortunately, squamous cell carcinomas tend to avidly utilize FDG, making whole body PET an excellent imaging choice with these cancers (Figure 11-17). Therapy and survival are mainly determined by the tumor location, its local or regional spread, and the presence (or absence) of lymph node metastases. Distant metastases occur fairly infrequently, but in about 15% of the cases, a second tumor develops in the esophagus or pulmonary bronchi.

Detection of lymph node involvement is very important when surgical dissection is contemplated because survival drops drastically when lymph node metastases are found. FDG PET distinguishes cancerous lymph node involvement better than CT or MRI.

Many head and neck tumors recur locally, usually within the first 2 years after the original resection. In these cases it can be very difficult to differentiate tumor recurrence from postoperative scarring or changes caused by radiation therapy. FDG PET accurately identifies tumor recurrences. When clinical evidence of local treatment failure exists, distant metastases can be identified in approximately 60% of these cases. Again, whole body FDG PET can be effectively used to screen for distant metastases because of the greatly increased FDG utilization in these tumors. Radiation therapy can cause local reactive inflammatory changes and increased local FDG metabolism, leading to the possible erroneous conclusion of local treatment failure. For this reason, it is advisable to wait at least 1 month, and preferably longer (3 months), after radiation therapy to assess for tumor recurrence.

Normal variants, such as salivary gland uptake and lingual, buccal, pharyngeal, laryngeal, and neck muscle activity can cause many diagnostic difficulties in the evaluation of head and neck tumors. Fortunately, correlation with complementary anatomic imaging and a physical examination usually determines the true tumor status.

Patients with esophageal cancer usually present with advanced disease and an unfavorable chance of survival. Accurate staging is important in selecting the appropriate individual therapies. Because esophageal cancers avidly utilize FDG, whole body PET is usually much more

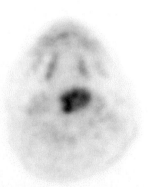

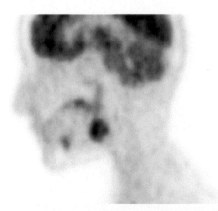

Figure 11-17 Head/neck cancer with tumor demonstrates intense activity, even more than the usual pharyngeal and salivary gland activity and equal to the activity in the brain.

accurate in staging local, regional, and distant disease than is conventional anatomic imaging. Whole body PET detects many more lymph node metastases than does CT or MRI. Since most treatment failures occur because of unknown distant metastases, whole body FDG PET permits better individual treatment planning through more accurate staging and helps dispense with unnecessary surgery.

BREAST CANCER

Breast cancer ranks as the number one malignant tumor in women. The most important prognostic factors in the long-term survival of breast cancer patients are the number and extent of axillary lymph node metastases. The survival rate drops precipitously if malignant axillary lymph nodes are present, and the rate drops even more if distant metastases are found.

Appropriate therapy depends mostly on accurate staging or on accurate re-staging after initial therapy. Currently, no anatomic imaging modality can accurately assess for lymph node metastases. Therefore axillary lymph node dissections are performed for prognosis and for determining the need of adjuvant chemotherapy and radiation therapy. Studies now underway are trying to determine the value of sentinel node biopsies. If these studies demonstrate that sentinel node biopsies accurately determine prognosis and the presence of lymph node metastases, breast cancer patients could be spared the morbidity of axillary lymph node dissections.

FDG PET detects axillary and mediastinal lymph nodes quite well, although micrometastases are frequently missed, which diminishes the utility of PET in these instances. For patients who have had previous lumpectomies, mammo-graphic assessment can be very difficult. Surgical scars mimic recurrent tumors. PET demonstrates an excellent ability to detect local recurrences, which helps prevent unnecessary repeat biopsies and further scarring. At the same time, PET can monitor for possible lymph node involvement and distant metastases, which would alter the planned therapies.

Finally, because FDG utilization is related to cellular metabolism, PET can help demonstrate responses to therapy. Figure 11-18 shows an example in which a significant reduction in FDG activity occurred in the metastatic nodes 3 months after therapy, and only very faint activity was seen after 5 months. Non-responders demonstrate little or no decreased FDG utilization after therapy. With newer therapy regimens, FDG PET may offer an effective method of determining which of the available therapy options would have the greatest chance of success.

BRAIN CANCER

Because the cerebral and cerebellar neurons utilize FDG avidly, primary and metastatic brain tumors can be, and are, missed. Figure 11-19 shows a brain tumor that cannot be identified with FDG imaging. However, after evaluation of the same patient using a synthetic amino acid (F-18-ACBC), a marker of protein synthesis, the tumor is easily recognized. This case reinforces the point that imaging of different cellular processes may be necessary in different individuals or in different types of cancer to assess each patient accurately.

Currently, FDG PET generally is used as an adjunct imaging tool to help differentiate residual tumor from radiation necrosis, and not as a screening tool for primary or

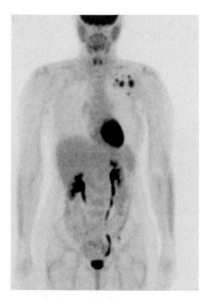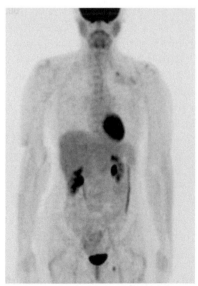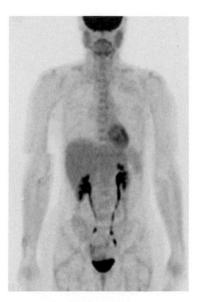

Figure 11-18 Serial FDG scans used to monitor breast cancer therapy. The left image shows increased activity in several left axillary lymph nodes. After 3 months of chemotherapy (*middle*), the nodes are still slightly visible. After 5 months (*right*), only very faint activity remains in the lymph nodes.

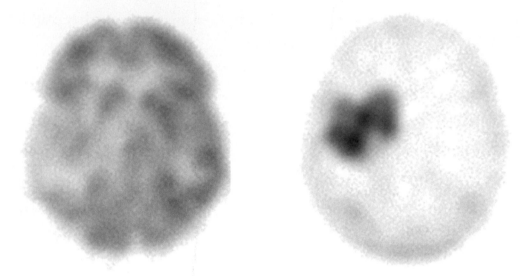

Figure 11-19   FDG PET imaging (*left*) of a low-grade brain cancer (grade II astrocytoma) demonstrates less glucose utilization than in normal brain. The FDG scan provides no information on the extent of the recurrent tumor. The F-18-ACBC PET scan (*right*), performed with a synthetic amino acid, shows limited utilization by normal brain tissue. The extent of the low-grade recurrent tumor is now clearly evident. This example dramatizes the value of imaging different metabolic processes with PET.

metastatic brain tumors. MRI is especially adept in the screening for and evaluation of primary or metastatic brain tumors.

PROSTATE CANCER

Apart from skin cancers, new cases of prostate cancer are diagnosed more frequently in men than any other form of cancer, and only lung cancer kills more often. An effective screening and staging tool, therefore, would be valuable. Unfortunately, whole body FDG PET does not detect the presence of local disease or distant metastases very well. This poor performance may be related to various factors but is probably due to the modest rate of FDG utilization in primary prostate tumors, involved lymph nodes, and bony metastases. Routine bone scintigraphy defines more lesions than FDG PET.

Because the prostate is situated just below the base of the bladder, the normal intense bladder activity may obscure small prostate tumors. However, primary tumors occasionally can be visualized (Figure 11-20). Although whole body FDG PET poorly demonstrates primary and metastatic prostate cancers, an abnormal FDG PET scan in patients with prostate cancer almost always indicates the presence of local or metastatic disease. Perhaps in the future a new PET radiopharmaceutical will allow this powerful imaging modality to become a much more effective tool in the evaluation of this common and deadly cancer.

OVARIAN CANCER

Ovarian cancer is a fairly common and deadly form of cancer in women. Approximately 25,000 new cases are diagnosed in the United States each year, accounting for about 15,000 deaths. Ovarian cancer usually strikes older women, and because the early symptoms are rather vague (and potentially misleading), the correct diagnosis is usually made when the disease is in an advanced stage.

Proper staging allows a correct prognosis. Patients in whom the cancer is confined to the ovary have a 5-year survival rate greater than 90%. However, in one third of the cases, distant metastases are present at the time of the original diagnosis. Another one third develop metastases within the first year after surgery, accounting for the fairly dismal overall survival rates.

Fortunately, ovarian cancers usually originate from the epithelium and commonly demonstrate quite noticeable FDG utilization (Figure 11-21). Ovarian cancers usually spread superficially over local structures (e.g., fallopian tubes, uterus, bladder, opposite ovary) and throughout the peritoneum, as well as to nearby pelvic and periaortic lymph nodes.

Correct staging with conventional anatomic imaging can be very difficult in ovarian cancers, and extensive surgical exploration usually is required. FDG PET offers a screening tool with the potential to obviate some primary laparotomies (because of the presence of unsuspected peritoneal studs, involved lymph nodes, or distant metastases) or second-look laparotomies in cases of possible tumor recurrence. PET may also prove helpful in the evaluation of tumor response to therapy and in patient management.

Potential pitfalls in FDG PET evaluation of ovarian cancers are the well-differentiated tumors with FDG utilization rates at background levels and microscopic peritoneal metastases, which may also be indistinguishable from the normal surrounding background tissues, especially when adjacent to the liver, spleen, or colon.

PET imaging in the pelvis occasionally may require bladder catheterization or administration of a diuretic (or both) to reduce bladder activity.

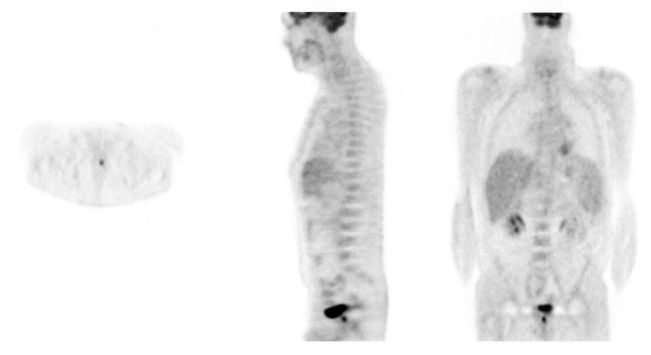

Figure 11-20   The increased FDG activity present on the transaxial, sagittal, and coronal images just below the bladder represents prostate cancer. However, normal activity in the bulbous urethra may appear in a similar manner.

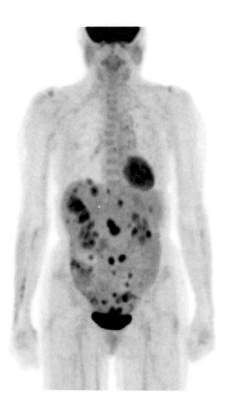

Figure 11-21   An FDG scan in a patient with ovarian cancer demonstrates extensive hepatic, peritoneal, and pelvic metastases. Most of these metastases were not demonstrated by either CT or MRI.

TESTICULAR CANCER

Testicular cancers are divided into two major categories: seminomas (50%), and non-seminomas (50%). Although rare, these tumors are the most common solid tumors in young males (15 to 40 years of age). When first diagnosed, a large percentage of these tumors have metastasized (approximately 30% of the seminomas and 70% of the non-seminomas). Metastases commonly occur in the periaortic, iliac, and inguinal lymph nodes and in the lungs.

These tumors are usually treated with a combination of surgery, radiation, and chemotherapy, depending on the histologic diagnosis and the tumor stage. It is important to stage these tumors accurately to determine the most effective therapies.

Testicular cancers, especially seminomas, avidly utilize FDG (Figure 11-22). Although few large studies exist to support the use of FDG PET in testicular cancers, it may be beneficial in the staging or re-staging of these tumors and in the evaluation of therapeutic response. This would allow more individualized therapies, with a possible reduction in the number of surgical interventions.

A substantial problem in the imaging of testicular tumors with PET is the varying degrees of FDG utilization by the different subsets of testicular cancers. Mature teratomas offer a dramatic example. Mature teratomas (tumors consisting of more than one tissue type) demonstrate a benign histology but arise from malignant precursors and must be removed surgically. These particular tumors show very little FDG activity and cannot be distinguished from necrotic or fibrous tissues. This makes assessment of these tumors with FDG ineffective and reemphasizes the point that if tumors do not

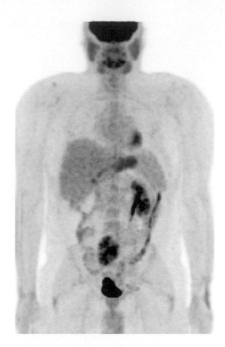

Figure 11-22 An FDG scan in a patient with testicular cancer shows a large collection above the bladder that represents a retroperitoneal metastasis. Note the commonly occurring, normally increased activity in the stomach and in the colon, especially in its descending portion.

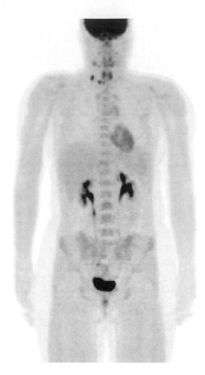

Figure 11-23 FDG accumulates in residual nests of the thyroid cancer on the right side of the neck. These lesions were not demonstrated on whole body ^{131}I scans.

utilize FDG more than the surrounding normal tissues, they are not identified, and a different metabolic process must be examined. Molecular imagers must be clearly advised about the clinical indications for each PET examination; also, they must know the particular tumors being evaluated and must understand the various PET presentations of these different tumors. For accurate assessment of each case, PET imaging requires meticulous attention to technical detail, to information gathering, and to scan interpretation. When a larger range of PET radiotracers and techniques becomes available, a much heavier burden will rest on the molecular imager to understand the unique characteristics of each "delivery system" and its interaction with the vast array of known cancers.

THYROID CANCER

An example of thyroid cancer is presented not to tout the strength of FDG PET in the evaluation of this particular type of cancer but to review the strengths and weaknesses of FDG PET imaging.

Thyroid cancers cover a wide range of histologic types, ranging from the most well-differentiated form (papillary) to the most deadly anaplastic form. They are divided in two main categories: follicular cell tumors, and C-cell tumors. Imaging protocols and treatments are fairly well established, although some controversies still exist. Iodine-131 (^{131}I) whole body imaging remains the diagnostic workhorse. Well-differentiated thyroid cancers usually continue to trap and organify iodine, allowing tumor detection with [131]I

whole body scanning. Poorly differentiated or anaplastic thyroid cancers do not normally organify iodine, rendering ^{131}I ineffective in the imaging or treatment of these cancers.

FDG utilization in thyroid cancers tends to follow the proliferative potential and metabolic activity of these tumors, with the more aggressive and poorly differentiated tumors utilizing FDG at a higher rate than the more well-differentiated forms. It would seem that the more common, well-differentiated forms of thyroid cancer would not utilize FDG to any noticeable degree and that the less common, more poorly differentiated forms would utilize FDG at much higher rates. Although this tendency exists, the correlation is weak. Aggressive and anaplastic tumors can be FDG negative, and well-differentiated thyroid tumors can be FDG positive (Figure 11-23). Normal variants and benign thyroid processes cause further confusion. Many thyroid nodules avidly accumulate FDG, whereas other nodules use FDG moderately if at all. This makes FDG evaluation of the thyroid difficult and treacherous.

Although imaging of the thyroid with FDG presents inherent diagnostic problems, the following two points should be emphasized:

1. In cases of recurrent thyroid cancer and negative ^{131}I whole body scans, whole body FDG PET imaging would be a reasonable diagnostic approach to search for more poorly differentiated forms of thyroid cancer.
2. When unexplained abnormal findings occur in the thyroid bed on FDG PET examinations obtained for other indications, additional conventional tests (e.g.,

US, ^{123}I scintigraphy, biopsies) should be performed to exclude unsuspected thyroid cancers (which occasionally have been identified first on whole body FDG PET imaging).

FUTURE TRENDS

It is to be hoped that the clinical examples detailed in this chapter demonstrate the nearly limitless future potential of PET imaging in oncology and the inherent power and weakness of FDG PET. The power of FDG PET lies in its ability to image a functional parameter (FDG utilization) rather than anatomic changes. Its weakness lies in the fact that FDG utilization does not necessarily distinguish between benign and malignant processes.

Functional imaging depends completely on effective "delivery systems" or radiopharmaceuticals to visualize the desired intracellular metabolic processes. Radioactive tracers arrive at their desired cellular locations through the actions of these "delivery systems" (e.g., FDG in the cellular cytosol by the increased facilitated diffusion and the increased hexokinase activity of cancerous cells). Because an enormous array of interesting and potentially useful metabolic pathways exists, the development of effective systems for delivering individualized PET radiotracers to specific targeted cells could transform PET into an extremely powerful clinical and research tool.

New PET radiotracers are becoming available to institutions with PET scanners: F-18-fluorothymidine (F-18-FLT) (cellular proliferation); F-18-fluoromisonidazol (F-18-FMISO) (hypoxia); F-18-fluorouracil (F-18-FU) (chemotherapy response); and F-18-fluorodeoxyphenylalanine (F-18-FDOPA) (movement disorders and neuroendocrine tumors). Even more PET radiotracers will be available soon to institutions with an on-site cyclotron: C-11-thymidine (C-11-dThd) (cellular proliferation); C-11-methionine (C-11-Met) (protein synthesis); C-11-tyrosine (C-11-Tyr) (protein synthesis); C-11-acetate (lipid synthesis, myocardial oxidation, and prostate cancer); C-11-choline (phospholipid synthesis and prostate cancer); O-15-H_2O, C-11, and N-13 ammonia (perfusion). On-site cyclotrons allow the production of positron emitters with very short half-lives (C-11, 20 minutes; N-13, 10 minutes; O-15, 2 minutes) and which fortuitously are also the building blocks of organic molecules.

Many novel radiopharmaceuticals will become available in the future, emerging from the imaginative efforts and ingenuity of biochemists, molecular biologists, biochemical and molecular engineers, cellular physiologists, geneticists, pharmacologists, and physicists. Indeed, PET will require the cooperation and expertise of many basic scientists and skilled technologists to expand its present utility and secure its place in the future of molecular medicine.

SUGGESTED READINGS

Gambhir SS et al: A tabulated summary of the FDG PET literature, *J Nucl Med* 42(suppl 5):1S–79S, 2001.

Ruhlmann J, Oehr P, Biersack H-J, editors: *PET in oncology,* Berlin, 1999, Springer-Verlag.

Schiepers C, editor: *Diagnostic nuclear medicine,* Berlin, 2000, Springer-Verlag.

von Schultess GK, editor: *Clinical positron emission tomography,* Philadelphia, 2000, Lippincott Williams & Wilkins.

Zsolt Szabo, Henry N. Wagner Jr., Jay K. Rhine,
Julia W. Buchanan

chapter **12**

Central Nervous System

Objectives

Diagram and describe the anatomy of the central nervous system.

Describe intercellular communication and neurotransmitters.

Diagram and describe the circulation of cerebrospinal fluid.

Discuss the properties of radiopharmaceuticals used in SPECT brain imaging.

Describe the technical parameters and instrumentation used for CSF studies.

Describe the use, dose, administration, and procedures for SPECT brain studies.

Describe the radionuclides used in PET imaging procedures.

Discuss PET imaging techniques for the brain.

All living systems require properly functioning communication and control processes. The information necessary for cells to function is stored and transferred by means of molecules, beginning with DNA and extending up through hormones, neurotransmitters, and other specific molecules. The DNA molecule contains 8,000 bits of information, whereas the average protein molecule contains 4,000 bits. A single cell contains about 10^{12} bits of information, which is equivalent to the information in 1,000 volumes of the *Encyclopædia Britannica*.

Neurons, the fundamental units of the nervous system, talk to each other in two ways: by means of electrical action potentials and by molecular messengers that carry information and modulate the electrical activity. Many of these molecules serve as receptors of molecular messages secreted into the synapses connecting dendrites and axons. They are involved in the movement of sodium, calcium, and potassium ions across cell membranes. Molecules such as adenosine triphosphate (ATP) provide energy that influences the overall activity of neurons.

Neuroreceptors are polymers that recognize specific messenger molecules that are released locally or circulate through the body until they encounter the appropriate biopolymer on the surface of neurons or other cells that fit their specific configuration. Molecular neurotransmitters, including amines, amino acids, and peptides, have the right shape, charge, and other physiochemical properties to bind to the receptor biopolymers. The patterns and quantities of these recognition sites integrate individual cells of the body to make the person a unique, whole individual. Disintegration results in disease or death.

The maintenance of life in all organisms, including human beings, requires intercellular communication, which in turn requires energy to generate the ion gradients that produce electrical action potentials and to synthesize transmitters and receptors. The rate of consumption of the principal source of energy for the brain—glucose—can be measured by means of positron emission tomography (PET) (Figure 12-1). Regional blood flow and intracellular communication within the brain can be examined with both PET and single photon emission computed tomography

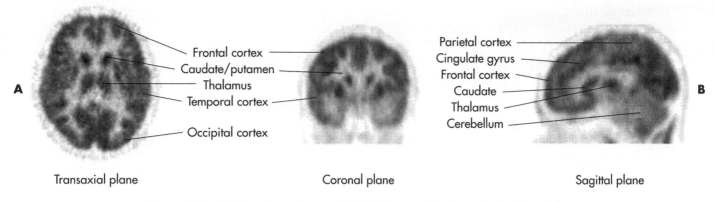

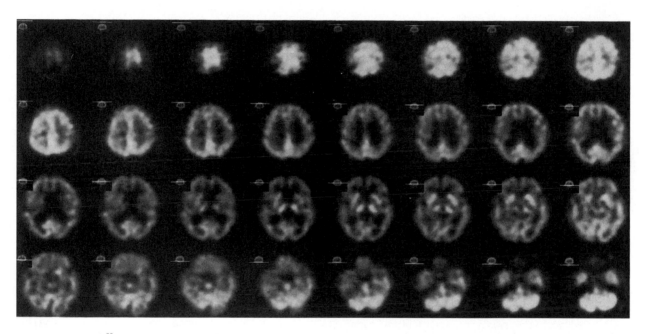

Figure 12-1   ¹⁸F-fluorodeoxyglucose (FDG) PET scan of the brain of a healthy subject.

Figure 12-2   Normal ^{99m}Tc HMPAO SPECT brain scan. (Courtesy Trionix Corp and Middleheim General Hospital, Antwerp, Belgium.)

(SPECT) (Figure 12-2). Since the 1950s more than 100 neurotransmitters, or chemical messengers, such as serotonin and dopamine, have been discovered. Acetylcholine stimulates skeletal muscle cells to contract but causes heart muscles to relax. Thus muscarinic acetylcholine receptors are excitatory; nicotinic acetylcholine receptors are inhibitory.

Enzymes in the cells of the body control the innumerable energy-transforming processes within cells, whereas membrane receptors control much of the transfer of information from one cell to another. The most highly specialized system for information transfer in the body is composed of the brain and nervous system. One neuron may interact with 1,000 to 10,000 other neurons. Molecular messengers, called neurotransmitters, include amines, amino acids, and peptides.

Neuronal membrane receptors respond to specific neurotransmitters and ignore other molecules that continually come in contact with them as they circulate through the body. Neurotransmitters secreted at the terminals of presynaptic neurons interact with receptors on postsynaptic neurons, which results in translation of information by means of changes in the state of ion channels or by formation of "second messenger" molecules. The most widely studied neurotransmission systems have been those involving dopamine, serotonin, norepinephrine, and acetylcholine.

Neurotransmitters are stored in vesicles at the terminal axonal branches of presynaptic neurons. When a sufficiently large number of impulses arrives at the nerve terminal, the molecules of the neurotransmitters are released in a burst and diffuse into the synaptic cleft, where they are bound to the specific molecular configuration of the receptor on the membranes of the postsynaptic neuron. Drugs may mimic the transmitter and bind to the receptor to produce the same action as the naturally occurring transmitter. Antibodies can block receptors, as in myasthenia gravis, and recent evidence suggests that abnormal metabolites can also block neuroreceptors.

Drugs, both licit and illicit, affect intercellular communication. Chemicals include amines, such as norepinephrine, dopamine, and serotonin; amino acids, such as gamma-aminobutyric acid (GABA), glutamic acid, aspartic acid, and glycine; and peptides, such as endogenous enkephalins. Neurotransmitters are secreted in varying amounts, depending on the number and rate of electrical impulses traveling down the axon of the presynaptic neuron from which the neurotransmitter is secreted.

In addition to involvement in neuron-to-neuron information transfer, neurotransmitters, including enkephalins, act as modulators of regional neuronal activity. Some chemical messengers act within fractions of a second, whereas others have an effect over hours or even days. Thousands of synapses, connecting with a single postsynaptic neuron, are integrated and determine whether the postsynaptic neuron fires an action potential. The availability of 20 different messenger amino acids means that a vast number of different combinations are possible and can encode a tremendous amount of information.

Radioactive tracers make it possible to detect and quantify molecular abnormalities, including those involved in intercellular communication. Positron-emitting radionuclides, particularly carbon (^{11}C) and fluorine (^{18}F), have been used to carry out studies with many receptor systems. Radioligands labeled with the single photon emitting radionuclides, such as iodine-123 (^{123}I) and technetium-99m (^{99m}Tc), have been developed, making it possible to perform these studies with SPECT systems.

In the care of patients with diseases of the central and peripheral nervous system, nuclear medicine techniques can be used to assess the effectiveness of surgery or radiation therapy, can document the extent of involvement of the brain by tumors, and can determine progression or regression of the lesions in response to different forms of treatment. Such data permit modification of the treatment plan sooner than can be determined by the patient's clinical response or by changes in the size of a lesion. Treatment, therefore, no longer needs to be based solely on clinical response, gross morphology of the lesions, and histopathologic examination of biopsies.

In addition to measuring blood flow to tumors, blood volume, glucose or amino acid incorporation into tumors, and DNA synthesis, PET and SPECT can be used to measure the number and affinity of hormone receptors that charac-terize certain tumors. Estrogen receptors are increased in many breast tumors in both the primary and metastatic sites. ^{18}F estradiol accumulation, as determined by PET, makes it possible to tailor the treatment of a specific patient on the basis of the number of estrogen receptors in a metastatic lesion from carcinoma of the breast. A brain metastasis containing estrogen receptors is more likely to be treated successfully with estrogen-receptor blocking drugs, such as tamoxifen, than are cancers that do not contain estrogen receptors. The presence of progesterone receptors as well as estrogen receptors is the best prognostic sign. Histopathology alone is no longer the only criterion for diagnosis, prognosis, and therapy.

Receptors are also found on pituitary tumors. Using the dopamine-receptor binding agent ^{11}C N-methylspiperone (NMSP), it is possible to classify pituitary adenomas according to whether they possess dopamine receptors. If the tumors contain such receptors, they can be treated chemically rather than surgically by administering the dopamine-receptor agonist bromocriptine. If a tumor contains somatostatin receptors, it can be treated with somatostatin analogs.

After treatment, measurement of the metabolic activity of the tumor makes it possible to detect persistence or recurrence of the tumor and damage to normal brain tissue, such as that resulting from radiation. For example, ^{11}C methionine is useful for delineating the boundaries of brain tumors, providing information of value in the planning and performance of brain surgery by permitting differentiation of the metabolizing brain tumor from simple disruption of the blood-brain barrier.[1]

ANATOMY AND PHYSIOLOGY

The most important clinical techniques of brain imaging are PET with fluorodeoxyglucose (FDG) and SPECT with ^{99m}Tc–labeled hexamethylpropylene amine oxime (HMPAO) or N,N-1,2-ethylenediylbis-L-cysteine diethylester (ECD). Although PET provides somewhat higher spatial resolution and more anatomic details, often the same information can be obtained with either technique. For example, both PET and SPECT show reduced temporal and parietal tracer accumulation in Alzheimer's disease, and both can be used to assess the severity of the disease. In healthy controls, both PET and SPECT demonstrate high tracer accumulation in the cerebral cortex, basal ganglia, thalami, and cerebellar cortex. This is based on the brain's high demand for delivery of oxygen and glucose and removal of its metabolic products.

An understanding of anatomy is as important for appropriate image acquisition as it is for efficient image interpretation. The central nervous system (CNS) consists of the brain and spinal cord. One of the body's largest organs, the brain is divided into four major parts: the cerebrum, the cerebellum, the diencephalon (thalamus and hypothalamus), and the brain stem (Figure 12-3).

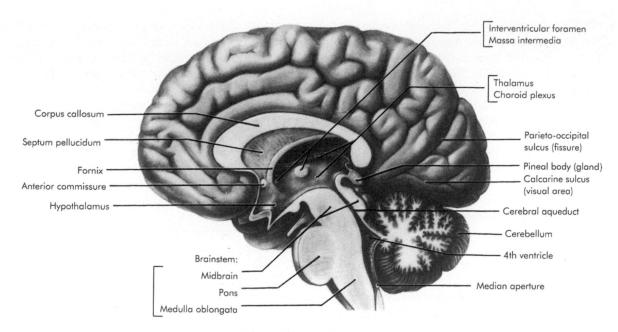

Corpus callosum

Septum pellucidum

Fornix

Anterior commissure

Hypothalamus

Interventricular foramen
Massa intermedia

Thalamus
Choroid plexus

Parieto-occipital
sulcus (fissure)

Pineal body (gland)
Calcarine sulcus
(visual area)

Cerebral aqueduct

Cerebellum

4th ventricle

Median aperture

Brainstem:

Midbrain

Pons

Medulla oblongata

Figure 12-3   Brain anatomy.

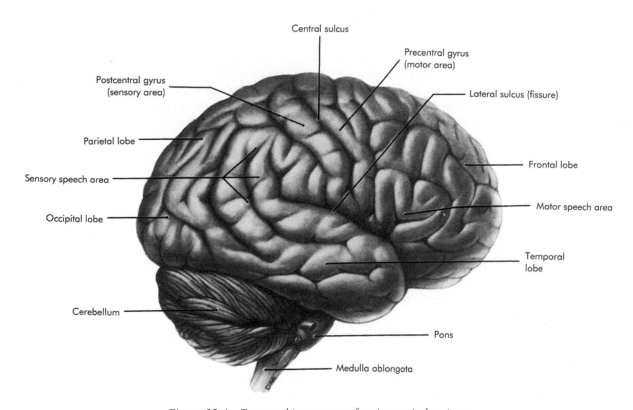

Central sulcus

Precentral gyrus
(motor area)

Postcentral gyrus
(sensory area)

Lateral sulcus (fissure)

Parietal lobe

Sensory speech area

Frontal lobe

Occipital lobe

Motor speech area

Temporal
lobe

Cerebellum

Pons

Medulla oblongata

Figure 12-4   Topographic anatomy of major cortical regions.

Cerebrum

The surface of the cerebrum is composed of gray matter (cerebral cortex). It contains primarily neurons with an underlying layer of white matter, which contains primarily nerve tracts. The two hemispheres of the cortex are connected by the corpus callosum. The cortex (Figure 12-4) is subdivided into four lobes, which are named for the cranial bones that overlie them: the frontal lobe, the temporal lobe, the parietal lobe, and the occipital lobe. The frontal lobe extends from the forehead posteriorly to the central sulcus and inferiorly to the lateral fissure. It is involved in higher mental activities such as planning, judgment, and personality. The prerolandic gyrus is involved in motor function, including speech. The temporal lobe is located below the lateral fissure and extends posteriorly along the sides of the brain. It is involved in hearing, language, memory, and learning. The parietal lobe is separated from the frontal lobe by the central sulcus and from the temporal lobe by the lateral sulcus. The postrolandic region involves sensory function. The occipital lobe is located posteriorly and forms boundaries with the parietal and temporal lobes. It contains the principal cortical areas involving vision.

Deep within each cerebral hemisphere are paired structures of gray matter, called the *basal ganglia,* which are responsible for the control of muscle tone and tremor, the initiation of movement, and emotions. Fibers extend from the basal ganglia to other parts of the cerebral cortex.

Cerebellum

The cerebellum is located in the inferior and posterior portion of the cranial cavity beneath the occipital lobes of the cerebrum. It is involved in the coordination of movement of skeletal muscle, or proprioception; however, other functions, such as memory, can also involve the cerebellum.

Diencephalon (Thalamus and Hypothalamus)

The diencephalon consists primarily of the thalamus and the hypothalamus. The thalamus is composed of two ovoid masses of gray matter, which are involved in the relay of sensory impulses from other parts of the central nervous system. The thalamus also aids in the sensations of pain and temperature. The hypothalamus, also composed of gray matter, is located beneath the thalamus. It is involved in autonomic functions such as regulating body temperature, water balance, pituitary function, hunger, and emotional expression.

Brain Stem

The brain stem consists of the medulla, the pons, and the midbrain. Cardiac and respiratory centers necessary for survival are located here, as are pathways connecting the cerebrum, the cerebellum, and the spinal cord.

Spinal Cord

The spinal cord, composed of both gray and white matter, is a cylindric structure that extends from the medulla and brain stem to the second lumbar vertebra. The spinal cord and its spinal tracts convey sensory impulses to the brain and motor impulses from the brain to the periphery. The spinal cord also contains reflex neuronal circuits.

Ventricular System and Cerebrospinal Fluid (CSF)

Cavities within the brain, called *ventricles,* are filled with cerebrospinal fluid, a transudate of blood formed by the secretion from the choroid plexus located in the lateral, third, and fourth ventricles of the brain (Figure 12-5). CSF is a clear, colorless liquid that protects the brain from shocks, delivers nutritive substances, and removes waste from the brain and spinal cord. The dynamics of CSF flow are demonstrated in Figure 12-6. CSF is produced in the choroid plexus of the lateral ventricles (first and second ventricle) and enters the third ventricle through the interventricular foramen (Monro), where it joins CSF produced in the choroid plexus of this ventricle. It is then transported into the fourth ventricle, which lies between the cerebellum and the pons. CSF leaves the fourth ventricle through the lateral apertures (Luschka) and the median aperture (Magendi) to enter the subarachnoid (thecal) space surrounding the spinal cord. In this space CSF descends along the posterior aspect of the spinal cord and then ascends along the anterior aspect of the cord to enter the system of basal, posterior, midline, and lateral cisterns. The largest posterior cistern is the cisterna magna, which can be punctured for injection of a radioactive tracer if more distal injections at the level of the lumbar spine are contraindicated or technically difficult. Finally, the CSF enters the outer convexities of the brain and is resorbed through the arachnoid granulations into the sagittal sinus.

Blood Supply

The brain is metabolically very active and requires a continual supply of oxygen and glucose. About 20% of the oxygen used by the entire body is consumed by the brain. If deprived of oxygen for more than several minutes, the brain can suffer permanent damage. Although the brain represents only 2% of the total body weight, it requires 20% of the total cardiac output. The brain's total blood is replaced with fresh oxygenated blood six times a minute, which corresponds to a mean perfusion time of 10 seconds. This parameter was previously measured with radionuclide angiography of the brain and currently is used to assess brain perfusion in CT or MRI contrast studies.

Glucose is the principal source of energy for the brain. In fact, measurement of regional glucose utilization is used to reflect neuronal activity of groups of neurons. Areas of the brain involved in mental functions show an increase in the utilization of glucose, as demonstrated with PET.

The right common carotid artery originates from the right subclavian artery, and the left common carotid artery originates from the aorta. At the level of the larynx, these arteries divide into the internal and external carotid arteries. Inside the cranium the right and left internal carotid arteries come together and, with the basilar artery, form the circle of Willis. From this circle of blood vessels arise the anterior and posterior cerebral arteries (Figure 12-7). These arteries are connected with the internal carotid arteries by the anterior and posterior communicating arteries, respectively. The circle of Willis tends to equalize blood pressure to the brain and provides collateral blood flow. Large dural sinuses (superior and inferior sagittal, straight, and transverse) drain

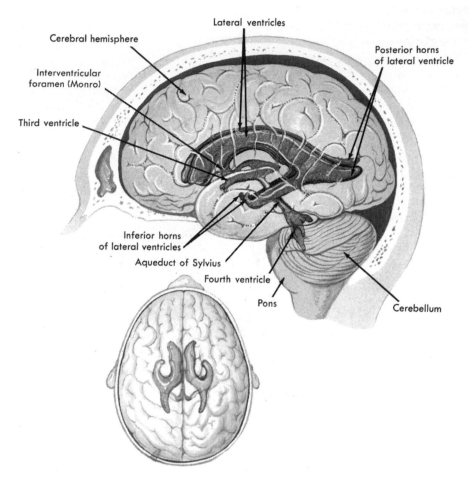

Figure 12-5   Cerebral ventricles projected on the lateral surface of the cerebrum. *Smaller drawing,* Ventricles from above.

blood into the internal jugular veins that descend on either side of the neck and join with the right and left subclavian veins. The joining of the internal jugular with the subclavian vein forms the right and left brachiocephalic veins, which deliver blood to the superior vena cava (Figure 12-8).

Blood-Brain Barrier

The blood-brain barrier (BBB) (Figure 12-9) protects the brain from potentially toxic substances from the diet or metabolic processes. The barrier exists because the brain's capillaries have tight endothelial junctions and continuous basement membranes, which prevent the exit of large molecules. The close approximation of the astrocyte foot processes also restricts the entry of material. Movement of substances across the blood-brain barrier is controlled by active transport or by the degree of lipophilicity of a substance (high lipophilicity enables a substance to cross the cells).

Injury to the brain related to disease, trauma, or toxins often causes the blood-brain barrier to lose its integrity, allowing normally restricted substances to enter the brain. Many of the radiopharmaceuticals used to examine the brain depend on lipophilicity or specific transport processes.

Neurons and Neuroglia

The nervous system consists of two major cell types: neurons and neuroglia. Neurons are highly specialized cells that carry either sensory impulses to the brain (afferent) or motor response impulses to the body with an appropriate response (efferent). There are millions of sensory neurons, tens of millions of motor neurons, and tens of billions of interneurons that connect the two and make complex human mental functioning possible.

Neurons consist of three major parts: the cell body, the dendrite, and the axon (Figure 12-10). Dendrites conduct nerve impulses (action potentials) toward the cell body, which contains the cell nucleus. Axons conduct the nerve impulses away from the cell body to other neurons or tissue. The interface between one neuron and another is called a *synapse.* At the synapse, chemicals called *neurotransmitters* are secreted from membrane-enclosed sacs, called *vesicles,* at the distal end of each axon. The actions of neurotransmitters impinging on a postsynaptic neuron are integrated to determine whether the postsynaptic electrical action potential will be passed to another neuron. Acetylcholine and the catecholamines norepinephrine and dopamine are examples of neurotransmitters. Each of these substances has a characteristic inhibitory or excitatory effect on the neurons. The effect

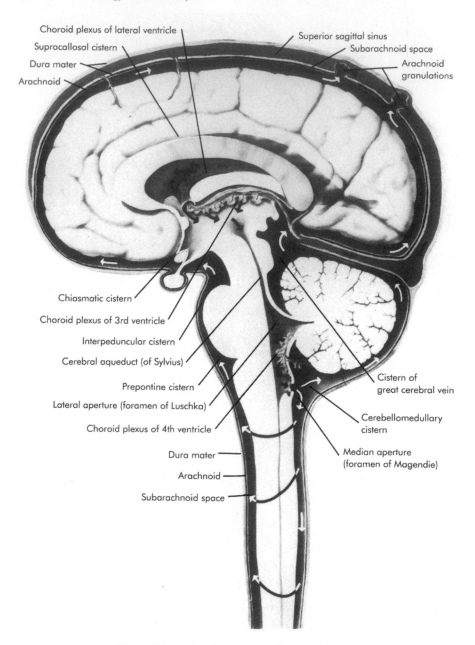

Figure 12-6   Circulation of cerebrospinal fluid.

of acetylcholine is excitatory in the brain and inhibitory in the heart. The repolarization of neurons after transmission of action potentials consumes much of the energy of the brain and accounts for about half of the glucose utilization.

Neuroglial cells do not transmit electrical impulses but instead are supportive and protective of neurons. Some contain neuroreceptors, such as benzodiazepine receptors of a type not found on neurons.

CLINICAL STUDIES

Cerebrovascular Disease

Clinical symptoms and signs often suggest the sites of cortical or subcortical injury in patients who have had an acute

stroke. However, lesions are not always found at the site suggested by clinical manifestations. The clinical picture may be the result of secondary effects, caused by lesions in other locations arising from deafferentation or other effects. The degree of mental dysfunction may be far greater than that suggested by the anatomic lesions seen in computed tomography (CT) or magnetic resonance imaging (MRI). Subcortical lesions, such as lacunar infarctions, can result in extensive cortical dysfunction on the affected side. The neurologic examination cannot effectively predict what the patient's eventual neurologic deficiency will be. CT often cannot reveal the extent of involvement until structural changes have developed several days after the onset of symptoms and signs. Arteriography can reveal the status of large vessels but does not provide information about cerebral

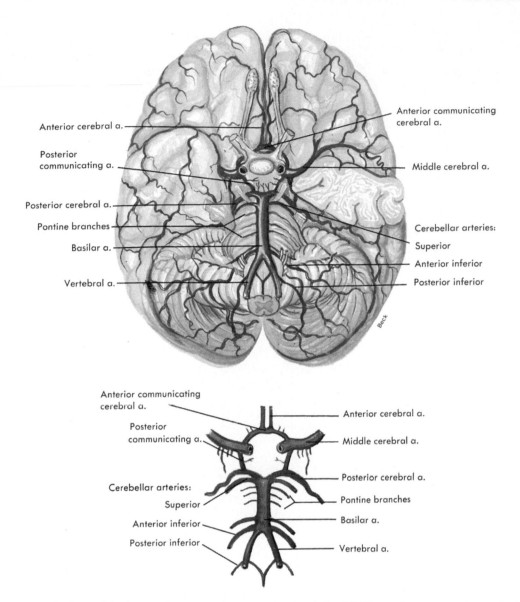

Figure 12-7   Arteries at the base of the brain. The arteries that comprise the circle of Willis are the two anterior cerebral arteries, which are joined to each other by the anterior communicating cerebral artery and to posterior communicating arteries.

perfusion through the microcirculation. SPECT and PET make it possible to delineate the severity and extent of the perfusion defects from the time of onset of the stroke (Figure 12-11).

PET makes it possible to measure cerebral blood flow, glucose and oxygen metabolism, or blood volume, thus providing a more complete understanding of the severity of the patient's illness. The area of lowest regional blood flow or metabolism usually predicts the region that will eventually develop radiolucency on CT, although the perfusion and metabolic lesions are often larger. The blood flow or metabolic abnormalities seen with PET or SPECT correlate better with the neurologic defects than do those seen with CT or MRI. The nuclear medicine images reflect function, whereas CT and MRI images reflect structure. Studies of the cerebral circulation are helpful in establishing a prognosis after acute cerebral ischemia. In stroke, metabolic abnormalities seen on PET frequently are more extensive than the corresponding CT findings. The pattern of metabolic abnormalities in PET correlates with the clinical syndrome and with the degree of eventual recovery.[11,7]

Tumors

Tumors involving the central nervous system are a treatable cause of neuropsychiatric dysfunction. Glioblastoma multiforme occurs in 15% to 20% of all intracranial neoplasms. Treatment includes surgical resection, external radiotherapy, and chemotherapy. At times, radiation necrosis of the brain occurs in patients who have received 5,000 to 6,000 rad of external radiation therapy. The use of nuclear medicine technology can define the precise localization of the extent of the tumor better than CT or MRI, which often reveal the response of the body to tumor, such as edema. Nuclear

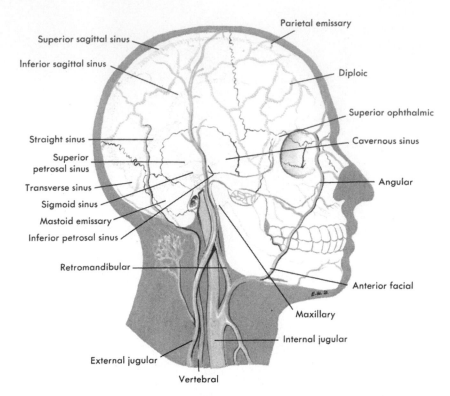

Figure 12-8 Semischematic projections of the large veins of the head. Deep veins and dural sinuses are projected on the skull. Note the connections (emissary veins) between the superficial and deep veins.

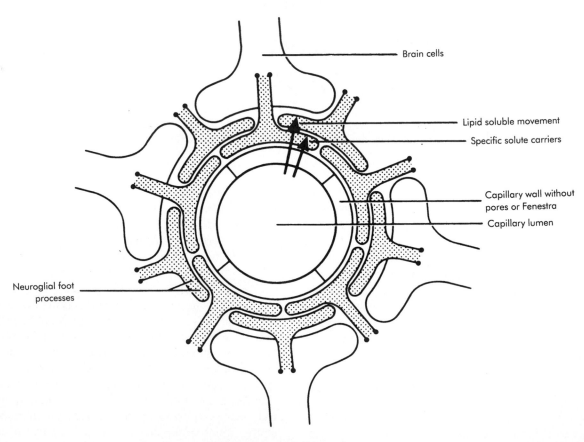

Figure 12-9 Blood-brain barrier.

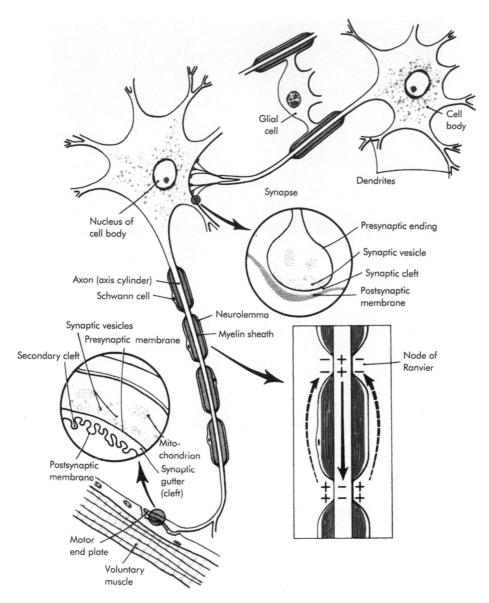

Figure 12-10   Neurons of the central nervous system. Neuron *A* is confined to the CNS and terminates on neuron *B* at a typical chemical synapse (*C*). Neuron *B* is a ventral horn cell; its axon extends to a peripheral nerve and innervates a voluntary muscle at the myoneural junction (*D*). In *E* the action potential is moving in the direction of the solid arrow inside the axon; the dashed arrows indicate the direction of flow of the action current.

studies also can help distinguish between the tumor and the effects of radiation (Figure 12-12).

When neurologic symptoms recur or change in patients treated with radiation, it is virtually impossible to distinguish radiation necrosis and gliosis from tumor recurrence by anatomic imaging techniques or clinical examination. Nuclear procedures often eliminate the need for a second craniotomy and tissue biopsy.[1,10,19] Cerebral blood flow and blood volume are not well correlated with the degree of malignancy, therefore metabolic studies are preferred.

Epilepsy

Epilepsy is one of the most common diseases of the brain. Approximately 800,000 Americans have focal seizures that do not progress to grand mal seizures (partial complex epilepsy). For most patients with partial epilepsy, diagnosis and classification are based on the use of surface electroencephalography (EEG), which records electrical activity associated with neuronal activity. However, for the approximately 20% of patients who are uncontrolled by medication (intractable epilepsy), additional information about localization of the epileptic focus is required if surgical therapy is anticipated. Radiologic techniques such as CT and MRI scanning usually show no abnormalities in these patients. Special localizing measures, including intraoperative electrocorticography and direct recordings from stereotaxically implanted depth electrodes, are valuable for improved localization, but these techniques can give rise to conflicting results and are accompanied by certain risks. In

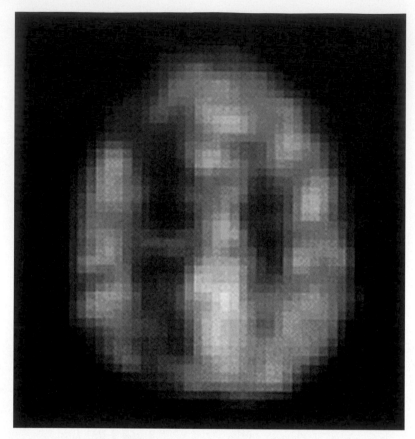

Figure 12-11 ECD SPECT scan of a subject with acute stroke. The most severe reduction of cerebral blood flow is seen in the right frontal lobe.

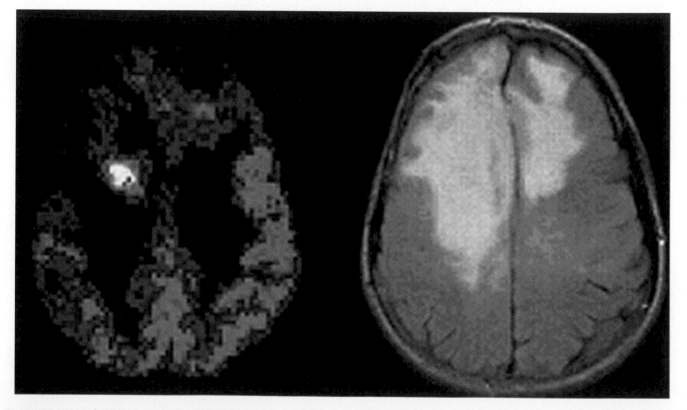

Figure 12-12 *Left,* MRI shows wide structural changes caused by radiation treatment that do not allow precise delineation of the tumor. *Right,* Recurrent brain tumor in the right frontal lobe clearly demonstrated with FDG PET.

such a setting the PET scan can provide independent, confirmatory information about the site of the epileptogenic lesion (Figure 12-13).

In the intraictal state (during seizures), brain metabolism and blood flow are increased at the site of onset of the seizures and in regions to which the seizure activity is propagated. In the interictal state (between seizures), both metabolism and blood flow are reduced at the site of onset. When PET was first applied in epilepsy, it was anticipated and subsequently confirmed that PET imaging would localize these focal changes in cerebral metabolism and perfusion and thus provide unique diagnostic information useful in the management of patients with epilepsy.[16]

PET scans obtained during partial complex seizures have shown marked increases in local brain metabolism and perfusion at the site of seizure onset, but because of propagated neuronal activity, the ictal scans are less useful in predicting epileptic origin than those made during the interictal state.[3-5] PET scans made during nonfocal seizures show a generalized increase in brain metabolism and perfusion. Unlike the typical PET scans found in partial epilepsy, no focal changes are found during interictal or ictal scans of patients with petit mal seizures. A diffuse increase of metabolism is seen at the time of the petit mal seizure.

PET scans obtained during the interictal state are most valuable in the management of the patient with partial complex seizures (older term: temporal lobe epilepsy or psychomotor epilepsy) in which consciousness is impaired. PET and SPECT are less useful in generalized seizures. The results of interictal PET scans in patients with complex partial seizures have been compared with the results of CT and EEG in multiple reports.[9,15,22] These studies showed that approximately 70% of the patients had zones of hypometabolism on interictal FDG scans in the involved regions.

PET and EEG are complementary methods of localizing areas in the brain causing epileptic activity. Focal abnormalities can be identified with PET even if EEG data are unable to reveal the focus. The combined use of surface EEG and PET has eliminated the need for depth electrodes in some surgical candidates. PET can aid in the localization of the site when the EEG findings are inconsistent. EEG can verify the epileptogenic nature of a zone of hypometabolism determined by PET. An excellent correlation has been obtained between the site of hypometabolism as determined by PET and the presence of a pathologic abnormality in the surgical specimen.

In patients with epilepsy, PET imaging provides information about local brain function that is quite different from the results of electrical measurements with EEG or structural assessments with CT. The combination of PET and EEG has been useful in presurgical evaluation for determining the site of seizure onset in patients with complex partial epilepsy

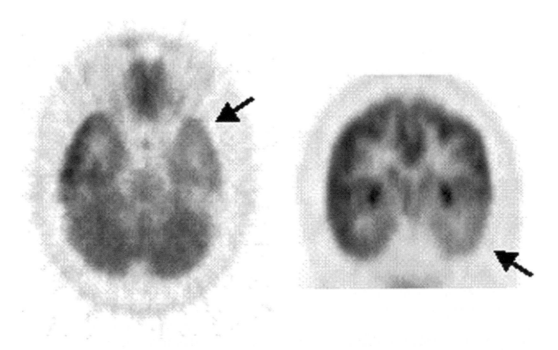

Figure 12-13 Transaxial and coronal slices of an F-18-fluorodeoxyglucose (FDG) PET scan of a patient with complex partial seizures. The arrows point to reduced metabolism in the left temporal lobe. An MRI study was unremarkable.

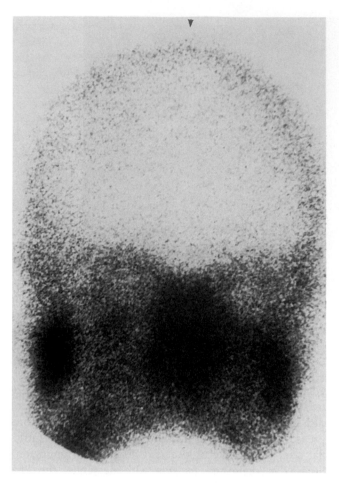

Figure 12-15 Brain death: early flow images demonstrated no intracranial blood flow. This image, obtained 1 minute after injection of the radiopharmaceutical, reveals an absence of tracer activity in the longitudinal sinus, indicating a complete absence of cerebral perfusion.

blood flow through the cerebral cortex; that is, no filling of the sagittal and transverse sinuses.

CSF Dynamics

CSF dynamics can be investigated after injection of indium-111 (^{111}In)-labeled diethylenetriamine pentaacetic acid (DTPA). The following three types of studies are used in nuclear medicine:

- *Radionuclide cisternogram,* which is used for the diagnosis of hydrocephalus. The tracer is injected into the subarachnoid space of the lumbar spine, and the head is imaged at 3 hours and 24 hours after injection.
- *Radionuclide shuntogram,* which is used for evaluation of the patency of ventriculoperitoneal shunts. The tracer is injected into the shunt reservoir, and images of the head and abdomen are obtained immediately after injection, 3 hours after injection and, if necessary, 24 hours after injection.
- *CSF leak imaging,* which is used for diagnosis of cerebrospinal fluid leaks. The tracer is injected into the

lumbar subarachnoid space, and images of the head are obtained 3 hours and 24 hours after injection.

A normal cisternogram (Figure 12-16) shows activity in the basal cisterns by 3 hours after injection, with flow over the convexities by 24 hours. No reflux into the ventricles is seen. In communicating hydrocephalus (Figure 12-17), reflux into the ventricles is seen with a delayed flow over the convexities. Noncommunicating hydrocephalus shows a lack of ventricular reflux and slow or normal flow over the convexities. Normal pressure hydrocephalus shows a ventricular reflux that persists 24 to 72 hours. The flow over the convexities is significantly delayed or absent.

In noncommunicating hydrocephalus, constant production of CSF and its inability to escape results in enlargement of the ventricles, which leads to compression and atrophy of the cerebral cortex and dementia. Ventriculoperitoneal (VP) shunts are used to divert the CSF from the ventricles. VP shunts consist of a proximal tubing, a reservoir, and a distal tubing. The proximal tubing connects the cerebral ventricle with the reservoir, and the distal tubing connects the reservoir with the peritoneal cavity. Less frequently, shunts are placed that connect the reservoir with the pleural space or the cardiac atrium.

There are two established tracer injection techniques for these cases. With the first, more popular technique, a small volume of the tracer is injected into the shunt reservoir and the injection tube is not flushed. This results in visualization of the reservoir and the distal tubing within minutes and spread of activity within the abdomen within an hour if both the proximal and the distal tubings are patent. Lack of tracer propagation is seen with obstruction of either the proximal or the distal tubing. With the second technique, a somewhat larger volume of the tracer is injected into the shunt reservoir, the distal tubing is compressed by a finger, and the radioactivity is forced to flow retrograde into the ventricles. This manipulation demonstrates whether the proximal tubing is patent. Subsequent spontaneous tracer clearance from the entire system into the abdomen demonstrates patency of the rest of the shunt. Delayed views are needed to show transport of the tracer and its dispersion in the pleural or peritoneal cavity.

In patients with injuries of the skull base and suspected CSF fluid leakage, the tracer is injected into the lumbar thecal space and its accumulation is imaged in the head. Pledgets are placed in the nostrils and removed when imaging shows that sufficient radioactivity has entered the basal cisterns. Sometimes the leak can be seen on the scintigraphic images; more often, however, leakage is discovered based on gamma counting of the pledgets and their comparison to plasma activity.

RADIOPHARMACEUTICALS

Both PET and SPECT are suited to investigation of the cerebral blood flow and receptor distribution in the brain. PET imaging of glucose metabolism with ^{18}F-labeled FDG

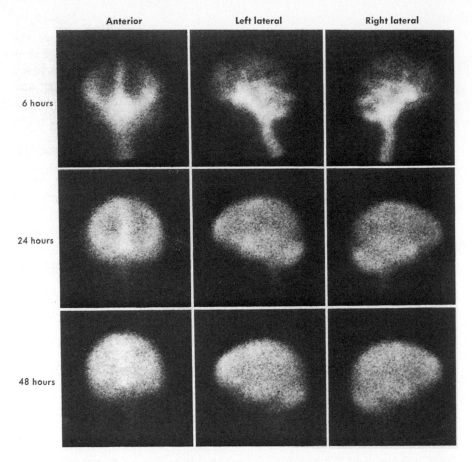

Figure 12-16   Normal cisternogram showing anterior and both lateral views at 6, 24, and 48 hours after intrathecal administration of the radiopharmaceutical.

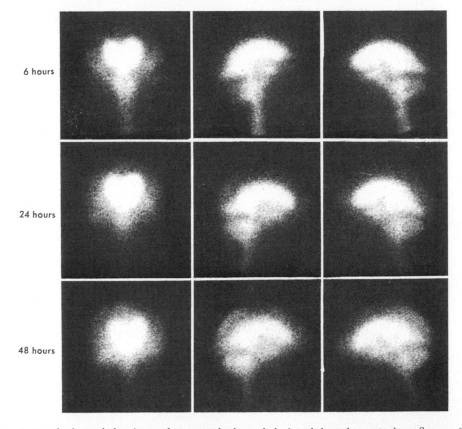

Figure 12-17   Communicating hydrocephalus (normal pressure hydrocephalus) with lateral ventricular reflux on 6-hour images and no significant ventricular clearing on 24- and 48-hour images.

provides better image quality than imaging of cerebral blood flow with SPECT. However, PET is less frequently used in the clinical routine because of its higher price and the lack of coverage by Medicare.

Before the development of contrast imaging techniques for MRI and CT of the brain, gamma camera brain imaging was used for the diagnosis of stroke and brain tumors. However, the mechanism of radiotracer accumulation involved damage of the blood-brain barrier and leakage of the tracer into the brain tissue. Single photon–emitting radiopharmaceuticals based on detection of a compromised blood-brain barrier included ^{99m}Tc pertechnetate and ^{99m}Tc DTPA.

Currently tumors of the brain are imaged either with FDG PET or with SPECT tracers such as thallium-201 (^{201}Tl). Like many radiopharmaceuticals, ^{201}Tl does not cross the blood-brain barrier in normal individuals, but it diffuses rapidly across an altered BBB. Thallium and SPECT have been used to diagnose brain tumors, clarify the nature of lesions found with CT or MRI, and detect tumor recurrence. The positive predictive value is much better than the negative predictive value, and thallium is usually not very helpful in determining the tumor type or predicting the clinical outcome. A dose of 2 mCi is used, and images may be obtained as soon as 10 minutes after injection.

Single photon radiopharmaceuticals used for the evaluation of regional brain perfusion include ^{99m}Tc HMPAO and ^{99m}Tc ECD.

^{99m}Tc HMPAO is a neutral lipid-soluble radiopharmaceutical that crosses the blood-brain barrier and remains trapped in the brain in a manner proportional to the cerebral blood flow. It can be used to reflect regional cerebral blood flow in a manner analogous to the use of microspheres that are trapped in cerebral capillaries. The relatively long retention time (24 hours) combined with the availability and superior imaging characteristics of ^{99m}Tc are attractive features. The average adult dose of ^{99m}Tc HMPAO is 20 mCi.[21,22] The most important application of ^{99m}Tc HMPAO is diagnosis of brain death.

^{99m}Tc ECD, which is more stable than ^{99m}Tc HMPAO, is the radiotracer most frequently used for imaging of the cerebral blood flow. It has a high first-pass extraction, and in vivo conversion of this lipophilic agent into nondiffusable metabolites occurs more slowly than for HMPAO.

PET extends the technology to include biologically important radiotracers that can be synthesized using radioactive forms of carbon (^{11}C), oxygen (^{15}O), nitrogen (^{13}N), and fluorine (^{18}F, a hydrogen substitute). Many of the radiotracers are identical to substances normally found in the body. These radionuclides are cyclotron produced and have short half-lives, therefore they require rapid synthesis and also quality assurance methods. Radiopharmaceutical doses range from 5 to 10 mCi for ^{18}F FDG to 20 mCi for ^{11}C compounds.

The development of regional pharmacies to distribute PET radiopharmaceuticals to hospitals and clinics unable to obtain and support a cyclotron will extend the benefits of PET to more patients.

^{111}In DTPA is an ideal radiopharmaceutical for the assessment of CSF dynamics. It satisfies the following criteria: (1) it is physiologically governed by CSF flow; (2) it has an adequate physical half-life of 2.8 days for the study; (3) it has a desirable photon emission for imaging (173 and 247 keV); (4) it has a relatively low radiation dose in the patient; (5) it has the least probable chemical toxicity; and (6) it has a controlled radiopharmaceutical quality.

A physician performing a lumbar puncture administers 500 μCi of ^{111}In DTPA intrathecally to the patient. A 21- to 22-gauge spinal needle connected to a three-way stopcock is often used to monitor CSF pressure, sample the CSF for routine cell and chemical tests, and administer the radiopharmaceutical flush. The patient is kept in a horizontal position for 2 hours after injection to minimize headaches caused by CSF leakage.

PLANAR, PET, AND SPECT IMAGING

Many problems can be solved by planar imaging alone, but the value of tomography in all types of medical imaging is now well established. For all imaging modalities, whether anatomic in orientation, as in CT, or physiologic and biochemical, as in nuclear medicine, viewing the body from a ring of viewpoints surrounding it increases contrast between lesions and normal tissues, which translates into improved diagnostic information.[2,14] For clinical problems in which the solution requires a high degree of spatial resolution (e.g., locating the point of origin of an epileptic seizure), PET or SPECT is always better than planar imaging.[17]

The most important difference between PET and SPECT lies in the radiotracers used with each. PET is based chiefly on the use of ^{11}C, ^{18}F, ^{15}O, and ^{13}N, the first two being the most commonly used.[12] The workhorse of SPECT is ^{99m}Tc. Other differences include the greater sensitivity of PET and the more accurate quantification, which results from the better ability to correct for attenuation. Generally, laboratories purchasing new equipment select SPECT rather than planar imaging systems. Although the image quality of PET is better than the image quality of SPECT, SPECT studies currently are performed much more frequently than PET studies because of the broader availability of SPECT scanners and SPECT tracers and because of the reluctance of health insurance companies to cover the costs of PET studies.

IMAGE ACQUISITION TECHNIQUES

Planar Imaging

The most important application of planar brain imaging is in the diagnosis of brain death. Two types of radiopharmaceuticals can be used, those that distribute in the cerebral parenchyma according to the blood flow (HMPAO and ECD) and those that distribute in the blood vessels (^{99m}Tc pertechnetate and ^{99m}Tc DTPA). Images are obtained during the blood flow phase and immediately after the accumulation of the tracers. For the blood flow phase, images are obtained at 3-second intervals for 1 to 2 minutes. These images demonstrate tracer present in the arteries and veins in subjects without brain death and absence of such activity in subjects with brain death, because brain death is equivalent to a complete absence of cerebral perfusion. This portion of the study provides identical information with both the vascular and parenchymal tracers, but it requires careful execution and may be uninterpretable if the injection site is infiltrated, if the camera is not set to the right energy window, or if image acquisition on the computer is not started immediately. In such situations delayed views are very helpful, because adequate time is available to correct the acquisition parameters and reposition the patient for this phase of the study.[20] Delayed views are particularly useful if tracers with parenchymal accumulation (HMPA and ECD) were injected, because they clearly show accumulation in the brain if brain death is absent and no accumulation if brain death is present.

CSF Imaging

The injection site is imaged immediately after radiopharmaceutical administration to rule out extravasation of the injected dose outside the subarachnoid space. If a wide segmental appearance is seen initially with no activity in the basal cisterns at 2 to 3 hours, re-injection is required.

Imaging is routinely performed at 2, 6, 24, and 48 hours after injection. Anterior and one or both lateral projections of the head and an anterior image of the abdomen are obtained 2 hours after injection for 200,000 counts. Positioning of these projections is the same as that used in planar brain imaging. Additional views of the head or spine may be indicated. No data processing is required unless CSF rhinorrhea is assessed.

The quantitative diagnosis of CSF rhinorrhea can begin 2 hours after intrathecal administration of ^{111}In DTPA. Cotton pledgets ($1\,cm^2$) are placed in each nostril by an otorhinolaryngologist in locations of suspected CSF leakage. A string is attached to each pledget to allow for retrieval and labeling of the anatomic location. A 5 ml heparinized blood sample is obtained from the patient when the pledgets are placed. The pledgets are removed 6 hours after injection of the radiopharmaceutical, and a second 5 ml heparinized blood sample is obtained. After centrifugation of both blood samples, 0.5 ml of plasma is withdrawn from each sample. A scintillation well counter with a 150 to 250 keV window is used to count each pledget and each blood sample. The results are expressed as the ratio of pledget activity (cpm) divided by the average plasma activity (cpm). Normal pledget to plasma ratios are 1 : 1.3. Anterior, posterior, and lateral images are obtained for 200,000 counts. Images should be obtained with the patient in a position that optimizes visualization of CSF leakage. Radiation safety and contamination precautions should be observed.

A variety of shunts are used to remove excess CSF from patients with hydrocephalus. A lumboperitoneal shunt consists of a tubing system placed in the lumbar subarachnoid space and extending into the abdominal cavity. A ventriculoperitoneal shunt consists of a ventricular catheter extending from the ventricles to a valve and distal tubing that drains into the peritoneal cavity. The Ommaya shunt is a system consisting of a reservoir and tubing used to deliver chemotherapeutic agents to the ventricles and the subarachnoid space. Nuclear medicine procedures are performed to evaluate the patency of the shunt and, in the case of the Ommaya shunt, to evaluate the distribution pattern of the radiotracer in the CSF to predict the distribution of chemotherapeutic agents.

Single Photon Emission Computed Tomography (SPECT)

The time required for a SPECT brain procedure, including patient preparation, is approximately 1 hour. The imaging room should be quiet and dimly lit to minimize the environmental effect on the distribution of the radiotracer. An intravenous (IV) line should be placed before injection of the radiotracer so that the patient does not experience pain when the radiotracer is injected. The patient is placed in a comfortable supine position with the head in a head holder and immobilized with a Velcro strap. Custom-fitted face masks are also available. Care must be taken to monitor the patient for motion during the imaging procedure. Often patients with certain neurologic disorders find it difficult to maintain a fixed position during the scanning procedure. The sagittal plane of the patient's head should be perpendicular to the table. The head is flexed so that the cerebellum is included in the field of view. The detector must be positioned as close as possible to the patient's head to ensure acquisition of high-quality images.

The rotating gamma camera is equipped with a low-energy, high-resolution parallel hole collimator. Fan beam collimators currently are used to improve the resolution of the images. A computer with SPECT capabilities is required for acquisition and processing of the imaging procedure.

The acquisition begins approximately 20 minutes after injection of the radiopharmaceutical. A general guideline for acquisition should include 64 images acquired for 20 to 40 seconds each through a range of 360 degrees. The patient's ability to endure the acquisition should be considered in the selection of the acquisition time. When choosing the acquisition matrix, the theory that each pixel should approximate half of the extrinsic full-width half-maximum (FWHM) provides a general rule. A 128×128 matrix, although providing good resolution, might not contain a statistically valid number of counts per pixel and requires longer reconstruction times and a greater need for computer disk space. Magnification can be used to keep both the matrix and pixel size small. A 64×64 matrix with a magnification factor (2.0) applied approximates a 128×128 matrix. This saves reconstruction time and reduces the amount of computer disk space used. Table 12-1 provides guidelines for brain SPECT acquisition on single-, dual-, and triple-head gamma cameras.

SPECT brain images are obtained using a filtered back-projection technique. To produce high-resolution, low-noise images, a combination of pre-processing, back-projection, and post-processing filters is used (Table 12-2). The selection of an appropriate SPECT processing protocol depends on the radiopharmaceutical, the imaging instrumentation, and the computer software being used. A knowledge of cross-sectional anatomy is essential for processing data for

subsequent interpretation by the nuclear medicine physician (Figure 12-18).

Center of rotation and field uniformity corrections should be performed during reconstruction to improve the overall quality of the SPECT images. Attenuation correction is accomplished using a computer-generated ellipse fitted to the brain image. Using existing calculations, the correction is performed within the ellipse. Failure to perform these corrections can result in the loss of detail of smaller structures located within the brain.

SPECT brain images can be reoriented along the x, y, or z axes or in a specific oblique plane; this allows for correc-

Table 12-1	SPECT acquisition parameters*			
Number of detectors	**Number of images per detector**	**Time per image**	**Matrix size**	**Collimator**
One detector	60	30 sec	64 × 64	High resolution
Two detectors	60	30 sec	128 × 128	High resolution/fan beam
Three detectors	40	45 sec	64 × 64	High resolution/fan beam

*30-Minute acquisition.

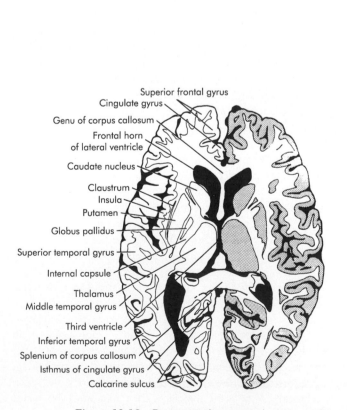

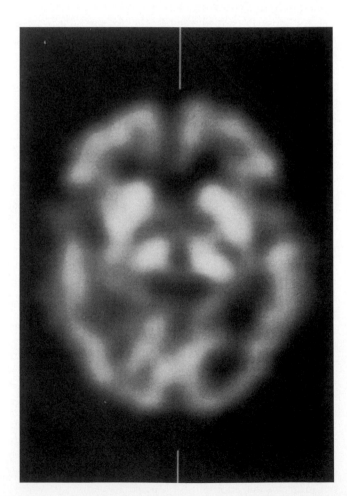

Figure 12-18 Representative anatomic cross sections of the brain and a PET study obtained at the same level.

tion of positioning errors as well. The images can be quantitated using left-to-right hemisphere ratio programs or by placing individual regions of interest over specific structures located in the brain.

A common method of display of SPECT brain images allows the sagittal, coronal, and transverse planes to be displayed simultaneously (Figure 12-19). This allows the physician to correlate images on one view with the other two tomographic planes. Volume and surface rendering programs allow three-dimensional display of brain SPECT images, which can be useful in localizing and determining the extent of disease.

Positron Emission Tomography (PET)

A radiopharmaceutical undergoing positron decay emits a positron with a range of energies characteristic of the radionuclide. Once emitted, a positron is an antimatter electron that travels several millimeters in tissue and encounters a free electron in the tissue, resulting in annihilation and subsequent release of two 511 keV photons at 180 degrees to each other. These photons are detected by a ring of opposing detectors surrounding the patient. When two 511 keV photons are detected by these electronically coupled detectors, an annihilation event is assumed to have occurred along the line joining the two detectors. The direction of travel of the photons is electronically determined without the need for a collimator.[12]

Upon acquisition of the raw data, the first step in PET image processing is reconstruction. The coincidence data are reoriented into a set of parallel projections. A standard

Table 12-2	Processing filters
Type of filter	**Use and effect**
Pre-processing	Two-dimensional filter applied to planar views before reconstruction, with resulting smoothing effect
Reconstruction	Simple back-projection technique of the ramp filter; range of filters used (high-frequency noise contribution to filters, which drastically smooth image)
Post-processing	Filter applied in all three dimensions of reconstructed image; smoothing

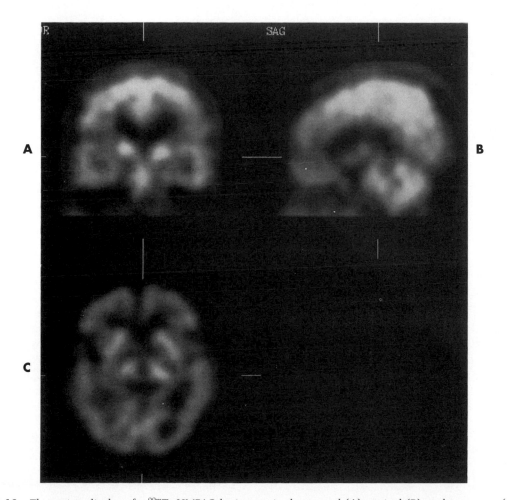

Figure 12-19   Three-view display of a ^{99m}Tc HMPAO brain scan in the coronal (**A**), sagittal (**B**), and transverse (**C**) planes.

back-filtered projection algorithm is used to reconstruct transverse slices. The final image obtained depends on the filter selected in the reconstruction process and the reconstruction algorithm. Once an image is obtained, further processing can be performed, depending on the purpose of the procedure.

Attenuation correction is routinely performed in PET and is accomplished by a calculated correction using an ellipse or by a measured correction using a transmission scan. Because of the short half-life of PET radiotracers, decay correction can also be performed. PET brain images can be quantitated by placing individual regions of interest over specific structures located in the brain.

With the so-called two-dimensional (2D) imaging technique, lead collimators are used ("septa out" technique) to limit the number of detector rings that can simultaneously detect the same positron decay event. In newer PET scanners with more powerful computers used for image reconstruction, the collimators can be removed ("septa in" technique) and images obtained in three-dimensional (3D) mode. This results in much higher photon density registration and higher image quality as a result of reduced noise. Patient throughput is also increased.

For FDG PET imaging the patient is injected with 10 mCi of FDG. Beginning 5 minutes before injection and for 30 minutes afterward, the patient is asked to sit quietly in an armchair with the legs and arms uncrossed. The patient is asked to refrain from talking and reading. The room lights are kept low, the patient's eyes are covered with a piece of black cloth, and the ears are plugged. The purpose of these preparations is to minimize sensory stimulation and activation of the patient's brain, particularly the auditory and visual centers.

With new PET scanners the entire brain can be covered with a single field of view. Three scans are required: an emission scan, an emission plus transmission scan, and a transmission-emission subtraction scan. Typically the 3D FDG emission scan is 20 minutes long, and the images are reconstructed in a 128×128 matrix, 25.6 cm diameter, using a ramp transaxial filter with a cutoff of 4 mm and an axial filter width of 8.5 mm. The transmission scan is obtained in 2D and is 10 minutes long.

With hybrid PET/CT scanners, instead of germanium-68, a CT scan is used for transmission imaging and attenuation correction. Typical CT parameters are helical high-speed acquisition, 1 second per rotation, 5 mm slice thickness, 22.5 mm per rotation, 140 kVp, 90 mA, 7.7 seconds total time (with a four-detector scanner), single field of view, and 35 slices. This CT protocol results in an average radiation exposure of 7.71 mGy.

REFERENCES

1. Conti PS: Brain and spinal cord. In Wagner HN Jr, Szabo Z, Buchanan JW, editors: *Principles of nuclear medicine,* ed 2, Philadelphia, 1996, WB Saunders.

2. Datz F: *Handbooks in radiology: nuclear medicine,* Chicago, 1988, Year Book Medical.

3. Engel J Jr, Ackermann RF, Kuhl DE et al: Brain imaging of glucose utilization in convulsive disorders. In Sokoloff L, editor: *Brain imaging and brain function: association for research in nervous and mental disease,* vol 63, New York, 1985, Raven Press.

4. Engel J Jr, Kuhl DE, Phelps ME: Regional brain metabolism during seizures in humans, *Adv Neurol* 34:141-148, 1983.

5. Engel J Jr, Lubens P, Kuhl DE et al: Local cerebral metabolic rate for glucose during petit mal absences, *Ann Neurol* 17:121-128, 1985.

6. Foster NL, Chase TN, Mansi L et al: Cortical abnormalities in Alzheimer's disease, *Ann Neurol* 16:649-654, 1984.

7. Frackowiak RSF: Pathophysiology of human cerebral ischemia: studies with positron tomography and ^{15}oxygen. In Sokoloff L, editor: *Brain imaging and brain function,* New York, 1985, Raven Press.

8. Friedland RP, Budinger TF, Ganz E et al: Regional cerebral metabolic alterations in dementia of the Alzheimer type: positron emission tomography with [^{18}F] fluorodeoxyglucose, *J Comput Assist Tomogr* 7:590-598, 1983.

9. Frost JJ, Mayberg HS: Epilepsy. In Wagner HN Jr, Szabo Z, Buchanan JW, editors: *Principles of nuclear medicine,* ed 2, Philadelphia, 1996, WB Saunders.

10. Glantz MJ, Hoffman JM, Coleman RE et al: Identification of early recurrence of primary central nervous system tumors by [^{18}F] fluorodeoxyglucose positron emission tomography, *Ann Neurol* 29:347-355, 1991.

11. Heiss W-D, Podreka I: Cerebrovascular disease. In Wagner HN Jr, Szabo Z, Buchanan JW, editors: *Principles of nuclear medicine,* ed 2, Philadelphia, 1995, WB Saunders.

12. Hubner K, Collmann J, Buonocore E et al: *Clinical positron emission tomography,* St Louis, 1992, Mosby.

13. Jones AG, Meltzer PC, Blundell P et al: Technepine: a technetium-99m SPECT agent for labeling the dopamine transporter in brain, *J Nucl Med* 37(suppl):17P, 1996.

14. Klingensmith W, Eshima D, Goddard J: *Nuclear medicine procedure manual,* Engelwood, Colo, 1991, Oxford Medical.

15. Kuhl DE, Engel J Jr, Phelps ME: Emission computed tomography in the study of human epilepsy. In Ward AA Jr, Penry JK, Purpura D, editors: *Epilepsy,* New York, 1983, Raven Press.

16. Kuhl DE, Engel J Jr, Phelps ME et al: Epileptic patterns of local cerebral metabolism and perfusion in humans determined by emission computed tomography of FDG and NH, *Ann Neurol* 8:348-360, 1980.

17. Links JM: Nuclear medicine physics, instrumentation, and data processing in pharmaceutical research. In Burns HD, Gibson RE, Dannals RF et al, editors: *Nuclear imaging in drug discovery, development, and approval,* Boston, 1993, Brikhäuser.

18. Meegalla SK, Plössl K, Kung M-P et al: Tc-99m labeled tropanes as dopamine transporter imaging agents, *J Nucl Med* 37(suppl):17P, 1996.

19. Patronas NJ, Di Chiro G, Kufta C et al: Prediction of survival in glioma patients by means of PET, *J Neurosurg* 62:816-822, 1985.

20. Rowell K, Harkness B, Christian P: *Clinical computers in nuclear medicine,* New York, 1992, Technologist Section, Society of Nuclear Medicine.

21. *SPECT brain imaging with Ceretec: a clinician's guide,* Arlington Heights, Ill, 1989, Amersham.

22. Theodore WH, Dorwart R, Holmes M et al: Neuroimaging in refractory partial seizures: comparison of PET, CT, and MRI, *Neurology* 36:60-64, 1986.

SUGGESTED READINGS

Sandler MP, Coleman RE, Patton JA et al, editors: *Diagnostic nuclear medicine,* ed 4, Baltimore, 2002, Lippincott Williams & Wilkins.

Wagner HN: Chemical neurotransmission in man, *Curr Conc Diagn Nucl Med* 3:14-18, 1986.

Wagner HN Jr, Szabo Z, Buchanan JW, editors: *Principles of nuclear medicine,* ed 2, Philadelphia, 1996, WB Saunders.

Stanley J. Goldsmith

chapter **13**

Endocrine System

Objectives

List the organs that comprise the endocrine system, describe their anatomy and physiology, and explain the relationships of their hormonal functions.

Discuss the choice of radionuclides that may be used for thyroid uptake and imaging procedures relative to their advantages and disadvantages for imaging.

Discuss the role of radioiodine uptake, thyroid scan, and whole body imaging in the planning of radioiodine therapy.

Discuss radionuclide therapy for the treatment of hyperthyroidism.

Describe procedures for treating thyroid carcinoma using radioiodine.

Explain procedures for parathyroid imaging using sestamibi-pertechnetate subtraction techniques and dual-phase sestamibi imaging.

Discuss the role of somatostatin-receptor imaging.

Describe the use of radiopharmaceuticals for imaging of the adrenal glands.

*T*he term *endocrine system* applies to the small group of organs that have the principal function of elaboration of hormones. Hormones are biologically active substances that have regulatory effects on diverse metabolic and biochemical processes throughout the body. The principal endocrine glands are the pituitary gland (anterior and posterior), the thyroid gland, the parathyroid glands, the islet cells of the pancreas, the adrenal glands (cortex and medulla), and the gonads (ovaries and testes).

Recent advances in cell biology have led to the recognition that biologically active substances are secreted by many cells scattered in tissues throughout the body. Many cells and tissues have specific receptors for these secretions. These observations have extended the scope of classic endocrinology into tumor, gastrointestinal, and vascular biology. For the purposes of this review, the definition of the endocrine system has been broadened from the classical list of individual organs to include the so-called neuroendocrine tissues, which are distributed throughout the organs that evolve from the primitive foregut (bronchus and lungs), midgut (stomach, small intestine, and pancreas), and hindgut (large bowel) and the chromaffin autonomic nervous system tissue (including the adrenal medulla).

In vivo nuclear medicine, both imaging and nonimaging applications, has played a significant role in the current understanding of the function and disorders of the endocrine glands, classically the thyroid, parathyroid, and adrenal glands and more recently the distributed neuroendocrine cells. Moreover, nuclear medicine diagnostic techniques are useful for monitoring treatment of the disorders that affect these organs and cells, as well as tumors arising from them. Iodine-131 (^{131}I) is used as a therapeutic agent in the clinical management of patients with hyperthyroidism or thyroid carcinoma. Clinical trials are underway to evaluate whether targeted radionuclide therapy can be used to treat tumors arising from the neuroendocrine cells based on the high degree of targeting possible using radiolabeled ligands.[17-19,46]

This chapter provides an overview of the endocrine system and describes the diagnostic in vivo imaging and radionuclide therapy procedures used in clinical nuclear medicine departments. It also discusses these procedures' current role in the diagnosis and management of patients with disorders of the organs and tissues that have the principal function of secreting compounds that regulate the function of other organs and tissues.

PITUITARY GLAND

Anatomy and Physiology

The pituitary gland is a small (0.5 g) pea-sized gland located at the base of the midbrain, just behind the optic chiasm. It is encased in its own bony vault at the base of the skull, the sella turcica. The pituitary has two distinctive portions, the anterior pituitary and the posterior pituitary, with the para intermedias, a small zone of specialized tissue, between the anterior and posterior secretory tissue (Figure 13-1). The anterior pituitary has a rich vascular network that includes the hypothalamic-hypophyseal portal venous system, which provides a means of communication with specialized neurosecretory tissue in the hypothalamus. The hypothalamus secretes peptides that control the synthesis and release of the anterior pituitary trophic hormones—thyrotropin-releasing hormone (TRH), corticotropin-releasing hormone

(CRH), and the corresponding releasing hormones for the gonadotrophins; these in turn affect distal organ function. Growth hormone (GH) release is modulated by somatostatin, a 14-amino-acid cyclic peptide that inhibits growth hormone synthesis, release, and action.

The anterior pituitary consists of two cell types, acidophils and basophils, so named based on their staining characteristics in histologic preparations (Table 13-1). Acidophils secrete growth hormone in response to the hypothalamic growth hormone–releasing hormone (GRH), or somatotropin, and prolactin in response to prolactin-releasing factor. The secretion of both growth hormone and prolactin also is controlled by specific inhibitory factors. Growth hormone has a widespread effect on body and organ growth and utilization of nutrients. Prolactin has effects on breast secretory gland function and on the corpus luteum in the female. In the male, increased prolactin secretion interferes with gonadal hormone response to stimulation by the gonadotrophins.

The basophil cells of the anterior pituitary elaborate several polypeptide hormones: thyrotropin (thyroid-stimulating hormone [TSH]), adrenocorticotropin (adrenal cortex–stimulating hormone [ACTH]), and the gonadotropins follicle-stimulating hormone (FSH) and luteinizing hormone (LH) or interstitial cell–stimulating hormone (ICSH), which exert their effects by stimulating other endocrine organs (the thyroid, adrenal cortex, and ovaries or testes, respectively). In turn, the hormones secreted by the thyroid, adrenals, and gonads have a negative feedback on the secretion of the hypothalamic-releasing hormones so that at elevated levels of the distal target gland hormone,

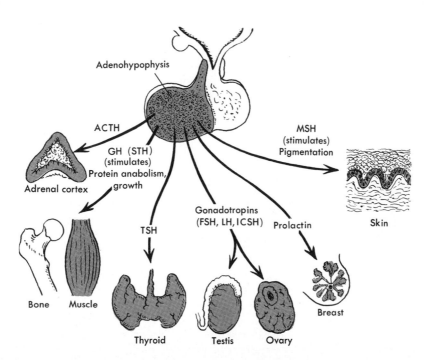

Figure 13-1 Anterior pituitary hormones and their target organs: adrenocorticotropic hormone (ACTH), thyroid-stimulating hormone (TSH), follicle-stimulating hormone (FSH), luteinizing hormone (LH), male analog of LH (ICSH), and melanocyte-stimulating hormone (MSH).

Table 13-1 Production, control, and effects of pituitary hormones

Pituitary gland (hypophysis cerebri)	Hormone	Source (cell type or location)	Control mechanism	Effect
Anterior pituitary gland (adenohypophysis)	Growth hormone (GH); somatotropin (STH)	Acidophils	GRH (growth hormone–releasing hormone) from the hypothalamus	Promotes body growth, protein anabolism, and mobilization and catabolism of fats; decreases glucose catabolism; increases blood glucose levels
Pars anterior	Prolactin (lactogenic or luteotropic hormone [LTH])	Acidophils	Prolactin-inhibitory factor (PIF); prolactin-releasing factor (PRF) from the hypothalamus and high blood levels of oxytocin	Stimulates milk secretion and development of secretory alveoli; helps maintain corpus luteum
	Thyrotropin (TH); thyroid-stimulating hormone (TSH)	Basophils	Thyrotropin-releasing hormone (TRH) from the hypothalamus	Growth and maintenance of the thyroid gland and stimulation of thyroid hormone secretion
	Adrenocorticotropin (ACTH)	Basophils	Corticotropin-releasing factor (CRF) from the hypothalamus	Growth and maintenance of adrenal cortex and stimulation of cortisol and other glucocorticoid secretions
	Follicle-stimulating hormone (FSH)	Basophils	Follicle-stimulating hormone–releasing hormone (FSH-RH) from the hypothalamus	In females stimulates follicle growth and maturation and secretion of estrogen
	Luteinizing hormone (LH in females, ICSH in males)	Basophils	Luteinizing hormone–releasing hormone (LHRH) from the hypothalamus	In females (LH) induces ovulation and stimulates formation of the corpus luteum and progesterone secretion In males (ICSH) stimulates interstitial cell secretion of testosterone
Pars intermedia	Melanocyte-stimulating hormone (MSH): intermedin	Basophils	Unknown in humans	May cause darkening of skin by increasing melanin production
Posterior pituitary gland (neurohypophysis)	Vasopressin (ADH)	Hypothalamus, mainly supraoptic nucleus	Osmoreceptors in the hypothalamus stimulated by an increase in the blood osmotic pressure, a decrease in extracellular fluid volume, or stress	Decreased urine output
	Oxytocin	Hypothalamus, paraventricular nucleus	Nervous stimulation of the hypothalamus caused by stimulation of the nipples (nursing)	Contraction of uterine smooth muscle and ejection of milk into lactiferous ducts

From Thibodeau GA: *Anthony's textbook of anatomy and physiology,* ed 13, St. Louis, 1990, Mosby.

hypothalamic and subsequently pituitary secretion of stimulating hormones is suppressed.

When the distal target gland (thyroid, adrenal cortex, or gonads) is absent or ineffective in hormone synthesis, resulting in low levels of circulating hormone, the hypothalamus is stimulated to secrete the specific releasing hormone that stimulates pituitary production and secretion of the appropriate stimulating hormone. Thyroid, adrenal, or gonadal end-organ failure, therefore, can be primary (i.e., the result of some inherent defect in the gland, such as in hypothyroidism secondary to chronic thyroiditis or genetic enzyme deficiencies or after ^{131}I therapy) or secondary (the result of failure of the hypothalamus or pituitary to adequately secrete one or more hormones that stimulate the end-organ). In primary end-organ failure, the pituitary-stimulating hormone concentration in the plasma is high; conversely, when the deficiency in end-organ function is the result of pituitary or hypothalamic disease, the pituitary hormone levels are inappropriately low or absent. The plasma concentrations of these hormones are measured using radioimmunoassay methods. The result should be compared with the end-organ hormone level. For example, if the TSH concentration is low and the thyroid hormone thyroxine (T_4) level is high, the patient is hyperthyroid. The TSH level is suppressed by the increased circulating T_4, regardless of whether the increase in T_4 is the result of increased ingestion of replacement T_4, Graves' disease, or autonomous nodule function. If both the TSH and T_4 levels are low, the patient is hypothyroid secondary to hypothalamic or pituitary disease. Hypothyroidism is more commonly due to primary failure of the thyroid gland in which case the T_4 is low but the plasma TSH level is elevated. In fact, the most sensitive marker of hypothyroidism is an elevated TSH. TSH is now routinely assayed in the newborn to evaluate the infants thyroid status before irreversible clinical sequelae of thyroid hormone deficiency. Isolated primary deficiency of pituitary hormones is rare. Pituitary hormone deficiency is commonly the result of a mass lesion affecting the pituitary or hypothalamus. Provocative and suppressive tests of pituitary hormone function have been described that measure the pituitary hormone concentration in plasma in response to known physiologic or pharmacologic stimuli.

The posterior pituitary communicates directly with hypothalamic nuclei and elaborates vasopressin (also known as antidiuretic hormone [ADH]), which promotes water resorption in the renal tubule, and oxytocin, which has a role in lactation and labor. Posterior pituitary failure (which usually is caused by a tumor, surgical trauma, or vascular insufficiency) that results in lack of ADH causes a disorder known as diabetes insipidus. In diabetes insipidus, the kidneys are unable to resorb water in the renal tubules, and the result is large volumes of dilute urine. This disease may appear suddenly as a result of infarction of the posterior pituitary during pregnancy or after an interval of hypotension (as may occur during surgery or shock after myocardial infarction).

Clinical Aspects

The clinical presentation of patients with pituitary disease takes several forms. Patients may present with symptoms and findings caused by increased secretion of metabolically active substances (the anterior pituitary hormones) or by deficiency of one or more of these hormones. In both instances, a tumor involving the hypothalamus or the pituitary itself may be the underlying cause of the problem. Anterior pituitary tumors may be functional or nonfunctional. Nonfunctioning tumors cause symptoms as a result of the tumor mass producing headache or visual disturbance, but they may manifest themselves clinically based on end-organ deficiency because of compromised pituitary function. Hence, pituitary tumors may present with hypogonadism, menstrual disturbances, galactorrhea, adrenal insufficiency, or, rarely, hypothyroidism. Widespread access to imaging techniques such as magnetic resonance imaging (MRI) permits identification of hypophyseal tumors such as microadenoma and macroadenoma before erosion of the osseous sella turcica occurs.

The most frequent and significant hyperfunctioning anterior pituitary tumor is associated with acromegaly caused by excess secretion of growth hormone. Diagnosis and management are usually based on the measurement of growth hormone levels by radioimmunoassay. Posterior pituitary hypofunction is the result of a tumor or infarction involving the hypothalamus. As mentioned previously, loss of the posterior pituitary hormone, ADH, results in diabetes insipidus.

Nuclear Medicine Procedures

Until indium-111–diethylenetriamine pentaacetic acid (^{111}In-DTPA) pentetreotide (Octreoscan, Mallinckrodt, St. Louis, Missouri) became available in the United States in 1994, there was no nuclear medicine technique available for clinical imaging of the pituitary. Given the proximity of the pituitary gland to the skull and soft tissues of the face, it is not surprising that nonspecific techniques such as imaging with gallium-67 (^{67}Ga), thallium-201(^{201}Tl), and technetium-99m 2-methoxy-2-methylpropyl isonitrile (^{99m}Tc-MIBI) were not used in the detection or management of pituitary tumors. Based on the increased amount of somatostatin receptors in the anterior pituitary, however, it is now possible to image the pituitary gland and tumors arising from it.

Somatostatin-receptor scintigraphy of the pituitary is performed with the usual dose of ^{111}In-DTPA pentetreotide (adult dose, 6.0 mCi). Patients may be imaged within hours after administration, but better contrast between the pituitary and background activity is achieved at 24 hours. When there is specific interest in the pituitary, single photon emission computed tomography (SPECT) imaging should be performed. If a high-resolution neuro-SPECT system is available, it should be used.

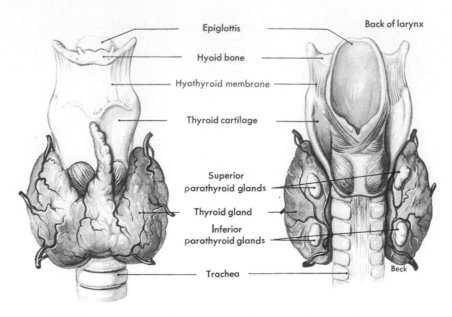

Figure 13-2 Thyroid and parathyroid glands in "normal" anatomic configuration. The thyroid is represented as a butterfly-shaped structure with a lobe of tissue on each side of the inferior portion of the thyroid cartilage. A prominent pyramidal lobe of the thyroid is depicted in the midline. Four parathyroid glands are illustrated in the classic superior and inferior symmetric distribution. In clinical nuclear medicine imaging of both the thyroid and parathyroid glands, considerable anatomic variation is encountered.

On whole body somatostatin-receptor scintigraphy with ^{111}In pentetreotide, variable but small amounts of tracer activity are seen in the region of the pituitary gland.[24,25] The ratio of pituitary to background activity (posterior to the pituitary activity) continues to increase after administration of the diagnostic tracer. At 24 hours, the ratio may be as high as 30:1 in normal subjects. Although patients with adenoma tend to have higher values than patients without pituitary disease, there is overlap among these populations.[45] Only limited results are available for somatostatin-receptor scintigraphy used for evaluation of viable residual tissue in post-operative or post-irradiation patients with nonfunctional tumors. These results have been disappointing, probably because of a reduced expression of somatostatin receptors on nonfunctioning tumors.

THYROID GLAND

Anatomy

The thyroid gland is located in the neck. It is usually somewhat butterfly shaped, with a lobe of tissue on each side of the thyroid cartilage joined to a variable degree in the lower portion by an isthmus of tissue (Figure 13-2). In the adult, each lobe weighs approximately 10 g. The embryonic origins of the thyroid gland involve evagination of tissue from the midline primordial gut, the base of the tongue, which then migrates caudally (downward) into the neck. Occasionally remnants of tissue remain along the migration path and are seen as an incidental finding during imaging. Asymmetry of the gland can also be observed. The most common evidence of the embryologic descent is a small amount of midline tissue arising from the isthmus, the pyramidal lobe. The thyroid gland tissue can even develop without migrating into the usual location astride the thyroid cartilage, resulting in a lingual thyroid, which is found at the base of the tongue. Another common but less frequently observed remnant of thyroid gland origin is the thyroglossal duct cyst, a midline cyst found superior to the thyroid, which evolves from a remnant of the embryonic duct that normally atrophies during fetal development. Most often, functioning thyroid tissue is not associated with the thyroglossal duct cyst. The diagnosis may be made clinically. Scanning is often performed to evaluate whether functional thyroid tissue is present before excision of the cystic remnant.

Physiology

The thyroid gland secretes the thyroid hormones thyroxine (T_4) and triiodothyronine (T_3). These hormones regulate tissue metabolism and are essential for normal body development and maintenance of function. Thyroid hormone synthesis depends on the trapping and organification of iodine ingested in food and water (Figure 13-3). Iodinated compounds are reduced to neutral iodine or iodide, which is actively trapped by the thyroid gland. This intrathyroidal iodine pool is in equilibrium with plasma iodine, but a gradient (intrathyroidal iodine/plasma iodine) is maintained. In the euthyroid state it is 6:1 and in the hyperthyroid state as high as 10:1 to 11:1. The net flux of iodine into the thyroid is continuous in the normal unblocked state because iodine in the intrathyroidal pool is rapidly organified; that is, bound to tyrosine to form monoiodotyrosine (MIT) and diiodotyrosine (DIT). Once iodine is bound to tyrosine (a component of the large intrathyroidal protein thyroglobulin), it is no longer a component of the gradient. This allows more

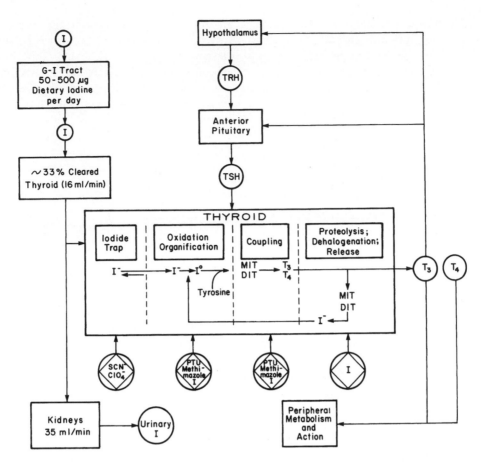

Figure 13-3 Schematic drawing of iodine metabolism and thyroid hormone regulation, synthesis, release, and biochemical site of pharmacologic effect of antithyroid drugs.

iodine to be trapped, maintaining the equilibrium gradient. After organification of the iodine (or iodination of tyrosine), the MIT and DIT molecules undergo an enzymatic step known as coupling to form T_3 or T_4. These T_3 and T_4 molecules are synthesized on the protein thyroglobulin, where they are stored until released into the circulation by proteolytic cleavage of thyroglobulin in response to TSH stimulation in the normal subject. In various forms of hyperthyroidism, T_3 and T_4 are released into the circulation without TSH stimulation.

After release into the circulation, T_3 and T_4 are bound to the specific binding protein, thyroxine-binding globulin (TBG). T_4 is bound with high affinity, whereas T_3 is more loosely bound. At the tissue level, T_4 is converted to T_3. T_3 has a direct effect on cellular metabolism, stimulating oxidation. Metabolic status is determined by the dissociated or free fraction of T_4 and T_3, which can be measured by determination of the so-called free T_4 and T_3. Alterations in the total TBG available, the fraction of TBG-binding sites available, or the affinity of binding of the T_4 and T_3 influence measured T_4 and the relationship between T_4 and T_3 measurements and the patient's metabolic state. In hyperthyroidism, T_4 and T_3 synthesis and secretion are increased, as are levels of TBG, resulting in increased plasma levels of total T_4 and T_3 and of free fraction of T_4 and T_3. Likewise, in

hypothyroidism thyroid hormone secretion is decreased, as is the absolute amount of TBG, and the T_4 and T_3 levels are low.

In the usual in vitro tests of thyroid function, plasma or serum total T_4 (or T_3) is measured, and these values are sufficient for diagnosis. Occasionally, abnormalities exist in the number of TBG-binding sites available because of an alteration either in the concentration of TBG or in the available binding sites. Drugs such as estrogens increase the amount of TBG, whereas androgens decrease TBG levels. Salicylates and the anticonvulsant drug phenylhydantoin (Dilantin) occupy binding sites on the TBG molecules, leaving fewer sites available for T_4 (or T_3) occupancy. In these instances, the measured T_4 value is artifactually increased or decreased, and the test result is incompatible with the clinical impression. Free T_4 and T_3 determine the body's metabolic level and remain consistent with the clinical status even if disturbances in TBG binding distort the serum total T_4 or T_3 levels.

A pharmacologic block at the organification step of iodine metabolism provides the basis for therapy of hyperthyroidism with antithyroid drugs, such as the sulfonylureas, methimazole, and propylthiouracil. These drugs also interfere with proteolysis and release of the thyroid hormone. Defects of this step also occur on a congenital basis (goitrous cretinism) as a result of enzyme deficiency and after irradiation and inflammation. The iodine organification defect can be demonstrated by either the perchlorate discharge test or the thiocyanate wash-out test. These techniques can be used also to demonstrate the degree of pharmacologic block produced by therapy with antithyroid drugs.

Direct measurement of TSH discriminates between physiologic variations in the T_4 concentration or variations in the T_4 concentration caused by a decreased or increased concentration of the binding protein TBG and pathologic low levels of T_4, which would result in elevation of serum TSH. Conversely, interpretation of borderline high T_4 or T_3 levels versus pathologic elevation in an individual is also augmented by knowledge of the serum TSH concentration, because abnormal elevation of T_4 or T_3 suppresses TSH levels. The use of serum TSH levels to determine or confirm clinical status has evolved in recent years with the availability of highly sensitive TSH radioimmunoassays, with assay sensitivity down to 0.01 mU/L. This assay permits differentiation of low levels from thoroughly suppressed values. Benign tumors (functioning adenomas) and malignant tumors (differentiated carcinoma) maintain the ability to synthesize thyroid hormones even without TSH stimulation. In Graves' disease, thyroid growth and hormone synthesis are stimulated by an immune globulin. Excessive production of thyroid hormone, which continues despite suppression of TRH or TSH, results in the clinical syndrome of hyperthyroidism. In autonomous nodules, areas of the thyroid gland function independent of TSH as a result of a biochemical defect in which the post-receptor signal persists without hormonal or other messenger activation of the receptor.

Clinical Aspects

Diseases of the thyroid gland can be classified into two types: disorders of function and disorders of structure (anatomy). In many instances both function and anatomy are involved; however, in other circumstances, derangement of only one or the other aspect exists. Accordingly, for proper evaluation it is necessary to integrate the findings from the clinical examination, laboratory results (in vitro procedures), and nuclear medicine procedures (uptake and scan).

The disorders of function are hyperthyroidism and hypothyroidism. Hyperthyroidism, or thyrotoxicosis, is a clinical disorder characterized by an increase in various metabolic processes and their effect on the entire body. The patient often has increased appetite and food intake but may nevertheless complain of weight loss. Classically, patients sleep poorly, feel tired upon awakening, have muscle weakness and wasting, and gastrointestinal disturbances, including increased bowel frequency. They report feeling warm and having increased sweating, emotional lability, tremors, rapid pulse, and palpitations (arrhythmias). All these findings are related to increased thyroid hormone levels in the blood. This, in turn, is the result of increased production and release of thyroid hormone by the thyroid gland. The most common etiology is Graves' disease, in which the thyroid is stimulated by an immunoglobulin that in some instances also stimulates receptors on the extraocular muscles, resulting in stare, lid lag, double vision, and other consequences known as orbitopathy. In extreme cases, vision may be threatened as a result of damage secondary to corneal dryness.

Alternately, a focal area of independent hormone production, either by an adenoma (toxic nodule or Plummer's disease) or by several areas of autonomous function within a multinodular goiter, may be the source of increased thyroid hormone. These foci of autonomous production are now believed to be clinical expressions of hormone synthesis that occurs without TSH or other receptor stimulation. Another basis for clinical hyperthyroidism may be subacute thyroiditis. In this instance there is an outpouring of thyroid hormone from the inflamed thyroid into the vascular space as a result of damage to the follicular structures and increased capillary permeability. Other, relatively rare causes of the syndrome include extrathyroidal sources of thyroid hormone, such as surreptitious ingestion of thyroid hormone, or the existence of struma ovarii, a gynecologic tumor in which ova differentiate and form functioning tissue without development of a fetus.

When the thyroid gland is the source of excessive thyroid hormone, the gland is usually diffusely enlarged, as in Graves' disease. Alternately, hyperthyroidism may occur secondary to overproduction of thyroid hormone by a solitary nodule (Plummer's disease) or multiple nodules (multinodular goiter). These nodules are usually identified on scintigraphy but may be palpable.

Hypothyroidism is a syndrome caused by thyroid hormone deficiency, usually as a result of failure of the thyroid gland to synthesize and release thyroid hormone. This is known as *primary hypothyroidism*. Occasionally the thyroid is intact, but TSH is deficient (so-called *secondary hypothyroidism*) either on a congenital basis or more commonly secondary to tumor (see Pituitary section). Primary thyroid failure has a number of causes. When the thyroid gland functions inadequately, TSH rises to stimulate further production of the thyroid hormones. If the gland has been removed surgically or damaged by ^{131}I therapy or chronic inflammation, including the long-term outcome of Graves' disease, there are no palpable findings. If, however, the receptors are intact but the gland cannot produce hormone, the gland enlarges while the subject develops hypothyroidism. Unless the TSH stimulation is aborted by thyroid hormone replacement therapy, TSH elevation continues, and further growth of the inefficient organ occurs. This is seen in children with inherited metabolic defects of thyroid hormone synthesis, the so-called goitrous cretins, but may be observed in older patients with acquired defects of these enzymes. Hence, an enlarged thyroid gland is seen in some cases of hypothyroidism as well as in hyperthyroidism (Graves' disease).

The second category of thyroid disorders is structural: palpable nodules or other findings without accompanying disturbances of function caused by thyroid hormone overproduction or underproduction. This category includes multinodular goiter, thyroid adenomas, thyroid carcinoma, and other tumors in or near the thyroid, including medullary carcinoma of the thyroid. Of course, over time, a patient with a functioning adenoma may progress from a euthyroid state to hyperthyroidism. Hyperthyroidism has even been observed in a patient with a large volume of metastatic thyroid carcinoma.[41] Accordingly, evaluation of the patient with thyroid disease involves review of the clinical status and palpable findings, laboratory tests of thyroid function, and nuclear medicine tests and imaging.

Nuclear Medicine Procedures

In vitro procedures. Radioimmunoassay is the most widely used procedure for measuring circulating serum T_4, T_3, TBG, and TSH and provides the most direct estimate of thyroid function. The TSH level is considered the most sensitive test of thyroid function. It is elevated in primary hypothyroidism and undetectable in hyperthyroidism. The currently available third-generation sensitive TSH assays are performed by the double-sandwich radioimmunoassay or the enzyme-linked immunosorbent assay (ELISA) method. The assay is sensitive to the 0.01 mU/L range. Sensitivity in this range permits differentiation of low values in the euthyroid population from patients with hyperthyroidism even if the T_4, free T_4, or T_3 values are in the borderline range.[22] TSH determinations are now widely available as a component of screening profile analyses. As a result, patients are identified with suppressed TSH as the only finding indicative of hyperthyroidism. When it is suspected that the management of coexisting medical conditions is complicated by subclinical hyperthyroidism, patients with minimal confirmatory evidence of hyperthyroidism are often referred for ^{131}I therapy.

T_4 and T_3 assays provide a direct measure of the thyroid hormone levels in plasma or serum. These hormone levels are elevated in hyperthyroid states and decreased in the hypothyroid state. They circulate primarily bound to the circulating protein TBG. When the assays are inconsistent with the clinical status, direct measurement of the TBG concentration is used to determine if alterations in serum T_4 or T_3 are caused by variations in the binding protein. Despite the availability of these assays, which explain laboratory results that are seemingly inconsistent with the patient's clinical status, TSH provides the single best evaluation of overall thyroid function and is relied upon as the definitive indicator of overall thyroid function.

Thyroglobulin assays are also performed using radioimmunoassay. Thyroglobulin is distinct from TBG. It is the intrathyroidal binding protein, whereas TBG is the circulating thyroxine-binding globulin. In the absence of disease, thyroglobulin is not detected in the plasma. Thyroglobulin is elevated when abnormal access to the vascular space exists as a result of tumor, inflammation, or trauma, usually surgical. It is most useful in following patients who have undergone total thyroidectomy for thyroid carcinoma. Detection of thyroglobulin after thyroidectomy indicates the presence of thyroid tissue, either a functioning remnant or a tumor. Because thyroglobulin is such a large protein, antisera from different sources recognize different portions of the protein molecule. This results in variation in the result obtained from laboratory to laboratory. In the past few years there has been considerable success in making this assay more specific and uniform.

Another confounding problem is the production of antibodies to thyroglobulin in individual patients. These antibodies compete with the antibodies used in the thyroglobulin immunoassay and lower measured values. Nevertheless, the thyroglobulin levels over time are a sensitive and useful method of monitoring patients for recurrence of thyroid cancer after thyroidectomy and radioiodine ablation. The truly athyrotic patient has no detectable thyroglobulin and no source of antibody-stimulating material.

In vivo function tests and imaging. In vivo tests for evaluating thyroid function are based on the usual association of the degree of iodine uptake and overall thyroid function. The most common of these is the thyroid uptake test. Thyroid gland imaging is performed to determine the size, location, and function of the thyroid gland and to evaluate palpable findings near, on, or within the thyroid gland[6] (Figures 13-4 to 13-9).

Choice of radionuclide. ^{131}I. The use of radioactive isotopes of iodine for thyroid in vivo function tests and imaging is based on the unique avidity of the thyroid gland for iodine.[24] For many years these procedures were performed with ^{131}I, an isotope of iodine that is readily produced in nuclear reactors. It is a product of nuclear fission but can also be produced by neutron bombardment. With a physical half-life of 8.1 days, ^{131}I was widely used for in vivo thyroid studies and became a mainstay of nuclear medicine in the 1960s. The long half-life made it convenient to transport and store. It is readily detected externally because of the energetic 364 keV gamma emission. In doses of 20 to 100 µCi, ^{131}I provided the foundation for contemporary nuclear medicine, permitting the development of reproducible techniques to quantify thyroid function (thyroid clearance and the 24-hour thyroid uptake) and to image the thyroid. In addition, ^{131}I decays by beta decay, which is useful for therapy.

Thyroid iodine uptake is most commonly performed using 5 to 10 µCi of ^{131}I. The uptake can be measured at any time after administration of radioiodine, but for a variety of reasons, 24 hours has evolved to be the most practical and reliable interval.[7] It provides better discrimination between hyperthyroid, euthyroid, and hypothyroid populations than earlier time points. In addition, 24 hours is long enough after oral administration to minimize differences caused by variations in the rate of gastrointestinal absorption. Uptake values do vary, however, depending on the type of radioiodine preparation used, because of bioavailability (e.g., liquid

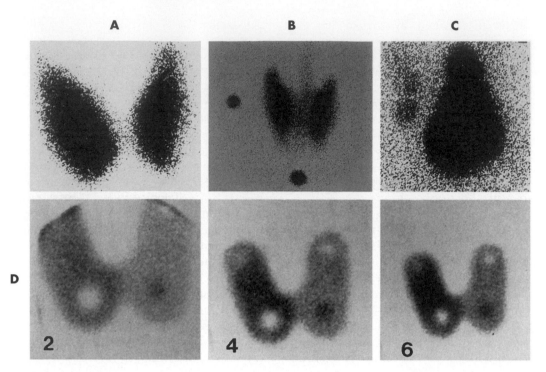

Figure 13-4 Thyroid gland scintigraphy (pinhole collimator technique). **A**, Normal, virtually symmetric thyroid gland, right and left lobes. No isthmus or pyramidal lobe activity. (4 mCi ^{99m}Tc pertechnetate.) **B**, Normal thyroid gland with isthmus and prominent pyramidal lobe. (400 μCi ^{123}I sodium iodide.) **C**, Marked asymmetry of thyroid gland after near-total thyroidectomy and compensatory enlargement of the left lobe. Asymmetry is secondary to surgical resection, but similar patterns are seen in congenital hemiagenesis of the thyroid. Interpretation requires correlation of scan findings with history and physical examination. (4 mCi ^{99m}Tc pertechnetate.) **D**, Effect of distance of pinhole collimator on scintigraphic thyroid gland size: images are shown at 2, 4, and 6 cm from the surface of the thyroid phantom. As the pinhole collimator comes closer to the imaged object, the recorded image becomes larger. Accordingly, conclusions about gland size require simultaneous imaging of a source of known size or correlation with findings on palpation.

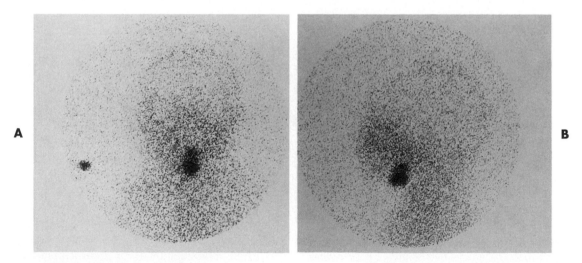

Figure 13-5 Lingual thyroid demonstrated in a 9-year-old child. (2 mCi ^{99m}Tc pertechnetate.) Anterior view **(A)** and left lateral view **(B)** demonstrate outline of skull, facial activity, and neck. A solitary focus of radiotracer uptake is seen in the midline of the neck near the base of the tongue. No uptake is seen in the thyroid bed.

is absorbed more rapidly than capsules).[36] There are variations in the degree of digestion and the rate of absorption of capsules from different manufacturers.[36] In the euthyroid subject, uptake is usually complete at 18 to 20 hours and stable for several hours thereafter.

^{123}I. As nuclear medicine evolved, other radionuclides became available as alternatives to ^{131}I. ^{123}I has been used for thyroid function studies and imaging. ^{123}I was introduced for clinical use in the late 1970s and early 1980s, when accelerator-produced radionuclides became available.

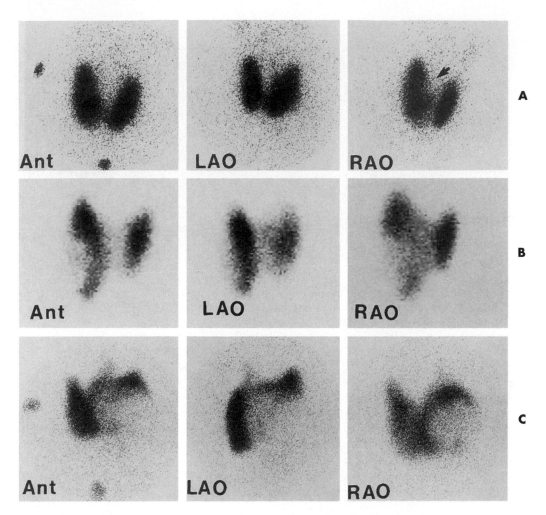

Figure 13-6 Three-view thyroid scintigraphy: anterior, left anterior oblique, and right anterior oblique views in three different patients demonstrating a solitary cold nodule of various sizes. (400 μCi ^{123}I sodium iodide.) **A**, Small defect (cold nodule) corresponding to a palpable nodule (*arrow*) is seen on the medial aspect of the right thyroid lobe in the right anterior oblique view. Oblique views increase the sensitivity of thyroid scintigraphy in the anterior view for the detection of small cold nodules, which might not be seen en face. **B**, Moderately large (3 × 1 cm) cold nodule in the lower portion of the right lobe. **C**, Large (5 × 4 cm) cold nodule replacing most of the left thyroid lobe.

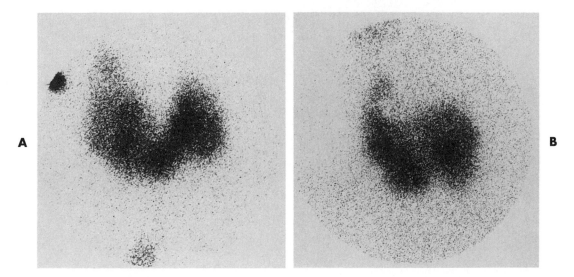

Figure 13-7 Multinodular goiter in a patient with Hashimoto's disease. Pinhole collimator, anterior views in the same patient, 9 months apart. Occasionally discrepancies are seen in areas that trap pertechnetate but do not organify iodine. **A**, 400 μCi ^{123}I. **B**, 4 mCi ^{99m}Tc pertechnetate.

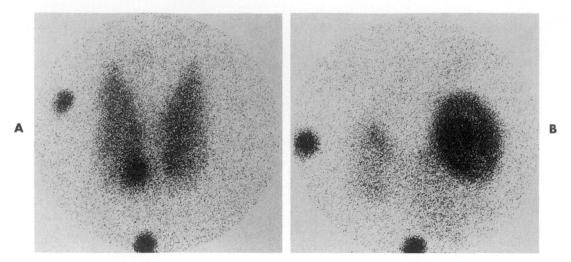

Figure 13-8 Thyroid imaging: hot nodule. **A,** Nonsuppressed thyroid and an area of hyperfunction seen overlying the medial aspect of the right thyroid lobe. The symmetric right and left thyroid lobes are readily seen. (400 μCi ^{123}I sodium iodide.) **B,** Large, somewhat heterogeneous area of activity is seen on the left, representing the dominant functioning thyroid nodule, with only faint activity representing the suppressed thyroid gland seen. (400 μCi ^{123}I sodium iodide.)

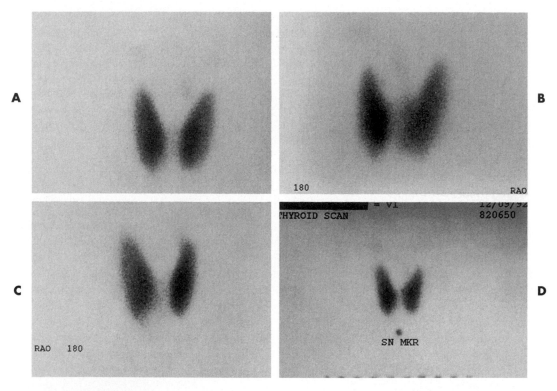

Figure 13-9 Thyroid imaging: normal thyroid gland, parallel hole collimator, electronic zoom technique. (10 mCi ^{99m}Tc pertechnetate.) **A,** Anterior. **B,** Left anterior oblique (LAO) view. **C,** Right anterior oblique (RAO) view. **D,** Anterior view with sternal notch markers (SN MKR) and size bar.

Despite the relatively short half-life of ^{123}I (13.3 hours), improved distribution networks provide this radionuclide at least 4 days a week throughout most of the United States, Canada, and Western Europe. Early methods to produce ^{123}I used the p,2n reaction, which resulted in a product with significant amounts of long-lived ^{125}I and ^{124}I as contaminants. These radiochemical impurities resulted in poorer image quality because of septal penetration of the high-energy gamma emissions from ^{124}I and loss of some of the dosimetry advantage of ^{123}I. ^{123}I is now produced by the p,5n reaction, which has a high degree of radiochemical purity.

^{123}I has a gamma emission of 159 keV and is therefore well suited for gamma camera imaging. Images of 100,000 counts can be obtained in less than 10 minutes at 20 hours

Table 13-2	Physical characteristics and absorbed doses of radionuclides used in thyroid imaging and diagnostic studies					
Nuclide	Dose Administered	$t_{1/2}$	Emission	Energy (keV)	Rad	
					Whole Body	Thyroid
^{131}I	5-10 µCi	8.1 days	Gamma, beta	364	1.2*	0.05-0.10
	100 µCi				20*	1
^{123}I	200 µCi	13 hr	Gamma	159	0.5-2.0	0.06
	400 µCi				1.0-4.0	0.12
^{99m}Tc	4 mCi	6 hr	Gamma	140	<1	<0.1

*Assumes average body and thyroid weight, thyroid turnover, and 20% uptake.

after ^{123}I administration.[6,22] A typical adult scanning dose is 300 to 400 µCi, resulting in a thyroid absorbed dose of 1 to 4 rad and a whole body absorbed dose of 0.12 rad. Imaging is best performed 2 to 4 hours after oral administration. Quantification of uptake can also be performed at that time. There are difficulties, however, in using ^{123}I to measure uptake at 24 hours. Because of the radionuclide's short half-life, a suitable standard and phantom must be available for counting in a geometric configuration approximating the patient's neck so as to provide corrections for attenuation and scatter. The ^{123}I gamma photon has a lower energy than that of ^{131}I (159 keV versus 364 keV), rendering it more sensitive to tissue attenuation. Consequently, relatively small variations in depth alter the counts obtained by an external probe. Nevertheless, imaging with ^{123}I is an improvement over ^{131}I.

In comparison studies, blinded observers regularly prefer ^{123}I images, probably because the images were obtained at 24 hours after ^{123}I administration and consequently they have better thyroid-to-background contrast.[2,6,22] The only significant limitations to ^{123}I are its availability and expense, which limit administered doses to 300 to 400 µCi. The 13.3-hour physical half-life makes storage prohibitive, and doses have to be ordered as a patient is scheduled.

As a diagnostic radionuclide, ^{123}I has several advantages over ^{131}I. In addition to its short half-life, it decays by electron capture with the release of a 159 keV gamma photon but no beta particle emission. This offers advantages in terms of less radiation absorbed dose to the thyroid. Consequently, doses of 300 to 400 µCi can be used. At the same time, these features of half-life and gamma energy are also disadvantages. Doses are usually ordered on a patient-by-patient basis. In the event a patient is delayed or cancels, the ^{123}I dose cannot be held over for another visit. Even though imaging is often performed within 3 or 4 hours after administration of ^{123}I, thyroid uptake is best performed at 24 hours. Because of the short half-life, the decay correction necessary is very sensitive to the interval. Finally, the "softer" gamma photon is attenuated by the neck tissue; variations in thyroid depth have a more profound impact on the uptake than when ^{131}I is used to quantify thyroid uptake (Table 13-2).

^{99m}Tc pertechnetate. Thyroid imaging is most often performed using ^{99m}Tc pertechnetate (TcO$_4$).[2,6,23] As was noted in the 1970s, its ionic charge and size allow the pertechnetate ion to be recognized by the thyroidal iodide trap and concentrated within the thyroid. It is an ideal choice for thyroid imaging because of its 6-hour half-life, 140 keV gamma emission, and ready availability either from a molybdenum generator or when purchased in bulk.[4] Pertechnetate is not organically bound, however, and cannot be used to measure uptake in the traditional sense. The plasma concentration decreases at about 20 minutes after intravenous injection because of renal and gastric excretion, and the pertechnetate begins to wash out of the thyroid. Thyroid uptake measurements shortly after injection have been reported but are not widely used.

Nevertheless, ^{99m}Tc pertechnetate has several advantages over ^{131}I as a thyroid imaging agent. The 140 keV gamma emission of ^{99m}Tc is more efficiently detected by the $^3/_8$- to $^1/_2$-inch scintillation camera crystal than is the 364 keV gamma photon of ^{131}I. The short physical half-life and isomeric transition mode of decay of ^{99m}Tc results in a more favorable patient radiation absorbed dose than ^{131}I and permits routine use of several millicuries of ^{99m}Tc pertechnetate for diagnostic studies. This dose provides better image quality than possible with ^{131}I. A typical scanning dose of ^{131}I (100 µCi) results in an absorbed dose to the adult thyroid of 20 rad, assuming a 20% uptake and typical turnover rate, and a 1 rad whole body dose, whereas a 4 mCi dose of ^{99m}Tc pertechnetate yields an absorbed dose of less than 1 rad to the thyroid and a whole body absorbed dose of 0.1 rad (see Table 13-2).

In summary, ^{99m}Tc pertechnetate provides excellent quality images at great convenience to the nuclear medicine service and the patient. These images identify the size and location of thyroid tissue. Images are obtained 15 to 20 minutes after ingestion. ^{99m}Tc pertechnetate is currently widely used for thyroid imaging. The concern that it is trapped but not organified and hence would provide misleading information about nodule function has proven to be less significant clinically than was initially thought to be the case.

In a patient with thyroid carcinoma, ^{99m}Tc pertechnetate may be used to detect remnants of the thyroid gland after surgery, but it is not useful to detect metastatic disease because of its short physical and biologic half-life in the thyroid.

There is no justification for using ^{131}I for diagnostic imaging of the thyroid gland itself. Whole body ^{131}I imaging is used in patients with known thyroid carcinoma to identify residual thyroid bed activity and distal metastases. Recently, it has been suggested that whole body ^{131}I imaging is less sensitive for the detection or exclusion of metastatic thyroid carcinoma than the post-recombinant TSH serum thyroglobulin level.[37] If confirmed, it is likely that the use of whole body ^{131}I scintigraphy will decline significantly, because patients may be treated with ^{131}I based on the elevation in serum of the tumor marker, thyroglobulin.

^{123}I also has been suggested for whole body imaging in thyroid cancer patients. Better imaging results have been obtained using several millicuries of ^{123}I, but this is prohibitively expensive in the United States and Europe. In the usual doses of 300 to 400 µCi of ^{123}I, the imaging results are no better than with ^{131}I.

^{18}F-FDG (fluorodeoxyglucose) PET (positron emission tomography) has been shown to detect thyroid carcinoma. Uptake appears to depend on the tumor's metabolic activity, so that some quiescent tumors that concentrate ^{131}I may not be seen with FDG PET, whereas others are. Of even greater value is the suggestion that thyroid tumors that have become more aggressive biologically can be identified even if they have lost the sodium-iodine symporter proteins necessary for thyroid tissue iodine uptake.[47,48] These observations make possible identification of a tumor that could be removed surgically if there is no evidence of inoperable disease. In fact, there have been reports of serendipitous finding of thyroid carcinoma in patients undergoing diagnostic FDG PET imaging for other indications.

^{131}I is used to treat hyperthyroidism (Graves' disease, multinodular toxic goiter, and toxic solitary nodule or adenoma) and to ablate normal thyroid tissue or treat thyroid carcinoma with local or distal metastases. The beta particle emission released during ^{131}I decay results in a profound radiobiologic effect.

Thyroid uptake. Despite the limitations arising from increased and variable iodine intake, thyroidal iodine uptake remains a frequently requested in vivo nuclear medicine procedure for assessing or confirming thyroid function. Even though the diagnosis of hyperthyroidism and hypothyroidism is currently based on TSH values, frequent measurement of TSH in routine clinical screening examinations has resulted in an increase in the number of patients referred for confirmatory diagnostic uptakes and treatment.

The role of thyroid uptake has evolved to confirming a diagnosis of hyperthyroidism or hypothyroidism, to calculating an ^{131}I dose before therapy of hyperthyroidism or ablation of a thyroid remnant, and to assessing residual uptake in a patient after thyroidectomy and/or ablation.

Thyroid iodine uptake is, in fact, nonspecific as a measure of thyroid function, because the value is influenced by total iodine intake. The 24-hour uptake is greater than normal in areas of dietary iodine deficiency, and it is low when patients have increased dietary iodine, take supplements or medication containing iodine, or have recently undergone studies using x-ray contrast material.

Over the past 50 years, ingestion of dietary iodine in the United States has increased as a result of the use of iodized salt, improved availability and increased preference for saltwater fish, use of iodinated preservatives in food (such as white bread), and widespread use of iodinated compounds in food dyes and medication. This has resulted in a decrease in 24-hour thyroid iodine uptake values at all levels of thyroid function. In 1960 the mean value for a group of euthyroid patients at a large medical center in New York was 25% ± 7%; in 1975 the mean value was 16 ± 8%.[22]

The wide regional variation in dietary iodine observed throughout the United States would seem to suggest that no single published figure or range can be accepted for the normal 24-hour thyroid iodine uptake. Nevertheless, if there is no history of exposure to excess dietary iodine (e.g., kelp, mineral supplements) or iodinated organic compounds (contrast media), the thyroid iodine uptake is expected to be increased in hyperthyroidism, reflecting increased thyroid function, and decreased in hypothyroidism, reflecting decreased thyroid function. In general, values below 12% are considered low at this time and require explanation. Any 24-hour thyroid uptake values in excess of 25% represent greater iodine uptake than is usually encountered in a normal population. In hyperthyroid patients, values of 35% to 95% are typically observed. Occasionally, a patient presents with rapid onset of symptoms of hyperthyroidism and abnormal elevations of serum T_3 and T_4 and appropriate suppression of TSH but is found to have very low iodine uptake. In these instances, so-called subacute thyroiditis should be considered. It is not appropriate to treat these patients with radioactive iodine.

The thyroid uptake probe contains a 1- to 2-inch sodium-iodide crystal with open-face collimation. Standards should be counted in an appropriate phantom. The Society of Nuclear Medicine has published consensus procedure guidelines on the issues involved in performing this procedure.[7]

The thyroid uptake test is billable as a stand-alone procedure or in combination with a thyroid scan. Most frequently, physicians request a thyroid uptake and scan. This is typically performed using 4.0 mCi of ^{99m}Tc pertechnetate for imaging, followed by 5 µCi of ^{131}I given orally with the patient returning the next day for the 24-hour thyroid iodine uptake.

Perchlorate discharge and thiocyanate wash-out tests. These procedures are infrequently performed in current practice. They can be used to demonstrate a thyroidal organification defect, which is now largely of academic interest. Patients with this disorder have clinical features of thyroid enlargement and elevated TSH levels. They can be treated with thyroid hormone replacement therapy based on these findings without the need to demonstrate an organification defect.

The test is performed after administration of radioactive iodine (5 to 20 μCi ^{131}I) given orally (or intravenously if sterile, pyrogen-free tracer is available). Counts are recorded over the thyroid bed with a thyroid uptake probe. When the radioiodine is administered by mouth, counts are usually taken every 15 to 30 minutes for approximately 2 hours. When sterile pyrogen-free material is available for IV administration, more frequent counting is performed: every minute if an automatic recording device is available or at 5-minute intervals if manual counting is done. These intervals allow sufficient time for thyroid uptake of the tracer iodine. At 2 hours, 600 to 1000 mg of potassium perchlorate is administered orally. The perchlorate ion competes with circulating iodide ion at the thyroid trap, blocking entry of additional radioactive iodine. In normal subjects the count rate remains stable over the next several measurements, because the trapped iodine will have been organified. If an organification defect is present, a significant decrease in the count rate (10% to 50% or more) is observed because the nonorganically bound iodine washes out of the trap and is replaced by perchlorate ion. Because the perchlorate results in removal of the nonorganically bound iodine, the procedure is called the *perchlorate discharge test.* The thiocyanate wash-out procedure is based on the same principle as the perchlorate discharge test except that the thiocyanate is injected intravenously, because it is available in sterile vials in poison control kits.

Thyroid imaging. Thyroid imaging is performed with a gamma camera and a pinhole collimator. It is possible to perform thyroid imaging with a parallel hole collimator and electronic zoom, but the resolution with this technique is less than that obtained with pinhole images. Zoomed images using a parallel hole collimator should not be used to evaluate thyroid nodules, because a small (1 cm) "cold" nodule (i.e., having decreased activity) will not be resolved. With pinhole collimation, image size varies with distance. The pinhole collimator should be used at a fixed distance from the surface so that some uniformity is established within a department (see Figure 13-4, *D*). Physicians and technologists become accustomed to the usual image size and recognize enlarged lobes or glands to get an objective measure of size. It is possible also to take additional images with a marker within the field of view. Regardless of the specific distance of the camera crystal surface to the thyroid, the marker provides an internal calibration by which estimates of organ dimensions and a calculation of area (or volume) can be made.

A variety of pinhole inserts are available. The diameter of the aperture of the insert determines the spatial resolution of the system. As usual, there is a tradeoff between sensitivity and resolution, with sensitivity decreasing as the aperture diameter decreases and the resolution improves.

The Society of Nuclear Medicine has published a consensus procedure guideline on technical recommendations for thyroid scintigraphy.[6] The thyroid has two lobes that straddle the thyroid cartilage. They are located just medial to the sternocleidomastoid muscle, 3 to 5 cm above the sternal notch. Oblique views better define nodules that may be on the anterior or posterior surface of the gland and thus obscured by activity within the normal lobe. It is customary to obtain an anterior image and both right and left anterior (45-degree) oblique views (see Figure 13-6). The sternal notch should be identified, usually by obtaining an additional image with a marker at the notch. In addition, right-left orientation should be identified by placing an additional marker on the right side. The images should be reviewed by the nuclear medicine physician before the patient leaves. The image findings should be correlated with the palpable findings. Activity in palpable nodules is compared to the remainder of the gland characterized as either increased ("warm" or "hot") or decreased ("cold") in activity (see Figures 13-6 to 13-8).

Although the thyroid is classically symmetric, various degrees of asymmetry in size between the two lobes are frequently observed. Asymmetry is usually a simple developmental anomaly and often not significant.

The principal reason to image a thyroid with palpable findings is to determine if a palpable nodule is cold, hot, or similar in function to the reminder of the thyroid. Of solitary cold nodules, 20% to 30% are malignant, most commonly differentiated thyroid carcinoma. Recently it was reported that even in multinodular goiters, 10% of the dominant cold nodules contained malignant cells. Accordingly, cold nodules should be biopsied and followed clinically even if the initial biopsy is benign. Depending on a number of factors, including age, gender, palpable findings, and patient anxiety, it is sometimes appropriate to have the nodule removed for thorough histologic examination. If it is found to be malignant, the patient should undergo subtotal or total thyroidectomy, depending on other risk factors and local surgical practice and skill.

In some settings it may be desirable to observe these nodules, in which case the patient should receive exogenous thyroid hormone to therapeutically suppress the gland. This course can be chosen in chronic thyroiditis (if thyroid antibodies are found) on the premise that the nodule represents a focal area of organification defect secondary to Hashimoto involvement, as opposed to malignancy. Multiple nodules can be uniformly active or can vary in activity, one from the other. In the clinically euthyroid patient, this usually represents a post-Hashimoto's thyroiditis. These patients may have elevated TSH, a compensatory response to the inefficient handling of iodine and thyroid hormone synthesis. The differential diagnosis of a cold nodule includes adenoma, cyst, focal thyroiditis, and hemorrhage.

A solitary warm nodule is likely to represent a functioning adenoma. The remainder of the thyroid gland may be visible, indicating that the adenoma is not functioning at a level sufficient to suppress TSH. Alternatively, the scan may reveal a warm nodule with suppression of the remainder of the gland even in the clinically euthyroid patient. The only evidence of hyperthyroidism may be a suppressed TSH. Of course, a solitary hot nodule may be found in a patient who is hyperthyroid. This is also called *toxic nodule*, or Plummer's disease (see Figure 13-8, *B*). Alternatively, a solitary area of thyroid tissue can represent a surgical remnant or an anatomic variant in which only one lobe or a portion of a lobe developed congenitally (Figure 13-4, *C*). After thyroidectomy for carcinoma, a solitary focus can represent residual thyroid tissue or tumor. For these reasons, the patient history contributes to the scan interpretation and differential diagnosis.

Significant discrepancies in the focal findings of pertechnetate and radioiodine images have been observed in Hashimoto's thyroiditis. Figure 13-7 shows nodules in a patient with Hashimoto's thyroiditis. Some nodules are perfused, trap pertechnetate, and appear warm on ^{99m}Tc pertechnetate images. Because they do not organify iodine, they are cold on ^{131}I imaging at 24 hours. The traditional view that ^{99m}Tc pertechnetate might not identify cold nodules is not consistent with a study that compared blind readings of ^{99m}Tc pertechnetate and ^{123}I scans in 316 patients and found agreement in 92% to 95%. In 12 patients with thyroid carcinoma, no discrepancy was found on images obtained with either radionuclide.[26]

Thyroid carcinoma. Thyroid carcinoma is the most common endocrine neoplasm, and mortality from thyroid carcinoma exceeds mortality from all other malignant endocrine tumors. At autopsy it is a common finding, detected in 3% to 10% of all cases. Nevertheless, thyroid cancer accounts for fewer than 1% of all deaths from malignancy. The challenge for nuclear medicine is to identify patients in whom the disease presents a greater risk of morbidity and mortality by providing evidence of metastases, to minimize morbidity, and to provide effective therapy using ^{131}I.

Differentiated thyroid carcinoma includes papillary carcinoma, follicular variant of papillary carcinoma, and follicular carcinoma.[1] Within the thyroid, these tumors are seen as cold areas because they generally function less efficiently than normal thyroid tissue (see Figure 13-6). After thyroidectomy, of course, the ability of differentiated thyroid carcinoma to trap and organify iodine provides the basis for identification of metastases, surveillance, and therapy. Other malignancies, such as medullary carcinoma, undifferentiated carcinoma, lymphoma, and metastases to the thyroid are also identified as cold nodules, but after detection and removal, ^{131}I is not used in management and therapy.

A nonfunctioning (cold) solitary nodule is an indication for needle biopsy.[35] If this procedure is unavailable or indeterminate, an excisional biopsy should be performed. In various series, 20% to 35% of the solitary cold nodules are malignant and usually represent differentiated carcinoma of the thyroid. Other noninvasive procedures, such as ultrasound, CT, or MRI or other radionuclide imaging procedures

with ^{201}Tl or ^{99m}Tc MIBI, may be useful. Frequently, however, patients with a palpable neck mass are referred directly to surgery for biopsy or removal without radionuclide thyroid scanning.

If a total thyroidectomy has been performed, many surgeons schedule the patient to have ^{131}I imaging to determine whether residual tissue or unsuspected local or distal metastases are present. If abnormal lymph nodes have been identified, if the surgical specimen reveals positive margins (tumor extending to the edge of the tissue removed), or if vascular invasion has occurred, ^{131}I imaging is a component of standard management.

After appropriate preparation, the patient is referred to the nuclear medicine service for diagnostic imaging to determine the amount and location of residual thyroid tissue or tumor based on the ability of this tissue to concentrate radioiodine. For effective evaluation and identification of residual thyroid tissue or tumor, steps should be taken to raise the plasma TSH before administration of the diagnostic tracer. This is accomplished in one of several ways: by not replacing thyroid hormone after total thyroidectomy; by discontinuing replacement thyroid hormone if the patient has been receiving it; or by injection of recombinant human TSH (rTSH) (Thyrogen, Genzyme, Cambridge, Massachusetts).

The patient should follow a low-iodine diet for 1 to 2 weeks before evaluation and should not undergo studies with iodinated contrast material during this interval. In patients who are not going to receive rTSH injections, several weeks should elapse to allow TSH levels to rise before radioiodine imaging is performed. The patient gradually develops symptoms and signs of hypothyroidism, including lethargy, soft tissue swelling, weight gain, constipation, coarsening of the skin, and bradycardia, as well as intolerance to cold. Serum T_4 and T_3 levels fall to the hypothyroid range. Serum for the TSH level should be obtained before a diagnostic radioiodine dose is administered even if a decision to proceed with the evaluation is based on clinical assessment. Failure of the TSH to rise might indicate that a significant functioning remnant exists. If the TSH has not risen and the patient has not developed signs of thyroid deficiency, the amount of residual tissue can be evaluated with a traditional thyroid uptake and scan or, alternatively, with a ^{99m}Tc pertechnetate scan.

In the event the patient has tissue or tumor producing enough thyroid hormone so that TSH is not stimulated or if the patient has an inadequate pituitary response, rTSH should be administered. In current practice, patients are often evaluated while hypothyroid after total thyroidectomy. In subsequent years, when the patient is receiving replacement thyroid hormone, evaluation can be performed with administration of rTSH before the ^{131}I tracer.[38]

The ^{131}I dose recommended for whole body imaging ranges from 1 to 10 mCi. The recently published *Procedure Guideline for Extended Scintigraphy for Differentiated Thyroid Cancer*, developed by the Society of Nuclear Medicine, recommends a 5.0 mCi dose of ^{131}I.[8]

Tumor foci are identifiable on gamma camera imaging when less than $10\,\mu$Ci of ^{131}I has accumulated in the focus. This represents 1% of a 1 mCi dose. Accordingly, administration of larger diagnostic doses (i.e., 10 mCi) permits identification of foci with a fractional uptake in the 0.1% range. In general, a lower dose is recommended when suspicion of residual thyroid tissue or tumor exists. Doses even less than 1 mCi may be used if it has already been determined that the patient will be treated subsequently with a dose of 29 mCi or more. Repeat imaging after a week or more is performed to take advantage of the incremental information available from images obtained with the therapeutic dose. If the patient has no known thyroid tissue and is being evaluated to exclude residual disease, a larger dose is recommended. Some centers use as high a dose as 10 mCi for this purpose, whereas others limit the dose administered to 3–5 mCi of ^{131}I. Clearly, the diagnostic yield increases with the imaging dose.

More recently, it has been suggested that ^{123}I should be used to determine if metastases are present. The advantage of this shorter-lived radionuclide is the increased photon flux available with less radiation absorbed dose to the patient. The problem with ^{123}I is that it is relatively expensive and not conveniently available because of its short half-life. It is principally used for this purpose in research centers that produce ^{123}I in on-site cyclotron facilities.

Another issue involved in dose selection is the concern about the phenomenon known as *stunning*. Thyroid stunning means impaired thyroid function as assessed by radioactive iodine uptake after prior administration of a ^{131}I dose. The significance of this phenomenon is that less of a subsequent therapeutic dose is localized in the thyroid tissue. If stunning exists, it is obviously an undesirable effect. The concern about stunning has fueled much debate for many years without a consensus as to whether the phenomenon is real or not. Reports appear at intervals that support one or the other side of the argument. A recent study reported no difference in outcome among patients receiving 3 to 5 mCi (111 to 185 MBq) with ^{131}I scans.[49] There are certainly documented cases of patients with less uptake of the therapeutic dose than would have been expected from the diagnostic or dosimetric uptake data. However, it is difficult to definitively ascribe this to stunning, because the images and measurements obtained are usually made at greater intervals after therapeutic dosing than after diagnostic doses because of the restrictions on patient access when the emitted radiation exceeds 5 mR/hr. In addition, it is not clear whether the different handling of the diagnostic and therapeutic ^{131}I dose is the result of the pre-treatment radionuclide administration or an effect of the sizable therapeutic dose itself.

Neck and whole body images are obtained at 24-hour intervals. Images obtained at 48 or 72 hours have been found to be optimal, because imaging at these intervals allows sufficient time for reduction of background activity through renal excretion.[8] Because radioiodine is secreted into the saliva and gastric fluids, activity in the gastrointestinal tract can be seen at 48 hours and can even be the source of background and bladder activity for several days, as the intestinal activity undergoes absorption and redistribution (Figures 13-10 to 13-12).

Even with diagnostic doses involving several millicuries of ^{131}I, the count rate in the images is poor. Accordingly, 10-minute image acquisition for static fields is recommended.

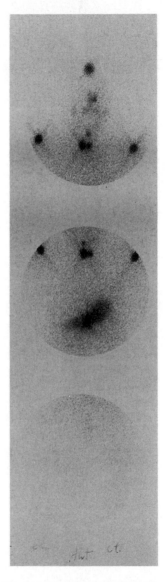

Figure 13-10 Whole body imaging in thyroid carcinoma; 1 to 10 mCi ^{131}I was used as the "diagnostic" tracer with high-energy collimation. This figure illustrates anterior images using gamma camera technique at 24 hours after tracer administration. Markers are placed at the top of the head and shoulders. Background activity is seen throughout the soft tissue, with secretion in the nasal and oral cavities, the parotid and submaxillary glands, and the salivary glands. Residual thyroid tissue is seen in the bed of both the right and left thyroid lobes. A small midline focus cephalad to the thyroid remnants is also seen, representing metastasis to a paratracheal lymph node. Prominent activity is seen in the stomach. No activity is seen in the bladder, although bladder activity is quite common, particularly at 24 hours after tracer administration. Posterior images are also obtained to evaluate possible osseous metastases.

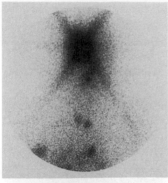
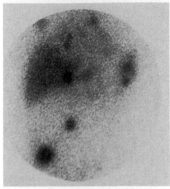
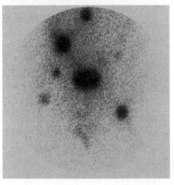

Figure 13-11   Whole body imaging in thyroid carcinoma. Gamma camera images at 72 hours after ^{131}I therapy (134 mCi); 30 sec/frame. Metastases are seen in the brain (with a star artifact caused by septal penetration, readily observed because of the large amount of activity concentrated in a brain metastasis). Additional metastases are seen in the cervical, mediastinal, hepatic, and femoral lymph nodes. Diffuse activity is seen in the liver parenchyma, representing hepatic excretion of radiolabeled thyroid hormone synthesized in the functioning metastases.

Radioactive makers may be placed to identify anatomic landmarks, such as the top of the skull and the axillae, umbilicus, iliac crests, and knees. If the sternal notch is to be marked, a repeat image without the marker should be obtained so as not to obscure a thyroid remnant or local tumor focus.

Radionuclide therapy.   Localization of iodine by thyroid tissue provides the basis for ^{131}I treatment of hyperthyroidism and thyroid cancer. The beta particle emission produces a profound radiobiologic effect. With appropriate doses of ^{131}I, normal as well as malignant thyroid tissue can be ablated.

^{131}*I treatment of hyperthyroidism.* ^{131}I has been used to treat hyperthyroidism regardless of whether the hyperthyroidism is secondary to a diffuse toxic goiter (Graves' disease), toxic multinodular goiter, or toxic nodule (adenoma). In the past, ^{131}I also was used to produce hypothyroidism in clinically euthyroid patients with severe coronary artery disease to reduce the metabolic needs of the myocardium. With the introduction of adrenergic blockers in the 1960s and, subsequently, other pharmacologic agents (e.g., calcium channel blockers), this indication has grown less frequent. More recently, however, it has been recognized that patients may present with suppressed TSH and normal T_4 and T_3 values. Because suppressed TSH is considered the most sensitive indicator of hyperthyroidism, these patients are also referred for treatment, particularly if a history of cardiac arrhythmias or other symptoms suggestive of hyperthyroidism are factors.

Treatment of hyperthyroidism with ^{131}I is simple, safe, effective, and relatively inexpensive and has minimal morbidity. Alternatives to ^{131}I therapy include antithyroid drugs or surgery. Before ^{131}I therapy is begun, the benefits and disadvantages of each therapeutic option should be discussed with the patient. In the United States, radioiodine therapy is the most frequently chosen treatment for adults with Graves' disease. Surgery is rarely used. Antithyroid drugs require 6 to 12 months of treatment and have a significant failure rate (i.e., recurrence of hyperthyroidism when the antithyroid medication is discontinued). In addition, both surgery and antithyroid drugs have rare but well-defined complications, whereas there is no demonstrable consequence to ^{131}I therapy other than hypothyroidism. ^{131}I has also been used to good effect in children and adolescents, but unfounded anxiety concerning long-term effects of radiation frequently leads to the choice of antithyroid drugs to control the disease in children. This often results in goiter, followed by surgery.

Hypothyroidism occurs frequently as a sequela of hyperthyroidism regardless of the treatment used (radioiodine, surgery, or drugs).[9,10] Because hypothyroidism is readily treatable with thyroid hormone replacement, there is less reluctance to treat vigorously with ^{131}I and to accept hypothyroidism as a natural outcome of hyperthyroidism. The effectiveness of replacement therapy, however, depends on patient compliance.

Although individual patient differences in therapeutic response to ^{131}I therapy has not been well characterized, it is recognized from clinical studies that toxic multinodular goiter (TMNG) is more resistant to ^{131}I than is Graves' disease and that a solitary toxic nodule is even more resistant. In addition, certain other clinical conditions have been associated with relative resistance to radiation, including increasing previous treatment with antithyroid medication and previous treatment with ^{131}I. Accordingly, regardless of

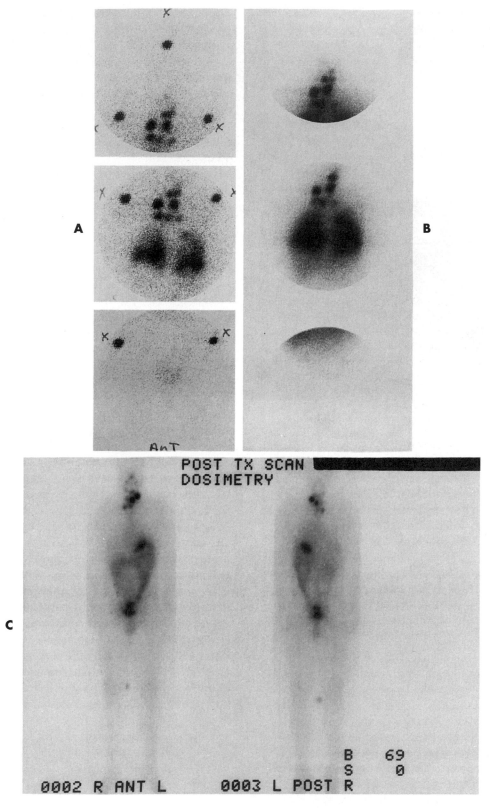

Figure 13-12   Whole body imaging in thyroid carcinoma. Gamma camera technique (**A**) 48 hours after administration of 10 mCi ^{131}I and (**B**) 72 hours after administration of 200 mCi ^{131}I (therapeutic dose). In **A**, markers are seen on the top of the skull, at the shoulders, and at the iliac crests. Focal metastases are seen at multiple sites in the neck and superior mediastinum and diffusely throughout the lungs. **C**, Scanning in a different patient at 72 hours after administration of 200 mCi ^{131}I (therapeutic dose). Prominent activity is seen in the left thyroid lobe remnant, a cervical lymph node lateral to the left lobe, and in two small foci in the superior mediastinum. Excreted activity is seen in the stomach, bowel, and bladder. A standard source has been placed between the knees.

the method used to select an ^{131}I dose, larger amounts of ^{131}I are usually used to treat patients with conditions associated with radiation resistance.

The three basic approaches to selecting the dose of radioactive iodine (^{131}I) to be administered as therapy for hyperthyroidism are as follows:

1. A relatively fixed dose can be administered, in which patients receive 3 to 7 mCi of ^{131}I; the dose chosen depends on a number of factors, such as gland size and the severity and etiology of the hyperthyroidism.
2. The dose can be based on microcuries delivered per gram, in which the estimated weight of the thyroid gland is taken into account. Based on experience, a choice is made as to whether a moderate amount of activity (50 to 80 μCi/g) or a more vigorous amount (160 to 200 μCi/g) should be administered. Factors such as the patient's age, whether nodules are present, and the severity of the hyperthyroidism are considered in selecting the amount of radioactivity per estimated gram of tissue. After this determination has been made, the amount to be administered is calculated corrected for the 24-hour uptake as follows:

$$(\mu Ci) = \frac{\mu Ci/g \text{ desired} \times \text{Gland weight (g)} \times 100}{\text{24-hr uptake (\%)}}$$

The term *μCi/g desired* allows the nuclear medicine physician to adjust the retained dose based on experience, the desire for disease control versus ablation, and the clinic's recent experience involving patient response to a particular microcurie per gram dose for the type of thyroid disease underlying the hyperthyroidism, which is a subtle correction for the average dietary iodine intake in the geographic area. Although not a sophisticated formulation, this method integrates physiologic observations into the selection of the therapeutic dose.

3. The dose can be based on the radiation absorbed dose (rad or centi-Grays [cGy]). This approach is slightly more sophisticated than the previous approach but in essence is quite similar. The physician selects the radiation absorbed dose (in cGy) for the given clinical setting. This choice is based in part on the type of underlying disease (i.e., 7,000 cGy [rad] for uncomplicated Graves' disease; 10,000 to 12,000 for toxic multinodular goiter; and 15,000 to 20,000 for toxic adenoma) (Table 13-3). The radiation absorbed dose is adjusted upward for factors such as age, disease severity, and prior therapy. Determination of the administered dose involves calculation of the number of microcuries that will deliver the selected radiation absorbed dose. The biggest advantage of this method is that it specifically measures the effective half-life and permits adjustment of the microcuries administered based on this measured factor, which is usually reflected in the degree of hyperthyroidism. The calculation can be performed using either the original

Table 13-3 Recommended radiation absorbed dose for various clinical conditions

Condition	Recommended radiation absorbed dose (cGy)
Graves' disease	7,000
Graves' disease with previous failed therapy	10,000 to 12,000
Toxic multinodular goiter	10,000 to 12,000
Toxic nodule	15,000
Ablation of remnant	30,000
Maximum blood dose	200

Quimby-Marinelli-Hine formula or the medical internal radiation dose (MIRD) formula. The Quimby-Marinelli-Hine formula has been simplified by Becker and colleagues for the geometry of the thyroid and combining constants.[9,10] The dose to be administered (in μCi) is calculated as follows:

$$\text{cGy(rad) desired} \times \text{Thyroid mass (g)} \times 6.67/t_{1/2e} \text{ (days)} \times \% \text{ 24-hour uptake}$$

in which $t_{1/2e}$ is the effective half-life. It is relatively easy to determine the thyroid gland mass by palpation, by estimate from scans, or by specific calculation based on measurement of areas of functioning tissue. A formula correlating mass and area has been reported: Mass (in grams) = 0.86 area (cm^2). Various methods to estimate weight give different results, and consistency is more important than accuracy. It is important that the nuclear medicine practitioner use a consistent method, because precision (reproducibility) is desired.

All patients must have a 24-hour radioactive iodine uptake scan before undergoing radioiodine therapy. The only additional element necessary for the calculation is determining the $t_{1/2e}$, which is accomplished by measuring the turnover of iodine in the thyroid gland by quantifying the amount remaining at a second and possibly a third time interval after the 24-hour uptake. The effective half-life is determined from a semilogarithmic plot of the thyroid counts versus time. In the determination of the effective half-life, counts should not be corrected for decay because the term *effective* includes both biologic turnover and physical decay. If decay-corrected values are determined at 24, 48, 72, and 96 hours, the half-value interval is the biologic half-life ($t_{1/2b}$). The effective half-life value can be determined by combining the value for the biologic half-life with the value for the physical half-life ($t_{1/2p}$; 8.04 days) as follows:

$$t_{1/2e} = (t_{1/2b})(t_{1/2p})/(t_{1/2b})(t_{1/2p})$$

The merit of calculating a radiation absorbed dose versus a simplistic, fixed millicurie dose is readily illustrated.[9,10] A 5 mCi ^{131}I administered dose can result in a thyroid radiation dose of 3,000 to 15,000 cGy (rad), a fivefold range depending on the percentage uptake, the effective half-life,

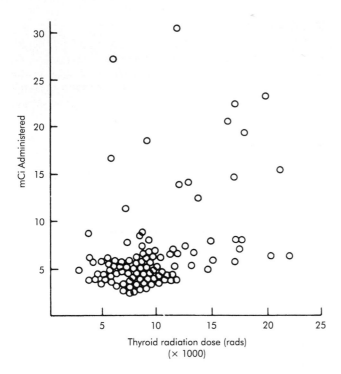

Figure 13-13 Relationship of radiation absorbed dose to the thyroid and the amount of ^{131}I administered in 92 hyperthyroid patients.

and the thyroid gland weight (Figure 13-13). Furthermore, to deliver 7,000 cGy (a frequently recommended radiation absorbed dose for patients with Graves' disease), doses from 3 to 27 mCi can be administered, depending on the variables described.

There is no evidence that the additional effort and calculation has a demonstrable clinical advantage in most patients. Many patients are in a narrow range for effective half-life values, and the individualized calculated dose to be administered is similar to the simpler calculation and sometimes to the fixed dose. The effective half-life can vary, however, from 1.5 to 6.0 days. Hence, it is recommended that the nuclear medicine practitioner make this measurement to select a patient-specific treatment dose. The minimal additional effort provides an opportunity to treat patients on a more rational basis by calculating the amount of radioactive material necessary to administer a specific radiation absorbed dose.

^{131}I treatment of thyroid carcinoma. In 1946 Seidlin and colleagues[41] reported the complete disappearance of multiple functioning metastases in a patient with thyroid carcinoma treated with ^{131}I. This report captured the imagination of the public and the press, leading to political support for and subsequent development of a civilian nuclear industry in the United States.

Radioiodine treatment using ^{131}I is involved at several points in the management of patients with thyroid carcinoma, including ablation of the residual thyroid remnant (after variable degrees of surgical thyroidectomy) and

treatment of local and distal metastases (see Figures 13-10 to 13-12). Despite 50 years of experience with ^{131}I as a therapeutic agent for thyroid carcinoma, the appropriate dose for therapy in specific clinical settings remains unresolved. For the most part, the therapeutic recommendations are generalizations from observations on a relatively small number of patients: 30 to 75 mCi of ^{131}I to ablate remnants, 75 to 150 mCi to treat local (cervical) metastases, and 150 to 300 mCi to treat distal metastases.

One of the reasons it has been difficult to determine a therapeutic dose is the relatively low frequency of thyroid carcinoma. In addition, the natural history of the disease is variable; many patients do well for long periods regardless of the therapeutic regimen. Some patients have an accelerated course with an unsatisfactory result despite aggressive therapy, whereas others have a slowly progressive course even if suboptimally treated.

Thyroid remnant ablation. Thyroid ablation is performed in patients with thyroid carcinoma who have had surgical removal of a significant portion of the thyroid gland. Although surgical practice and skill vary, it is well established that many patients have residual thyroid tissue in the region of the thyroid bed (see Figure 13-10). Thyroid ablation refers to elimination of this tissue. It had been the practice to administer 75 to 100 mCi of ^{131}I for this purpose.[22,29,30,42] Successful ablation in 87% of patients studied has been reported. In 1983 Snyder and colleagues at the Mayo Clinic reopened the controversy of dose selection by reporting the effectiveness of 30 mCi doses of ^{131}I in remnant ablation.[42] They observed complete ablation in 42 of 69 patients (61%) with a single dose of 29 mCi and minimal residual thyroid tissue in another 14. Four more patients responded to a second 29 mCi dose. Some centers routinely administer 75 mCi as an ablative dose. In the past, patients receiving greater than 30 mCi of ^{131}I were classified as radiation sources by the Nuclear Regulatory Commission (NRC). These patients were hospitalized until their body burden (radioactivity) fell to less than 30 mCi. In general, this is no longer an issue. Maxon and colleagues at the University of Cincinnati Medical Center have reported the results of quantitative dosimetry of thyroid remnants.[28,29] They report ablation with ^{131}I in 122 of 142 thyroid remnants (86%) in 57 of 70 patients (81%) by delivering 30,000 rad. The range of activity administered was 26 to 246 mCi. Twenty-six of 70 patients (37%) received less than 30 mCi of ^{131}I. This impressive study speaks forcefully for individualized dosimetric determinations in patients undergoing radionuclide thyroid remnant ablation. The results are as good as those achieved in the high-dose protocols. This method makes it possible to identify patients "likely to respond to outpatient therapy with a higher chance of success" and "those who will require greater administered activities and inpatient treatment."[29]

Local and distal metastases. Cervical lymph nodes and metastases to sites such as mediastinal lymph nodes, pulmonary parenchyma, and bone require larger doses of ^{131}I, usually 150 to 300 mCi (see Figures 13-11 and 13-12) than does ablation of normal thyroid gland remnant. Of course, the nuclear medicine physician has no influence over the percentage uptake in each metastatic lesion except to ensure that the TSH is elevated. Accordingly, it is not feasible to administer a selected radiation absorbed dose to each tumor site.

Classically, a dose of 150 to 300 mCi is selected, depending on the location and extent of the metastases. Indeed, Leeper,[28] Beierwaltes,[13] and other researchers[29,30,39] have reported satisfactory resolution of lymph node metastases in patients receiving 150 mCi of [131]I. These patients, of course, were followed with radioiodine scans and re-treated with similar doses if necessary. Beierwaltes and co-workers [13] reported 80%, 97%, and 100% ablation of cervical lymph node metastases in patients receiving 150 to 174, 175 to 199, and 200 mCi or more in a series of 35, 37, and 9 patients, respectively, at each level of administered activity. As metastases became more distant, ablation of the functioning tissue was somewhat less successful, but results as good as 75% total ablation of mediastinal nodes were observed in patients receiving less than 200 mCi of [131]I. It is interesting to note that patients receiving 175 to 199 mCi had an 89% ablation success rate. It seems likely that the larger administered dose was selected for patients with greater tumor burdens, but this is not documented in the report. It does support the contention, however, that any single variable (e.g., tumor mass or percentage uptake of administered dose) is an insufficient basis for dose selection.

In a small number of patients reported by Beierwaltes and colleagues,[13] patients with lung metastases had a 67% success rate when greater than 200 mCi was administered (3 patients) versus a 20% response rate in patients receiving 175 to 199 mCi (5 patients) and a 60% response rate in patients receiving 150 to 174 mCi (5 patients). In patients with bone metastases, the response rates were 60% in patients receiving 150 to 174 mCi (5 patients), 71% in patients receiving 175 to 199 mCi (7 patients), and 80% in patients receiving greater than 200 mCi (5 patients).

In 1980 Leeper and co-workers[28] at the Memorial Sloan-Kettering Cancer Center in New York proposed a different approach; determination of a maximum permissible dose for patients with metastases beyond the cervical lymph nodes based on limiting pulmonary parenchymal exposure to less than 80 mCi and bone marrow exposure to less than 200 rad per administered dose, which was further limited to one therapeutic dose per year. Through determination of the bone marrow exposure radiation dose, bone marrow depression was avoided despite administration of doses in excess of 300 mCi. One patient was reported who was free of disease or complications 3 years after a 320 mCi administered dose.

Recently Maxon and colleagues[29,30] reported the results of a larger series of thyroid cancer patients who underwent quantitative radiation dosimetry. This group had previously reported successful ablation of thyroid remnants at 30,000

rad and of nodal metastases at 8,000 rad.[29,30] When the radiation dose to the involved nodes was greater than 8,000 rad, 98% of patients responded to treatment, whereas only 20% responded at less than this radiation absorbed dose. In the recent series they observed a success rate of 86% of patients and 90% of involved nodes in situations in which 14,000 rad or more was administered.

In summary, a rational basis exists for the use of quantitative dosimetry for the selection of a therapeutic dose of [131]I. Bone marrow dose is determined as a worst-case calculation, with the assumption that the radiation absorbed dose is equivalent to the blood dose. This is determined by measuring the blood disappearance rate of a tracer dose and assuming a blood volume for the functioning marrow space of 20% of the total blood volume. A maximum "safe" dose is thus determined that will limit the calculated marrow exposure to 200 rad. Tumor dosimetry is problematic. Although it would be of value to know the radiation absorbed dose at various tumor sites, this is not readily accomplished, particularly in a clinical setting. Nevertheless, calculation of the maximum safe dose to be administered provides a basis for administering doses greater than 150 mCi of [131]I.

An additional category of patients to consider for therapy are those without demonstrable foci of ^{131}I uptake but with elevated serum thyroglobulin levels (>10 ng/ml). The generally accepted approach had been to continue observation of these patients and not to treat them with radioactive iodine unless iodine-concentrating tissue is identified. Two well-documented groups of thyroid carcinoma patients were found to have elevated serum thyroglobulin and negative body ^{131}I scans after total removal of the thyroid gland. Of 83 patients treated at the University of Pisa, Italy, one third had positive scans after a therapeutic dose of 100 mCi of [131]I.[34] Many of the patients had a significant lowering of serum thyroglobulin after radioiodine treatment. At the National Institutes of Health (NIH), nine of 10 patients with similar diagnostic results (elevated thyroglobulin levels and negative ^{131}I diagnostic scans) had abnormal scans when imaged after a therapeutic dose.[1]

With the advent of ^{18}F-FDG imaging, it has been demonstrated that thyroid carcinoma is identified by FDG PET imaging even if the ^{131}I imaging is negative. This information provides the physician and the patient with several therapeutic options. Improved anatomic localization and exclusion of other sites of known tumor involvement make it feasible to consider surgical resection or even limited external beam radiation therapy.[47,48]

PARATHYROID GLANDS

Anatomy and Physiology

The parathyroid glands are located in the neck. They are multifocal (usually four) and found alongside the thyroid gland, lying either adjacent, beneath, or within the substance of the thyroid (see Figure 13-2). The parathyroids migrate from their embryologic origins in the branchial clefts into the neck to their usual location alongside the thyroid. Considerable variation may occur, however, in their ultimate location. They can be found within the thyroid gland, elsewhere in the neck, in the mediastinum, within the thymus, among the great vessels (within the carotid sheath above the level of the thyroid to the area around the subclavian and innominate vessels in the thorax), and within the mediastinum.

The parathyroid glands synthesize, store, and secrete parathyroid hormone, a polypeptide hormone that regulates calcium and phosphorus metabolism via action on the bone, kidneys, and gastrointestinal tract. In bone, parathyroid hormone directly stimulates osteoclastic activity, increasing bone resorption and thereby making calcium (and phosphorus) available to the plasma and tissues. In the kidneys, parathyroid hormone increases urinary excretion of phosphorus by inhibiting tubular resorption of phosphate. In the gastrointestinal tract, calcium absorption from the bowel lumen is enhanced by parathyroid hormone.

Synthesis and secretion of parathyroid hormone are regulated by the plasma ionized calcium level, which is maintained in a physiologic range by means of a negative feedback loop: a decline in plasma ionized calcium stimulates the release of parathyroid hormone, making the calcium ion available.

Clinical Aspects

Failure of the parathyroid tissue to produce parathyroid hormone results in hypoparathyroidism, causing a gradual reduction in serum calcium (hypocalcemia). Clinical manifestations of hypocalcemia are a consequence of delayed repolarization of cell membrane electrical potential, which results in muscle spasm and irritability and cardiac conduction abnormalities.

Excessive secretion of parathyroid hormone (inappropriate secretion despite normal or elevated calcium levels) is known as hyperparathyroidism. A principal component of this disorder is elevation of the serum calcium (hypercalcemia). This is associated with increased urinary excretion of calcium, which can cause renal stones and calcification of the kidney (renal calcinosis) and other soft tissues. Because the bones provide a storage source for calcium, orthopedic complications arise from bone mineral loss. This condition, known as *primary hyperparathyroidism*, is most frequently associated with a functioning parathyroid adenoma arising from one of the parathyroid glands (80% to 90% of cases). Hyperplasia of the parathyroid glands accounts for the remaining 10% to 20% of cases. The underlying mechanism for diffuse hyperplasia with loss of normal feedback suppression is unknown but probably is a result of receptor autonomy.

In chronic renal disease, the kidneys fail to excrete the phosphate ion adequately and serum phosphate levels rise. Because an upper limit exists for the production of serum calcium and the phosphate ion concentration, calcium is deposited in soft tissues or excreted. Lowering of the serum calcium in this manner stimulates parathyroid hormone secretion and parathyroid gland growth, leading to a clinical condition known as *secondary hyperparathyroidism*. The clinical picture is a mixed one, expressing the underlying chronic renal disease, the secondary hyperparathyroidism (hypocalcemia and increased bone resorption). Therapy should be directed to the underlying renal disease. At times the hyperparathyroidism is so severe that a transplanted kidney would be at risk. Surgical removal of the excess parathyroid tissue is also necessary. Although the excessive parathyroid hormone synthesis and secretion in chronic renal disease begins as a homeostatic response to the hypocalcemia (secondary to the hyperphosphatemia), the hyperactivity may persist after correction of the renal disorder as a consequence of a functioning parathyroid adenoma. This is so-called *tertiary hyperparathyroidism*.

In the modern era, routine serum calcium determinations result in earlier clinical recognition of hypercalcemia, leading to earlier detection of hyperparathyroidism. This presents an opportunity for nuclear medicine to assist in the localization of the functioning adenoma, because with earlier recognition comes the challenge of locating smaller adenomas.

Nuclear Medicine Procedures

In clinical situations in which abnormalities of parathyroid gland function are suspected, direct measurement of serum parathyroid hormone by radioimmunoassay provides the basis for the diagnosis.

The principal role of the nuclear medicine service for patients with confirmed hyperparathyroidism is identification of the site of parathyroid hormone production, usually a single parathyroid adenoma.[5] Parathyroid adenomas are found in diverse locations alongside, behind, and within the thyroid and in areas somewhat distant from the thyroid, such as high or low in the neck or mediastinum (see Figure 13-2). The surgeon is aided and total operative time is reduced by localization of the site of excess hormone production before surgery. Despite the availability of CT and MRI to locate parathyroid adenomas, parathyroid scintigraphy performs well with a high degree of accuracy.[5]

In the past few years, ^{99m}Tc-MIBI has emerged as the radionuclide of choice for the localization of parathyroid adenomas.[32,33,43,44] Two methods are currently available. First, ^{99m}Tc pertechnetate is used as part of a dual radionuclide subtraction technique in which thyroid tissue is initially identified. Subsequently, ^{99m}Tc-MIBI is administered to identify both thyroid and parathyroid tissue. The initially acquired ^{99m}Tc pertechnetate distribution map of thyroid tissue is normalized to the total counts in the ^{99m}Tc-MIBI images and subtracted from the secondarily acquired ^{99m}Tc-MIBI thyroid and parathyroid image. The residual image represents parathyroid tissue.

Other abnormalities, such as thyroid adenoma, that poorly trap ^{99m}Tc pertechnetate are also identified as pertechnetate-poor, perfused ^{99m}Tc-MIBI–positive areas that cannot be differentiated from parathyroid adenomas.

In late 1992 Taillefer and colleagues[44] described a so-called double-phase study in which anterior cervical images are obtained at 15 to 20 minutes after injection of 20 to 25 mCi of ^{99m}Tc-MIBI and again at 2 to 3 hours after injection. Ten-minute acquisition was obtained using a parallel hole, low-energy, high-resolution collimator with a 1.5 zoom factor. The differential wash-out of the ^{99m}Tc-MIBI (with retention by the parathyroid tissue) resulted in preferential visualization of parathyroid in 19 of 21 instances[44] (Figure 13-14). Another advantage of the Taillefer technique is the convenient acquisition of mediastinal images at both the early and late acquisition sessions because the patient is already positioned under a camera with a parallel hole collimator.

This procedure has been modified somewhat since the initial description. ^{99m}Tc-MIBI is injected and the images of the neck are acquired after approximately 30 minutes, the so-called early phase. Repeat imaging of the neck follows at 90 to 120 minutes with comparison of the two image sets. Identification of the parathyroid tissue is based on greater retention of the ^{99m}Tc-MIBI in the metabolically active, mitochondrial dense parathyroid adenoma. However, this mode of identification is not completely parathyroid tissue specific either, because other focal lesions, specifically thyroid adenomas and carcinomas, preferentially retain ^{99m}Tc-MIBI compared with the surrounding thyroid and other tissue. Nevertheless, in an appropriate clinical setting of elevated parathyroid hormone levels, it is most likely that the mitochondria-rich tissue represents the functioning parathyroid adenoma.

In the dual radionuclide technique, 4 to 5 mCi of ^{99m}Tc pertechnetate is injected first. After acquisition of images of the neck at about 20 minutes, 20 to 25 mCi of ^{99m}Tc-MIIBI is injected, and imaging is done approximately 30 minutes later. The patient must remain in position, assisted by pillows or sandbags to maintain location. It is recommended that markers be placed in the field of view. Current digital imaging display equipment allows repositioning of acquired images to ensure superimposition before subtraction. For the dual phase ^{99m}Tc-MIBI technique, 20 to 25 mCi also is used. Obviously, the two techniques can be combined; that is, the dual radionuclide method followed by acquisition of a delayed-phase ^{99m}Tc-MIBI image. Because the amount of ^{99m}Tc-MIBI activity administered is four to five times that of the ^{99m}Tc pertechnetate, the ^{99m}Tc pertechnetate component can be ignored when viewing the ^{99m}Tc-MIBI images. Nevertheless, to prepare subtraction images, the initial ^{99m}Tc pertechnetate image must be normalized for count density before it is subtracted from the ^{99m}Tc-MIBI images.

Before the patient is released, an image of the mediastinum or chest should be obtained to detect ectopic parathyroid adenoma. Lesions in this area are quite distinct and can readily be identified, because the surrounding tissue is relatively poorly perfused (mediastinum) or less dense (lung) (see Figure 13-14).

Several embellishments for parathyroid scintigraphy with ^{99m}Tc-MIBI have been described. It has been suggested that SPECT imaging may provide additional information helpful in the surgical location of the hyperfunctioning parathyroid tissue.[16] This has met with limited acceptance because of the difficulty in assigning location to the anatomy-poor images. Most recently, however, image fusion instrumentation has become available that combines CT images with scintigraphic data, allowing precise identification of anatomic location. Even-Sapir reported an experience with eight patients with this technique and demonstrated no difference in the overall high degree of accuracy but greater confidence and precision in identification of the site of the hyperfunctioning tissue.[21] Zwas and colleagues[50] recently reported a series demonstrating that an intraoperative probe is effective for reducing operative time.

A number of other ^{99m}Tc tracers for myocardial perfusion imaging are available and have been used in place of ^{99m}Tc-MIBI for identification of parathyroid adenomas. These compounds (e.g., ^{99m}Tc tetrafosmin) have extraction efficiencies and efflux rates that are slightly different from those of

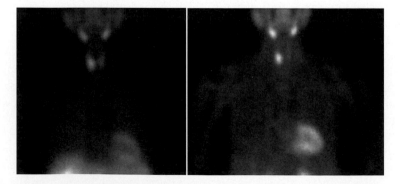

Figure 13-14   Anterior neck and upper thorax region images at 10 minutes and 2 hours after administration of 20 mCi ^{99m}Tc MIBI. In the early images, activity is seen throughout both thyroid lobes. The delayed image shows prominent activity in the lower pole of the right thyroid lobe. This focus of persistent activity is characteristic of a parathyroid adenoma and has a high degree of accuracy in predicting the location of this lesion in an appropriate at-risk population (patients with hyperparathyroidism). False-positive results may be associated with thyroid abnormalities.

^{99m}Tc-MIBI. Although satisfactory images have been obtained in many instances, the few comparison studies available suggest that ^{99m}Tc-MIBI is superior to its competitors for the localization of parathyroid adenomas.[22] The use of ^{99m}Tc-MIBI has supplanted the use of ^{201}Tl with ^{99m}Tc pertechnetate or ^{123}I subtraction of thyroid tissue.

The sensitivity (and specificity) of ^{99m}Tc-MIBI (and ^{99m}Tc tetrafosmin) subtraction scintigraphy appears to exceed that of the results obtained with ^{201}Tl subtraction scintigraphy.[3,22] In the initial report comparing the ^{201}Tl–^{99m}Tc pertechnetate subtraction technique with ^{99m}Tc-MIBI scintigraphy, O'Doherty and collagues[32] reported that 37 of 40 adenomas were detected with ^{201}Tl and 39 of 40 were detected with ^{99m}Tc-MIBI.[32] In 15 patients with hyperplastic glands, ^{99m}Tc-MIBI identified 32 glands, whereas ^{201}Tl localized 29 hyperplastic glands. In a direct comparison of ^{99m}Tc tetrafosmin–^{99m}Tc pertechnetate subtraction to ^{201}Tl–^{99m}Tc pertechnetate subtraction, the ^{99m}Tc agent subtraction scintigraphy had a sensitivity, specificity, and accuracy of 76%, 92%, and 83% compared with 52%, 85%, and 65% for ^{201}Tl–^{99m}Tc pertechnetate subtraction.[3] The improvement in overall accuracy is partly the result of superior imaging characteristics (lower energy) and greater photon flux (larger dose, shorter half-life) and also of the pharmacology-biochemistry of the ^{99m}Tc-MIBI and other ^{99m}Tc tumor perfusion agents. Because it binds efficiently to mitochondrial proteins, wash-out from the mitochondria-rich parathyroid adenoma is reduced. This results in a greater parathyroid-to-thyroid and parathyroid-to-background ratio than was observed with ^{201}Tl.

PANCREAS

Anatomy and Physiology

The pancreas is a somewhat serpentine-shaped organ found between the inferior (greater) curvature of the stomach and loops of small bowel. Most of the organ consists of acinar cells that secrete digestive enzymes into the proximal small bowel. The endocrine pancreas consists of the islets of Langerhans, small foci of cells that synthesize, store, and secrete insulin and other peptide hormones.

Insulin is the principal product of the beta cells. It is the major regulator of glucose homeostasis, principally through promotion of the active transport of glucose at the cell membrane. Many other metabolic effects occur as a consequence of this biochemical action, such as preferential utilization of glucose with preservation of stored glycogen, adipose tissue, and protein. In the normal subject, blood glucose is regulated and body energy metabolism is efficiently maintained. By contrast, in insulin-dependent diabetes mellitus, beta cells atrophy and fail to secrete sufficient insulin to maintain the homeostatic mechanisms just described. Blood glucose rises but is not used effectively by the tissues. The amount of glucose that appears in the glomerular filtrate exceeds the capacity for resorption, resulting in loss of glucose (and water) in the urine. Glycogen stores are depleted, and adipose tissue is mobilized for energy. All these metabolic consequences produce the dramatic clinical picture of insulin deficiency, culminating in diabetic ketoacidosis, hyperglycemia, dehydration, and death if insulin, fluids, electrolytes, and glucose are not replaced.

Both benign and malignant tumors of the beta cells secrete insulin in excess of the amount needed for glucose regulation and thus produce hypoglycemia (low blood glucose). Because glucose is the principal substrate for the brain, hypoglycemia produces mental confusion, metabolic and cardiovascular signs of stress, and loss of consciousness.

Other islet cell tumors elaborate excessive amounts of other peptide hormones such as gastrin, glucagon, vasoactive intestinal peptide (VIP), or somatostatin.

Nuclear Medicine Procedures

Radioimmunoassay initially was developed Berson and Yalow[14,15] as a method to measure insulin. In 1977 Roslyn Yalow, a medical physicist, was awarded the Nobel Prize in Medicine and Physiology for the discovery of this powerful technique. Her colleague, Solomon Berson, had died earlier that decade. Radioimmunoassay of insulin in small volumes of plasma provided investigators with a method that revolutionized the understanding of insulin physiology. Once validated for the measurement of insulin, radioimmunoassay was applied to virtually any substance of biologic interest. With appropriate choice of reagents, radioimmunoassay has been used to quantify peptides of pancreatic and nonpancreatic origin, including growth hormone, parathyroid hormone, calcitonin, glucagon, gastrin, and other less commonly studied peptides. These assays, however, are not routinely performed as clinical procedures in nuclear medicine departments.

Islet cell tumors may be benign or malignant and functional or nonfunctional. Functional tumors present early as a consequence of the metabolically active substances, usually peptides, that they elaborate, such as insulin, glucagon, gastrin, VIP, or somatostatin. Both normal islet cell function and tumors arising from islet cells are regulated in part by somatostatin, a 14-amino-acid peptide initially identified as a hypothalamic regulator of pituitary function. It is now known that somatostatin is produced in small quantities in many tissues and that it regulates these tissues by means of interaction with somatostatin receptors that are also present on many cell types. Tumors arising from these cell types, including islet cell tumors, have increased expression of somatostatin receptors and hence are detected with somatostatin-receptor scintigraphy using ^{111}In-DTPA pentetreotide, a somatostatin analog.

SOMATOSTATIN-RECEPTOR IMAGING

Anatomy and Physiology

Somatostatin is a 14-amino-acid regulatory neuropeptide initially identified as a hypothalamic hormone that inhibited the release of growth hormone from the anterior pituitary.

Somatostatin has effects on many tissues, most specifically the neuroendocrine secretory cells distributed throughout the gastrointestinal tract and respiratory passages. At these sites somatostatin inhibits the release of the islet cell hormones insulin and glucagon, the release of gastrin and other internal secretions that regulate bowel function, and the secretion of digestive enzymes in response to other localized regulatory secretions. It has complex effects on the immune system and generally seems to inhibit cell proliferation.

Rather than reflecting classic *endocrine* function (i.e., an internal secretory product of one organ that affects a distal organ or tissue), somatostatin is usually a local regulator of tissue function manifesting *paracrine* (nearby) and *autocrine* (self) regulatory function.

The effects of somatostatin are modulated by specific somatostatin receptors. Knowledge of somatostatin-receptor biology is still evolving; human beings have at least five receptor subtypes. Different subtypes are expressed on different tissues. The significance of receptor subtypes is this: somatostatin binds to all receptor subtypes and initiates whatever biologic effect is so regulated; drug analogs, however, react with the receptor subtypes in some tissues but not those in others. Receptors may decrease in affinity or number per cell; indeed, a tumor may de-differentiate to a point where it no longer expresses a receptor. This may account for the abrupt acceleration of the clinical course as the tumor de-differentiates, because if a tumor had decreased receptor expression, it would no longer be receptive to the inhibiting effect of somatostatin.

Clinical Aspects

The clinical significance of the discovery of somatostatin is the development of drug analogs such as octreotide (Sandostatin, Sandoz), which binds to somatostatin receptors and is useful for inhibiting the release of metabolically active materials such as growth hormone in acromegaly or a variety of vasoactive amines in carcinoid syndrome. Octreotide is an 8-amino-acid analog of somatostatin. It retains an affinity for somatostatin receptors but has a longer plasma and biologic half-life than native somatostatin. Octreotide has a high binding affinity for somatostatin receptor (SSTR) subtype 2, subtype 5, and to a lesser extent subtype 3.

Somatostatin receptors have increased expression on tumors arising from cells that have evolved from the embryonic neural crest. This includes pituitary tumors; medullary carcinoma of the thyroid; pancreatic islet cell tumors; carcinoid tumors; and tumors of the chromaffin tissue, pheochromocytomas, neuroblastomas, and paragangliomas. Because of the distributive nature of the cell types from which these tumors arise, the tumors themselves may have an idiosyncratic distribution. These tumors frequently present as a result of the symptoms produced by their metabolically active products. Metastatic carcinoid tumors, pituitary tumors, and functioning islet cell tumors (insulinomas, gastrinomas, and glucagonomas) and pheochromocytomas are in this category. Carcinoid tumors may be discovered as an incidental finding during a surgical procedure or CT. These are usually benign, but differentiation of benign and malignant carcinoid tumors frequently is difficult. Symptoms such as flushing, diarrhea, hives, asthma, and heart valve problems arising from the carcinoid secretory products do not occur unless liver metastases are present, because the portal circulation detoxifies secretions from the primary bowel site. Carcinoid tumors are found in the appendix (38%), the ileum of the small intestine (23%), the rectum (13%), the bronchus (11.5%), at sites throughout the gastrointestinal tract, and rarely in other organs. Nonfunctioning islet cell tumors and medullary carcinoma of the thyroid do not cause metabolic symptoms, therefore they usually do not become manifest until extensive metastases are present, unless they are identified coincidentally during surgery.

Nuclear Medicine Procedures

Somatostatin-receptor scintigraphy is performed with ^{111}In-DTPA pentetreotide, a radiolabeled derivative of octreotide to identify tumors that arise from the widely distributed specialized secretory cells with somatostatin receptors, the so-called *neuroendocrine tumors*.[24,25]

Much of the early clinical evaluation of somatostatin-receptor scintigraphy was performed by Krenning and co-workers, who first evaluated an ^{123}I tyrosyl derivative of octreotide.[24] Although it was shown to be of value for detection of neuroendocrine tumors, the utility of ^{123}I tyrosyl octreotide was impaired by the relatively high cost and short shelf life of ^{123}I, deiodination of the product, and the significant fraction of the administered dose secreted into the bile that appeared as intestinal activity. Subsequently, a DTPA derivative of the 8-amino-acid octreotide was prepared. This derivative, Octreoscan (Mallinckrodt, St. Louis, Missouri), is available in kit form to be labeled with [111]In.

The adult dose of ^{111}In-DTPA pentetreotide (Octreoscan) is 6.0 mCi. The usual approach to pediatric dosage can be used. Despite the cost of the radiotracer and the excellent results frequently obtained, the dose should not be reduced in adult patients because receptor affinity for this agent varies from tumor type to tumor type and from patient to patient.

[111]In pentetreotide should be slowly injected intravenously because the pentetreotide (octreotide) component is pharmacologically active. Although the amount of octreotide injected is only a fraction of the usual pharmacologic dose, instances of a drop in blood pressure and other consequences have been observed in patients whose clinical state is dominated by the secretory products of the neuroendocrine tumor.

Because plasma is rapidly cleared of ^{111}In pentetreotide, it would be expected that imaging at 4 hours would be sufficient. Many lesions can be identified at this point, but image quality and lesion detection are better at 24 hours because of enhancement of the tumor-background contrast. Nevertheless, areas suspected of involvement should be imaged at 4 hours initially, because it is frequently necessary to have these early images for comparison with the 24-hour images to decide whether abdominal foci of activity represent bowel contents (often seen at 24 hours despite bowel preparation) or bowel wall activity, indicating tumors (Figures 13-15 and 13-16).

Approximately 10% of the ^{111}In-DTPA pentetreotide administered is cleared through the hepatobiliary system. Accordingly, a gentle laxative should be administered the evening after the injection. Better results are obtained by pre-treating the patient with a laxative before injection of the tracer and again the evening after the injection but before the 24-hour images are taken.

Dual energy acquisition is performed with 20% windows centered on the 179 and 267 keV photopeaks. In most instances (except pituitary or other cranial tumors), high-count static acquisitions should be obtained of the thorax and abdomen in the anterior and posterior projections for at least 10 minutes each. These images should be stored digitally for further manipulation if necessary.

Scanning gamma cameras produce good-quality whole body images but can be misleading. A negative study does not exclude disease or even provide a complete picture of the extent of disease involvement. High-quality SPECT imaging of appropriate areas (thorax or abdomen or both) should be obtained. In patients suspected of having carcinoid or functioning or nonfunctioning islet cell tumors,

as well as pheochromocytomas or other chromaffin tissue tumors, complete evaluation includes SPECT imaging of the abdomen. Scintigraphy of patients with ectopic ACTH syndrome (frequently the result of a bronchial carcinoid) also should include SPECT of the thorax unless the somatostatin-receptor–positive focus has been identified in the abdomen.

After intravenous administration of ^{111}In-DTPA pentetreotide, the material is cleared rapidly from the plasma, with a plasma half-time of 20 minutes. On whole body images obtained at 4 hours, activity is seen in the liver, spleen, kidneys, and bladder. Approximately 50% is cleared by the kidneys and appears in the urine. On 24-hour images, the bladder is usually clear, and a variable amount of activity is seen in the bowel (see Figures 13-15 and 13-16).

Activity that appears on planar images in the region of the gallbladder activity or bowel or bladder activity cannot be dismissed as physiologic activity. Although that conclusion may be correct, SPECT imaging or re-imaging after an even longer interval is necessary to differentiate physiologic excretion from tumor localization. Similarly, medullary carcinoma of the thyroid may involve mediastinal lymph nodes that are not visible on standard displays. If plasma markers are present indicating the presence of tumor, the nuclear medicine physician and technologist would be remiss in accepting a negative study.

The recent clinical availability of fusion imaging serves to provide even better localization of accumulated activity. Even-Sapir has reported her initial results in 10 patients with neuroendocrine tumors.[20] Although there are not yet sufficient studies to determine the impact on overall accuracy, if any, fusion imaging provides greater confidence and credibility in the interpretation.

Activity in the kidneys remains an obstacle to interpretation because these organs occupy a large portion of the abdomen. The right kidney obscures part of the right hepatic lobe and may both interfere with the identification of metastases in that region and confuse the identification of right adrenal masses and lesions in the head of the pancreas. Tumors in the tail of the pancreas may be obscured by the left kidney. Once again, SPECT imaging provides an opportunity to identify lesions that otherwise would be obscured, but there is a limit to the ability of this technique to reconstruct the distribution of activity found in small lesions near the kidneys, which are relatively large and contain a considerable fraction of the administered dose of radioactivity.

In addition to the technical factors considered above, a number of biologic features of somatostatin-receptor imaging may contribute to false-negative and false-positive findings. Certain drugs may down-regulate or cross-react with the receptor so that it can no longer be occupied by the labeled octreotide. For example, it currently is a subject of controversy whether a patient receiving octreotide therapeutically should have this medication discontinued before therapy. It has been shown that tumors can be identified in patients who receive such treatment and that, in fact,

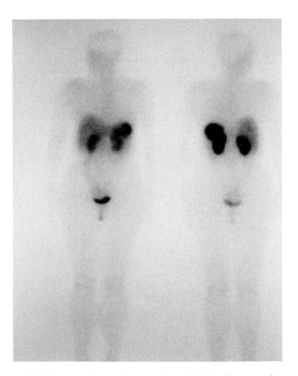

Figure 13-15 Anterior and posterior whole body scan obtained 4 hours after IV injection of 6.0 mCi ^{111}In pentetreotide. Although patient was referred to locate residual medullary carcinoma of the thyroid, this figure was interpreted as normal. Scan speed is 10 cm/min; at 24 hours, the scan speed is reduced to 8 cm/min. Normal distribution includes mild hepatic uptake and marked spleen and renal uptake. At 4 hours, excretion into the bladder is also seen.

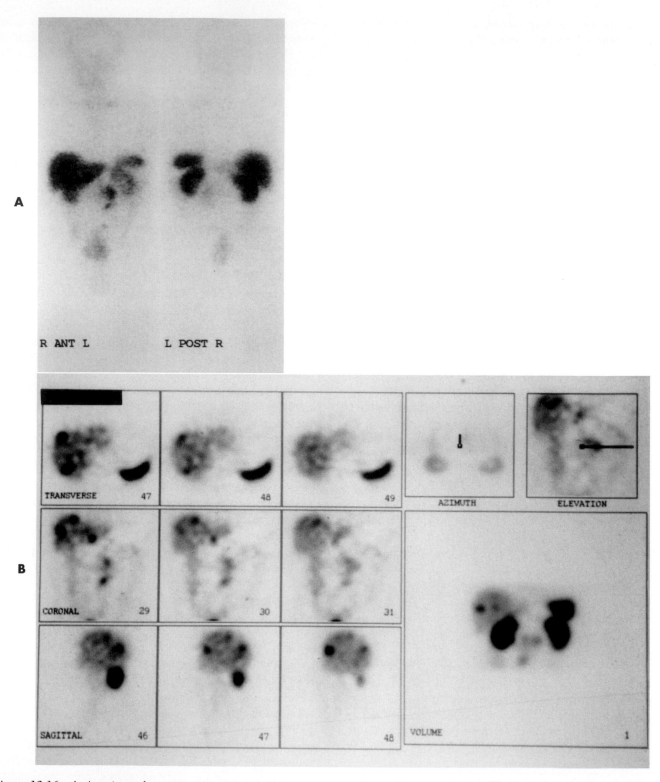

Figure 13-16   A, Anterior and posterior scanning gamma camera images obtained at 24 hours after ^{111}In pentetreotide administration in a patient subsequently confirmed to have metastatic carcinoid tumor. Acquisition was stopped below the pelvis. Uptake in the liver, spleen, and kidneys is seen. Bladder activity is minimal at 24 hours. In addition to the usual organ distribution, two foci are seen in the abdomen slightly to the left of the midline. These represent a primary carcinoid tumor in the wall of the small bowel and a regional nodal metastasis. Neither lesion was identified on abdominal CT or contrast studies. The image is too dark to reveal several metastatic foci in the liver. **B,** Transverse, coronal, and sagittal slices after SPECT acquisition of the same patient. Three distinct foci are seen within the hepatic parenchyma. The bowel and lymph node foci are confirmed.

octreotide therapy up-regulates the receptors in various cell lines. It is believed that if it is desirable to evaluate the extent and location of disease involvement, octreotide therapy should be discontinued. This belief is based on the conclusive demonstration that the uptake of the labeled agent is specific and readily blocked by unlabeled peptide administered before the labeled form.

False-positive image interpretation is a result either of misreading normal distribution of activity as lesions (e.g., interpreting gallbladder, bowel, or bladder activity as lesions) or of increased expression of somatostatin receptors on other tissue. Activated lymphocytes express somatostatin receptors. Consequently, positive foci of activity are seen in a variety of disorders with lymphocytic responses such as Graves' orbitopathy, tuberculosis or other pulmonary granulomatous disorders, pulmonary and nonpulmonary sarcoid, changes in the pleura after irradiation, activation of respiratory tract lymph nodes during viral upper respiratory infections, and rheumatoid arthritis or tumors other than neuroendocrine tumors (e.g., lymphomas, breast carcinoma) that express somatostatin receptors.[27]

SSTR imaging also has been particularly useful for identifying functional and nonfunctional islet cell carcinomas. Increased receptor density and the subtype seem to vary somewhat with the type of islet cell tumor. Gastrin-secreting tumors (gastrinomas) have virtually 100% detectability, whereas insulin-producing tumors (insulinomas) have a 50% detection sensitivity. Of course, identification of the tumor is not tumor type specific. [111]In pentetreotide scintigraphy also detects somatostatin-positive, nonfunctional islet cell tumors. The presence of somatostatin receptors has anecdotally been reported to be a more reliable means of differentiating nonfunctioning islet cell tumors from adenocarcinoma of the pancreas than histopathologic examination of the tumor. Surgical tissue from patients who have had a prolonged survival despite a pathologic diagnosis of adenocarcinoma of the pancreas was reevaluated for somatostatin receptors. All of the prolonged survivors had somatostatin receptors, which demonstrates immunohistology. Because adenocarcinoma of the pancreas is known not to have somatostatin receptors, it is concluded that the classic microscopic examination (with immunohistology or radioautographic identification of somatostatin receptors) was inaccurate or at least not capable of differentiating between islet cell tumors and adenocarcinoma of the pancreas.

^{111}In-DTPA pentetreotide is also useful for the detection and localization of pheochromocytoma and neuroblastoma.

Medullary carcinoma of the thyroid may also be identified with ^{111}In-DTPA pentetreotide. The frequency of somatostatin receptors on radioautographic examination is reported to be about 33%, which is less than ideal. In small series, tumors have been identified in 50% to 70% of cases. Results are better in de novo patients. This is probably because it is earlier in the course of the disease, before the tumor has de-differentiated. The initial diagnosis, however, usually is made serendipitously after surgical removal of a thyroid nodule that is reported as a medullary carcinoma. More frequently, the nuclear medicine facility is asked to identify the source of the recurrent elevation of thyrocalcitonin in a patient who has undergone total thyroidectomy for medullary carcinoma. The task is complicated at that time because the tumor may have decreased receptor expression or saturation of the receptors as a result of synthesis of somatostatin by the tumor. In these instances, iodine-131 metaiodobenzylguanidine (^{131}I-MIBG) is often of greater value in identifying the site or sites of functioning tissue.

Somatostatin-receptor scintigraphy can be either a gratifying, relatively easy technique or an exceedingly frustrating, challenging procedure. In many instances the tumor is readily identifiable. This should not lead to a false degree of confidence. To achieve the greatest possible diagnostic yield, the nuclear medicine department should be prepared to perform a full set of images of the highest quality and to modify the protocol to suit the particular clinical and scintigraphic setting. Clinical trials are currently in progress to evaluate the therapeutic potential of targeted radionuclide therapy using radiolabeled peptides for the therapy of tumors expressing high-affinity receptors.[17-19,46]

ADRENAL GLANDS

The adrenal glands consist of an outer adrenal cortex and an interior neurosecretory adrenal medulla. They are located in the retroperitoneum, superior to the kidneys (suprarenal), lying approximately below the eleventh rib. The right adrenal is higher and more posterior than the left (even though the left kidney is frequently higher than the right); the right adrenal is triangular, sitting astride the upper pole of the right kidney. The left adrenal is more crescent shaped and lies anteromedial to the upper pole of the left kidney. The adrenal cortex contains 6% cholesterol by weight, the highest fraction per organ in the body. This cholesterol is the principal metabolic precursor in the synthesis of the adrenal corticosteroids.

ADRENAL CORTEX

Anatomy and Physiology

The adrenal cortex is further classified on histologic section into three zones: the glomerulosa, the intermedia, and the fasciculata, each having specific secretory products. The zona glomerulosa is the site of synthesis of the glucocorticoids, cortisone and hydroxycortisone. These corticosteroids have profound effects on body function, metabolism, and the inflammatory and immune responses. Although these compounds have salt-retaining properties also, another steroid, aldosterone, with more potent effects on sodium retention and potassium loss, is synthesized in and secreted by the zona intermedia. The zona fasciculata is the site of adrenal androgen synthesis in both men and women.

Destruction of the adrenal glands by tumor, inflammation, or spontaneous atrophy results in adrenal insufficiency, marked by profound sodium loss, inability to respond to external stressors, hypotension, and death. Overproduction of one or more steroid species is caused by adrenal hyperplasia, adenoma, or carcinoma and results in a number of well-characterized and dramatic syndromes. An excess of glucosteroids results in Cushing's syndrome, a clinical complex of moon facies, weight gain with central obesity, hypertension, diabetes, purple abdominal striae, and emotional lability. Conn's syndrome (hypertension and hypokalemia) is the result of excess aldosterone.

Masculinizing syndromes occur secondary to excess adrenal elaboration of androgens. In addition to benign adenomas, the adrenals also can exhibit a focal or diffuse microadenomatous or even macroadenomatous histologic configuration. This observation is significant because it complicates the diagnostic workup; bilateral hyperplasia is caused by excess production of ACTH, usually from the pituitary, although ectopic ACTH production by carcinoids or other tumors sometimes may be the underlying cause. Therapy is directed to the source of the ACTH overproduction. Bilateral macroadenomas require surgical removal of the functioning adrenal adenomas. Accordingly, it is important that an accurate diagnosis be established in order to select the appropriate intervention. Despite the availability of high-resolution imaging techniques, differential diagnosis frequently requires the use of physiologic imaging using a radiotracer to demonstrate the pattern and location of adrenal steroid overproduction.

The availability of high-resolution imaging techniques such as CT and MRI also has resulted in a new clinical observation, the incidental identification of adrenal masses. These *incidentalomas* sometimes require further evaluation with functional imaging to assess if they are truly incidental or actually elaborating inappropriate amounts or patterns of secretory products.

Nuclear Medicine Procedures

Adrenal cortical imaging is indicated in clinical situations characterized by increased cortisolism, increased aldosteronism, and increased virilization when the source of the hypersecretion of the appropriate hormone is not clear. Identification of the site of adrenal hormone synthesis is the basis for adrenal cortical imaging with radiotracers. The unique dependence on cholesterol as the biochemical precursor of the steroid hormones provides the tool for accomplishing this task. Because it had been demonstrated that ^{14}C cholesterol injected intravenously in animals is incorporated into newly synthesized steroids, Sarkar, Beierwaltes, and colleagues[40] evaluated the utility of ^{131}I iodocholesterol as a marker of the site of cholesterol synthesis. This compound resulted in adrenal to liver ratios of 168:1 and adrenal to kidney ratios of 300:1. Subsequently, a number of analogs were produced during the labeling process. One of these, ^{131}I-6-beta-iodomethyl-19-norcholesterol (^{131}I NP-59), had even greater avidity for adrenal cortical functioning tissue than the original compound. In addition, it had greater in vivo stability and less deiodination.[12]

Because the need for an adrenal cortical imaging agent is limited, no commercial source for this agent is available. In addition, the costs associated with pre-market evaluation and the FDA approval process are prohibitive. The Radiochemistry Section of the Nuclear Medicine Department at the University of Michigan supplies ^{131}I NP-59 as a radiochemical to investigators with appropriate radionuclide possession licenses. Human use in the United States requires physician-sponsored investigational new drug (IND) status and approval by an institutional human use committee for use as an investigational agent.

^{131}I NP-59 is available in 3 mCi batches and is administered as a 1 mCi dose to the average adult patient (1.7 m^2), correcting for size if necessary on a weight or body surface basis. ^{131}I NP-59 is a cholesterol derivative, insoluble in aqueous solutions, and therefore prepared in an alcohol-saline solution with the solubilizing agent Tween-80, a polyoxyethylene sorbitol fatty acid ester. The material should be used as soon as possible after receipt to minimize aliquot volume. It should be injected slowly (over 2 to 5 minutes), because the Tween-80 can release endogenous histamine, resulting in characteristic manifestations—shortness of breath, chest tightness, palpitations, vasodilatation, nausea, and dizziness for 5 to 20 minutes after injection. In susceptible patients, pre-treatment with oral Benadryl might be indicated.

Clinical facilities are expected to confirm radiochemical purity with a simple, thin-layer chromatography (TLC) procedure using silica gel and chloroform. The ratio of solute migration to solvent flow (e.g., the relative flow [R$_f$] of ^{131}I NP-59 in this system is 0.4, and the R$_f$ of free iodide ion is 0.0) indicates no elution with chloroform. Preparations with more than 10% free iodide should be rejected. Nevertheless, some elution of iodine bound to ^{131}I NP-59 occurs, and patients should be pretreated with Lugol's solution: 3 drops daily for 2 days before tracer administration. Lugol's solution should be administered daily for 6 days throughout the study.

Whether a patient requires pretreatment with dexamethasone depends on the degree of hypercortisolism and the clinical indication for ^{131}I NP-59 imaging. Patients with clinical Cushing's syndrome need not receive pretreatment with corticosteroids if the hypercortisolism is confirmed, because the elevated level of endogenous cortisol indicates that the visualized tissue is nonsuppressible. Patients who are being evaluated to determine the site of excess production of aldosterone or adrenal androgens should receive steroid suppression. Dexamethasone (1 mg four times a day for 7 days before ^{131}I NP-59 administration) is recommended. The dose is continued until imaging is complete.

Patients should be injected in a fasting state (overnight). Fatty food ingestion interferes with absorption, lipoprotein transport, and receptor uptake, as does an elevated serum cholesterol in excess of 400 mg/dl.

Patients are imaged at 72 hours with a gamma camera with a high-energy collimator and 20% energy window centered at 364 keV for 10 to 15 minutes. At 72 hours there usually is sufficient plasma clearance to provide good-quality images with 75,000 to 150,000 counts in 10 to 15 minutes (Figures 13-17 to 13-19). If the right adrenal location is obscured by gallbladder or colonic activity, additional images can be obtained at 96 hours or later. Cleansing enemas may be necessary. A lateral view can be obtained to assist interpretation and evaluation of asymmetric activity. Asymmetry of greater than 2:1 is indicative of adenoma. Most clinical users do not quantify uptake, but even if symmetric, adrenal uptake greater than 0.3% of injected dose is abnormal.

The normal distribution of ^{131}I NP-59 reflects lipoprotein-receptor uptake, with a significant fraction being removed by the liver, excreted into the bile, and subsequently appearing in the bowel. In the presence of elevated cortisol levels, normal adrenal tissue is not visualized. The appearance of activity bilaterally usually indicates or confirms bilateral adrenal hyperplasia. This is usually associated with elevated plasma ACTH levels, but ACTH radioimmunoassay might not be available. Bilateral functioning adrenal tissue in the absence of elevated ACTH suggests bilateral adrenal microadenomas or macroadenomas. Unilateral uptake identifies the site of a functioning adenoma, whereas failure to identify functioning adrenal tissue despite proper technique in a hypercortisol patient increases the

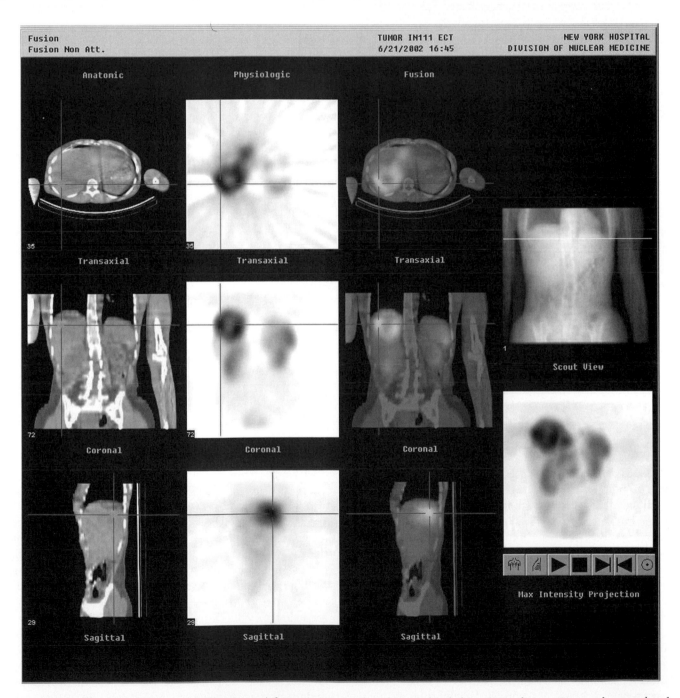

Figure 13-17 ^{111}In-DTPA pentetreotide (Octreoscan) fusion imaging. Selected triangulated slices: *Top to bottom:* Transaxial, coronal and sagittal. *Left to right:* CT (anatomy), scintigraphy (physiology), fused anatomy and physiology. *Extreme right:* Scout CT (*upper*) and volume reconstruction (*lower*).

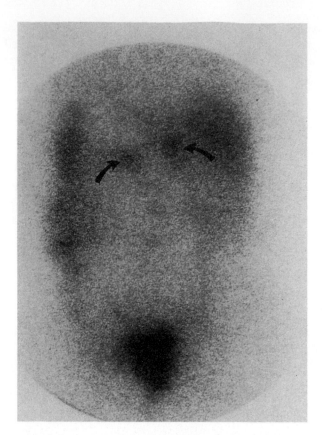

Figure 13-18 Adrenal cortical imaging. Bilateral adrenal activity 72 hours after administration of 1 mCi ^{131}I NP-59 in a 63-year-old woman with clinical Cushing's syndrome and normal CT of the adrenals. A CT scan of the brain and skull revealed a small intrapituitary adenoma that was caused bilateral adrenal hyperplasia. Excreted radiotracer is also seen in the liver, large bowel, and rectum.

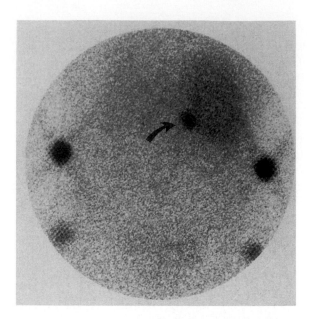

Figure 13-19 Adrenal cortical imaging using 1 mCi ^{131}I NP-59. Posterior abdominal view in a 67-year-old woman who received oral dexamethasone (1 mg daily for 7 days) before radiotracer administration and throughout the study. Intense activity is seen in the right adrenal bed (*arrow*). At surgery an adrenal adenoma was resected. No increased activity is seen in the region of the left adrenal. A faint outline of hepatic parenchyma is seen. The other foci represent markers at the lower margin of the rib cage and superior iliac crests.

likelihood that functioning adrenal carcinoma is the underlying pathologic lesion. These tumors are capable of enormous rates of steroid synthesis even though they may not be identified with ^{131}I NP-59.

Benign adenomas weighing less than 1 g have been identified with ^{131}I NP-59 scintigraphy. In patients suspected of having hyperaldosteronism, low-renin hypertension, and virilization syndromes, ^{131}I NP-59 uptake in a dexamethasone-suppressed patient is indicative of the site or sites of excess steroid synthesis. Although adenomas are typically unilateral, bilateral uptake suggests either hyperplasia or a bilaterally adenomatous process. [131]I NP-59 imaging has been particularly useful in clinical management by providing direction to the surgeon as to whether a unilateral or bilateral approach is necessary, because CT or MRI may not identify small microadenomas or macroadenomas (see Figure 13-19).

The technique has been reported to be 81% to 100% accurate in the diagnosis of adrenal hyperplasia and adenoma in Cushing's disease. In patients with aldosterone-producing lesions, the overall sensitivity is relatively low (approximately 50%), but correct lateralization is high. Because the sensitivity of the procedure in hyperaldostero-

nism is only 50%, the failure to detect an adenoma in a patient suspected of hyperaldosteronism does not exclude the possibility of such disease.

In one series of 37 patients evaluated because of excessive androgen production, 15 had bilateral uptake identified in less than 5 days. All were confirmed to have bilateral adrenal hyperplasia. Five of the 37 had unilateral uptake, and four of the five had adenoma. The remaining 17 patients had only minimal uptake, which was not clearly apparent until at least 5 days after injection; all had normal adrenals.[12]

ADRENAL MEDULLA

Anatomy and Physiology

The adrenal medulla is typically located within the adrenal gland surrounded by the adrenal cortex. The medullary tissue is quite small; on sectioning, the area of the adrenal cortex–adrenal medulla is approximately 10:1. The adrenal medulla tissue synthesizes and secretes the catecholamines epinephrine and norepinephrine, hormones that maintain (or increase) smooth muscle tone, heart rate and force of contraction, and other physiologic responses associated with stress.

Benign or malignant functioning tumors of this tissue are known as *pheochromocytomas*, which are hyperplastic nodules 1 cm in diameter or larger. Below this size the entity is defined as macronodular hyperplasia. Despite their

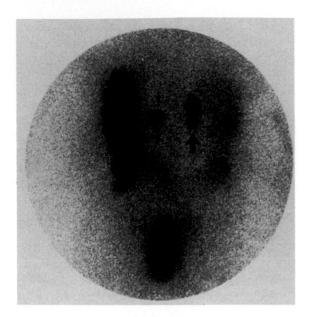

Figure 13-20 Adrenal cortical imaging using 1 mCi ^{131}I NP-59. Posterior abdominal view in a 55-year-old woman with Cushing's syndrome. The patient had a mass in the right adrenal cortex on CT. The scintigraphic study demonstrates a large area of uptake in the right adrenal and a second area in the left adrenal (*arrows*). These findings suggested a bilateral surgical exploration. At surgery a 1.7 cm² macroadenoma was found on the right adrenal and a 0.67 cm² macroadenoma was found in the left adrenal. A significant amount of excreted radiotracer is seen in the ascending, transverse, and (most prominent) descending colon and rectum (midline).

small size, these tumors elaborate excessive amounts of epinephrine or norepinephrine, producing a classic picture of undesirable symptoms, particularly hypertension and other consequences of excessive catecholamine product. Pheochromocytomas occur as an apparently spontaneous benign or malignant tumor of the adrenal medulla but may arise from any site of autonomic nervous tissue. They are a frequent component of the hereditary syndrome multiple endocrine neoplasia (MEN) types IIa and IIb. Despite advances in clinical chemistry that make direct assay of catecholamines and even specific assays of plasma and urinary epinephrine and norepinephrine more readily available, the disease is often a clinical enigma, frequently not diagnosed until postmortem examination. The small size of the adrenal medullary tissue and a propensity for ectopic sites make diagnosis even by CT and MRI unreliable. The aberrant distribution pattern is documented in Figure 13-20, in which 24 of 107 pheochromocytomas were found outside the adrenal glands.[31]

Nuclear Medicine Procedures

The role of nuclear medicine is to identify the location of the hypersecreting tumor with a physiologic imaging technique that identifies the site or sites of excessive neurosecretory activity. ^{131}I-MIBG has been approved by the FDA for clinical use as a diagnostic imaging agent to identify normal, ectopic, or hyperfunctioning adrenal medullary tissue. This material is the product of many years of dedicated research by chemists at the University of Michigan. The development is documented in several reviews.[11,12] More recently, ^{123}I-MIBG has been synthesized, but the short half-life of ^{123}I precludes availability of this material except at institutions prepared to synthesize the radiotracer and confirm the pharmaceutical purity, sterility, and apyrogenicity. The product still requires IND and institutional review board (IRB) review and approval on an individual user basis for clinical use.

After secretion, norepinephrine is resorbed at the presynaptic site and stored in adrenergic granules. MIBG has little or no pharmacologic effect and does not bind significantly at postsynaptic receptors, but it is incorporated into the adrenergic storage granules because of structural similarities to norepinephrine.

Although ^{123}I-MIBG would seem to be advantageous in terms of increased photon and hence information flux, the short half-life limits delayed imaging to 24 hours after injection; with ^{131}I-MIBG, it is possible to image patients at 3 to 5 days after administration of the radiopharmaceutical. The longer interval provides for an improved target-to-background ratio and hence images of potentially greater diagnostic accuracy. Because the blood flow to the adrenal medulla is only a small fraction of the circulation, a considerable interval is necessary for sufficient material to be taken up and for plasma and soft tissue activity to fall sufficiently to identify localization. Studies comparing the two tracers ([131]I- and ^{123}I-labeled MIBG) have shown equivalent performance in terms of detecting pheochromocytoma and neuroblastoma (which also localizes MIBG).

Lugol's solution should be given to the patient to block thyroid uptake of released iodine at least 1 day before ^{131}I-MIBG (or ^{123}I-MIBG) administration and continued for 7 days thereafter. The adult dose of ^{131}I-MIBG is 0.5 mCi, injected slowly intravenously over 15 seconds. Patients under 18 years of age receive a reduced dose based on body weight, but the dose is calculated based on a full adult dose of 1.0 mCi; that is, 1.0 mCi/70 kg, with a maximum dose of 0.5 mCi.

Patients are imaged with a gamma camera fitted with a collimator suitable for the 364 keV gamma emission from [131]I. There is considerable difference in the sensitivity and resolution of collimators designed to image in the 364 keV range. If a choice is available, the nuclear medicine department should opt for a greater count rate; the use of a collimator with greater sensitivity provides some soft tissue background activity that is helpful in interpretation, because it provides anatomic landmark information. [131]I collimators, which are ideal for imaging after high doses of ^{131}I, actually produce uninterpretable images and should not be used. A 15% to 20% energy window centered at 364 keV is used. For detection of pheochromocytoma, the entire thorax, abdomen, and pelvis should be imaged anteriorly and posteriorly with markers. [131]I capsules (approximately 5 μCi) are

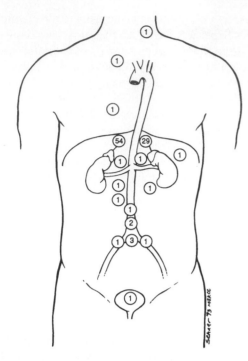

Figure 13-21 In a large surgical series, pheochromocytoma was found in the adrenal bed in 83 of 100 patients (three patients had bilateral pheochromocytoma) and in extra-adrenal sites in 17 patients. These sites were distributed principally along the paraaortic tissue as far caudally as the bifurcation and iliac vessels and cephalad above the aortic arch. In one patient a pheochromocytoma was found in the bladder wall.

useful for this purpose. The axillae, lower rib markings, and iliac crests should be marked. The patient should void before imaging begins. Because the total number of counts per view depends on many factors, acquisitions for a reasonable time interval (i.e., 20 minutes per view) are appropriate. The images should be digitized in at least a 128 × 128 matrix to allow subsequent optimization of images. Imaging should be performed on day 1 (24 hours after injection of the tracer), day 3, and day 7 if necessary.

The normal distribution of ^{131}I-MIBG includes the heart (because of the rich neural innervation), the liver, spleen, salivary glands, and bladder (the latter two sites because of excretion of free iodine eluted from the tracer). In normal subjects the adrenal medulla is either not visualized or is seen only transiently on the first day of imaging. Activity that persists on subsequent images is abnormal. The lesion-to-background contrast improves with time. Day 3 (72-hour) images usually provide the most useful information, with maximum contrast between abnormal foci of activity and background.

Intense tracer uptake is seen in pheochromocytomas, which can be identified in the adrenal bed or elsewhere in the abdomen or thorax (Figure 13-21; also see Figure 13-20). Persistent or increased uptake bilaterally suggests bilateral pheochromocytoma, although this diagnosis should not be considered if only faint uptake is seen at 24 hours

that does not increase in activity or contrast. In malignant pheochromocytoma, uptake is seen in metastases in the liver, bone, lymph nodes, heart, lungs, mediastinum, and other sites. At the University of Michigan, analysis of a 400-patient series with malignant pheochromocytoma demonstrated a sensitivity of 92.4% and a specificity of 100%.[11,12] ^{131}I-MIBG is also useful for determining the extent of involvement of neuroblastoma, a malignant tumor of childhood that can be widely disseminated.

^{111}In-DTPA pentetreotide (Octreoscan) has also been used to image pheochromocytoma. In initial studies it was reported to be equally sensitive for the detection of pheochromocytomas, but this is no longer considered to be the case. ^{131}I-MIBG is currently considered to be the preferred radiotracer for detection of pheochromocytoma. If ^{111}In-DTPA pentetreotide is used subsequent to negative results with ^{131}I-MIBG scintigraphy, sufficient time should be allowed for clearance and decay of the ^{131}I-MIBG.

GONADS

Anatomy and Physiology

The gonads are the principal source of sex hormones, accounting for the differentiation of male and female sexual characteristics.

In the female, the ovaries are found in the pelvis, one on each side, near the termination of the fallopian tubes. As a result of complex endocrine orchestration, an ovum matures and is released from one of the ovaries to the opening of the fallopian tube each month during a 35- to 40-year interval after sexual maturity. The ovaries produce estrogens, several structurally related steroid hormones that control and maintain secondary sexual characteristics and other metabolic effects, such as skeletal osteoid.

In the adult male, the testes produce sperm and elaborate testosterone, which produces the male secondary characteristics. The testes are normally found in the scrotum, but one or both can fail to descend adequately from the pelvis.

Currently there are no routine scintigraphic procedures for either the ovaries or testes. In the evaluation of the female patient with masculinizing syndromes with ^{131}I NP-59 (iodocholesterol), anterior views of the lower abdomen and pelvis should be obtained to identify a possible focus of activity representing increased ovarian steroid synthesis. There have been only random reports of this application.

Finally, it should be recalled that certain ovarian neoplasms (struma ovarii) may contain functioning thyroid tissue. There are rare reports of hyperthyroidism arising from this ectopic source and of thyroid carcinoma developing at this site.

SUMMARY

The elements of endocrine organ anatomy and physiology and the major clinical syndromes have been reviewed, as have the basis and description of the nuclear medicine

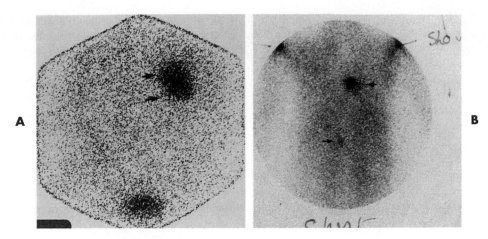

Figure 13-22   Imaging at 72 hours after 500 μCi ^{131}I MIBG. **A**, Gamma camera view of the anterior abdomen in a patient with a pheochromocytoma arising from the left adrenal medulla (*arrows*). **B**, Gamma camera view of the posterior thoracolumbar region in another patient with a recurrent malignant pheochromocytoma. A small residual focus is seen in the left adrenal bed region, and a prominent intense focus is seen in the right thoracic paraspinal region (*arrows*).

procedures available for the evaluation of these glands and the disorders affecting them. Except for radioiodine therapy of hyperthyroidism and thyroid carcinoma, the role of nuclear medicine is diagnostic; that is, imaging and in vivo assessment of function. Nuclear medicine is a medical discipline and technology that requires specific training and experience for the technologists and physicians involved in the use of these procedures for patient care. The physiologic basis for the technology has been discussed in detail, as have the technologic aspects of the nuclear medicine procedures currently used to characterize human endocrine physiology in health and disease.

REFERENCES

1. Ain KB: Thyroid cancer: a lethal endocrine neoplasm—biology and management of differentiated thyroid carcinoma of the follicular cells, *Ann Intern Med* 115:133-147, 1991.
2. Andros G, Harper PV, Lathrop KA et al: Pertechnetate-99m localization in man with applications to thyroid scanning and the study of thyroid physiology, *J Clin Endocrinol Metab* 35:250-256, 1972.
3. Apostolopoulos DJ, Houstoulaki E, Grannakenas E et al: Technetium-99m-tetrofosmin for parathyroid scintigraphy: comparison with thallium-pertechnetate scanning, *J Nucl Med* 39:1433-1441, 1998.
4. Atkins HL, Richards P: Assessment of thyroid function and anatomy with ^{99m}Tc-pertechnetate, *J Nucl Med* 9:7-9, 1968.
5. Attie JN, Kahn A, Rumancik WM et al: Preoperative localization of parathyroid adenomas, *Am J Surg* 156:323-326, 1988.
6. Becker DV, Charkes ND, Dworkin H et al: Procedure guideline for thyroid scintigraphy: 1.0, *J Nucl Med* 37:1264-1266, 1996.
7. Becker DV, Charkes ND, Dworkin H et al: Procedure guideline for thyroid uptake measurement: 1.0, *J Nucl Med* 37:1266-1268, 1996.
8. Becker DV, Charkes ND, Dworkin H et al: Procedure guideline for extended scintigraphy for differentiated thyroid cancer: 1.0, *J Nucl Med* 37:1269-1271, 1996.
9. Becker DV, Hurley JR: Current status of radioiodine (^{131}I) treatment of hyperthyroidism. In Freeman L, Weissmann HS, editors: *Nuclear medicine annual 1982*, New York, 1982, Raven Press.
10. Becker DV, Hurley JR: Radioiodine treatment of hyperthyroidism. In Gottschalk A, Hoffer PB, Potchen EJ, editors: *Diagnostic nuclear medicine*, vol 2, Baltimore, 1988, Williams & Wilkins.
11. Beierwaltes WH: Clinical applications of 131-I labeled metaiodobenzylguanidine. In Hoffer PB, editor: *1987 Year Book of nuclear medicine*, Chicago, 1987, Year Book Medical.
12. Beierwaltes WH: Endocrine imaging: parathyroid, adrenal cortex and medulla, and other endocrine tumors, part II, *J Nucl Med* 32:1627-1639, 1991.
13. Beierwaltes WH, Nishiyama RH, Thompson NW et al: Survival time and "cure" in papillary and follicular carcinoma with distant metastases: statistics following University of Michigan therapy, *J Nucl Med* 23:561-568, 1982.
14. Berson SA, Yalow RS: Immunoassay of endogenous plasma insulin in man, *J Clin Invest* 35:170-177, 1960.
15. Berson SA, Yalow RS, Glick SA et al: Immunoassay of protein and peptide hormones, *Metabolism* 13:1135-1140, 1964.
16. Billotey C, Sarfati E, Aurengo A et al: Advantages of SPECT in technetium-99m-sestamibi parathyroid scintigraphy, *J Nucl Med* 37:1773-1778, 1996.
17. Chinol M, Bodei L, Cremonisi M et al: Receptor-mediated radiotherapy with ^{90}Y-DOTA-$_D$Phe^1-Tyr^3, *Semin Nucl Med* 32: 141-147, 2002.

18. de Jong M, Bakker WH, Breeman WAP et al: Phase I study of peptide receptor therapy with [^{111}In-DTPA[0]] Octreotide: the Rotterdam experience, *Semin Nucl Med* 32:110-122, 2002.

19. de Jong M, Valkema JF, Kvols LK et al: Somatostatin receptor–targeted therapy of tumors: preclinical and clinical findings, *Semin Nucl Med* 32:133-140, 2002.

20. Even-Sapir E, Keidar Z, Sachs J et al: The new technology of combined transmission and emission tomography in evaluation of endocrine neoplasms, *J Nucl Med* 42:998-1004, 2002.

21. Fjeld JG, Ericksen K, Pfeffer PF et al: Technetium-99m-tetrafosmin for parathyroid scintigraphy: a comparison with sestamibi, *J Nucl Med* 38:831-834, 1997.

22. Goldsmith SJ: Thyroid: in vivo tests of function and imaging. In Rothfield B, editor: *Nuclear medicine: endocrinology*, Philadelphia, 1978, JB Lippincott.

23. Hertz S, Roberts A, Evans RD: Radioactive iodine as an indicator in the study of thyroid physiology, *Proc Soc Exp Biol Med* 38:510-514, 1938.

24. Krenning EP, Bakker WH, Kooij PPM et al: Somatostatin receptor scintigraphy with indium-111 DTPA-D-phe-1-octreotide in man: metabolism, dosimetry and comparison with iodine-123-tyr-3-octreotide, *J Nucl Med* 33:652-658, 1992.

25. Krenning EP, Kwekkeboom DJ, Bakker WH et al: Somatostatin receptor scintigraphy with [In-111 DTPA-D-Phe-1]- and [I-123-Tyr3] octreotide: the Rotterdam experience with more than 1000 patients, *Eur J Nucl Med* 20:716-731, 1993.

26. Kwekkeboom DJ, Krenning EP: Somatostatin receptor imaging, *Semin Nucl Med* 32:84-91, 2002.

27. Kusic Z, Becker DV, Saenger EL et al: Comparison of technetium-99m and iodine-123 imaging of thyroid nodules: correlation with pathologic findings, *J Nucl Med* 31:393-399, 1990.

28. Leeper RD, Shimaoka K: Treatment of metastatic thyroid cancer, *J Clin Endocrinol Metab* 9:383-404, 1980.

29. Maxon HR, Englaro EE, Thomas SR et al: Radioiodine-131 therapy for well-differentiated thyroid cancer: a quantitative radiation dosimetric approach—outcome and validation in 85 patients, *J Nucl Med* 33:1132-1137, 1992.

30. Maxon HR, Thomas SR, Hertzberg VS et al: Relation between radiation dose and outcome of radioiodine therapy for thyroid cancer, *N Engl J Med* 309:937-941, 1938.

31. Melicow MM: One hundred cases of pheochromocytoma (107 tumors) at the Columbia-Presbyterian Medical Center, *Cancer* 40:1987-2004, 1977.

32. O'Doherty MJ, Kettle AG, Wells P et al: Parathyroid imaging with technetium-99m-sestamibi: preoperative localization and tissue uptake studies, *J Nucl Med* 33:313-318, 1992.

33. Okerland MD, Sheldon K, Corpuz S et al: A new method with high sensitivity and specificity for localization of abnormal parathyroid glands, *Ann Surg* 200:381-383, 1984.

34. Pacini F, Lippi L, Formica N et al: Therapeutic doses of iodine-131 reveal undiagnosed metastases in thyroid cancer patients with detectable serum thyroglobulin levels, *J Nucl Med* 28:1888-1891, 1987.

35. Ridgeway EC: Clinician's evaluation of a solitary thyroid nodule, *J Clin Endocrinol Metab* 74:231-235, 1992.

36. Rini JN, Vallabhajosula S, Zanzonico P et al: Thyroid uptake of liquid versus capsule ^{131}I tracers in hyperthyroid patients treated with liquid ^{131}I, *Thyroid* 9:347-52, 1999.

37. Robbins RJ, Chon JT, Fleisher M et al: Is the serum thyroglobulin response to recombinant human thyrotropin sufficient, by itself, to monitor for residual thyroid carcinoma? *J Clin Endocrinol Metab* 87: 3242-3247, 2002.

38. Robbins RJ, Tuttle RM, Sharaf RN et al: Preparation by recombinant human thyrotropin or thyroid hormone withdrawal is comparable for the detection of residual differentiated thyroid carcinoma, *J Clin Endocrinol Metab* 86:619-625, 2001.

39. Samaan NA, Schultz PN, Haynie TP et al: Pulmonary metastases of differentiated thyroid carcinoma: treatment results in 101 patients, *J Clin Endocrinol Metab* 60:376-381, 1985.

40. Sarkar SD, Beierwaltes WH, Ice RD et al: A new and superior adrenal scanning agent, NP-59, *J Nucl Med* 16:1038-1042, 1975.

41. Seidlin SM, Marinelli LD, Oshry E: Radioactive iodine therapy: effect on functioning metastases of adenocarcinoma of the thyroid, *JAMA* 132:838-841, 1946.

42. Snyder J, Gorman C, Scanlon P: Thyroid remnant ablation: questionable pursuit of an ill-defined goal, *J Nucl Med* 24:659-665, 1983.

43. Strashun A, Vaquer RA, Goldsmith SJ: Localization of parathyroid adenomata by thallium-201 and technetium-99m subtraction scintigraphy, *Mt Sinai J Med* 55:171-175, 1988.

44. Taillefer R, Boucher Y, Potvin C et al: Detection and localization of parathyroid adenomas in patients with hyperparathyroidism using a single radionuclide imaging procedure with technetium-99m sestamibi (double-phase study), *J Nucl Med* 33:1801-1807, 1992.

45. van Royen EA, Verhoeff NPLG, Meylaerts SAE, et al: Indium-111 DTPA octreotide uptake measured in normal and abnormal pituitary glands. *J Nucl Med* 37:1449-1451, 1996.

46. Virgolini I, Britton K, Buscombe J et al: [111]In and ^{90}Y-DOTA-lanreotide: results and implications of the MAURITIUS trial, *Semin Nucl Med* 32:148-155, 2002.

47. Wang W, Larson SM, Fazzari M et al: Prognostic value of [^{18}F] fluorodeoxyglucose positron emission

tomographic scanning in patients with thyroid cancer, *J Clin Endocrinol Metab* 85:1107-1113, 2000.

48. Wang W, Macapinlac H, Larson SM et al: [^{18}F]-2-fluoro-2-deoxy-D-glucose positron emission tomography localizes residual thyroid cancer in patients with negative diagnostic ^{131}I whole body scans and elevated serum thyroglobulin levels, *J Clin Endocrinol Metab* 84:2291-2302, 1999.

49. Waxman A, Ramanna L, Chapman N et al: The significance of I-131 scan dose in patients with thyroid cancer: determination of ablation—concise communication, *J Nucl Med* 22:861-865, 1981.

50. Zwas ST, Mintz Y, Rotenberg G et al: The value of pre- and intra-operative 99mTc-sestamibi parathyroid SPECT with radio-guided probe in focused parathyroidectomy, *J Nucl Med* 43:125P, 2002.

William L. Hubble, David J. Phegley,
Roger H. Secker-Walker

chapter 14

Respiratory System

Objectives

Possess a general understanding of normal lung anatomy and physiology.

Understand how the blood flow within the lung is altered by pathology.

Understand the mechanism of perfusion imaging.

Be aware of the special care needed for perfusion imaging of patients with severe pulmonary hypertension.

Understand the patient preparation requirements for lung imaging.

Know the importance of the number of particles administered for perfusion imaging.

Understand the effect of time and decay on particle count.

Be aware of the effects of gravity on particle distribution in the lung.

Know the importance of communicating the method of injection to the interpreting physician.

Be aware of the various techniques for ventilation studies.

Understand the limitations and advantages of the various ventilation radiopharmaceuticals.

Possess an understanding of the advantages of the combined diagnostic information of ventilation and perfusion imaging studies.

Understand how lung imaging studies are used to diagnose disease.

Possess a knowledge of the general applications of lung imaging.

Be aware of the various references on the subject of lung imaging.

*R*egional ventilation was first studied by Knipping and colleagues using radioactive xenon almost 50 years ago.[29] Much of our present understanding of regional lung function, both in health and in disease, is based on the use of this gas and other radionuclides by respiratory physiologists working in London and Montreal.[6,46] During this time considerable advances were also made in understanding the detailed anatomy of the lung[50] and in appreciating the mechanical interrelationships of airways, alveoli, and the thoracic cage.[32] Nonrespiratory functions have also been studied, particularly those dealing with lung defense mechanisms[18] and the metabolic activity of the lung.[15]

The development of macroaggregated albumin, at first labeled with iodine-131[44] (^{131}I) and later with technetium-99m (^{99m}Tc), led to the widespread use of perfusion scanning for the diagnosis of pulmonary embolism. The use of radioactive xenon to study regional ventilation has spread from the research laboratory to routine use in the past 30 years. This combined insight into regional ventilation and regional blood flow allows more accurate assessment of the disturbed physiology and, at the same time, increases both the diagnostic sensitivity and the specificity of the procedure.[3,33]

NORMAL ANATOMY AND PHYSIOLOGY

The lungs, shown diagrammatically in Figure 14-1 and schematically in Figure 14-2, lie within the thorax, protected by the rib cage. The ribs offer support to the intercostal muscles and the diaphragm. It is the action of these muscles that enlarges the chest during normal breathing. Air enters the lungs, first passing through the nose or mouth and then the pharynx, larynx, and trachea. It is warmed, moistened,

and filtered during this time. The trachea divides into right and left mainstem bronchi, and these in turn divide into lobar bronchi (upper, middle, and lower on the right, and upper and lower on the left). The airways continue to divide in a somewhat irregular fashion, about 16 times from the trachea to the terminal bronchioles and a further four to seven times as respiratory bronchioles, alveolar ducts, and alveolar sacs (Figure 14-3). Bronchi have cartilage in their walls, which distinguishes them from bronchioles. Smooth muscle, collagen, and elastic fibers encircle the airways from the trachea to the alveolar ducts. The collagen and elastic fibers continue to the periphery of the lung as a

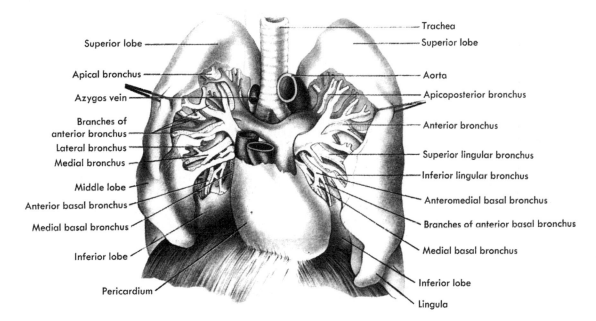

Figure 14-1   Anatomic diagram showing the relationships of the heart, pulmonary vessels, airways, and lungs.

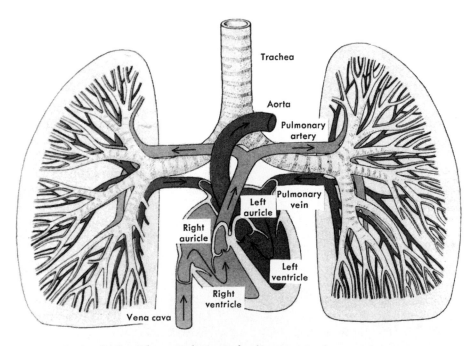

Figure 14-2   Schematic diagram of pulmonary circulation and airways.

three-dimensional latticework in the walls of the alveoli. Alveoli first appear in the respiratory bronchioles but are most numerous around the alveolar sacs.

The alveoli are packed together like the cells of a honeycomb (Figure 14-4). Each alveolus offers some support to its neighbors, as well as through the collagen and elastic fibers to the airways. This structural arrangement and the surfactant that lines the surface of the alveoli are responsible for the elastic properties of the lungs and provide the main force for expiration during normal breathing.

The bronchial epithelium is lined by ciliated cells interspersed with a few goblet cells and the openings of bronchial glands.[9] The alveoli, where oxygen and carbon dioxide are exchanged, are lined by alveolar type I cells. These are very thin and spread over the surface of the alveoli. Pulmonary capillaries lie in contact with these cells (see Figure 14-4). Two other important cells are found in the alveoli: alveolar type II cells, which make surfactant, and alveolar macrophages, which remove particulate matter that reaches the alveoli.

The pulmonary artery divides to form the right and left pulmonary arteries. These vessels follow the bronchi and bronchioles, dividing with them until they reach the alveoli (see Figure 14-2). Each alveolus, and there are about 250 million to 300 million in an adult, is supplied by a terminal pulmonary arteriole, which has a diameter of about $35\,\mu m$ and which gives rise to about 1000 capillaries per alveolus. The capillaries are 7 to $10\,\mu m$ in diameter. The distance between the alveolar surface and the capillaries is only about 0.05 to $0.1\,\mu m$. The pulmonary capillaries drain into the pulmonary veins and from there into the left atrium.[50]

The lungs also receive blood from the aorta through the bronchial arteries. These are small but also follow the bronchial tree as far as the respiratory bronchioles. They supply nourishment to the bronchi, surrounding blood vessels, nerves, and lymphatics. Anastomoses are formed between the bronchial and pulmonary circulations at the capillary level around the respiratory bronchioles. Most of the blood from the bronchial circulation drains into the left atrium through the pulmonary veins.[13]

The lungs are richly supplied with lymphatics. Some course over the pleura and pass into the lungs, whereas others arise in the interstitial spaces of the lungs. Lymphatic vessels travel toward the hilum of the lung, with airways and blood vessels, reaching lymph nodes there and continuing into the mediastinum.

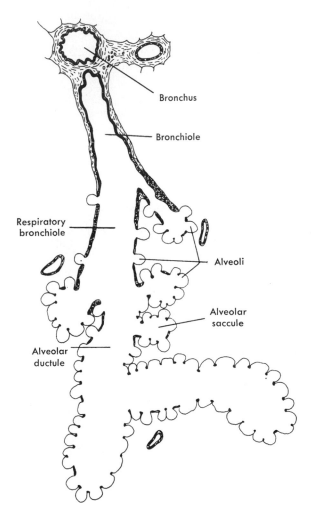

Figure 14-3 Schematic cross section of branching of airways from terminal bronchiole to alveolar ductules, saccules, and alveoli.

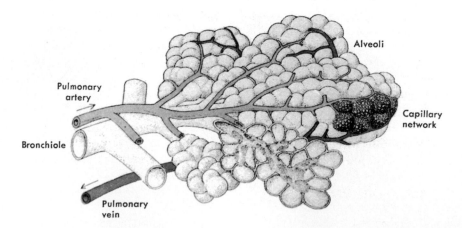

Figure 14-4 Schematic drawing of peripheral airways and alveoli and their accompanying blood vessels.

The volume of air breathed out in a normal breath is called the *tidal volume,* and the volume of air in the lungs at the end of a normal breath is called *functional residual capacity.* *Total lung capacity* is the volume of air in the lungs when as much air has been inhaled as possible, whereas *residual volume* is the volume of air left in the lungs after a complete exhalation. These volumes are measured by standard pulmonary function tests.[49]

During tidal breathing only a small proportion of the air in the lungs (about 10% to 15%) is exchanged with each breath. More is exchanged with deeper breaths or a faster rate of breathing. About one third of each breath is wasted because the air in the bronchial tubes at the end of the breath does not reach the alveoli. This is called *anatomic dead space* because it takes no part in gas exchange.

The structure of the lung is well suited to its chief function of gas exchange; that is, delivering oxygen to the bloodstream and removing carbon dioxide so that the body's cellular metabolism can continue. Despite the numerous divisions of the bronchial tree, the resistance to air flow is low. Most of this resistance (80% to 90%) is found in the larger bronchial tubes, where air flow is turbulent. Only small pressure changes in the chest are required for normal breathing. The change in volume for a change in pressure is called *compliance,* which is a measurement of the ease with which air enters or leaves the lungs. The pressure in the pulmonary artery is considerably lower than that in the systemic circulation, and there is very little resistance to blood flow. The entire cardiac output passes through the pulmonary capillaries, in an almost continuous sheet, in the alveolar walls. These thin walls, which have a surface area of 70 to 80 m², offer an almost negligible barrier to the diffusion of gases from alveoli to blood or vice versa.

As the lung ages, its elastic properties diminish and the smaller bronchial tubes tend to collapse during a full expiration. The volume of air in the lungs when closure begins is the *closing capacity.* Both radioactive xenon and nonradioactive tracer gases (e.g., nitrogen, helium, and argon) have been used to measure this volume. Early damage to the small airways from any cause increases this volume, an increase that therefore is a sensitive but nonspecific indication of small-airway disease.[4,10]

In the 1960s it was shown that both ventilation and blood flow are not evenly distributed within the lungs. Posture and the direction of gravity or of acceleration play an important part in healthy lungs.

In the upright position, ventilation of the upper parts of the lung increases about one and one half to two times from the upper third of the lung to the lower third.[6,28,48] In the supine position, the distribution is more uniform from top to bottom, but there is then a gradient from front to back. If a person lies on one side, more air is exchanged in the lower part of the lungs compared with the upper part. The distribution is modified by exercise, the rate of breathing, and diseases that affect the bronchial tubes or the lung parenchyma.

In the upright position, blood flow increases threefold to fivefold from the upper parts of the lung to the base. In fact,

the upper one fourth of the lungs gets very little blood flow at rest while a person is sitting upright.[5,48] In the supine position, blood flow is more uniform from apex to base, but then a gradient exists from front to back. Lying on one side causes more blood to flow to the lower-most part of the lung. Apart from the disease states that usually alter blood flow within the lung, exercise results in a more even distribution. Lowering the oxygen tension in the bronchial tubes also alters blood flow by causing local constriction of the pulmonary arterioles and diverting blood flow away from this region.

The distribution of blood flow within the upright lung shows the largest gradient from top to bottom when the measurements are made at total lung capacity. At functional residual capacity, blood flow increases from the apex to about the level of the fourth or fifth rib and then decreases a little toward the base. If the distribution of blood flow is measured at residual volume, it is almost even throughout the lungs.[23]

The ratio in which ventilation and blood flow are mixed is not uniform from top to bottom in the upright position. Ventilation exceeds blood flow by about 2:1 to 3:1 in the upper zones. In the midzones they are more closely matched, whereas in the lower parts of the lung blood flow exceeds ventilation. The closer the matching of ventilation and blood flow, the better the oxygenation of the blood. Whenever ventilation is reduced in comparison to blood flow, the oxygenation of the blood is also reduced. If ventilation exceeds blood flow, the red cells quickly take up their maximum load of oxygen (4 molecules per hemoglobin molecule, or 1.34 ml of O_2 per gram of hemoglobin), and the excess ventilation is then wasted.[49]

PATHOPHYSIOLOGY

The distribution of blood flow within the lungs is altered by many disease processes that affect the lungs, the heart, the chest wall, or the diaphragm. The mechanisms underlying these disturbances are outlined schematically in Figure 14-5. *A* to *C* in Figure 14-5 represent disease processes that affect the pulmonary vasculature. The most obvious cause, represented by *A,* is pulmonary embolism, in which the embolus (usually a small blood clot) blocks one of the branches of the pulmonary artery so that no blood can flow past this obstruction. The defect produced on the perfusion scan corresponds to the anatomic segment or lobe of the lung involved.

Other causes of defects in blood flow from disease processes that affect the pulmonary vessels are shown in Figure 14-5, *B* and *C. B* represents enlarged lymph nodes at the hilum of the lung, as might be seen in advanced lung cancer, causing compression of the pulmonary vessels and hence alterations in blood flow. *C* represents disease processes that involve the smaller pulmonary arterioles, such as a vasculitis or multiple small pulmonary emboli.

D to *F* in Figure 14-5 represent diseases in which the initial problem is in the airways (or bronchial tubes), and

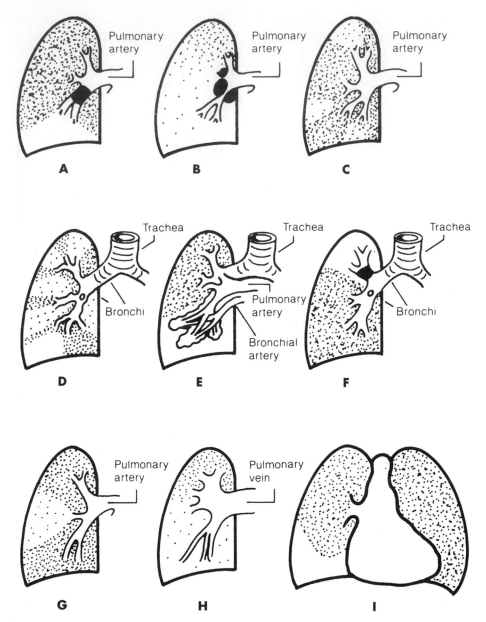

Figure 14-5 Schematic representation of major mechanisms of abnormal perfusion scans (**A** to **I**). *Spotted areas,* Blood flow; *clear areas,* regions with absent blood flow.

blood flow is reduced as a result of the diminution in ventilation. *D* is a composite diagram that represents the changes seen in chronic bronchitis, emphysema, and asthma. *E* represents bronchiectasis in which there is dilatation of the peripheral bronchi and surrounding inflammation. The bronchial arteries to the affected region are often greatly enlarged. There is virtually no blood flow through the pulmonary artery and very little exchange of air in the bronchiectatic segment. *F* represents obstruction of a bronchus by a tumor or foreign body. Blood flow is reduced in part by the local hypoxia.

G to *I* in Figure 14-5 represent miscellaneous conditions. In *G* the lung parenchyma is filled with inflammatory exudate, as is seen in pneumonia, or with blood, as is seen in a pulmonary infarction. Blood flow is greatly reduced, and there is no ventilation of the affected region. *H* represents the interesting phenomenon of a reversal of the normal gradient of blood flow. This is seen when the pressure in the left atrium is elevated, such as in mitral stenosis or left ventricular failure. *I* represents a condition in which a pleural effusion or a large heart is compressing lung tissue, reducing blood flow in that region.

The mechanisms responsible for the disturbances in ventilation are shown in Figure 14-6. Figure 14-6, *A,* represents diseases that cause obstruction to air flow by narrowing or distorting the airways. Chronic bronchitis, for example, is marked by excess mucus production and some inflammatory swelling of the bronchial walls. Both processes narrow

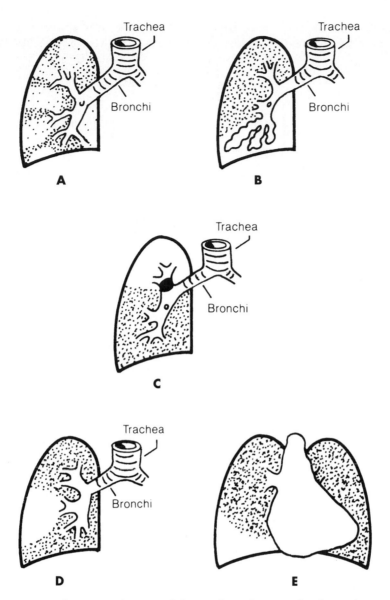

Figure 14-6   Schematic representation of major mechanisms of abnormal ventilation studies (**A** to **E**). *Spotted areas,* Ventilation; *clear areas,* regions of abnormal ventilation.

the lumen of the airways, usually in an irregular fashion, producing variable patterns of airway obstruction. In emphysema the main damage is in the alveoli, which are steadily destroyed, resulting in loss of surface area and capillaries. The small airways are not properly supported; they become kinked and distorted and collapse readily on expiration, which leads to inefficient exchange of air. Chronic bronchitis and emphysema are usually found together because both diseases are caused, for the most part, by cigarette smoking.

Bronchial asthma is marked by spasm of the bronchial smooth muscle, which causes narrowing of the airways and increased mucus production and edema of the bronchial mucosa. Severe abnormalities of ventilation and blood flow may be seen.

Figure 14-6, *B,* represents bronchiectasis. Little or no air exchange takes place in the dilatated bronchi, which are often the seat of chronic infection. Figure 14-6, *C,* represents narrowing or complete obstruction of a bronchus because of a tumor or foreign body. The worse the obstruction, the more obvious the abnormality in ventilation. If the obstruction is in a lobar bronchus, the affected lobe of the lung collapses as its lumen closes off. If the obstruction is in a segmental or smaller bronchus, collateral ventilation through the pores of Kohn can prevent complete collapse by allowing air to enter the segment from a neighboring segment.

Figure 14-6, *D,* represents the condition in pneumonia or pulmonary infarction, in which the alveoli are filled with exudate or blood and hence do not exchange any air.

Figure 14-6, *E,* represents pleural fluid or a large heart, both of which occupy lung volume, thus reducing ventilation.

PERFUSION IMAGING

The distribution of pulmonary arterial blood flow is usually demonstrated by intravenous injection of radioactive particles. The method was shown to be effective by Haynie and colleagues, who injected labeled ceramic microspheres into dogs.[21] The development of macroaggregated albumin (MAA), labeled with ^{131}I by Taplin and colleagues[44] and Wagner and colleagues[47] in 1964, led to the first successful lung scans in human beings. After intravenous injection the particles, which measure 30 to 40 μm in diameter, pass through the right atrium and right ventricle, where they are well mixed with blood, and then into the pulmonary artery. They pass into the blood vessels of the lung until they become impacted in the terminal arterioles and capillaries because they are too large to pass through them. The usual diameter of human albumin microspheres corresponds to the size of the smallest pulmonary arterioles. The distribution of particles has been shown experimentally to be closely related to the distribution of pulmonary arterial blood flow,[37] by comparison of their relative distribution to the uptake of oxygen by each lung and also by comparison of the distribution of particles to that of labeled red blood cells.[46] A normal perfusion scan is shown in Figure 14-7.

It is important to remember that the distribution is that which exists at the time of injection.

Macroaggregated albumin, human albumin microspheres, and other particles break up and pass through the pulmonary capillaries and are removed from the circulation in the liver and spleen. These particles have variable biologic half-lives in the lung, which depend not only on the nature of the particles but also to some extent on the underlying disease processes. Clearance is delayed in chronic lung disease and heart failure.

With the usual dose of particulate material of the appropriate size, fewer than 1 in 1000 pulmonary arterioles is blocked.[19,44] No abnormalities of pulmonary function can be demonstrated after such an injection.[16,38] Perfusion scanning has a reputation for great safety, but special care should be taken in patients known to have severe pulmonary hypertension because the available vascular bed is reduced in diameter.[12] Special care should also be taken in patients with right-to-left shunts[36] because the particles pass through to the systemic circulation and embolize to the brain, kidneys, heart, and other organs. Half the usual dose should be given to patients who have had a pneumonectomy.

Radioactive xenon dissolved in saline solution is occasionally used to demonstrate the distribution of blood flow. It is given intravenously, and because the gas is relatively insoluble, it comes out of solution as it reaches the air contained in the alveoli. Its distribution can be measured during breath holding and corresponds to pulmonary capillary blood flow. Regions of the lung that are collapsed or con-solidated, as in pneumonia, appear to have no blood flow because the alveoli contain no air.

Preparation

No special patient preparation is required for either ventilation or perfusion lung imaging. However, a few things should be done in advance of the examination. A recent chest radiograph (within 4 hours) should accompany the patient to the nuclear medicine facility. The radiograph allows the physician to be more specific when interpreting the images. A few physicians also require that a blood gas or D-Dimer assay report accompany the patient. Again, this additional information can provide another clue to the correct diagnosis of the patient. Spiral CT is another modality being used to diagnose pulmonary emboli.[52] It is not the technologist's responsibility to set laboratory policy with regard to this type of advance information. However, it generally is the technologist's responsibility to enforce it.

Dosage

In addition to the amount of radioactivity given, the number of particles and the amount of albumin injected are of special importance. Because, as previously discussed, a small percentage of the capillary bed is obstructed so that the perfusion image can be performed, care must be taken to ensure that the patient's respiratory ability is not further impaired by a test intended to help him.[19] In a normal patient, a satisfactory perfusion image can be obtained with 125,000 to 350,000 particles.[22,51,54] An appropriate reduction in the number of particles should be applied for pediatric patients, those with pulmonary hypertension, and those who have had a pneumonectomy. To help control the number of particles used in perfusion imaging, aggregated albumin kits should be prepared to the same volume every day, and patients should be scheduled as close as possible to the preparation time. Every technologist in the laboratory should know the total number of particles in whichever kit the laboratory uses.

If too few particles are given, the scans have an obvious blotchy appearance. An even more blotchy appearance is seen if small blood clots or incompletely separated particles are inadvertently injected.

Method of Injection

The patterns of perfusion are different, depending on whether the particles are injected with the patient in the upright or the supine position. As indicated earlier, gravity plays an important role in the pressure relationships within the lungs. Patients injected when upright tend to have a larger proportion of the particles distributed toward the bases. Patients injected when supine demonstrate a more homogeneous distribution of particles from the bases to the apices. There are arguments and situations favoring each position for injection. As long as both the technologist and

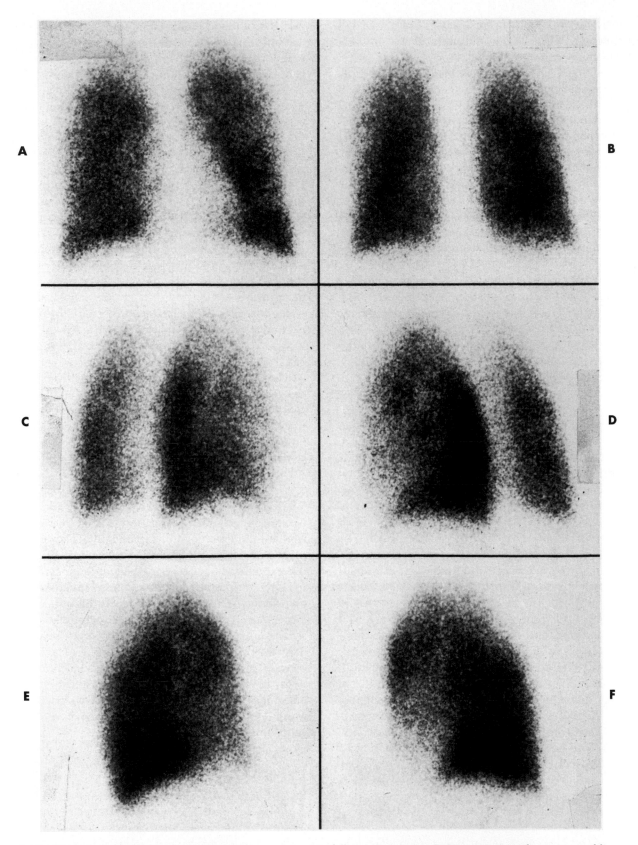

Figure 14-7 Normal six-view perfusion scan. Images are arranged as follows: **A,** Anterior. **B,** Posterior. **C,** Right posterior oblique. **D,** Left posterior oblique. **E,** Right lateral. **F,** Left lateral.

the physician are aware of the difference, either method is satisfactory. The method of injection should be noted somewhere on the film or film jacket. Albumin appears to have an affinity for the plastic tubing of intravenous sets, catheters, and syringes. If these avenues of administration are used, a variable proportion of the dose never reaches the patient. We recommend a saline syringe, three-way stopcock, and dose syringe setup (Figure 14-8) for aggregated albumin injections. This arrangement also eliminates the drawing of blood back into the dose and prevents the possible formation of small thrombi as a result of the mixing of whole blood and MAA.

Labeled particles are always injected slowly over 30 seconds or longer. Some physicians recommend having the patient take a few deep breaths during the injection to assist the homogeneous distribution of the particles.[53]

Positioning

Standard perfusion imaging includes the six basic views: posterior, anterior, right and left laterals, and right and left posterior obliques.[11,34,40] We recommend doing the posterior view first, for 500,000 counts, and then each of the other views for the same time that it takes to do the posterior view. The lateral views can then be compared more easily. About one third of the counts from the contralateral lung are included during lateral imaging.

Unlike in many radiographic procedures, the radionuclide images provide the physician with very few landmarks that indicate rotation or distance from the collimator face.[42] The responsibility for good positioning in the nuclear medicine area is basically in the hands of the technologist.

VENTILATION IMAGING

Table 14-1 shows some of the radiopharmaceuticals used to study regional ventilation. Xenon-133 (^{133}Xe) has been used for quasistatic measurement of regional ventilation and blood flow, for dynamic measurement of regional ventilation, for measurement of regional lung volumes, for closing volume, and for studying factors that influence the distribution of a single breath. Clinical studies of regional ventilation are usually done with ^{133}Xe.

Table 14-1 Radiopharmaceuticals used for ventilation lung imaging

	Agent		
	^{99m}Tc DTPA aerosol	^{133}Xe	^{81m}Kr
Physical half-life	6.0 hr	5.3 days	13 sec
Principal gamma energy	140 keV	80 keV	190 keV
Radiation absorbed dose per millicurie in lungs	112.5 mrad*	12 mrad†	7.5 mrad†

*Actual dose delivered to lung is approximately one fifth because lung deposition is on the order of 200 μCi.
†Radiation absorbed dose has been estimated with a rebreathing time of 3 minutes.

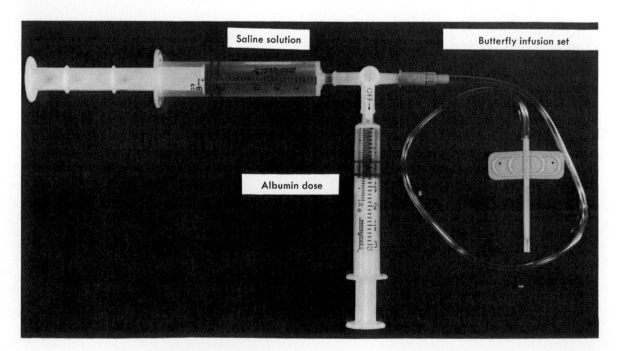

Figure 14-8 Arrangement of recommended injection set for albumin particles.

Techniques for ventilation studies are not yet standardized, but three aspects of ventilation are often examined: (1) the distribution of a single breath, (2) the distribution of lung volume, and (3) the distribution of the efficiency of ventilation from the clearance of radioactive xenon. Single-breath studies show the distribution of a bolus of radioactive xenon inhaled, with air, to total lung capacity—a somewhat unphysiologic situation (Figure 14-9, *A*). If the tracer gas is rebreathed to equilibrium (i.e., until the concentration of xenon in the lungs and in the rebreathing system is constant), the distribution of xenon within the lungs corresponds to lung volume (Figure 14-9, *B*). Measurements made during a wash-in of xenon to equilibrium reflect the efficiency of ventilation; the faster a region reaches equilibrium, the better its ventilation and vice versa. When air is breathed after a wash-in, the subsequent wash-out provides excellent evidence of the regional variations in ventilation (Figure 14-10). The best-ventilated regions clear fastest, and the poorly ventilated ones stand out by contrast as regions where the clearance of radioactivity is delayed.[1]

Xenon-133 (^{133}Xe) Ventilation Imaging

Currently the most readily available nuclide for performing ventilation studies is ^{133}Xe. Although it is not an ideal nuclide for this study because of its low energy, beta emission, and solubility in fat and blood, its price and ready availability have forced it into prominence. The energy, 80 keV, is not optimal for the Anger camera because so much scattered activity is included in the window.

Ideally, the perfusion study should be done first so that if a ventilation study is necessary, the patient can be positioned for it on the basis of the perfusion scan. Several institutions do the perfusion image first, using only 1 mCi of ^{99m}Tc-labeled particles, and then proceed with a ventilation study using 20 to 30 mCi of ^{133}Xe or more. However, because the energy of ^{133}Xe is lower than that of ^{99m}Tc and because of the importance of the wash-out phase, it is technically more satisfactory to perform the ventilation study before the perfusion examination.

A number of commercial gas delivery and rebreathing units are available for ventilation studies, but with a little imagination and some engineering skill, you can build your own[41] (Figure 14-11). An additional problem with xenon ventilation studies is disposal of the xenon when the study is finished. Many laboratories, if suitably located, simply vent the diluted xenon (half-life of 5.27 days) into the atmosphere. The Nuclear Regulatory Commission (NRC) requires that the average yearly concentration be less than 5×10^{-7} µCi/ml. There are some arguments against this practice, but from a pragmatic standpoint, it is the simplest solution. An alternative is to trap the xenon. Several commercial units are available for this purpose, most of which use activated charcoal.[31]

Several methods can be used to do a ventilation study. Some laboratories use the single-breath technique, which is to have the patient inhale a bolus of 10 to 20 mCi of ^{133}Xe and hold the breath for 10 to 20 seconds while a static image is taken. Serial wash-out images are then made at 30- to 60-second intervals as the xenon clears from the lungs. This method works well but requires a good deal of patient

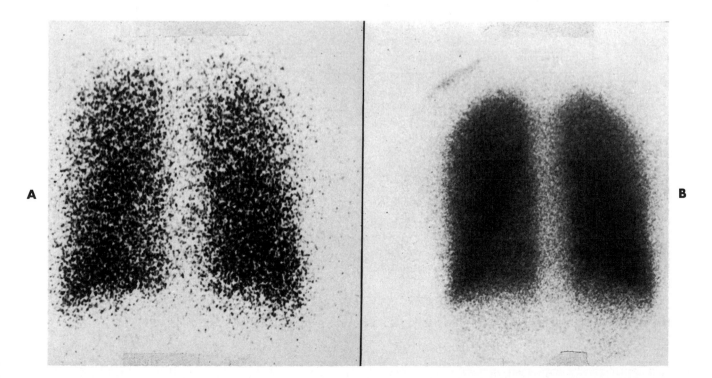

Figure 14-9   **A,** Normal distribution of a single breath of ^{133}Xe in the posterior projection. **B,** Wash-in equilibrium image of the same patient.

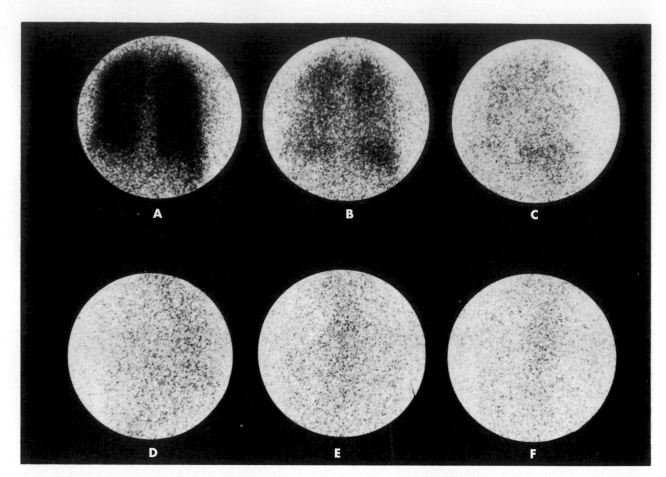

Figure 14-10   Posterior projection of wash-out of xenon from the lungs. **A,** Equilibrium image. **B** through **F,** Wash-out images of 1, 2, 3, 4, and 5 min.

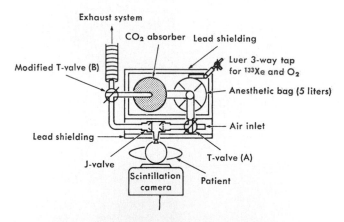

Figure 14-11   Diagram of simple rebreathing apparatus that can be constructed from commercially available parts.

cooperation in taking a deep breath and then holding it for 10 to 20 seconds.

We favor the more straightforward wash-in-wash-out method, which can be used even on comatose patients. In this method, 10 to 20 mCi of ^{133}Xe diluted in 2 L of oxygen are rebreathed from a simple rebreathing apparatus for

approximately 3 minutes while a static wash-in image is taken. Air is then breathed, and serial images are taken at 30- to 60-second intervals as the xenon clears from the lungs. With the variety of mouthpieces, respiratory masks, and harnesses available, a technologist can perform a ventilation study without assistance from the patient. We have successfully completed this type of examination on many patients and feel confident in saying that if the patient is breathing, a ventilation study can be done. Such studies can also be done on patients using mechanical ventilation.

The ventilation study may be done in any position. Routinely we use the posterior view in the upright position because this provides the best view of the greatest area of lung. The patient should be seated comfortably with the back to the scintillation camera and should be encouraged to keep as still as possible during the study. The first few breaths of xenon, which are seen on the monitor, can be used to adjust the position of the camera before the wash-in images are started.

Krypton-81m (^{81m}Kr) Ventilation Imaging

Krypton-81m is being used in some centers. This gas has such a short half-life that when inhaled continuously during normal breathing, an equilibrium count rate that is proportional to ventilation is reached. This means that images can be made in the same projections used for perfusion imaging and are directly comparable. Images made in this way show the distribution of regional ventilation, whereas images made with ^{99m}Tc human albumin microspheres show the distribution of regional blood flow. Therefore visual comparisons of the matching of ventilation and blood flow are considerably easier with ^{81m}Kr than with radioactive xenon[14,17] (Figure 14-12).

This gas is obtained by elution of a rubidium-81 (^{81}Rb) generator with a stream of moist air. ^{81m}Kr generators are delivered containing 5 mCi of ^{81}Rb at the time of calibration and have a useful life of approximately 6 hours. ^{81m}Kr has a 13-second half-life and an energy of 190 keV so that the examinations can be performed in the preferred order. This short half-life also eliminates any problems of trapping, venting, or contamination. Because ^{81m}Kr decays almost immediately, four- or six-view ventilation studies to match the perfusion images can be done routinely.[14,17]

Aerosol Ventilation Imaging

Aerosols are deposited in the bronchial tree in relation to particle size, air flow rates, and turbulence. The delivery tubing effectively filters out larger particles, 10 to 15 μm in diameter. Smaller ones are deposited in the larger airways during both inspiration and expiration. Particles less than 2 μm can reach the alveoli and be deposited there, whereas even smaller particles, less than 0.1 μm, probably escape in the expired air. Radioactive aerosols have been used for more than three decades to study the patency of the airways. It is important that aerosol particle size be well controlled for reproducible studies. Many radionuclides have been used, specifically ^{99m}Tc diethylenetriamine pentaacetic acid (^{99m}Tc DTPA), ^{99m}TcO$_4$, ^{99m}Tc sulfur colloid, ^{99m}Tc HSA, and ^{113m}In Cl$_2$.

The aerosol is generated from an ultrasound nebulizer or a positive-pressure nebulizer. It is inhaled through a mouthpiece or a face mask. If older systems are used, exhaled material must be collected, and the procedure is best done near a fume hood with an extraction fan. This is not necessary, however, with the newer systems that incorporate a bacterial filter at the outlet. Three to 5 ml of fluid containing up to 35 mCi of the nuclear pharmaceutical are inhaled. Only 10% to 15% actually reaches the lungs. Images can then be made in the six standard views (Figure 14-13). Normal aerosol scans look much like perfusion scans except that the trachea and mainstem bronchi usually can be seen, as well as the esophagus and stomach because of swallowed material.

With obstructive disease of the airways, central deposition in the larger bronchial tubes, with little or no peripheral filling, may occur, a pattern seen in severe bronchial asthma and emphysema. Less central but definitely patchy peripheral filling tends to be seen in chronic bronchitis, cystic fibrosis, and mild bronchial asthma. Delayed views, 4 to 6 hours after the initial images, can help resolve some

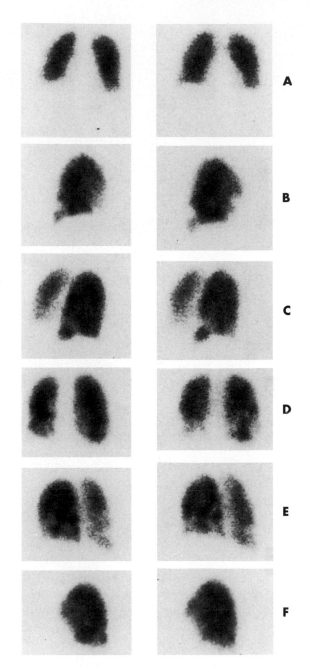

Figure 14-12   Side-by-side comparison of blood flow with ^{99m}Tc MAA (*column I*) and ventilation utilizing ^{81m}Kr (*column II*). Images are arranged as follows: **A,** anterior; **B,** right lateral; **C,** right posterior oblique; **D,** posterior; **E,** left posterior oblique; **F,** left lateral.

central deposition. This is cleared by mucociliary transport in otherwise normal subjects, leaving normal delayed images. Aerosol scans are almost as sensitive as xenon studies in detecting early disease of small airways. Sequential images for several hours after aerosol inhalation have been used to measure mucociliary clearance rates in smokers, nonsmokers, and children with cystic fibrosis.[39]

The development of small, disposable nebulizers has renewed interest in the use of aerosols for lung imaging.[20]

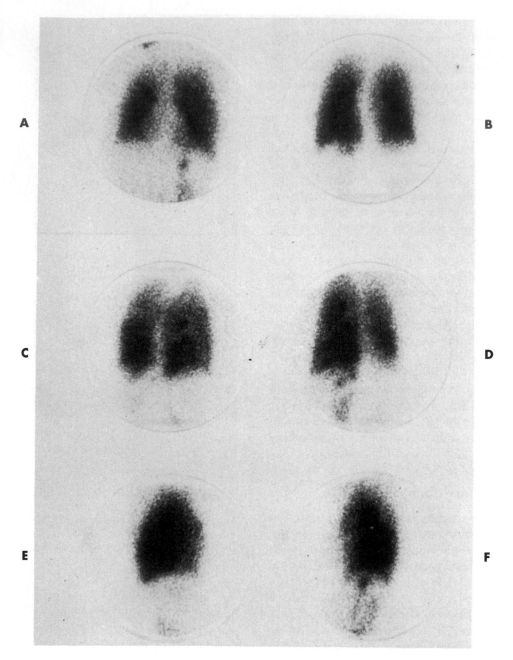

Figure 14-13   Six views of aerosol ventilation scan using ^{99m}Tc DTPA. Images are arranged as follows: **A,** anterior; **B,** posterior; **C,** right posterior oblique; **D,** left posterior oblique; **E,** right lateral; **F,** left lateral.

These light, portable units have been greatly improved over the cumbersome systems designed during the development of this technique. Bedside procedures are possible with a cooperative patient. Even with these improvements, however, the aerosol technique remains one of the more difficult nuclear medicine procedures. It requires detailed attention to variables such as tubing length and diameter, air flow, and pressure.

Technegas and Pertechnegas

Technegas is an ultrafine or gaslike microaerosol of a graphite-coated technetium atom that was developed at the Australian National University. Technegas is a derivative of the "buckyball" family with a cross section of 5 to 30 nm and a thickness of 3 nm. The particle is a hexagonal crystal of native ^{99m}Tc metal within a "shrink-wrap" of graphite that completely encloses it. Technegas is produced by placing 7 to 10 mCi of sodium pertechnetate (USP) into a pure graphite crucible within a 6 L lead-shielded chamber (Figure 14-14). The crucible is warmed to evaporate all the liquid as the chamber air is replaced with pure argon. After 6 minutes, the unit is ready to create Technegas. The patient rehearses the ventilation procedure during this preparation phase, preferably in a supine position on the imaging table with the camera set for a posterior view. The "start" button

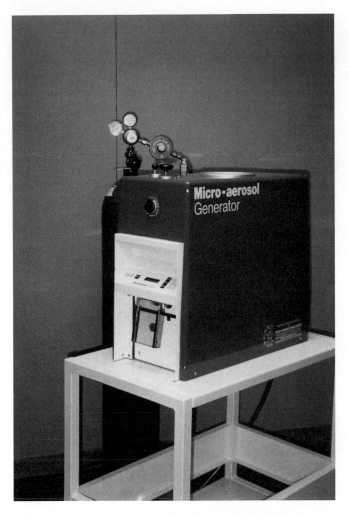

Figure 14-14 Technegas crucible device, which is labeled a "microaerosol generator" for its U.S. Food and Drug Administration (FDA) trials in the United States, with a standard tank of argon behind it. (Courtesy William M. Burch, Ph.D.)

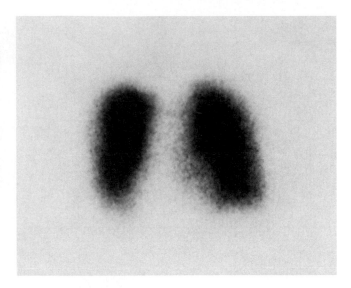

Figure 14-15 Anterior lung microaerosol scan with Technegas. (Courtesy William M. Burch, Ph.D.)

heating cycle of the machine. The addition of oxygen to the blanket gas prevents the formation of the graphite "shrink-wrap," leaving technetium oxides only in the chamber. On inhalation, these oxides hydrolyze rapidly in the high water vapor of the lungs' airways, reverting immediately to TcO_4^-.

Clinically, Pertechnegas is identical to an inhaled pertechnetate aerosol but with the significant advantage that it is delivered in one or two breaths, even in patients with severe respiratory distress. Again, the administration may be controlled by having the technologist load more activity into the crucible and allowing only a predefined level of activity to enter the patient's lungs.

VENTILATION-PERFUSION STUDIES

By combining studies of ventilation and perfusion, it can be determined whether defects in blood flow are associated with defects in ventilation. The pulmonary diseases commonly seen in clinical nuclear medicine tend to fall into two categories: (1) those with abnormal regional pulmonary blood flow but normal (or almost normal) regional ventilation (pulmonary embolism is by far the most important of these, but early heart failure, interstitial lung diseases, some lung cancers, and other abnormalities of the pulmonary vasculature may show this pattern) and (2) those with abnormal ventilation and abnormal blood flow. The most common conditions are chronic bronchitis, emphysema, and asthma; however, cystic fibrosis and bronchiectasis cause similar patterns. Cancers of the bronchus, other bronchial tumors, or foreign bodies obstructing a bronchus can all produce localized abnormalities of ventilation and blood flow. In general, the disturbance of ventilation is more pronounced than that of blood flow and is detected as a regional delay in the clearance of xenon. When this delay is great, a corresponding defect is usually visible on the wash-in image as an area of

on the machine is pressed, and the crucible in its argon atmosphere heats to 2550°C in less than 0.5 second and holds that temperature for 15 seconds before switching off. The machine is then wheeled into the camera room, and the Technegas is administered to the patient by means of a self-contained breathing apparatus. Usually only two or three breaths are needed to deliver a suitable dose (1 mCi) for ventilation imaging (Figure 14-15).

Technegas microaerosol images are performed from several projections before lung perfusion images from the same views. The Technegas particle is hydrophobic and chemically inert, therefore once it lodges in the alveoli, it remains there indefinitely. As a consequence, it is becoming more common for SPECT studies to be routinely performed, particularly as the newer multihead cameras are used. Outside the United States, Technegas imaging has become a common means of assessing ventilation.

Pertechnegas is a derivative of Technegas formed by the simple expedient of using 3% to 5% oxygen in the argon in the 6 L chamber of the generator during the main 15-second

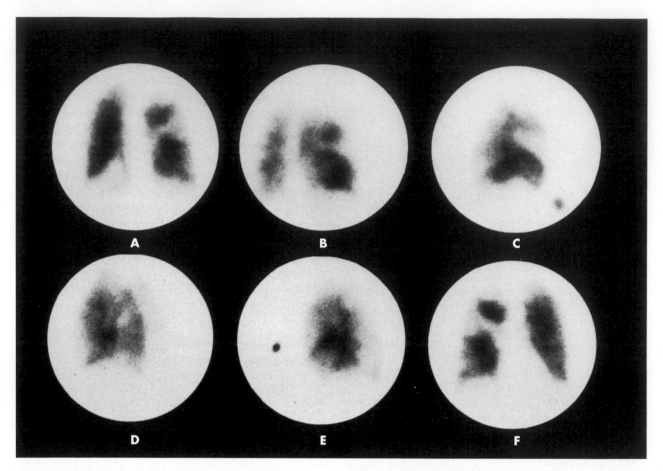

Figure 14-16 Markedly abnormal perfusion scan of the lungs demonstrating multiple segmental defects. Images are arranged as follows: **A,** Posterior. **B,** Right posterior oblique. **C,** Right lateral. **D,** Left posterior oblique. **E,** Left lateral. **F,** Anterior.

diminished activity, where this part of the lung has not reached equilibrium with the tracer gas.

Pneumonias, pulmonary infarctions, and severe pulmonary edema are all associated with defects in the equilibrium images, which correspond to the infiltrates seen on the chest radiograph. No retention of radioactive xenon is seen during the wash-out because no radioactive xenon can enter the fluid-filled alveoli.

Normal perfusion scans show an even gradation of activity, with more activity visible in the lower lobes than in the upper lobes, if the injection is given with the patient in the upright posture. The outline of the lungs and mediastinum corresponds closely to that seen on the chest radiograph. A normal wash-in image shows an even distribution of activity throughout the lungs, and a normal wash-out is usually complete within 3 to 4 minutes of breathing air. Occasionally the bases can clear a little faster than the upper zones.

Computer Processing of Ventilation-Perfusion Images

The ready access to digital computer processing of image data has led to several different ways of processing the information from ventilation-perfusion imaging. The parti-

tioning of ventilation, lung volume, and blood flow between the lungs can be obtained with considerable ease; however, measurements of regional ventilation and regional ventilation-perfusion ratios are less readily obtained. In most instances the numeric values obtained do not correspond to how much air is exchanged or to the physiologic ventilation-perfusion ratios.[42]

Pulmonary Embolism

In pulmonary embolism the defects in blood flow correspond to anatomic subdivisions of the lung, such as segments or lobes, in 75% of patients. The remaining 25% have ill-defined nonsegmental defects. If the patient had previously healthy lungs, ventilation is usually well maintained to the affected parts of the lung because their bronchial tubes are patent (Figures 14-16 and 14-17). Only a small proportion (10% to 15%) of patients with emboli develop pulmonary infarction, with its associated infiltrates, as seen on the chest radiograph.

Interpretation is more difficult and less reliable when the patient already has chronic obstructive pulmonary disease (COPD), such as chronic bronchitis, emphysema, or asthma.[2] Retrospective studies from the 1970s suggested that the true positive rate, or sensitivity, and the true

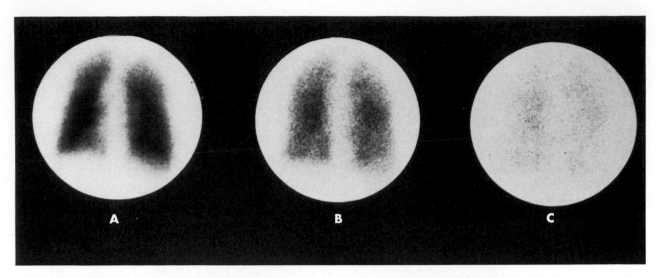

Figure 14-17   Essentially normal ^{133}Xe ventilation scan. Images are arranged as follows: **A**, Equilibrium image. **B**, One-minute wash-out. **C**, Three-minute wash-out.

negative rate, or specificity, of ventilation-perfusion scanning were more than 90%.[3,33] Subsequent studies have not shown this to be true.[2,7,8]

Two recent prospective studies of the accuracy of ventilation-perfusion scanning in comparison to pulmonary angiography showed pulmonary embolism to be present in about 90% of patients with high probability lung scan interpretations.[24,35] However, for other interpretations, such as intermediate, indeterminate, or low probability, the proportion of patients with angiographically proven pulmonary emboli ranged from 14% to 40%. When the perfusion scan was completely normal, pulmonary emboli were rarely found.[24,27]

For patients with ventilation-perfusion scans that are neither high probability nor normal, further diagnostic studies are indicated. Noninvasive tests for proximal vein thrombosis, such as B-mode ultrasound or impedance plethysmography, should be considered, or even the more invasive venography if these noninvasive tests are not available.[26,30] Finding evidence of venous thrombosis would lead to treatment for venous thromboembolism.[26] If the diagnosis is still in doubt, pulmonary angiography, if available, may be needed to resolve the problem.[7,8,25] Most but not all pulmonary emboli are eventually lysed by the body's own fibrinolytic systems, therefore defects in blood flow tend to disappear with time. Most improvement is seen in the first few days. Further improvement occurs more slowly over the next 3 to 4 weeks and can continue for several months.[43] Anticoagulant treatment is important; it prevents the formation of new blood clots and the extension of those already present in the lungs.

Chronic Obstructive Pulmonary Disease

Radioactive ventilation studies provide one of the most sensitive ways of detecting damage to the small airways.[45]

Patients with chronic bronchitis and emphysema show an endless variety of defects in blood flow and ventilation. Eighty percent of the time the defects in blood flow cannot be strictly related to anatomic subdivisions of the lung. In general, both lungs tend to be affected to a similar although rarely identical degree. In some patients most of the damage is in the lower zones, in others in the upper zones, and in yet others the damage is scattered throughout both lungs. It is by no means rare for one lung to be distinctly more severely affected than the other (Figures 14-18 and 14-19).

In chronic bronchitis, ventilation tends to be more severely affected than blood flow, and some changes in the pattern of ventilation and blood flow can be seen with exacerbations of this disease. In emphysema, the defects in ventilation and blood flow correspond more closely and tend to be more stable from year to year.

Patients with bronchial asthma also show considerable changes in both ventilation and blood flow, with ventilation being more severely affected. If just a perfusion scan is done, often the defects are recognizably segmental, or even lobar, leading to a false diagnosis of pulmonary embolism.

In cystic fibrosis, the upper lobes usually are the more severely affected, and fissure signs are often seen on the lateral views. This sign is attributable to a defect in blood flow along the greater fissure. It is also seen in other obstructive airway diseases, as well as in pulmonary edema with pleural fluid and occasionally in pulmonary embolism. The segments or lobes of lung involved with bronchiectasis are clearly outlined by lack of ventilation and absent pulmonary arterial blood flow.

Lung Cancer

In cancer of the bronchus, ventilation-perfusion studies can be used to determine individual lung function when a pneumonectomy is planned. The relative distribution of blood

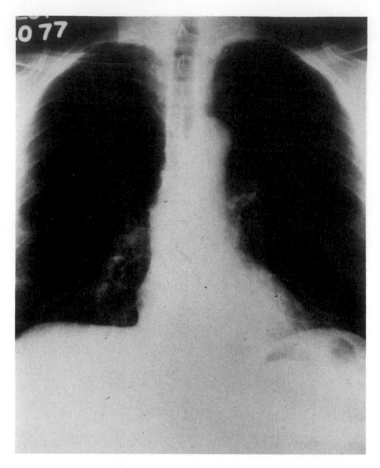

Figure 14-18 Chest radiograph of a 64-year-old man with severe emphysema. He has large lungs and bullous areas in the upper lobes.

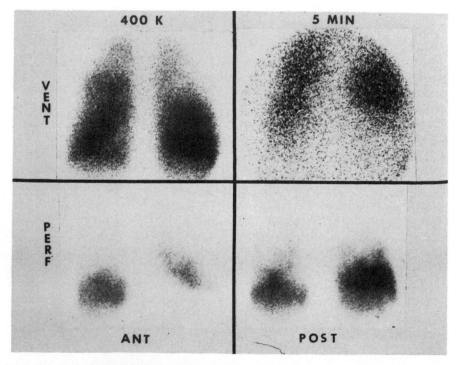

Figure 14-19 Selected ventilation and perfusion images of the patient in Figure 14-18. Perfusion images show decreased perfusion in the upper half of both lung fields. Diminished filling of both upper lung fields is seen on equilibrium (wash-in) images *(upper left)* and delayed clearance from both lungs during wash-out *(upper right)*.

flow calculated from an upright perfusion scan enables post-operative lung function to be predicted with considerable accuracy. A successful resection of the tumor tissue is less likely if the affected lung receives less than about 25% to 30% of the total pulmonary blood flow. Occasionally the site of a tumor can be identified by ventilation-perfusion scanning when it cannot be found by conventional means. After radiation treatment for lung cancer, ventilation usually improves, but blood flow is restored in a much smaller proportion of such patients.

The most important indication for ventilation-perfusion scanning is in the differential diagnosis of pulmonary embolism. Lesser indications are for the follow-up of this condition and for the assessment of regional and individual lung function in the preoperative assessment of patients with lung cancer or other conditions in which lung tissue may be resected. Ventilation-perfusion scans can sometimes be helpful in the management of patients with COPD. They may also play some part in the follow-up of patients who have had surgical correction of certain congenital heart defects.

REFERENCES

1. Alderson PO, Biello DR, Khan AR et al: Comparison of ^{133}Xe single-breath and washout imaging in the scintigraphic diagnosis of pulmonary embolism, *Radiology* 137:481-486, 1980.
2. Alderson PO, Biello DR, Sachariah KG et al: Scintigraphic detection of pulmonary embolism in patients with obstructive pulmonary disease, *Radiology* 138:661-666, 1981.
3. Alderson PO, Rujanavech N, Secker-Walker RH et al: The role of ^{133}Xe ventilation studies in the scintigraphic detection of pulmonary embolism, *Radiology* 120:633, 1976.
4. Anthonisen NR, Danson J, Roberson PC et al: Airway closure as a function of age, *Respir Physiol* 8:58, 1969.
5. Anthonisen NR, Milic-Emili J: Distribution of pulmonary perfusion in erect man, *J Appl Physiol* 21:760, 1966.
6. Ball WC Jr, Stewart PB, Newham IGS et al: Regional pulmonary studies with xenon 133, *J Clin Invest* 41:519, 1962.
7. Biello DR, Mattar AG, McKnight RC et al: Ventilation-perfusion studies in suspected pulmonary embolism, *Am J Roentgenol* 138:661-666, 1981.
8. Biello DR, Mattar AG, Osei-Wusu A et al: Interpretation of indeterminate lung scintigrams, *Radiology* 133:189-194, 1979.
9. Breeze RG, Wheeldon EB: The cells of the pulmonary airways, *Am Rev Respir Dis* 116:705, 1977.
10. Buist AS, Van Fleet DL, Ross BB: A comparison of conventional spirometric tests and the test of closing volume in an emphysema screening center, *Am Rev Respir Dis* 107:735, 1973.
11. Burdine JA, Murphy PH: Clinical efficacy of a large-field-of-view scintillation camera, *J Nucl Med* 16:1158, 1975.
12. Child JS, Wolfe JD, Tashkin D et al: Fatal lung scan in a case of pulmonary hypertension due to obliterative pulmonary vascular disease, *Chest* 67:308, 1975.
13. Daly I de B, Hebb C: *Pulmonary and bronchial vascular systems,* Baltimore, 1966, Williams & Wilkins.
14. Fazio F, Jones T: Assessment of regional ventilation by continuous inhalation of radioactive krypton-81m, *Br Med J* 3:673, 1975.
15. Fishman AP, Pietra G: Handling of bioactive materials by the lung, *N Engl J Med* 281:884, 953, 1974.
16. Gold WM, McCormack KR: Pulmonary function response to radioisotope scanning of the lungs, *JAMA* 197:146, 1966.
17. Goris ML, Daspit SG, Walter JP et al: Applications of ventilation lung imaging with ^{81m}krypton, *Radiology* 122:399, 1977.
18. Green GM: The Amberson Lecture: in defense of the lung, *Am Rev Respir Dis* 102:691, 1970.
19. Harding LK, Horsfield K, Singhal SS et al: The proportion of lung vessels blocked by albumin microspheres, *J Nucl Med* 14:579, 1973.
20. Hayes M, Taplin GV, Chopra SK et al: Improved radioaerosol administration system for routine inhalation lung imaging, *Radiology* 131:256-258, 1979.
21. Haynie TP, Calhoon JH, Nasjleti CE et al: Visualization of pulmonary artery occlusion by photoscanning, *JAMA* 185:306, 1963.
22. Heck LL, Duley JW: Statistical considerations in lung imaging with Tc-99m albumin particles, *Radiology* 113:657, 1974.
23. Hughes JMB, Glazier JB, Maloney JE et al: Effect of lung volume on the distribution of pulmonary blood flow in man, *Respir Physiol* 4:78, 1968.
24. Hull RD, Hirsh J, Carter CJ et al: Diagnostic value of ventilation-perfusion lung scanning in patients with suspected pulmonary embolism, *Chest* 88:819-828, 1985.
25. Hull RD, Hirsch J, Carter CJ et al: Pulmonary angiography, ventilation lung scanning, and venography for clinically suspected pulmonary embolism with abnormal perfusion lung scan, *Ann Intern Med* 98:891-899, 1983.
26. Hull RD, Raskob GE, Coates G et al: A new noninvasive management strategy for patients with suspected pulmonary embolism, *Arch Intern Med* 149:2549-2555, 1989.
27. Hull RD, Raskob GE, Coates G et al: Clinical validity of a normal perfusion lung scan in patients with suspected pulmonary embolism, *Chest* 97:23-26, 1990.
28. Kaneko K, Milic-Emili J, Dolovich MB et al: Regional distribution of ventilation and perfusion as a function of body position, *J Appl Physiol* 21:767, 1966.

29. Knipping HW, Bolt W, Vanrath H et al: Eine neue Methode zur Prüfung der Herz- und Lungenfunktion, *Deutsch Med Wochenschr* 80:1146, 1955.

30. Lensing AWA, Prandoni P, Brandjes D et al: Detection of deep-vein thrombosis by real-time b-mode ultrasonography, *N Engl J Med* 320:342-345, 1989.

31. Luizzi A, Keaney J, Freedman G: Use of activated charcoal for the collection and containment of Xe-133 exhaled during pulmonary studies, *J Nucl Med* 13:673, 1972.

32. Mead J, Takishima T, Leith D: Stress distribution in lungs: a model of pulmonary elasticity, *J Appl Physiol* 28:596, 1970.

33. McNeil BJ: A diagnostic strategy using ventilation-perfusion studies in patients suspect for pulmonary embolism, *J Nucl Med* 17:613, 1976.

34. Nielsen PE, Kirchner PT, Gerber FH: Oblique views in lung perfusion scanning: clinical utility and limitations, *J Nucl Med* 18:967, 1977.

35. PIOPED investigators: Value of the ventilation/perfusion scan in acute pulmonary embolism: results of the prospective investigation of pulmonary embolism diagnosis, *JAMA* 263:2753-2759, 1990.

36. Rhodes BA, Stem HS, Buchanan JA et al: Lung scanning with Tc-99m microspheres, *Radiology* 99:613, 1971.

37. Rogers RM, Kuhl DE, Hyde RW et al: Measurement of the vital capacity and perfusion of each lung by fluoroscopy and macroaggregated albumin lung scanning, *Ann Intern Med* 67:947, 1967.

38. Rootwelt K, Vale JR: Pulmonary gas exchange after intravenous injection of ^{99m}Tc sulphur colloid albumin macroaggregates for lung perfusion scintigraphy, *Scand J Clin Lab Invest* 30:17, 1972.

39. Sanchis J, Dolovich M, Rossman C et al: Pulmonary mucociliary clearance in cystic fibrosis, *N Engl J Med* 288:651, 1973.

40. Sasahara AA, Belko JS, Simpson RC: Multiple view lung scanning, *J Nucl Med* 9:187, 1968.

41. Secker-Walker RH, Barbier J, Weiner SN et al: A simple ^{133}Xe delivery system for studies of regional ventilation, *J Nucl Med* 15:288, 1974.

42. Secker-Walker RH, Evens RG: The clinical application of computers in ventilation-perfusion studies, *Progr Nucl Med* 3:166, 1973.

43. Secker-Walker RH, Jackson JA, Goodwin J: Resolution of pulmonary embolism, *Br Med J* 4:135, 1970.

44. Taplin GV, Johnson DE, Dore EK et al: Lung photoscans with macroaggregates of human serum radioalbumin: experimental basis and initial clinical trials, *Health Phys* 10:1219, 1964.

45. Taplin GV, Tashkin DP, Chopra SK et al: Early detection of chronic obstructive pulmonary disease using radionuclide lung imaging procedures, *Chest* 71:567, 1977.

46. Tow DE, Wagner HN, Lopez-Majano V et al: Validity of measuring regional pulmonary arterial blood flow with macroaggregates of human serum albumin, *Am J Roentgenol Radium Ther Nucl Med* 96:664, 1966.

47. Wagner HM, Sabiston DC, McAfee JG et al: Diagnosis of massive pulmonary embolism in man by radioisotope scanning, *N Engl J Med* 271:377, 1964.

48. West JB: Pulmonary function studies with radioactive gases, *Ann Rev Med* 18:459, 1967.

49. West JB: *Respiratory physiology: the essentials,* Baltimore, 1975, Williams & Wilkins.

50. Weibel ER: *Morphometry of the human lungs,* New York, 1963, Academic Press.

51. Dworkin HJ, Gutkowski RF, Porter W et al: Effect of particle number on lung perfusion images: concise communication, *J Nucl Med* 18:260-262, 1977.

52. Kleine JA, Johns KL et al: New diagnostic tests for pulmonary embolism, *Ann Emerg Med* 35:2, 2000.

53. Parker JA, Coleman RE, Siegel BA et al: *Procedure guideline for lung scintigraphy,* Reston, Va., 1977, Society of Nuclear Medicine.

54. Swanson DP, Chilton HM, Thrall JH: *Pharmaceuticals in medical imaging,* Colombus, Ohio, 1990, Macmillan.

Neeta Pandit, Arvind Sinha, H. William Strauss

chapter 15

Cardiovascular System

Objectives

Diagram the structures of the heart.

Describe the mechanical and electrical activity of the heart.

List the acquired abnormalities of the cardiovascular system that can be evaluated with radionuclide techniques.

State the preparation, dosage, and injection technique for radionuclide evaluation of ventricular function.

Discuss the tracer requirements for first-pass studies.

Explain how an ejection fraction is calculated.

Describe an exercise and a pharmacologic stress test and explain when each is used.

Discuss radiopharmaceuticals used for myocardial perfusion imaging.

Describe the imaging techniques for planar and SPECT myocardial perfusion imaging.

Discuss the advantage of PET radionuclides for cardiac imaging.

Radionuclide studies of the cardiovascular system are primarily used to detect and characterize acquired heart diseases, such as coronary artery disease, cardiotoxicity of antineoplastic drugs, and congestive heart failure. Although nuclear procedures can quantitate shunts in patients with congenital diseases, such as atrial and ventricular septal defects, those assessments generally are made by a combination of echocardiography and magnetic resonance imaging. This chapter focuses on the clinical applications of nuclear techniques; the reader is referred to other sources for procedures of historic importance.

Most nuclear medicine laboratories use single photon radiopharmaceuticals and multiple-detector gamma cameras to record clinical data. Positron emission tomographs (PET scans) have higher spatial resolution than single photon systems and can be used to acquire a repertoire of measurements similar to those obtained with single photon devices; PET, however, has the added capability of absolute quantitation (e.g., expressing myocardial perfusion as milliliters/minutes/gram of myocardium). Advances in multidetector gamma camera design have led to the creation of hybrid cameras that can record both single photon and coincidence images, making positron imaging techniques available to users who do not have dedicated positron tomographs. Because most imaging is carried out with single photon techniques, we first devote our attention to these techniques.

CLINICAL PROBLEM

Approximately 62 million people in the United States have one or more forms of acquired disease of the heart or blood vessels. Elevated blood pressure

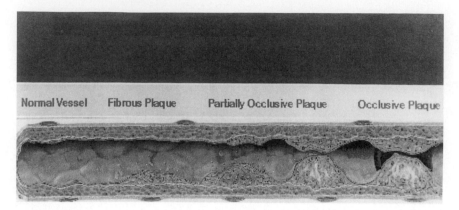

Normal Vessel   Fibrous Plaque   Partially Occlusive Plaque   Occlusive Plaque

Figure 15-1 Progression of atherosclerosis. As a result of factors that are not well defined but are associated with hyperlipidemia and probably injury to vessels, lipids such as cholesterol and fatty acids accumulate in the area beneath the endothelium. These lipids are irritating, leading to invasion by monocytes and macrophages, which over many years enlarges the lesion. The lesion may then break through the endothelial cells, resulting in the formation of a clot at the site of rupture and often myocardial infarction.

(hypertension) occurs in 50 million adults; coronary artery disease occurs in 12.6 million (6.4 million have *angina,* or chest pain of cardiac origin); rheumatic heart disease occurs in approximately 1.3 million; and stroke occurs in 4.6 million. Coronary artery disease (CAD) caused about 1 million deaths in the United States in 1999, making CAD the number one killer in the United States. About 1.5 million people will suffer a new or recurrent heart attack each year. In addition to CAD, heart failure (inability of the heart to pump sufficient blood to meet the demands of the body) is becoming increasingly prevalent as the population ages.

In the United States almost 4.8 million patients have heart failure, and about 550,000 new cases occur each year. Heart failure often occurs in the final phase of an underlying heart disease. Cardiomyopathy, a disorder of the heart muscle itself, is a category of diseases associated with abnormal enlargement of the myocardium (hypertrophic myopathy) or with inability of the heart to contract effectively despite an adequate blood supply; this results in thinning of the muscle and dilation of the chambers (dilated myopathy), which results in altered function.

Coronary artery disease causes myocardial ischemia and infarction. Myocardial ischemia is a *reversible* condition caused by a temporary deficiency in the supply of oxygen to the myocardium, usually as a result of narrowing of a coronary artery. Myocardial infarction is an *irreversible* condition that leads to the death of a portion of the myocardium caused by occlusion of a coronary artery. In patients with infarction, early identification of the process is important, because restoration of blood flow within the first 6 hours after onset often results in preservation of myocardium and improved function.

Although myocardial infarction can occur with no warning and can cause sudden death, the underlying disease of the coronary arteries has evolved over decades. The arterial lesions progress from small lipid deposits in the wall of the vessel that begin around puberty, called *fatty streaks,* to raised lesions that intrude on the arterial lumen over about 20 to 30 years (Figure 15-1). The rate of progression can be controlled to some degree by the patient's diet, cholesterol and homocysteine levels, genetic heritage, and lifestyle. Atheromatous narrowings that occupy more than 50% of the lumen diameter restrict the maximum amount of blood that can flow through a vessel; these lesions may not be associated with any symptoms.

When patients exercise or when certain drugs are administered, the demand for blood flow (oxygen) through the coronary arteries increases. If this increased demand cannot be met, the myocardium becomes *ischemic.* Ischemia is associated with decreased tissue perfusion and decreased contraction in the affected area. These changes can be readily detected by radionuclide imaging studies.

ANATOMY

The adult heart (Figure 15-2) weighs about 300 g and holds approximately 500 ml of blood. The heart is located in the lower portion of the thoracic cavity between the lungs. It is covered by a clear, double-layered, fibrous sac, the pericardium, which contains a minimal amount of fluid. The fluid acts as a lubricant between the moving surface of the heart muscle (myocardium) and the other structures in the chest. The heart is actually two pumps (the right heart and left heart) operating in parallel to eject the same amount of blood with each beat. The right heart accepts blood from the body and pumps this blood to the lungs, where it is oxygenated. The left heart accepts blood returning from the lungs and pumps it to the body. There is no direct communication of blood between the left and right sides of the heart. Each side has two chambers, a thin-walled atrium, which holds about 100 ml, and a more muscular ventricle, which has a capacity of about 150 ml. Atria serve as temporary reservoirs for blood being returned to the heart, and the ventricles do the major work of pumping the blood away from the heart. The right ventricle (RV), which is shaped like a pyramid with the tricuspid valve at its base, pumps blood into a low-resistance vascular bed in the lungs. This pumping demand requires relatively little force, which can

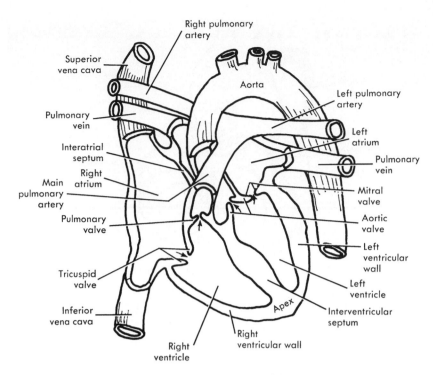

Figure 15-2   Gross anatomy of the heart.

be met by a 5 mm thick myocardium. The left ventricle (LV) is a football-shaped structure. Pumping blood to the higher resistance systemic circulation requires more force per beat, which is generated by the 10 mm thick LV myocardium. The right and left atria are separated by a thin muscular wall, the interatrial septum; the ventricles are separated by the thicker, muscular interventricular septum.

Valves separate the atria from the ventricles and the ventricles from the arteries. The purpose of the valves is to prevent back flow of blood from the ventricles to the atria during ventricular contraction or from the arteries to the ventricles during ventricular relaxation. The tricuspid valve (named for its three leaflets, or cusps) separates the right atrium from the right ventricle, and the mitral valve separates the left atrium from the left ventricle. The pulmonary valve separates the right ventricle from the pulmonary artery, and the aortic valve separates the left ventricle from the aorta. The valves in the heart play no role in propelling or initiating flow, only in preventing back flow. The design of the mitral and tricuspid valves is different from that of the pulmonic and aortic valves: the leaflets of the tricuspid and mitral valves are much larger and require "anchors" in the ventricle to prevent blow back during ventricular systole. To ensure that the leaflets of the valves stay in contact when the valves are closed, the leaflets are anchored by tendinous strands, the *chordae tendineae* to the papillary muscles, which are integrated into the ventricular walls. The aortic and pulmonic valves are smaller and function without the need for special leaflet support.

The aorta distributes blood via a branching network of arteries to the organs. Within an organ the arteries branch to form arterioles, which branch further at the cellular level to form capillaries, where the nutrients and oxygen are exchanged for waste products and carbon dioxide. From the aorta to the capillary, the blood vessels branch more than 20 times. As blood exits the capillaries, it is carried by venules, which coalesce to form veins, back to the heart.

Although the heart pumps blood, it receives its blood supply, as do all other organs, through arteries that specifically supply its needs. Oxygen and nutrients are delivered to the myocardium by the left and right coronary arteries (Figure 15-3). The left main coronary artery divides into two main branches. The left anterior descending artery supplies oxygen and nutrition to the interventricular septum and the anterior wall of the left ventricle; the left circumflex artery supplies the left atrium and the posterior and lateral walls of the left ventricle. The right coronary artery supplies the inferior wall of the left ventricle, the free wall of the right ventricle, and the right atrium. Blood drains from the myocardium to the coronary veins, which run alongside the coronary arteries and terminate in the coronary sinus of the right atrium.

PHYSIOLOGY

Circulation

Blood flows unidirectionally through each blood vessel under normal physiologic conditions. Deoxygenated venous blood, loaded with carbon dioxide and waste products, returns from the tissues toward the heart via the superior and inferior venae cavae veins (Figure 15-4). Although venous pressure is low, resistance to blood flow is also low, and blood flows through the large veins at 40 cm/sec on its

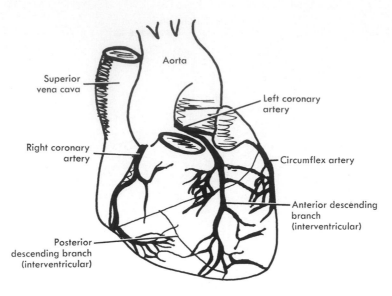

Figure 15-3 Anterior view of the heart, showing the coronary arteries.

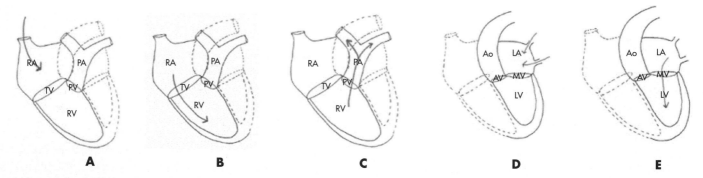

Figure 15-4 Poorly oxygenated blood returning to the heart from the organs enters the right atrium (RA) and is stored there until the right atrium contracts. When the right atrium contracts, the tricuspid valve (TV) opens, allowing blood to enter the right ventricle (RV). When the right ventricle contracts, the pulmonic valve (PV) opens, and blood is propelled into the pulmonary artery (PA). The pulmonary artery carries the blood to the lungs, where it picks up oxygen. Well-oxygenated blood returning to the heart from the lungs enters the left atrium and is stored there until the left atrium contracts. When the left atrium contracts, the mitral valve opens, allowing the blood to enter the left ventricle, from which it is pumped into the aorta during systole and distributed to various organs and tissues.

way to emptying into the right atrium at a pressure of less than 5 mm. Blood traverses the tricuspid valve to enter the right ventricle, which contracts with a plungerlike motion to expel blood through the pulmonic valve into the pulmonary artery and lungs for oxygenation. Blood is expelled from the right ventricle into the lungs at a pressure of 25 mm Hg. In the enormous capillary bed of the lungs, the velocity of blood slows to 1 mm/sec in the capillaries of the alveoli, where carbon dioxide is eliminated and oxygen is taken up.

The oxygenated blood returns to the left atrium via the pulmonary veins at a pressure of less than 5 mm Hg. The blood then flows through the mitral valve to the left ventricle, which contracts with a complex wringing motion; this provides sufficient kinetic energy to expel blood through the

aortic valve, at a velocity of about 15 m/sec, into the aorta at a systolic pressure of about 120 mm Hg, which permits the blood to travel to the farthest capillary bed. The velocity of the blood slows in the pulmonary capillaries to allow the exchange of gases (oxygen and carbon dioxide) and in the tissue capillaries to permit the exchange of nutrients for waste products.

Mechanical Activity of the Heart

Each cardiac cycle (one beat) consists of *systole,* the period of ventricular contraction, and *diastole,* the period of ventricular relaxation (Figure 15-5). The two sides of the heart contract in unison, but for clarity our discussion follows the left heart through a contraction cycle starting in late dias-

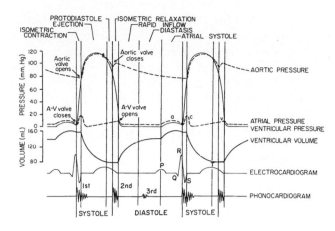

Figure 15-5 Events in the cardiac cycle, showing the simultaneous relationship of the electrocardiogram and phonocardiogram to the measured pressures in the left atrium, the left ventricle, and the aorta and the volume of the ventricles.

Table 15-1	Cardiac output at rest and exercise	
Organ	**Fraction of cardiac output**	
	Rest (5 L/min)	**Exercise** (15 L/min)
Brain	15%	4%
Heart	4%	5%
Kidneys	20%	5%
Liver	10%	1%
Gastrointestinal tract	15%	1%
Skeletal muscle	20%	70%
Skin	6%	10%
Other	10%	4%

From McCardle WD et al: In *Exercise, physiology, energy, nutrition and human performance,* Philadelphia, 1981, Lea & Febiger.

tole. During this period both the left atrium and the left ventricle are relaxed. Left atrial pressure is slightly higher than left ventricular pressure, the mitral valve is open, and blood passes from the left atrium through the mitral valve into the ventricle. Most ventricular filling (80% to 90%) takes place in this passive fashion. The aortic valve is closed during this time because aortic pressure is higher than left ventricular pressure. At the end of diastole the atrium contracts, adding 10% to 20% more volume to the left ventricle. The quantity of blood in the ventricle at the end of diastole is called the *end-diastolic volume* (about 150 ml in an average 70 kg adult).

During systole, the myofibrils of the ventricular myocardium shorten and left ventricular pressure rises, causing the mitral valve to close. As the myofibrils continue to shorten, left ventricular pressure rises rapidly. The interval after mitral valve closure but before the generation of sufficient pressure to open the aortic valve is called the *interval of isovolumetric* (i.e., no change in volume) *contraction.* Continued shortening of the myofibrils causes the left ventricular pressure to exceed aortic pressure; the aortic valve opens, and ventricular ejection begins. During the 250- to 300-msec interval when the myofibrils shorten to their minimal length, approximately one half to two thirds of the end-diastolic volume is ejected. Blood returning to the left heart during the interval of ventricular ejection, when the mitral valve is closed, is stored in the left atrium. As a result, both left atrial volume and pressure rise during the interval of ventricular ejection. At the conclusion of left ventricular ejection, the myofibrils rapidly relax, left ventricular pressure falls, the aortic valve closes, the mitral valve opens, and the ventricle starts to fill with blood that has returned to the left atrium during the interval of ventricular ejection. Filling occurs rapidly during early diastole and slows as atrial pressure and volume decrease. This filling pattern ensures the heart's ability to function unimpaired during times of increased heart rate (as with exercise and emotional stress),

when the length of diastole is shortened. In a relative sense the atrial contribution to end-diastolic volume is greater during exercise, when cardiac output and heart rate are increased, than at rest.

The amount of blood ejected from the left ventricle over a 1-minute interval is the *cardiac output* (usually expressed in liters per minute). A normal 70 kg adult has a cardiac output of approximately 5 to 6 L/min at rest. The amount of blood ejected in a single beat is the *stroke volume* (usually expressed in milliliters). The normal adult stroke volume is approximately 80 to 100 ml. The cardiac output is distributed to the organs in proportion to their oxygen requirements, which change from rest to exertion (Table 15-1).

Electrical Activity of the Heart

The myocardial muscle has an intrinsic rhythm of contraction. The sinoatrial node, a small mass of specialized cells embedded in the wall of the right atrium near the entrance of the superior vena cava, has the fastest inherent rhythm and supersedes other similar sites in the heart (Figure 15-6). Consequently, the sinoatrial node usually serves as the impulse generator for the remainder of the heart. The wave of electrical depolarization spreads to the surrounding atrial muscle cells and stimulates mechanical contraction. There are no specialized conduction fibers within the atria, and the impulse spreads from cell to cell to cover the entire atria within 0.08 second. Mechanical contraction requires approximately 0.1 second, much longer than the spread of the electrical signal.

To maximize the amount of blood in the ventricles before the onset of ventricular contraction, atrial systole must be completed before the ventricles begin to contract. This requires a delay in the transmission of the electrical signal from the atria to the ventricles. The electrical signal enters the atrioventricular node, where it is held for over 0.1 second before entering the specialized conduction system (the *bundle of His*) to signal ventricular systole. The electrical signal for the ventricles to contract, therefore, starts at the conclusion of mechanical atrial systole. Rapid conduction along the bundle of His results in depolarization of the right and left ventricular myocardium almost simultaneously. The electrical signal is followed by the onset of mechanical systole, which requires approximately 0.3 second.

Unlike the atria, the ventricular muscle needs a specialized conduction system to propagate the impulse through the thick myocardium. If the signal were to propagate through the muscle fibers without the specialized conduction system, it would cause each area to contract as it is depolarized, resulting in sequential contraction rather than simultaneous contraction. A series of specialized muscle fibers in the ventricular walls, called the *conducting system,* carries the electrical impulse from the atrioventricular node to the far reaches of the ventricular myocardium.

An electrocardiogram (ECG) reflects the electrical activities of the heart (Figure 15-7). It typically consists of a P wave, QRS complex, and T wave. The P wave is the electrical signal to the atria to contract, the QRS complex serves the same function in the ventricles, and the T wave identi-

fies an electrical reset of the ventricles for the next cardiac cycle. During much of diastole the heart is electrically silent.

Irregularities or abnormalities of conduction are quite common and can have substantial effects on ventricular function and radionuclide studies. Some of the more common conduction abnormalities are listed in Box 15-1.

RADIONUCLIDE IMAGING CONSIDERATIONS

Tracers Used for Cardiac Imaging

Radiopharmaceuticals determine which aspect of the heart is depicted in the image. The five major categories of radio-

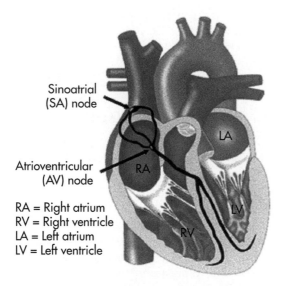

Figure 15-6 Conduction system of the heart.

> **Box 15-1** | Common Conduction Abnormalities
>
> - **Premature systoles** may originate in the atria (premature atrial contractions [PACs]) or ventricles (premature ventricular contractions, [PVCs]) or may be coupled. If the extrasystoles occur every other beat, the rhythm is called *bigeminy.*
> - **Ventricular tachycardia** originates in a focus in the ventricle. This type of rapid rate is potentially life-threatening and should be treated immediately. Ventricular tachycardia can proceed to ventricular fibrillation, which if left untreated results in death.
> - **Atrial fibrillation** is defined as a totally disorganized firing at multiple sites in the atria that causes a rapid, irregular ventricular rate.
> - **Left bundle branch block** is an abnormal conduction pattern associated with slower depolarization of the conducting pathway through the left ventricle than through the right ventricle.
> - **Right bundle branch block** is an abnormal conduction pattern associated with slower depolarization of the conducting pathway through the right ventricle than through the left ventricle.
>
> From Zipes DP: In *Heart disease: a textbook of cardiovascular medicine,* Philadelphia, 1984, WB Saunders.

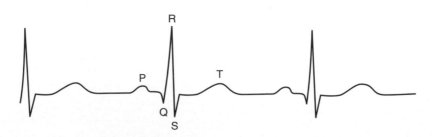

Figure 15-7 A normal electrocardiogram (ECG) tracing showing the P, Q, R, S, and T waves.

pharmaceuticals involved in clinical cardiac imaging include agents used for evaluation of perfusion, measurement of ventricular function, detection of acute myocardial necrosis, measurement of metabolism, and measurement of sympathetic innervation (Box 15-2).

| **Box 15-2** | Radiopharmaceuticals for Clinical Cardiac Imaging |

Evaluation of myocardial perfusion

Single photon emitters
Thallium-201 (^{201}Tl) chloride
Technetium-99m (^{99m}Tc) sestamibi
^{99m}Tc tetrafosmin
^{99m}Tc teboroxime
Positron-emitting tracer
Rubidium-82 (^{82}Rb)

Measurement of ventricular function

^{99m}Tc-labeled red blood cells
^{99m}Tc albumin

Detection of acute myocardial necrosis

^{99m}Tc pyrophosphate
Indium-111 (^{111}In) antimyosin

Measurement of myocardial metabolism

Iodine-123 (^{123}I) fatty acids
^{18}F fluorodeoxyglucose (^{18}F-FDG)
^{11}C-labeled fatty acid

Meaurement of sympathetic innervation

Iodine-123 metaiodobenzylguanidine (^{123}I-MIBG)

Planar and SPECT Data Acquisition

Data can be recorded with planar or single photon emission computed tomography (SPECT) techniques with any of the radiopharmaceuticals. However, it is best to use planar imaging when studies have a low count rate or when data must be recorded within a short interval. Planar images can sample the major surfaces of the left ventricle (usually in three views). SPECT imaging should be used when high count rates or longer imaging times are available. Images are recorded with a single-detector or a multidetector scintillation camera with extrinsic resolution better than 5 mm full width at half maximum (FWHM). Digital image data are typically recorded in a computer, usually in a 64 × 64 matrix for a standard field of view detector or a 128 × 128 matrix for a large-field detector (see Chapter 4).

SPECT cardiac images are recorded as a series of planar images obtained at 3- to 6-degree steps in an arc spanning at least 180 degrees, beginning at 30 degrees right anterior oblique (RAO) and moving to 30 degrees left posterior oblique (LPO). Data are reconstructed into transverse tomographic slices. The planar projections are reconstructed into a series of transverse slices through the imaged volume. The transverse slices are reoriented to permit additional reconstructions oriented along the long and short axes of the left ventricle. This reorientation permits depiction of the myocardium or blood pool in a standard presentation, which simplifies interpretation (see Chapter 9 for details of SPECT acquisition and processing). Short axis images depict the myocardium from the apex to the base; vertical long axis images slice the volume from the anterolateral wall to the inferior wall; and horizontal long axis images depict the right ventricle, septum, and posterior wall (Figure 15-8).

Reconstruction can be done with mathematical techniques (see Chapters 4 and 9) using either filtered back-

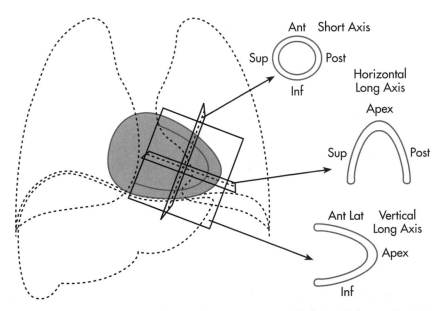

Figure 15-8 Schematic representation of the heart in the chest. SPECT data are reoriented to present the myocardium in views that are orthogonal to the major cardiac axes. The slices are called *short axis views* (cut from the apex to the base of the left ventricle), *horizontal long axis views* (cut from the septum to the posterior wall rotated with the apex pointing to the top to differentiate this view from the vertical long axis), and *vertical long axis views*. The specific walls depicted in each view are indicated with the representative slice.

projection or iterative algorithms. When filtered back-projection is used, the filter should have sufficient spatial resolution to permit visualization of the myocardial borders (a frequency of 0.5 to 0.7 cycle/cm usually is used). Transverse section images should provide six to eight slices through the heart (typical reconstructions are 1 to 2 pixels thick with no spaces between the slices). Before reconstruction the projection images should be reviewed as a cinematic display to detect patient motion, major changes in cardiac position during acquisition, and technical problems, such as missed or duplicated angles. Single episodes of motion of less than 2 pixels can usually be tolerated. Although motion correction software is available in many of the reconstruction software programs, the corrections are often incomplete and may result in artifacts in the reconstructed data. Multiple episodes of motion, movement greater than 2 pixels, or loss of more than one set of projection data creates artifacts in the reconstructed tomograms that may result in an erroneous interpretation. If these situations occur, a repeat acquisition should be recorded.

SPECT images should be recorded with a multidetector rotating scintillation camera to reduce the acquisition time (compared with a single-detector instrument). The most common multidetector (multiheaded) cameras have two detectors (which can assume positions ranging from 90 to 180 degrees apart). Three-detector instruments, which are much less common, have detectors in a fixed orientation spaced 120 degrees apart. To record the 180-degree imaging arc, a dual-detector system with the detectors oriented 90 degrees to each other is preferable, because the detector is closest to the heart for each image. This maximizes collimator resolution and eliminates the highly attenuated photons arising from the back of the patient that would be recorded if a full 360-degree acquisition were used. The 180-degree limited imaging reduces both the noise that comes from recording data from the patient's back (which is far from the heart) and the attenuation artifacts that may be caused by the spine.

An alternative to recording data with 180-degree sampling is to record information from a full 360 degrees. Although 360-degree acquisitions are the standard from a physics perspective, the data recorded in this fashion incorporate information from the back and right posterior oblique positions, which are far from the heart. The 360-degree data generally show lower contrast between lesions and normal myocardium than do data recorded in 180 degrees. If data are to be recorded with 360-degree sampling, a three-detector system is preferred.

Sensitivity is a function of the total number of detectors. For example, a two-detector system at 90 degrees can acquire a cardiac SPECT in half the time of a single-detector system for the same total counts in a 180-degree acquisition. A three-detector system, however, does not save as much time because the third detector generally is recording data far from the heart. The time required for a three-detector cardiac acquisition is similar to that for a dual-detector 90-degree instrument. The increased sensitiv-

ity of multidetector instruments can be used to reduce the examination time (while maintaining study quality), increase study quality by doubling the count density, or slightly shorten the time to accomplish some of both. The differences in image quality between 180- and 360-degree acquisitions are reduced when a technetium-labeled radiopharmaceutical is used.

To maximize spatial resolution, the detectors should be as close as possible to the surface of the patient when recording each image. Mechanically, it is easiest to rotate the detector through a circle when recording data for 15 to 60 seconds at each step. Inadequate sampling (step angles greater than 6 degrees or gaps between steps) can result in an artifact that resembles the spokes of a wheel (star artifact). To avoid this, angular sampling of about 3 degrees or continuous data acquisition is recommended. Common angular projections for imaging range from 32 to 64. When fewer than 30 projections are used, degradation of the image quality results. However, doubling the number of projections while holding the acquisition time constant also leads to a reduction in the count density and an increase in noise. This requires more filtering and use of a lower filter cutoff frequency, which blurs details in the image and diminishes resolution.

A circular orbit maximizes the distance between the collimator and the body surface in the anterior and posterior positions, resulting in a spatial resolution of approximately 12 to 19 mm in the reconstructed data. Moving the detector through an ellipse as it traverses the chest keeps the detectors closer to the heart, resulting in some improvement in resolution. However, setting up a noncircular acquisition is more complex, and even though the detector is closer to the body surface, the heart is not in the center of the body. Because the gain in resolution is small, especially for large patients, a circular orbit generally is used.

SPECT data are acquired in a step-and-shoot or continuous acquisition mode. The step-and-shoot mode has greater resolution (no detector motion blurring during acquisition) but requires more time for acquisition, because it takes 1 to 2 seconds to incrementally move several thousand pounds of detector and bring it to a full stop before the next image is acquired. During the 20- to 30-minute acquisition, the patient lies supine with the left arm above the head (a fairly uncomfortable position). In some clinics SPECT images are recorded with the patient prone to minimize attenuation from the diaphragm. Prone patients also elevate the left arm to minimize attenuation. Although prone image acquisition provides better images, the improvement comes at a cost of marked patient discomfort.

To maximize spatial resolution, SPECT images should be recorded with high- or ultrahigh-resolution collimation.

Data can be recorded with or without synchronization to the patient's cardiac cycle (physiologic [e.g., ECG] gating). However, adding the key cardiac parameters of regional wall motion and ejection fraction makes the procedure more valuable than imaging perfusion alone. As a result, all myocardial perfusion scans should be recorded with gating.

Even studies recorded with thallium-201 (^{201}Tl) can be analyzed to make these determinations. Because of the increased photon flux available from technetium-99m (^{99m}Tc)–labeled perfusion agents, which allows higher quality gated myocardial perfusion SPECT studies to be recorded, ^{99m}Tc agents are preferred for these studies. In addition to regional wall motion and the ejection fraction, ventricular volume data from gated perfusion scans may be helpful in distinguishing attenuation artifacts from significant perfusion abnormalities.

Attenuation correction. The soft tissue of the chest musculature, breast, and diaphragm is known to cause attenuation of the signal and to lead to artifacts that resemble perfusion defects. Sometimes the pattern is very difficult to separate from true defects and real abnormalities. It generally is perceived that attenuation is more pronounced for the lower energy photons of thallium and not significant for technetium. However, this is not true. Technetium has only 20% less attenuation than thallium.

Attenuation can be corrected by measuring the attenuation coefficients using a transmission source (as is done in x-ray computed tomography). The information is incorporated into the reconstruction data to compensate for the attenuation. Transmission scans are used to develop the attenuation map. Gadolinium-153 (^{153}Gd; 48 and 100 keV) and cobalt-57 (^{57}Co; 122 keV) are sources used for ^{99m}Tc; americium-241 (^{241}Am; 60 keV) is used for ^{201}Tl attenuation correction. An x-ray source can be used as an alternative to a radioactive source for the attenuation information. The abundant photons from the x-ray make the x-ray-determined attenuation map much more precise than that available from a radioactive source.

RADIONUCLIDE EVALUATION OF VENTRICULAR FUNCTION

The heart's ability to function as a pump can be measured by recording data with gating during myocardial perfusion imaging or by imaging a radiopharmaceutical that is retained in the blood pool. As an alternative to recording data with electrocardiographic synchronization, rapid data (20 to 50 msec/frame) can be recorded during the first pass of the radiopharmaceutical through the heart, a first-pass acquisition. The typical gated study is recorded over hundreds of beats, whereas the first-pass study usually is completed within 30 seconds of injection of the radiopharmaceutical.

Although the recording techniques are different, the measurements made from the data are similar. These include the size and shape of the chambers, the motion of the walls during each beat, and the ejection fraction. The most common measurement made is the left ventricular ejection fraction (LVEF), a value calculated by dividing the amount of blood ejected by the ventricle during systole by the amount of blood in the ventricle at the end of diastole. The first-pass and equilibrium techniques place different constraints on the radiopharmaceutical. For equilibrium blood pool images, the tracer must remain in the bloodstream for at least 30 minutes.

First-Pass Studies

Because first-pass data are recorded in less than 60 seconds, the tracer can be cleared rapidly from the blood, allowing repeat studies in the same imaging session if necessary. Various tracers used for these studies are listed in Table 15-2.

First-pass studies performed with injection of about 740 MBq (20 mCi) of activity challenge the maximum count rate of the gamma camera. For most of the data acquisition, the entire 20 mCi is in the field of view. In the average 70 kg person, the distance between the center of the cardiac chamber and the anterior chest wall is about 8 cm of water-equivalent density, for a peak photon flux (through a high-resolution collimator) of about 83,000 counts/sec.* Most Anger cameras can image maximum count rates of more than 100,000 counts/sec with dead time losses of less than 20% and no image distortion. Phantom studies should be performed before first-pass imaging to determine the count rate characteristics of the camera/computer. Typically these studies are performed with a series of sources of increasing intensity.

Data recording. Data should be recorded with an all-purpose or a high-resolution collimator. High-sensitivity collimation provides about twice the count rate of an all-purpose collimator (and about four times the count rate of a high-resolution collimator), but resolution falls off rapidly as the distance between the heart and the face of the collimator increases. As a result, for patients with a soft tissue thickness greater than 5 cm, an all-purpose or high-resolution collimator is preferred. Acquisition is done in the anterior (for assessment of overall cardiac function) or the 45-degree left anterior oblique (LAO) position for optimum separation of the right and left ventricles, then data recording is started at 25 msec/frame and the tracer is injected. About 1 minute of data (2,400 frames) is collected.

Injection technique. The quality of the examination is determined by the characteristics of the bolus. The radiopharmaceutical should be administered in a small volume, typically less than 1 ml, into a jugular or basilic vein, followed by a flush of about 5 to 10 ml of saline. Injection via the external jugular vein provides the shortest, most direct

---

*Peak count rate calculation: (1) 740 MBq = 740 million disintegrations/sec. (2) For every 100 disintegrations of ^{99m}Tc, 90 photons occur. (3) Half the photons are going away from the detector, which reduces the photon flux by a factor of 2. (4) The high-resolution collimator eliminates about 1000 photons for each photon that passes through to the detector. (5) The half-value distance for 140 keV photons (the distance where half the photons will be absorbed) in tissue-equivalent material is about 4 cm. Therefore: $(740 \times 10^6) \times 0.5 \times 0.9 \times 10^{-3} \times (0.25) = 83,250$ counts/sec.

Table 15-2	Tracers used for first-pass evaluation of ventricular function

Tracer	Comments
Technetium based tracers	
Overall long half-life is not optimal for repeated studies of first pass.	
^{99m}Tc-DTPA	Most commonly used; rapid clearance through kidneys; multiple studies possible
^{99m}Tc pertechnetate	Accumulates in gastric mucosa, which interferes with evaluation of inferior wall; multiple studies not possible
^{99m}Tc sulphur colloid	Multiple studies not possible because of accumulation in liver and spleen
^{99m}Tc-MAA	Preferred when only right ventricular (RV) assessment is needed
Non-technetium-based short-life isotopes	
These isotopes are expensive and have lower energies. They are generator produced and need elution close to patients at the imaging areas, which limits quality control assessment. They are not very widely used.	
^{133}Xe in saline	RV function assessment
^{81m}Kr in saline	^{81}Rb/^{81m}Kr generator produced; $t_{1/2}$ is 13 sec; absorbed in alveoli when it passes through the lungs; only 15% enters left heart; rubidium buildup in eluant causes radiation burden
^{195m}Au	^{195}Hg/^{195m}Au generator produced; $t_{1/2}$ is 30 sec; a blood pool agent, it can be used both for RV and left ventricular (LV) function; ^{195}Hg buildup in eluant causes radiation burden
^{191m}Ir	^{191}Os/^{191}Ir generator produced; $t_{1/2}$ is 4.7 sec; a blood pool agent that traverses the lung; not useful in patients with heart failure; low radiation burden makes it preferable for infants
^{178}Ta	^{178}W/^{178}Ta generator produced; $t_{1/2}$ is 10 min; binds to plasma proteins; suitable for obtaining multiple views

^{99m}Tc-DTPA, Technetium-99m diethylenetriamine pentaacetic acid; *^{99m}Tc-MAA,* ^{99m}Tc macroaggregated albumin; *^{133}Xe,* xenon-133; *^{81m}Kr,* krypton-81m; *^{81}Rb,* rubidium-81; *^{195}Hg,* mercury-195; *^{195m}Au,* gold-195m; *^{191}Os,* osmium-191; *^{191m}Ir,* iridium-191m; *^{178}W,* tungsten-178; *^{178}Ta,* tantalum-178.

path and produces optimum results. The laterally located cephalic vein takes a less direct path to the subclavian vein and tends to produce a fragmented bolus, making the data difficult to analyze. Injection into an indwelling line placed in the basilic (medial) vein of the forearm is frequently used. Typically an 18-gauge needle or intracath is placed in the basilic vein. A three-way stopcock is placed at the end of the line, a syringe containing the tracer is connected to one port, and a syringe containing 10 to 20 ml of a flushing solution (sterile saline) is connected to the other. A blood pressure cuff is placed proximal to the catheter. While the radial pulse is palpated, the cuff is inflated until the pulse just disappears; the pressure then is reduced by about 10 mm Hg. Inflation is maintained for 1 minute and then increased above the systolic pressure; the radiopharmaceutical is slowly injected through the stopcock into the occluded vein, the computer is started, the cuff is rapidly removed (not deflated), and the flushing dose is administered. The injection should be given during normal respiration, and care should be taken to ensure that the patient does not alter the normal breathing pattern during the study.

Framing interval. To determine the ejection fraction, both end-systole and end-diastole must be accurately sampled. End-systole is shorter and defines the framing interval. At a heart rate of 70 beats/min, end-systole lasts less than 80 msec. To ensure that this interval is properly measured, data are recorded at 40 msec/frame or preferably 25 msec/frame.

Total data recording. The normal transit time through the heart and lungs is 15 seconds, but in patients with heart disease, bolus transit may take 45 seconds. Because additional time is needed to start the camera/computer before injection, at least 60 seconds of data should be obtained (1,500 to 2,400 frames). It may be necessary to have two people work together to record these studies: one to start the camera/computer and the other to perform the bolus injection.

Data analysis. Sequential groups of 20 to 40 frames are added together to help identify the structures, and data are reviewed in intervals of 0.5 to 1 second. Reformatted frames are displayed as an endless loop movie to identify the superior vena cava, right and left ventricles, and lungs. Regions of interest are drawn over each of these, and a time-activity curve is generated from the original short-duration frame data.

The superior vena caval curve is evaluated for the duration of the bolus. The FWHM transit time of activity through this curve should be less than 2.5 seconds. If the transit time is longer than this, activity enters the left ventricle before it has completely cleared the right, and the calculated left ventricular ejection fraction may be erroneous.

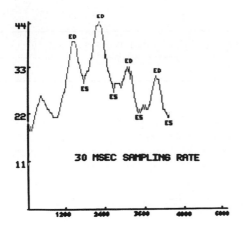

Figure 15-9   Right ventricular time-activity curve in the first-pass method.

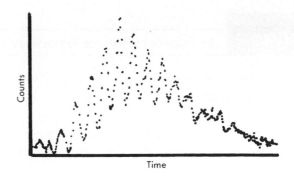

Figure 15-10   Corrected left ventricular time-activity curve in the first-pass method.

The right ventricular (RV) curve should appear as a sawtooth, with one or two peaks (end-diastole) and comparable minima (end-systole) (Figure 15-9). A second series of sawtooth peaks occurs as activity enters the left ventricle, because the ventricles overlap in the anterior position. Frames with activity in the left ventricle should be excluded from analysis of right ventricular function. The counts at the peak points selected from the early part of the curve, when activity is only in the right heart, should be added together, and the counts at the minimal points should be added together to give end-diastolic (ED) and end-systolic (ES) counts, respectively. The right ventricular ejection fraction (EF) is calculated as follows:

Ejection fraction = (End-diastolic counts −
          End-systolic counts)/End-diastolic counts

For most clinical applications, background can be ignored for the right ventricular data because the surrounding activity is negligible. On the other hand, background must be determined and subtracted from the left ventricular data.

The lung curve (obtained from a region of interest placed adjacent to the left ventricle) should appear smooth, rising as the RV curve falls and falling before the rise of the left ventricular (LV) curve. The counts per pixel of the lung curve are determined to permit correction of the left ventricular curve for background.

The curve obtained from the left ventricular region of interest should appear as a sawtooth, starting after the peak of the lung curve. A series of small peaks can be seen in synchrony with transit of the bolus through the right ventricle as a result of overlap of the chambers, as just described. These peaks should not be used to calculate the ejection fraction of the left ventricle. The LVEF should be calculated from a minimum of three beats occurring near the peak of the LV time-activity curve, when lung activity is decreasing. The left ventricular curve must be corrected for background activity in the lungs (lung counts/pixel in a region adjacent to the LV, multiplied by the number of pixels in the left

ventricular region of interest) (Figure 15-10). The counts at the peak of each cardiac cycle (end-diastole) are then added together; the corresponding end-systoles are similarly added; and the ejection fraction is computed as described for the right ventricle.

Wall motion may be assessed by viewing a cinematic display of the summed end-diastolic and end-systolic frames; by examining the stroke volume image (produced by subtracting the end-systolic image from the end-diastolic image); or by outlining the blood pool at end-systole and end-diastole based on count thresholds. Because of the low counts involved, the first-pass approach is relatively insensitive for the detection of modest abnormalities of wall motion.

Gated Blood Pool Studies

Radiolabeled autologous red blood cells are the preferred tracer for determining cardiac function with gated blood pool imaging. Other tracers used for this study are listed in Table 15-3.

Because multiple points in the cardiac cycle are recorded, the technique is often called MUGA (for multiple gated acquisition). After the tracer has equilibrated in the blood pool (about 5 to 10 minutes after administration of the labeled red cells), data are recorded in synchrony with the patient's cardiac cycle. The R wave of the patient's electrocardiogram is used as a fiducial marker for the end of diastole. The heart rate is computed, and the result is expressed in milliseconds per cycle. The length of the cardiac cycle is divided by the number of points (frames) necessary to calculate the ejection fraction or regional wall motion (usually 16 frames). This number of frames is derived from the fact that end-systole lasts 80 msec in an adult with a resting heart rate of 80 beats/min. To sample an 80 msec interval, the computer should be collecting data at about 40 msec/frame. At 80 beats/min, the cardiac cycle lasts 750 msec. Dividing this interval by 16 requires 46 msec/frame—about right for really sampling end-systole.

The computer is instructed to record data from the first portion of the cardiac cycle into the first frame, the second

Table 15-3 Evaluation of ventricular function: gated blood pool/multiple gated acquisition (MUGA) studies

Technique	Comments
Red blood cell labeling techniques	
In vivo labeling: Give stannous pyrophosphate intravenously (10 mg ion/kg weight). Wait 15 to 30 min. Use separate IV access to inject 20 mCi of ^{99m}Tc pertechnetate.	Overall poor labeling is seen in patient with a hematocrit <30%. Plasma characteristics may be altered with lower temperature, very sick patient. Stannous citrate/stannous diphosphonate, stannous pyrophosphate/stannous glucoheptonate produce good labeling results. Separate IV access prevents adherence of tracer to catheter. Labeling efficiency is 60% to 90%. Heart to background ratio is 2:1. Radiation dose to bladder is 2.2 rad.
In vitro labeling: Draw 12 ml of blood into syringe with heparin/ACD plus stannous ion. Incubate 10 to 20 min at room temperature. Centrifuge and remove supernatant plasma. Add 20 mCi of pertechnetate to RBCs. Incubate 10 min and centrifuge again. Remove supernatant and inject RBCs.	Labeling efficiency is 95%. Ultratag (Mallinckrodt, St. Louis, Missouri), a kit available for tagging RBCs, is simple and easier to use.
Modified in vivo labeling: Inject stannous pyrophosphate intravenously. Wait 15 to 30 min. Withdraw 1 to 5 ml of blood into a heparin syringe with 20 mCi of pertechnetate. Mix. Incubate syringe 10 min at room temperature. Reinject whole blood.	Labeling efficiency is 90 to 95%.
Labeled albumin	
A commercial kit is available in Europe but not in the United States. The albumin is reconstituted and labeled with pertechnetate.	Albumin is available immediately and requires minimal handling or exposure to blood. The kit can be used for multiple doses. Disadvantages include diffusion out of the vasculature and high background and liver activity.

portion of the cycle into the second frame, and so on until the last frame is reached or the next R wave is sensed, which resets the recording to the first frame to repeat the process (Figure 15-11). Data from about 500 to 1,000 cycles are added to obtain an "average" cardiac cycle.

Equilibrium-gated blood pool imaging can be done as a planar or tomographic acquisition. It differs from first-pass studies in several respects:

1. The time required to acquire the data is much longer, typically 8 to 10 minutes for each planar view.
2. The overlap of the chambers makes it difficult to distinguish portions of the right ventricle from the left ventricle in the anterior view (this can be partly overcome by using SPECT, but complex cardiac motion often moves chambers in and out of the slice during the cycle).
3. The count density of the images is much greater, permitting minimal abnormalities of wall motion to be readily detected.
4. Images can be recorded over several hours without the need to reinject the patient, which permits assessment of several short-acting drug interventions.

5. Images are usually recorded in multiple views. The views typically obtained are the anterior view (to examine right atrial size and motion, tricuspid valve motion, and right ventricular and pulmonary artery size and motion); the 45-degree LAO (optimized to separate the right and left ventricles and to determine the timing and motion of the anterior wall of the right ventricle, posterior wall of the left ventricle, and overall motion and thickening of the septum); and either the left lateral or left posterior oblique view (to view the inferior and posterior surfaces of the left ventricle and the size and motion of the left atrium).

Gated blood pool SPECT imaging has the advantage that, using the same acquisition time, the heart is viewed from 360 degrees. This eliminates the anatomic overlap that occurs in planar imaging, in which the left atrium overlaps the left ventricle posteriorly in LAO view and the right ventricle obscures the inferior wall of the left ventricle in the RAO or anterior view. Because the left atrium and left ventricle beat out of phase with each other (i.e., the atrium fills while the ventricle empties and vice versa), including the left atrium in the left ventricular region of interest

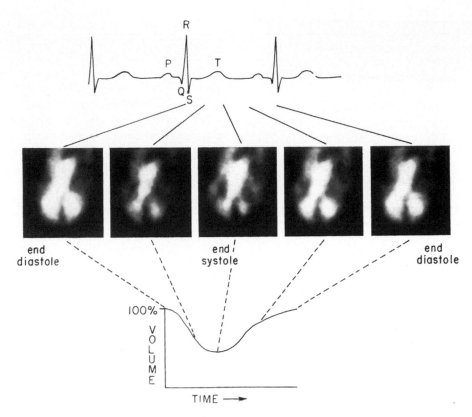

Figure 15-11 Sequential scintiphotos of the heart during a cardiac cycle shown in relation to the ECG waveform and left ventricular volume.

reduces the calculated LVEF. SPECT eliminates the need for obtaining a single view that optimizes RV/LV separation. Instead, after the data have been reconstructed, they can be reoriented to display this information, which then can be used to calculate the LVEF. In addition, the regional wall motion assessment is better. SPECT imaging also permits more accurate assessment of the right ventricular ejection fraction (RVEF).

Radiopharmaceuticals Used for Blood Pool Imaging

Table 15-3 shows the tracers and labeling techniques used for red blood cells (RBCs). The in vivo method is simple and does not require the handling of blood outside the body; however, the average labeling efficiency is lower, and the noncardiac blood pool counts are higher than that with the in vitro or modified in vitro methods.

Patient preparation. ECG electrodes should be placed (Figure 15-12), and a baseline recording should be evaluated. Good electrode contact with the skin is ensured if the skin is lightly abraded by rubbing it with alcohol or very fine sand paper before the electrodes are applied. Meticulous attention to skin preparation can reduce the resistance between the electrodes and the skin from 50,000 to 5000 ohms. Usually, four electrodes are placed to record one of the standard limb leads of the electrocardiogram. The

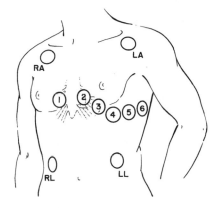

Figure 15-12 Placement of ECG leads. **Limb leads:** Both supraclavicular and abdominal regions (adjacent to the pelvic crest) bilaterally. **Chest leads:** These leads are placed in the following sequence and positions:
V_1: Second intercostal space to the immediate right of the sternum
V_2: Second intercostal space to the immediate left of the sternum
V_4: Left midclavicular line in the fifth intercostal space
V_3: Halfway between V_2 and V_4
V_6: Left midaxillary line in the fifth intercostal space
V_5: Midway between V_4 and V_6

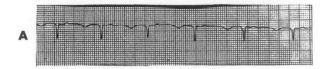

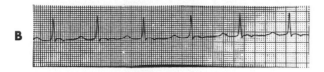

Figure 15-13 **A,** Negative QRS complex. **B,** Positive QRS complex.

ECG waveform should be reviewed to determine that the initial portion of the QRS complex is positive (Figure 15-13). Although gating occurs with either negative or positive waveforms, some triggers seek the positive deflection, creating a slight temporal offset in the data when the initial waveform is negative. Consequently, it is best to standardize on one polarity. If the initial waveform is negative, the electrodes should be moved or the leads reversed to provide a positive complex.

To maximize image quality, the waveform should be reviewed to make certain that only a single, well-defined QRS complex is observed with each cardiac cycle. The gate may trigger twice on a single beat in patients with pacemakers or tall, peaked T waves or less frequently in patients with tall P waves. If more than one complex per cycle is seen, the electrodes should be moved until the waveform of one complex is maximized and the other minimized; this ensures that only a single triggering signal is obtained for each cardiac cycle.

If the patient has a markedly irregular heart rate (greater than 10% variation in the R-R interval in more than 10% of the beats), as occurs in atrial fibrillation or with multiple premature contractions, the rates of filling and emptying of the heart change substantially from beat to beat. As a result, it is not physiologically correct to add these data together to calculate rates of filling or emptying. However, it is possible to calculate the ejection fraction from these data, because diastolic function is generally affected more by such phenomena than is systolic function.

Data recording: planar imaging. Data recording can begin within 5 to 10 minutes of administration of the radiopharmaceutical. However, if absolute ventricular volumes are measured either by a count-based method or by comparison to a blood sample, the tracer must be allowed to equilibrate for at least 15 minutes before data acquisition. The 5 to 10 minutes needed to record high-quality, equilibrium blood pool images in each projection requires that the data be recorded with the patient lying on a stretcher and

the heart centered in the field of view. Typically, the heart is evaluated from three perspectives at least 45 degrees apart. The anterior view usually is recorded in preference to the RAO because the collimator can be positioned closer to the patient's chest, which maximizes resolution. Although the anterior view does not allow the left ventricle to be viewed in its long axis, the left ventricle is not totally obscured by the right ventricle. Using the persistence mode on the computer, the LAO view is optimized to separate the left ventricle from the right. Some cranial angulation of the camera (the body of the camera is tilted cranially, with the crystal pointing caudally) may be necessary to accomplish this. At the conclusion of the LAO view, the patient is rotated into either the left lateral or left posterior oblique position, and the last view is recorded (Figure 15-14).

Data recording: SPECT imaging. Data may be acquired using a single head or a dual head (90-degree angle or variable angle detectors). The acquisition may be in the 180- or 360-degree arc. For 180-degree acquisition, data recording starts at RAO, 45-degree angle and goes to 45 degrees LPO. High-resolution, low-energy collimators should be used. The acquisition matrix is 128×128. Zoom may be applied to a factor of 1.2 to 1.5, depending on the size of the detectors. Thirty-two views are acquired at 30 sec/frame. Typical counts acquired may be in the range of 30 million to 40 million.

Data analysis. Data from equilibrium images are evaluated visually and quantitatively. Initially, the images are reviewed as a cinematic display for adequacy of count density over the cardiac blood pool and for appropriateness of positioning. The total counts in each frame are determined to ensure that the last useful frame of the sequence has less than 15% drop-off in counts compared with the beginning of the study. Count rate drop-off occurs when a significant change in the rhythm or heart rate occurs during acquisition. If there is no apparent motion of the cardiac chambers or if the counts decrease by more than 15%, the electrodes and ECG-triggering apparatus should be rechecked, and if necessary the images should be repeated.

The LAO or best septal view is analyzed to calculate the ejection fraction from the total counts in the left ventricle at end-systole and end-diastole (after background correction) (Figure 15-15). Regions of interest can be drawn over the LV automatically (using either a second derivative or threshold algorithm) or manually. Identification of the ventricular border often is facilitated by smoothing the data spatially and temporally or by applying a resolution recovery (Wiener) filter before analysis. Temporal smoothing should be used only when the heart rate is regular. If the R-R interval has significant variation, temporal smoothing causes errors. The latter frames of the acquisition, which contain fewer counts, are averaged with the initial frames, thereby lowering the counts in the early frames. If these data are used to calculate the ejection fraction, the end-diastolic counts in the left ventricle are lower than they should be, resulting in a calculated ejection fraction that is too low.

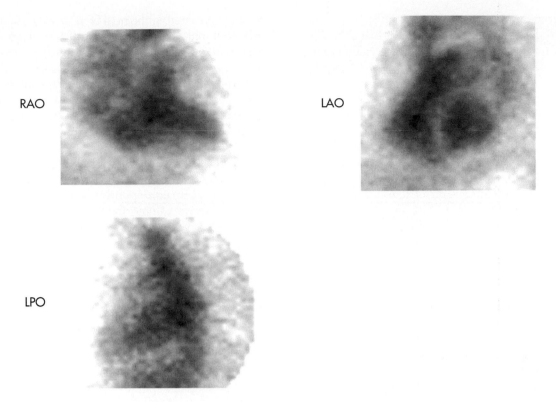

RAO

LAO

LPO

Figure 15-14 Planar multiple gated acquisition (MUGA) images showing the three views of the heart.

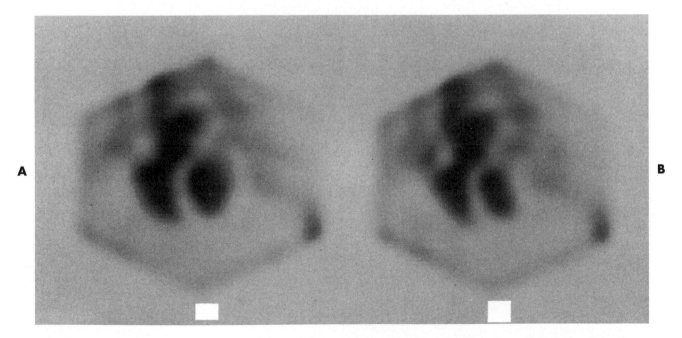

A

B

Figure 15-15 End-diastolic (**A**) and end-systolic (**B**) ventricular images demonstrating optimum ventricular separation.

A background region is selected, located at about 3 to 6 o'clock from the left ventricle and free of branches of the pulmonary artery, left atrium, and spleen (Figure 15-16), and the counts per pixel in the lung are determined. A typical value for lung background is 40% to 60% of the left ventricular end-diastolic counts (depending on the radio-pharmaceutical, window setting, and collimator). This value is then subtracted from each pixel in the left ventricular region of interest. The background subtraction step is crucial to the subsequent calculation of the ejection fraction. Subtraction of too much background results in a falsely elevated ejection fraction, and subtraction of too little produces a falsely depressed EF.

The total background-corrected counts in the left ventricle on each frame are then normalized to the counts in the end-diastolic frame, and the time-activity curve from the left ventricular region of interest is displayed. The EF is calculated from the time-activity curve. Normal values for the left ventricular ejection fraction range from 50% to 75%. In addition to the ejection fraction, the time of filling and emptying and the ejection and filling rates of the ventricles can be readily computed from these curves.

An alternative approach to calculation of the ejection fraction uses a single region of interest, based on the end-diastolic frame, to measure the time-activity curve. Calcu-lated by this approach, the LVEF is usually about 5% lower than that obtained with the variable region of interest method. This method has the advantage of producing a smoother curve, which is useful for calculating the filling and emptying rates. A hybrid approach is to use this fixed region of interest method to select the end-diastolic and end-systolic frames from the time-activity curve and then draw individual regions of interest on these frames to calculate the ejection fraction.

Regional motion of the left and right ventricles can be readily appreciated from visual assessment of the cinematic display. An alternative approach to depicting regional function is the stroke-volume image, obtained by subtracting the end-systolic image from the end-diastolic image. Similarly, a "dyskinesis" image can be recorded by subtracting the end-diastolic image from the end-systolic image. The stroke-volume image demonstrates ventricular motion and does not demonstrate the atria. The dyskinesis image shows atrial function but does not demonstrate any activity in the region of a normally contracting ventricle.

The high count density of the equilibrium images permits another approach to the evaluation of regional wall motion, *phase* and *amplitude* images. Phase analysis assumes that the heart contracts in a specific pattern that resembles the wave-form of a cosine function. Each pixel in the image can be

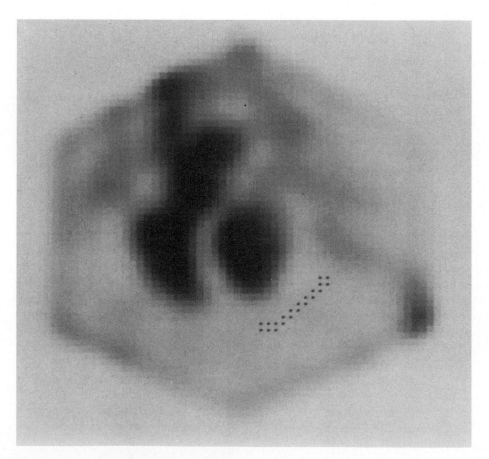

Figure 15-16 Background region of interest (ROI) selection (*light dots adjacent to posteroinferior margin of left ventricle*) from end-diastolic image of equilibrium-gated study.

evaluated for the timing (phase) of these changes in activity and for its amount of change (amplitude) between the maximum and minimum count values in the pixel. This information can be calculated and presented as a functional image, in which specific colors or brightness represent information about amplitude or phase. An advantage of this approach is that the data are analyzed without operator interaction (Figure 15-17).

MUGA SPECT images are reconstructed with standard techniques of back-projection. Generally, the filters used are the ramp/Butterworth, with an order approximately of 3, and a two-dimensional (2D) reconstruction filter using a cut-off of 0.55 to 0.65. Generally, if the image is noisy, the cut-off frequency may be adjusted and lowered. Similarly, if the image is too smooth, the frequency may be increased. The total reconstruction time is about 1 to 2 minutes. Software programs that process the data automatically are available and easy to use. Three-dimensional (3D) cine volume rendering display can be obtained for visual analysis. The ejection fraction is calculated using ED and ES counts on all frames. The EF can also be calculated manually by creating boundaries on short axis and oblique axis slices on 16 frames. The RVEF can also be calculated by defining the RV regions (Figure 15-18). The automated program also gives

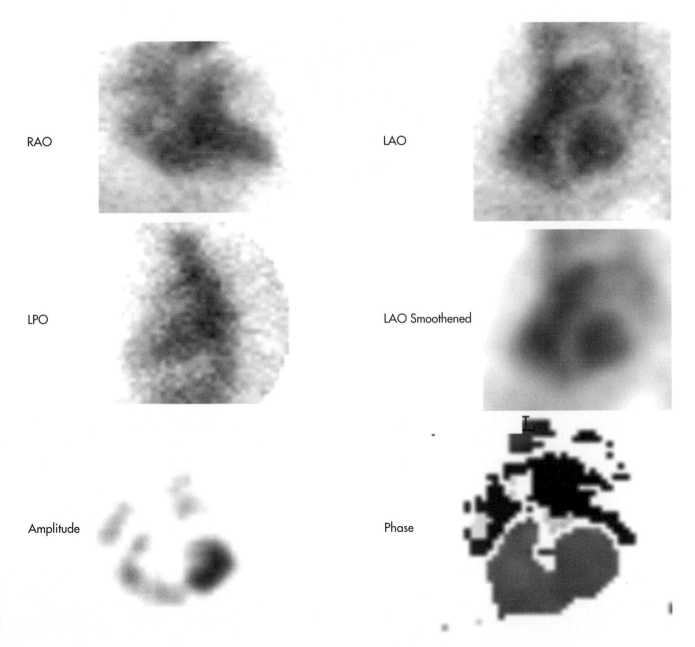

RAO

LAO

LPO

LAO Smoothened

Amplitude

Phase

Figure 15-17 MUGA amplitude and phase analysis image.

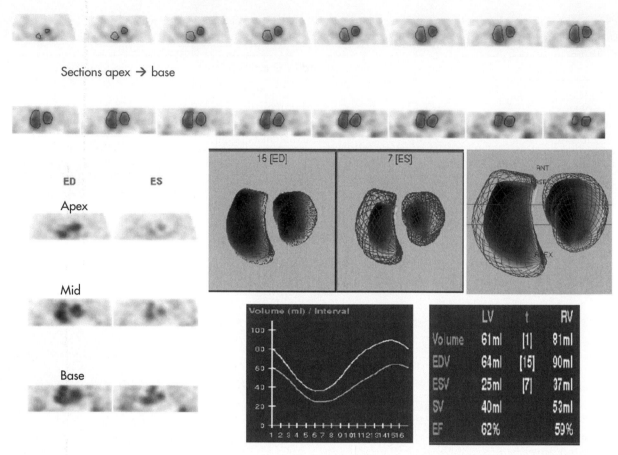

Sections apex → base

Figure 15-18 MUGA SPECT images showing the slices from apex to base, end-diastolic and end-systolic frames, calculated left ventricle (LV) and right ventricle (RV) ejection fraction (EF), and 3D images.

the LV and RV volumes; however, there may be considerable underestimation, and the data generally should not be used as absolute values. SPECT reconstruction requires corrections for flood nonuniformity and center of rotation that should be performed on a routine basis.

Chemotherapy cardiotoxicity. A major application of rest gated blood pool images is the evaluation of left ventricular function in patients receiving potentially cardiotoxic chemotherapy (Table 15-4). Patients frequently are evaluated before administration of these agents and at the conclusion of a course of therapy. Patients who show a decrease in the LVEF below 50% or a drop in the LVEF of 5% or greater from a prior determination are likely to be experiencing significant cardiotoxicity from the therapy. Patients with antecedent heart disease are at particular risk.

General Stress Studies (MUGA or Perfusion)

Measurement of cardiac function at rest is valuable for evaluating cardiac function in patients with a history of myocardial infarction, valvular disease, shortness of breath, and suspected heart failure. Recording of information about cardiac function while the subject is undergoing an exercise stress test adds both prognostic and diagnostic information.

The basics of exercise stress testing are outlined here, with further details provided as they apply to myocardial perfusion imaging in the following section.

As the heart does more work (pumping more blood per minute, pumping the same amount of blood at a higher pressure, or both), the amount of oxygen delivered to the myocardium must increase. In some organs the amount of oxygen extracted as blood traverses the capillaries can increase to deliver more oxygen without an increase in blood flow. In the heart, however, oxygen extraction is very high even under basal conditions. The only way to deliver additional oxygen is to increase blood flow to the myocardium.

Normal coronary arteries are 3 mm in diameter at the origin of the vessel. The three coronary arteries are capable of supplying the myocardium with 0.6 to 1 ml/min/g of left ventricular muscle under basal conditions. When the myocardial oxygen demand increases, the coronaries dilate by an additional 1 to 1.5 mm, the precapillary arteriolar

Table 15-4   Cardiotoxic chemotherapeutic drugs

Agent	Cardiac toxicity
Anthracycline agents (e.g., doxorubicin)	Cardiomyopathy
Cyclophosphamide	Cardiomyopathy and myocardial necrosis
Cisplatin	Cardiomyopathy
Fluorouracil (rare)	Ischemia and angina
Trastuzumab (Herceptin)	Cardiomyopathy
Aldesleukin (Proleukin)	Pericarditis, myocarditis; rarely cardiomyopathy and endocarditis
Arsenic	Prolonged QT and QT intervals
Capacitabine (Xeloda)	Cardiomyopathy, dysrhythmias
Fludarabine	Angina and heart failure
Pacitaxol	Hypertension, bradycardia, congestive failure
Pegaspargase	Cardiomyopathy
Pentostatin	Electrocardiographic abnormalities, chest pain, and hypertension
Procarbazine	Tachycardia, hypertension

sphincter relaxes, and coronary blood flow increases by threefold to fivefold. If a coronary artery is narrowed by more than 50%, blood flow cannot increase sufficiently to meet the maximum demand for oxygen. When myocardial oxygen demand exceeds the oxygen supply, myocardial ischemia results. The inadequately perfused zone of myocardium stops contracting within a few seconds (if the mismatch is severe, or contraction is reduced if the mismatch is less severe), causing a regional wall motion abnormality on images recorded during ischemia. If the area supplied by the stenosed coronary artery is extensive, overall function of the ventricle may be impaired, reducing the ejection fraction.

A typical exercise test increases the workload in a graduated fashion. Most blood pool exercise studies are performed on a bicycle ergometer. The initial workload is 20 to 25 watts, with increments every 3 minutes. Gated blood pool data are recorded as planar images in the LAO view during the last 2 minutes of each stage. Data are not recorded during the first minute of each stage because the heart rate is changing as the patient adjusts to the increased workload. In 2 minutes only about 70,000 to 100,000 counts are recorded from the left ventricle (about 4,000 to 6,000 counts/frame). The limited count density makes edge detection difficult; this limits the resolution for detection of small reductions in wall motion but still provides adequate data for analysis of overall (global) function (ejection fraction). Hence, lesions are detected only when they affect overall ventricular function and result in a reduced ejection fraction.

Patient preparation. As part of the patient preparation (Box 15-3), all pertinent questions must be asked before the

Box 15-3   Patient Preparation for Stress Studies

1. Instruct the patient to fast for at least 4 hours before the stress study.
2. Obtain a detailed cardiac history in order to plan the exercise and to be aware of what to expect.
3. Inform the patient about the procedure and obtain consent.
4. If contraindications to physical stress are found, switch to pharmacologic stress.
5. Prepare the chest and place the leads (12 leads should be placed for the stress test).
6. Obtain baseline ECG and blood pressure values.
7. Check resting images.
8. Ensure that a crash cart is available in case of an emergency.

stress test to ensure that no contraindications exist. Stress tests can cause severe ischemia, arrhythmias, hypotension, infarction, and death. For these reasons, these examinations should be performed only by personnel familiar with the procedure and with cardiopulmonary resuscitation. Nuclear medicine technologists work with the exercise team of physicians and nurses to perform the stress procedure. In addition to certification in advanced life support (to assist in case of a catastrophe, an event that occurs in about 1 in every 300 stress tests), technologists should be aware of the indications to terminate the tests. The baseline ECG is reviewed before the stress procedure.

For MUGA studies, the subject is seated on the bicycle ergometer, the pedals are adjusted, and the resting radionuclide examination is recorded as previously described using the first-pass or equilibrium technique. The baseline images and EF should be checked to ensure that no contraindications exist. Exercise is begun at a constant number of revolutions per minute (rpm) of the pedals, with subsequent adjustment of the workload (usually in 25 watt increments every 3 minutes). The ECG is monitored continuously and blood pressure is recorded at least once every stage throughout the procedure. Good venous access should be available to facilitate administration of drugs if necessary, and a crash cart should be kept in the immediate vicinity of the stress laboratory.

For the first-pass technique, the radiopharmaceutical is administered at peak exercise and data are recorded over the next 60 seconds as described in the rest procedure. Typically, a dose of 5 to 10 mCi is used for the rest study and 10 to 20 mCi for the exercise examination. The first-pass approach is well suited to the exercise test, because patients can maintain their maximum effort for only a short interval.

For an equilibrium study, an LAO view at rest is recorded in the same position that the patient will use for exercise. Data usually are acquired for each stage of exercise. At the conclusion of the exercise procedure, the data are analyzed as described for equilibrium studies. Normal subjects should have at least a 5% increase in the ejection fraction from rest to the maximum level of exercise achieved. However, in normal patients with an ejection fraction of 65% or greater at rest, the EF might not increase with exercise.

When patients cannot exercise, a pharmacologic stress test can be performed. To increase myocardial oxygen consumption, agents such as dobutamine typically are infused at an initial dose of 10 μg/min, which is increased gradually to 40 μg/min, and data are recorded at each phase of the infusion. Figure 15-19 shows the changes in ventricular function between rest and stress that occur in a normal patient undergoing a pharmacologic stress test. Typically, a rise of more than 5% is expected between the rest and the stress LVEF.

MYOCARDIAL PERFUSION IMAGING

Perfusion imaging is performed to detect myocardial ischemia and to determine its location and extent. Perfusion imaging with injection of a radiotracer during stress detects a relative decrease in blood flow to the myocardium directly. The first myocardial perfusion agent used to detect exercise stress–induced myocardial ischemia, potassium-43, has

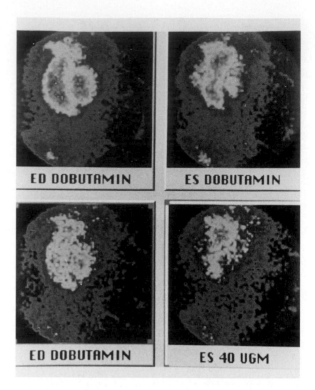

Figure 15-19 Planar gated blood pool scans in the 45-degree LAO position recorded at rest (*top panels*) and during dobutamine infusion (*bottom panels*) at end-diastole (*left*) and end-systole (*right*). The right and left ventricles and great vessels are seen. Note the marked reduction in right and left ventricular size and volume from diastole to systole. During dobutamine stress, the end-systolic size of the ventricle is smaller than at rest, suggesting an increase in the ejection fraction.

major photons at 390 and 640 keV, which are not well suited for use with the thin crystal of the scintillation camera. As a result, this agent was replaced by 201Tl, with its 80 keV mercury x-ray, as the major photon. This agent has been in wide clinical use since it was initially approved for that purpose in 1974 and is still preferred by many laboratories. Two 99mTc-labeled agents, tetrafosmin and sestamibi, are gaining popularity. The shorter physical and biologic half-lives of these two agents result in a lower radiation burden per millicurie, which allows doses up to 30 mCi per examination, much higher than the 4 mCi dose usually used with thallium. The technetium agents do not redistribute, allowing images to be recorded at some time after tracer administration. Each of these agents has some features that require specific tailoring of the examination. As a result, a laboratory should gain experience with one or two of these agents and become proficient in its use.

A treadmill is usually used for exercise tests in the United States, whereas a bicycle is preferred in Europe. The patient's heart rate, ECG, blood pressure, and symptoms are continuously monitored as described for blood pool imaging. The exercise test is performed to the same endpoints. The perfusion tracer is administered at the *peak of exercise,* and the patient is urged to continue exercising for at least 1 to

2 additional minutes to permit the tracer to deposit in the tissues.

Perfusion images are acquired after injection of tracer with the patient at rest and injection of tracer with the patient at stress. A uniform pattern of myocardial perfusion at rest and stress makes it very unlikely that a patient has a significant risk of sudden death or myocardial infarction within the next 2 years. An abnormal scan with injection at stress and a normal scan with injection at rest suggests myocardial ischemia. Depending on the site and extent of the abnormality, the risk of a significant cardiac event (myocardial infarction, angina, or sudden death) varies from 1% to 2% up to about 15% in the next 2 years. An abnormality on both the rest and stress examinations suggests myocardial scarring, which is less likely to cause a significant event than ischemia.

Radiopharmaceuticals Used for Perfusion Imaging

[201]Tl is a monovalent cationic radiopharmaceutical with biologic behavior similar to that of potassium-43 (see Box 15-2 for a list of agents used for perfusion imaging). It is a cyclotron-produced agent with a physical half-life of 74 hours, and it decays by electron capture with the production of mercury x-rays of about 80 keV. Thallium is minimally excreted through the bowel and kidneys (only 10% is lost from the body over 10 days), resulting in a long biologic half-life. After intravenous injection about 3.5% of the injected dose localizes in the myocardium.* In myocardium that is ischemic, the relative amount of thallium in the zone of diminished perfusion is lower than that of the normally perfused zone (in direct proportion to that difference in tissue blood flow to the two regions). If serial images are recorded over several hours, the relative loss of thallium from the normally perfused zone is greater than that of the ischemic zone. At about 3 to 4 hours the relative concentration of thallium in the two areas may appear similar. This phenomenon, called *redistribution,* has made thallium very useful for identifying ischemic myocardium.

In contrast to its behavior in the myocardium, about 10% of each dose of thallium localizes in each kidney. Once in the kidney, the tracer is retained for days, resulting in a radiation burden of about 1.7 rad/mCi to the kidney and the small intestine. The combination of a long effective half-life, which limits the dose that can be injected to about 4 mCi, and the low energy, which makes attenuation artifacts particularly prominent, resulted in a search for a technetium-labeled heart agent. [201]Tl decays by means of electron capture to stable mercury-201 ([201]Hg), with the production of the 69 to 80 keV mercury x-rays (100% abundant) and gamma photons of 135 and 167 keV (2% and 8% abundance,

respectively). Images are usually recorded with the x-ray or a combination of the x-ray and gammas.

Once deposited in the myocardium, thallium clears at different rates from normal and ischemic tissue, with faster clearance from normal tissue. Maximum contrast between normal and ischemic tissue occurs immediately after injection and persists for about 20 minutes. Thereafter contrast gradually decreases, with the normal and ischemic tissues achieving similar concentrations over intervals ranging from 4 to 24 hours. The differential clearance of thallium from these zones of myocardium defines a need for immediate imaging of stress-injected thallium perfusion studies to optimize the detection of altered perfusion. If imaging is delayed longer than 20 minutes after injection, subtle lesions may be missed in patients with ischemia. When the tracer is injected at rest, however, the changes in myocardial uptake are less of a problem; imaging can be postponed for some time to maximize the likelihood that redistribution has occurred and that all viable myocardium is visualized.

Although three technetium-labeled perfusion tracers have been approved by the U.S. Food and Drug Administration (FDA)—teboroxime, sestamibi, and tetrafosmin (Table 15-5)—only two of these agents, sestamibi (MIBI) and tetrafosmin, are in wide clinical use. There are several reasons for this. First, sestamibi and tetrafosmin have lower myocardial extraction (about 60% for MIBI and 50% for tetrafosmin, versus 88% for thallium), therefore a smaller fraction of the injected dose per millicurie of injected activity localizes in the myocardium. Second, these agents have slightly slower blood clearance than thallium, making it particularly important to continue the exercise for about 2 minutes after injection instead of the 1 minute usually used for thallium. Third, tetrafosmin and MIBI have more favorable dosimetry (20 mCi of sestamibi delivers 3.6 rad to the large bowel, and 20 mCi of tetrafosmin delivers only 1.5 rad to the large bowel), which permits administration of doses up to 30 mCi. The higher administered dose results in a much greater photon flux from the myocardium and allows recording of first-pass data at the time of injection. Although gated SPECT studies can be recorded with thallium, they pale in comparison with the high-quality gated SPECT of the technetium-labeled tracers.

Because technetium agents are not redistributed, separate injections are required to define perfusion at rest and with stress. Teboroxime, which has a biologic half-life of about 5 minutes in the myocardium, requires completion of myocardial images within 10 minutes of tracer administration. For effective use of this agent, patients must be injected in the immediate vicinity of the imaging device or while actually on the imaging table.

Some clinics perform adenosine or dobutamine stress imaging with the patient positioned on the gamma camera table, recording first-pass data during injection, followed immediately by SPECT. In contrast to the typical SPECT acquisition, in which the camera rotates through a 180-degree arc over a period of 20 to 30 minutes, in a teboroxime SPECT study, the camera records data continuously as

---

*The myocardium receives 4% of cardiac output. Thallium has a myocardial extraction of 88%, resulting in the myocardial uptake of about 3.5% of the administered dose.

Table 15-5	Technetium-labeled perfusion tracers		
Agent	**Myocardial concentration**	**Myocardial t_{1/2}**	**Comments**
Teboroxime	3.6%	5 min	Imaging must be completed within 10 min of injection
Sestamibi	2.4%	6 hr	Slight redistribution (not nearly as much as with thallium, but images should be recorded within 90 min of injection to maximize detection of ischemic lesions); myocardial images can be recorded with gating, allowing an estimate of left ventricular ejection fraction and regional myocardial thickening
Tetrafosmin	2.0%	8 hr	Does not redistribute; myocardial images can be recorded with gating to estimate ventricular function and regional thickening

it rotates through a 180-degree arc in 20 seconds, reverses direction, and repeats the process until at least 3 minutes of post-injection data have been obtained. This data acquisition averages the rapid myocardial tracer loss and bowel excretion, limiting artifacts on reconstruction of the teboroxime data. Conventional acquisition, on the other hand, limits the utility of teboroxime for routine imaging. In contrast, sestamibi and tetrafosmin have biologic half-lives of longer than 5 hours in the myocardium, allowing images to be recorded up to 90 minutes after injection. When possible, earlier images are preferred, and most laboratories image these agents 15 to 30 minutes after injection.

Imaging protocols. Table 15-6 presents the commonly used protocols. Thallium imaging is done with stress injection first and redistribution imaging at 3 to 4 hours later. Also, 24-hour imaging may be done for additional information with or without reinjection.

Imaging with technetium-labeled tracers can be done with either a 1- or a 2-day protocol. In the 2-day protocol, the rest and stress examinations are done on separate days, each with a dose of 20 to 30 mCi. For the 1-day study, patients can have either the rest or stress study performed first, typically with a dose of 10 mCi, followed about 4 to 6 hours later (to permit both physical decay and biologic loss of radiopharmaceutical from the myocardium) by the rest or stress examination at a dose of 20 to 30 mCi. In summary, patients can be injected first at rest and then at stress, or vice versa, with a larger dose of tracer used for the second study.

A dual isotope technique is an alternative approach that uses thallium for the rest-injected tracer and one of the technetium agents for the stress-injected agent. The advantages of this approach are that delayed/rest images can be recorded with thallium to detect viable myocardium, and the stress test can be performed at the conclusion of rest imaging with only minimal residual activity in the technetium window (caused by a 12% incidence of gamma photons from ^{201}Tl). This eliminates the waiting time needed to image with a single isotope.

Perfusion Imaging with Technetium-Labeled Agents

The technetium-labeled agents can be substituted for thallium in the rest or stress or both portions of the examination. These agents have significant differences in selected aspects of their behavior compared with [201]Tl. The technetium-labeled agents are lost very slowly from the myocardium, with comparable clearance from normal and ischemic tissue. Separate injections are required for the rest and stress portions of the study. The question of whether the rest or stress study should be performed first has been the subject of great debate. Optimally, the rest and stress examinations are performed on separate days, which eliminates the problem of any residual background activity. Often, however, patients prefer to have the studies completed on a single day. Same-day studies usually use 10 to 15 mCi for the first examination and 25 to 30 mCi for the second. There appears to be little difference in the sensitivity or specificity of perfusion imaging between the 1-day and the 2-day protocol.

Technetium-labeled agents are somewhat less sensitive than thallium for the detection of viable ischemic myocardium. The reason for this is unclear, but it may relate to the lack of redistribution. When there is a high likelihood of severe stenosis and limited collateral blood flow to a region of potentially viable myocardium, the combination of a rest-injected thallium scan and a stress-injected technetium-labeled tracer study may be useful. In this circumstance the dose of thallium is administered first, and images of the rest distribution of perfusion are recorded. Thereafter, the patient is stressed, the technetium-labeled tracer is administered, and stress technetium images are recorded.

With single-radiopharmaceutical studies, the data should be carefully reviewed for technical adequacy before the SPECT data are reconstructed. When doses of 3.5 to 4.5 mCi are used for the thallium study (and the patient's weight is less than 180 pounds), useful data can be reconstructed using a Butterworth filter with a frequency of 0.55

| Table 15-6 | Imaging protocols |

Protocol	Comments
Technetium agents: ^{99m}Tc sestamibi or ^{99m}Tc tetrafosmin	
Two-day stress-rest: Inject 15 to 30 mCi at peak exercise. Begin imaging at 15 to 30 min after injection during exercise. On day 2, give same dose at rest. Begin imaging at 45 to 60 min after injection at rest.	Observing a waiting period after injection allows adequate hepatobiliary clearance. For sestamibi, the recommended wait after injection is at least 15 to 20 min for exercise stress, 60 min for pharmacologic stress, and 45 to 60 min for rest. For tetrafosmin, the recommended wait after injection is at least 10 to 15 min after exercise stress, 45 min after pharmacologic stress, and 30 to 45 min after rest.
One-day rest-stress: This is a same-day imaging protocol using a low-dose (8 to 10 mCi) resting study followed by a high-dose (20 to 25 mCi) stress study. This protocol is preferred over the stress-rest technique.	
One-day stress-rest: Give stress injection of 10 to 15 mCi, followed by an interval of 2 to 4 hr; then give rest injection of 20 to 25 mCi.	
Thallium-201 (^{201}Tl)	
Stress and delay (standard): Inject 2.5 to 3.0 mCi at peak stress and wait 2 to 4 hr (3 hr is preferred) for rest imaging. Waiting time is only 5 to 10 min. After stress 1.5 mCi may be re-injected. Imaging and re-imaging may be done again after 1 to 4 hr.	Delay should be avoided, because redistribution occurs early.
Rest redistribution: Inject 3 mCi at rest and obtain initial image. Delayed image is acquired at 3 hr. Further imaging may be done at 24 hr without re-injection.	
Dual isotope	
^{201}Tl rest and ^{99m}Tc sestamibi/tetrafosmin stress studies are performed the same day. Inject 3 mCi of thallium and image. Later inject 20 to 25 mCi of technetium agent at stress. Image at appropriate times.	Cross-talk occurs between the energies of thallium and technetium; however, when imaging is done in this sequence, the energy spill is minimal compared with imaging thallium after technetium.

cycles/cm. The technetium data should be reconstructed with a filter of about 0.65 cycles/cm to take advantage of the higher photon flux. These combined tracer data are interpreted in similar fashion to that recorded when a single radiopharmaceutical is used. If the rest and stress data appear similarly abnormal, the patient can return for imaging at 24 hours and no additional radiopharmaceutical administration is required. These delayed rest-injected images are particularly helpful for the detection of viable myocardium, especially in patients with a diminished ejection fraction.

For the detection of ischemia, thallium and technetium agents perform equally well. When there is a question of severe myocardial ischemia and the issue is myocardial viability, thallium is preferred. If it is important to review myocardial function and perfusion at the same time, a gated myocardial SPECT study can be recorded, which is less noisy with the technetium agents. Gated SPECT studies also

can be recorded with thallium, but the higher photon flux of the technetium-labeled agents provides better quality data (Figure 15-20). The sensitivity of planar ^{201}Tl imaging for coronary artery disease is greater than 85% despite the requirement for at least 25% difference in the distribution of perfusion between adjacent areas for impaired tissue to be visible as a lesion on the scan. The specificity of this test also is high, typically in the 80% to 90% range.

Imaging techniques. In contrast to ventricular function measurements, for which imaging is performed during exercise, myocardial perfusion studies are recorded after exercise has concluded. For stress images a treadmill or bicycle exercise is usually done. Preliminary preparation and questions should be asked as described earlier (see Box 15-3). A complete medication history should be recorded to determine if any medication would alter the sensitivity of the procedure. To determine if medical therapy

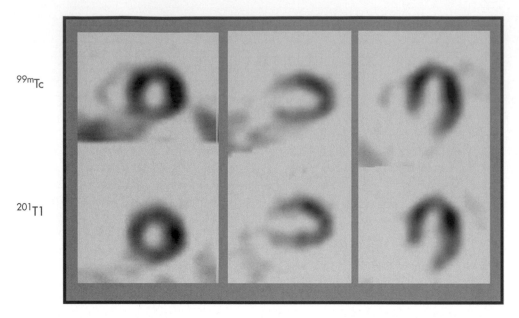

Figure 15-20 Effect of photon energy on images. Thallium images demonstrate slightly less activity in the inferobasal, anterobasal and posterobasal segments compared with technetium images because of attenuation caused by the overlying right ventricle in the vertical long axis view and the attenuation effect in the horizontal long axis view.

Table 15-7	Drugs that can affect exercise test response and interpretation
Drug	**Discontinuation before exercise test**
Antiarrythmics	48 hr
Antihypertensives	4 days
Beta-adrenergic blockers	48 hr
Calcium channel blockers	48 hr
Digitalis/digoxin	1 to 2 wk
Diuretics	4 days
Long-acting nitrates	At least 12 hr
Sedatives and tranquilizers	1 day
Sublingual nitroglycerin	2 hr

Table 15-8 Bruce protocol

Stage	Duration (min)	Speed (mph)	Grade (%)
I	3	1.7	10
II	3	2.5	12
III	3	3.4	14
IV	3	4.2	16
V	3	5.0	18
VI	3	5.5	20
VII	3	6.0	22

reduces the incidence of ischemia, it is helpful to perform the procedure while the patient is taking the medication. If the test is done to make the diagnosis of coronary disease, beta-blocking medication and calcium channel blocking medication should be stopped for at least 24 hours (Table 15-7).

The standard Bruce protocol (Table 15-8) is usually applied, although modifications can be used when indicated. To maximize the likelihood of detection of coronary artery disease with perfusion imaging, the radiopharmaceutical should be administered at the peak of exercise and the exercise should continue for an additional 1 to 2 minutes to permit the tracer to localize in the myocardium in proportion to perfusion at the peak of exercise. Stress is stopped when indicated (Box 15-4). If exercise is terminated prematurely, particularly in patients with small zones of ischemia (which may normalize rapidly), part of the dose is delivered at a time when the tissue has decreased flow and part of the dose is delivered when perfusion is normal. This phenomenon reduces contrast between the normal and ischemic tissue, making detection of the lesion difficult.

An intravenous (IV) line is placed to facilitate injection at the peak of stress. Because glucose alters the clearance rate of ^{201}Tl from the myocardium, the IV line should be kept open with saline. Injection of the radiopharmaceutical

1. Marked arrhythmia induced by exercise (e.g., ventricular tachycardia, PVCs in pairs or triplets, and atrial fibrillation)
2. Decrease in blood pressure or heart rate as exercise progresses
3. Extreme elevation in blood pressure (systolic pressure >200 or diastolic pressure >120 mm Hg)
4. Severe chest pain
5. Achievement of greater than 85% (preferably 100%) of predicted heart rate for age, computed as 220—Age (yr)
6. Severe ST depression (>3 mm) or elevation
7. Onset of advanced atrioventricular block
8. Onset of bundle branch block
9. Failure of monitoring system
10. Severe fatigue, leg pain, or breathlessness

should be followed by a flush of 10 ml of saline to minimize the time that the radiopharmaceutical is in contact with the veins of the arm. After injection, exercise should continue for at least 1 minute with thallium and preferably 2 minutes with the technetium-labeled tracers (because they have slightly slower blood clearance than thallium). If the patient has difficulty maintaining peak exercise levels, the workload can be reduced markedly to maintain the heart rate and blood pressure elevation during the brief interval of tracer clearance.

After exercise the patient is placed supine on an imaging table; ECG and blood pressure monitoring continue until the heart rate has decreased to within about 20% of baseline, transient ECG changes and arrhythmias have resolved, and blood pressure is near normal. Imaging should commence within 10 minutes of injection with thallium and within 15 minutes for sestamibi and tetrofosmin. Imaging within a short time of the conclusion of stress increases the likelihood of detection of transiently increased lung uptake, enlarged left ventricular cavity size, and a fall in the ejection fraction.

SPECT myocardial perfusion imaging is generally recorded with gating to provide information about regional perfusion and function simultaneously. Ventricular dilation and increased lung uptake may normalize within 10 to 15 minutes after injection and can be missed if images are not recorded soon after injection.

Thallium images are recorded using the mercury x-ray (centered at 80 keV) and the gamma photons. A low-energy, all-purpose or high-resolution collimator is used. Data are recorded digitally in a 64×64 or 128×128 matrix (depending on the detector's field of view) to permit review of the images with contrast enhancement and quantification

of the regional distribution of ^{201}Tl. SPECT imaging is recorded as described above.

If thallium is the only tracer used for recording myocardial perfusion images, the stress examination is performed first and followed by immediate imaging. Because thallium redistributes (has differential clearance from normal and ischemic tissue), delayed images are obtained 3 to 4 hours later. The patient should be instructed not to eat any food containing carbohydrates, because ingestion of glucose accelerates the rate of ^{201}Tl clearance from both normal and ischemic myocardium, minimizing the differential clearance necessary to detect ischemia. When the patient returns, images are recorded as described above. Occasionally, to improve count statistics, an additional 1 mCi dose of thallium is administered at rest before the delayed images are recorded. In the case of re-injection, the tracer is measuring the regional distribution of perfusion at rest, a circumstance markedly different from that at stress (and similar to the conditions used for the technetium-labeled tracers). The potential problem with a rest injection is that under some circumstances of severe coronary disease, the perfusion to the tissue is markedly reduced even at rest, yet the tissue is alive. The "viability" of this tissue is best detected by redistribution imaging without additional tracer administration.

Pharmacologic stress. Some patients cannot exercise because of peripheral vascular disease, neurologic problems, or musculoskeletal abnormalities. In these patients, instead of the exercise test, myocardial blood flow may be increased by using drugs to cause vasodilation of the coronary bed or to increase myocardial oxygen demand. The vasodilator method is used more often, using *dipyridamole* or *adenosine*. By increasing the local tissue level of adenosine, both agents cause relaxation of precapillary sphincters in the arterioles, resulting in a marked decrease in peripheral resistance and an increase in regional blood flow to the myocardium. These agents cause a generalized vasodilation, and neither is specific for the heart.

Dipyridamole reduces the metabolism of endogenously produced adenosine by inhibiting an enzyme called adenosine deaminase. Adenosine that is infused, on the other hand, exerts a direct effect by occupying the adenosine receptors. Dipyridamole lasts for several hours after administration, whereas adenosine has a biologic half-life of only 10 seconds.

When the drugs are infused, coronary arteries free of atherosclerosis dilate to increase myocardial blood flow uniformly to all areas of the myocardium. If tracer is administered at the time of the maximum effect of the drug, all areas of the myocardium show normal uptake. If a vessel is markedly narrowed, flow distal to the narrowing does not increase to the same degree as that in myocardial territories supplied by normal coronary arteries, and areas of low uptake can be seen (Figure 15-21). Although this phenomenon does not usually cause ischemia, as in exercise tests, the underlying basis for detection of abnor-

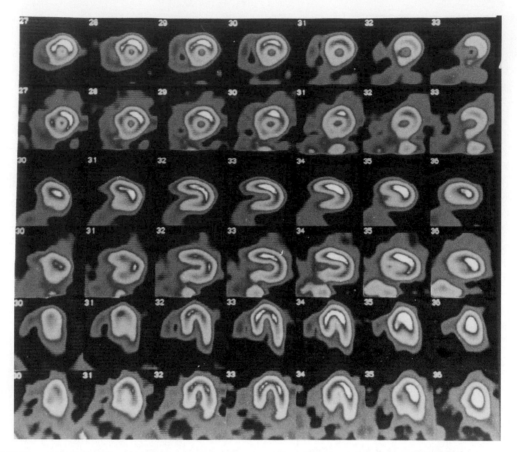

Figure 15-21   SPECT myocardial perfusion scan reconstructed in the short axis *(top two rows)*, vertical long axis *(middle two rows)*, and horizontal long axis views *(bottom two rows)* after administration of adenosine *(upper row of each pair)* and at rest *(bottom row of each pair)*. Perfusion to the inferior portion of the left ventricle is reduced after adenosine stress (best seen on the short axis images). The distribution of perfusion improves at rest, suggesting an ischemic lesion in the myocardium, usually supplied by the right coronary artery.

malities (the stenosis of a coronary artery) remains the same.*

The effects of dipyridamole and adenosine can be reversed by administration of aminophylline. Because the vasodilator properties of adenosine and dipyridamole result in decreased blood pressure, patients should be studied while they are lying supine on a stretcher, and the blood pressure and ECG should be monitored continuously. Typically hypotension is mild, causing a reduction in blood pressure of 10 to 15 mm Hg. In some patients, however, the reduction in blood pressure can be profound, leading to death if not treated. In the unlikely event that a patient develops serious complications during the test, a syringe of aminophylline should be available. As with exercise tests, serious side effects such as arrhythmias, severe hypotension, cerebral ischemia, stroke, and death have been reported with the pharmacologic stress test. Therefore the examina-

tion should be performed only in facilities equipped to handle medical emergencies.

Before the pharmacologic stress test is performed, patients should be asked if they have asthma (a relative contraindication for the use of either dipyridamole or adenosine). Patients should prepare for the test by fasting for at least 4 hours, abstaining from food containing caffeine (e.g., coffee, tea, and many soft drinks) for at least 24 hours, and discontinuing all xanthine-containing medications 36 hours before the study. Caffeine and xanthine-containing medications reduce the effectiveness of the vasodilator and may produce a negative test result in patients with coronary stenoses.

The blood pressure and ECG must be monitored throughout the procedure. The drugs are injected intravenously using an infusion pump. The test is performed after administration of 0.56 mg/kg dipyridamole over 4 minutes or 140 μg/kg/min of adenosine for 6 minutes while serial blood pressure and ECG recordings are made. The perfusion tracer is administered approximately 3 to 4 minutes after the conclusion of the dipyridamole infusion or during the third minute of adenosine infusion. Imaging commences about 10 minutes later.

---

*Vasodilation can cause ischemia, particularly if the territory is perfused primarily by collateral vessels. Collateral vessels are relatively narrow and require normal blood pressure to maintain adequate flow. When blood pressure decreases, as often occurs during infusion of adenosine or dipyridamole, flow through collaterals may also decrease, resulting in myocardial ischemia.

Administration of adenosine or dipyridamole often is accompanied by a pounding headache, a sensation of heaviness in the chest, nausea, and a feeling of breathlessness. These symptoms can be minimized with low-level exercise, either by walking on the treadmill at about 1 mile/hr or using arm weights of 2 to 5 pounds during the infusion.

Dobutamine is a sympathomimetic drug that increases the heart rate and blood pressure. This agent increases myocardial work and hence the need for increased flow in the coronary arteries. In contrast to other drugs in this category, dobutamine has a low incidence of cardiac arrhythmia. The drug has a half-life of about 1 to 2 minutes, which limits the duration of effect. As with the vasodilator agents, the heart rate, ECG, and blood pressure should be monitored continuously during administration of the drug. Because the drug causes increased oxygen consumption, it can cause ischemia, similar to exercise.

Dobutamine is infused at a graduated rate, which is started at $10 \mu g/min$ and increased every 3 minutes to a maximum of $40 \mu g/min$. If the heart rate has not achieved 85% of maximum and the blood pressure is still in an acceptable range, atropine is administered in divided doses up to a total of 1 mg to produce a tachycardia. The perfusion agent is administered, and the dobutamine infusion is continued for an additional 2 minutes.

Although pharmacologic testing is useful in patients who cannot exercise, the vasodilator agents cause a marked increase in blood flow to the liver, which can make it difficult to see lesions of the inferior wall. Neither the vasodilators nor dobutamine provide the breadth of information about cardiac performance that is available with an exercise study. Exercise testing offers information about the overall status of the patient's cardiovascular fitness, the duration and severity of exercise that causes symptoms, and the timing of symptoms versus objective indicators of ischemia (ST segment changes or perfusion scan abnormalities). This information frequently plays a key role in the planning of therapy.

Nitrates. Nitroglycerin is often used to relieve myocardial ischemia. The drug works by causing both venodilation and arterial dilation. As a result of the venodilation, the amount of blood returning to the heart is reduced, decreasing myocardial oxygen requirements. The arterial dilation results in increased blood flow to the myocardium. The combination is very effective. In the case of patients with coronary artery disease, some lesions are so severe that blood flow through the vessel is reduced even at rest. This occurs when lesions narrow more than 95% to 99% of the vessel lumen. Administration of nitroglycerin to patients with severe coronary disease enhances the detection of viable but ischemic myocardial tissue in 10% to 15% of subjects. Typically, nitroglycerin is administered as a single, 0.4 mg sublingual tablet 2 to 4 minutes before the rest tracer injection. The patient should be seated for the procedure, and the pulse and blood pressure should be recorded at baseline and at the time of tracer administration.

SPECT Imaging

SPECT imaging results in a marked improvement in image contrast compared with planar imaging. However, this improvement comes with a significant price—artifacts in the data may be difficult to appreciate. Two types of artifacts occur fairly frequently: attenuation (caused by breast or stomach tissue) and motion (caused by slight patient movement during the lengthy acquisition). Both these artifacts tend to cause areas of decreased counts in the reconstructed data that can be mistaken for zones of decreased perfusion. These artifacts can be readily appreciated if the projection data are reviewed in a cinematic display. When attenuation is seen, its impact on the data can be anticipated, and the images can be interpreted correctly. Attenuation correction methods may be used, but these sometimes can produce artifacts caused by overcorrection (Figure 15-22). Motion, on the other hand, is difficult to correct. If multiple motion episodes are seen or if a discrete movement changes the data by more than 2 pixels, the reconstructed data (which presumes that the data are consistent) probably will have focal artifacts. If this is seen, another acquisition should be recorded rather than an attempt made to eliminate the motion by shifting the data in the computer.

It is recommended that SPECT imaging begin about 10 minutes after high-level exercise (>10 metabolic equivalents [METS]) to avoid the phenomenon of myocardial motion caused by a change in the degree of diaphragmatic excursion as the patient's respiration returns to normal. This phenomenon has been referred to as *myocardial creep* or *upward creep* and is seen mostly in patients who achieve high levels of exercise. It typically results in an artifactual lesion in the inferior or inferoseptal regions of the left ventricle. After positioning the patient with the heart in the center of the field, the detectors are rotated through an acquisition orbit in an effort to bring the camera heads as close to the patient as possible without touching at the angle with the greatest body diameter. Some devices can collect data in an elliptical orbit, allowing the detector to remain closer to the patient (enhancing resolution) during rotation.

If data are collected in a 360-degree orbit, the patient should have both arms elevated and supported to alleviate fatigue and minimize movement. If a 180-degree orbit is chosen, only the left arm needs to be out of the field of view, and the right arm can be at the side and held in place with an elastic chest binder. Data acquisition for the 180-degree orbit typically begins at 45 degrees RAO and ends at 45 degrees LPO.

Image acquisition time varies from 20 to 30 minutes, depending on several factors: (1) whether a single-detector or a multidetector camera is used; (2) whether a 180-degree or a 360-degree acquisition is performed; (3) the dose of radiopharmaceutical used; (4) whether a 3- or a 6-degree step angle is used; and (5) the number of counts collected at each increment. A typical SPECT protocol requires 32 (or 64) stops for 180 degrees or 64 (or 128) stops for 360 degrees. A technologist should be present in the room

Attenuation correction

No attenuation correction

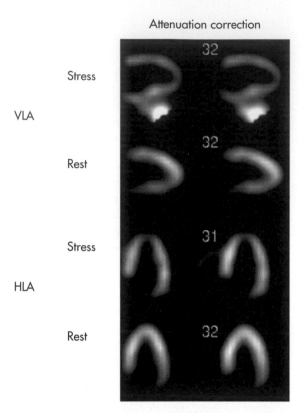
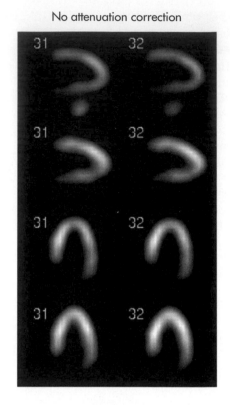

Figure 15-22 Effects of attenuation correction. Although attenuation correction is helpful for overcoming attenuation artifacts, it sometimes can lead to artifactual defects as a result of overcorrection caused by count distribution techniques. On the left is an image corrected for attenuation that shows a defect in the apex with adjacent activity in the liver. Images not corrected for attenuation show no defect.

throughout SPECT data collection to prevent possible injury from a malfunction of the moving detector.

Gated Perfusion Imaging

Gated perfusion SPECT typically is recorded using 8 instead of 16 frames per cardiac cycle because of the enormity of the data set. When 64 angles are recorded with 8 frames/cycle at each location, a total of 512 images are obtained. Although end-systole is not correctly identified under this circumstance, the apparent loss of ejection fraction is typically on the order of 5% and is most apparent in patients with high ejection fractions at rest. This type of study has sufficient precision to differentiate patients with normal ejection fractions from those with depressed ejection fractions.

Data analysis. Myocardial perfusion data are evaluated by viewing the images to detect zones of diminished tracer localization and by quantification of the relative regional distribution of the agent. Qualitative interpretation reviews the images for the factors listed in Box 15-5 (Figure 15-23). Data

are quantified by region of interest analysis to express the regional concentration of thallium in the myocardium graphically (Figure 15-24). Although planar and SPECT images can be quantified, planar quantification is rarely used. SPECT images are usually quantified by stacking the reconstructed/reoriented short axis slices onto a bull's-eye display, where the apex is at the center and the basal slice is at the periphery.

The basis of interpretation is that perfusion abnormalities that appear less severe on rest or delayed images than they do on the stress studies indicate areas of stress-induced myocardial ischemia (Figures 15-25 and 15-26), whereas those that remain fixed on delayed imaging most likely reflect sites of myocardial scarring (Figure 15-27).

Interpretation is facilitated by presentation of the images in a standard format, realigned along the major cardiac axes (see Figure 15-23). Realignment is performed by reconstructing the projection data by filtered back-projection into transverse slices. The long and short axes of the heart are determined, and the data are reoriented and reconstructed into short and long axis images of the myocardium. Quantitative analysis of these slices is most sensitive for the

Box 15-5	Myocardial Uptake Patterns with Perfusion Agents

- *Homogeneity of tracer distribution in the left ventricular (LV) myocardium.* Adjacent areas of normally perfused tissue should vary by <15% (with the exception of an occasional papillary muscle that may have markedly increased activity). Focal zones of decreased or absent tracer concentration are the hallmark of diminished perfusion.
- *Visualization of the right ventricular (RV) myocardium.* The intensity of RV myocardial activity should be ~50% that of the LV. Failure to see RV myocardial activity may indicate RV ischemia or infarction. Excess RV activity may indicate hypertrophy.
- *Size and shape of the LV and RV cavities.* The LV cavity should have the shape of a football in the anterior and left lateral views. A round shape suggests disease of the myocardium. The RV cavity should have the shape of a crescent moon in the left anterior oblique (LAO) view. If the borders appear rounded, dilation of the RV cavity should be considered.
- *Thallium used for an exercise stress test.* Activity in the left lung adjacent to the heart should be <60% of the peak LV myocardial activity (assuming the peak heart rate is >120 beats/min). If the lung concentration is elevated, pulmonary congestion associated with exercise should be considered. This finding is usually associated with severe coronary disease, which causes left ventricular dysfunction with exercise.

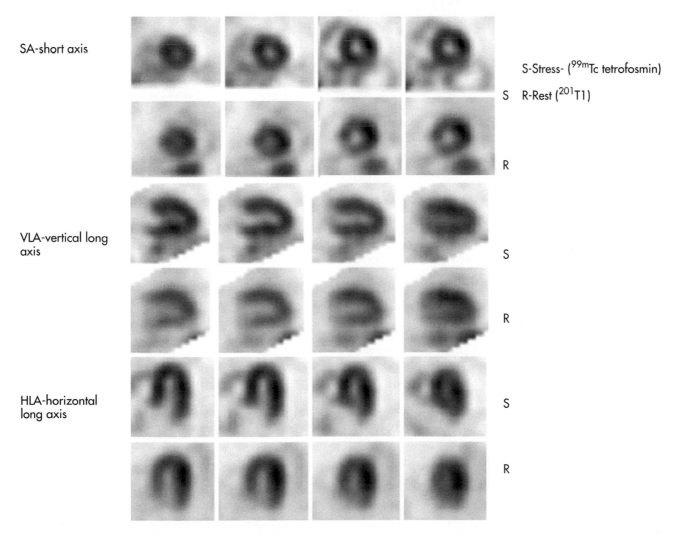

Figure 15-23   Normal myocardial perfusion with dual isotope. Slices in three reconstructed axes.

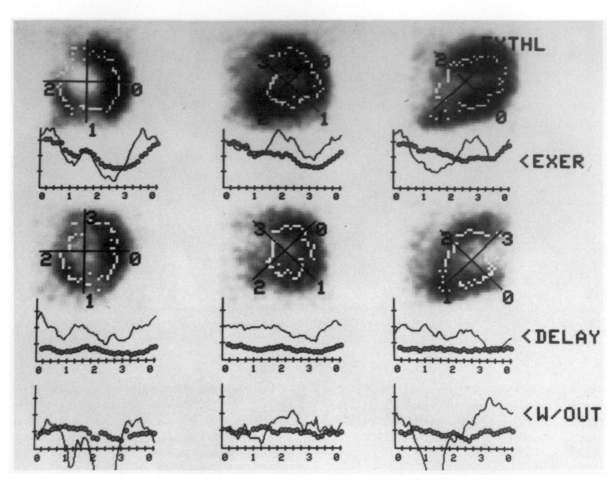

Figure 15-24 Quantitative circumferential profile analysis of planar thallium scintigrams. Upper row shows immediate post-exercise images (35 degrees LAO; anterior; 70 degrees LAO), which have been smoothed and corrected for background by an interpolative background-subtraction technique. The white pixels displayed in each image represent maximum pixel values located by the computer along each line of radial searching from the center of the left ventricular cavity (determined by operator-positioned superimposed crosshairs; on each image position, 1 corresponds to the apex). Beneath each exercise image, the corresponding plot of circumferential profile values is expressed as a percentage of the maximum pixel value in that image (*solid line*). The lower limit of normal for circumferential profile values is shown by the small boxes. In this patient, both the images and circumferential profiles demonstrate subnormal activity in the inferoapical region, interventricular septum (35-degree LAO view), and anteroseptal wall (70-degree LAO view). Borderline abnormal activity is seen in the anterolateral wall (anterior view). Background-subtracted delayed images with their circumferential profiles are displayed below each stress image. Displayed profile values are the normalized maximum pixel value in the corresponding immediate post-exercise image. Bottom row shows wash-out profile curves expressed as the percentage wash-out in each radius between exercise and delay. In this patient, subnormal values, indicative of redistribution and therefore ischemia, are apparent in inferoapical and septal regions on the 35-degree LAO view, in the anterolateral wall on the anterior view, and in the apical and anteroseptal walls on the 70-degree LAO view.

identification of alterations in regional perfusion. Long axis slices through the left ventricle, in both the vertical and horizontal planes, also are generated for visual analysis, which is useful for confirmation of findings noted on the short axis images and for assessment of the apex. Artifacts can occur as a result of attenuation from adjacent tissues (breast or stomach) or intense areas of adjacent activity (liver or loops of bowel). Although quantitation is valuable, the quantitative approaches in use cannot distinguish artifacts from significant areas of ischemia. The quantitative data, therefore, can serve as a guide rather than as a primary means of interpreting SPECT data.

Tomographic images also can be analyzed using the bull's-eye type of display. For this display, the short axis

SPECT images are arranged concentrically from the apex of the ventricle (center) to the base (periphery), and the three-dimensional myocardium is thus flattened into a single-plane map of the left ventricle. Bull's-eye maps of both the stress and rest studies also can be used to quantify the tomographic data.

Gated image display. After reconstruction of the data, the gated slices usually are displayed as multiple cine loops on the screen for visual assessment. Thereafter the endocardial borders of the midventricular horizontal and vertical long axis slices are defined, and the ejection fraction and ventricular volumes are calculated. These data can be appended to the evaluation of myocardial perfusion and are

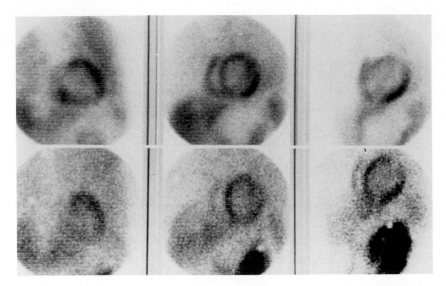

Figure 15-25   Planar thallium myocardial perfusion images recorded immediately after injection at stress *(top panels)* and at 24 hours *(bottom panels)* in the anterior view *(left)*, 45-degree LAO view *(middle)*, and left lateral view *(right)*. The left ventricle is markedly dilated. On the LAO view, the thallium concentration is decreased in the septum but improves on the 24-hour images, indicating an area of myocardial ischemia.

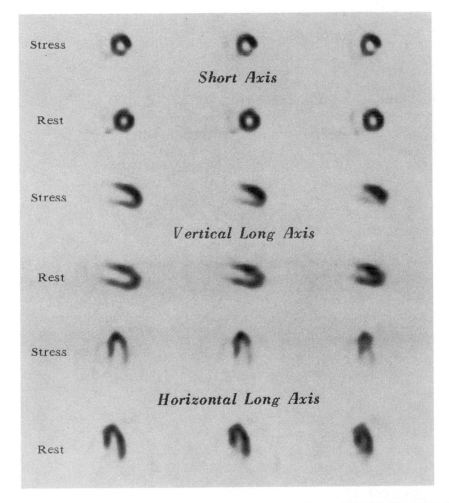

Figure 15-26   Selected short axis, vertical long axis, and horizontal long axis slices from a SPECT thallium-201 (^{201}Tl) study of a patient with exercise-induced ischemia of the inferolateral and inferior walls. Images obtained immediately after ^{201}Tl injection at peak exercise (stress) reveal a focal, marked decrease in ^{201}Tl activity within the inferolateral myocardial segment (seen best on the short axis and horizontal long axis views), with a milder decrease in activity within the inferior wall (seen best on the short axis and vertical long axis views). Repeat images obtained after a 4-hour delay (rest) demonstrate complete redistribution, with normal ^{201}Tl activity in these regions.

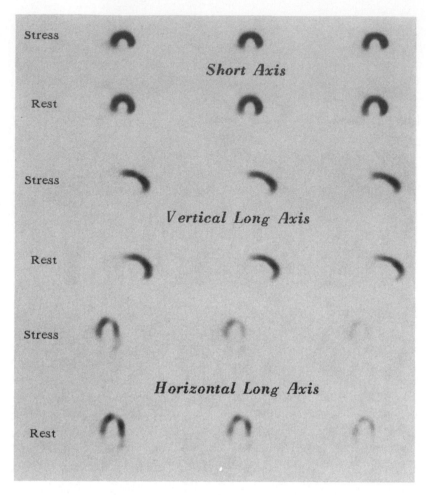

Figure 15-27   Selected slices from a ^{201}Tl SPECT study of a patient with a previous inferior wall myocardial infarction. Images obtained immediately after injection of ^{201}Tl at peak exercise (stress) demonstrate a large inferior region of markedly decreased myocardial uptake of ^{201}Tl. Repeat imaging after a 4-hour delay (rest) shows no significant redistribution of activity into this region.

particularly useful for determining the appearance of regional function in areas of diminished perfusion (Figure 15-28). Because the gated study is performed at rest, after the ischemic episode is over, zones of ischemia should have normal function (i.e., appear as areas of decreased intensity with normal thickening). Areas of scar, on the other hand, should have decreased perfusion and diminished function.

All the above-described techniques and procedures using single photon agents can also be done using positron emitters and a PET camera (see Positron Emission Tomography below).

POSITRON EMISSION TOMOGRAPHY

Myocardial Perfusion

Perfusion tracers. Positron-emitting radionuclides used for the assessment of regional perfusion can be classified into two groups: tracers that are only partly extracted by the myocardium (rubidium-82 [^{82}Rb] chloride and nitrogen-13 [^{13}N] ammonia) and tracers that are freely diffusible (oxygen-15 [^{15}O] water) (see Box 15-2).

^{82}Rb chloride, an FDA-approved radiopharmaceutical, is available from a strontium-82 (^{82}Sr) generator (there is no need for a cyclotron) and has a physical half-life of 75 seconds. ^{82}Rb behaves physiologically in a fashion similar to ^{201}Tl and is initially concentrated in the myocardium in proportion to regional myocardial perfusion, with an extraction of 65%. Retention of ^{82}Rb chloride depends at least partly on sodium-potassium adenosine triphosphatase (Na$^+$/K$^+$-ATPase) transport. Myocardial accumulation of ^{82}Rb chloride depends partly on the metabolic state of the myocardium. The short half life of this tracer permits repeat imaging.

^{13}N ammonia, produced by deuteron bombardment of oxygen-^{16} in a cyclotron, localizes in the myocardium in approximate proportion to regional myocardial perfusion, with the same practical limitations as ^{82}Rb chloride. Because of its 9.9-minute physical half-life and favorable myocardial kinetics, image quality with ^{13}N ammonia generally is superior to that obtained with the shorter half-life of ^{82}Rb chloride.

^{15}O is a cyclotron-produced radionuclide with a physical half-life of 122 seconds that can be used to label water

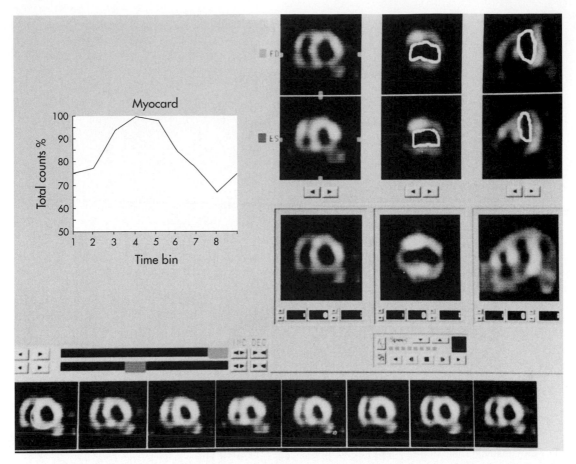

Figure 15-28   Gated myocardial perfusion SPECT in a patient with myocardial infarction. Images in the top row are midventricular slices at end-diastole (ED) in the short axis *(left),* vertical long axis *(middle),* and horizontal long axis *(right).* The next row shows the same slices at end-systole (ES). Cine displays in the third row allow the viewer to see the thickening of each slice (when viewed on the computer display). The bottom row illustrates eight gated images of the midventricular short axis slice. The graph depicts regional changes in counts in the short axis slice, demonstrating regional wall thickening. Endocardial outlines are drawn on the long axis images to permit calculation of left ventricular volumes and the ejection fraction.

($H_2{}^{15}O$). Because water is virtually freely diffusible into myocytes, extraction of this tracer by myocardial tissue is nearly 100% and does not depend on the flow rate. In addition, this tracer is metabolically inert, therefore its accumulation in the myocardium does not depend on the metabolic state of the tissue. However, because ^{15}O water resides in both the tissue and the blood pool, a second tracer (usually ^{15}O carbon monoxide, which is inhaled by the patient and subsequently binds avidly to erythrocytes) must be administered to permit correction for ^{15}O water activity emanating from the intravascular compartment.

To detect ischemia with PET radiopharmaceuticals, two injections are required: one set of images is recorded at rest, and a second set is recorded after stress, usually produced by pharmacologically induced vasodilation with dipyridamole or adenosine. All these tracers yield accurate estimates of regional myocardial perfusion in relative terms. Although quantification of myocardial perfusion in absolute terms can be most accurately performed with ^{15}O water, ^{82}Rb chloride and ^{13}N ammonia can also be used (Figures 15-29 and 15-30).

Detection of coronary artery disease. Most of the studies designed to assess the accuracy of myocardial perfusion imaging with PET in the detection of coronary artery disease have used either ^{82}Rb chloride or ^{13}N ammonia. PET and SPECT have sensitivities ranging from 80% to 95%, depending on the patient population studied. However, because PET has higher energy of annihilation radiation and improved correction for attenuation, its specificity tends to be about 10% to 15% higher than that of SPECT.

Ischemia is assessed by evaluation of glucose utilization with suppressed fatty acid metabolism after oral glucose administration (and if necessary, insulin infusion). These studies usually are performed with oral glucose loading (producing release of endogenous insulin from the patient's pancreas) or by using the glucose/insulin clamp approach, in which a continuous infusion of glucose and insulin is administered at the time of fluorodeoxyglucose (FDG) injection. The infusion is maintained during the interval of FDG blood clearance, before myocardial imaging.

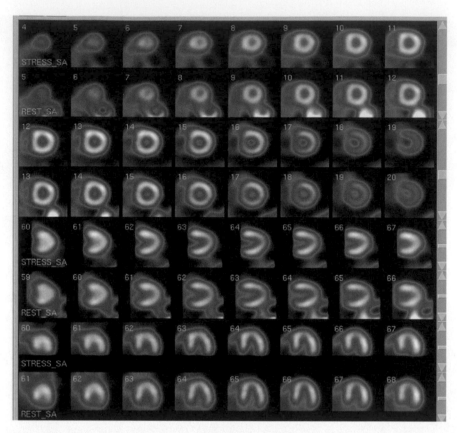

Figure 15-29 Normal myocardial perfusion with PET. A 47-year-old male with no risk factors presented with a history of atypical chest pain. A rest/stress dipyridamole rubidium-82 (^{82}Rb) PET study was done. The stress and rest images are shown in the short, vertical, and long axes. Uniform tracer distribution is seen in all segments, with no perfusion defects. (Courtesy J. Machac, MD, Mount Sinai School of Medicine.)

Myocardial Metabolism

A fundamental characteristic of the myocardium is its continuous requirement for oxygen and metabolic substrates to meet its energy needs. The heart meets its energy demands largely by oxidizing fatty acids and glucose. Under normal conditions, fatty acids are the preferred energy source for overall oxidative metabolism. When blood flow is reduced to the heart muscle and ischemia ensues, fatty acids can no longer be oxidized and glucose becomes the preferred energy source. This metabolic phenomenon is useful for the identification of myocardium that is underperfused but still viable. Such tissue is often hypokinetic or akinetic but returns to normal or near-normal function if blood flow is restored. Consequently, in patients with severely impaired ventricular function, combined measurements of myocardial perfusion and glucose metabolism have been advocated.

Metabolic tracers. ^{18}F fluorodeoxyglucose (^{18}F-FDG), ^{11}C palmitate, and ^{11}C acetate are typical examples of PET radiopharmaceuticals used for metabolic cardiac studies. Deoxyglucose is an analog of glucose that can be labeled with ^{18}F, a cyclotron-produced radionuclide, to form ^{18}F-FDG. Its myocardial uptake reflects overall myocardial utilization of glucose. Palmitate is a naturally occurring fatty acid that can be chemically synthesized and labeled with ^{11}C,

a cyclotron-produced radionuclide with a physical half-life of approximately 20.4 minutes. Its myocardial uptake and clearance reflect the myocardial utilization of fatty acids. The utilization of fatty acids and glucose by the heart is exquisitely sensitive to the level of glucose, fatty acids, and insulin in the blood, as well as the level of blood flow to the myocardium. Consequently, the substrate environment must be standardized when these two tracers are used to study myocardial metabolism. Acetate labeled with ^{11}C has recently emerged as a promising tracer of overall oxidative metabolism. The myocardial uptake and clearance of ^{11}C acetate is directly related to regional myocardial oxidative metabolism under diverse loading conditions and levels of blood flow. Unlike ^{11}C palmitate and FDG, the myocardial kinetics of ^{11}C acetate are relatively insensitive to changes in the substrate environment (Figure 15-31).

Detection of viable myocardium. Under conditions of glucose loading, a relative excess of myocardial FDG, compared with perfusion, is indicative of viable ischemic myocardium (Figure 15-32). Persistence of metabolic activity (demonstrated by PET with FDG) occurs in up to 50% of ^{201}Tl myocardial perfusion defects, defined as fixed on 1- and 4-hour imaging. However, the percentage of fixed myocardial perfusion lesions on 1- and 4-hour ^{201}Tl imaging that demonstrate accumulation of FDG is similar to the

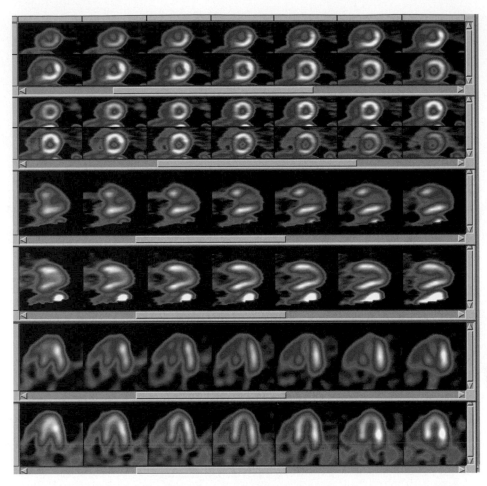

Figure 15-30 A 68-year-old asymptomatic obese male with a history of smoking, hypertension, and hyperlipidemia and a family history of heart disease had a rest/stress dipyridamole ^{82}Rb PET study. The images show severe apical, anterior, and septal defects during stress and a normal perfusion pattern at rest, indicating severe ischemia and high-grade occlusion of the left anterior descending (LAD) coronary artery. Angiography showed a 95% proximal LAD lesion, which was treated with stent placement. (Courtesy J. Machac, MD, Mount Sinai School of Medicine.)

percentage of segments with fixed defects that ultimately show improvement with ^{201}Tl re-injection. Although thallium imaging is very useful for the detection of viable myocardium, FDG imaging appears to be slightly more sensitive in patients with severely depressed ejection fractions (LVEF <30%). A general method for cardiac imaging with FDG is outlined in Table 15-8.

IMAGING OF MYOCARDIAL NECROSIS

Acute Infarct Imaging

Two agents have been proposed for the imaging of acute myocyte necrosis: ^{99m}Tc pyrophosphate and indium-111 (^{111}In) antimyosin. Myocardial infarction (irreversible damage) occurs when a zone of heart muscle is deprived of an adequate supply of oxygen for longer than 15 minutes. Infarction usually occurs when an artery becomes occluded by a clot. A clot usually forms at the site of an atheromatous lesion that has ruptured, releasing thrombogenic material into the blood. The sudden cessation of perfusion usually is associated with typical symptoms and ECG changes. In the

process of irreversible damage, the cell membrane of the myocardial cell (myocyte) loses its integrity, becomes permeable to macromolecules or charged substances that ordinarily are confined to the interior of the cell, and finally develops microscopic holes. The loss of integrity of the cellular envelope leads to loss of the intracellular contents into the surrounding extracellular fluid; this is detectable as elevations of serum enzymes such as creatine phosphokinase (CPK), lactate dehydrogenase (LDH), and a number of other substances such as troponin and myoglobin. In the emergency room, elevations of these markers usually are used as indicators of acute necrosis because the assays can be done quickly, often at the bedside. Cell necrosis causes local inflammation (arising from the irritation caused by leakage of these unusual substances into the extracellular environment); this is followed by infiltration of the area with white blood cells, which ingest the debris, and finally by the presence of fibroblasts, which produce the fibrous tissue (scar) that replaces the dead myocytes.

Increased permeability of the cell membrane not only allows substances usually confined to the cell to escape but also allows substances that are ordinarily excluded from the

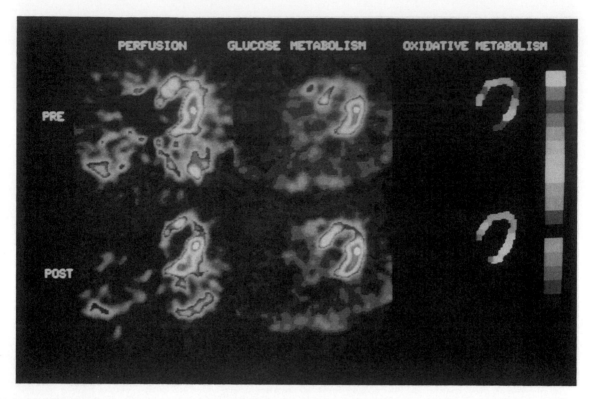

Figure 15-31 Midventricular PET images of myocardial perfusion and metabolism in a patient with an anterior myocardial infarction that contained nonviable myocardium, before and after coronary artery bypass surgery. Images of relative perfusion are at left, and those depicting relative glucose metabolism are shown in the middle. Images on the right reflect regional differences in myocardial oxidative metabolism, as measured with the ^{11}C acetate clearance technique. White represents peak activity, and black represents lowest activity. Orientation in images is the septum to the left and the anterior structures on top. Before surgery (*top row*), myocardial perfusion and glucose metabolism were concordantly reduced in the anterior wall compared with values in the functionally normal posterolateral wall. Moreover, myocardial oxidative metabolism in the anterior wall was severely depressed, to approximately 30% to 40% of that in the normal posterolateral wall. After coronary artery bypass grafting (*bottom row*), regional myocardial perfusion, glucose metabolism, and oxidative metabolism in the anterior wall remain diminished compared with normal myocardium.

cell to enter. In the case of pyrophosphate, the cell loses its ability to regulate the amount of calcium. Extracellular calcium enters the cell, establishing a condition similar to that found when bone is formed. If ^{99m}Tc-labeled pyrophosphate is administered at that time, it localizes in the zone of necrosis. Conditions that lead to localization of pyrophosphate start to occur within hours of the onset of occlusion and persist for about 8 to 10 days. Thereafter little localization of pyrophosphate occurs.

An alternative, elegant approach to the detection of acute necrosis uses an antibody raised against the heavy chain of cardiac myosin. One of the least soluble elements in the myocyte is the heavy chain of cardiac myosin, a key protein of the heart's contractile apparatus. When the cell membrane is intact, antimyosin antibody cannot come in contact with its antigen, and no localization occurs in the heart. Loss of cell membrane integrity in irreversibly damaged cells permits antimyosin to enter the damaged cell and combine with the antigen, resulting in localization in areas of acute necrosis. Antimyosin antibody is administered as an Fab fragment, which has a blood clearance half-time of 10 to 12 hours compared with about 18 to 20 hours for the intact antibody. The antibody fragment is labeled with ^{111}In using

a bifunctional chelate. Localization of antimyosin can be seen within hours of occlusion and occurs in most patients with acute infarction if the antibody is administered within 10 to 14 days of the event. Thereafter the incidence of localization decreases, such that after 9 months, patients with acute infarction rarely localize antimyosin at the site of necrosis.

Although imaging with these agents provides definitive information about the site and extent of acute necrosis, these procedures are rarely used for clinical purposes because other, less expensive approaches, such as serial electrocardiograms and serum enzymes, provide similar information.

^{99m}Tc Pyrophosphate

Data recording. No special patient preparation is required. ^{99m}Tc pyrophosphate is administered intravenously in a dose of 20 mCi between 12 hours and 10 days after the suspected acute event. Images are recorded 4 to 6 hours after injection to minimize the possibility of residual radiopharmaceutical in the blood pool. Planar and SPECT images are recorded; planar images are recorded for at least 500,000 counts with

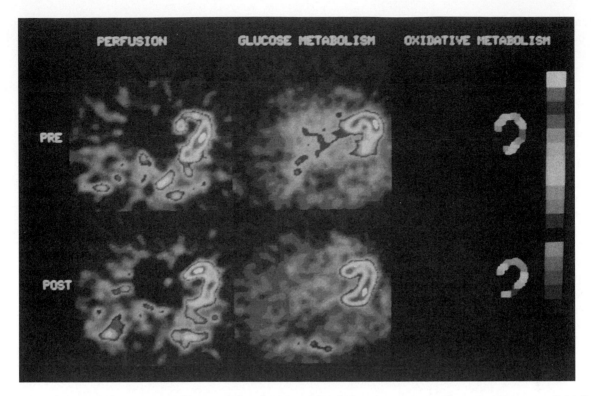

Figure 15-32 Midventricular PET images of myocardial perfusion and metabolism in a patient with an anterior myocardial infarction that contained viable myocardium, before and after coronary artery bypass surgery. Before revascularization, glucose metabolism in the anterior wall was increased relative to that in the normal posterolateral wall. With anterior wall hypoperfusion, this finding indicates augmented glucose metabolism relative to flow (metabolism-flow mismatch). After coronary artery bypass grafting, regional myocardial perfusion, glucose metabolism, and oxidative metabolism in the anterior wall are comparable with values in normal myocardium.

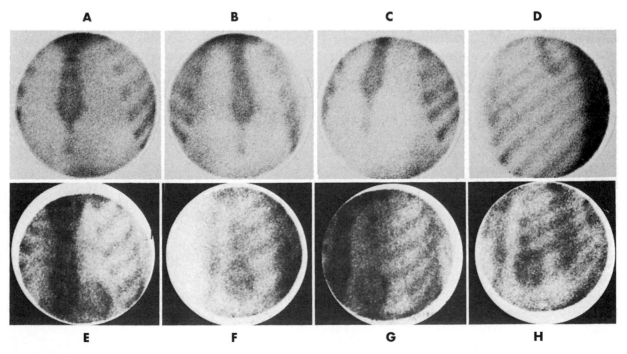

Figure 15-33 Normal ^{99m}Tc pyrophosphate myocardial images. **A**, Anterior. **B**, RAO. **C**, LAO. **D**, Left lateral. An abnormal concentration of radiopharmaceutical is seen in the anterior (**E**), left lateral (**F**), 40-degree LAO (**G**), and 70-degree LAO (**H**) views.

a high-resolution or all-purpose parallel hole collimator in at least four positions: anterior, 30-degree RAO, 45-degree LAO, and left lateral (Figure 15-33). The ribs and sternum provide anatomic landmarks but also can be sources of difficulty for detection of small sites of necrosis. SPECT imaging is particularly helpful for visualizing small or faint focal areas of myocardial ^{99m}Tc pyrophosphate uptake despite normal thoracic cage activity.

Data analysis. The images usually are interpreted subjectively by comparing the intensity of the lesion with rib and sternal intensity. Zones of increased activity in the region of the myocardium that are seen on at least two views are considered significant.

Studies have shown that some patients have a persistently positive scan result long after myocardial infarction. Occasionally such uptake reflects the formation of a ventricular aneurysm or continued ischemia of the surviving tissue. In other cases the cause of this phenomenon is unknown, but it usually signifies a poor prognosis. The intensity of uptake in these patients typically is low, and the radiopharmaceutical uptake can diffusely involve the myocardium or may be concentrated in the area of previous damage.

SUGGESTED READINGS

Beller GA: *Clinical nuclear cardiology,* Philadelphia, 1995, WB Saunders.

Bergmann SR: Quantification of myocardial perfusion with positron emission tomography. In Bergmann SR, Sobel BE, editors: *Positron emission tomography of the heart,* Mount Kisco, NY, 1992, Futura.

Gerson MC, editor: *Cardiac nuclear medicine,* ed 2, New York, 1991, McGraw-Hill.

Goris ML, Bretille JA: *Colour atlas of nuclear cardiology,* London, 1992, Chapman & Hall.

Heart facts, Dallas, 1996, American Heart Association.

Wackers F, Soufer R, Zaret BL: Nuclear cardiology. In Braunwald EB, editor: *Heart disease,* ed 5, 1996, WB Saunders.

Zaret BL, Beller GA, editors: *Nuclear cardiology: state of the art and future directions,* St Louis, 1993, Mosby.

Zipes DP: Specific arrhythmias: diagnosis and treatment. In Braunwald EB, editor: *Heart disease: a textbook of cardiovascular medicine,* Philadelphia, 1984, WB Saunders.

Leon S. Malmud

Gastrointestinal System

Objectives

Diagram and describe the organs and structures of the gastrointestinal system.

Describe the physiology of the gastrointestinal system, including the esophagus, stomach, liver, hepatobiliary collecting system and gallbladder, small intestine, and large intestine.

Describe the technique for parotid imaging.

Describe various techniques for evaluating esophageal transit using computerized regions of interest studies.

Discuss gastroesophageal reflux procedures and imaging techniques for esophageal reflux, pulmonary aspiration, and calculation of a gastroesophageal reflux index.

Explain the clinical aspects of performing radionuclide gastric emptying studies.

Diagram the hepatobiliary system (e.g., common duct, cystic duct, gallbladder, and bile duct).

Describe the procedure for liver and spleen scintigraphy using colloidal materials.

Describe imaging procedures using labeled red cells to detect hepatic hemangioma.

Discuss imaging procedures for the hepatobiliary system and identification of cholecystitis.

Explain procedures that can be used for the determination of enterogastric reflux.

Differentiate the advantages of sulfur colloid imaging from labeled red cell imaging for the identification of gastrointestinal bleeding.

Describe the principles of performing breath test studies with ^{14}C-labeled compounds.

The gastrointestinal system consists of the gastrointestinal tract, or alimentary canal, and several accessory organs. The alimentary canal is a continuous tube running through the ventral body cavity; it originates at the mouth and is followed by the pharynx, esophagus, stomach, small intestine, and large intestine (Figure 16-1).

The purpose of the alimentary canal is to provide a route of intake for nourishment, to digest and absorb nutrients, and to eliminate waste products. For the purpose of this chapter, the accessory organs involved are the salivary glands, pancreas, liver, and gallbladder. Although not a part of the gastrointestinal system, the spleen is mentioned, but only its morphology is considered.

A variety of radionuclide techniques are available for evaluation of the gastrointestinal tract, including techniques for imaging specific organs and those that

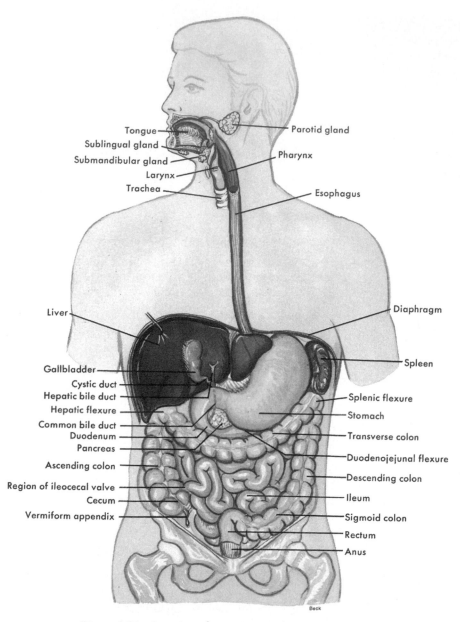

Tongue
Sublingual gland
Submandibular gland
Larynx
Trachea

Parotid gland
Pharynx
Esophagus

Liver
Gallbladder
Cystic duct
Hepatic bile duct
Hepatic flexure
Common bile duct
Duodenum
Pancreas
Ascending colon
Region of ileocecal valve
Cecum
Vermiform appendix

Diaphragm
Spleen
Splenic flexure
Stomach
Transverse colon
Duodenojejunal flexure
Descending colon
Ileum
Sigmoid colon
Rectum
Anus

Beck

Figure 16-1 Location of gastrointestinal system organs.

characterize function. In this chapter, methodologies are described in detail for procedures used to study the movement of luminal contents in the gastrointestinal tract. These techniques take advantage of the unique features offered by the use of radiotracers in the study of physiologic processes; that is, they permit quantitative measurement of gastrointestinal function but do not disturb the process under study. The newer methodologies include evaluation of the swallowing function and esophageal transit, detection and quantitation of gastroesophageal reflux, measurement of gastric emptying, and qualitative and quantitative evaluation of gallbladder function and enterogastric reflux. Other techniques include detection of pulmonary aspiration and ^{14}C breath testing. Techniques that long have enjoyed clinical acceptance, such as colloid liver and spleen scanning, gas-

trointestinal bleeding studies, and salivary gland imaging, are also reviewed in detail.

SALIVARY GLANDS

The salivary glands consist of three paired exocrine glands that produce saliva. Saliva, a fluid that initiates the chemical breakdown of food, is continuously secreted into the mouth. The primary set of salivary glands is the parotid glands, which are located in the cheeks, below and in front of the ears (see Figure 16-1). The parotid glands empty into the oral cavity through Stensen's ducts. The second pair of salivary glands is the submandibular glands, which are located beneath the tongue in the posterior aspect of the floor of the mouth; these empty directly into the oral

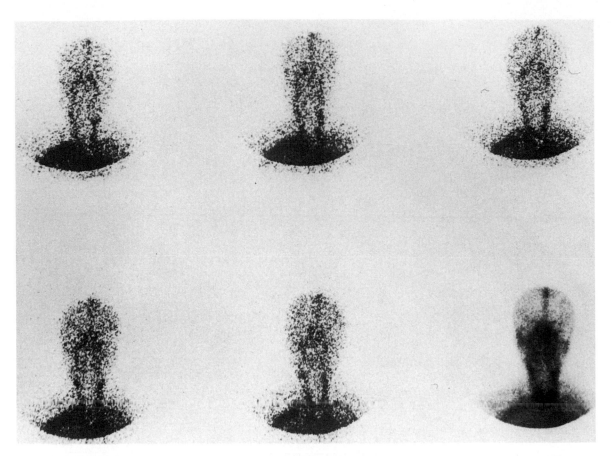

Figure 16-2   Rapid sequential images of the head and neck in the anterior projection at 2-second intervals. There is symmetric perfusion with simultaneous and rapid localization in the salivary glands.

cavity. The third pair of sublingual glands is also located beneath the tongue and is anterior to the submandibular glands.

Salivary gland imaging, also known as nuclear sialography,[31] is used primarily to determine the size, location, and function of the salivary glands.

The salivary glands indiscriminately trap a number of ions, among them the iodides and the technetium-99m (^{99m}Tc) pertechnetate ion. Also, these ions are actively excreted by the glands into the saliva. Hence, the production and excretion of saliva can be evaluated using ^{99m}Tc pertechnetate.

The indications for salivary gland imaging include detection and evaluation of mass lesions involving the salivary glands and evaluation of the symptom of dryness of the mouth, or *xerostomia*. Xerostomia is a difficult clinical symptom to assess, because it may have a psychosomatic origin. However, the possibility must be considered that the xerostomia is caused by blockage of one or several of the salivary gland ducts by a benign or neoplastic mass. Xerostomia is also an important feature and often a presenting complaint in several systemic disease complexes, notably the collagen-vascular diseases, particularly Sjögren's syndrome.[31] Xerostomia can also be associated with thyroiditis and should be taken into account in the interpretation of salivary gland images. Xerostomia occurs in sarcoidosis, after

radiation therapy to the head and neck, during states of dehydration, and as a result of administration of certain drugs and pharmacologic agents.

Imaging Procedure

No patient preparation is necessary. Rinsing of the mouth before the examination may reduce pertechnetate excretion into the oral cavity. The patient is seated comfortably facing the scintillation camera. The camera is peaked for ^{99m}Tc with a 20% energy window and fitted with a low-energy parallel hole collimator. To prevent superimposition of the thyroid gland on the salivary glands, the patient's head should be tilted backward with the neck extended as far as possible, allowing the chin to make contact with the camera face.

^{99m}Tc pertechnetate (1 to 5 mCi) is administered intravenously after the patient has been properly positioned. Rapid sequential anterior images of the face and neck are obtained at 1- to 2-second intervals (Figure 16-2). These should demonstrate simultaneous and symmetric uptake of the radiotracer in the parotid, submandibular, and sublingual glands. Thereafter, the study often is useful for obtaining anterior and lateral views of the head and neck (Figure 16-3) to confirm the normal presence of radiotracer in the saliva in the oral cavity.

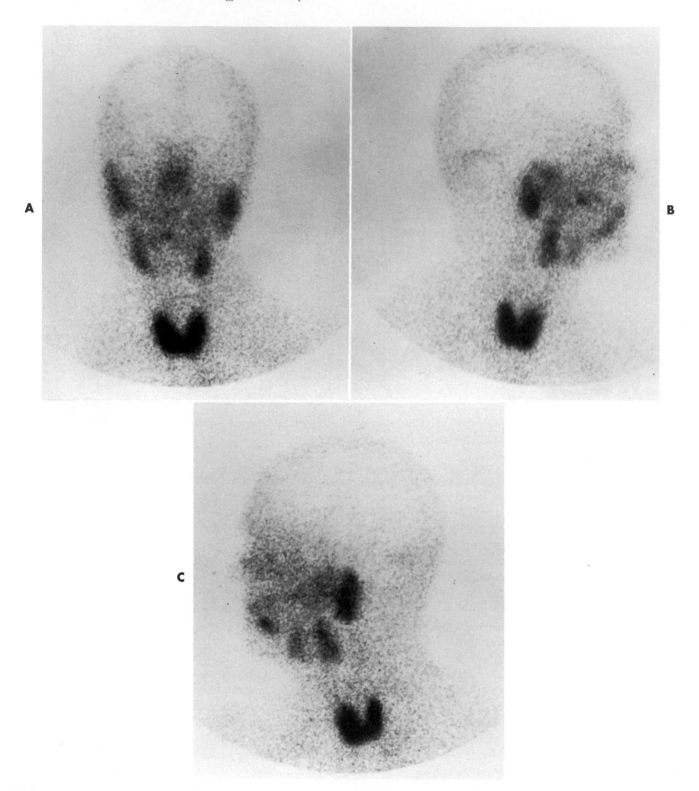

Figure 16-3   **A,** Anterior view of the head 15 minutes after injection. Normal salivary glands display homogenous distribution of ^{99m}Tc pertechnetate. Localization is symmetric in the parotid, submandibular, and sublingual glands. Uptake is also seen in the thyroid gland. **B,** Right lateral view of the head and neck. **C,** Left lateral view of the head and neck. The parotid and submandibular glands are seen particularly well in these lateral views.

It may be useful at this point to test the salivary gland response to gustatory stimulation.[4] A 1:1 dilution of commercial lemon juice (pH approximately 2.6) may be used; alternatively, fresh-squeezed lemon juice diluted equally with tap water may be substituted. The patient is instructed to take a mouthful of the lemon juice solution, swish it throughout the mouth for approximately 5 seconds, and then expectorate fully into a disposable beaker. The patient may then be repositioned in front of the camera and imaged for an additional 20 minutes. In normal individuals a rapid, symmetric, and profound diminution in radiotracer localization in the salivary glands usually is seen (Figure 16-4).

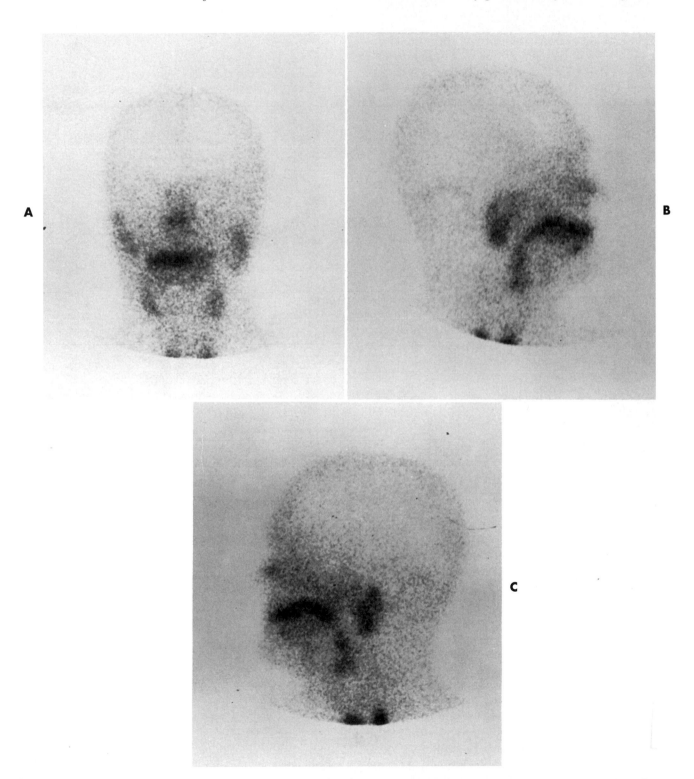

Figure 16-4   Anterior (**A**), right lateral (**B**), and left lateral (**C**) views of the head 20 minutes after oral administration of dilute lemon juice. Rapid, symmetric, and profound diminution of radiotracer localization in the salivary glands has occurred. Compared with Figure 16-3, most of the activity is now in the oral cavity.

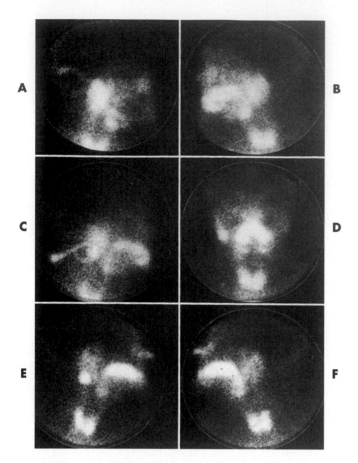

Figure 16-5 Warthin's tumor of the right parotid gland. Immediate right (**A**) and left lateral (**B**) views. **C,** Delayed right lateral view with radioactive string marker around palpable nodule. One-hour delayed views taken in the anterior (**D**), right (**E**), and left lateral (**F**) positions.

Prior administration of perchlorate should be avoided, because it would partly block salivary gland uptake of the radiotracer.

The estimated radiation dose to the normal parotid gland is 0.6 rad/mCi of ^{99m}Tc pertechnetate.

Clinical Aspects

Normally, simultaneous, rapid, and symmetric localization of the radiotracer occurs in all three pairs of salivary glands (see Figure 16-2), with homogeneous distribution of the pertechnetate (see Figure 16-3). It originally was hoped that this examination could be used to discern a wide variety of mass lesions in the salivary glands, but this has not been the case. Only two types of neoplasm have a consistent appearance on nuclear sialography: Warthin's tumors, which appear as focal areas of increased uptake (Figure 16-5), and metastatic lesions, which are characteristically cold focal areas. Benign mixed tumors of the salivary glands may appear as focal areas of increased or decreased uptake. Focal cold areas are seen with other types of malignancy, cysts, some mixed tumors, enlarged lymph nodes, and inflamma-

tory diseases. Decreased or absent uptake in a single gland or set of glands may be seen in congenital aplasia or obstructive sialolithiasis and after sialectomy, trauma, or radiotherapy. In Sjögren's syndrome and other types of vascular and connective tissue diseases, either asymmetric arrival of the radiotracer in the salivary glands is seen, or radiotracer uptake in the salivary glands is delayed compared with radiotracer uptake in the thyroid. On delayed images, bilaterally decreased uptake can be seen in these diseases, and a response after administration of a gustatory stimulant may be absent or blunted.[4] Bilaterally decreased uptake in the salivary glands can also be seen in acute suppurative parotitis and multicentric sialoangiectasis and in some aged individuals.

Poor response to gustatory stimulation is seen in the systemic connective tissue diseases, acute parotitis (mumps), and after radiotherapy of the head and neck. If a single salivary gland or group of salivary glands fails to excrete, this is suggestive of stenosis or blockage of the salivary duct.

Despite lack of anatomic detail, salivary gland imaging plays a useful clinical role in the evaluation of certain morphologic and functional diseases. In some situations contrast sialography can differentiate neoplasm from inflammation, benign from malignant masses, and extrinsic from intrinsic masses.

OROPHARYNX

The oropharynx lies posterior to the mouth and is a complex organ composed of numerous small muscles, cartilage, and tendons. Because the oropharynx functions in both a respiratory and digestive capacity, its components must function in a coordinated manner to accept food from the mouth and propel it from the esophagus while suspending respiration. Although radiographic studies of swallowing have been in use for some time, they are accompanied by a relatively high radiation burden and do not readily provide quantitative information of the swallowing function. Because radionuclide studies generally are very sensitive and provide information that is both physiologic and quantitative in nature, the radionuclide oropharyngeal study was developed as a method of measuring clearance of liquids from the oropharynx. This technique may be combined with esophageal transit and gastroesophageal reflux studies.

Imaging Procedure

Cold tap water (10 ml) is mixed with 1 mCi of ^{99m}Tc sulfur colloid by shaking for 30 seconds immediately before this study. A liquid sample of approximately 10 ml is used, because this volume is easily swallowed as a bolus.

A large field of view scintillation camera fitted with a high-sensitivity collimator is used. Images should be acquired on a computer. The patient is seated erect in front of the camera in the anterior position with the neck rotated to the left. The right cheek is positioned at the surface of the collimator, as is the chest, such that a right lateral view of

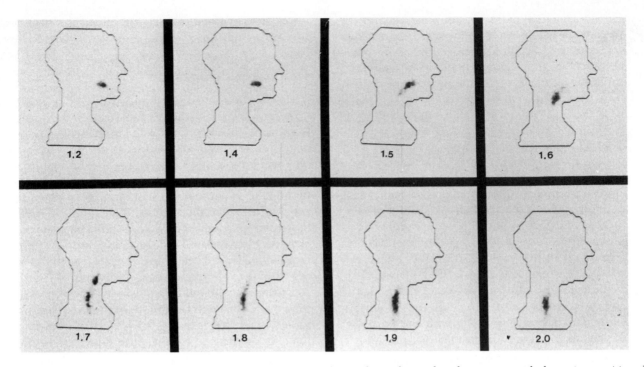

Figure 16-6 Normal oropharyngeal 0.1-second images obtained on-line and stored on a digital computer with the patient positioned with the right side of the face at the surface of the collimator.

the mouth and oropharynx and an anterior view of the chest are obtained.

The patient is instructed to sip the fluid through a straw and to hold the entire amount of the material in the mouth. On command the patient is instructed to swallow all the material at once. It may be useful to review the procedure with the patient using sips of plain water before administration of the test dose. After swallowing the radiopharmaceutical, the patient is instructed to dry swallow every 15 seconds on command. The patient should breathe quietly through the nose during the remainder of the study.

Images are acquired for 5 minutes in the computer for subsequent analysis. The initial 30 seconds of the examination are acquired at 0.1 sec/frame, and the following 270 seconds are acquired at 15 sec/frame (Figure 16-6).

Images for the first 30 seconds are added by the computer to yield a composite image for anatomic definition of the oropharynx. From this summed image a manually outlined region of interest is drawn and stored in the computer. The region of interest is used to generate a time-activity curve from the raw data. The time-activity curve, representing the oropharyngeal count rate, is fitted to a biexponential clearance model, which consists of fast- and slow-clearing components (Figure 16-7), each associated with an amplitude and half-life.

Clinical Aspects

This radionuclide imaging procedure is useful for documenting the swallowing function and pharyngeal transit time. The test may be useful to document and quantify

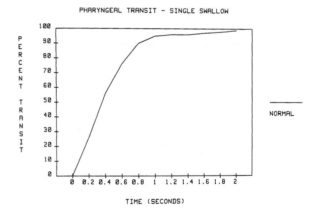

Figure 16-7 Normal time-activity curve representing oropharyngeal function. Function is biexponential with a fast- and slow-clearing component.

abnormalities of the swallowing function in patients in whom no demonstrable abnormality can be seen either by direct inspection or by other methods, such as the barium swallow. A prolonged high-amplitude slow component appears to be characteristic of an abnormal swallowing function.

ESOPHAGUS

The esophagus is a muscular tube extending from the pharynx to the stomach. Its function is to transport a swallowed food bolus from the pharynx to the stomach, which is accomplished by coordinated contractions of its muscular layers, termed *peristalsis*. The esophagus is located posterior to the trachea in the thorax and in its resting state remains collapsed (see Figure 16-1).

The esophagus is slightly narrowed, or pinched, just above the stomach as it passes through the respiratory diaphragm. This narrowing, along with the muscular layer of the diaphragm, constitutes the physiologic lower esophageal sphincter, or gastroesophageal sphincter. Proper relaxation of the lower esophageal sphincter is necessary to allow the passage of the food bolus into the stomach. Incoordinate lower esophageal sphincter function has been implicated in a number of disorders that affect esophageal transit, as well as in gastroesophageal reflux.

Esophageal Transit

Radionuclide esophageal transit studies[13] are useful as a noninvasive screening test for suspected disorders of esophageal motility. Usually an individual with dysphagia (any difficulty or discomfort associated with swallowing) has a more conventional examination, such as a barium swallow or endoscopy, before or after a radionuclide examination. Scintigraphic studies do not provide information about anatomic detail, and more conventional examinations must be performed to exclude any structural lesions. Scintigraphic studies are more sensitive for detecting esophageal motor disorders and provide quantitative information.

In the act of swallowing, a bolus of solid or liquid food moves through the length of the esophagus by the forces of peristalsis and gravity. This movement is defined as esophageal transit, different from esophageal clearance, which refers to the emptying from the esophagus of refluxed material from the stomach.

Difficulty or discomfort associated with swallowing can be associated with anatomic lesions of the esophagus or an esophageal motor disorder. Severely painful swallowing can be associated with mucosal destruction of the esophagus from infection, reflux esophagitis, ulcerations, or tumor. Esophageal studies are also useful for evaluating patients with suspected regurgitation or aspiration pneumonias. Motility disorders of the esophagus may be the result of innate muscular or innervation disorders or can occur secondary to a systemic disease, such as a connective tissue disease. Amotility, which is seen in achalasia and scleroderma, may be a factor. Hypomotility, or decreased pressure of swallowing, can be seen in aged individuals, and hypermotility can be seen in diffuse esophageal spasm.

Imaging procedure. The patient should fast for at least 2 hours before the examination. The radiopharmaceutical is prepared by mixing 300 μCi of ^{99m}Tc sulfur colloid in 15 ml of tap water.

The patient is placed supine under the camera for an anterior view of the thorax. The camera is fitted with a high-sensitivity or low-energy all-purpose collimator and interfaced to a computer. The patient is positioned with the stomach at the bottom of the field of view. The radiophar-

maceutical is administered orally through a straw, and the patient is instructed to take the entire volume into the mouth but not to swallow until instructed to do so. The computer is started, and the patient is instructed to swallow the contents of the mouth as a single compact bolus. The patient is instructed to dry swallow every 15 seconds for the next 10 minutes. Images are acquired every 0.25 second for the first minute and at 15-second intervals for the remaining 9 minutes (Figure 16-8). At the conclusion of the study, the data are retrieved from the computer for analysis.

Currently, two methods of data analysis are used to measure esophageal transit. A global measure of esophageal emptying can be made by recording the counts present in the total esophagus after multiple swallows using a computer-generated rectangular region of interest over the entire esophagus (Figure 16-9). The count rate in the esophageal region of interest is used to determine the rate of esophageal transit according to the following formula[13]:

$$C_t = (E_{max} - E_t)/E_{max} \times 100$$

where C_t represents the esophageal transit at time t; E_{max} is the maximum count rate in the esophagus; and E_t is the esophageal count rate at time t.

The second method analyzes regional esophageal transit by dividing the esophagus into proximal, middle, and distal regions of interest. Three equal-size rectangular regions of interest are drawn. A plot of counts against time is used to describe the transit of the bolus through each esophageal region (Figure 16-10).

Clinical aspects. Esophageal activity decreases rapidly, usually within 5 to 10 seconds after the first swallow, and the activity is no longer visible (see Figure 16-8), although count rates of approximately 10% of peak activity may be found until the eighth swallow (2 minutes) (Figure 16-11). As the initial bolus passes through the esophagus, a smooth progression of sequential peaks of activity in the proximal, middle, and distal esophagus are demonstrated (see Figure 16-10). By the fortieth swallow (10 minutes), less than 5% of peak activity remains in the whole esophageal region of interest (see Figure 16-11). Using these methods, it is possible to differentiate patients with achalasia (see Figure 16-11; Figure 16-12) from those with scleroderma, because in scleroderma most of the bolus activity is able to enter the stomach, whereas in achalasia a more marked delay in esophageal emptying is seen. With diffuse esophageal spasm, the radionuclide study shows incoordinate activity, which is different from patients with nonspecific abnormalities.

The radionuclide method has demonstrated 100% sensitivity for detecting achalasia, diffuse esophageal spasm, and scleroderma. Radionuclide esophageal transit studies can also be useful in the evaluation of esophageal strictures and esophageal diverticula and after radiotherapy for carcinoma of the esophagus.

A routine esophageal transit study may be combined with delayed images of the thorax in the anterior and posterior

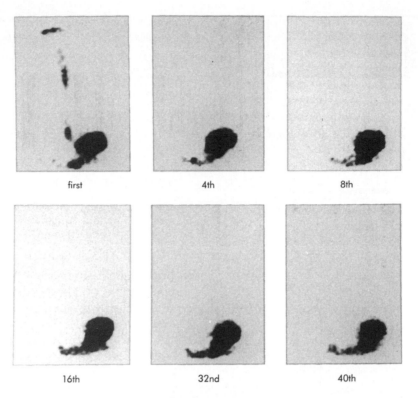

first   4th   8th

16th   32nd   40th

Multiple swallow technique—normal subject

Figure 16-8 Normal esophageal images. Images of the esophagus are acquired in the anterior projection at the initial swallow and then every 15 seconds with each "dry swallow" for the next 10 minutes. Individual images are shown for the initial swallow, first, fourth, eighth, sixteenth, thirty-second, and fortieth swallows. Images are acquired on-line, stored on a digital computer, and later retrieved for analysis. NOTE: In normal subjects, no activity is seen in the esophagus after the initial swallow.

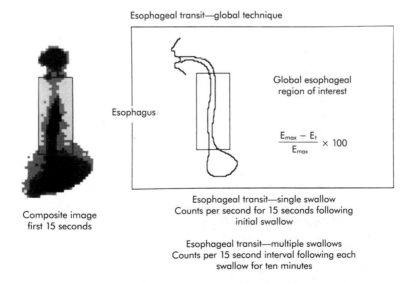

Esophageal transit—global technique

Esophagus

Global esophageal region of interest

$$\frac{E_{max} - E_t}{E_{max}} \times 100$$

Composite image
first 15 seconds

Esophageal transit—single swallow
Counts per second for 15 seconds following
initial swallow

Esophageal transit—multiple swallows
Counts per 15 second interval following each
swallow for ten minutes

Figure 16-9   The esophageal region of interest when esophageal transit is measured as a global function.

projections for the detection of aspirated radionuclide. Delayed images of the thorax can be particularly useful in an adult patient with nonspecific pulmonary symptoms in whom the diagnosis of pulmonary aspiration is often difficult to confirm. Overnight pulmonary aspiration of a radionuclide from the stomach, when demonstrable, is seen as a highly specific, though insensitive, method for detecting this disorder (Figure 16-13). Unfortunately, a pulmonary aspiration scan result can be negative, even in patients with clear symptoms.

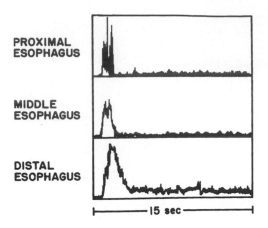

Figure 16-10 Normal esophageal transit. Three equal-size rectangular regions of interest are used to generate time-activity curves through each of three esophageal regions.

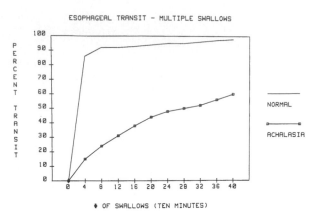

Figure 16-11 Time-activity curves of percentage transit versus the number of swallows for 10 minutes. Both a normal individual (patient in Figure 16-8) and a patient with achalasia (patient in Figure 16-12) are illustrated.

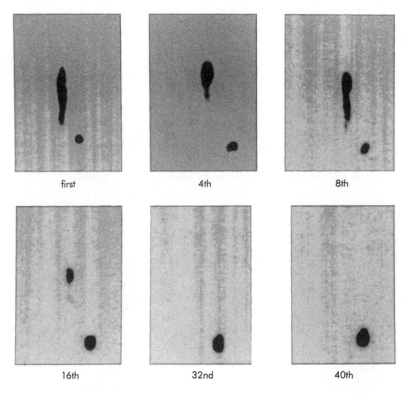

Multiple swallow technique in a patient with achalasia

Figure 16-12 Anterior views of the esophagus in a patient with achalasia. Note poor passage of liquid bolus in the esophagus (retention) despite repeated "dry swallows." Percentage transit is illustrated in Figure 16-11.

Gastroesophageal Reflux

Gastroesophageal reflux refers to the symptom complex of heartburn, regurgitation, and chest pain. Esophageal reflux occurs when either gastric or duodenal contents enter the esophagus. Some of the anatomic abnormalities that can result in incompetence of the lower esophageal sphincter and symptomatic gastroesophageal reflux include enlargement of the diaphragmatic hiatus, disruption of the phrenoesophageal ligament, loss of the acute cardioesophageal angle of Hiss, loss of the gastric mucosal rosette, and a change in the distal paraesophageal pressure from an intraabdominal to an intrathoracic level. In short, lower esophageal sphincter incompetence must be present for acid reflux to occur.

A number of nonradionuclide studies are available for the detection of gastroesophageal reflux, including barium esophagography, barium cine-swallow, endoscopy, mucosal biopsy, manometry, acid-perfusion, clearance, and reflux testing. Of these available studies, none is as sensitive as gas-

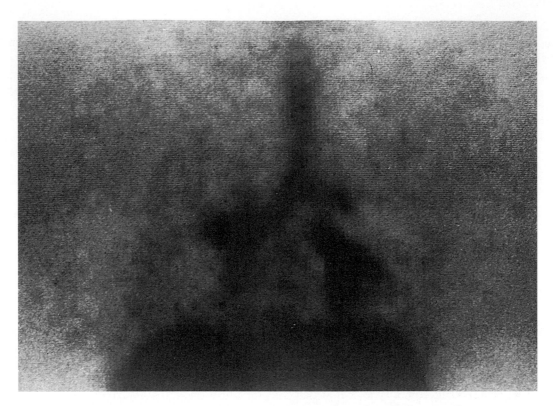

Figure 16-13 Pulmonary aspiration. Anterior view of the thorax obtained 24 hours after instillation of ^{99m}Tc sulfur colloid into the stomach via nasogastric tube. Activity is seen in the trachea, bronchi, and peripheral lung fields, indicating overnight aspiration of gastric contents.

troesophageal scintigraphy in the detection of reflux.[13,25] Furthermore, only gastroesophageal scintigraphy is quantitative and can be used both to determine the severity of reflux and to evaluate the patient's response to therapy.

The clinical significance of minimal degrees of esophageal reflux is questionable at best. It has been suggested that diminished muscle tone in the lower esophagus, rather than hiatal hernia, is the cause of most reflux.[29] Simple, inexpensive regimens, such as the use of antacids and changes in the diet to include more protein, may resolve symptoms in most patients (only 5% of whom may eventually require surgery). Small degrees of reflux are hardly grounds for surgery, and a trial of therapy (known to be innocuous) can satisfy both patient and referring physician much more than the results of complicated diagnostic tests.[7]

Anatomically, the gastroesophageal sphincter of the distal esophagus has not been convincingly demonstrated. The concept of a physiologic sphincter is based on the fact that the proximal esophagus functions differently from the distal esophagus. The upper third of the esophagus has striated muscle, and the remaining two thirds consists of smooth muscle. The body of the esophagus contracts in response to swallowing, during which time the lower esophageal sphincter relaxes. This reciprocity of esophageal function, proximally versus distally, constitutes evidence for a physiologic sphincter mechanism. Many esophageal disorders disrupt neural and muscular mechanisms that control this normal sphincter activity.

Fat, alcohol, chocolate, and cigarette smoking are some of the factors that commonly cause depression of the lower esophageal sphincter pressure, and these have also been associated with symptomatic gastroesophageal reflux. Consequences of recurring gastroesophageal reflux are esophagitis, unrelenting heartburn, and eventual dysphagia. Often these symptoms are associated with abnormalities in esophageal clearance, and it may be beneficial routinely to perform esophageal and gastroesophageal scintigraphic studies as a single examination.

Imaging procedure. The patient must fast at least 8 hours before the examination; then, the esophageal transit study should be performed first. This allows the technologist to note all the obvious abnormalities that can impair esophageal clearance. After these data for the esophagus have been stored for later processing, the gastroesophageal reflux study may be performed.

The patient is given an oral solution containing 300 µCi of ^{99m}Tc sulfur colloid mixed with 150 ml of orange juice and 150 ml of 0.1 normal hydrochloric acid. The entire 300 ml of solution should be administered, because this volume of liquid in the stomach opposes induced abdominal pressure. The patient then is fitted with an abdominal binder similar to a large blood pressure cuff (Baum-Velcro Abdominal Binder). The patient is positioned supine under the camera, and the abdominal binder is readjusted so that the inflatable bladder within it is centered over the stomach and below the costal margin. In female patients, care should be taken not to pinch the breasts. The binder should be positioned carefully so as to induce a pressure that forces the stomach superiorly. Compression of the lower ribs should be avoided because this forces the stomach inferiorly, away from the diaphragm.

Four factors are required to successfully cause an induced reflux in a patient who is prone to gastroesophageal reflux: oral administration of an acidified solution; successive, increased applied pressure to the abdomen; maintenance of a supine position; and at least a 300 ml volume in the stomach to oppose the applied pressure.

No longer than 10 minutes after oral administration of the ^{99m}Tc sulfur colloid solution, the patient is centered under the camera so that the stomach is positioned at the bottom of the field. The entire stomach must be included on all images. As pressure is increased with the abdominal binder, the stomach image is seen to rise, but immediate repositioning is not necessary unless the esophageal region is excluded from the field of view. If activity is seen in the esophagus during positioning, either a delay in esophageal clearance or a spontaneous reflux has occurred. An additional 30 ml of tap water should clear this activity.

Use of a parallel hole collimator on a large field of view camera is best, although a diverging collimator with a small-field-of-view camera may be used. Images are acquired for 30 seconds at the following pressure points, which are obtained by inflating the abdominal binder: 0, 20, 40, 60,

80, and 100 mm Hg. A post-deflation image also is obtained. Increments of 20 mm Hg on the abdominal binder are successively applied while the sphygmomanometer attached to the binder is monitored (increments of 20 mm Hg applied externally have been shown to increase the pressure across the lower esophageal sphincter in increments of 5 mm Hg) (Figure 16-14). Images should be acquired as quickly as possible so that patient discomfort is not prolonged. It is important not to deflate the binder between successive stages of pressure. Most patients can tolerate pressure of 100 mm Hg, but it should be kept in mind that some patients cannot withstand this level because of debilitating surgery or their present symptoms.

It is best that an oscilloscope with a high persistence be used as a visual aid during the performance of the examination. Reflux can be visualized during the course of the test (Figure 16-15). Computer images might warrant adjustment of contrast in cases of subtle reflux. Subtly visualized activity in the esophagus has been shown to correspond to 3% to 4% of the 300 μCi ^{99m}Tc dose and can be used to confirm reflux. (NOTE: In patients in whom the esophageal transit study is done before the gastroesophageal reflux study, a greater amount of activity will be noted in the stomach at the beginning of the examination.)

Patients with known esophageal motor disorders or with a large hiatal hernia should have an endogastric tube placed before performance of the reflux study. In this way the radiopharmaceutical solution can be delivered into the stomach

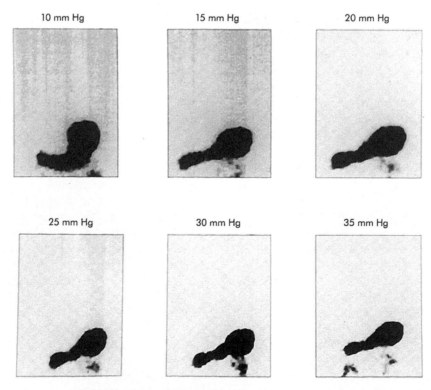

Figure 16-14 Serial scans of a gastroesophageal reflux study in a normal individual. The resting pressure across the lower esophageal sphincter is 10 mm Hg, and with each successive inflation of the abdominal binder, a corresponding pressure increase of 5 mm Hg is seen across the lower esophageal sphincter. Throughout the study no gastroesophageal reflux is visualized.

through the tube, bypassing the esophagus. The tube can be flushed with 10 to 15 ml of tap water and removed before the imaging study is begun. This technique prevents retention of activity in the esophagus, which can be related to the motor disorder or to a hiatal hernia.

Patient with reflux

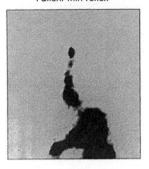

Normal subject

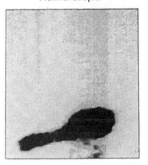

Figure 16-15 Anterior images of the thorax obtained in a patient with reflux and in a normal subject, respectively. An oscilloscope with a high persistence should be used as a visual aid during the performance of this examination, because reflux can be readily visualized on the oscilloscope face.

Computer analysis of this study is accomplished by recalling the separate images and drawing regions of interest for the stomach and esophagus (Figure 16-16). The counts in the stomach region of interest and in the esophageal region of interest are noted and used to calculate a gastroesophageal reflux index for each level of abdominal pressure using the following formula:

$$GERI = (E_p / G_{max}) \times 100$$

where *GERI* is the gastroesophageal reflux index in percent, E_p is the esophageal counts at a specific pressure point *p*, and G_{max} is the maximum gastric count obtained for one image in this study.

Clinical aspects. A normal gastroesophageal reflux study has a reflux index of less than 4%; this is the level at which gastroesophageal reflux cannot be visualized (see Figure 16-15). An index greater than 4% is considered to be abnormal and usually can be visualized in the images (Figure 16-17). This quantitative feature is unique to the scintigraphic study and permits the evaluation of patients before and after medical or surgical therapy for gastroesophageal reflux.

Delayed images of the thorax can be obtained up to 24 hours to detect reflux leading to pulmonary aspiration (see Figure 16-13). This is particularly useful in children and infants, in whom the radionuclide solution can be delivered through intubation or by placing the radiopharmaceutical in a bottle with the infant's formula or juice. Radionuclide studies are superior to barium studies for diagnosing reflux in children, not only because of the lower radiation burden, but also because reflux occurs intermittently, and fluoroscopy cannot be performed continuously because of its associated high-radiation exposure.

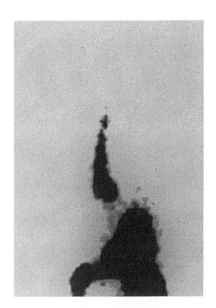

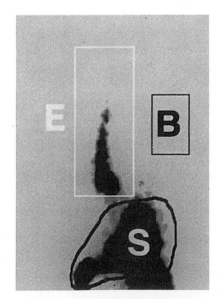

Figure 16-16 Anterior view of the thorax is recalled from the computer for analysis. Regions of interest are drawn for the esophagus (*top left*), the stomach (S), and the background (B). Counts in each region of interest are recorded for each pressure level and then used to calculate the gastroesophageal reflux indices.

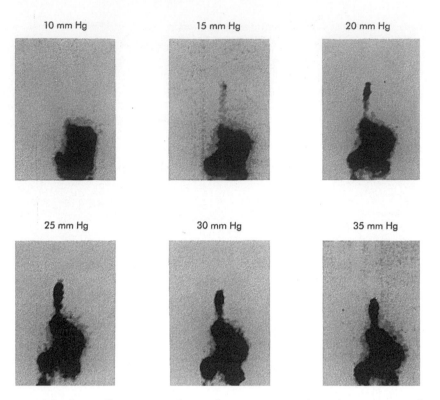

Figure 16-17 Anterior views of the thorax illustrating an abnormal examination result. With progressive inflation of the abdominal binder, causing incremental pressure increases of 5 mm Hg across the lower esophageal sphincter, an increase in the amount of induced gastroesophageal reflux is seen.

STOMACH

The stomach is a crescent-shaped, pouchlike organ that lies just below the diaphragm (Figure 16-18). Its proximal connection is the esophagus, and its distal connection is the duodenum, the first portion of the small intestine. The stomach consists of three muscular coats, and its inner surface is lined with a membrane responsible for secreting both a protective mucous layer and the hydrochloric acid used in the digestion of swallowed food particles. The stomach is divided into three anatomic regions: the fundus, the corpus (or body), and the antrum. The coordination of muscular function in the stomach is mediated by both extrinsic and intrinsic nervous pathways and is also mediated by a number of hormones (e.g., gastrin, secretin, and cholecystokinin). The proximal portion of the stomach acts as a reservoir for ingested food, and its muscular layers generate a low-level pressure gradient to propel food toward the more distal portion of the stomach. In the antrum, intense muscular contractions act to grind food particles and mix them with digestive enzymes. These contractions also propel food out of the stomach through the pyloric sphincter.

Control of gastric emptying of food depends on the meal's volume and energy density (amount of carbohydrates and fats). Hormones such as cholecystokinin and gastrin are known to inhibit gastric emptying.

Gastric emptying studies are used when standard radiographic or endoscopic examinations cannot adequately explain clinical signs and symptoms such as nausea, vomiting, abdominal fullness, distention, and weight loss. Such symptoms may be the result of mechanical obstruction by an anatomic lesion (e.g., ulceration, edema, tumor, or foreign body), or they may arise from a gastric motility disorder. Mechanical and nonmechanical causes of gastric motility disorders are summarized in Table 16-1.

With the advent of radionuclide techniques for accurate and noninvasive assessment of gastric motility, symptoms such as unexplained nausea and vomiting now can be shown to have an organic cause; furthermore, new medications have been introduced to treat disorders of gastric emptying. Emptying of both liquids and solids is significantly decreased in patients with impaired gastric emptying; rapid gastric emptying (dumping syndrome) also occurs, especially after gastric surgery. Duodenal ulcer disease, Zollinger-Ellison syndrome, Chagas' disease, and malabsorption syndromes, including pancreatic insufficiency, have been reported to increase gastric motility.

The stomach accepts a variety of both liquid and solid food, functions as a storage and mixing chamber for digestion, and then propels digested foods into the duodenum. Gastric emptying is a complex process affected by the physical and chemical composition of the ingested meal, the intrinsic and extrinsic nervous innervation of the stomach, and circulating neuroendocrine transmitters. In terms of functional gastric emptying, the stomach can be divided into the proximal region (fundus), which controls liquid emptying, and the distal region (antrum), which controls the rate

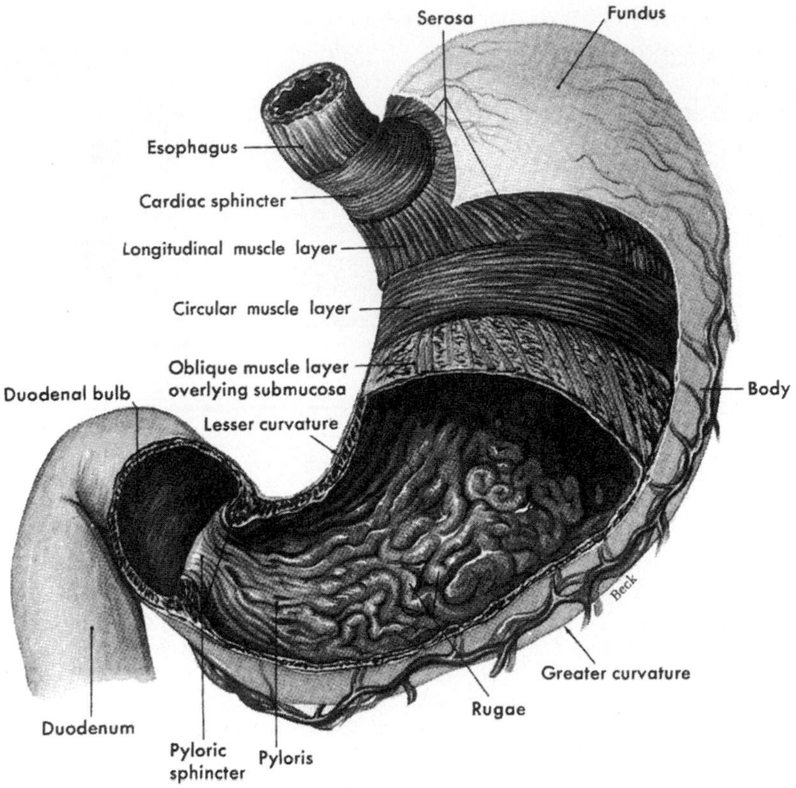

Figure 16-18   Stomach regions and structure.

| **Table 16-1** | Causes of gastric motility disorders |

Mechanical causes	Nonmechanical causes
Peptic ulceration	Metabolic causes
Duodenal ulcer	Diabetes
Pyloric channel ulcer	Uremia
	Hypotension or hypertension
	Gastrinoma
Postsurgical causes	Neurologic causes
Pyloroplasty	Vagotomy
Hemigastrectomy	Neuropathy
	Gastroparesis
Hypertrophic pyloric stenosis	Systemic diseases
	Scleroderma
	Amyloidosis
	Smooth muscle disorders
	Anorexia nervosa
Cancer of the stomach	Drug-induced causes
	Anticholinergics
	Opiates
Post-radiotherapy	
Trauma	

of emptying for solids. Tonic contractions generated in the proximal portion of the stomach produce a pressure gradient between the stomach and duodenum, forcing liquid material into the distal stomach and through the pylorus. In the distal portion of the stomach, digestible solids are churned and liquefied before leaving the stomach. Solid particles are retained in the body of the stomach until they are smaller than 1 to 2 mm. The pylorus helps break down large solid particles not ready for digestion and restricts the rate of gastric emptying while preventing reflux of duodenal contents back into the stomach.

Numerous methods[10,11,26] have been proposed for a simultaneous radionuclide study of the liquid and solid components of a meal using different radionuclide labels for the solid and liquid portions of the test meal and dual isotope counting. Because the rate of gastric emptying varies with meal size, each laboratory must standardize meal size and composition according to the amount of carbohydrate, fat, protein, nondigestible solids, and caloric content. A wide variety of meals, including meat, potatoes, porridge, pancakes, cornflakes, chicken liver, eggs, French toast, and chemical resins, have been used.[8,19,27,36] Indium-111 (^{111}In) and ^{99m}Tc are the radionuclides most often used, because they are well suited for imaging with the scintillation camera. Adequate images and good counting statistics can be achieved with small doses, and the radiation burden to the patient is kept to a minimum.[34]

The simplest approach to measurement of gastric emptying with the scintillation camera involves giving a dual

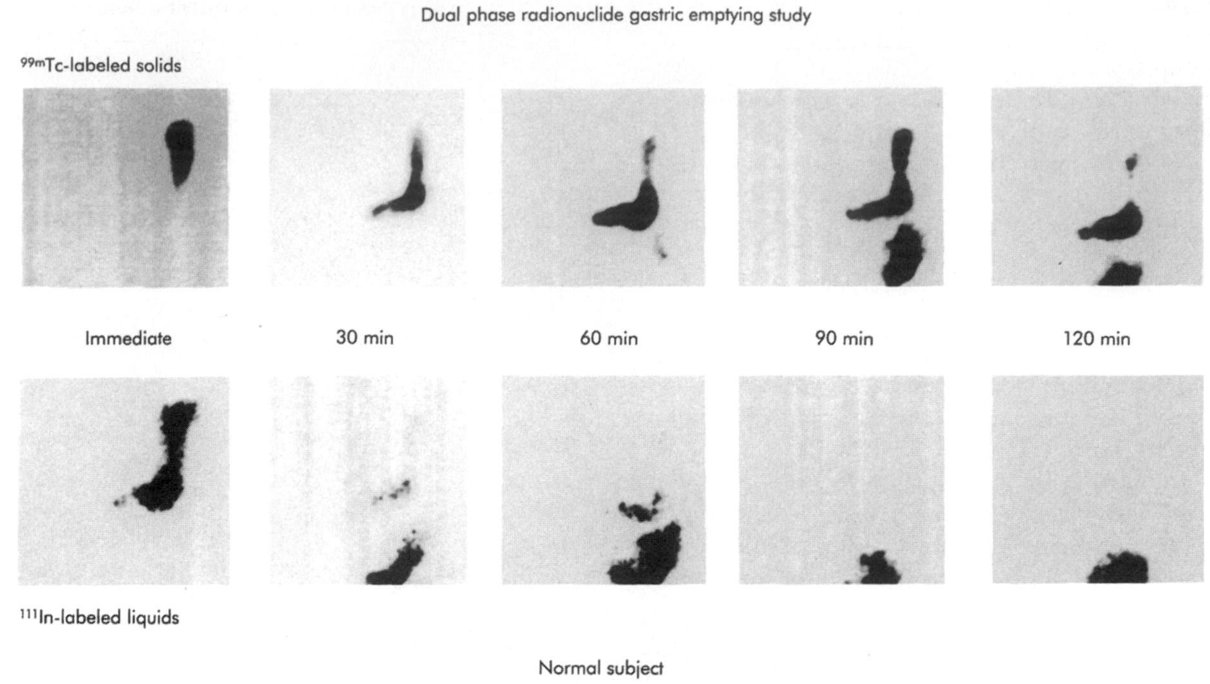

Figure 16-19   Dual isotope gastric scintigraphy. Anterior images of the abdomen obtained in a normal subject after oral administration of a scrambled egg sandwich prepared with ^{99m}Tc sulfur colloid and the liquid portion consisting of ^{111}In-DTPA in water. Images were obtained for 1 minute at 30-minute intervals at both ^{99m}Tc and ^{111}In window settings. Note the emptying of both liquids and solids from the stomach.

solid/liquid labeled test meal and serially measuring anterior count rates from the stomach with the patient either upright or supine. Corrections for attenuation, physical decay, and downscatter from ^{111}In in the ^{99m}Tc window may be necessary to measure accurately the amount of activity remaining in the stomach during the study.[10] This is particularly true in light of the fact that the examination may continue over several hours. Therefore each laboratory must perform its own phantom studies to determine the appropriate correction factors.

Imaging Procedure

In preparation for the study, the patient should fast for at least 8 hours.

A number of techniques are available for preparation of a solid test meal. Among them is in vivo labeling of chicken liver; in vitro–labeled chicken liver may also be prepared. However, a simple method that provides a stable in vivo solid label involves an egg sandwich. Two raw eggs are gently broken into a disposable beaker and are injected with 500 µCi of ^{99m}Tc sulfur colloid. The eggs are allowed to incubate for 5 minutes behind a lead shield; then they are scrambled well with a disposable stirrer and fried in an electric skillet until firm and dry. The eggs are placed between two slices of toasted white bread. The liquid portion of the meal is prepared by using 125 µCi of indium-111 diethylenetriamine pentaacetic acid (^{111}In-DTPA)[19] in 300 ml of tap water.

The patient is instructed to eat the egg sandwich within 5 minutes and then to drink the liquid portion of the meal. A large field of view camera is fitted with a medium-energy collimator and interfaced to a computer. The camera system is peaked for both ^{99m}Tc and ^{111}In using a pair of 20% energy windows. As soon as the patient finishes the radiolabeled meal, images of the abdomen are acquired in the anterior and posterior projections with the stomach in the center of the field of view. Images are acquired for 60 seconds with the camera peaked first on the technetium setting and then on the 247 keV setting of indium. The two images are repeated every 15 minutes for at least the next 2 hours for both the ^{99m}Tc and the ^{111}In windows (Figure 16-19). The study may be extended beyond 2 hours if the stomach does not appear to empty.

The stored images are retrieved from the computer, a region of interest is drawn around the stomach, and the counts are generated for each image (both the ^{99m}Tc and ^{111}In images for each 15-minute interval). The total counts for each region at each time are recorded. The ^{99m}Tc counts are corrected for radioactive decay. The geometric mean of counts (anterior × posterior) is calculated, and the technetium and indium curves are each normalized to 100%. Other correction factors may be necessary,[10] and resultant values represent the percentage of gastric retention.

The most common method for displaying gastric emptying data is to plot the normalized percentage of stomach retention for each radionuclide on linear graph paper, with the y axis representing the percentage of retained activity and the x axis representing the time elapsed at each 15-

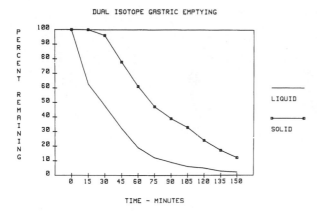

Figure 16-20 Normal dual isotope gastric emptying. Time-activity curves for both liquids and solids are graphed as percentage remaining as a function of time. Note emptying of both liquids and solids. This is the same individual as Figure 16-19.

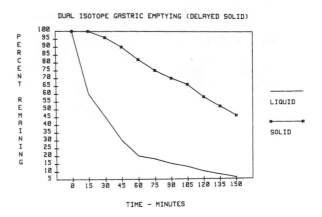

Figure 16-21 Abnormal dual isotope gastric emptying curves, generated for the patient in Figure 16-23. When compared with the normal curve study, liquids empty normally, whereas solids are delayed.

minute interval[26] (Figure 16-20). The most popular measure of gastric emptying is the half-emptying time ($t_{1/2}$), which is found by taking the 50% retention point from the plot and noting the time to reach this point. The $t_{1/2}$ emptying times for liquids and solids may be compared among groups of patients and between one series of examinations and another. However, the $t_{1/2}$ emptying time does not fully characterize the complex process of gastric emptying, and other methods have been described to characterize the entire pattern of gastric emptying.

Clinical Aspects

Detection of abnormally delayed or rapid emptying of liquids or solids depends on the test meal used. Patient data, therefore, are most conveniently displayed by superimposition on a normal plot for that particular test meal. For the test meal previously described, liquids may be expected to have a $t_{1/2}$ ranging from 10 to 45 minutes and a $t_{1/2}$ for solids ranging from 60 to 105 minutes (see Figure 16-20). The overall appearance of the emptying curves may be more useful in the detection of abnormalities than simple $t_{1/2}$ emptying times (Figures 16-21 and 16-22).

Abnormally delayed emptying of solids and liquids may be seen in peptic ulceration, diabetic gastroparesis, scleroderma, amyloidosis and smooth muscle disorders and after radiotherapy (Figures 16-23 and 16-24). Rapid emptying of solids and liquids may be seen after gastric and duodenal surgery and in Zollinger-Ellison syndrome, duodenal ulcer disease, and some malabsorption syndromes. A variety of medications also cause rapid gastric emptying.

PANCREAS

The pancreas is an oblong gland, 13 cm long and 3 cm thick (see Figure 16-1), that lies behind the stomach. Its proximal portion abuts the duodenum, and its more distal portion, the tail, is nestled in the splenic hilum. The pancreas'

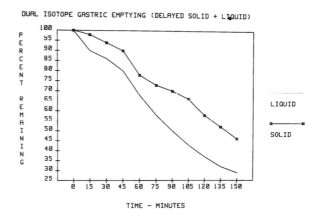

Figure 16-22 Abnormal dual isotope gastric emptying curves (same patient as Figure 16-24). Retention of both liquids and solids is seen during the course of the examination. Compare with normal subject in Figure 16-20.

exocrine function entails the excretion of potent digestive enzymes, which are carried into the duodenum through a central duct. The opening of the central duct into the duodenum is the ampulla of Vater.

The pancreas also performs endocrine functions that mediate the digestive process; for example, it secretes the hormone gastrin into the bloodstream, which inhibits gastric emptying and stimulates gastric production of acid. The pancreas also secretes both insulin and glucagon, which regulate the levels of circulating blood glucose in both the fasting and sated states.

Scintigraphy of the pancreas has been performed using selenomethionine (^{75}Se). However, the superior anatomic resolution of ultrasound and computed tomography have replaced radionuclide imaging of the pancreas.[2]

LIVER AND SPLEEN

The liver is a solid, lobulated organ located in the right upper quadrant of the abdomen beneath the right side of

Dual phase radionuclide gastric emptying study

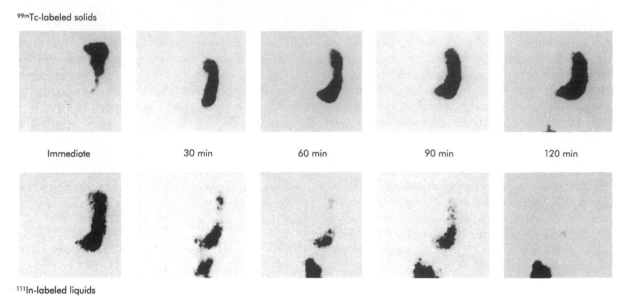

Figure 16-23   Abnormal dual isotope gastric scintigraphy. Anterior images of the abdomen were obtained in this patient with delayed emptying of solids and normal emptying of liquids. Compare images with normal individual in Figure 16-19.

Dual phase radionuclide gastric emptying study

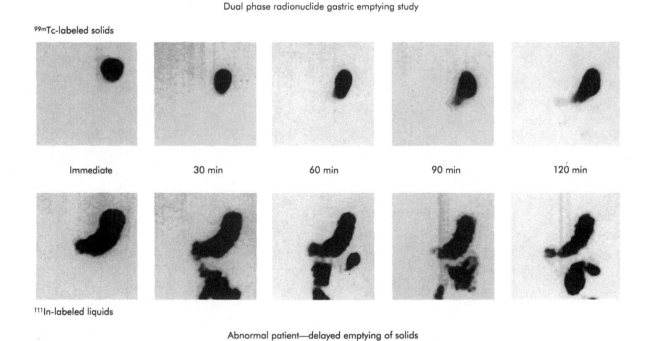

Figure 16-24   Abnormal dual isotope gastric scintigraphy. Anterior images of abdomen obtained at 30-minute intervals reveal delayed emptying of both liquids and solids. Compare with normal individual in Figure 16-19.

the diaphragm (Figure 16-25). In an adult male the liver weighs about 1800 g and is divided into two principal lobes, the right lobe and the left lobe, which are separated by the falciform ligament. The inferior quadrate and posterior caudate lobes are associated with the right lobe. The con-

figuration of the normal liver varies widely; however, the right lobe generally is larger than the left.

The liver is composed of two major cell populations, the reticuloendothelial cells (Kupffer's cells) and hepatocytes. The hepatocytes perform a variety of functions, among them

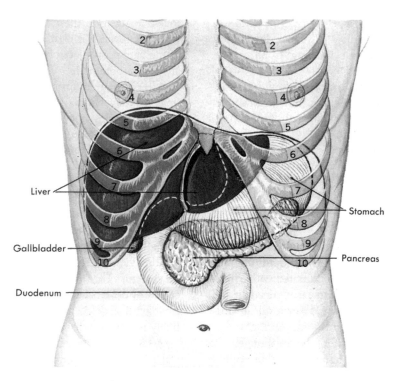

Figure 16-25 Liver in its normal position relative to the rib cage, diaphragm, stomach, and pancreas.

the conversion of bilirubin to bile. The hepatocytes secrete bile into small canaliculi that empty into the intrahepatic ducts, which merge to become the common hepatic duct. The common hepatic duct joins the cystic duct of the gallbladder to form the common bile duct, which drains into the duodenum via the ampulla of Vater (Figure 16-26).

The liver possesses a dual blood supply: arterial oxygenated blood is received from the hepatic artery, which is a branch of the abdominal aorta; venous blood draining from the intestines is carried through the hepatic portal vein into the liver. The hepatic portal system carries nutrients absorbed from the intestines into the liver for processing by hepatocytes.

The spleen is an oval mass of lymphatic tissue located in the left upper quadrant of the abdomen. It is situated between the fundus of the stomach and the left half of the diaphragm. The spleen is part of the reticuloendothelial system but not part of the gastrointestinal system.

Liver and Spleen Scintigraphy

Liver and spleen scintigraphy is the only imaging modality available for the evaluation of functional liver disease, such as cirrhosis, hepatitis, and metabolic disorders. Liver and spleen scintigraphy is also useful for the detection of hepatic lesions for biopsy and for the evaluation of hepatomegaly, jaundice, ascites, and liver enzyme abnormalities of uncertain cause.

The large field of view scintillation camera allows simultaneous imaging of the liver and spleen in most patients. A density of at least 2000 counts/cm² should be

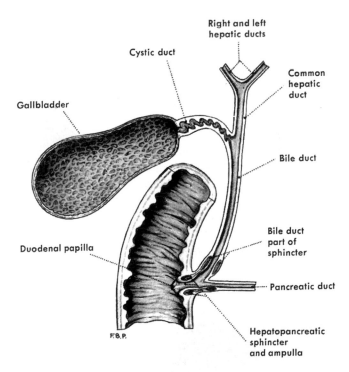

Figure 16-26 Schematic representation of extrahepatic biliary apparatus.

obtained, which corresponds to approximately 1 million counts/image.

^{99m}Tc sulfur colloid and ^{99m}Tc albumin colloid are the radiopharmaceuticals most commonly used for imaging the liver and spleen. However, this study can be combined with

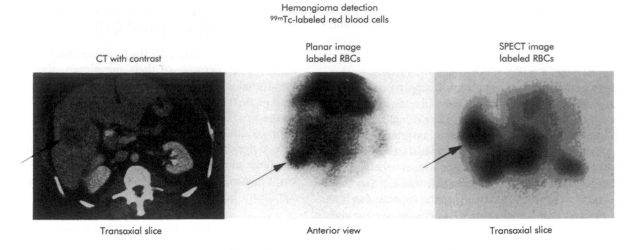

Hemangioma detection
99mTc-labeled red blood cells

CT with contrast

Transaxial slice

Planar image
labeled RBCs

Anterior view

SPECT image
labeled RBCs

Transaxial slice

An ill-defined mass is seen on CT (arrow), which is seen to collect
the labeled red-cells on planar and SPECT images obtained
at least two hours post-dose (arrows).

Figure 16-28   Example of the use of 99mTc-labeled red blood cells to detect hepatic hemangioma. The initial image is a transaxial CT slice revealing a space-occupying lesion in the right lobe of the liver (arrow). Planar and SPECT images obtained at least 2 hours after in vivo labeling of the patient's red blood cells show accumulation of the radiolabeled cells in the lesion (arrows), indicating a hemangioma.

SPECT images. Other types of lesions, such as hepatic carcinoma and metastatic disease, can show increased blood flow and early accretion of the radiolabeled cells, but they do not retain the cells for long. Only hemangiomas retain red cells until the 2-hour interval. Adequate time must be allowed for the hemangioma to accumulate a sufficient quantity of the radiolabeled cells to be identified (Figure 16-28).

GALLBLADDER

The gallbladder is a hollow, pear-shaped organ about 7 to 10 cm long (see Figure 16-26). It is located against the visceral surface of the liver, where it occupies a small indentation, the gallbladder fossa. The gallbladder concentrates and stores bile, which it receives from the common hepatic duct through the cystic duct. After ingestion of a fatty meal, the gallbladder is stimulated to contract, and it discharges the stored bile into the duodenum. Bile is useful in digestion in the breakdown and emulsification of fats.

Hepatobiliary Imaging

Radiopharmaceutical agents that localize in the hepatobiliary system can be extremely valuable in several clinical situations.[16,17,38] The most commonly used radiopharmaceuticals are derivatives of 99mTc iminodiacetic (99mTc-IDA) such as 99mTc hepatoiminodiacetic acid (99mTc-HIDA), 99mTc-DISIDA, and 99mTc mebrofenin. These agents are superior to iodine-131 (131I) rose bengal, because 99mTc-IDA derivatives provide a relatively low radiation dose to the patient,[39] have a 6-hour half-life, and provide very high count images.

Cholescintigraphy is a valuable method for investigating patients with upper abdominal pain. Because acute chole-

cystitis generally is caused by cystic duct obstruction, visualization of the gallbladder with the radionuclide tracers virtually excludes the diagnosis of acute cholecystitis. Conversely, lack of gallbladder visualization with these agents carries a high probability of acute cholecystitis. In this way, obstructive causes of clinical jaundice may be differentiated from hepatocellular causes. In the neonate, suspected biliary atresia can be evaluated with these agents. 99mTc-IDA derivatives are selectively removed from the blood circulation by hepatocytes, therefore these agents are specific for liver tissue. This high specificity allows cold defects demonstrated on colloidal liver and spleen scans to be identified as anatomic variants of the biliary anatomy. However, if the defect is not adequately explained by hepatobiliary imaging, other causes, such as benign or malignant mass lesions, must be considered.

The clinical indications for biliary tract imaging are summarized in Box 16-1.

Imaging procedure. It is preferable to have the patient fast for at least 2 hours before the study; prolonged fast (longer than 24 hours) should be avoided. Failure to follow this guideline may result in nonvisualization of the gallbladder. Pain medications that contain opium or morphine derivatives or their synthetic counterparts should be discontinued 2 to 6 hours before the study, because these medications can prevent transit of the radiotracer through the biliary system.

The usual adult dose is 1 to 5 mCi of the 99mTc-IDA given intravenously. Imaging may begin immediately, with the patient supine under a large field of view scintillation camera with a low-energy, all-purpose parallel hole collimator. The patient is positioned so that the liver appears in the upper left corner of the field of view. Sequential images are

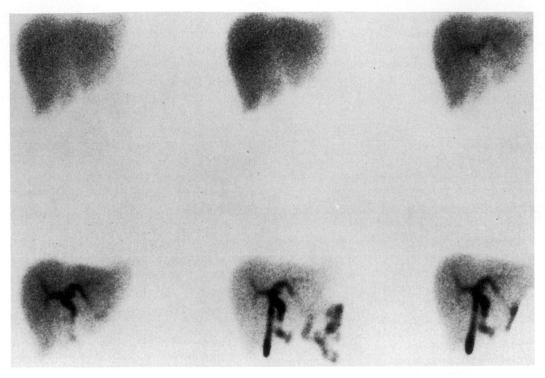

Figure 16-29   Normal hepatobiliary scan. Anterior images of the abdomen obtained at approximately 10-minute intervals after intravenous administration of 5 mCi ^{99m}Tc-IDA. Rapid uptake of the radiotracer by the liver is seen, with excretion into the biliary ducts, gallbladder, and small bowel.

Box 16-1	Hepatobiliary Imaging: Clinical Indications

- Acute (or chronic) cholecystitis
- Calculation of gallbladder ejection fraction
- Evaluation of enterogastric reflux (bile reflux
- Evaluation of the biliary system after surgery
- Jaundice (obstructive versus nonobstructive)
- Pediatrics (biliary atresia versus neonatal hepatitis; presence of choledochal cyst)
- Evaluation of cold defects seen on radiocolloid liver images

---

obtained in the anterior projection for time or total counts (1 million) for at least 1 hour (Figure 16-29). Supplemental views in the anterior oblique or right lateral projection may be useful for separating underlying structures such as the kidneys.

If the gallbladder or biliary ducts fail to visualize by 1 hour, imaging should be continued for up to 4 hours or longer, because delayed visualization of the gallbladder and biliary tree could indicate chronic cholecystitis.

The count rate of the liver changes constantly during the study because of the metabolism and excretion of the radiotracer into the bile ducts. Cameras with good resolution can

delineate the path of the biliary ducts and the gallbladder. Supplemental pinhole views may be useful for further evaluation.

Clinical aspects. In the normal individual, the radiopharmaceutical begins to concentrate in the liver during the first few minutes after injection. By 15 to 30 minutes after injection, most of the radiopharmaceutical has been removed from the bloodstream and is concentrated in the liver. This is followed by concentration of the tracer in the biliary ducts and gallbladder (see Figure 16-29). The gallbladder is typically well visualized by 45 to 60 minutes, and radioactivity is identified in the gastrointestinal tract (duodenum and proximal jejunal loops) by 30 minutes after injection (Figure 16-30).

In acute cholecystitis the liver, common bile duct, and gastrointestinal tract are visualized within 60 minutes after injection. However, the gallbladder is not visualized at 60 minutes and if further imaging is obtained, it will still fail to visualize up to 4 hours after injection (Figure 16-31). The lack of visualization of the gallbladder is the result of functional or anatomic obstruction of the cystic duct of the gallbladder, which is the basis for acute cholecystitis. In chronic cholecystitis the liver, common bile duct, and gastrointestinal tract may visualize by 60 minutes; there usually will be delayed visualization of the gallbladder after 60 minutes, usually 2 to 4 hours after injection.

The use of pharmacokinetic agents, such as cholecystokinin (CCK) analogs[15] and morphine sulfate, has been

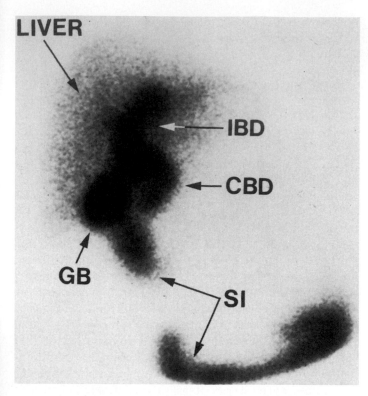

Figure 16-30   Normal hepatobiliary scan. This is a single anterior image of the abdomen obtained at 60 minutes after intravenous administration of a ^{99m}Tc-IDA compound. The scan shows normal visualization of the gallbladder (*GB*), intrahepatic biliary duct (*IBD*), common bile duct (*CBD*), and small intestine (*SI*).

advocated by some practitioners to separate patients with acute cholecystitis from those with chronic cholecystitis without the need for imaging to 4 hours. In general, if administration of either of these agents during a study in which the gallbladder does not visualize by 60 minutes causes gallbladder visualization to occur, cystic duct obstruction is not present.

Occasionally the liver, common bile duct, and gallbladder visualize within 60 minutes after injection but no radiotracer is seen in the gastrointestinal tract. In these instances it might be necessary to obtain delayed views of the abdomen up to 24 hours after injection. Absence of excretion of the radiotracer into the gastrointestinal tract is evidence of common bile duct obstruction, either functional or anatomic.

In the evaluation of cold defects seen on a ^{99m}Tc sulfur colloid liver and spleen scan, use of a biliary agent can answer the question of whether the cold defect seen on the sulfur colloid liver image is the result of normal anatomic structures of the biliary system. This is particularly useful when the defect is in the region of the porta hepatis or when it must be determined whether an apparent lesion is caused by an intrahepatic gallbladder.

In pediatric and congenital abnormalities, ^{99m}Tc-IDA agents are extremely helpful in the detection of choledochal cysts, biliary atresia, and other congenital abnormalities. The

radiation dose to the child is minimal, the study can be performed without sedation or restraints, and there is no danger of morbidity.

A common problem in performing this examination is the presence of profound jaundice in the patient. When the serum bilirubin approaches 15 to 20 mg/dl, extraction of the ^{99m}Tc-IDA compounds by the hepatocytes is severely reduced. Spurious excretion of the radiotracer through the urinary system may occur, causing circulating background-level activity to be high. In these instances delayed images may be useful up to 24 hours.

Hepatobiliary imaging is not a useful method for detecting gallstones in the gallbladder or common bile duct. Oral cholecystography, ultrasonic examination, and computed tomography are the methods of choice for detecting gallstones, although the presence of gallstones alone is not a true indicator either of acute or chronic cholecystitis.

Enterogastric Reflux (Bile Reflux) Imaging

Functional scintigraphy can help detect and quantitate enterogastric reflux with the use of hepatobiliary (^{99m}Tc-IDA) agents.[35] Enterogastric scintigraphy can confirm the reflux of bile into the stomach in patients with symptoms of bile reflux gastritis.

Both alkaline gastritis and bile reflux gastritis have been used to describe patients with symptoms of nausea, bile vomiting, abdominal fullness, heartburn, gastric pain, weight loss, and anemia. In severe cases the patient may vomit bile-stained fluid that does not contain food. These patients also have high concentrations of bile acid in fasting gastric aspirates, gastritis or esophagitis, and no peptic ulcerations.

The enterogastric reflux study is particularly useful in individuals who have undergone gastric surgery in which the pyloric sphincter mechanism was rendered incompetent, removed, or bypassed. Although gastric endoscopy may confirm the presence of bile in the stomach in these individuals, the scintigraphic study has the advantage of being noninvasive and can also quantitate the amount of refluxed bile.

Imaging procedure. The patient fasts overnight, and any medication that might affect gastrointestinal motility is stopped. Although patients can be imaged standing, sitting, or supine, supine imaging is preferred because there is less chance of patient movement, repositioning is easier, and overlap of the stomach and small bowel is minimal.

For identifying the stomach, a dual radiopharmaceutical imaging technique with a radiolabeled test meal is helpful. A 2 to 5 mCi dose of ^{99m}Tc-IDA is prepared for intravenous injection, and a fatty meal is prepared by mixing 100 to 250 µCi of ^{111}In-DTPA with a commercial fatty meal preparation of 250 cc. Any fatty meal preparation may be used, although it is most convenient to use one of the several bottled or canned preparations available on the market (e.g., Meritene).

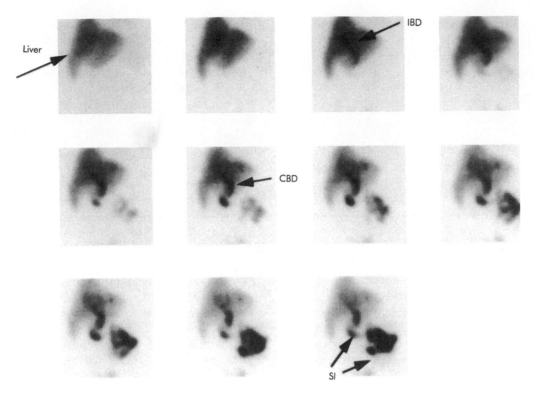

Figure 16-31   Abnormal hepatobiliary study. Multiple anterior views of the abdomen obtained over 60 minutes after intravenous administration of a ^{99m}Tc-IDA compound. Normal excretion of the radiotracer through the intrahepatic biliary ducts *(IBD)*, common bile duct *(CBD)*, and small intestine *(SI)* is seen. However, no radiotracer localization is seen in the expected area of the gallbladder. Compare with Figure 16-29.

After intravenous injection of the ^{99m}Tc-IDA, the patient is immediately positioned under a large field of view camera with a low-energy, all-purpose collimator. The patient is positioned so that the liver appears in the left upper quadrant of the image. Images are recorded for 45 minutes until peak filling of the gallbladder is seen on the persistence scope. At this point the patient is instructed to drink the fatty meal labeled with the ^{111}In-DTPA. At this time the liver and biliary tree are identified by imaging the technetium window, and the stomach is identified by imaging the indium window (Figure 16-32). Images are obtained at 15-minute intervals for 2 hours at both the technetium and the indium window settings for 1 minute each. Between imaging intervals the patient is permitted to assume the upright position, to sit, or to stand. At each imaging interval the liver, gallbladder, and biliary tree are identified by the pattern of ^{99m}Tc activity seen before the meal was given (Figure 16-33).

At the conclusion of the study the images are recalled from the computer, and regions of interest are created for the stomach and for the hepatobiliary area, which includes the liver, bile ducts, and gallbladder (Figure 16-34). The counts for both the ^{111}In and the ^{99m}Tc images are recorded in both regions of interest for time zero (ingestion of the fatty meal) and for each subsequent 15-minute interval (Figure 16-35). Corrections must be made for the ^{111}In downscatter

into the ^{99m}Tc window, and the technetium counts must be decay corrected.

Enterogastric reflux is defined as the increase in ^{99m}Tc activity in the stomach area of interest divided by the decrease in ^{99m}Tc activity in the hepatobiliary tree, using the following formula:

$$EGRI_t = (S_t - S_o)/(HB_o - HB_t) \times 100$$

where $EGRI_t$ is the enterogastric reflux index at time t, S_o represents the ^{99m}Tc activity in the stomach at time zero (immediately after ingesting the fatty meal), HB_o represents the activity in the hepatobiliary area of interest immediately following the fatty meal, and S_t and HB_t indicate the activity in the stomach and hepatobiliary area at subsequent time intervals.

Clinical aspects.   In the normal individual without previous gastric surgery, very little, if any, of the ^{99m}Tc counts can be expected in the stomach, usually less than 15% at 15 to 30 minutes. In patients who have undergone previous peptic ulcer surgery in which a portion of the stomach was removed and the pyloric sphincter mechanism was removed, rendered incompetent, or bypassed, enterogastric reflux usually is observed, even in asymptomatic patients. In studies with asymptomatic post-surgical patients, an enterogastric reflux index of approximately 25% at 15 to 30

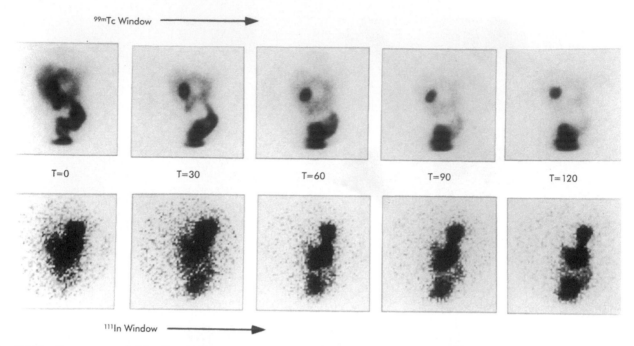

Figure 16-32 Enterogastric (bile) reflux study. Anterior images of the abdomen were obtained after intravenous administration of one of the ^{99m}Tc-IDA compounds and after oral ingestion of a fatty meal containing ^{111}In-DTPA. Images are shown for the ^{99m}Tc window and the ^{111}In window. The presence of ^{99m}Tc tracer in the stomach is evidence of enterogastric reflux.

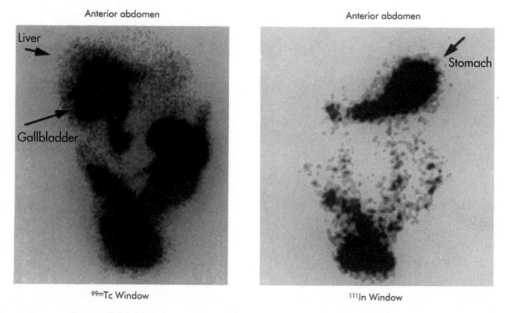

Figure 16-33 Enterogastric reflux study. Anterior images of abdomen were obtained after intravenous administration of one of the ^{99m}Tc-IDA compounds and oral ingestion of a fatty meal labeled with ^{111}In-DTPA. The liver, gallbladder, and stomach are seen.

minutes may be expected. In post-surgical patients with symptoms of nausea, bile vomiting, and abdominal burning, the enterogastric reflux index can be greater than 80% at 15 to 30 minutes. This study is useful in post-surgical patients in whom the degree of enterogastric reflux can be used to determine the response to therapy. A trial of medical therapy can be instituted and followed by repeat examination to determine if the degree of enterogastric reflux has diminished.

Several variations in the performance of this particular examination have been proposed, in particular the use of cholecystokinin analogs to replace the fatty meal. Also, several sources of error are inherent in the scintigraphic determination of enterogastric reflux. Each laboratory must establish methods for background-level correction, tissue attenuation, scatter correction, and correction for interference from liver and small bowel overlap. Normal values must be established for each laboratory. Simple visual inter-

Anterior abdomen

Anterior abdomen

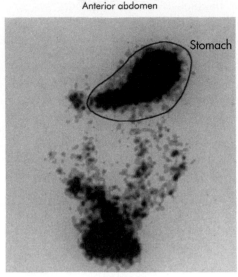

⁹⁹ᵐTc Window

¹¹¹In Window

Figure 16-34 Calculation of the enterogastric reflux index. Anterior images of the abdomen are recalled from the computer, and regions of interest are created for the stomach, liver, and gallbladder (*GB*). The hepatobiliary area includes the liver, bile ducts, and gallbladder. Both the ¹¹¹In and the ⁹⁹ᵐTc counts are recorded in both regions of interest at each 15-minute interval.

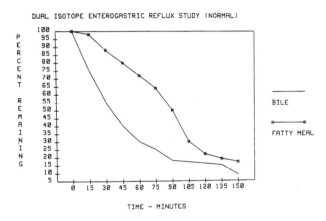

Figure 16-35 Normal dual isotope enterogastric reflux study. The percentage normalized remaining ¹¹¹In counts and ⁹⁹ᵐTc counts are graphed as a function of time. Smooth emptying of the fatty meal from the stomach area is seen, with a nearly parallel decrease in the labeled bile.

pretation of the images can be used to determine if reflux is present (see Figure 16-32).

INTESTINAL TRACT

The small intestine is a lengthy, hollow tube extending from the pyloric sphincter of the stomach to the ileocecal valve at the large intestine. The small intestine is divided into the duodenum, the jejunum, and the ileum (see Figure 16-1). It is responsible for digestion and absorption of all nutrients in the body. The inner lining of the small intestine contains glands that secrete intestinal digestive enzymes. The lining is also especially adapted for absorption of all needed nutrients; microvilli cover the entire 20-foot length of the

small intestine. These microvilli are also known as the *brush border.*

The large intestine extends from the ileocecal valve to the anus. The large intestine is divided into the cecum, ascending colon, transverse colon, descending colon, sigmoid colon, and rectum (see Figure 16-1). Very little absorption of nutrients occurs in the large intestine, with the notable exception of some vitamins. The major function of the large intestine is resorption of water; this results in the formation of fecal material, which is expelled through the anus.

Gastrointestinal Bleeding

Evaluation of gastrointestinal bleeding using radionuclide methods is now a routine procedure in most clinical nuclear medicine facilities.[24] Initial studies using ⁵¹Cr-labeled red blood cells demonstrated the feasibility of detecting and localizing sites of gastrointestinal hemorrhage using radiolabeled markers. ⁹⁹ᵐTc-labeled agents are now widely used to detect gastrointestinal bleeding; however, controversy over the selection of the labeled agent exists. Two groups of agents have been proposed, based on whether they are extracted rapidly or slowly from the intravascular space. Of the rapidly extracted agents, ⁹⁹ᵐTc sulfur colloid and ⁹⁹ᵐTc-labeled heat-treated red blood cells are commonly used, with the former being preferred because it can be rapidly and simply prepared. Slowly extracted agents include ⁹⁹ᵐTc-labeled albumin and non–heat-treated ⁹⁹ᵐTc-labeled red blood cells. Non–heat-treated ⁹⁹ᵐTc-labeled red blood cells can be labeled using either in vivo or in vitro techniques.

⁹⁹ᵐTc sulfur colloid has the advantage of minimizing background-level activity and promoting the highest contrast ratios. However, its rapid clearance requires that the

patient be actively bleeding at the time of injection (or within minutes after injection). Non–heat-treated ^{99m}Tc-labeled red blood cells, with their prolonged retention in the intravascular pool, are preferred by investigators who maintain that gastrointestinal bleeding is most often intermittent and slow. Furthermore, non–heat-treated ^{99m}Tc-labeled blood cells allow repetitive imaging for up to 36 hours after injection with a far lower radiation dose to the liver and spleen and have the ability to better detect gastrointestinal bleeding in the upper abdominal region. The theoretical disadvantage of higher background-level activity with the labeled red blood cells in the heavily vascularized abdominal organs does not appear to be a significant factor in several clinical comparisons.

The methods using the rapidly extracted ^{99m}Tc sulfur colloid and the slowly extracted non–heat-treated ^{99m}Tc-labeled red blood cells follow.

Imaging procedure

^{99m}Tc sulfur colloid technique. The patient is placed supine under a large field of view scintillation camera equipped with a low-energy parallel hole collimator so as to include the inferior margin of the liver to the symphysis pubis. Freshly made ^{99m}Tc sulfur colloid (7 to 10 mCi) is injected as an intravenous bolus, and an anterior flow study of the abdomen is obtained at 1 to 2 sec/frame for 2 to 3 minutes. Thereafter 500,000- to 750,000-count anterior images of the abdomen are obtained every 1 to 2 minutes for 20 to 30 minutes at intensity settings such that the bone marrow can be visualized. If an area of bleeding is identified, more detailed views of that area can be obtained with oblique, lateral, or posterior views. If no bleeding site is identified at the end of 30 minutes, a 1 million-count image of the upper abdomen is obtained with oblique views to better delineate the hepatic and splenic flexures. If these views are negative, repeat lower abdominal views can be obtained in 15 to 20 minutes to check for activity that may have been obscured in the areas of the hepatic and splenic flexures by liver and spleen activity. Any bowel movements by the patient during the course of the study should be scanned in the bedpan to ensure that a very low rectal source of bleeding has not been obscured by genital activity. If the scan result is negative, repeat injections of the tracer may be necessary, if clinical evidence exists of renewed active bleeding.

The flow study clearly delineates the aorta and other vascular structures, including the liver, spleen, kidneys, and small and large bowel. As the ^{99m}Tc sulfur colloid clears the intravascular space, it accumulates in the liver and spleen and bone marrow and fades from the vascular structures. The genital areas have a significant accumulation of the ^{99m}Tc sulfur colloid, and a lateral view may be helpful to avoid confusion with a possible source of lower rectal bleeding. If a fresh preparation of ^{99m}Tc sulfur colloid is used, renal and bladder activity will be minimized, because the amount of free ^{99m}Tc will be less than 2%.

Care should be taken in positioning the patient so that only small margins of the liver and spleen are seen in the images. This brings out any activity in the abdominal cavity.

Non–heat-treated ^{99m}Tc-labeled red blood cell method. ^{99m}Tc-labeled red blood cells provide a long-lived blood pool tracer that can identify areas of upper and lower gastrointestinal bleeding. This method may be able to image bleeding rates of 0.2 to 0.4 ml/min.

Although several methods are available for labeling red blood cells with ^{99m}Tc, either the in vitro technique (Brookhaven kit) or a modified in vivo method offers a high degree of labeling efficiency. This minimizes the amount of free ^{99m}Tc that can accumulate in the stomach and ultimately collect in the colon. A modified in vivo method is described below.

Initially the patient is injected intravenously with 6 to 12 mg of cold stannous pyrophosphate. After a 10- to 20-minute wait, the patient is placed supine under a large field of view camera fitted with a low-energy, parallel hole collimator. The patient is positioned in such a way that the xiphisternum is at the top of the field of view and the symphysis pubis is at the bottom. The patient is then given 15 to 25 mCi of ^{99m}Tc pertechnetate as an intravenous bolus (pediatric dose is 240 μCi/kg with a minimum dose of 2 mCi). An immediate flow study of the abdomen is acquired at 1 to 3 sec/frame for the next 2 to 3 minutes. This is primarily used to identify normal abdominal structures. After this, 1 million-count anterior abdominal views are obtained at 1- to 5-minute intervals for the next 60 minutes to include the inferior aspect of the heart to the symphysis pubis. Oblique, lateral, and posterior views can be obtained as necessary.

The images can be stored on a computer and displayed in the cine mode to help visualize both normal and abnormal movement of the tracer. If active bleeding is not identified during the first hour, delayed views at 2-, 4-, and 6-hour intervals can be obtained as clinically suggested by changes in vital signs or evidence of recurrent bright red blood per rectum. Delayed views for up to 36 hours after injection can be obtained with good results.

Normally, with this method the vascular structures of the abdomen are well visualized, including the great vessels and the highly vascular kidneys, spleen, bowel, and genital organs (Figure 16-36). It may be necessary to obtain supplemental views with lead shielding placed over certain vascular structures, because the degree of background-level activity can obscure small foci of gastrointestinal bleeding.

Clinical aspects. Using ^{99m}Tc sulfur colloid, areas of active bleeding may be seen on the flow study, but they are more commonly identified after the first 5 minutes. They usually appear as focal areas of increased activity that can become more intense with time as background-level activity decreases. Because blood is both a stimulant and an irritant in the bowel, the activity can pass more quickly through the colon. Retrograde motion that can occur may make

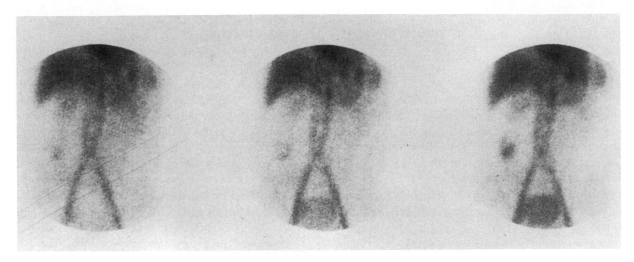

Figure 16-36 ^{99m}Tc-labeled red blood cell study. Anterior views of the abdomen were obtained to visualize an intermittent bleeding site. Images were obtained at approximately 5-minute intervals. Progressive accumulation of the tagged red cells is seen in the right lower quadrant of the abdomen, with apparent tracking of these cells in the ascending colon toward the hepatic flexure. Note the structures normally visualized with this method: the liver, spleen, abdominal vessels, kidneys, bladder, and stomach.

localization of the site of bleeding difficult. Both arterial and venous bleeding can be identified from both small and large bowel sources. False-positive study results can occur if there is asymmetric bone marrow accumulation of the tracer, as can be seen with replacement of marrow by tumor, after radiation therapy, or as a result of some other pathologic process, such as Paget's disease. In such cases the area of involvement has decreased uptake, and the more normal-appearing area on the other side of the abdomen can be misinterpreted as an area of bleeding. False-positive study results can also occur in renal transplants, which accumulate ^{99m}Tc sulfur colloid during rejection.

Using the non–heat-treated ^{99m}Tc-labeled red blood cell method, the flow study outlines the great vessels of the abdomen and the general position of the kidneys, spleen, small and large bowel, and genital organs (particularly in women when the uterus may be well vascularized). Occasionally, if marked bleeding is occurring, it can be seen on the flow study. Additionally, vascular tumors can be seen as abnormal tracer collections on the arterial phase that disappear during the venous phase. An abnormal scan demonstrates a focus of tracer activity, which usually becomes more intense with time and is not related to normal abdominal structures (see Figure 16-36). Generally speaking, the tagged red cell method can identify colonic bleeding more easily than small bowel bleeding sites. It is important to get frequent images for accurate localization of the bleeding site. If early views are negative and only delayed views show activity in the cecum, it may be difficult to pinpoint the site of bleeding, because bleeding may have occurred in the upper small bowel, right side of the colon, or transverse colon and merely collected in the cecum. This is especially true if suboptimum red cell labeling has occurred and gastric activity is noted on the initial views. False-positive study results may occur if anatomic variants of vascular structures are present in the abdomen.

Meckel's Diverticulum

Meckel's diverticulum is a common cause of gastrointestinal tract bleeding in children, and Meckel's diverticulum imaging is most frequently done in children. The acute remnant is a small invagination of the intestine that can contain gastric mucosa. Bleeding is the presenting symptom in almost three fourths of patients, but other symptoms may include inflammation, obstruction, intussusception, or perforation of the bowel. Most Meckel's diverticula are located in the ileum, usually within 1 m of the ileocecal valve. Most patients with gastrointestinal bleeding are found to have gastric parietal cells in the Meckel's diverticulum. These cells cause peptic ulceration of the bowel by acid secretion.

^{99m}Tc pertechnetate concentrates in gastric mucosa and can be used to detect and localize a symptomatic Meckel's diverticulum (Figure 16-37). Details of this procedure may be found in Chapter 21.

Barrett's Esophagus

The presence of ectopic gastric mucosa in the distal esophagus is called *Barrett's esophagus*. Scintigraphic detection of this ectopic gastric mucosa in the distal esophagus was proposed because the parietal cells contained in gastric mucosa are known to concentrate ^{99m}Tc pertechnetate. However, scintigraphy can only support the diagnosis of Barrett's esophagus; mucosal biopsy still is necessary to confirm it. With the widespread use of fiberoptic endoscopy, use of this examination has declined. However, it may still serve as an aid in locating a more specific region for biopsy.

Imaging procedure. The patient should fast for 2 hours before the examination. ^{99m}Tc pertechnetate (5 mCi) is given intravenously. Dental sponges are placed in the oral cavity to prevent the patient from swallowing pertechnetate

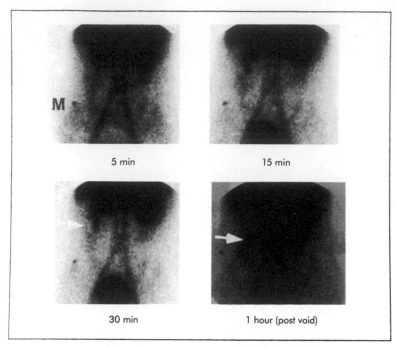

Anterior views of abdomen following premedication with
H-2 blocker and pentagastrin, and 25 mCi ^{99m}Tc pertechnetate I.V.

Figure 16-37   Meckel's diverticulum in the right side of the abdomen. The patient received H_2 blockers for 2 days before the study and 20 minutes before the examination pentagastrin was given. Progressive accumulation of the radiotracer is seen in the diverticulum (*arrow*). M, Marker at right iliac crest.

excreted in the saliva and to avoid confusion of the origin of esophageal activity. The patient then is placed in a sitting position with the anterior chest against a large field of view camera with a parallel hole collimator. Images are acquired for 5-minute intervals for the next 30 minute.

Prior administration of atropine or atropine-like compounds or administration of potassium perchlorate is to be avoided. These agents are known to reduce uptake of pertechnetate ions by gastric mucosa.

Clinical aspects.   Normally, activity is visualized only in the stomach and salivary glands. Pertechnetate activity above the level of the diaphragm suggests the presence of ectopic gastric mucosa in the distal esophagus. Barrett's esophagus is associated with dyspepsia, esophagitis, and upper gastrointestinal bleeding.

Gastric mucosal imaging has also been used for preoperative diagnosis of pulmonary and mediastinal enterogenous cysts containing gastric mucosa.

BREATH TESTING WITH ^{14}C-LABELED COMPOUNDS

Breath testing is used to diagnose bacterial overgrowth and carbohydrate malabsorption. Breath testing also shows potential in the evaluation of sucrose-isomaltose malabsorption, fat malabsorption, and liver function.

Gas, produced in the bowel lumen by various acid-base or metabolic reactions, diffuses to some degree into the

body circulation and is excreted by respiration into the breath. Of the five principal colonic gases (carbon dioxide, hydrogen, methane, nitrogen, and oxygen), carbon dioxide and hydrogen are the two most important for breath analysis.

The isotopic carbon dioxide breath tests[33] use ^{14}C-labeled substrates, which are given orally. Labeled carbon dioxide is then excreted in the breath as a result of carbon dioxide production from absorption and breakdown of ^{14}C-labeled material.

^{14}C carbon dioxide can be measured directly by passing the expired breath through plastic filament detectors or by liquid scintillation counting of specimens in which ^{14}C carbon dioxide breath is trapped as labeled carbonic acid by a known amount of alkali such as hyamine hydroxide.

Liver Function Analysis

Measurement of ^{14}C-labeled carbon dioxide after either oral or intravenous administration of ^{14}C-labeled aminopyrine provides an estimate of hepatic mixed oxidase function.[3,20] The radiolabeled aminopyrine breath test has the clinically useful potential for differentiating patients with the cholestatic form of chronic active hepatitis from those with primary biliary cirrhosis. Correct categorization of such patients is not easily accomplished by other means, and simple blood tests do not measure actual liver function. Therefore the aminopyrine test has important therapeutic implications.

Xylose Breath Test

The most sensitive and specific breath test for bacterial overgrowth of the small intestine uses 1 g of ^{14}C-labeled D-xylose. This test has greater than 95% sensitivity and specificity for detecting abnormal proliferation of the small bowel microflora.

Breath excretion of labeled carbon dioxide is measured from 30 to 60 minutes after the patient drinks a solution containing 1 g of xylose with 5 to 10 μCi of ^{14}C-labeled D-xylose mixed in 500 ml of water. Rapid results make this test clinically practical and ensure that analysis occurs during the period when the test solution is still only in the small intestine. In the rare patient with extremely slow gastric emptying, it may be necessary to make a delayed analysis at 180 minutes to ensure bacterial content with the test substrate.

The ^{14}C-labeled D-xylose breath test is even more sensitive than a single jejunal culture. The breath test integrates the findings over a long segment of the small intestine, whereas a single culture can be made only from one site, which may not reflect the true state of the surrounding flora.

^{14}C-Labeled Bile Acid Test

The ^{14}C-labeled bile acid breath test was the first developed for detecting abnormal contact of intestinal bacteria with substrate. It relies on deconjugation of ^{14}C-labeled cholylglycine by anaerobic bacteria, which produces ^{14}C carbon dioxide from the labeled glycine.

Because conjugated bile salts are absorbed in the distal rather than the proximal small bowel, even normal subjects display substantial contact of the labeled substrate with their colonic flora. This contamination creates a background of labeled carbon dioxide, produced by colonic flora, against which small intestine bacterial-labeled carbon dioxide must be measured.

The ^{14}C-labeled bile acid test, used concomitantly with another test to rule out bacterial overgrowth, may be useful for detecting bile acid malabsorption. This condition, which can lead to vexing diarrhea, is often difficult to diagnose.

Fat Absorption Test

One of the earliest reported uses of the labeled carbon dioxide breath test was breath analysis after oral administration of fat labeled with isotopic carbon.[30] Despite earlier encouraging reports, simple carbon dioxide testing does not adequately distinguish those with moderate fat malabsorption from normal subjects. The steps between ingestion of labeled fat and excretion of labeled carbon dioxide are much more complicated than those encountered with other labeled carbon dioxide breath tests. Hence, the clinical use of these tests remains elusive.

REFERENCES

1. Alfidi RJ, Haaga J, Meaney TF et al: Computed tomography of the thorax and abdomen: a preliminary report, *Radiology* 117:257, 1975.
2. Barkin J, Vining D, Miale AJ Jr, et al: Computerized tomography, diagnostic ultrasound and radionuclide scanning: comparison of efficacy in diagnosis of pancreatic carcinoma, *JAMA* 238(19):2040, 1977.
3. Bircher J, Kupfer A, Gikalov I, et al: Aminopyrine demethylation measured by breath analysis in cirrhosis, *Clin Pharmacol Ther* 20:484, 1976.
4. Blue PW, Jacison JH: Stimulated salivary clearance of technetium-99m pertechnetate, *J Nucl Med* 26:308, 1985.
5. Brodsky RI, Friedman AC, Maurer AH, et al: Hepatic cavernous hemangioma: diagnosis with ^{99m}Tc-labeled red cells and single-photon emission computed tomography, *Am J Roentgenol* 148:125-129, 1987.
6. Bryan PJ, Dunn WM, Grossman ZD: Correlation of computerized tomography, gray scale ultrasonography and radionuclide imaging of the liver in detecting space-occupying processes, *Radiology* 124:387, 1977.
7. Castell DO: The lower esophageal sphincter: physiologic and clinical aspects, *Ann Intern Med* 83:390, 1975.
8. Chaudhuri TK, Heading RC, Greenwald A, et al: Measurement of gastric emptying (GET) of solid meal using ^{99m}Tc DTPA, *J Nucl Med* 15:483, 1974.
9. Christian PE, Coleman RE, Harris CC: An accessory for estimating organ size from gamma camera images, *J Nucl Med Technol* 8:211, 1980.
10. Christian PE, Datz FL, Sorenson JA, et al: Technical factors in gastric emptying studies, *J Nucl Med* 24:264, 1983.
11. Cooperman AM, Cook SA: Gastric emptying: physiology and measurements, *Surg Clin North Am* 56(6):1277, 1976.
12. Crandell DC, Boyd M, Wennemark JR, et al: Liver-spleen scanning: the left lateral decubitus position is best for lateral views, *J Nucl Med* 13:720, 1972.
13. Datz FL: The role of radionuclide studies in esophageal disease, *J Nucl Med* 25:1040, 1984.
14. DeNardo GL, Stadalnik RC, DeNardo SJ, et al: Hepatic scintiangiographic patterns, *Radiology* 111:135, 1974.
15. Freeman LM, Sugarman LA, Weissman HS: Role of cholecystokinetic agents in ^{99m}Tc IDA cholescintigraphy, *Semin Nucl Med* 11:186, 1981.
16. Fonseca C, Greenberg D, Rosenthall L, et al: Assessment of the utility of gallbladder imaging with ^{99m}Tc-IDA, *Clin Nucl Med* 3:437, 1978.
17. Fonseca C, Rosenthall L, Greenberg D, et al: Differential diagnosis of jaundice by ^{99m}Tc-IDA hepatobiliary imaging, *Clin Nucl Med* 4:135, 1979.

18. Garcia AC, Yeh SDJ, Benua RS: Accumulation of bone-seeking radionuclides in liver metastasis from colon carcinoma, *Clin Nucl Med* 2:265, 1977.

19. Heading RC, Tothill P, Laidlaw AJ, et al: An evaluation of [113m]indium DTPA chelate in the measurement of gastric emptying by scintiscanning, *Gut* 12:611, 1975.

20. Hepner GW, Vesell ES: Quantitative assessment of hepatic function by breath analysis after oral administration of (^{14}C) aminopyrine, *Ann Intern Med* 83:632, 1975.

21. Kranzler JK, Vollert JM, Harper PV, et al: The diagnostic value of hepatic pliability as assessed from inspiration and expiration views on the gamma camera, *Radiology* 97:323, 1976.

22. Kumar B, Coleman RE, Alderson PO: Gallium citrate Ga-67 imaging in patients with suspected inflammatory processes, *Arch Surg* 110:1237, 1975.

23. Lomas F, Dibos PE, Wagner HN Jr: Increased specificity of liver scanning with the use of [67]gallium citrate, *N Engl J Med* 286:1323, 1972.

24. Lull RJ, Morris GL: Scintigraphic detection of gastrointestinal hemorrhage: current status, *J Nucl Med Technol* 14:79, 1986.

25. Malmud LS, Fisher RS: Quantitation of gastroesophageal reflux before and after therapy using the gastroesophageal scintiscan, *South Med J* 71(suppl 1):10, 1978.

26. Malmud LS, Fisher RS, Knight LC, et al: Scintigraphic evaluation of gastric emptying, *Semin Nucl Med* 12:116, 1982.

27. Meyer JH, MacGregor IL, Gueller R, et al: ^{99m}Tc-tagged chicken liver as a marker of solid food in the human stomach, *Am J Dig Dis* 21:296, 1976.

28. Oppenheimer BE, Hoffer PB, Gottschalk A: The use of inspiration-expiration scintiphotographs to determine the intrinsic or extrinsic nature of liver defects, *J Nucl Med* 13(7):554, 1972.

29. Pope CE II: Pathophysiology and diagnosis of reflux esophagitis, *Gastroenterology* 70:445, 1976.

30. Ruttin JM, Shingelton WW, Baylin GJ, et al: [131]I labeled fat in the study of intestinal absorption, *N Engl J Med* 225:594, 1956.

31. Schmitt G, Lehmann G, Strotges W, et al: The diagnostic value of sialography and scintigraphy in salivary gland diseases, *Br J Radiol* 49:326, 1976.

32. Selby JB: Radiological examination of subphrenic disease process, *CRC Crit Rev Diagn Imaging* 9(3):229, 1977.

33. Shreeve WW: Labeled carbon breath analysis. In Rocha AFG, Harbert JC, editors: *Textbook of nuclear medicine: basic science,* Philadelphia, 1978, Lea & Febiger.

34. Siegel JA, Wu RK, Knight LC, et al: Radiation dose estimates for oral agents used in upper gastrointestinal disease, *J Nucl Med* 24:835, 1983.

35. Tolin RD, Malmud LS, Stelzer F, et al: Enterogastric reflux in normal subjects and patients with Bilroth II gastroenterostomy, *Gastroenterology* 77:1027, 1979.

36. van Dam APM: The gamma camera in clinical evaluation of gastric emptying, *Radiology* 110:155, 1974.

37. Waxman AD, Apaw R, Siemsen JK: Rapid sequential liver imaging, *J Nucl Med* 13:522, 1972.

38. Wistow BW, Subramanian G, Van Heertum RL, et al: An evaluation of ^{99m}Tc-labeled hepatobiliary agents, *J Nucl Med* 18:455, 1977.

39. Wu RK, Siegel JA, Rattner Z, et al: Tc-99m HIDA dosimetry in patients with various hepatic disorders, *J Nucl Med* 25:905, 1984.

SUGGESTED READINGS

Maurer AH, editor: Gastrointestinal nuclear imaging. I. Functional studies, *Semin Nucl Med* 25:4, 1995.

Maurer AH, editor: Gastrointestinal nuclear imaging. II. *Semin Nucl Med* 26:1, 1996.

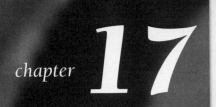

Henry D. Royal

chapter 17

Genitourinary System

Objectives

Describe the anatomy and physiology of the genitourinary system.

List the radiopharmaceuticals used for renal studies and discuss their characteristics.

Describe the excretion methods for renal radiopharmaceuticals.

List common renal nuclear medicine studies and their indications.

Describe the performance of functional renal study.

Discuss the procedure for diuretic renal scintigraphy.

Describe the procedure for performing renal scintigraphy with ACEI augmentation.

Describe the performance of scintigraphy for morphologic renal imaging.

Discuss the anatomy, physiology, and indications for testicular scintigraphy.

Define ERPF and GFR and describe methods to obtain these measurements.

ANATOMY

The top of the kidneys usually is located just underneath the lowest ribs in the back (Figure 17-1), spanning the distance from about the twelfth thoracic vertebra to the third lumbar vertebra. In the adult the kidneys measure about 11 to 12 cm (long axis) and are 5 to 7.5 cm wide and 2 to 3 cm thick.[14] Because it is displaced by the liver, the right kidney usually is slightly lower than the left kidney.

Determining the size of the kidney by planar scintigraphy is less accurate than determining the size of the kidney by ultrasound. With planar scintigraphy, the kidney may appear smaller than its actual size if the long axis is not parallel to the surface of the crystal of the gamma camera. This artifact is called *foreshortening* (Figure 17-2). Single photon emission computed tomography (SPECT) imaging using a morphologic renal imaging agent such as dimercaptosuccinic acid (DMSA) is a more accurate technique for measuring renal size.[20]

Normally the kidneys are about an equal depth from the skin of the back, but in some patients the depths of the kidneys may be unequal. When the kidneys are at unequal depths, measurement of the relative activity in each kidney is inaccurate because of greater attenuation of the radiation from the deeper kidney. Consequently, the relative function of the deeper kidney is underestimated. One way to tell whether asymmetric activity in the kidneys is related to a difference in kidney depth is to obtain an anterior view of the kidneys. If relatively more activity is seen on the anterior view in the kidney that has decreased activity in the posterior view, a difference in kidney depth is at least partly responsible for the difference in kidney activity.

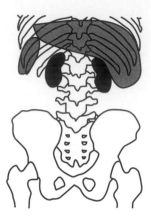

Figure 17-1   Location of the kidneys on the posterior view. The right kidney is normally slightly lower than the left kidney because it is displaced by the liver. The background activity for the right kidney is usually higher than that for the left because of activity that accumulates in the liver. Blood flow to the spleen can be misinterpreted as blood flow to the left kidney, especially when the blood flow to the left kidney is reduced.

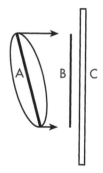

Figure 17-2   Foreshortening. The true length of the long axis of the kidney (**A**) will be underestimated (**B**) if the long axis of the kidney is not parallel to the plane of the gamma camera crystal (**C**).

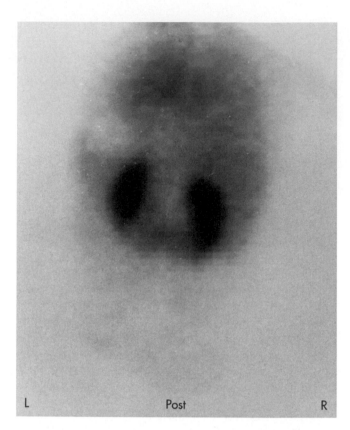

Figure 17-3   Horseshoe kidney. Posterior image of the kidneys of a 10-month-old girl acquired 0 to 2 minutes after injection of ^{99m}Tc-MAG3. Ultrasound examination had shown bilateral hydronephrosis. Hydronephrosis is frequently seen with horseshoe kidneys because the connecting band of tissue compresses the ureters. The decreased activity noted superior and lateral to the left kidney is caused by a full stomach. This decrease in activity is often seen in infants after feeding.

When a kidney study is obtained in the intensive care unit, imaging must be performed by placing the patient in a lateral decubitus or prone position. Either of these positions may exaggerate the asymmetric depth of the kidneys, because one kidney may fall forward more than the other. It is sometimes tempting to perform a mobile study in the anterior view; however, anterior images of normally positioned kidneys are rarely satisfactory.

Sometimes the bottoms of the two kidneys are joined; this congenital abnormality is called a *horseshoe kidney* (Figure 17-3). Because the spine attenuates the activity coming from the thin band of tissue connecting the lower poles of the kidneys, this congenital abnormality may be missed if only posterior views are obtained. An anterior view often clearly shows the band of functioning tissue that connects the lower poles of the kidneys. Another clue to the presence of a horseshoe kidney is the orientation of the kidneys. The lower ends of horseshoe kidneys are closer together than in normal kidneys.

Another disease that can grossly distort the anatomy of the kidney is polycystic kidney disease. Patients with this inherited disease have multiple large cysts in the kidneys and liver (Figure 17-4). These cysts increase in size as the patient ages, often resulting in renal failure.

Occasionally a kidney may be in an unusual location. Sometimes a kidney is located in the pelvis, particularly if the patient is sitting or standing. When the patient is imaged in the supine position, the kidney may return to a more normal position. A mobile kidney in an abnormal position is called *ptotic*. Transplanted kidneys are most often placed in the anterior pelvis. Before beginning a kidney study, the technologist should inquire whether it is likely that the patient's kidneys are in an unusual location so as to make certain that the camera is optimally positioned.

Another important clinical determination in some cases is what proportion of renal function can be ascribed to a transplanted kidney and what proportion to the patient's native kidneys. This question is best answered by obtaining simultaneously an anterior view of the transplanted kidney and a posterior view of the native kidneys, using a large field of view, dual-headed camera.

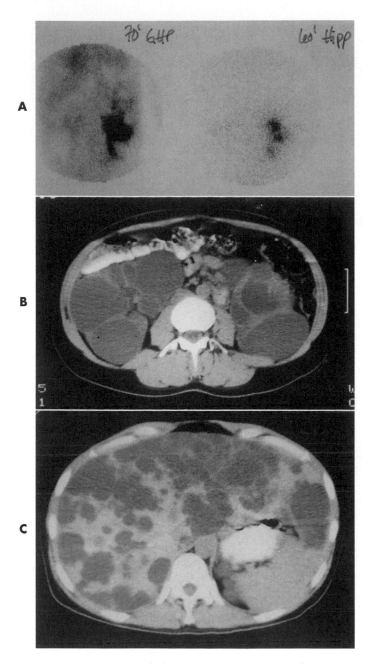

Figure 17-4   Polycystic kidneys. **A,** Posterior images of the kidneys obtained 70 minutes after injection of ^{99m}Tc glucoheptonate *(left)* and 60 minutes after injection of ^{131}I hippuran *(right)*. Both images are very abnormal (this patient had polycystic kidney disease and renal failure). The function of the left kidney is considerably worse than that of the right kidney. The areas of decreased activity seen on the glucoheptonate images are caused by the renal cysts. Despite the poor renal function, most of the hippuran is in the collecting system at 60 minutes. The glucoheptonate is cleared from the rest of the body more slowly than hippuran and is retained in the renal parenchyma. **B,** CT scan of the kidneys shows nearly complete replacement of the renal tissue by cysts. **C,** CT scan of the liver shows extensive cystic disease of the liver. Patients with polycystic kidney disease often have cysts in the liver.

The urine produced by the kidneys is excreted into the renal pelvis and then transported to the bladder through the ureters (Figure 17-5). Dilation of the renal pelvis and ureters is called *hydronephrosis*. This condition can occur with obstruction of the collecting system, or it may be the result simply of a dilated but not obstructed collecting system.

The bladder is a distensible bag that stores urine until it is eliminated through the urethra. Sometimes a patient's bladder is removed to treat bladder cancer. A new "bladder," called an *ileal loop,* can be made from a portion of the small bowel (ilium) (Figure 17-6). Barium in the rectum can cause an artifact that overlies the bladder (Figure 17-7).

The scrotum is a skin pouch suspended from the lower pelvis that contains the testes, epididymis, and vas deferens. The testes produce spermatozoa and the hormone testosterone. The epididymis is a tortuous tubular structure in which spermatozoa mature and are stored before they are transported. The vas deferens is contiguous to the epididymis and is the excretory duct of the testes.

The blood flow to and from the kidney usually is through a single artery and vein that subsequently divide into interlobar arteries. A common variation of normal anatomy of the renal artery is to have two main renal arteries to a kidney, usually one to the upper pole of the kidney and one to the lower pole. These arteries subdivide until they form the afferent arteriole to a web of capillaries called *glomeruli*. The blood leaves the glomerulus through the efferent arteriole, which courses deep into the medulla, forming the peritubular capillaries and the vasa recta.

PHYSIOLOGY

The kidney has several major functions, including excretion of waste products, resorption of important body constituents, maintenance of acid-base balance, and maintenance of fluid balance. To accomplish these functions, the kidney requires a large blood flow. Approximately 20% to 25% of the cardiac output goes to normally functioning kidneys. Because the resting cardiac output is 5 L/min, total renal blood flow is about 1.2 L/min (Table 17-1). Because plasma constitutes about 50% of the total blood volume, the effective renal plasma flow (ERPF) is about 600 ml/min. When the plasma and red cells pass by the glomerulus, approximately 20% of the plasma passes through the glomerulus into the renal tubules, resulting in a glomerular filtration rate (GFR) of 120 ml/min. Most of the filtrate is

Table 17-1	Normal physiology flow rates
Cardiac output	5 L/min
Renal blood flow	1.2 L/min
Effective renal plasma flow	600 ml/min
Glomerular filtration rate	125 ml/min
Filtration fraction	25%

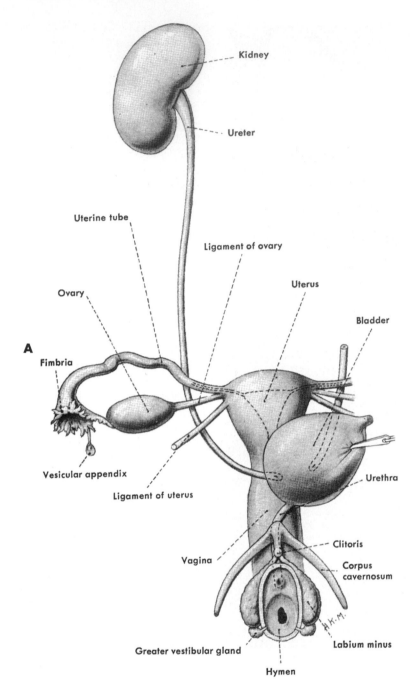

Figure 17-5   Schematic representation of urogenital organs in the female (**A**) and the male (**B**).

reabsorbed. The proportion of plasma that reaches the kidney and is filtered by the glomerulus is called the *filtration fraction*. Normally, the filtration fraction is equal to about 20% (GFR/ERPF).

Only 1000 to 1500 ml of urine are produced each day. More than 170 L of urine would be produced per day if none of the plasma that was filtered through the glomerulus was reabsorbed by the tubular cells. On average, the body contains only about 42 L of water, therefore tubular cell dysfunction that prevents resorption of the filtrate would rapidly result in death from dehydration. Fortunately, when tubular dysfunction occurs, a number of reflex mechanisms cause a dramatic decrease in renal blood flow and glomeru-

lar filtration. Although these compensatory mechanisms have significant long-term adverse effects, rapid death from acute dehydration is prevented.

The basic functional unit of the kidney is called a *nephron* (Figure 17-8). A normally functioning kidney has millions of nephrons. The nephron consists of an afferent arteriole that delivers blood to a web of capillaries (vascular tuft) in the glomerulus. The blood leaves the glomerulus through the efferent arteriole. Between the afferent and efferent arterioles is an important hormone-producing mass of cells called the *juxtaglomerular apparatus*.

The porous surface of the glomerulus permits filtration of water and solutes into Bowman's capsule (Figure 17-9).

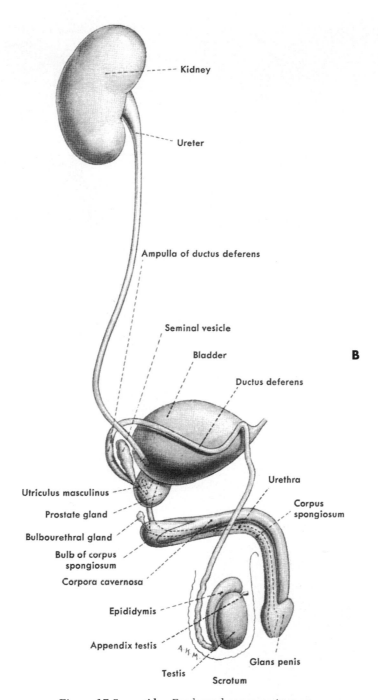

Kidney

Ureter

Ampulla of ductus deferens

Seminal vesicle

Bladder

B

Ductus deferens

Urethra

Utriculus masculinus

Corpus
spongiosum

Prostate gland

Bulbourethral gland

Bulb of corpus
spongiosum

Corpora cavernosa

Epididymis

Appendix testis

Glans penis

Testis

Scrotum

Figure 17-5, cont'd.   For legend see opposite page.

The major factor that determines whether a substance is filtered is its molecular size. Substances with a molecular size of less than 150,000 daltons are freely filterable if they are not protein bound. Filtration is a passive process, and the rate is primarily determined by the perfusion pressure. The large volume of filtrate (125 ml/min) is transported to the proximal and distal renal tubules. More than 99% of the filtrate is selectively reabsorbed by the tubular cells. The nephron is oriented with the glomerulus in the cortex of the kidney, whereas the tubules are primarily in the medulla.

The kidney produces a number of important hormones. The physiology of the renin-angiotensin system is important for understanding renovascular hypertension. When renal artery stenosis is present, the perfusion pressure decreases (Figure 17-10). This results in a decrease in pressure in the afferent renal arteriole and thus a decrease in filtration pressure and the glomerular filtration rate. Fortunately, the kidney has an important reflex mechanism to maintain the glomerular filtration pressure even with renal artery stenosis. The decrease in perfusion pressure in the afferent renal arteriole is a potent stimulus for the release of renin from the juxtaglomerular apparatus. Renin converts angiotensinogen to angiotensin I, which subsequently is converted to angiotensin II by the angiotensin-converting enzyme (ACE).

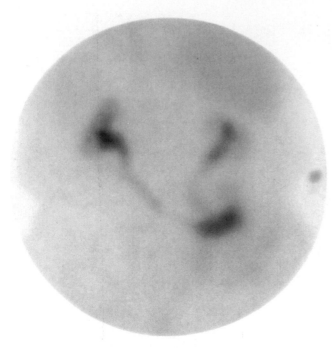

Figure 17-6   Ileal bladder. This patient's bladder has been removed. Excreted activity collects in an artificial bladder that has been created using a section of ilium. The ileal bladder usually drains into a collecting bag.

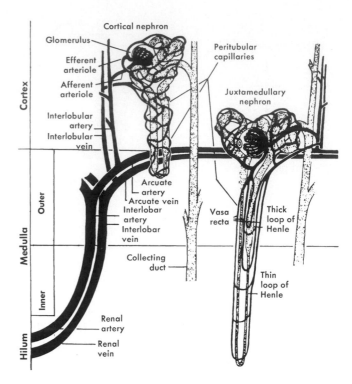

Figure 17-8   Schematic representation of a nephron, circulation, and respective locations in the kidney.

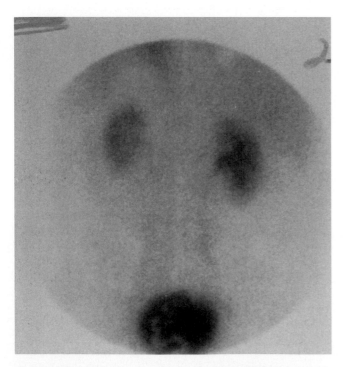

Figure 17-7   Barium in the rectum. The serpiginous area of apparent decreased activity overlying the bladder is caused by barium in the rectum.

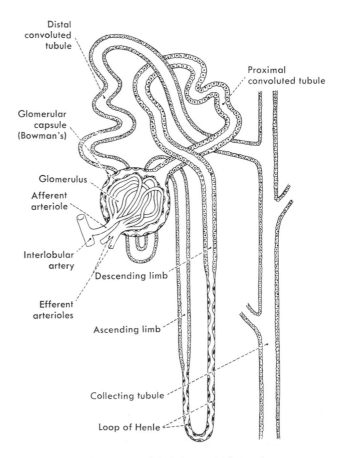

Figure 17-9   Simplified diagram of a nephron.

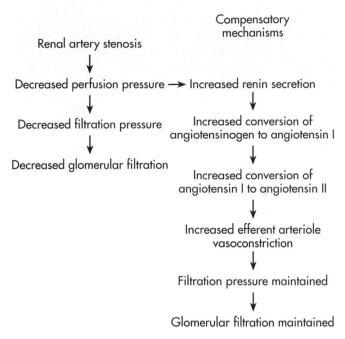

Renal artery stenosis
↓
Decreased perfusion pressure → Increased renin secretion
↓   ↓
Decreased filtration pressure   Increased conversion of
↓   angiotensinogen to angiotensin I
Decreased glomerular filtration   ↓
                                 Increased conversion of
                                 angiotensin I to angiotensin II
                                         ↓
                                 Increased efferent arteriole
                                 vasoconstriction
                                         ↓
                                 Filtration pressure maintained
                                         ↓
                                 Glomerular filtration maintained

Compensatory mechanisms

Figure 17-10 Renovascular hypertension.

Angiotensin II causes vasoconstriction of the efferent glomerular arteriole, thus helping to preserve filtration pressure and the GFR. In addition, angiotensin II increases the secretion of aldosterone, which in turn causes increased sodium resorption by the tubular cells. The increased salt retention increases the systemic blood pressure, and the increased blood pressure helps preserve the perfusion/filtration pressure of the kidney.

When a patient with renal artery stenosis is given an ACE inhibitor (ACEI), the conversion of angiotensin I to angiotensin II is blocked and the compensatory mechanisms are lost. The loss of efferent glomerular arteriolar vasoconstriction results in decreased filtration pressure and a subsequent decrease in the GFR. ACE inhibitors decrease the vascular resistance of abnormal kidneys, therefore blood flow to the kidney is maintained or may increase despite the decrease in the GFR. For this reason, when an ACE inhibitor is given, the initial uptake of a blood flow agent, such as technetium-99m mercaptoacetyl-triglycerine (^{99m}Tc-MAG3), may be preserved even though the initial uptake of a GFR agent, such as ^{99m}Tc diethylenetriamine pentaacetic acid (^{99m}Tc-DTPA), may be markedly decreased. Both agents show prolonged retention of the radiopharmaceutical because of the decrease in the GFR.

RADIOPHARMACEUTICALS

Conceptually, it is best to divide renal radiopharmaceuticals into two categories, functional agents and morphologic agents (Table 17-2).[10,39,41] Functional radiopharmaceuticals are rapidly taken up and excreted by the kidneys by a single, simple physiologic mechanism such as ERPF or the GFR. Morphologic tracers are also rapidly taken up by the kidney but by more complicated mechanisms that usually involve

a complex interaction of the ERPF, GFR, tubular secretion, and tubular resorption. The hallmark of a morphologic tracer is that some of the tracer is retained in the renal parenchyma for a prolonged period. Prolonged retention of the tracer in the kidney makes relatively high-resolution imaging of the renal parenchyma possible, even several hours after injection of the tracer.

Functional agents (see Table 17-2) include iodine-131 (^{131}I) hippuran, ^{99m}Tc-MAG3,[41] and ^{99m}Tc-DTPA. [131]I hippuran is used infrequently because a high-energy collimator is required, and the amount of ^{131}I hippuran administered is limited to 100 µCi because of the high radiation dose to the patient. The small amount of administered activity and use of a high-energy collimator compromise the quality of the images that can be obtained. [123]I hippuran has better imaging characteristics but is not readily available because of the short half-life of [123]I (13 hours). Also, ^{123}I hippuran currently is not available in the United States.

Hippuran is the classic agent that has been used to measure effective renal plasma flow. The ideal characteristics of an agent to measure ERPF or the GFR are listed in Box 17-1. Hippuran fulfills these requirements because first-pass extraction of this agent is high as it passes through the kidney. A high first-pass extraction means that almost all of the agent delivered to the kidney remains in the kidney. For hippuran the ratio of activity in the renal vein to the activity in the renal artery is about 0.15, because about 85% of the activity is retained in the kidney. The most accurate blood flow agent is microspheres, because they have the highest first-pass extraction (about 100%). Hippuran has such high first-pass extraction because it is efficiently secreted by the renal tubule cells and is not reabsorbed from the tubular lumen.

^{99m}Tc-MAG3 has largely replaced hippuran as a functional agent.[41] Like hippuran, MAG3 has a high first-pass extraction fraction. Unlike hippuran, MAG3 is taken up by red blood cells, therefore it clears the plasma even more rapidly than hippuran. ^{99m}Tc-MAG3 is preferred over hippuran because of its superior imaging characteristics.

^{99m}Tc-DTPA is cleared from the plasma almost exclusively by glomerular filtration by the kidney. Several other radiopharmaceuticals (e.g., ^{125}I iothalamate) also have the

necessary characteristics for measuring the GFR,[25] but optimum imaging is possible only with ^{99m}Tc-DTPA.

^{99m}Tc-DMSA and ^{99m}Tc glucoheptonate are considered morphologic imaging agents (see Table 17-2), because accumulation in the kidney is the result of a complex interaction of blood flow, the GFR, tubular secretion, and tubular resorption. Approximately 30% of DMSA is retained in the renal parenchyma, compared with 5% to 10% of glucoheptonate.

Although the choice of radiopharmaceutical for renal imaging is somewhat arbitrary, a few major factors guide selection. A technetium-labeled agent is required to obtain a flow study (Figure 17-11). For evaluation of the renal collecting system for obstruction, an agent that is rapidly excreted into the collecting system is best. For optimum visualization of the renal parenchyma, an agent that is retained in the renal parenchyma is preferred.

Before the introduction of ^{99m}Tc-MAG3 in 1989, different radiopharmaceuticals and different combinations thereof were chosen for different indications. Since the introduction of MAG3, a functional radiopharmaceutical, our institution has used it for most indications. With MAG3 it is even possible to evaluate the morphology of the renal parenchyma, because very good images of the kidney can be obtained within the first few minutes after injection of the tracer (Figure 17-12).

RADIONUCLIDE PROCEDURES

Practical Considerations

To maximize the clinically relevant information obtained from radionuclide renal imaging, the reasons for doing the study must be determined before it is started. Major

Table 17-2	Renal radiopharmaceuticals
Functional radiopharmaceuticals	**Comments**
[131]I hippuran	Effective renal plasma flow agent; paraaminohippuric acid analog
	High first-pass extraction
	Freely filtered; near-total tubular secretion; no tubular resorption
	High target to background even with poor renal function
	[131]I has poor imaging characteristics and gives a relatively high radiation dose to patient
	^{123}I-labeled hippuran has much better imaging characteristics and gives a relatively low radiation dose to patient; however, it is expensive and not readily available because of its short half-life (13 hr)
^{99m}Tc-DTPA (diethylenetriamine pentaacetic acid)	Glomerular filtration agent; inulin analog
	Freely filtered; no tubular secretion; no tubular resorption
	Readily available
	Very good imaging characteristics; low radiation dose to patient
^{99m}Tc-MAG3 (mercaptoacetyl-triglycerine)	Effective renal plasma flow agent; biokinetics are different from those of hippuran
	High first-pass extraction
	Freely filtered; near-total tubular secretion; no tubular resorption
	High target to background even with poor renal function
	Very good imaging characteristics; low radiation dose to patient
	Recently introduced; likely to replace all other renal radiopharmaceuticals for most applications
Morphologic radiopharmaceuticals	**Comments**
^{99m}Tc-DMSA (dimercaptosuccinic acid)	Hepatobiliary excretion with poor renal function can interfere with delayed imaging of renal parenchyma
	Physiologic mechanisms for uptake; excretion and retention are complex
	66% of dose is excreted; 34% is retained by renal cortex at 6 hr after injection
[99m]Tc glucoheptonate	Physiologic mechanisms for uptake; excretion and retention are complex
	More than 90% of dose is excreted; 6% to 10% is retained by renal cortex

indications for radionuclide imaging are listed in Box 17-2. Pertinent clinical information includes the number and size of the kidneys, the results of other imaging tests, the patient's creatinine level and current medications, and any specific instructions regarding the physiologic conditions under which the test is to be performed.

Common physiologic variables include the state of hydration and the position of the patient. Normally patients are hydrated by having them drink two or three 8-ounce glasses of water. Renal imaging usually is performed with the patient in the supine position, except for diuretic renal imaging, which is performed with the patient in the upright position. Less common but potentially important physiologic variables include whether various draining tubes (e.g., Foley catheter, nephrostomy tubes, wound drains) should be clamped.

In general, no patient preparation is necessary. A number of drugs can significantly affect the function of the kidney or directly interfere with the uptake of the radiopharma-ceuticals.[28] If a renal arteriogram is performed a few days before the radionuclide renal study, an inaccurate impression of renal function (absolute and relative) may be obtained because of transient contrast-induced acute tubular necrosis (ATN). Drugs that block tubular secretion (e.g., probenecid) may interfere with the uptake of certain tracers despite normal renal function.

Technologists should reassure patients about the safety of the examination. Reactions to iodinated hippuran are extremely rare, even in patients with a history of iodine contrast hypersensitivity. These agents are extremely safe because such small amounts are injected. The amount of iodine in labeled hippuran is about one billionth of the iodine injected with iodinated contrast. Patients often express concern about having a radioactive material injected into their bodies. The radiation dose is similar to that from contrast intravenous urography.[37] The overall risk of a radionuclide examination is much less than the risk from urography because of the extreme rarity of hypersensitivity reactions with radiopharmaceuticals.

Common Procedures

Functional renal imaging. Functional renal imaging using ^{99m}Tc-MAG3 or ^{99m}Tc-DTPA is the most common radionuclide renal imaging study performed at most medical centers. Common indications for this study include (1)

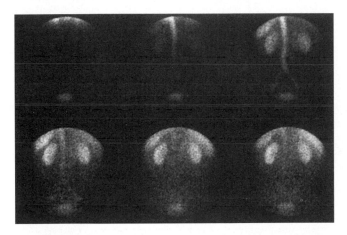

Figure 17-11   Radionuclide flow study of the kidneys. A flow study of the kidneys is obtained as the tracer is being injected. These images have been added on the computer so that each image contains 10 seconds of data. Activity initially is seen in the descending aorta, then in the kidneys and the spleen. Note that the activity in the liver does not appear until well after the activity in the spleen, because most of the hepatic blood flow is from the portal circulation.

Box 17-2	Major Indications for Radionuclide Renal Scintigraphy

Relative renal function
Renal transplant evaluation
Acute renal failure
Obstructive uropathy
Renovascular hypertension
Infection and inflammation
Vesicoureteral reflux

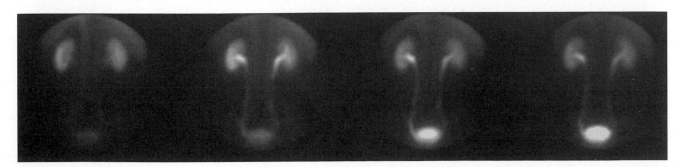

Figure 17-12   Evaluation of the renal parenchyma with ^{99m}Tc-MAG3. Relatively high-quality images of the renal parenchyma can be obtained using MAG3. Images from the dynamic study have been added so that each image contains 5 minutes of data. Evaluation of the renal parenchyma is not compromised by collecting-system activity on the earliest images.

measurement of relative renal function, (2) evaluation of a renal transplant, and (3) evaluation of acute renal failure.[40]

A typical protocol for functional renal imaging consists of a rapid sequence of blood flow images (e.g., one 64×64 image every 2 to 3 seconds for 1 minute), followed by a sequence of functional images obtained at a slower rate (e.g., one 128×128 image every 20 to 30 seconds for 19 minutes). Functional renal imaging can be used to determine both absolute and relative renal function. Most medical centers do not measure absolute renal function (ERPF or the GFR) because the most accurate methods are time-consuming and cumbersome, requiring several timed blood samples.[32] Measurements of absolute renal function based on imaging alone are done infrequently because in most clinical settings, serum creatinine is a satisfactory indicator of absolute renal function.

Much more useful is the ability of radionuclide renal imaging to provide an index of relative individual kidney function. A major factor in the decision to treat or remove a diseased kidney is the degree to which the diseased kidney contributes to total renal function. Usually little effort is expended to repair a kidney that contributes less than 10% of total renal function.

Functional renal imaging also has been used to predict post-operative renal function after removal of a kidney for a renal malignancy. In this setting, post-operative renal function may be underestimated because of compensatory mechanisms.[18]

Relative renal function is calculated using an early image of the kidneys (1 to 3 minutes or 2 to 3 minutes after injection). The relative renal function is calculated by dividing the background-corrected kidney counts by the sum of the background-corrected counts from both kidneys. An early image is used because the radiopharmaceutical is primarily in the parenchyma (functioning tissue) of the kidney at this time. In later images the radiopharmaceutical may be retained in the collecting system. Collecting system activity does not correspond to relative renal function. To measure relative renal function, whole kidney regions of interest are drawn. Partial kidney regions of interests (in an attempt to avoid collecting system activity) would be unsatisfactory.

The time-activity curve (renogram) (Figure 17-13, A) from a normal hippuran or MAG3 study shows prompt uptake of the tracer, with the activity in the kidney peaking at 3 to 5 minutes after injection and decreasing to less than 50% of peak value by 20 minutes. Abnormal curves can result because of abnormal renal function, retention of activity in the collecting system, or patient movement. The cause of an abnormal curve usually can be easily determined from visual inspection of the images, with careful attention paid to the fate of activity seen in the peripheral parenchyma of the kidney. A carefully drawn crescent-shaped region of interest that excludes the collecting system may be helpful if significant retention of activity is seen in the renal pelvis.

Several caveats attend the determination of relative renal function. First, calculation of the relative renal function requires estimates of the number of counts in each kidney and the number of counts in a background region of interest (Figure 17-13, B).[16] Normally, this calculation is quite robust; however, as renal function deteriorates, the number of counts in the background region of interest increases and becomes much more important in the calculation. Under

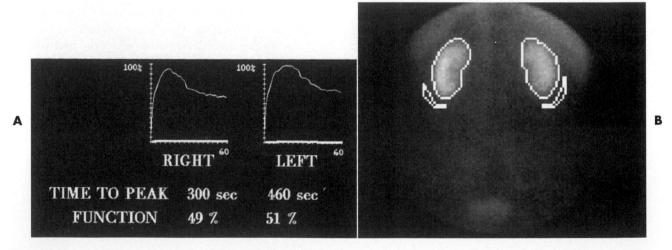

Figure 17-13 **A,** Renogram. The background-corrected activity versus the time curve from the kidney regions of interests is called the renogram. The renograms from the right and left kidneys are shown. The renogram represents only the function of the kidney when there is no significant retained activity in the collecting system. Retained activity in a dilated collecting system can give the false impression of decreased renal function. To avoid this error, both the images and the curves must be examined. **B,** Relative renal function. The percentage of renal function contributed by each kidney is calculated by drawing a region of interest around each kidney. In addition, a background region of interest is drawn for each kidney. The contribution of each kidney to total renal function is calculated by dividing the background-corrected counts for each kidney at 1 to 3 (or 2 to 3) minutes after injection by the background-corrected counts at 1 to 3 (or 2 to 3) minutes from both kidneys. The results usually are expressed as a percentage.

these circumstances (high background counts), the choice of the background region of interest can significantly change the measured contribution of the diseased kidney, therefore a subjective estimate of the relative function may be just as accurate. Unfortunately, no universally accepted standards have been adopted for defining regions of interests.

A second source of error for the measurement of relative renal function is attenuation. Some of the radiation coming from the kidneys is absorbed by the soft tissue between the kidney and the gamma camera. If there is a significant difference in the depths of the kidneys, the contribution of the deeper kidney will be underestimated.

Finally, under some conditions (e.g., acute urinary obstruction, especially in young children) the loss of renal function may be reversible.

The role of functional renal imaging in the routine post-operative management of renal transplant patients is controversial.[9] Routine post-operative radionuclide imaging is not performed at most medical centers because unexpected surgical complications from renal transplantation are rare. In selected patients, radionuclide imaging can be useful for identifying urine leaks, obstruction of the urinary collecting system, and renal infarctions (Figures 17-14, 17-15, and 17-16). Differentiation of acute tubular necrosis, rejection, and cyclosporine toxicity with radionuclide imaging is imperfect.[8]

Treatable causes of acute renal failure include dehydration (hypovolemia), infection, urinary collecting-system obstruction, and acute vascular obstruction. Radionuclide renal imaging is most helpful in excluding acute vascular obstruction as the etiology of acute renal failure. Acute vascular obstruction is an uncommon cause of acute renal failure. One clinical setting in which vascular obstruction is likely to be considered is the aftermath of abdominal aortic aneurysm repair. Decreased renal function after surgery is most likely caused by the transient ischemia of the kidneys that commonly occurs during repair of the aorta; however, an alternative cause is vascular obstruction, especially if the renal arteries had to be reimplanted at the time of surgical repair. If the kidney failure is the result of transient ischemia, renal function probably will improve; if it is the result of vascular obstruction, the loss of renal function likely is permanent.

Another potential use for radionuclide renal imaging in patients with acute renal failure is prognosis. Patients with little or no detectable renal activity on radionuclide renal imaging with hippuran (and presumably with ^{99m}Tc-MAG3) are unlikely to recover significant renal function.[36] Determination of the likelihood of recovery of renal function is helpful in deciding whether an arteriovenous shunt should be placed for future hemodialysis.

Diuretic renal imaging. The standard method used to differentiate a dilated renal collecting system from an obstructed renal collecting system is called the Whitaker test.[43] This invasive test requires placement of an infusion catheter percutaneously into the collecting system proximal to the suspected point of obstruction. Saline is infused at high, nonphysiologic flow rates (about 25 ml/min) while the pressure in the proximal collecting system is monitored. If no significant increase in pressure is seen, no urodynamically significant obstruction is present. Because it is invasive, the Whitaker test cannot be used routinely to follow patients for urinary tract obstruction. In addition, some question the significance of increased pressure at high, nonphysiologic flow rates.

Diuretic renal imaging is particularly useful for differentiating a dilated renal collecting system from an obstructed renal collecting system (Figure 17-17, A).[2,4,23,27,29] Many dilated but unobstructed collecting systems empty spontaneously during routine radionuclide renal imaging. If collecting-system activity persists on a sitting post-void image of the kidneys obtained 20 minutes after injection of the radiopharmaceutical, intravenous injection of furosemide (Lasix) (e.g., 0.5 mg/kg) is very useful. After injection of the furosemide, an additional 20 to 30 minutes of functional images are obtained. If a urodynamically significant outflow obstruction is present, the affected kidney is unable to increase its urine flow rate significantly in response to the furosemide injection. Because the urine flow rate does not increase, wash-out of the activity from the collecting system is prolonged (clearance half-time [$t_{1/2}$] of longer than 20 minutes). A dilated but unobstructed kidney can increase its urine flow rate in response to furosemide, therefore the wash-out of activity from the collecting system is in the normal range ($t_{1/2}$ of less than 10 minutes) (Figure 17-17, B). When the $t_{1/2}$ for wash-out is 10 to 20 minutes, the results are equivocal.

Compared with the Whitaker test, diuretic renal imaging has a high sensitivity for the urodynamic detection of significant lesions. False-positive results and equivocal interpretation may arise when (1) a diseased kidney is not responsive to furosemide injection (such as with immature renal function in neonates, severe dehydration, and poor baseline renal function); (2) the collecting system is grossly dilated; and (3) vesicoureteral reflux or a fully distended bladder (e.g., neurogenic bladder) is present.

ACEI-augmented renal scintigraphy. The relationship between renal artery stenosis (RAS) and renovascular hypertension is complex.[6,34] Patients with hypertension may be classified into three groups: (1) those with hypertension and no significant RAS, (2) those with hypertension in whom RAS is a major contributor to the hypertension, and (3) those with hypertension in whom RAS is an insignificant contributor to the hypertension. Renal imaging with and without an ACE inhibitor is intended to identify patients in whom RAS is a major contributor to the hypertension (group 2 above) These patients have renovascular hypertension,[1] and the hypertension is likely to be more easily controlled if the RAS is repaired.

The physiology of renovascular hypertension has been reviewed. If an ACE inhibitor is given, less efferent arteriolar constriction occurs, the glomerular filtration pressure

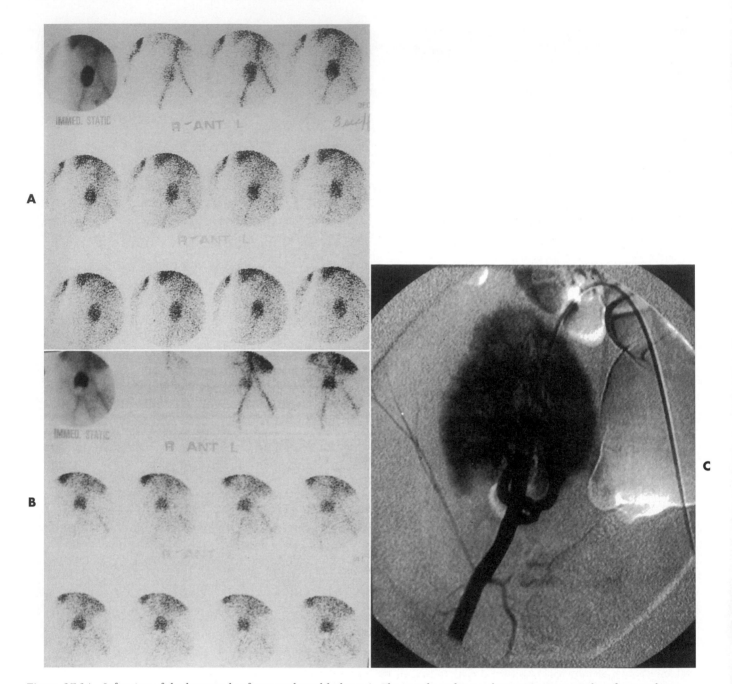

Figure 17-14 Infarction of the lower pole of a transplanted kidney. **A,** Flow study and immediate static image 1 day after renal transplant. The donor kidney was supplied by two renal arteries. **B,** Flow study and immediate static image 7 days after renal transplant when the patient was having pain and swelling of the transplanted kidney. **C,** Arteriogram of the transplanted kidney confirming the occlusion of the artery to the lower pole of the transplanted kidney.

decreases, and the GFR declines. The ACE-dependent change in renal function can be detected using radionuclide imaging with and without an ACE inhibitor (Figure 17-18).

A number of different parameters can be used to document the change in renal function, including a decrease in renal uptake, prolongation of renal parenchymal transit, a decrease in the relative function of the affected kidney, and an increase in the time to peak activity.[33] Different investigators have used different parameters and combinations of parameters to detect renovascular disease.[12,39] Recent studies

have documented the accuracy of this test in the prediction of normalization of blood pressure after revascularization.*

Morphologic renal imaging. Morphologic renal imaging after injection of ^{99m}Tc glucoheptonate or ^{99m}Tc-DMSA can be used to document global and regional changes in renal function. In patients with acute pyelonephritis, areas of decreased function may improve with appropriate

*References 7, 13, 15, 22, 30, and 42.

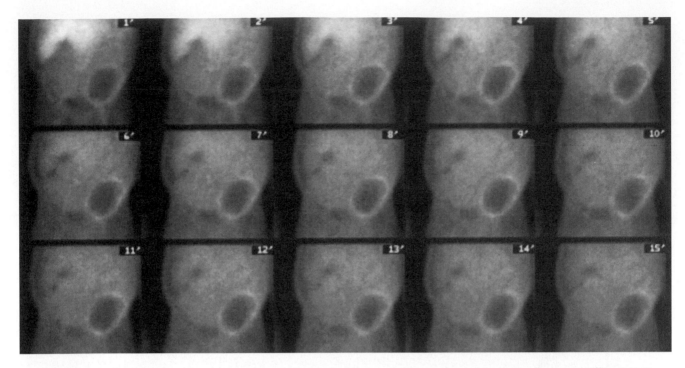

Figure 17-15   Infarction of a transplanted kidney. A 20-minute dynamic study (1 minute per image) after injection of ^{99m}Tc-MAG3 reveals decreased activity and no function of the renal transplant. The ring of increased activity is caused by an inflammation surrounding the infarcted kidney.

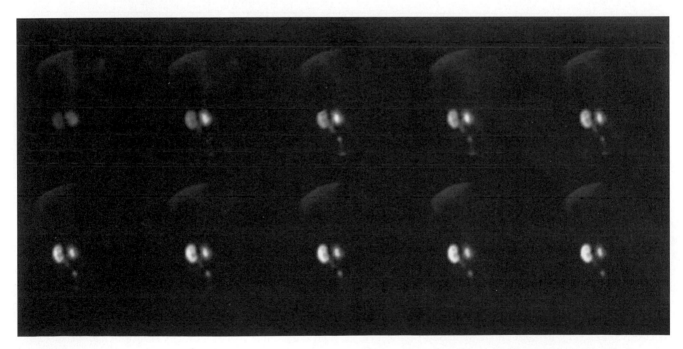

Figure 17-16   Two pediatric kidneys. Shown is a 20-minute dynamic study (2 minutes per image) done after injection of ^{99m}Tc-MAG3 in an adult patient who received both kidneys from a child donor. The kidney at the iliac bifurcation is functioning normally; the other kidney has prolonged retention of activity consistent with acute tubular necrosis (ATN), probably caused by a longer ischemic time.

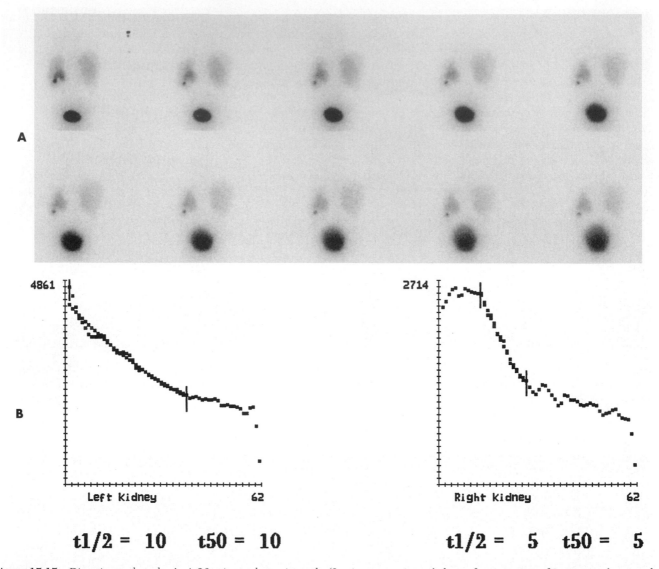

$$t1/2 = 10 \qquad t50 = 10 \qquad\qquad t1/2 = 5 \qquad t50 = 5$$

Figure 17-17 Diuretic renal study. **A,** A 20-minute dynamic study (2 minutes per image) done after injection of Lasix reveals normal wash-out of the radiopharmaceutical from the dilated but unobstructed left renal collecting system. **B,** Renogram reveals that both kidneys have a normal response to Lasix ($t_{1/2} \leq 10$ minutes).

treatment. In children with vesicoureteral reflux and a history of urinary tract infections, the decision to repair the ureters may be influenced by the presence or absence of persistent renal cortical defects as demonstrated by radionuclide imaging.* SPECT imaging also may be useful.[5,24]

Morphologic renal imaging may also be used to detect the presence or absence of small renal infarctions. These infarctions may occur in patients at increased risk of systemic emboli, such as patients with atrial fibrillation or a left ventricular aneurysm. Infarctions that can occur as the result of a complicated renal procedure, such as percutaneous angioplasty of a stenotic renal artery or repair of an abdominal aortic aneurysm, also can be detected with renal imaging.

Vesicoureteral reflux study. A conventional contrast-voiding cystourethrogram is the initial investigation of choice in selected children with urinary tract infections. The anatomic information provided by this study is far superior to the functional information provided by the radionuclide vesicoureteral reflux (VUR) study. Because of its lower radiation dose, a VUR study is preferred for follow-up when the primary concern is the severity and presence (or absence) of reflux rather than anatomy.[11,38] Radionuclide cystography can be performed by catheterizing the patient and directly instilling the radionuclide into the bladder (Figure 17-19) or by injecting the patient with the tracer and allowing the bladder to fill with the tracer as it is excreted from the kidneys. Direct catheterization has a higher sensitivity and specificity than the indirect method and is the preferred method for radionuclide cystography. The clinical importance of reflux in children is its association with chronic

---

*References 3, 19, 21, 26, 29, 31, 35, and 36.

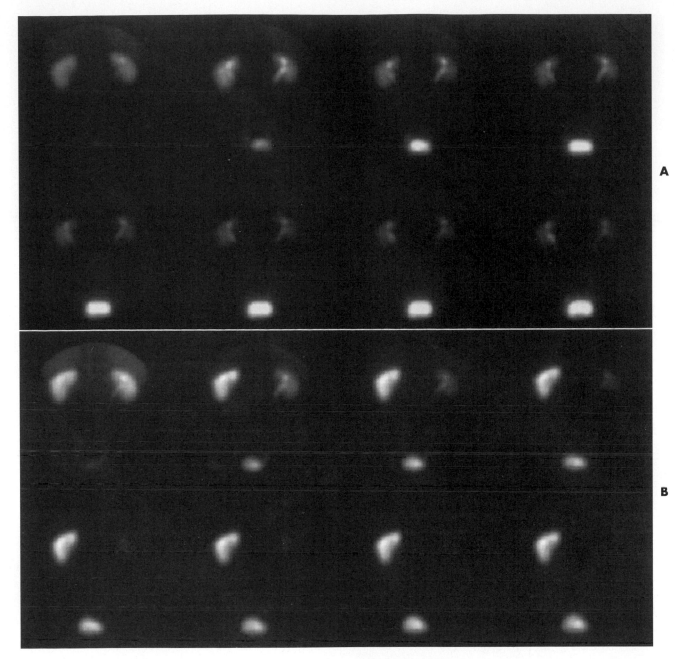

Figure 17-18 Renovascular hypertension. **A,** Baseline renal imaging (2.5 min/image) shows prompt symmetric uptake of ^{99m}Tc-MAG3. A small amount of retained activity is seen in the renal collecting system bilaterally. Little retained activity is seen in the renal parenchyma. **B,** Renal imaging (2.5 min/image) after administration of an ACE inhibitor shows prompt uptake of activity in both kidneys. There is marked prolonged retention of activity in the left kidney. The patient had left renal artery stenosis.

pyelonephritic scarring and subsequent increased risk of hypertension in later years.

TESTICULAR IMAGING

Anatomy and Physiology

The testicles develop in the abdomen and descend to their normal position in the scrotum at about the time of birth. During their descent, the testicles are draped with a fold of parietal peritoneum called the *tunica vaginalis* (Figure 17-20). Normally the tunica vaginalis covers only the antero-lateral surface of the testicle. The blood supply enters the posterior aspect of the testicle and prevents it from rotating in the scrotum. In a common variant of this normal anatomy, the tunica vaginalis more fully envelops the testicle. The blood supply that normally would enter posteriorly enters superiorly and no longer tethers the testicle, preventing it from rotating. This common variant, called the *"bell clapper" deformity,* is always present in cases of acute testicular

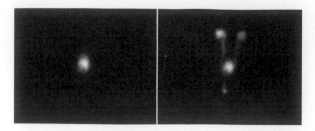

Figure 17-19   Vesicoureteral reflux (VUR) study. Two images from the first 2 minutes of a VUR are shown. Activity initially is seen only in the bladder (*left*). There is prompt, severe reflux of activity to the level of both renal collecting systems (*right*).

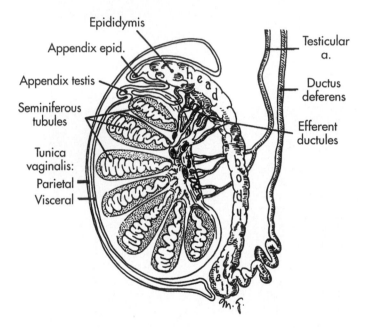

Figure 17-20   Testicular anatomy.

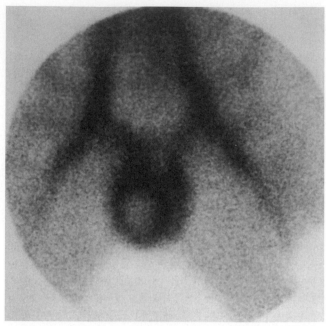

Figure 17-21   Delayed torsion. Testicular scintigraphy reveals a central area of decreased activity with a surrounding area of increased activity. The increased activity is caused by inflammation that occurs after the testicle becomes nonviable.

Other diseases that can cause testicular pain include epididymoorchitis, tumor, torsion of the appendix testis, trauma, and abscess. These causes of testicular pain usually can be differentiated from acute torsion by the patient's history and a physical examination.

Testicular Scintigraphy

Use of testicular scintigraphy to diagnose testicular torsion has largely been replaced by Doppler ultrasound examination of the testicles. In addition to morphologic information, Doppler ultrasound is able to measure blood flow to the testicles.

Testicular scintigraphy consists of a flow study and immediate static images.[17] 99mTc pertechnetate is the most commonly used radiopharmaceutical. The penis of the supine patient should be taped over the pubis. A tape sling should be used to support the testicles between the thighs. Cephalic angulation of the camera can help separate the activity from the thighs and pelvis from the activity from the testicles. Lead shielding can be used on the immediate static images but may make interpretation of the flow study more confusing. When lead shielding is used on the immediate static images, it must be carefully placed to shield both testicles symmetrically.

The blood flow study is primarily used to detect asymmetric blood flow. It usually is impossible to distinguish low testicular blood flow from normal testicular blood flow. The main purpose of the flow study is to detect areas of increased blood flow that would be seen with diseases such as epididymoorchitis, delayed torsion, tumor, trauma, and

torsion. Because the "bell clapper" deformity is usually bilateral, corrective surgery on the unaffected testicle is indicated when testicular torsion has been diagnosed.

Torsion, which most commonly occurs in males between 10 and 19 years of age, usually is marked by a sudden onset of testicular pain. Because the torsed testicle remains viable only for several hours, it is imperative that the diagnosis be suspected and the patient undergo surgery quickly. Some testicles are no longer salvageable after 4 hours of torsion. None are salvageable after 12 to 24 hours of torsion. When testicular torsion lasts longer than 24 hours (delayed torsion), the testicle becomes necrotic and an inflammatory reaction occurs (Figure 17-21). Occasionally, testicular torsion can be intermittent, and the patient can have recurrent episodes of pain. Because acute testicular torsion is a surgical emergency, surgery should not be delayed. Patients suspected of having acute torsion should be sent directly to the operating room. Testicular scintigraphy should be reserved for patients who are unlikely to have acute testicular torsion.

abscess. Acute torsion probably will produce normal-appearing blood flow images. In acute torsion, the immediate static images reveal a central area of decreased activity with normal surrounding activity. A central area of decreased activity can also be seen with a hydrocele (fluid in the space formed by the tunica vaginalis). Hydroceles usually are painless and can be identified by transillumination on physical examination. Abscesses, necrotic tumors, hematomas, and delayed torsion usually have a central area of decreased activity surrounded by an area of increased activity caused by the surrounding inflammatory reaction.

MEASUREMENT OF EFFECTIVE RENAL PLASMA FLOW AND THE GLOMERULAR FILTRATION RATE

Effective renal plasma flow and the glomerular filtration rate can be quantified by measuring the plasma clearance of the selected radiopharmaceutical (see Table 17-2). Plasma clearance of substances can be measured using two fundamentally different approaches. The first approach is called the UV/P (UV divided by P) method (Table 17-3). This method requires (1) measurement of the plasma concentration of the substance (P [mg/ml]), (2) the rate of urine production (V [ml/min]), and (3) the concentration of the substance in the urine (U [mg/ml]). The units of clearance are milliliters per minute. Conceptually, clearance is how much plasma is completely cleared of the substance (ml) per unit time (min).

The UV/P method has two major limitations. First, it works best with a steady plasma concentration of the substance of interest. In practice this requires that the patient be given a constant infusion of the substance over a few hours. Second, although the plasma and urine concentrations of the substance are readily measured, accurate measurement of urine production requires timed, complete urine collections. Hydration (to increase urine production) and bladder catheterization are needed to increase the reliability of the method.

A second way to determine how well the kidneys clear a substance from the plasma is to measure the plasma disappearance curve. This method produces reliable results only when the kidneys are the only significant pathway for excretion. This important requirement is adequately met by only

a few radiopharmaceuticals. Typically the plasma clearance curve is modeled as two compartments (Figure 17-22). The first compartment is the intravascular compartment (plasma), and the second compartment is the extravascular compartment. Initially, the concentration of the tracer in the plasma is very high. The initial rapid clearance of the tracer from the plasma (often called the *fast component*) is primarily the result of diffusion into the extravascular compartment. During this time a small amount of tracer is also cleared from the intravascular space by kidney excretion. Once the tracer reaches equilibrium in the two compartments, any decrease in activity in the intravascular compartment is the result of kidney excretion alone. Mathematically, the clearance curve that results from this model consists of the sum of two monoexponential equations. The plasma clearance curve method does not require the urine collections that are needed for the UV/P method. However, the plasma clearance curve method also is laborious because at least eight blood samples collected over a 4-hour period are needed to estimate accurately the biexponential clearance of the tracer. Methods using only one or two blood samples have been described.[32]

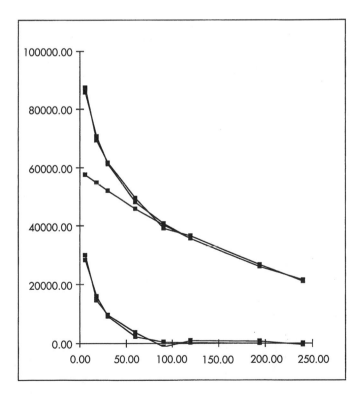

Figure 17-22 GFR plasma clearance curve and plasma clearance curve after intravenous injection of ^{99m}Tc-DTPA. The *x* axis is minutes and the *y* axis is counts per milliliter. The GFR is calculated by fitting a monoexponential to the slow component (the last four points) of the plasma clearance curve. The fitted curve is subtracted from the original data. A monoexponential curve is then fitted to the first four points of the resulting curve (the curve on the bottom of the graph). The GFR can be calculated based on the results of the two fitted monoexponential equations.

Table 17-3	UV/P method

U (urine concentration) = 4,000 cpm/ml
V (timed urine collection) = 60 ml urine produced/20 min
P (plasma concentration) = 100 cpm/ml

$$GFR = \frac{UV}{P} = \frac{60\,ml * 4,000\,cpm * 1\,ml}{20\,min * 1\,ml * 100\,cpm}$$

$$= \frac{240,000\,ml}{2,000\,min} = 120\,ml/min$$

REFERENCES

1. Black HR: Captopril renal scintigraphy: a way to distinguish functional from anatomic renal artery stenosis, *J Nucl Med* 33:2045-2046, 1992.
2. Conway JC: The principles and technical aspects of diuresis renography, *J Nucl Med Tech* 4:208-214, 1989.
3. Chiou YY et al: Renal fibrosis: prediction from acute pyelonephritis focus volume measured at ^{99m}Tc dimercaptosuccinic acid SPECT, *Radiology* 221(2):366-370, 2001.
4. Conway JJ, Maizels M: The "well tempered" diuretic renogram: a standard method to examine the asymptomatic neonate with hydronephrosis or hydroureteronephrosis: a report from combined meetings of the Society for Fetal Urology and members of the Pediatric Nuclear Medicine Council, the Society of Nuclear Medicine, *J Nucl Med* 33(11):2047-2051, 1992.
5. Craig JC et al: Reliability of DMSA for the diagnosis of renal parenchymal abnormality in children, *Eur J Nucl Med* 27(11):1610-1616, 2000.
6. Davidson RA, Wilcox CS: New tests for diagnosis of renovascular disease, *JAMA* 268:3353-3358, 1992.
7. Dondi M et al: Prognostic value of captopril renal scintigraphy in renovascular hypertension, *J Nucl Med* 33:2040-2044, 1992.
8. Dubovsky EV, Russell CD: Radionuclide evaluation of renal transplants, *Semin Nucl Med* 3:181-198, 1988.
9. Dubovsky EV et al: Report of the Radionuclides in Nephrourology Committee for evaluation of transplanted kidney (review of techniques), *Semin Nucl Med* 29(2):175-188, 1999.
10. Eshima D, Fritzberg AR: Radiopharmaceuticals for renal imaging. In Henkin RE et al, editors: *Nuclear medicine,* St Louis, 1996, Mosby.
11. Fettich JJ, Kenda RB: Cyclic direct radionuclide voiding cystography: increasing reliability in detecting vesicoureteral reflux in children, *Pediatr Radiol* 22:337-338, 1992.
12. Fine EJ: Interventions in renal scintirenography, *Semin Nucl Med* 29(2):128-145, 1999.
13. Fommei E, Volterrani D: Renal nuclear medicine, *Semin Nucl Med* 25(2):183-194, 1995.
14. Gates GF: Glomerular filtration. In Henkin RE et al, editors: *Nuclear medicine,* St Louis, 1996, Mosby.
15. Geyskes GG et al: Renovascular hypertension identified by captopril-induced changes in the renogram, *Hypertension* 1:36-42, 1987.
16. Harris CC et al: Effect of region assignment on relative renal blood flow estimates using radionuclides, *Radiology* 151:791-792, 1984.
17. Holder LE et al: Testicular radionuclide angiography and static imaging: anatomy, scintigraphic interpretation, and clinical indications, *Radiology* 125:739-752, 1977.
18. Johansson M, Moonen M: Prediction of postoperative glomerular filtration rate after nephrectomy for renal malignancy, *Clin Physiol* 21(6):688-692, 2001.
19. Konda R et al: Ultrasound grade of hydronephrosis and severity of renal cortical damage on 99m-technetium dimercaptosuccinic acid renal scan in infants with unilateral hydronephrosis during follow-up and after pyeloplasty, *J Urol* 167(5):2159-2163, 2002.
20. Lin E et al: Reproducibility of renal length measurements with ^{99m}Tc-DMSA SPECT, *J Nucl Med* 41(10):1632-1635, 2000.
21. Majd M, Rushton HG: Renal cortical scintigraphy in the diagnosis of acute pyelonephritis, *Semin Nucl Med* 22:298-311, 1992.
22. Marks LS, Maxwell MH: Renal vein renin: value and limitation in the prediction of operative results. *Urol Clin North Am* 2:311-317, 1975.
23. Niemczyk P et al: Use of diuretic renogram in evaluation of patients before and after endopyelotomy, *Urology* 53(2):271-275, 1999.
24. Peng NJ et al: ^{99m}Tc dimercaptosuccinic acid renal scintigraphy for detection of renal cortical defects in acute pyelonephritis: posterior 180-degree SPECT versus planar image and 360-degree SPECT, *Nucl Med Commun* 22(4):417-422, 2001.
25. Perrone RD et al: Utility of radioisotopic filtration markers in chronic renal insufficiency: simultaneous comparison of ^{125}I iothalamate, ^{169}Yb-DTPA, ^{99m}Tc-DTPA, and inulin, *Am J Kid Dis* 16(3):224-235, 1990.
26. Piepsz A et al: Consensus on renal cortical scintigraphy in children with urinary tract infection, Scientific Committee of Radionuclides in Nephrourology, *Semin Nucl Med* 29(2):160-174, 1999.
27. Pohl HG et al: Early diuresis renogram findings predict success following pyeloplasty, *J Urol* 165(6 part 2):2311-2315, 2001.
28. Prescott MC, Johnson WG: Influence of drugs on the renogram. In O'Reilly PH, Shields RA, Testa HJ, editors: *Nuclear medicine in urology and nephrology,* Boston, 1989, Butterworth.
29. Rossleigh MA: Renal cortical scintigraphy and diuresis renography in infants and children, *J Nucl Med* 42(1):91-95, 2001.
30. Roubidoux MA et al: Renal vein renins: inability to predict response to revascularization in patients with hypertension, *Radiology* 178:819-822, 1991.
31. Rushton HG et al: Renal scarring following reflux and nonreflux pyelonephritis in children: evaluation with ^{99m}technetium-dimercaptosuccinic acid scintigraphy, *J Urol* 147:1327-1332, 1992.
32. Russell CD, Dubovsky EV: Measurement of renal function with radionuclides, *J Nucl Med* 30:2053-2057, 1989.
33. Setaro JF et al: Simplified captopril renography in diagnosis and treatment of renal artery stenosis, *Hypertension* 18:289-298, 1991.

34. Sfakianakis GN et al: Single-dose captopril scintigraphy in the diagnosis of renovascular hypertension, *J Nucl Med* 28:1383-1392, 1987.

35. Shapiro E et al: Optimal use of ^{99m}technetium-glucoheptonate scintigraphy in the detection of pyelonephritic scarring in children: a preliminary report, *J Urol* 40:1175-1177, 1988.

36. Sherman RA, Sherman B: Clinical significance of nonvisualization with I-131 hippuran renal scan. In Hollenberg NK, Lange S, editors: *Radionuclides in nephrology,* Stuttgart, 1980, Thieme.

37. Snyder WS et al: *Absorbed dose per unit cumulated activity for selected radionuclides and organs,* MIRD Pamphlet No 11, New York, 1975, Society of Nuclear Medicine.

38. Stork JE: Urinary tract infection in children, *Adv Pediatr Infect Dis* 2:115-134, 1987.

39. Taylor A: Radionuclide renography: a personal approach, *Semin Nucl Med* 29(2):102-127, 1999.

40. Taylor A Jr, Nally JV: Clinical applications of renal scintigraphy, *Am J Roentgenol* 164(1):31-41, 1995.

41. Taylor A et al: Clinical comparison of I-131 orthoiodohippurate and the kit formulation of Tc-99m mercaptoacetyl-triglycine, *Radiology* 170:721-725, 1989.

42. Van Bockel JH et al: Renovascular hypertension: collective review, *Surg Gynecol Obstet* 169:471-478, 1989.

43. Whitaker RH: Methods of assessing obstruction in dilated ureters, *Br J Urol* 45:15-22, 1973.

Paul E. Christian, R. Edward Coleman

chapter **18**

Skeletal System

Objectives

Explain the composition of bone and list the general types of bones.

Name the major bones and joints of the skeleton.

Explain the accumulation mechanism of bone-imaging agents.

Discuss the advantages of whole body imaging techniques versus spot imaging.

Describe adequate acquisition parameters for static bone imaging using spot-film and whole body imaging devices.

Explain the advantages of performing SPECT bone scans.

Describe imaging techniques and acquisition parameters for obtaining flow studies and blood pool imaging.

Explain the advantages of performing delayed imaging in the diagnosis of osteomyelitis.

Discuss the use of gallium and white cell imaging techniques in correlation with bone scans.

Describe the principles of bone therapy and discuss the characteristics of radioactive strontium.

Identify the appropriate radiopharmaceutical dose and administration technique for strontium bone therapy.

---

*T*he skeleton performs several functions for the body, including support, protection, movement, and blood formation. Bone, like other connective tissues, consists of living cells and a predominant amount of nonliving intercellular substance that is calcified. It is a metabolically active tissue with large amounts of nutrients being exchanged in the blood supplying the bone. Thus the skeleton and body fluids are in equilibrium. Tracer techniques have been used for many years to study the exchange between bone and blood.[5] Radionuclides have played an important role in the understanding of normal bone metabolism, in addition to the metabolic effects of pathologic involvement of bone.

Radionuclide imaging of the skeleton is being used with increasing frequency in the evaluation of abnormalities involving bones and joints.[7] Several studies have demonstrated that different information can be obtained from radionuclide bone imaging compared with radiography and blood chemistry analysis.[18,22,28,37,44] Radionuclide joint imaging has been used for a shorter period than bone imaging and is still being evaluated in many diseases involving the joints.*

---

*References 15, 31, 38, 39, 53, and 54.

A thorough knowledge of the anatomy and physiology of bones and joints is necessary to fully understand the technical and clinical aspects of radionuclide imaging of the skeletal system. The first part of this chapter reviews skeletal anatomy and physiology. The remainder of the chapter discusses radionuclide imaging of the bones and joints, with an emphasis on the technical aspects and applications of the imaging procedure.

COMPOSITION OF BONE

Bone is no different from other tissues in the body in that it is maintained by living cells in addition to having amorphous ground substance and fibers, as does other connective tissue. The main difference between bone and other connective tissue is that it is calcified; thus it is harder. Bone matrix, the other major constituent of bone, consists of collagen, amorphous ground substance, and mineral.

The composition by weight of normal adult cortical bone is approximately 5% to 10% water, 25% to 30% organic matter (collagen, ground substance, and cellular elements), and 65% to 70% inorganic matter (bone mineral). Collagen is the main protein constituent and accounts for 90% to 95% of the organic matter of bone. Collagen is present in the form of fibrils bunched together into bundles of fibers. The ground substance is the interfibrillar cement substance in which the fibrils are embedded.

The bone salt mineral (inorganic matter) has the crystalline form of an apatite, and chemical analysis reveals the following ions: calcium, phosphate, hydroxyl, carbonate, and citrate, with lesser amounts of sodium, magnesium, potassium, chloride, and fluoride. Approximately 27% of the weight of cortical bone is calcium. The main anion constituent of bone is phosphorus (as phosphate), which contributes approximately 12% of the weight of cortical bone. The bone mineral consists of individual crystals so small that the electron microscope is needed for visualization of the crystals. The crystalline structure is hydroxyapatite, $Ca_{10}(PO_4)_6(OH)_2$. This formula represents the ratio of the constituent elements and is not necessarily the molecular formula.

GROSS STRUCTURE OF BONE

Bones have obvious differences in size and shape but also certain features in common. They have a *cortex* (compact bone) surrounding various amounts of *cancellous* (spongy or trabecular) *bone,* which contains blood-forming (*myeloid*) elements or fatty marrow (Figures 18-1 and 18-2). In the adult most of the myeloid marrow is in the bones of the trunk, with some in the calvarium and upper ends of the humeri and femora. Bones are also similar in that they are covered by periosteum, except in areas of articulation or where tendons and ligaments connect them. The gross structure of bones is discussed in respect to their general archi-

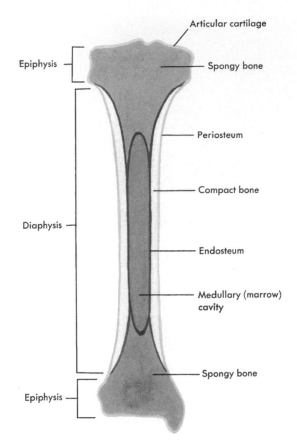

Figure 18-1   Structure of long bone in longitudinal section.

tecture in the following groups: tubular, short, flat, and irregular.

Tubular Bones

The long tubular bones include the humerus, radius, ulna, femur, tibia, and fibula. The short tubular bones include the metacarpals, metatarsals, and phalanges. Often the tubular bones are all classified as long bones. The tubular bones have a shaft (*diaphysis*) consisting of a cortex of compact bone surrounding the medullary cavity, which contains bone marrow (see Figure 18-1). In the adult this is mainly yellow, or fatty, marrow, except for the proximal humerus and femur, where it is red (blood-forming) marrow (see Figure 18-2). The cortex is thickest at the midshaft and tapers toward the ends of the shaft. The end of a bone that previously had an epiphysis is known as an *epiphyseal bone end.* The juncture of the cancellous bone of the epiphyseal bone end and the spongy bone of the diaphysis is called the *metaphysis.*

Short Bones

The short bones include the wrist (carpals), ankle (tarsals), sesamoids (small bones forming in a tendon or joint capsule), and other anomalous or extra bones. These bones are generally cubic and have spongy osseous tissue covered by a shell of compact bone.

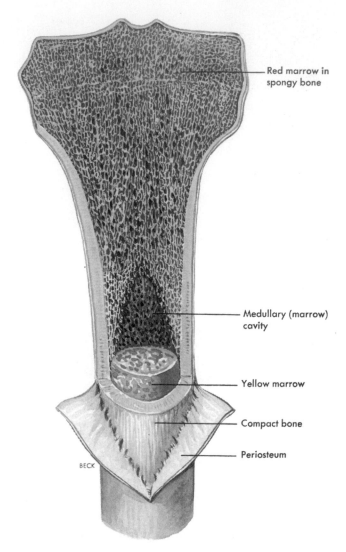

Figure 18-2 Cutaway section of long bone.

Table 18-1	Skeletal system
Skeletal parts	**Number of bones**
Axial skeleton	
Skull and hyoid	29
Vertebrae	26
Ribs and sternum	25
	80
Appendicular skeleton	
Upper limbs	64
Lower limbs	62
	126
Total	**206**

SKELETON

The skeletal system (Figures 18-3 and 18-4) usually contains 206 bones; it provides a supporting framework for the body and forms protective chambers, such as the skull and thorax. The skeleton is divided into two main parts, the axial skeleton and the appendicular skeleton (Table 18-1). The axial skeleton is composed of the bones of the skull, thorax, and vertebral column, which form the axis of the body. The appendicular skeleton is composed of the bones of the shoulder, upper extremities, hips, and lower extremities. A detailed structure of the vertebrae is shown in Figure 18-5.

JOINTS

Joints (articulations) are spaces where bones come into contact and are bridged in some manner. The articulations have variable amounts of movement and have been classified into two main types according to the amount of movement: rigid (synarthroses) or freely movable (diarthroses).

With a synarthrosis there is absence of a joint space, with little or no movement allowed. In the formation of a synarthrosis the tissue connecting the bones is replaced by the ends of the bone growing together. The sutures of the skull are examples of synarthroses, with only a thin, fibrous membrane separating the ends of the bones (Figure 18-6, *A*). In some synarthroses, cartilage grows between the articular surfaces of the bones and may allow some motion. Examples of the cartilaginous synarthroses are the symphysis pubis and the joints between the vertebral bodies (Figure 18-6, *B* and *C*).

A diarthrosis permits freedom of movement and is the most common type of joint in the body. A diarthrosis has a well-defined articular cavity that contains fluid (synovia) and is lined by a synovial membrane (Figure 18-6, *D* and *E*). Intraarticular structures such as ligaments and menisci

Flat Bones

The flat bones include the ribs, sternum, and scapulae and several of the skull bones. These bones are thin and have little spongy bone between two layers of compact bone. The flat bones of the skull consist of an inner and outer table (layers of cortical bone) separated by a thin layer of spongy bone (*diploë*). The spongy layer of the ribs and sternum contains considerable red marrow.

Irregular Bones

The irregular bones include the bones of the spine and pelvis and some of the skull. Part of an irregular bone may fit into one of the other categories, but the entire bone does not fit into any of the previous categories. The largest part of these bones often consists of large amounts of spongy osseous tissue with a very thin surrounding cortex, whereas another part of the same bone may have no spongy tissue and may be composed of two layers of compact bone.

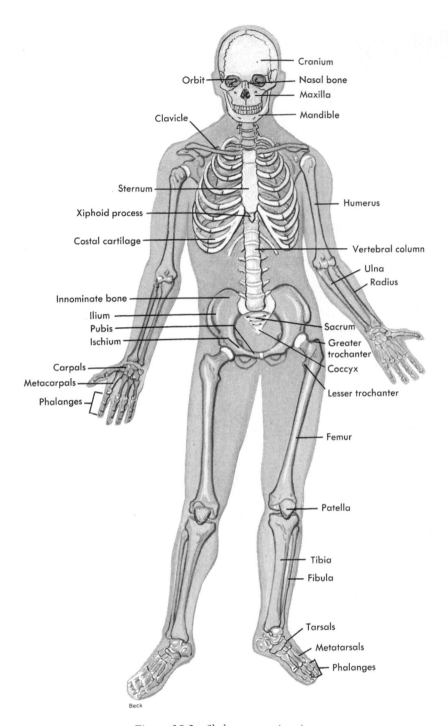

Cranium

Orbit

Nasal bone

Maxilla

Mandible

Clavicle

Sternum

Xiphoid process

Costal cartilage

Humerus

Vertebral column

Ulna

Radius

Innominate bone

Ilium

Pubis

Ischium

Sacrum

Greater trochanter

Coccyx

Lesser trochanter

Carpals

Metacarpals

Phalanges

Femur

Patella

Tibia

Fibula

Tarsals

Metatarsals

Phalanges

Beck

Figure 18-3   Skeleton, anterior view.

may be present. A thin layer of hyaline cartilage, known as *articular cartilage,* cushions the ends of each bone in the joint. The synovial joint develops from undifferentiated mesenchyme between the bone rudiments. Part of the undifferentiated mesenchyme differentiates into synovial mesenchyme and subsequently into synovial membranes, menisci, and ligaments. The outer portion of the undifferentiated mesenchyme condenses and forms the joint capsule, which attaches to the bone ends of the joints beyond their articular cartilages.

RADIONUCLIDE IMAGING

Of the many different imaging procedures performed in clinical nuclear medicine, radionuclide bone and joint studies especially require the technologist to be thoroughly knowledgeable of anatomy and imaging techniques so that excellent images of the radiopharmaceutical distribution can be obtained. Because early disease involvement of bone initially may be subtle, improper positioning of the patient for imaging or improper exposure of the film may lead to an

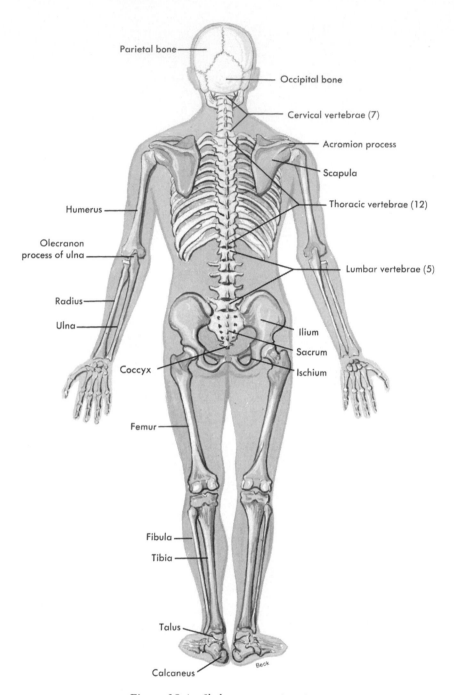

Figure 18-4   Skeleton, posterior view.

inaccurate interpretation. Furthermore, because these studies frequently are used to follow therapy, the technique must be reproducible to allow careful comparison with a previous study. Several different types of radionuclide studies can be performed in the evaluation of bone and joint disorders. The most commonly performed procedure is radionuclide bone imaging with a technetium-99m (^{99m}Tc) phosphate compound. Joint imaging is used in the evaluation of suspected inflammatory processes involving bones and joints.

Past and Present Radiopharmaceuticals

The earliest applications of radionuclides to the study of bone were performed with phosphorus-32 and calcium-45 for observation of bone structure and function.[2,40] These radionuclides are pure beta particle emitters and accumulate in regions of increased bone mineral deposition, but their lack of gamma radiation limits external measurement. Clinical application became possible only with the use of strontium-85 (^{85}Sr), a calcium analog that produced gamma

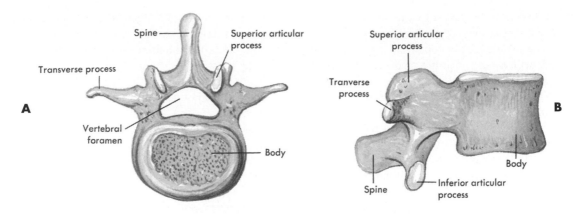

Figure 18-5   Third lumbar vertebra from above (**A**) and the side (**B**).

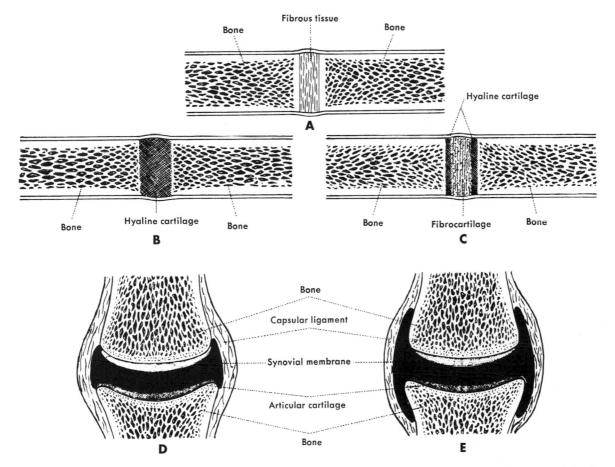

Figure 18-6   Classification of joints. **A,** Fibrous synarthrosis. **B** and **C,** Cartilaginous synarthroses. **D** and **E,** Synovial diarthrosis.

rays that could be detected externally.[4,12,13] The introduction of the rectilinear scanner and [85]Sr in the early 1960s made bone scanning possible; however, because of the high radiation dose involved, its use was limited to patients with documented malignancy. [85]Sr has a half-life of 65 days and emits a gamma ray at 513 keV. The long effective half-life of this radionuclide limits the amount of activity injected to 100 μCi. With this small amount of activity, scanning time was extensive and the information density of the image was extremely low. Although the accumulation of strontium in bone is rapid, blood and gastrointestinal clearances are slow, therefore a 2- to 7-day interval between the times of injection and scan was needed.

Another isotope of strontium used for bone scanning is [87m]Sr, which has a half-life of 2.9 hours and a gamma ray energy of 388 keV.[51] This short half-life allows the administered dose to be increased to a range of 1 to 4 mCi, and scans can be performed 2 to 3 hours after injection. ^{87m}Sr is a generator-produced isotope from a parent product of yttrium-87, which has a half-life of 80 hours. Unfortunately, ^{87m}Sr was rather expensive.

Fluorine-18 (^{18}F) was the first bone-seeking radiopharmaceutical that gave an acceptable radiation dose to the patient and provided a higher quality scan than the strontium isotopes; this permitted a wider application of bone imaging in the late 1960s and early 1970s.[10] The rapid blood clearance of ^{18}F is advantageous for the performance of bone scans because the blood and tissue activity levels are low compared with that of bone at the time of imaging and therefore give a high ratio of bone to soft tissue. The disadvantage of using ^{18}F is its half-life of 1.87 hours, which makes it very expensive to manufacture and deliver to a large number of hospitals at any great distance from the production facility. The annihilation radiation (511 keV) from its positron emission is suitable for imaging with a rectilinear scanner but not a scintillation camera because of the high-energy photons.

The development of ^{99m}Tc-labeled phosphate complexes for bone imaging was introduced by Subramanian in 1971.[52,53] ^{99m}Tc in the form of pertechnetate does not localize to any useful extent in bone. ^{99m}Tc has excellent physical properties for nuclear medicine imaging because of its ideal characteristics for use with the Anger scintillation camera. The short half-life of ^{99m}Tc allows several millicuries of activity to be injected; allowing images with high information density to be obtained.

Because ^{99m}Tc is the current radionuclide of choice, the phosphate compound that produces the best image needs to be determined. Figure 18-7 shows the structure of four phosphate compounds that have been used in routine clinical bone imaging. To evaluate these various phosphate compounds, their distribution in the body relative to the rate and amount of accumulation in various organ systems and bone must be determined.

Polyphosphate was the first commercially available ^{99m}Tc-labeled compound for bone imaging. The structural formula of polyphosphate includes a group of phosphates with a chain length of approximately 40 to 55. Extremely long phosphate chains can result in the formation of a radiocolloid in the bloodstream, causing hepatic localization of the pharmaceutical. Further development of this agent moved from longer phosphate chains toward shorter, more stable phosphate complexes. Among these were pyrophosphate and ethylenehydroxydiphosphonate (EHDP). Pyrophosphate is a naturally occurring compound in the body, and its P—O—P bond is subject to breakdown by phosphatase enzymes. The carbon-carbon bond of EHDP is believed to offer greater stability than pyrophosphate. Both pyrophosphate and EHDP have a faster blood and tissue clearance than polyphosphate.

Methylene diphosphonate (MDP) and hydroxymethylene diphosphonate (HMDP) are similar to pyrophosphate and EHDP but have faster blood clearance.[33] The blood clearance of MDP and HMDP in the initial 3 to 4 hours after administration is very similar to that of fluorine. MDP and HMDP labeled with ^{99m}Tc provide a better image of the bones, because the lower blood and tissue concentrations give a higher ratio of bone to tissue. MDP and HMDP give comparable quality bone images.

Mechanism of Accumulation

The accumulation of radionuclides in bone is related both to vascularity and to the rate of bone production.[19,52]

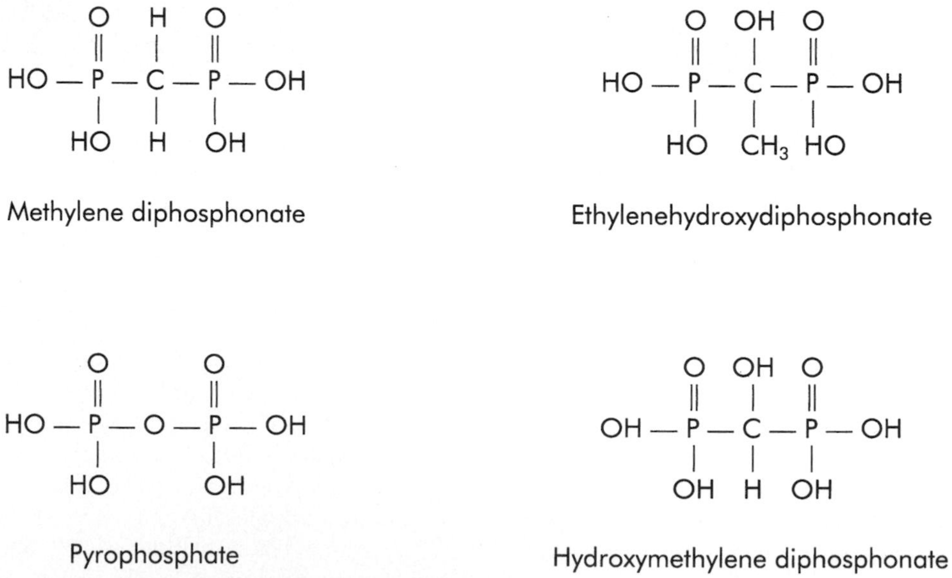

Figure 18-7   Structural formulas of various phosphate pharmaceuticals in acid form.

Increased blood supply to an area of bone results in a blood pool image (obtained immediately after radiopharmaceutical administration) with increased activity.

Localization of various bone-imaging agents is related to exchange with ions in the bone. The process of exchange of an ion native to bone for a labeled, bone-seeking ion is termed *heterionic exchange*.[11,27] Calcium phosphate is the main inorganic constituent of bone; however, calcium is also found in the form of carbonate and fluoride. Calcium is located in microcrystals of hydroxyapatite.[42] Analog elements of calcium, such as strontium, are believed to exchange with the calcium. ^{18}F exchanges with the hydroxyl (OH) ion in the hydroxyapatite. The accumulation of labeled phosphate compounds probably is related to the exchange of the phosphorus groups onto the calcium of hydroxyapatite. Although these mechanisms are not completely understood, the principle of bone imaging is fairly basic. Calcium analogs or phosphate compounds have a low concentration in blood and tissue.

Radiopharmaceuticals used for bone imaging can localize in soft tissue areas, demonstrating not only calcification but also infarction, inflammation, trauma, and tumor. The portion of any radiopharmaceutical that does not accumulate in bone and tissue or that stays in the circulation is eliminated from the body by various routes, depending on the radiopharmaceutical. ^{85}Sr has some concentration in the gastrointestinal tract for several days. ^{18}F and phosphate scans labeled with ^{99m}Tc demonstrate activity in the kidneys and bladder, because these agents are excreted through the urinary tract.

Technical Considerations

The physical characteristics of the radionuclides that have been used for bone imaging present several important factors in radiopharmaceutical selection. These factors relate primarily to the amount of activity that may be administered to the patient, the gamma ray energy, and the amount of accumulation of radiopharmaceutical in the bone.

Before the introduction of ^{18}F and ^{99m}Tc phosphate compounds, bone imaging was a time-consuming procedure associated with a high radiation dose to the patient and poor information content in the images. The subsequent development of better radiopharmaceuticals and improved instrumentation produced images of higher quality with better information about bone physiology. In conjunction with the improved information in the images, the need for carefully controlling the technical aspects of the procedure became apparent.

Selection of the best radionuclide for bone imaging currently is a simple choice based on the physical characteristics. The strontium and fluorine isotopes have high-energy gamma rays and require the use of coarse-resolution collimators with thick lead septa. The high-energy gamma rays have a low attenuation coefficient, resulting in a poor detection efficiency in the thin, sodium iodide crystal of the Anger scintillation camera. Also, these radionuclides must be administered in amounts of activity smaller than those of ^{99m}Tc, yielding lower information-density images. ^{18}F is an excellent agent for bone imaging, but its short half-life and high cost limit its general availability. ^{99m}Tc-labeled compounds allow larger quantities of activity to be administered with a resultant lower radiation dose than do the other radionuclides. The monoenergetic gamma ray emission of 140 keV and the absence of particulate radiation make ^{99m}Tc well suited for use with the scintillation camera. ^{99m}Tc is also readily available to all laboratories at a very low cost, unlike other radionuclides for bone imaging.

Patient Preparation

Preparation of the patient for bone imaging is minimal when any of the ^{99m}Tc-labeled agents are used, but several factors must be taken into consideration. The patient needs to have a complete understanding of the procedure, especially the reason for the delay between radiopharmaceutical administration and imaging. A delay of approximately 3 hours is generally an adequate time to achieve good bone accumulation and a low soft tissue level of the radiopharmaceutical. Radiopharmaceuticals with fast blood and tissue clearance, such as MDP and HMDP, allow imaging as early as 2 hours after administration. Unless contraindicated, patients should be hydrated to aid clearance of the radiopharmaceutical from the body. Administration of four to six glasses of liquid during the delay period is adequate, and the patient should be encouraged to void frequently to reduce the radiation dose. Patients must also void immediately before imaging begins so that the image of the pelvis is not obscured by a large amount of radioactivity in the bladder. Because of the high concentration of radioactivity in the urine, care must be taken to avoid contamination of the patient, the patient's clothing, or the bed sheets, which can lead to a false-positive result on the study.

INSTRUMENTATION

Several types of instruments have been used for bone imaging. Wider application of this procedure has been responsible for the design of new instruments and accessories.

The Anger scintillation camera is currently the most versatile and most commonly used imaging device for ^{99m}Tc-labeled compounds. Because the skeleton is one of the most extensive organ systems in the body, application of the mobile camera with an approximately 10-inch standard field of view requires 25 to 30 separate views for complete imaging. Performing bone imaging by this technique requires a large amount of the technologist's time and effort in positioning the patient for all these views. High-resolution or medium-resolution (140 keV) collimators are well suited for bone imaging with a standard-field camera (high-sensitivity collimators should not be used). However, a 140 keV diverging collimator can maintain good resolution

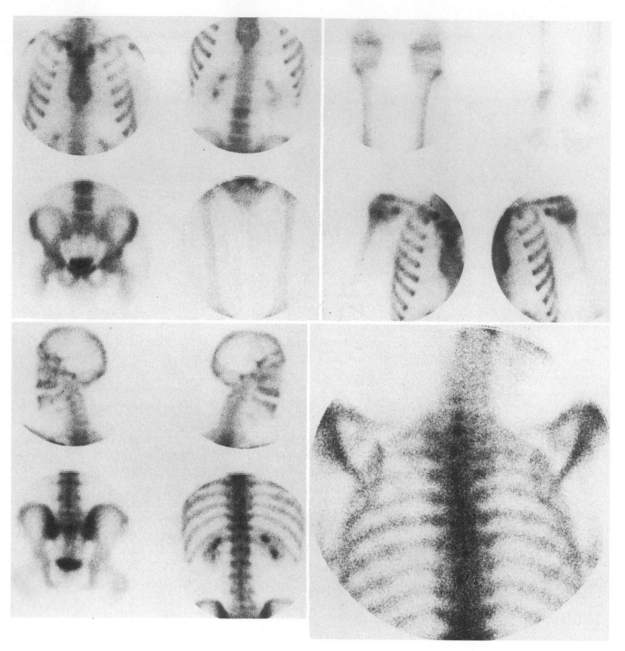

Figure 18-8 Thirteen images necessary to cover whole body with large-crystal camera. Forearms and hands are still omitted with these images.

and allow reduction of the total number of images because of the larger effective field of view. The currently used diverging collimators result in slight spatial distortion and loss of resolution at the image edges. Use of a large-crystal (15-inch) scintillation camera with a parallel hole collimator allows inclusion of a larger area of the body in each view, reducing the total number of images to approximately 13 to 16 views (Figure 18-8). Newer cameras with extra large crystals, either square, rectangular (Figure 18-9), or circular, can image larger areas of the body, and fewer images are needed for whole body imaging.

The bone area and activity in the field of the camera can be highly variable for different portions of the body, and some images may require a long imaging time to achieve high information density (ID). Commonly, multiple individual images are taken for an equal amount of time. This equal-time technique allows comparison of the film density in one image with that in another image, because the exposure is made for equal amounts of time. This method is effective as long as adequate statistics are achieved. First, one area of the body (e.g., the anterior or posterior view of the chest) is imaged for a preset number of counts. Between 400,000 and 600,000 counts are accumulated for a standard-field camera and between 500,000 and 1 million for a large-crystal camera. After this first exposure, all subsequent images are taken for the same interval. An alternative

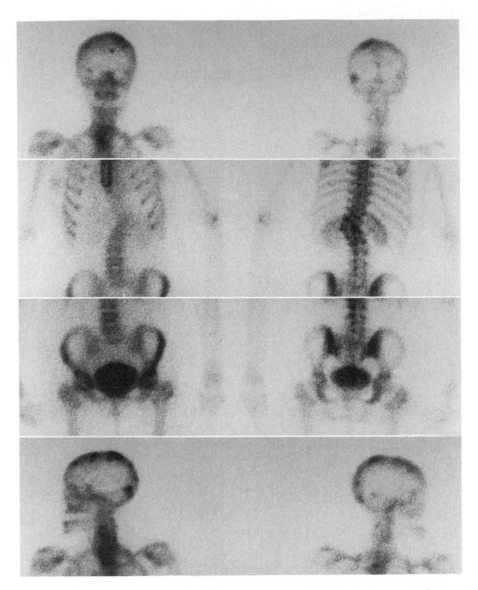

Figure 18-9   Images from a 24-inch rectangular-field gamma camera. *Left*, Anterior images. *Right*, Posterior images.

method of performing equal-time imaging is to use the ID feature available on some scintillation cameras. An area of normal bone in the sternum or spine is selected with the ID marker, and an exposure is made until the ID in this region reaches a range of 2500 to 4000 counts. The time for this exposure is then used to obtain the other images.

Individual images of certain areas can be obtained with the scintillation camera after the initial image of the total skeleton on another type of instrument has been performed. The spot films provide detailed images of areas that were not well visualized on the whole body imaging instruments or supply additional views that aid the determination of the presence (or absence) of abnormality. A detailed view of the pelvis can be degraded by whole body imaging devices because of activity accumulated in the bladder before the imaging device reaches the pelvis. Images of the pelvis should be obtained immediately after the patient has voided, which can be before or after the whole body image.

WHOLE BODY IMAGING

The production of an image of the total body area (Figure 18-10) onto one film is accomplished by an accessory that moves either the camera detector or the patient through the camera field of view. As the body moves past the detector, the area seen by the camera is minified and advances across the film at a speed proportional to that of the patient. Some large-crystal cameras can cover the body in two passes or, when equipped with a special diverging collimator, in one pass. When multiple passes are required to produce the image, faint longitudinal lines appear on the image. This "zipper" is created because of the slight separation of each pass over the body.

When a scintillation camera is used with a whole body imaging accessory, a portion of the crystal may be masked either electronically or by collimation into a rectangular field of view. It is essential that this region of the detector be

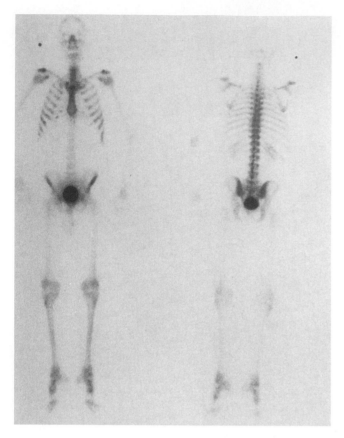

Figure 18-10 Normal whole body bone scan with extra-large-crystal camera. Anterior views (*left*) and posterior views (*right*) are obtained simultaneously using two detectors.

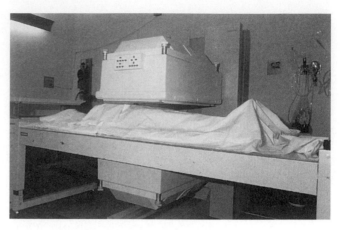

Figure 18-11 Dual-detector extra large field of view (24 inches wide) for whole body image.

proportional in its speed over the patient compared with the motion of the minified image area that moves across the cathode ray tube (CRT).

The technique for establishing imaging parameters is determined by monitoring the count rate or ID or by selecting the total time for the whole body scan. A region for measuring the count rate usually is selected anteriorly over the chest or posteriorly over the spine. The same scan speed should be used for both the anterior and the posterior images. The scan speed is determined by one of several techniques. Most camera manufacturers supply a table, chart, or nomogram for determining the proper scan speed, based on the desired ID in the image and the count rate from the patient. Some systems may have a microcomputer for automatically calculating the scan speed, determined from monitoring the count rate from the patient. All these methods are basically the same, but some additional variations from the manufacturer's method may give improved image quality. Digital cameras record the whole body scan in a high-resolution matrix for photographing after data acquisition.

It is recommended that the whole body image include more than 2.5 million counts. The best positioning of the patient is to have the detector under the table and have the patient lie prone and supine to produce the anterior and posterior images, respectively. Using this technique, the detector can be nearer the patient during imaging.

Whole body imaging with the scintillation camera provides a good esthetic relationship of overall radiopharmaceutical distribution with only a small loss in resolution generated from the motion synchronization of the table and the CRT recording. Less manipulation of the patient is necessary, and little effort is required of the technologist during the imaging procedure.

Figure 18-11 shows a dual-detector, large-field camera for performing whole body imaging. Anterior and posterior scans are obtained simultaneously using detectors that cover the full body width.

SPECT IMAGING

The potential use for single photon emission computed tomography (SPECT) in bone imaging is in the examination of areas in which substantial superimposition of bony structures occurs. Bone studies using SPECT have mainly involved patients with suspected disease of the hips, lumbar spine, temporomandibular joints, and facial bones. Bone SPECT has been demonstrated to be the most sensitive noninvasive test for evaluation of the extent of arthritis in patients with chronic knee pain examined by conventional radiography, bone scanning, and subsequent arthroscopy. SPECT offers advantages over planar imaging in the evaluation of patients with suspected avascular necrosis of the hip. A photopenic area is frequently seen on SPECT imaging that is not seen on planar imaging. SPECT has also been shown to be more sensitive than planar imaging in the evaluation of patients with evidence of spondylolysis or spondylolisthesis. SPECT is better than planar imaging in identifying the site of abnormality in symptomatic patients with defects in the pars interarticularis. SPECT is also superior to planar imaging in the evaluation of patients with temporomandibular joint dysfunction who undergo pre-operative evaluation.

Bone SPECT imaging of the axial skeleton should be performed with high-resolution collimators. As with usual SPECT imaging, the detector to patient distance should be minimized. High-quality images can be obtained only with an adequate imaging time (i.e., 30 to 45 minutes). Imaging of the lumbar spine should be done with the patient's legs slightly elevated to make the spine straight. Imaging with a single-head camera is most commonly performed using a 64 × 64 image matrix; some newer cameras have high enough resolution to warrant the use of a 128 × 128 matrix. Studies should be acquired using a large number of views (120 to 128) in 360 degrees to obtain good angular sampling. SPECT studies acquired with these parameters have very high counts and very high resolution and therefore should be reconstructed with high-resolution pre-filtering and reconstruction filters. Reconstructed images should be reviewed by the technologist for proper orientation and should be free of artifacts. Reconstructed transverse, coronal, and sagittal slices should be oriented to the patient's anatomy for interpretation and comparison with planar images.

The importance of quality control in SPECT is stressed in Chapter 9. SPECT studies of poor quality or those per-formed improperly are inferior to quality planar images. The improved image contrast for lesions makes SPECT of inter-est for bone imaging. The utility of SPECT in bone imaging is now being determined. Furthermore, removal of super-imposition of bony structures results in better localization of abnormal accumulation. The widespread use of SPECT for bone imaging will determine its appropriate role in radionuclide bone imaging.

Figure 18-12 shows a SPECT study of the lumbar spine compared with planar images. SPECT applications to bone scintigraphy can add clinically useful information in nearly all parts of the skeleton, particularly the spine, skull, knees, and hips. The primary advantage is to add three-dimensional information about the extent of disease. SPECT also occasionally shows lesions not seen on planar images.

CLINICAL ASPECTS

The skeleton is a complex organ system subjected to many different types of adversities. Bone disease can be generally classified into two broad categories, congenital and acquired. In the congenital bone diseases, radionuclide imaging has essentially no role, because most of these

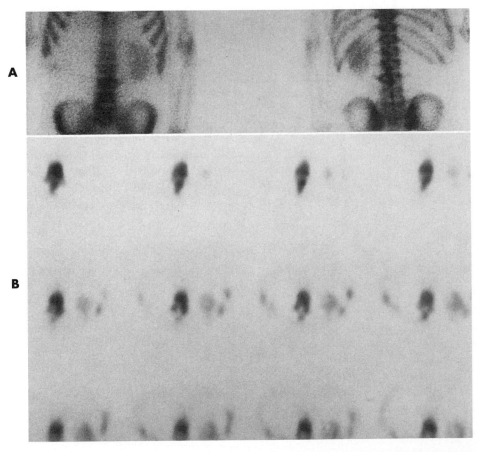

Figure 18-12   **A,** Planar images of lumbar spine with abnormal radiopharmaceutical accumulation in the L2-3 region. **B,** Reconstructed superior-to-inferior transverse slices show increased uptake in the transverse and spinous process of these vertebrae.

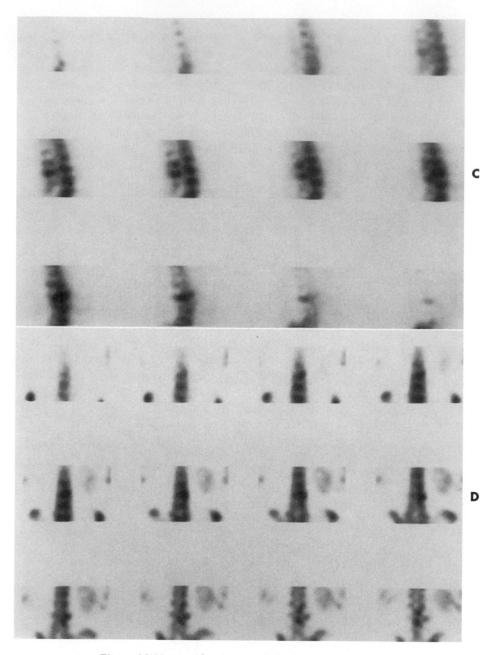

Figure 18-12, cont'd C, Sagittal slices. **D,** Coronal slices.

diseases have a characteristic radiographic appearance. However, radionuclide bone imaging is important in the evaluation of several acquired bone diseases. These can be classified as traumatic, neoplastic, inflammatory, metabolic, degenerative, vascular, and other bone diseases that do not fit into these listed categories.

Localization of the bone-seeking radiopharmaceuticals depends mainly on two factors, bone blood flow and bone production. The relative importance of each of these parameters is not well defined, but frequently both are increased. Increased radiopharmaceutical deposition accompanying increased bone production is well exemplified by the epiphyseal growth plate in bone imaging in children (Figure 18-13). Occasionally an abnormality is detected as

a focal area of decreased pharmaceutical accumulation (Figure 18-14). This decreased accumulation can be related to impaired blood flow or to complete destruction or replacement of bone by a tumor, an inflammatory mass, or radiation.

The indications for bone imaging are as follows:

1. Staging of malignant disease (screening of high-risk patients and localization of biopsy sites)
2. Evaluation of primary bone neoplasms
3. Diagnosis of early skeletal inflammatory disease
4. Evaluation of skeletal pain of undetermined etiology
5. Evaluation of elevated alkaline phosphatase of undetermined etiology

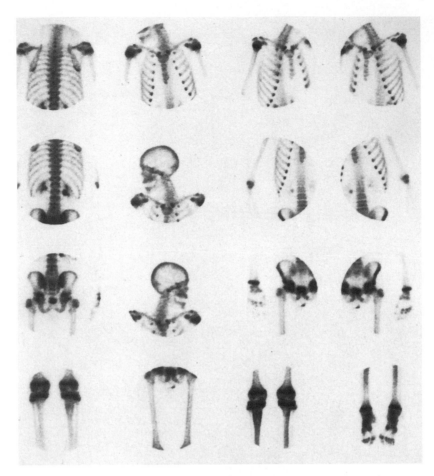

Figure 18-13 Multiple gamma camera images from a large-crystal camera of a 15-year-old boy with an aneurysmal bone cyst of the right tibia. The epiphyseal activity in multiple areas is apparent.

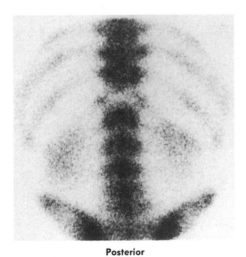

Posterior

Figure 18-14 Absent accumulation of radiopharmaceutical in vertebral body.

6. Determination of bone viability
7. Evaluation of painful total joint prostheses

The most frequent reason for ordering a bone scan is to stage malignant disease by determining whether spread to bone has occurred. The other indications are used less frequently but are important reasons for bone imaging.

Anterior and posterior images of the whole body generally are obtained (see Figure 18-10). The anterior skull, facial bones, mandible, clavicle, sternum, anterior ribs, anterior iliac spine, and pubic rami are best visualized on the anterior images. The posterior skull, spine, posterior ribs, scapulae, sacroiliac joints, and ischia are best visualized on the posterior images. The shoulders, hips, and extremities are commonly seen well on both views, primarily depending on patient positioning.[12] The activity in the skeleton is usually symmetric from side to side. However, some asymmetry may be seen in the skull, shoulders, sternoclavicular joints, and anterior ends of the ribs without a pathologic condition present.[55] The activity in the kidneys is variable. With ^{99m}Tc-MDP or ^{99m}Tc-HMDP, kidney activity is usually less than the surrounding bone activity. Kidney disease may be associated with pronounced asymmetry of renal activity, a focal area of absent activity (cyst or tumor),

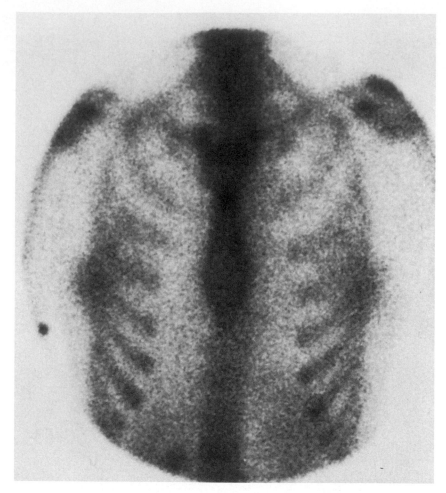

Figure 18-15 Anterior chest image in a bone scan of a 37-year-old woman demonstrating bilateral accumulation of the radiopharmaceutical in normal breasts.

or ureteric visualization, suggesting ureteric obstruction.[9,34] Accumulation of the bone-imaging radiopharmaceutical can occur in the normal female breast and with various diseases of the breast[3] (Figure 18-15).

In most institutions radionuclide bone imaging has replaced the radiographic skeletal survey for evaluation of skeletal metastatic disease. Metastases to bone are common in several primary malignancies, including lung, breast, and prostate carcinomas. Metastases to the spine are difficult to detect radiographically, because loss of approximately 50% of the mineral content of the bone must occur before lytic lesions are detected.[16] Whereas 10% to 40% of adult patients with metastatic bone disease and an abnormal bone scan may have normal radiographs, fewer than 5% of bone scans are negative when the radiograph demonstrates metastatic disease.[29,50] In the pediatric population one study has demonstrated 68% of metastases identified by radionuclide imaging alone.[23] False-negative scans have been related to several factors. If the skeleton is diffusely involved with metastatic disease, the focal nature of the lesions might not be apparent.[17] A diffusely abnormal scan may be difficult to differentiate from a normal scan, but with quality images

from the scintillation camera, irregularities of radiopharmaceutical deposition can generally be noted (Figure 18-16). Metastatic lesions may have no associated osteoblastic activity and thus may not be detected by bone scan or may be detected as a photon-deficient area.[24] An example of a disease in which the lesions might not produce an abnormality on the bone scan is multiple myeloma, which has a high false-negative rate. After the bone images are performed, radiographs of the abnormal areas are often recommended for a more definitive diagnosis and to exclude other etiologies of an abnormal scan in the patient with suspected metastatic disease.

The usual pattern of skeletal metastatic disease is multiple focal lesions throughout the skeleton, with the greatest involvement generally in the axial skeleton[26,28] (Figure 18-17). The area of abnormal radiopharmaceutical deposition represents the edge of the metastatic deposit where osteoblastic repair is attempted. Some primary cancers that metastasize to tissue other than bone accumulate bone-seeking radiopharmaceuticals (Figure 18-18). These tumors generally tend to be calcified on radiographs, but the bone scan is abnormal before the radiographs. A few bone-

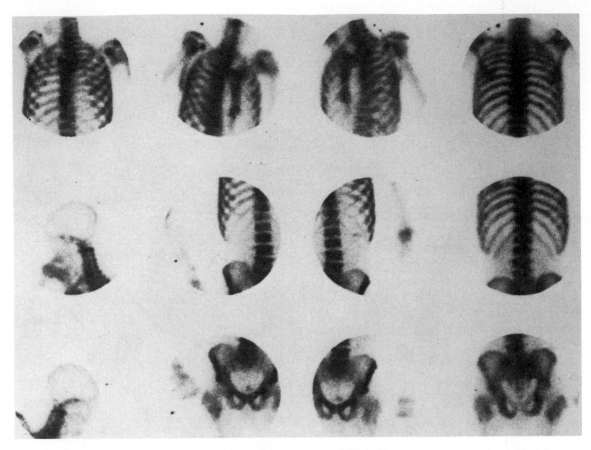

Figure 18-16   Bone scan in a 61-year-old man with prostate cancer demonstrating diffusely increased activity in the ribs, spine, and pelvis. Irregular distribution of activity is noted in the ribs and minimal activity in the soft tissue and kidneys. This is a "superscan" from widespread metastatic disease.

producing metastatic lesions do occur, such as those attributable to osteogenic sarcoma (Figure 18-19). Accumulation of the agent in soft tissue metastases may prove helpful in detecting extra-skeletal involvement.[46]

The malignancies in which bone imaging has demonstrated importance for the staging of the disease are breast, lung, and prostatic carcinomas.[28,37,45] These are common malignancies with a high incidence of bony metastatic disease. Other malignancies are now evaluated with bone imaging, and there is a higher incidence of bony metastases than previously suspected. Therefore most patients with malignancies now have a bone scan as part of their evaluation.

Bone scanning is also used for the evaluation of primary bone neoplasms. Usually the patient has already had radiographs of the primary tumor, and the bone scan offers no additional information about that area. The extent of the abnormality on the bone scan is generally not much different from that of the radiographically apparent lesion. The value of bone scanning in patients with primary bone malignancy lies in the detection of the disease elsewhere.[23] As many as 30% of patients with Ewing's sarcoma may have lesions in other bones, a finding that significantly alters the therapy of the disease.[8,23,56] Metastatic deposits in soft tissue

from osteogenic sarcoma can be detected by scan before the appearance of radiographic abnormalities.[46]

Radionuclide bone imaging also is used in the evaluation of several nonmalignant processes. Bone imaging has been demonstrated to be useful in the evaluation of patients with suspected osteomyelitis and diskitis.[20,30,47,57] The bone scan may be positive within 24 hours after the onset of symptoms, whereas the radiographic changes are not apparent for 10 to 14 days.

Early images are important in the evaluation of inflammatory processes, therefore a three- or four-phase bone scan should be performed. A three-phase bone scan is performed by acquiring a rapid flow sequence of images over the area of interest during radiopharmaceutical injection. Flow images are taken every 2 to 4 seconds for 40 to 60 seconds. Static images are then immediately obtained for 300,000 to 500,000 counts without moving the patient, and additional projection images are taken as necessary. Both osteomyelitis and cellulitis cause early increased activity as a result of an increased vascular response to the affected area. The second phase is routine scanning at 2 to 3 hours after injection. The third phase is to evaluate persistent increased activity at 5 hours. A fourth phase can be added by taking images after a 24-hour delay. The third- and fourth-phase images should

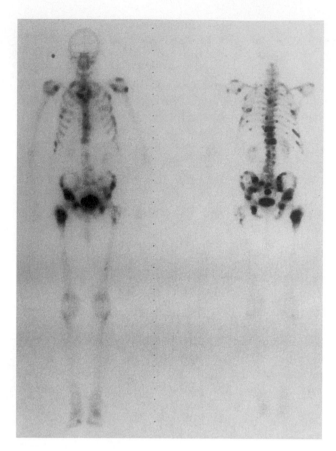

Figure 18-17 Multiple focal lesions in the bone of a patient with prostate carcinoma.

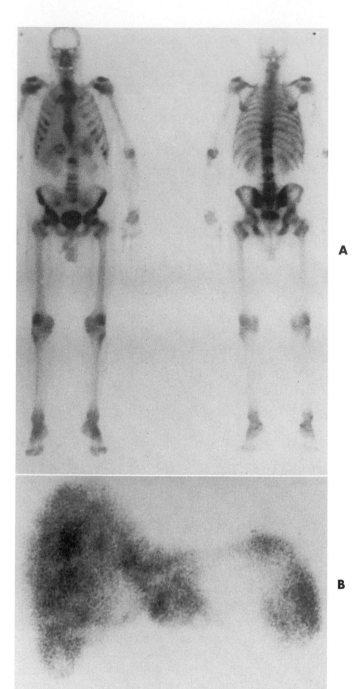

A

B

Figure 18-18 Metastatic colon cancer. **A,** Anterior whole body scan reveals a doughnut-shaped area of abnormal accumulation in the right upper quadrant. **B,** ^{99m}Tc sulfur colloid liver-spleen scan reveals areas of diminished colloid localization. This abnormality is a metastatic lesion from a primary colon cancer.

be taken for 100,000 to 250,000 counts to allow comparison of these delayed images with respect to changes in activity in the affected area (Figure 18-20).

With cellulitis, increased blood pool activity may be seen diffusely throughout the area of involvement, as well as some diffusely increased activity on the regular bone images obtained 2 to 3 hours after injection. Osteomyelitis, however, demonstrates focally increased activity in the involved bone on both the blood pool and routine images (see Figure 18-20). Since bone imaging came to be used for detecting osteomyelitis, it has been found that several patients do not subsequently develop the typical radiographic changes because the early treatment prevents the development of radiographic abnormalities.

Diskitis, an inflammatory process of the disk space, usually occurs secondary to a bacterial infection. The bone scan reveals increased activity in the vertebral bodies on each side of the disk space (Figure 18-21).

In some instances trauma is being evaluated with bone scanning.[44] Immediately after a fracture, for the first day or two, there may be decreased activity visualized at the site. After day 3, there is generally diffusely increased activity in the area of fracture, which becomes focally increased by day 10. Depending on the angulation of the fracture and stress, for example, the activity decreases with time but may remain

abnormal for years if the fracture is complicated and bone remodeling continues. The bone scan has been used to evaluate patients with normal radiographs suspected of having fractures (Figure 18-22). Some of these patients have normal radiographs at the time the bone images are abnormal.

Radionuclide bone imaging is also used with several other conditions. Paget's disease is associated with greatly abnor-

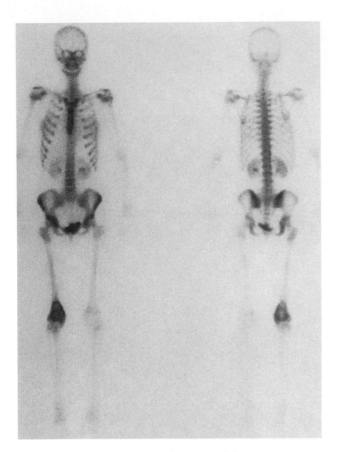

Figure 18-19 Osteogenic sarcoma of distal femur in a 16-year-old girl shows tumor restricted to femur without evidence of metastatic disease.

mal radiopharmaceutical accumulation typically involving the greater part of a bone[1,48] (Figure 18-23). The bone scan has been used to evaluate therapy for this disease.[1] Determination of the cause of pain after a total joint replacement is frequently difficult, and radionuclide imaging has been demonstrated to be a sensitive method of detecting a complication, such as loosening or infection of the prosthetic implant[21] (Figures 18-24 and 18-25). Radionuclide imaging is also very sensitive for the detection of osteoid osteomas, a cause of skeletal pain that may go undetected for years.[32]

Avascular necrosis of the hip is difficult to diagnose by clinical examination and radiographs of the hips, and radionuclide imaging frequently is used in the evaluation of these patients. Early in the course of the disease, a decrease in the blood flow and blood pool, in addition to decreased accumulation of the bone-scanning radiopharmaceutical on delayed images, can be seen. Magnetic resonance imaging (MRI) may also detect abnormalities before radiographic changes (Figure 18-26).

Joint Imaging

Radionuclide imaging of the joints has been used in several institutions for the evaluation of inflammatory joint disease.* This imaging has been performed with either ^{99m}Tc pertechnetate or ^{99m}Tc phosphate compounds. The ^{99m}Tc pertechnetate images are obtained immediately after injection of the radiopharmaceutical, and abnormal accumulation is noted in areas of increased blood flow, such as are found in synovitis. ^{99m}Tc phosphate compounds localize in areas of joint inflammation, which show an increased turnover rate and vascularity of the adjacent bone, as well as increased synovial vascularity (Figure 18-27). Either of these radiopharmaceuticals can be used to detect early joint inflammation, often before radiographic abnormalities occur. Compared with a physical examination, radiographs, and arthrography, joint imaging with the ^{99m}Tc phosphate complex is the most sensitive indicator of early degenerative disease of the knee.[54]

Several recent studies have demonstrated the utility of ^{99m}Tc phosphate imaging in the early detection of sacroiliac inflammatory disease[15] (Figure 18-28). Detection of the inflammatory process before radiographic changes have occurred has been demonstrated. The technique uses a computer to quantify areas of bone activity and compares the activity in the sacroiliac joint region with an area of equal size in the midsacrum.

Radionuclide Therapy of Painful Bone Metastases

Some neoplasms, such as those of the breast, lung, prostate, kidney, and thyroid, frequently spread to bone and cause pain.[35] The method of treatment for painful bone metastases is a dilemma for the oncologist. Narcotic medication is widely used in the treatment of bone pain, but lethargy and constipation are major side effects of these drugs that limit their usefulness. Biphosphonites originally were used to treat the hypercalcemia resulting from bone metastases, and they are now used alone or in combination with cytotoxic agents in the palliation of painful bone metastases.[35] External beam radiotherapy is used to treat focal sites of painful disease. Hemibody radiation has been used in patients with multiple sites of painful metastases. In some patients with multiple focal sites of painful metastases, external beam radiation therapy is not an option.

Unsealed sources of radiopharmaceuticals have been shown to be beneficial in the treatment of some patients who have painful bone metastases.[41] These radiopharmaceuticals are beta emitters and have a chemical affinity for sites of formation of new bone using differing mechanisms.[49] The radiopharmaceuticals used to treat painful bone metastases include ^{89}Sr chloride ($t_{1/2}$ of 50.5 days), and samarium-153 (^{153}Sm) EDTMP ($t_{1/2}$ of 1.9 days). Other radiopharmaceuticals are in clinical trials. The results of studies using these radiopharmaceuticals have been similar. The response rates for pain relief have varied in the different studies, with a range of 37% to 91%. Complete remission of the bone pain

*References 6, 15, 31, 36-39, 53, and 54.

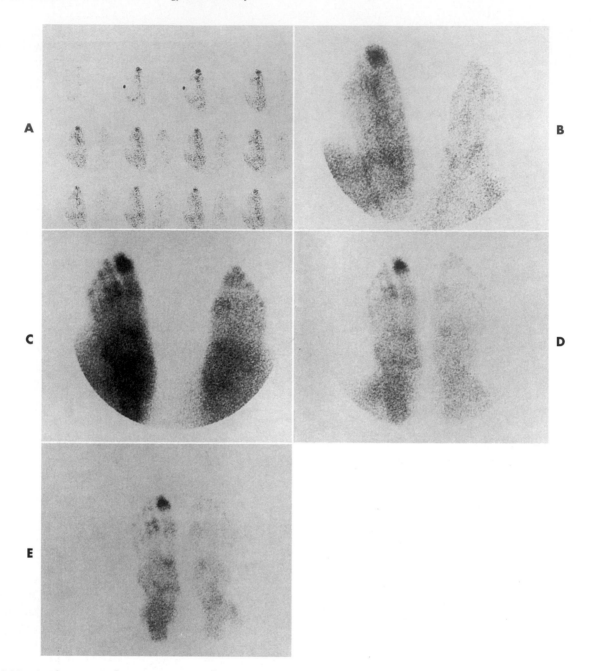

Figure 18-20 **A,** Plantar view flow images at 4 sec/frame show increased perfusion to the first right distal phalanx. **B,** Blood pool images also demonstrate abnormal accumulation. Images at 2 hours (**C**), 5 hours (**D**), and 24 hours (**E**) show persistent radiopharmaceutical collection consistent with osteomyelitis.

is less common than partial remission. Twenty percent to 30% of patients show no response to systemic radionuclide therapy. The side effects, including the effects on the production of blood cells, are not significantly different for any of the radiopharmaceuticals and are uncommon.

^{89}Sr is a pure beta emitter with a half-life of 50.6 days that is capable of delivering a high radiation dose to cortical and trabecular bone. Patients may be considered candidates for ^{89}Sr chloride therapy on confirmation that metastatic disease is the cause of the bone pain. ^{89}Sr may be administered in conjunction with external beam radiother-

apy or chemotherapy or both. Patients should have platelet counts above 60,000/mm^3 and white cell counts greater than 2400/mm^3. Any patient with impending pathologic fractures or spinal cord compression should not be considered a candidate for this therapy. As part of the screening process, bone scans should be performed with ^{99m}Tc-MDP to document that abnormal bone turnover has been identified at the site of pain.

The dose of ^{89}Sr is 40 to 60 μCi/kg or 4 mCi.[43] Good radiation safety practices should be used in the handling of the therapeutic radiopharmaceutical, including gloves, plastic

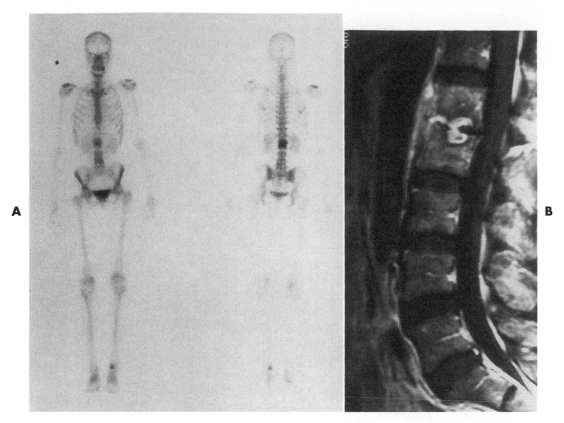

Figure 18-21   **A,** Whole body bone scan reveals diffusely increased radiopharmaceutical accumulated in T10 and L2 vertebral bodies. **B,** T$_2$-weighted MRI image reveals abnormal signal intensity in disk space between L1 and L2 with the abnormal signal extending into the vertebral bodies. This patient had diskitis.

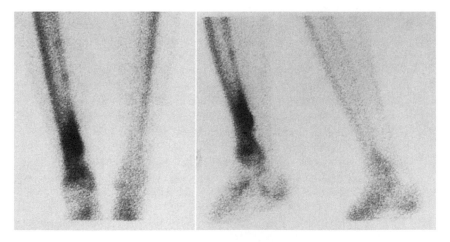

Figure 18-22   Delayed static images of the lower extremities of a 20-year-old male athlete with pain in the tibia (plain radiographs were normal). The bone scan shows marked abnormal accumulation in the distal tibia (anterior and lateral) with the abnormality extending through the cortex, characteristic of a stress fracture.

syringe shields, and an absorbent pad under the injection area. The dose should be injected into an indwelling catheter using a three-way stopcock and at least a 10 ml saline flush to ensure complete delivery of the radiopharmaceutical intravenously. The syringe, three-way stopcock, and catheter should be disposed of appropriately, and the area where the dose was administered should be monitored with a Geiger counter. The patient should be routinely monitored for 30 minutes after administration of the radiopharmaceutical in case of rare adverse reactions such as nausea or tachycardia. The radiation dose to metastatic sites may be in the range of 300 to 2500 rad/mCi.

Patient follow-up is important for monitoring the individual's hematologic status and the effectiveness of pain

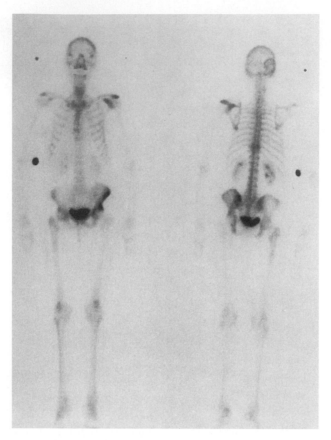

Figure 18-23 Paget's disease. Whole body images demonstrate abnormal uptake in the left ilium, left scapula, thoracic spine, right proximal femur, and skull.

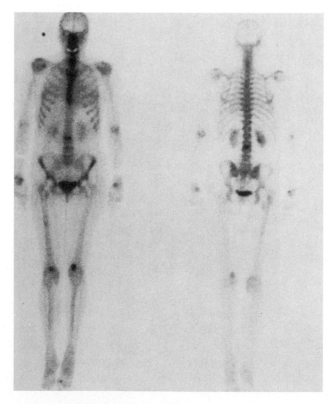

Figure 18-24 Loosened total hip prosthesis. Patient with bilateral hip prostheses has focal abnormal accumulation in the right femoral lesser and greater trochanters and the tip of the prosthesis, typical of loosening.

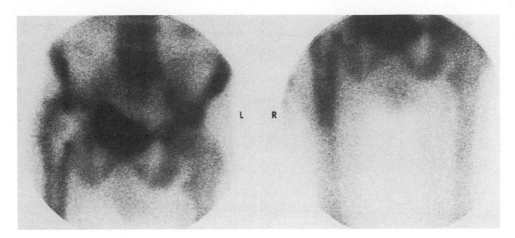

Figure 18-25   Infected total hip prosthesis. Diffusely abnormal accumulation around the entire prosthesis in right hip is characteristic of an infected implant.

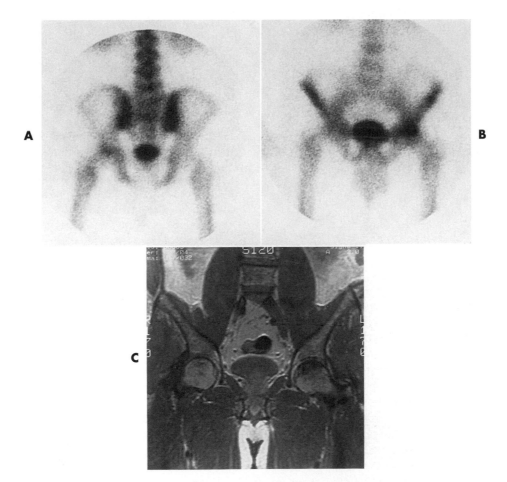

Figure 18-26   Patient with left hip pain from aseptic necrosis. **A** and **B,** Anterior and posterior bone scan demonstrates increased uptake in left femoral head with slightly increased uptake in right femoral head. **C,** Coronal magnetic MRI demonstrates decreased signal in 30% to 40% of left femoral head and 10% to 15% of right femoral head.

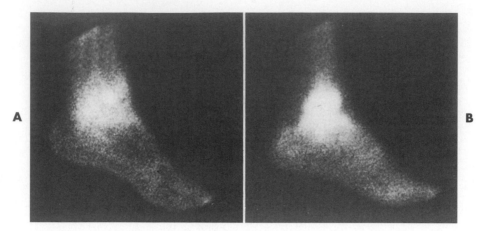

Figure 18-27 Septic arthritis of tibiotalar joint. **A,** Blood pool image obtained after administration of ^{99m}Tc methylenediphosphonate (^{99m}Tc-MDP) demonstrates abnormal accumulation in ankle joint area. **B,** Routine image obtained 2½ hours later demonstrates focal accumulation in distal tibia and talus. Joint fluid was aspirated, and the aspirate grew pathogenic organisms. Radiographs revealed no joint abnormality.

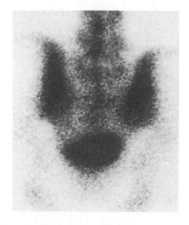

Figure 18-28 Sacroileitis. Posterior pelvic image in a patient with low back pain. Quantification revealed ratio of activity in sacroiliac area to midsacrum to be greater than 2 (normal is less than 1.5).

relief. Radiostrontium relieves pain in approximately 80% of patients. Some reports indicate that an increase in bone pain during the first week after injection is a positive prognostic indicator for later pain relief. Depending on the patient's hematologic status, repeat therapeutic injections may be given at 3-month intervals. Although the cost of a single radiostrontium treatment may exceed $3000, this is a cost-effective treatment in bone pain patients compared with the cost of radiotherapy, chemotherapy, and analgesic palliative strategies.

The response with serial injections can be similar to or better than the response seen after the first injection.[41] A painful flare reaction is noted in 10% to 20% of patients and is predictive of a good response to the therapy. Radionuclide

therapy should not be given to a patient with an impending or current pathologic fracture or to a patient suspected of having medullary epidural compression.

^{67}Ga and ^{111}In White Blood Cell Imaging in Bone and Joint Disease

Several studies have recently demonstrated the value of gallium-67 (^{67}Ga) citrate scanning in patients with inflammatory bone and joint disease.[25,30-32] Some patients with osteomyelitis or septic arthritis may have normal ^{99m}Tc phosphate complex images but abnormal ^{67}Ga images.

Indium-111 (^{111}In)-labeled white blood cells (see Chapter 20) have also been used in the evaluation of patients with suspected bone and joint infections.[14] The results of using ^{111}In white cells have varied, which is most likely related to the patient populations studied. One study had only a 50% sensitivity in detecting skeletal infection (Figure 18-29), but the patient population included many individuals with chronic infection. Another study reported a 98% sensitivity in patients with suspected bone and joint infection. Although ^{111}In white cell imaging can be comparable to ^{67}Ga citrate imaging in detecting inflammatory bone and joint disease, ^{67}Ga citrate imaging does not require the handling of blood products and is the preferred procedure at some institutions. Recent reports of patients with diabetes mellitus and skin ulcers of the feet have demonstrated a high frequency of osteomyelitis and a high accuracy of ^{111}In white cell imaging in this patient population.

^{67}Ga citrate imaging is used to stage certain malignancies, such as Hodgkin's lymphoma and malignant melanoma. The study typically is used to detect the soft tissue involvement of these malignancies, but skeletal involvement can be detected (Figure 18-30).

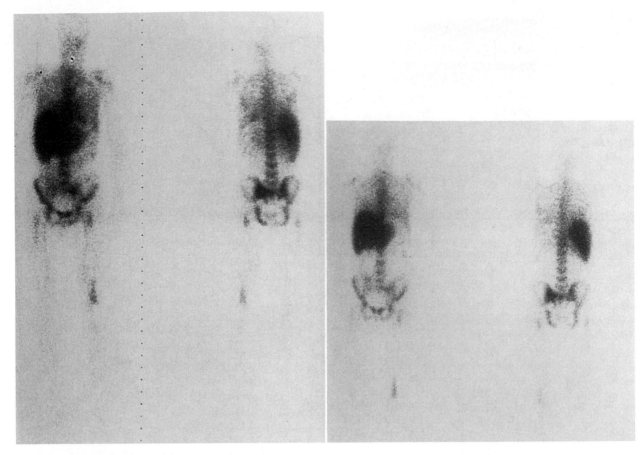

Figure 18-29   Osteomyelitis. Whole body images obtained 4 hours *(left)* and 18 hours *(right)* after administration of ¹¹¹In leukocytes in a patient after splenectomy. Abnormal accumulation is seen in the left sacroiliac joint, left ischium, left proximal femur, and left distal femur in this patient with multifocal osteomyelitis.

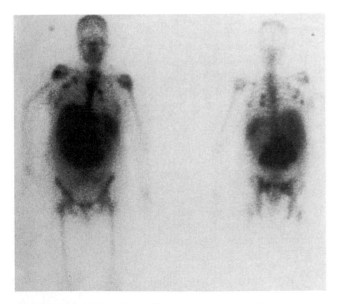

Figure 18-30   Whole body ⁶⁷Ga citrate imaging demonstrates markedly abnormal accumulation in abdominal lymphadenopathy and in multiple ribs in this patient with Hodgkin's lymphoma.

REFERENCES

1. Altman RD, Johnston CC, Khairi MRA et al: Influence of disodium etidronate on clinical and laboratory manifestations of Paget's disease of bone (osteitis deformans), *N Engl J Med* 28:1379, 1973.
2. Anderson J, Emergy EW, McAlister JM et al: The metabolism of a therapeutic dose of calcium-45 in a case of multiple myeloma, *Clin Sci Mol Med* 15:567, 1956.
3. Bassett LW, Gold RH, Webber MM: Radionuclide bone imaging, *Radiol Clin North Am* 19:675, 1981.
4. Bayer GCH, Wendeberg B: External counting of Ca-47 and Sr-85 in studies of localized skeletal lesions in man, *J Bone Joint Surg* 41B:558, 1959.
5. Belchier J: An account of the bones of the animals being changed to a red color by aliment only. In Bauer GCH, editor: Tracer techniques for the study of bone metabolism in man, *Adv Biol Med Phys* 10:228, 1965.
6. Bekerman C, Genant HK, Hoffer PB et al: Radionuclide imaging of the bones and joints of the hand, *Radiology* 118:653, 1975.

7. Bernier DR, Coleman RE: Impact of computed cranial tomography on radionuclide imaging and cisternography, *J Nucl Med Technol* 4:180, 1976.

8. Bhansali SK, Desai PB: Ewing's sarcoma: observations in 107 cases, *J Bone Joint Surg* 45A:541, 1963.

9. Biello D, Coleman RE, Stanley RJ: Correlation of renal images on bone scan and intravenous pyelogram, *Am J Roentgenol Radium Ther Nucl Med* 127:633, 1976.

10. Blau M, Nagler W, Bender MA: Fluorine-18: a new isotope for bone scanning, *J Nucl Med* 3:332, 1962.

11. Charkes ND, Philips CM: A new model of ^{18}F-fluoride kinetics in humans. In *Medical radionuclide imaging,* vol 2, Vienna, 1977, International Atomic Energy Agency.

12. Charkes ND, Sklaroff DM: Early diagnosis of metastatic bone cancer by photoscanning with strontium-85, *J Nucl Med* 5:168, 1964.

13. Charkes ND, Valentine G, Cravitz B: Interpretation of the normal ^{99m}Tc polyphosphate rectilinear bone scan, *Radiology* 107:563, 1973.

14. Coleman RE, Welch DM, Baker WJ et al: Clinical experience using indium-111–labeled leukocytes. In Thakur ML, Gottschalk A, editors: Indium-111–labeled neutrophils, platelets, and lymphocytes, New York, 1980, Trivirium.

15. Davis P, Thomson ABR, Lentle BC: Quantitative sacroiliac scintigraphy in patients with Crohn's disease, *Arthritis Rheum* 21:234, 1978.

16. Edelstyn GA, Gillespie PJ, Grebbel FS: The radiological demonstration of osseous metastases: experimental observations, *Clin Radiol* 18:158, 1967.

17. Frankel RS, Johnson KW, Mabry JJ et al: "Normal" bone radionuclide image with diffuse skeletal lymphoma, *Radiology* 111:365, 1974.

18. Galasko CSB: The detection of skeletal metastases for mammary cancer by gamma camera scintigraphy, *Br J Surg* 56:757, 1969.

19. Galasko CSB: The mechanisms of uptake of bone-seeking isotopes by skeletal metastases. In *Medical radionuclide imaging,* vol 2, Vienna, 1977, International Atomic Energy Agency.

20. Gelfand MJ, Silberstein EB: Radionuclide imaging: use in diagnosis of osteomyelitis in children, *JAMA* 237:245, 1977.

21. Gelman MI, Coleman RE, Stevens PM et al: Radiography, radionuclide imaging, and arthrography in the evaluation of total hip and knee replacement, *Radiology* 128:467, 1978.

22. Gerber FH, Goodreau JJ, Kirchner PT et al: Efficacy of pre-operative and post-operative bone scanning in the management of breast carcinoma, *N Engl J Med* 297:300, 1977.

23. Gilday DL, Ash JM, Reilly BJ: Radionuclide skeletal survey for pediatric neoplasms, *Radiology* 123:399, 1977.

24. Goergen TG, Alazraki NP, Halpern SE et al: "Cold" bone lesions: a newly recognized phenomenon of bone imaging, *J Nucl Med* 12:1120, 1974.

25. Handmaker H, Giammona ST: The "hot joint": increased diagnostic accuracy using combined ^{99m}Tc phosphate and [67]Ca citrate imaging in pediatrics, *J Nucl Med* 17:554, 1976.

26. Hart G, Hoerr SO, Hughes CP: Detection of bone metastases from breast cancer: an accurate, four film roentgenographic survey, *Cleve Clin Q* 38:1, 1971.

27. Jones AG, Francis MD, Davis MA: Bone scanning: radionuclide reaction mechanisms, *Semin Nucl Med* 6:1, 1976.

28. Krishnamurthy GT, Tubis M, Hiss J et al: Distribution pattern of metastatic bone disease: a need for total body skeletal imaging, *JAMA* 237:2054, 1977.

29. Legge DA, Tauxe WN, Pugh DG et al: Radioisotope scanning of metastatic lesions of bone, *Mayo Clin Proc* 45:755, 1970.

30. Lisbona R, Rosenthall L: Observations on the sequential use of ^{99m}Tc-phosphate complex and ^{67}Ga imaging in osteomyelitis, cellulitis, and septic arthritis, *Radiology* 123:123, 1977.

31. Lisbona R, Rosenthall L: Radionuclide imaging of septic joints and their differentiation from periarticular osteomyelitis and cellulitis in pediatrics, *Clin Nucl Med* 2:337, 1977.

32. Lisbona R, Rosenthall L: Role of radionuclide imaging in osteoid osteoma, *Am J Roentgenol Radium Ther Nucl Med* 132:77, 1979.

33. Littlefield JL, Rudd TG: Tc-99m hydroxymethylene diphosphonate and Tc-99m methylene diphosphonate: biologic and clinical comparison: concise communication, *J Nucl Med* 24:463, 1983.

34. Maher FT: Evaluation of renal urinary tract abnormalities noted on scintiscans, *Mayo Clin Proc* 50:370, 1975.

35. Maisano R, Pergolizzi S, Cascini S: Novel therapeutic approaches to cancer patients with bone metastases, *Crit Rev Oncol Hematol* 40:239, 2001.

36. Merkel KD, Brown ML, Fitzgerald RH et al: Prospective In-111 WBC scan versus Tc-99m-MDP–Ga-67 scan for low-grade osteomyelitis, *J Nucl Med* 24:72, 1983.

37. Merrick MV: Review article: bone scanning, *Br J Radiol* 48:327, 1975.

38. Namey TC, Rosenthall L: Periarticular uptake of [99m]technetium disphosphonate in psoriatics, *Arthritis Rheum* 24:607, 1976.

39. Park HM, Terman SA, Ridolfo AS et al: A quantitative evaluation of rheumatoid arthritic activity with Tc-99m HEDP, *J Nucl Med* 18:973, 1977.

40. Pecher C: Biological investigations with radioactive calcium and strontium, *Proc Soc Exp Biol Med* 46:86, 1941.

41. Pons F, Fuster D: Underutilization of radionuclide therapy in metastatic bone pain palliation, *Nucl Med Commun* 23:301, 2002.

42. Rasmussen H: Parathyroid hormone, calcitonin, and calciferols. In Williams RH, editor: *Textbook of endocrinology,* ed 5, Philadelphia, 1974, WB Saunders.

43. Robinson RG, Preston DF, Schiefelbein M et al: Strontium-89 therapy for the palliation of pain due to osseous metastases, *JAMA* 274:420, 1995.

44. Rosenthall L, Hill RO, Chuang S: Observation on the use of ⁹⁹ᵐTc-phosphate imaging in peripheral bone trauma, *Radiology* 119:637, 1976.

45. Schaffer DL, Pendergrass HP: Comparison of enzyme, clinical, radiographic, and radionuclide methods of detecting bone metastases from carcinoma of the prostate, *Radiology* 121:431, 1976.

46. Schall GL, Zeiger L, Primack A et al: Uptake of ⁸⁵Sr by an osteosarcoma metastatic to lung, *J Nucl Med* 12:131, 1971.

47. Shirazi PH, Rayudu GVS, Fordham EW: ¹⁸F bone scanning: review of indications and results in 1500 cases, *Radiology* 112:361, 1974.

48. Shirazi PH, Rayudu GVS, Ryan WG et al: Paget's disease of bone: bone scanning experience with 80 cases, *J Nucl Med* 14:450, 1973.

49. Silberstein EB: Treatment of pain from bone metastases employing unsealed sources. In Sandler MP, Coleman RE, Wacker FJTh et al, editors: *Diagnostic nuclear medicine,* ed 3, Baltimore, 1996 Williams & Wilkins.

50. Sklaroff DM, Charkes DN: Diagnosis of bone metastasis by photoscanning with strontium 85, *JAMA* 188:1, 1964.

51. Spencer R, Herbert R, Rish MW et al: Bone scanning with ⁸⁵Sr and ¹⁸F: physical and radiopharmaceutical considerations and clinical experience in 50 cases, *Br J Radiol* 40:641, 1976.

52. Subramanian G, McAfee JG, Blair RJ et al: Radiopharmaceuticals for bone and bone-marrow imaging. In *Medical radionuclide imaging,* vol 2, Vienna, 1977, International Atomic Energy Agency.

53. Sy WM, Bay R, Camera A: Hand images: normal and abnormal, *J Nucl Med* 18:419, 1977.

54. Thomas RJ, Resnick D, Alazraki NP et al: Compartmental evaluation of osteoarthritis of the knee: comparative study of available diagnostic modalities, *Radiology* 116:585, 1975.

55. Thrall JH, Ghaed N, Geslien GE et al: Pitfalls in ⁹⁹ᵐTc polyphosphate skeletal imaging, *Am J Roentgenol Radium Ther Nucl Med* 121:739, 1974.

56. Wang CC, Schulz MD: Ewing's sarcoma: a study of 50 cases treated at the Massachusetts General Hospital, 1930-1952 inclusive, *N Engl J Med* 284:571, 1953.

57. Waxman AD, Bryan D, Siemsen JK: Bone scanning in the drug abuse patient: early detection of hematogenous osteomyelitis, *J Nucl Med* 14:647, 1973.

SUGGESTED READINGS

Probst-Proctor SL, Dillingham MF, McDougall IR et al: The white blood cell scan in orthopedics, *Clin Orthop Rel Res* 168:157, 1982.

Subramanian G, McAfee JF: A new complex of ⁹⁹ᵐTc for skeletal imaging, *Radiology* 99:192, 1971.

Helen H. Drew, Ursula Scheffel, Patricia A. McIntyre

chapter *19*

Hematopoietic System

Objectives

List the normal components of blood in the plasma compartment and cellular compartments.

Define a hematocrit value, how it is derived, and how to interpret it.

Describe the function, life span, and survival problems of a red blood cell.

Describe how to label platelets with indium-111 (^{111}In) oxine.

State the isotope dilution principle.

Explain the ascorbic acid technique for labeling red blood cells with chromium-51 (^{51}Cr).

Describe the correct procedure and calculation for performing a total red cell volume measurement, including sample collection, processing, and counting.

Describe the correct procedure and calculation for performing a total plasma volume measurement, including sample collection, processing, and counting.

Describe the limitations imposed when attempting to compare measured red cell and plasma volumes to normal volumes.

Describe the technique used to perform a red cell survival, and calculate the results.

Describe the technique used to perform a splenic sequestration.

Describe the technique of performing an in vivo cross match.

Describe the calculations and interpretation of an in vivo cross match.

Describe the performance and calculate the results of a stage I, II, and III Schilling test, including patient preparation, test administration, sample collection, sample processing, and counting.

List the sources of errors in performing a Schilling test and explain the role of the "flushing" doses.

BLOOD COMPONENTS

Circulating blood is an extraordinarily complex mixture. Some of the representative components are listed in Box 19-1. When blood is collected with an anticoagulant (a substance that prevents normal clotting), the whole blood divides into a plasma compartment and a cellular compartment. If it is collected without an anticoagulant, the fluid that can be separated from the clot is known as serum. The clot contains most of the cellular elements and the proteins consumed in the coagulation process. It is important to recognize this fundamental difference between the terms *plasma* and *serum*. Many of the anticoagulants routinely used by hematologists are not applicable to nuclear hematologic studies because they prevent clotting by chelating calcium (a requirement for normal clotting) and other heavy ions such as tracer iron, which is used in some nuclear medicine studies.

Box 19-1	Selected Representative Components of Blood

1. Plasma compartment
   a. Water
   b. Simple solutes (e.g., Na^+, K^+, Cl^-, Mg^{2+}, Ca^{2+}, HCO_3^-, and sugar)
   c. Proteins
      (1) Albumin
      (2) Immunoglobulins (e.g., gamma globulin [IgG] and macroglobulins [IgM])
      (3) Transport proteins (e.g., transferrin, transcobalamin I, and transcobalamin II)
      (4) Lipoproteins (and other lipids)
      (5) Precursors and active components of the complex coagulation-fibrinolysis system
2. Cellular compartment
   a. Erythrocytes (red blood cells [RBCs]): about $5 \times 10^6/mm^3$
   b. Leukocytes (white blood cells [WBCs]): about $5 \times 10^3/mm^3$
      (1) Granulocytes
      (2) Lymphocytes
      (3) Monocytes
      (4) Plasma cells and fragments of or whole megakaryocytes (rarely present in routine preparations of peripheral blood for microscopic examination)
   c. Platelets (thrombocytes), about $3.5 \times 10^5/mm^3$

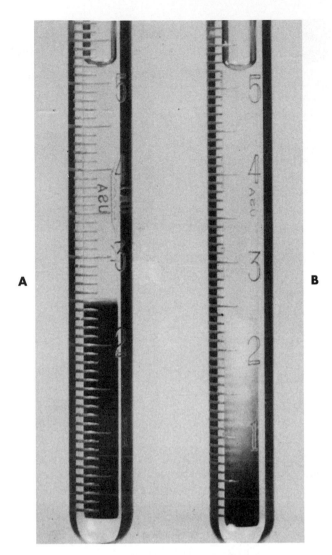

Figure 19-1 **A,** Normal blood sample. **B,** Sample of blood from a patient with a basic hematologic abnormality. Cellular elements have been separated from plasma by centrifugation.

The relative numbers of the basic cellular types present in circulating blood are listed in the lower portion of Box 19-1. Only rarely is the number of red blood cells in a given volume of blood measured to assess whether a patient has anemia, although this value may be included with the information routinely printed out by an automated electronic particle counter. A much simpler method is to measure the hematocrit value. This is done by placing a well-mixed sample of anticoagulated blood in a suitable tube and centrifuging it for an appropriate period to use G force (multiples of gravity) to separate the cellular elements from the plasma phase. When hematocrits are performed on normal blood, the red cells comprise most of the volume of packed cells (Figure 19-1, *A*) because of their relatively great number and size. The layer just above the red cells, known as the *buffy coat,* is slightly grayish; this is the white cell population in that sample of blood. Just above the buffy coat is an even more minute layer of creamy-colored cells, representing the platelets. Because of their smaller number (and, in the case of platelets, minute size), the hematocrit value cannot be relied on to measure the quantity of white cells and platelets, which must be counted separately, preferably with an electronic particle counter. Figure 19-1, *B*,

shows the blood of a patient with a basic hematologic abnormality. The overwhelming majority of packed cells are made up of platelets and white cells, and the lower portion is a poorly separated mixture of white and red cells. If only a casual glance were given to this hematocrit value, especially if it were done as a routine in a microcapillary tube, the serious error of overlooking the severe degree of anemia and greatly abnormal increase in white cells and platelets could easily be made.

Two important facts must be remembered about the interpretation of a hematocrit value. First, it represents merely the ratio of the cellular compartment volume to the total volume of a given sample of blood. Accordingly, alterations in the plasma compartment (e.g., dehydration) can make the hematocrit value seem falsely elevated. Second, very careful examination of the hematocrit tube is necessary to make sure that in fact a normal red cell population is present in the packed cells and not a preponderance of white cells or platelets. Should the latter condition prevail and go

Table 19-1	Circulating cellular elements: origin, function, approximate life span		
	Erythrocytes	**Granulocytes**	**Monocytes**
Tissue of origin in normal adults	Red (hematopoietically active) marrow	Same as erythrocytes	Same as erythrocytes; monocytes circulate through blood to become tissue macrophages
Earliest recognizable precursor cell in the bone marrow	Proerythroblast	Myeloblast	Promonocyte
Function of mature cell	Oxygen transport to tissues	Phagocytosis	Phagocytosis and processing of antigens
Life span	90 to 110 days	50% to 60% of mature granulocytes in blood adhere to vascular endothelium, the so-called marginal pool, and are freely exchangeable with those circulating; half-life in blood is 6 to 7 hr; cells may survive up to 5 days after migration into tissues	Probably very similar to life span of granulocytes in blood; once macrophages enter and are converted to tissue, they may survive months to years

unrecognized, tracer-labeling studies will give false and misleading results. A hand-held magnifying glass or the magnifier supplied with the reading equipment should be used with microhematocrit tubes.

Table 19-1 presents a summary of the important features of the cellular elements of the blood. Because most clinical nuclear medicine laboratories perform cell-labeling studies of the erythrocytes, this chapter chiefly discusses tests that deal directly or indirectly with the mature red blood cells and factors that may influence their production. Random platelet labels and white cell labels are also discussed.

Because of their oxygen transport function, mature circulating red blood cells (RBCs), or erythrocytes, are critical to the survival and proper function of each cell in each tissue of the body. RBCs survive for approximately 100 days, even though with each complete transit of the circulation they are shot out of the aorta during left ventricular contraction at speeds approaching those of a jet airliner. At the other extreme, RBCs are required to weave their way slowly through the tiny, intricate openings in the splenic sinusoids, which are much smaller than the cells themselves. In their transit through the spleen, RBCs actually are required to deform themselves, with only a tiny portion initially emerging through an opening and the rest being pulled slowly after it; after this they nevertheless are able regain their normal biconcave shape and maintain their normal functions.

The RBC life span of approximately 100 days has a profound implication; every day the bone marrow must replace 1% of the total circulating mass of RBCs that have died of

old age. Considering that the mean hematocrit value is approximately 45% and the total blood volume in adults averages 5 L, it can be seen that the normal bone marrow performs a most efficient assembly line function to maintain homeostasis; the same is obviously true for the production by the marrow of all the other cellular elements of the blood. Furthermore, normal marrow contains reserves of mature cells, which can be quickly released into the circulation when needed; also, with continuing stress, normal marrow can gradually increase its daily rate of production manyfold (up to eight times normal in the case of RBCs).

A complete list of all known causes and types of anemia would require several pages of this textbook; however, the following list summarizes the basic mechanisms by which anemia may be caused:

1. Excessive rate of removal of RBCs from the circulation
2. Blood loss
3. Hemolysis
4. Deficient production of RBCs
5. Lack of proper building blocks (e.g., iron, vitamin B_{12}, folic acid)
6. Suppression of marrow activity by a wide variety of acute and chronic diseases
7. Primary disorders of the bone marrow

Obviously anemia can result either from an excess rate of removal of RBCs or from deficient production. Blood loss, be it chronic or acute, remains high on the list of causes of anemia. Accelerated destruction of the RBCs in the patient's body, a process known as *hemolysis,* has the same end result

Platelets	Lymphocytes	Plasma cells
Same as erythrocytes	Same as erythrocytes	Some if not all are derived from immunologically stimulated lymphocytes.
Megakaryocyte	Certain small marrow lymphocytes are morphologically indistinguishable from pluripotential stem cells; however, other evidence suggests that lymphocytes are not derived from the same stem cell as the erythrocytes, granulocytes, and platelets.	
Vital components of normal coagulation process	After release from marrow, lymphocytes differentiate into (1) B lymphocytes (precursors of plasma cells) with production of circulating humoral antibody and (2) T lymphocytes (participants in cellular immunity). B lymphocyte: Unknown T lymphocyte: Long live; continue to recirculate	Plasma cells produce a humoral antibody specifically directed against the antigen to which they are exposed Highly variable; some may persist for many months

as blood loss, provided that either occurs at a rate that exceeds the ability of the normal bone marrow to compensate. Deficient production can result from a lack of proper building blocks, suppression of marrow activity by a wide variety of acute and chronic diseases, or, least commonly, a primary disorder of the bone marrow. Iron deficiency anemia, a simple and rapidly curable condition, remains the most common worldwide hematologic disorder. Vitamin B_{12} and folic acid are included in the list above not because they represent the only other building blocks of importance, but because nuclear medicine can provide useful information about the differential diagnosis in patients with manifestations of deficiency of these two components.

Acute, self-limited, or rapidly cured disorders, such as the common cold or acute pneumonia, cause temporary, essentially complete, cessation of marrow RBC production. Because normal RBCs live approximately 100 days, such a short-term illness does not result in a recognizable degree of anemia. Certain patients who have a compensated hemolytic anemia (i.e., RBCs with a significantly shortened life span but a very active marrow that maintains a normal hematocrit value by an increased rate of erythrocyte production) may very rapidly develop a severe degree of anemia because of marrow suppression from such otherwise mild illnesses. A wide variety of chronic diseases (e.g., rheumatoid arthritis, malignant disorders) may cause chronic suppression of marrow activity and consequent anemia.

Primary disorders of the bone marrow are complex hematologic problems, and in these cases the judicious choice of nuclear medicine procedures often provides unique and valuable information that could not be gathered in any other fashion.

ISOTOPIC LABELING OF CELLULAR ELEMENTS

All isotopic labels of the cellular elements of the blood are of two general types: cohort, or pulse, labels and random labels. It is important to recognize the fundamental difference in the information to be gained with each of them.

Cohort (Pulse) Labels

Cohort (pulse) labeling is available only to the marrow precursors of a given cell type for a specific and limited length of time; it therefore does not label cells already circulating. Incorporation of this type of label in the marrow erythroid precursors results in the appearance in the circulation of mature labeled RBCs of the same age. An ideal cohort label that met all these necessary criteria and that had the appropriate gamma-emitting nuclide would permit study of the rate of production of RBCs, their kinetics, longevity, manner of death, and ultimate disposal in the body. However, none of the currently available radioisotopes for cohort labeling of RBCs satisfies all these requirements, and none is used in routine clinical studies.

Random Labels

Random labels are radiopharmaceuticals applied to the circulating cells of the peripheral blood in vitro. This process labels all cells in the sample, that is, from the youngest to the oldest circulating blood cells or, as classically expressed, blood cells of random age; thus these are applicable to the study of mean cell survival or other direct measurements of the circulating cells of the blood. It is important to emphasize that isotopic labeling of circulating blood cells provides reasonably precise data only if separation, labeling, and reinfusion of these cells are performed so as to minimize damage to them. Strict adherence to aseptic techniques is also obligatory.

PLATELET KINETICS

The only isotopic labels available for platelets are of the random type; that is, applicable to determination of the fate of platelets already circulating in the blood. [51]Cr chromate has been extensively used as a random platelet label and was recommended in 1977 by the International Panel on Diagnostic Application of Radioisotopes in Hematology[3] as the only available satisfactory agent for studies in humans. The major limitations of ^{51}Cr arise from the physical characteristics of the radionuclide. Only 9% of the emissions of ^{51}Cr are useful gamma photons. Furthermore, the 27.8-day half-life of ^{51}Cr is long for studies of human platelets, which have a mean survival of approximately 10 days. These studies also are limited by the low platelet labeling efficiency of ^{51}Cr chromate; large amounts of blood (up to 500 ml) must be drawn even from normal subjects to maximize the final platelet-bound ^{51}Cr activity. Even with optimum harvesting and labeling procedures, the amount of ^{51}Cr infused labeled to platelets is limited to approximately 10 to 30 μCi. As a consequence of this low labeling efficiency and the 9% gamma emission of ^{51}Cr, the circulating platelet-associated measurable radioactivity is low, particularly in the latter days of the study. External quantitative organ localization or imaging studies cannot be performed with adequate statistics despite the 320 keV energy of ^{51}Cr because of the restricted number of photons available for such studies.

The discovery of ^{111}In oxine as a random cellular label has made possible precise platelet kinetic and organ distribution studies.[19] In 1988 the International Panel on Diagnostic Application of Radioisotopes in Hematology recommended the use of ^{111}In as a random label for platelets.[11] Platelet labeling with ^{111}In is possible at lower platelet counts than with [51]Cr.

The ^{111}In oxine complex easily penetrates the cell membrane because of its lipophilic nature, and the ^{111}In label has been shown to possess great stability. The viability of the cells reportedly is not affected by the ^{111}In oxine labeling procedure if care is taken to avoid cell damage during separation and washing procedures and if labeling is carried out in the presence of plasma.

Because all cellular elements of the blood (red and white cells, leukocytes, and platelets) are labeled with ^{111}In oxine, platelets must first be separated by differential centrifugation before the ^{111}In labeling complex is introduced. After incubation of the platelets with ^{111}In oxine, the unbound

[111]In radioactivity must be removed. For this purpose, the cells are washed with plasma, centrifuged, and resuspended in fresh plasma.[17,18,20]

[111]In has a half-life of 2.8 days. Its gamma photon energies of 173 and 247 keV and their relatively high yield (84% and 94%, respectively) allow quantitative external imaging of sites of platelet distribution and deposition and precise determination of platelet survival.

Clinical Application

[111]In-labeled platelets are used for the study of platelet kinetics and for in vivo quantification of sites of platelet distribution and deposition. They have also been used extensively in the investigation of thrombotic and vascular disorders and in monitoring the therapeutic effectiveness of platelet-active drugs in these conditions.

Platelet Survival Studies

The mean platelet survival time (MPST) in a normal person is 8 to 10 days. The normal recovery of the labeled platelets (i.e., the percentage of ^{111}In platelets in the circulation shortly after injection) is approximately 60%; the rest of the dose (about one third) accumulates in the splenic pool. To determine the mean platelet survival, multiple venous blood samples must be drawn. If a normal or nearly normal platelet life span can be expected, blood samples are obtained at 90 minutes after infusion and daily thereafter for 10 days. In patients with idiopathic thrombocytopenia (ITP), in which the MPST can be as short as 1 day or even less, blood samples must be drawn much more frequently (e.g., at 10, 30, and 60 minutes after injection) and then at 2-hour intervals until whole blood indium activity is approximately 10%.

The hematocrit value and platelet count are determined in each sample. Duplicate samples of 5 ml of whole blood, lysed with saponin, and 2 ml of platelet-free plasma (PFP) diluted with 3 ml of water are prepared for measurement of the radioactivity. Standards are made by adding 20 μl of the injectate to 5 ml of water. All samples are counted with less than 3% statistical error in a scintillation-detector system. The results are expressed as a percentage of the injected dose in circulating platelets as follows:

$$\% \text{ Injected dose in circulating platelets} = \left[\frac{[cpm(1\,ml\,WB) - (cpm[1\,ml\,plasma] \times Plct)}{cpm(Std) \times \text{Dilution factor}]} \right] \times (BV) \times (100)$$

where cpm is counts per minute, Plct is decimal plasma-crit (1.00—decimal hematocrit), and WB is whole blood.

The data are then subjected to computer analysis. Several mathematical models have been proposed for formal curve fitting. Of these models, the maximum likelihood estimate of the integer-ordered gamma function is preferred.

[111]In oxine–labeled white blood cells (WBCs) are used routinely in nuclear medicine departments for imaging of inflammatory lesions. Simple sedimentation techniques are routinely used to separate the WBCs from the RBCs. This technique yields a variety of labeled WBCs, including polymorphs, lymphocytes, and monocytes. The mixed cell types cannot be used to study the kinetics of a specific cell type but are acceptable for abscess location. Detailed labeling techniques for WBCs are outlined in Chapter 20.

ERYTHROKINETICS

Measurement of Circulating Red Blood Cell Mass

The determination of the RBC mass and plasma volume is based on the simple radioisotope dilution technique.[4] The larger the volume into which the label is mixed, the lower the counts in the sample withdrawn; conversely, the smaller the volume, the higher the counts in the sample. This dilution technique is true only when a closed system is used and no radiopharmaceutical is allowed to leak out of the system being measured. Also, the volume of the unknown must not change significantly during the measurement. RBC volume measurements are performed in a closed system using ^{51}Cr-labeled RBCs.

Whole blood is collected by use of the appropriate anticoagulant in the correct ratio to the volume of whole blood. If citric acid, trisodium citrate, and dextrose (ACD)-NIH solution A or Strumia ACD solution is used, the ratio is 1 : 5. Because of the wide variance in the composition of the many citric acid, sodium citrate, sodium biphosphate, and dextrose (CPD) solutions, now judged to be at least as good and in some instances preferable, it is imperative to consult the manufacturer's recommendation as to the proper ratio of whole blood to CPD. Heparin and ethylenediaminetetraacetic acid (EDTA) are unsatisfactory for use in this procedure. Several satisfactory methods are available both for preparing the ^{51}Cr-labeled RBCs and for performing the necessary measurements. We describe in detail the one we routinely use, but readers interested in other methods should refer to a publication of the International Panel on Diagnostic Applications of Radioisotopes in Haematology.[1]

[51]Cr is not an entirely ideal label for RBC mass measurements. Only 9% of its emissions are gamma rays, therefore a substantially larger amount of radioactivity must be injected to obtain statistically significant counting rates compared with an isotope having 100% gamma emission. Furthermore, the relatively long half-life of [51]Cr (27.8 days), coupled with its relatively slow rate of removal from circulating RBCs (1% per day), means that serial RBC volume measurements require undesirable increases in the amount of ^{51}Cr injected for each subsequent study. For these reasons, labeling of RBCs with technetium-99m (^{99m}Tc) and trace amounts of stannous ion is a useful alternative method of measuring RBC mass.[7,8,12] [99m]Tc has a 6-hour half-life and for practical purposes can be considered a pure gamma ray emitter. Therefore physically it is nearly ideal for RBC mass

measurements. It can be used in amounts that greatly reduce the radiation dose to patients who undergo serial RBC mass measurements. Because of the more rapid loss of the ^{99m}Tc label, however, ^{51}Cr-labeled RBCs should be used when sampling times for a single study must extend beyond 60 minutes after injection.

[51]Cr Ascorbic Acid Method for Labeling Red Blood Cells

For the ^{51}Cr ascorbic acid method of labeling RBCs, 10 ml of venous blood is withdrawn from the patient into a 20 ml syringe containing 2 ml of Strumia ACD formula and is transferred into a sterile 20 ml vial. About 30 μCi of ^{51}Cr in the form of chromate ion is added to the vial. About 80% to 95% of the chromate ion is promptly transported across the RBC membrane and binds to the beta chain of the hemoglobin molecule. During labeling within the RBCs, the hexavalent chromate ion is reduced to a trivalent chromic ion. After 15 minutes of incubation, ascorbic acid (50 mg) is added to reduce the free chromate to chromic ion, which immediately stops the tagging procedure, because the chromic ion is unable to penetrate the RBC membrane.

Exactly 5 ml of the labeled blood is drawn into a syringe, and the remainder is kept to make a standard. The 5 ml is injected intravenously, with care taken not to infiltrate any of the dose. After adequate time to ensure complete mixing of the labeled RBCs in the circulation, a sample is drawn from a vein other than that used for the injection. In normal subjects 10 minutes is sufficient to ensure complete mixing. However, in disease states, such as splenomegaly or severe polycythemia, mixing may be greatly delayed. In such cases case serial samples should be taken until no significant difference in counts is seen.

In other seriously ill patients, a less pronounced delay of mixing may occur. For this reason, the routine in our clinic is to wait 30 minutes to obtain the post-injection sample (with use of a heparinized syringe).

Hematocrit (Hct) value determinations are performed on the well-mixed standard and blood samples. Four counting tubes are prepared to contain 1 ml volumes of the following:

Whole blood from the standard = Std WB
Plasma from the standard = Std Plas
Whole blood from the sample = Samp WB
Plasma from the sample = Samp Plas

The standards and samples are counted in a well counter with the spectrometer centered about the 320 keV photopeak of ^{51}Cr and counted for sufficient time to ensure a counting accuracy of 1% error or less. Usually there are so few counts in the post-injection plasma sample that a shorter counting time is acceptable for this tube.

$$RBC\ volume\ (ml) =$$

$$\frac{[cpm\ Std\ WB - (cpm\ Std\ Plas \times Std\ Plct)]}{[cpm\ Samp\ WB - (cpm\ Samp\ Plas \times Samp\ Plct)]} \times Volume\ injected \times Samp\ Hct$$

where *Plct* is decimal plasma-crit (1.00—decimal hematocrit) and *Samp Hct* is decimal hematocrit of sample.

Falsely high results are found if a faulty intravenous injection technique is used and the entire dose is not injected into a vein. Damaged RBCs or excessive binding of the ^{51}Cr by WBCs or platelets when these are abnormally elevated also yields spuriously high values. Falsely low values are caused by failure to obtain a pre-injection blood sample in a patient who has had previous administration of radioactive tracers. Contamination of equipment with radioactivity also yields spuriously low results.

The ^{51}Cr should not be added to the ACD solution before the patient's blood is added to the vial. Dextrose contained in the ACD solution acts as a reducing agent.

For measurement of the circulating RBC mass, $10\,\mu$Ci of ^{51}Cr is an adequate amount of activity and provides enough counts so that statistically significant sample counting can be performed in a reasonable time. The specific activity of the ^{51}Cr chromate must be such that less than $2\,\mu$g of chromium ion is present per milliliter of packed RBCs. This becomes particularly critical when this technique is used for RBC survival studies that require larger doses of ^{51}Cr.

Plasma Volume

Iodinated human serum albumin is the conventional agent used for estimation of plasma volume. Albumin does not remain in the intravascular space but diffuses rapidly into extravascular compartments. Because this vascular space is now an open system, use of the closed-system isotope dilution principle for calculations causes errors in the plasma volume measurement. An extrapolation procedure can be used to calculate the volume if the injected tracer leaves the open system at a rate that is slow compared with the rate of mixing uniformly within that system, and samples are taken only after mixing has been completed.[22]

Iodine-125 (^{125}I)-labeled human serum albumin is provided by radiopharmaceutical manufacturers in a concentration of $10\,\mu$Ci per 1.5 ml. Not more than 2% of the radioactivity can be in the free form (the free form is removed from the intravascular space more rapidly than the labeled albumin, causing an overestimation of plasma volume). ^{99m}Tc-labeled albumin can also be used but must be 98% bound on injection.

The patient should be at rest or supine for at least 10 to 15 minutes before the study is started; this is done because in the standing position, plasma volume decreases because of an increase in venous pressure in the legs, which causes water to move from the intravascular to the extravascular space.[22] It is recommended that thyroid blockage of radioiodine be performed at least 30 minutes before injection of the radiotracer by means of oral administration of 5 drops (150 mg) of a supersaturated solution of sodium iodide (SSKI).

The dose of $10\,\mu$Ci of ^{125}I-labeled human serum albumin is injected intravenously, with care being taken that it all enters the vein. A site different from the injection site is used

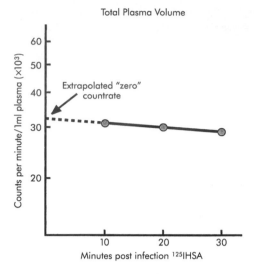

Figure 19-2 Extrapolation graph used to determine zero-time activity for calculation of plasma volume.

to collect three timed heparinized samples of blood at 10, 20, and 30 minutes. These samples are centrifuged, and 1 ml aliquots of plasma are counted.

The radioactivity in each of these samples is measured and plotted against time on semilogarithmic paper (Figure 19-2). The best straight line is drawn through these points, and only the earlier points are used if the later points deviate from the initial linear slope. The zero-time activity is estimated by extrapolation and used to calculate the plasma volume. A standard is prepared and counted. All counts are performed with the spectrometer adjusted to count ^{125}I (20 to 50 keV) for a time long enough to ensure a 1% error or less. The plasma volume is calculated as follows:

Plasma volume (ml) =

$$\frac{\text{Volume injected} \times \text{cpm in 1 ml Std} \times \text{dilution factor}}{\text{cpm of plasma sample obtained by extrapolation}}$$

With a precisely measured RBC or plasma volume and the venous hematocrit value, the volume of the other compartment can be safely calculated and the total blood volume estimated only in normal subjects. The reason is that in normal subjects a fixed relationship exists between the whole body hematocrit (Hct_b) and the venous hematocrit (Hct_v); the ratio of Hct_b to Hct_v on the average is 0.90. It is believed that two factors are responsible for the difference observed between the Hct_b and the Hct_v: (1) the hematocrit value of blood in small capillaries is lower than that found in larger vessels and (2) the iodinated albumin used to measure the plasma space is immediately distributed into a space larger than that of the vascular space in which the RBCs are distributed.

It is important to recognize, however, that most of the patients referred to the clinical nuclear medicine service for measurement of either RBC or plasma volume are severely ill, and the predictable normal relationship most likely will not be present in these individuals. For instance, in patients

Table 19-2	Normal blood volume compartment values (ml/kg)	
	Males	**Females**
Total blood volume	55 to 80	50 to 75
Red blood cell volume*	25 to 35	20 to 30
Plasma volume†	30 to 45	30 to 45

*95% Confidence limits.

†Because of the many variables that may influence plasma volume in normal subjects, it is not possible to place confidence limits on these values.

with moderate or gross splenomegaly, the ratio of Hct_b to Hct_v may be substantially and unpredictably increased to greater than 1; in patients with severe polycythemia, abnormalities may be present in the plasma volume as well as the RBC mass. In clinical circumstances, therefore, total blood volume can be reliably estimated only by measuring red cell mass and plasma volume simultaneously.

A limitation in the interpretation of these studies is that normal values for blood volume in any given individual cannot be simply predicted from such parameters as height and weight despite the many elaborate formulas that have been proposed. In interpreting studies in adults, the simplest method of calculating the values in milliliters per kilogram is probably at least as reliable as using any of the various formulas or nomograms. The normal values published by the International Panel on Standardization in Haematology are shown in Table 19-2. Note the wide range in plasma volume observed in normal subjects; this immediately tells us that this is less than a precise test. The undesirable rapid diffusion of the radiolabeled albumin from the vascular space is but one factor making this procedure less than precise, even in normal subjects. Body position, recent exercise, and a number of other factors cause rapid, significant changes in plasma volume. Therefore although we can precisely measure the circulating RBC mass, it is best always to report the plasma volume as estimated.

Other factors seen in patients referred for study, such as obesity, recent weight loss, and prolonged bed rest, may make it impossible to estimate the RBC and plasma volume solely from height and weight measurements. Because the RBC mass is related to lean body mass, the measured values of patients who are exceptionally obese or who have had a recent significant weight loss should be compared with values based on ideal or recent body weight.

Blood volume measurements have proved to be of considerable value in several specific circumstances. Use of ^{51}Cr-labeled RBCs to measure the RBC mass allows a precise determination of whether true polycythemia is present or the patient has an elevated hematocrit because of a reduced plasma volume. Hematologists see several patients each year who have a persistent elevation of the hematocrit, but the RBC mass is normal when measured by the ^{51}Cr technique. Usually these are normal subjects whose RBC mass is near

the upper limits of normal and whose plasma volume is near the lower limits of normal. The performance of this one, simple, relatively inexpensive test, which proves that the RBC mass is normal, spares these patients an elaborate, expensive, and prolonged series of other diagnostic procedures.

Patients with polycythemia vera and myelofibrosis may have pronounced expansion of the plasma volume, which is apparent only if this parameter is directly measured. Because of the combined abnormality of plasma volume and red cells, serial measurements of both the RBC and plasma volume may become essential to the management of patients with polycythemia vera. In these circumstances the availability of ^{99m}Tc-RBCs becomes invaluable.

Paradoxically, in an acutely hemorrhaging patient or a patient suffering from recent severe trauma, the hematocrit may remain normal or disproportionally high for some time. In these circumstances direct measurement with ^{51}Cr-labeled RBCs reveals the true RBC mass.

Erythrocyte Survival and Splenic Sequestration Studies

RBCs are labeled using the same technique as that for RBC volume determination except that the dose of ^{51}Cr is adjusted to $1.5\,\mu Ci$ per kilogram of body weight. After labeling, the cells are reinjected, and the first sample is obtained 24 hours later. (To permit removal from the circulation of any cells accidentally damaged during the labeling procedure; during this same interval, any injected plasma radioactivity is cleared from the circulation). Samples are then obtained every other day for the next 3 weeks; a 6 ml sample of blood is drawn and placed in a tube containing an anticoagulant (preferably solid EDTA or concentrated heparin).

Five milliliters of whole blood is pipetted from the tubes as it is collected. (To ensure thorough mixing, the tubes should be inverted 12 to 15 times before samples are pipetted and hematocrit values are determined.)

Hematocrit determinations are made on each sample on the day of collection. A tiny amount of saponin powder then is added to each tube, and the tubes are gently tilted several times to ensure mixing and complete lysis of the RBCs. Care is taken not to allow the sample to touch the cap of the counting tube.

On the last day of the study, all the samples are counted on the gamma spectrometer with settings of 280 to 360 keV for ^{51}Cr. The samples are counted to give a sample error of 1% or less (for approximately 10 minutes each).

For calculation of the half-time ($t_{1/2}$) of disappearance of the labeled RBCs, the net counts per minute of each sample are plotted on semilogarithmic paper as a function of time (Figure 19-3). The best straight line is drawn through all the points. The $t_{1/2}$ is obtained as follows:

1. The line to time zero is extrapolated; this is the y intercept.
2. The y intercept value is divided by 2. At this value on the y axis, a straight line is drawn parallel to the x axis

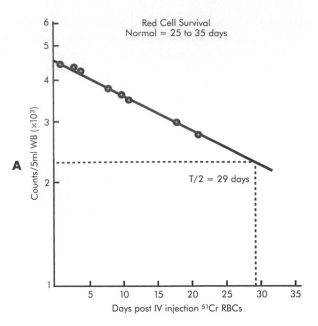

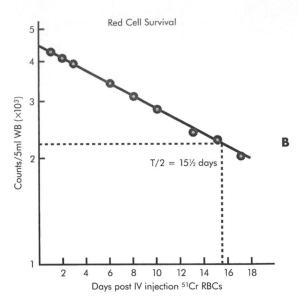

Figure 19-3   Red cell survival graph showing a normal $t_{1/2}$ of 29 days **(A)** compared with an abnormal $t_{1/2}$ **(B)**, which indicates a hemolytic process resulting in shortened survival of ^{51}Cr-labeled erythrocytes.

until it intersects the best straight line drawn through the observed data points.

3. A perpendicular line is dropped to the *x* axis; this is the labeled RBC half-time disappearance rate or survival time as measured by the ^{51}Cr technique, not corrected for elution of the isotope.

Occasionally a patient's data do not permit a satisfactory "eye fit" of a single straight line to the data points. The publication on RBC survival studies by the International Panel on Diagnostic Applications of Radioisotopes in Haematology[2] describes alternative methods, including computer programs for handling such data. Now that most clinical nuclear medicine laboratories have one or more dedicated computers, it is suggested that the appropriate programs be added to their software for use as needed.

The mean half-life of normal ^{51}Cr-labeled RBCs is 25 to 35 days. Normal RBCs are removed from the circulation when they become senescent at a rate approximating 1% per day; the true mean life span of the normal RBC, therefore, is 50 to 60 days. However, this approximately 1% per day removal of senescent RBCs from the circulation coupled with the approximately 1% per day elution of the ^{51}Cr label from the RBCs gives a mean half-life of 25 to 35 days when measured with this technique. Tables are available for correcting for this elution, but they were derived from studies in normal subjects, and their relevance in disease states in which the elution rate is known to vary is uncertain. However, the more severe the hemolytic process or bleeding, and thus the more rapid the rate of removal of the ^{51}Cr-labeled RBCs, the less significant this ^{51}Cr elution becomes.

Determination of the mean RBC life span from a label randomly applied to cells of all ages is meaningful only in a patient who is in a steady state with regard to the rate of production and destruction of RBCs. If either of these rates changes, the mean age of the circulating RBCs is changed and the ^{51}Cr results will be affected, even though the actual longevity of the individual RBC has not changed. A constant hematocrit value before and during the period of study is one index of a steady state. Obviously, inaccurate results are obtained in a patient who is being or has recently been transfused.

The study of splenic sequestration should be a routine part of any ^{51}Cr-RBC survival study. Organ counting is begun 24 hours after labeled cells are reinjected and is continued approximately every other day for the next 3 weeks.

The counting probe should be equipped with a flat-field collimator designed to exclude radiation from areas other than the organs of interest but that still permits sampling of a large enough organ volume to give adequate count rates. The spectrometer is adjusted to count gamma rays from 280 to 360 keV.

The patient is positioned on the examining table as follows:

Precordium: The patient is placed in the *supine* position, and the detector is centered over the left third intercostal interspace at the sternal border.

Liver: The patient is placed in the *supine* position, and the detector is placed over the ninth and tenth ribs on the right, in the midclavicular line. In elderly subjects and patients with chronic obstructive pulmonary disease, the exact location of the liver should be checked by percussion.

Spleen: The patient is placed in the *prone* position, and the detector is placed two thirds of the distance from the spinous process to the lateral edge of the body at the level of the ninth and tenth ribs.

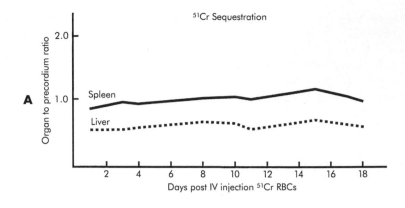

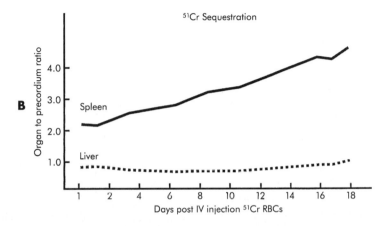

Figure 19-4   Organ localization of ^{51}Cr-labeled erythrocytes. Normal liver-to-precordium and spleen-to-precordium ratios (**A**) compared with increasing spleen-to-precordium ratios (**B**), showing active splenic sequestration.

The skin is marked with indelible ink, which in turn is covered by transparent nonallergenic tape to indicate the position of the external detector from one day to the next. Each area must be counted with the same geometry each time by having the detector touch the patient's skin. The areas are counted to give a sample error of 5% or less.

The results are expressed as the ratio of the count rate over the spleen to the count rate over the precordium. The count rate over the liver is also expressed relative to the count rate over the precordium. These ratios are graphed as a function of time on linear graph paper (Figure 19-4).

In normal subjects the spleen-to-liver ratio is less than or may approximate 1:1. In patients with active splenic sequestration of cells, this ratio often rises to 2:1 or even to 4:1. The spleen-to-precordium ratio is judged to be clearly abnormal if the ratio is greater than 2:1. An initial and persistent elevation of the spleen-to-precordium ratio is attributable to an increased splenic blood pool. A progressive gradual increase indicates active sequestration of the labeled cells.

Sources of Error

Sources of error include the following:

1. Inaccurate probe positioning, which causes spurious results

2. Blood loss from the gastrointestinal tract or surgical sites, which results in a shortened half-life
3. Blood transfusions during the procedure, which also cause an apparent shortening of the half-life (by increasing the volume of the unlabeled cells)

Obviously neither blood loss from the gastrointestinal tract or surgical sites nor blood transfusions during the procedure would affect the outcome of the splenic sequestration study; they therefore do not warrant discontinuation of the test unless the hemorrhage is truly massive, leaving an insignificant amount of circulating radioactivity.

Quantitation of Blood Loss

Occult blood loss is difficult to demonstrate with sensitivity and specificity. Over the years many methods of stool collection, homogenization, and counting have been devised by a great number of technologists to make this procedure more esthetic. Our current procedure has been demonstrated to be sensitive, specific, and acceptable to the technical staff. RBCs are labeled as in the RBC survival and sequestration study and returned to the patient intravenously. The patient is instructed to collect all stools for 4 days in clean paint cans and to avoid contaminating the collection with urine. Five milliliters of concentrated phenol in water is added to the stool collections as they arrive in the laboratory. The total weight of the can containing the fecal specimen and phenol is then brought to 2 kg by the addition of tap water, and the lid is tightly shut on the can. The stool is homogenized in the can by shaking the can on a commercial paint shaker for about 10 minutes. Blood samples are drawn on the first and third days, counted with identical geometry, and compared with the counts of the homogenized stool samples to determine blood loss.

$$\frac{\text{Total net cpm in 24-hour stool}}{\text{Net cpm in 1 ml of WB}} = \text{Blood loss (ml)}$$

Normal values are 1.2 ± 0.5 ml with a range of 0.3 to 2.8 ml/24 hr. Any blood in the stools in excess of this amount suggests enteric blood loss.

In Vivo Cross Matching

In rare instances blood banks are unable to identify a satisfactory donor for a patient requiring transfusion.[4] In these unusual circumstances, use of chromium-labeled *donor* RBCs for an in vivo cross match may provide a life-saving service.

The general principle is to infuse the patient with no more than 1 ml of donor cells after they have been labeled with ^{51}Cr. Carefully timed serial blood samples are then taken from the recipient at 3, 10, and 60 minutes, and both whole blood and plasma radioactivity are measured in the samples. The technique follows:

1. With sterile technique, 50 μCi of sodium ^{51}Cr chromate is added to 5 ml of the donor blood in a sterile test tube. This mixture is inverted gently several times to ensure proper mixing and then allowed to incubate for 15 minutes at room temperature, with occasional inverting.
2. The tube is centrifuged, and the supernatant plasma is aseptically withdrawn with an 18-gauge spinal needle. The tube then is filled with sterile isotonic saline, gently inverted several times, and centrifuged as before.
3. The washing procedure is repeated, and the cells then are resuspended in isotonic saline to the initial volume.
4. One milliliter of the ^{51}Cr-tagged, washed cells is drawn into a 3 ml syringe, and the remaining labeled cells are kept to make a standard.

Technique and Sample Preparation

A hematocrit value is determined on the 3-minute sample; 1 ml of whole blood is pipetted from each of the blood samples into tubes, which are then labeled. The remaining whole blood from the 10- and 60-minute samples is centrifuged, and 1 ml of the plasma is pipetted into the tubes, which are then labeled. Two milliliters of labeled whole blood is pipetted from the dose tube into a 100 ml volumetric flask containing 50 to 60 ml of distilled water. The flask is then filled to the mark with water and mixed. A 1 ml sample is pipetted from the flask into counting tubes, which are labeled. All samples are then counted in a well counter with spectrometer settings for ^{51}Cr (280 to 360 keV); the samples are counted long enough to achieve a counting accuracy of 1% error or less.

Interpretation. The estimated RBC mass is obtained from tables based on the sex, body weight, and venous hematocrit value of the recipient. The predicted RBC mass is compared with the calculated value by use of the 3-minute sample.

$$\text{Red blood cell mass (ml)} =$$

$$\frac{\substack{\text{Volume injected} \times \text{cpm in 1 ml Std} \times \\ \text{Dilution factor} \times \text{Samp Hct}}}{\text{cpm of 1 ml blood sample at 3 minutes}}$$

If immediate removal of a significant portion of the donor RBCs from the circulation does not occur, the estimated and the calculated RBC masses should be the same order of magnitude.

When compatible RBCs have been injected, about 99% of the radioactivity in the 3-minute whole blood sample is found in the 60 minute sample (range, 94% to 104%) and no radioactivity is seen in any of the plasma samples. In cases of urgency or if great difficulty is encountered in finding completely compatible RBCs, donor cells may be transfused with minimal hazard when 70% of the radioactivity in the 3-minute sample is found in the 60-minute sample and the amount of radioactivity in the 10- and 60-minute plasma samples is less than 5% of the radioactivity injected.

MEASUREMENT OF ABSORPTION AND SERUM LEVELS OF ESSENTIAL NUTRIENTS

Vitamin B$_{12}$ (Cyanocobalamin) Absorption

Nuclear medicine has furnished important tools for the diagnosis of vitamin B$_{12}$ deficiency. The consequences of untreated vitamin B$_{12}$ deficiency include anemia, thrombocytopenia, leukopenia, crippling spinal cord degeneration, and death.

The importance of measuring vitamin B$_{12}$ absorption in patients with unexplained anemia deserves emphasis, because the principle that anemia is not a disease per se but only a symptom of some underlying disorder is not always reflected in practice. The onset of clinical symptoms from vitamin B$_{12}$ deficiency is notoriously insidious, and the initial complaints of patients often are vague; in the early stages the classic RBC changes are not present.

Box 19-2 summarizes the causes of vitamin B$_{12}$ deficiency. Box 19-3 summarizes factors important in vitamin B$_{12}$ nutrition and absorption in humans. Absorption of this vitamin through the terminal ileum depends on secretion by the stomach of intrinsic factor, which exists as a dimer and binds two molecules of B$_{12}$. Intrinsic factor itself is not absorbed at the sites in the terminal ileum, but it is required in an

Box 19-2 Causes of Vitamin B_{12} Deficiency

I. Inadequate intake
II. Malabsorption
   A. Caused by gastric abnormalities
      1. Absence of intrinsic factor
         a. Congenital
         b. Addisonian pernicious anemia
         c. Total gastrectomy
         d. Subtotal gastrectomy
      2. Excessive excretion of hydrochloric acid (Zollinger-Ellison syndrome)
   B. Caused by intestinal malabsorption
      1. Destruction, removal, or functional incompetence of ileal mucosal absorptive sites
      2. Competition with host for available dietary vitamin B_{12}
         a. *Diphyllobothrium latum* (fish tapeworm)
         b. Small bowel lesions associated with stagnation and bacterial overgrowth (e.g., jejunal diverticula, strictures, blind loops)
      3. Drug therapy*
         a. Para-aminosalicylic acid (PAS)
         b. Neomycin
         c. Colchicine
         d. Calcium-chelating agents
   C. Caused by genetic abnormality in the transport protein transcobalamin II

*Although any of these agents may cause abnormalities in vitamin B_{12} absorption, only patients undergoing long-term PAS therapy have been reported to develop clinical evidence of vitamin B_{12} deficiency.

active transport mechanism. Ionic calcium and a pH of ileal contents greater than 6 are also required. Once absorption takes place, a normal transport protein, transcobalamin II, must be present in the bloodstream to convey the B_{12} to areas of the body for utilization or storage.

Isolated "pure" dietary deficiency (apart from severe prolonged protein deprivation) is very rare. Therefore the overwhelming number of cases of vitamin B_{12} deficiency are caused by some underlying disorder attributable to malabsorption. The most common cause of vitamin B_{12} malabsorption is a deficiency in intrinsic factor, a protein secreted by the parietal cells of the stomach that is an obligatory requirement for normal vitamin B_{12} absorption by the terminal ileum.

The availability of radioactive vitamin B_{12} for specific testing of a patient's ability to absorb physiologic amounts of this essential nutrient has been of great clinical value. Vitamin B_{12} is a complex corrinoid compound (Figure 19-5), the central ligand of which is cobalt; several radioactive isotopes of cobalt are available. The earliest in use was cobalt-60 (^{60}Co), but ^{57}Co and ^{58}Co are now preferred for routine clinical studies because of their shorter half-lives and smaller radiation doses (Table 19-3).

The Schilling test of urinary excretion is generally accepted as the standard method of measuring absorption of radioactive vitamin B_{12}. This test requires (1) oral administration and retention of a tracer dose of vitamin B_{12} (it is

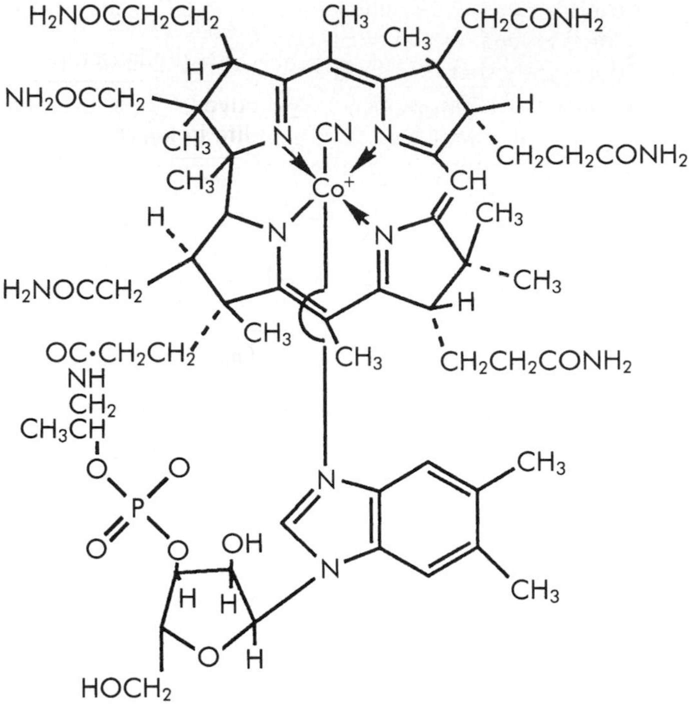

Figure 19-5 Structure of cyanocobalamin, the most widely administered form of vitamin B_{12}.

Box 19-3 Absorption of Dietary Vitamin B_{12} in Humans*

1. Vitamin B_{12} is available for human nutrition only from animal food sources.
2. Vitamin B_{12} is bound to the intrinsic factor by the gastric mucosa.
3. Normal ileal mucosal absorptive sites depend on the presence both of ionic Ca^{2+} and of ileal contents with a pH higher than 6.
4. Normal transport protein (transcobalamin II) conveys vitamin B_{12} from ileal absorptive sites to areas of active utilization and storage.

*The same factors apply to absorption of tracer amounts of the radioactive vitamin B_{12} used in absorption studies.

Table 19-3   Characteristics of selected radioisotopes of cobalt

Isotope	Physical half-life	Effective half-life in liver*	Radiation	Principal photon energies (meV)	Relative dose to liver
^{57}Co	270 days	161 days	Electron capture	0.122 (87%)	1[†]
^{58}Co	72 days	60 days	Electron capture, β^+, γ	0.810 (99%) 0.511 (30%)	2
^{60}Co	52 years	331 days	β^-, γ	1.17 (100%) 1.33 (100%)	29

Compiled from McIntyre PA: *Textbook of nuclear medicine: clinical applications,* Philadelphia, 1979, Lea & Febiger; adapted from Heinrich HC, editor: *Vitamin B-12 und intrinsic factor. II. Europäisches Symposium über Vitamin B-12 und Intrinsic Factor,* Hamburg, 1961, Stuttgart, 1961, Ferdinand Encke Verlag, p. 306.
*Assuming a biologic half-life of 400 days after administration as radioactive cobalt-labeled vitamin B_{12}.
[†]Approximately 0.051 rad per 0.5 μCi of ^{57}Co-labeled vitamin when parenteral dose of 1 mg of vitamin B_{12} is given, resulting in renal excretion of approximately 30% of the absorbed dose of radioactive vitamin B_{12}.

important that this oral dose be in the range of 0.25 to 2 μg, an amount similar to one that might be present in a normal meal, because amounts above this level may be absorbed by mechanisms not dependent on intrinsic factor) and (2) transient saturation of normal binding sites in the plasma, which is achieved by injection of a flushing dose of 1 mg of nonradioactive vitamin B_{12}.

Patients may drink water before and after the test; however, they should have nothing to eat after midnight on the day before the test and should remain fasting for 2 hours after the oral dose of ^{57}Co vitamin B_{12}. The patient's physician should be instructed not to give enemas or laxatives or to schedule the patient for a barium enema or intravenous pyelogram for the duration of this study. The patient should be questioned before the dose is given regarding medications that may interfere with the results (e.g., vitamin B_{12} injections, colchicine corticosteroids, and adrenocorticotropic hormone [ACTH]). Because of hepatobiliary recirculation, it is theoretically possible to block all the absorptive sites (in the terminal ileum) if large (1 mg or greater) daily doses of vitamin B_{12} are administered. If the patient has normal renal function, however, all excess vitamin B_{12} is promptly excreted in the urine, and the test needs to be delayed only 24 to 48 hours after discontinuation of the vitamin B_{12} injections.

If the patient has previously been given radioactive materials, a 24-hour urine collection is obtained for background. The dose of 0.5 μCi of ^{57}Co vitamin B_{12} is administered orally, and 2 hours later 1 mg of stable vitamin B_{12} is given intramuscularly. Two 24-hour urine collections are obtained, one for each 24-hour period. The patient is instructed to collect all urine during this period and avoid losing any urine during defecation.

The total volume and specific gravity of each 24-hour collection are measured. The urine samples and a standard are counted in a well counter with the spectrometer set to count gamma rays from 105 to 145 keV.

% of ^{57}Co vitamin B_{12} in 24-hour urine =

$$\frac{cpm\ in\ urine \times \dfrac{Urine\ volume}{Sample\ volume} \times 100}{cpm\ in\ Std \times Dilution\ factor}$$

Malabsorption of vitamin B_{12} can be documented by the appearance of less than 9% of the administered dose in the first 24-hour urine collection.

The major problem with this test is its dependence on a complete 24-hour urine collection. The loss of just one urine specimen may cause falsely low results. The 24-hour test also requires that urinary function be intact. Erroneously low values result from abnormal urinary retention, as in men with benign prostatic hypertrophy or in patients with renal disease. In such patients the amount excreted in the first 24 hours is reduced, but significant radioactivity continues to be excreted for the next 24 to 48 hours; total excretion eventually is within normal limits. For this reason and because it often indicates when the first 24-hour collection was incomplete, our routine is to have the patient collect two separate 24-hour urine specimens after the single flushing dose. We measure volume, specific gravity, and the percentage of the administered dose of radioactivity separately in each 24-hour specimen. Table 19-4 gives some typical patient results and illustrates the value of this minor modification of the Schilling test.

If less than 6% of the dose is excreted in 24 hours, a stage II Schilling test should be performed with 10 mg of intrinsic factor given along with the ^{57}Co-labeled vitamin B_{12}. About 3 to 7 days must elapse before the stage II test. A normal urinary excretion value after administration of intrinsic factor is seen with intrinsic factor deficiency.

Several factors can contribute to a false-negative result on the stage II Schilling test. When radioactive vitamin B_{12} and intrinsic factor are given in separate capsules, incomplete binding of the two in the stomach may result. Before administration, the radioactive vitamin B_{12} and intrinsic factor

Table 19-4 Representative results of Schilling test using two 24-hour urine collections (single nuclide without intrinsic factor)

Patient	First 24-hr urine collection			Second 24-hour urine collection		
	Volume	Specific gravity	Dose excreted (%)	Volume	Specific gravity	Dose excreted (%)
A	640	1.010	3.0	1230	1.010	0.8
B	1210	1.012	3.0	1120	1.012	0.8
C	1200	1.010	3.0	1150	1.010	3.0
D (normal)	1210	1.012	14.0	1200	1.012	0.3

Patient A had an incomplete first 24-hr urine collection because of inadvertent loss of urine during cleansing enemas.
Patient B subsequently had normal excretion when the test was repeated with the addition of a potent intrinsic factor. Other studies confirmed the diagnosis of addisonian pernicious anemia.
Patient C was recognized on reexamination to have benign prostatic hypertrophy with significant bladder retention. The delayed pattern of excretion of the radioactive vitamin B_{12} was the first clinical indication of this condition.
Patient D was a cooperative, normal volunteer.

should be mixed together in water.[16] If hog intrinsic factor is used, a negative result does not completely rule out intrinsic factor–dependent malabsorption. Some patients who have previously been exposed to hog intrinsic factor (as present in many multivitamin preparations) may have antibodies against it. Vitamin B_{12} deficiency can produce small bowel megaloblastosis with atrophy, which can cause ileal malabsorption. Vitamin B_{12} therapy may be necessary to allow the ileum to heal before a stage II study is performed.[10]

If it is determined that the stage II study result is truly abnormal, other causes of malabsorption must be investigated and treated if possible, followed by another stage I Schilling test.

Dual-isotope method for measuring vitamin B_{12} absorption. The conventional Schilling test for vitamin B_{12} absorption is done in two stages, requiring at least 1 week for a final result if stage I is abnormal. A dual-isotope method is available in which vitamin B_{12} labeled with two different isotopes of cobalt is administered. One form, [57]Co vitamin B_{12}, is bound to intrinsic factor by prior incubation with normal human gastric juice; the other form contains non-protein-bound [58]Co vitamin B_{12}.

The two capsules are ingested orally by a fasting patient, after which a flushing injection of 1 mg of nonradioactive vitamin B_{12} is given. Two 24-hour urine samples are collected. Differential isotope counting is performed to determine the percentage of administered dose of each isotope that has been excreted in the urine. A patient with normal vitamin B_{12} absorption excretes equal amounts of the two isotopes, whereas a patient lacking intrinsic factor excretes greater amounts of intrinsic factor–bound [57]Co vitamin B_{12}. In patients with bacterial overgrowth or bowel lesions resulting in vitamin B_{12} malabsorption, both isotopes are excreted in abnormally low amounts.

The dual-isotope Schilling test has several advantages over the conventional method. The advantage of taking only 2 days compared with 1 week to obtain results leads to

earlier diagnosis and treatment and saves money. The use of [57]Co vitamin B_{12} bound to human gastric juice eliminates the use of hog intrinsic factor preparations, against which some patients may have developed antibodies.

Although the same conditions in the patient for comparing the absorption of free and bound vitamin B_{12} are present in this method, small bowel changes caused by vitamin B_{12} deficiency are not considered. The absorption of the [57]Co vitamin B_{12} bound to gastric juice will be falsely low, along with a low [58]Co vitamin B_{12} absorption. This leads to a false-negative result.[9]

Serum vitamin B_{12} assays. The first assay for vitamin B_{12}, introduced in the early 1950s, used the microorganisms *Lactobacillus leichmannii* and *Euglena gracilis*. The rate of growth of these organisms in the appropriate media is directly related to the concentration of vitamin B_{12} in the sample added. An assessment of organism growth thus provides an estimate of vitamin B_{12} concentration. These methods were tedious and time-consuming, and antibiotics introduced in the patient's sample interfered with the assay.

In the early 1960s the first radioisotopic dilution assay was introduced using competitive protein-binding principles. Radioactive and non-radioactive vitamin B_{12} compete for the binding sites on protein-purified intrinsic factor, and separation of the protein-bound vitamin B_{12} from the free vitamin follows. The accuracy of these first radioassays for serum levels of vitamin B_{12} was questioned for several years. In the late 1970s Cooper and Whitehead[6] reported that 10% to 20% of patients diagnosed with pernicious anemia had normal serum B_{12} levels using these assays. At the same time, studies by Kolhouse and colleagues[13] showed that the intrinsic factor used in these assays contained contaminants called R-proteins, which can bind to biologically inactive vitamin B_{12} analogs, causing erroneously elevated levels in vitamin B_{12}–deficient patients.

In 1980 the National Committee for Clinical Laboratory Standards (NCCLS), under direction from the U.S. Food and Drug Administration (FDA), published standards for manufacturers and laboratories to follow to validate their assay and ensure correct measurement of serum vitamin B_{12} levels. Serum vitamin B_{12} radioassays using competitive protein-binding techniques are still in widespread use. A highly purified intrinsic factor is used as the binder. Recently, an enzymatic nonisotopic-binding protein assay for measuring serum vitamin B_{12} levels was reported to be equal to the conventional competitive protein-binding radioassay.[21]

Serum vitamin B_{12} levels, when measured by a reliable assay, are an early indicator of vitamin B_{12} deficiency before macrocytosis, megaloblastic changes, or neuropathy occurs.[15]

Although current assays are reliable, normal results obtained in any patient who otherwise has clinical evidence suggestive of vitamin B_{12} deficiency should be confirmed by a radioactive vitamin B_{12} absorption study. A single injection of vitamin B_{12} results in a normal serum value that can persist for many weeks despite the patient's inability to absorb dietary vitamin B_{12}.

Antiintrinsic factor–blocking antibodies. The most common cause of vitamin B_{12} malabsorption is pernicious anemia. Approximately 51% to 76% of affected patients have antiintrinsic factor–blocking antibodies in the serum.[5] A diagnosis of pernicious anemia can be made if these antibodies are present.

Blocking antibodies interfere with the formation of the intrinsic factor–B_{12} complex in the stomach. A commercially available assay for measuring blocking antibodies uses a highly purified intrinsic factor covalently bound to microscopic glass particles. Blocking antibody in the patient's serum combines with intrinsic factor to form a solid phase complex. This complex is separated from endogenous B_{12} binding proteins by centrifugation before the addition of ^{57}Co B_{12}.

The blocking antibodies prevent binding of the tracer to intrinsic factor. A second centrifugation step separates the bound complex from the free ligand. The presence of blocking antibodies in serum is extremely suggestive of pernicious anemia. The combination of megaloblastic anemia, low serum vitamin B_{12} levels, and serum-blocking antibodies to intrinsic factor is diagnostic of pernicious anemia.

Serum Folate Assays

Serum folate concentrations traditionally were measured microbiologically using *Lactobacillus casei*. As with vitamin B_{12} microbiologic methods, these assays were tedious, time-consuming, and inhibited by antibiotics present in blood specimens. A competitive protein-binding (CPB) assay of serum folate, using a folate-binding protein (β-lactoglobulin) present in cow's milk, has been developed and forms the basis for commercially available kits. Commercial folate CPB assays vary in the selection of the folate form used as standards and the folate form for tracer and in the methods used to denature endogenous folate binders.[14]

Because serum folate deficiency can be caused by several mechanisms, including vitamin B_{12} deficiency, and serum levels respond quickly to dietary intake of folate, RBC folate levels are a much better indicator of folate stores. Folate is incorporated into RBCs during their formation and remains there during the cell's life span. Serum folate and RBC folate levels are both low in folate deficiency megaloblastic anemia; red cell folate levels are also low in vitamin B_{12} deficiency. Because serum folate levels can be either elevated or normal in vitamin B_{12} deficiency, both must be measured before a diagnosis of folate deficiency is rendered. RBC folate and serum vitamin B_{12} levels reflect the status of tissue stores. The serum folate level reflects fluctuations caused by intake and changes in body demand.[17]

The most important recent development in the folate radioassay was its combination with the vitamin B_{12} radioassay into a simultaneous procedure. Because both assays are routinely requested on the same patient sample, this combination reduces performance time by half, lowering the cost of folate and vitamin B_{12} assays. Mixtures of ^{57}Co cyanocobalamin and ^{125}I folate are used as the tracers, mixtures of folic acid and vitamin B_{12} are used as standards, and a mixture of intrinsic factor and milk-binding protein is used as binders. The assays can be simultaneously counted in a dual-channel gamma counter with the appropriate window settings.

Serum Ferritin Assays

Ferritin is an iron-binding protein that contains virtually all the soluble iron stores in the body. Serum ferritin concentrations in normal subjects parallel the body iron stores; levels reflect iron deficiency and iron overload states and are clinically useful in the diagnosis and management of patients with these disorders. Serum ferritin measurements are a useful screening test for early iron deficiency and can be substituted for bone marrow biopsy.

Serum ferritin assays are done with immunoradiometric techniques using the ^{125}I-labeled antibody and a second antibody attached to a solid support. This two-site principle involves sandwiching the ferritin molecule (either in the patient sample or the standard) between the two antibodies generated against different portions of the ferritin molecule. As the concentration of ferritin increases, the amount of radioactivity increases in direct proportion. This technique allows accurate laboratory measurement of body iron stores over a wide concentration range.

Serum ferritin levels must be interpreted with caution because the direct relationship between serum ferritin and iron stores is not always reliable. Disorders that cause a disproportionate elevation in ferritin levels include liver disease, anemia of chronic disease, and disorders associated with increased or abnormal erythropoiesis.

REFERENCES

1. Belcher EH, Berlin NI, Dudley RA et al: Recommended methods for measurement of red

cell and plasma volume, *J Nucl Med* 21:793-800, 1980.

2. Belcher EH, Berlin NI, Dudley RA et al: Recommended methods for radioisotope red-cell survival studies, *Br J Haematol* 21:241-250, 1971.

3. Belcher EH, Berlin NI, Eernisse JG et al: Recommended methods for radioisotope platelet survival studies by the panel, *Blood* 50:1137-1144, 1977.

4. Belcher EH, Berlin NI, Eernisse JG et al: Standard techniques for the measurement of red cell and plasma volume, *Br J Haematol* 25:801-814, 1973.

5. Chanarin I: *The megaloblastic anaemias,* ed 2, Oxford, 1979, Blackwell.

6. Cooper BA, Whitehead VM: Evidence that some patients with pernicious anemia are not recognized by radiodilution assay for cobalamin in serum, *N Engl J Med* 299:816-818, 1978.

7. Ducassou D, Arnaud D, Bardy A et al: A new stannous agent list for labeling red blood cells with ^{99m}Tc and its clinical application, *Br J Radiol* 49:344-347, 1979.

8. Eckelman W, Richards P, Hausen W et al: Technetium-labeled red blood cells, *J Nucl Med* 12:22-24, 1971.

9. Fairbanks JF, Wahner HW: Clinical interpretation of the DICOPAC test of B_{12} absorption, *Nucl Med Commun* 5:47-51, 1984.

10. Haurani FI, Sherwood N, Goldstein F: Intestinal malabsorption of vitamin B_{12} in pernicious anemia, *Metabolism* 13:1342-1348, 1964.

11. International Committee for Standardization in Hematology: Panel on diagnostic applications of radionuclide (ICSH), *J Nucl Med* 4:564-566, 1988.

12. Jones J, Mollison PL: A simple and efficient method of labeling red cells with ^{99m}Tc for determination of red cell volume, *Br J Haematol* 38:141, 1978.

13. Kolhouse JF, Kondo H, Allen NC: Cobalamin analogues are present in human plasma and can mask cobalamin deficiency because current radioisotope dilution assays are not specific for true cobalamin, *N Engl J Med* 299:785-792, 1978.

14. Kubasik NP, Volosin MT, Sine HE: Comparison of commercial kits for radioimmunoassay. III. Radioassay of serum folate, *Clin Chem* 21:1922-1926, 1975.

15. Lindenbaum J: Status of laboratory testing in the diagnosis of megaloblastic anemia, *Blood* 4:624-627, 1983.

16. McDonald JW, Barr RM, Barton WB: Spurious Schilling test results obtained with intrinsic factor enclosed in capsules, *Ann Intern Med* 83:827-829, 1975.

17. Nickoloff EL, Drew H, Hagan J: *In vitro techniques: radionuclides in haematology,* London, 1986, Churchill Livingstone.

18. Scheffel U, Tsan MF, McIntyre PA: Labeling of human platelets with (^{111}In)-8-hydroxyquinoline, *J Nucl Med* 20:524-531, 1979.

19. Scheffel U, Tsan MF, Mitchell TG et al: Human platelets labeled with In-111-8-hydroxyquinoline: kinetics, distribution, and estimates of radiation dose, *J Nucl Med* 23:149-156, 1982.

20. Tsan MF, Hill-Zobel RL: Should platelets be radio-labeled in plasma medicine? *Am J Hematol* 25:355-359, 1987.

21. Vander Weide J, Homan HC, Rheenen EC et al: Nonisotopic binding assay for measuring vitamin B_{12} and folate in serum, *Clin Chem* 5:766-768, 1992.

22. Wright RR, Tno M, Pollycove M: Blood volume, *Semin Nucl Med* 5:63-77, 1975.

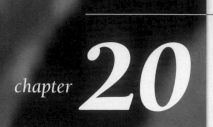

David F. Preston

chapter 20 Inflammatory Process and Tumor Imaging

Objectives

Discuss the pathogenesis of cancer cells.

Discuss the formation and pathogenesis of an abscess.

Describe the properties of carrier-free gallium citrate and its biodistribution.

Describe the technical considerations and instrumentation used for gallium imaging.

Explain the labeling methods for white cells using indium-111.

Describe the imaging techniques for performing indium-111 white blood cell scans.

Describe the principles of imaging using radiolabeled antibodies.

Describe positron emission tomography (PET) imaging in oncology.

---

*C*arrier-free gallium-67 (^{67}Ga) citrate is the radiopharmaceutical most frequently used for the detection and staging of cancer and for identifying inflammation and abscess. Imaging for inflammation with indium-111 (^{111}In)-labeled white blood cells (leukocytes) has proved to be an excellent alternative to ^{67}Ga citrate. Recently, white cell labeling with technetium-99m hexamethylpropylene amine oxime (^{99m}Tc-HMPAO) has been shown to be useful in searching for inflammation.

PATHOGENESIS

Cancer

Cancer is an uncontrolled overgrowth of cells often associated with the development of tumor nodules at sites remote from the original tumor. It is these remote tumor nodules, called *metastases,* that usually lead to the death of the patient. Over the past two decades, a remarkable improvement in life expectancy has been achieved for victims of several types of cancer. Early stages of Hodgkin's disease, choriocarcinoma, and some leukemias are now considered curable. The concept of cancer as a systemic process, one that involves the entire body possibly through altered immune mechanisms, has gained acceptance only in the past several years. The increasing success of chemotherapy, radiation therapy, and surgery to a great extent depends on early diagnosis. Staging and defining the extent of the disease at the time of diagnosis have permitted appropriate therapy to be instituted. The stage of the disease, the type of treatment, and the tumor's response to treatment are recorded in a database, and the results of innovations in therapy are measured against the recorded results of established therapeutic modalities.

No one is sure when a cancer begins. Biochemical changes must precede the histologic changes by years. Currently cancer is defined by cellular changes seen by the pathologist. A premalignant lesion is a progressive cellular change in which the final outcome is frank cancer. An incomplete list of organs in which premalignant lesions have been identified includes the skin, breast, lung, cervix, and colon. The pathologist identifies the premalignant lesions by unusual changes in the nuclei of the cells, by changes in the cytoplasm, and by loss of the usual orientation of cells. If the atypical cells have invaded the surrounding tissue or blood vessels, a malignancy is considered to exist. The initial site is considered the primary cancer. The primary site often can be excised by surgery. For cancer to kill a human being, it must be in a critical location or must disseminate to distant parts of the body, as when a colon cancer establishes itself in the liver or lymph nodes. This is metastatic cancer.

For cancer to continue to grow, new blood vessels must develop. When a cancer reaches a certain size (e.g., about 1 cm in diameter for breast cancer), capillaries from surrounding tissue grow toward the cancer and provide it with an adequate blood supply. Cancer implants in the anterior chamber of rabbits' eyes appear to release a substance that causes local capillary proliferation. The increased blood supply permits increased nutrients, white cells, and antibodies to be exposed to the cancer. Many cancers are associated with large accumulations of serum proteins.[24]

On many occasions the center of a cancer becomes necrotic because the central blood flow is insufficient to maintain cellular life. Often these fast-growing cancers usurp the blood at the periphery that is needed centrally. The anoxic center has implications for radiation therapy. Decreased oxygenation is associated with decreased radiation responsiveness. The surface of a tumor cell contains antigens that are characteristic of the tumor. Antibodies to these antigens have been labeled with gamma ray–emitting radionuclides.[25] Labeled antibodies have been approved by the U.S. Food and Drug Administration (FDA) to localize colon cancer and ovarian cancer. Labeled antibodies are available but unapproved by the FDA for localization of breast cancer and melanoma.

Abscess

A pyogenic abscess is a localized collection of dead white cells and bacteria. Typically an abscess begins with a small nidus of inflammation, increased capillary permeability, capillary leakage of serum proteins, and increasing concentrations of white cells. The increased permeability of the surrounding capillaries is caused by release of histamine and the capability of some bacteria to release toxins. Pyogenic abscesses may be found in any part of the body.

The two major types of white cells are granulocytes and lymphocytes. The neutrophil is the granulocyte most involved in the defense against pyogenic (pus forming) bacteria. If the blood supply does not bring adequate neutrophils to the nidus of infection, the bacteria increase in number. The process of inflammation causes release of certain substances called *leukotaxines,* which cause neutrophils to migrate to the area of inflammation. Some bacteria, such as staphylococci, release a toxin, a coagulase, that

causes deposition of fibrin, thereby walling off the bacteria from neutrophils and antibiotics. Streptococci produce hemolysins, which cause destruction of red blood cells (erythrocytes). A large cluster of vigorously growing bacteria can produce toxins that destroy neutrophils. As local blood flow brings more neutrophils to the scene, the neutrophils attempt to engulf the bacteria and digest them with packets of enzymes called *lysosomes.* The mixture of dead bacteria, dead granulocytes, and fluid is commonly known as pus. If the pus accumulates faster than the local circulation can remove it, the inflammatory volume expands and its center becomes a small volume of pus with viable bacteria. This is an abscess. At the periphery of the abscess new neutrophils arrive, fibrinogen and other serum proteins accumulate, fibrin is deposited, and the abscess becomes walled off. This wall is called the *pyogenic membrane*. The pyogenic membrane helps to isolate the abscess and limit its spread. Unrecognized abscesses are a common cause of death in seriously ill hospitalized patients.

There are five major areas of localized infection in which ^{67}Ga imaging can play a major role. Bacterial endocarditis is a serious medical emergency in which bacteria colonize a heart valve, usually the aortic or mitral valve. If the infection is not detected in time, the valve can be destroyed or scarred to the point of deformity and incompetence. Additionally, small particles of fibrin and bacteria can break off the valve and be carried by the bloodstream to embolize any area. Embolization of the brain, eyes, and kidneys is most common. The diagnosis of bacterial endocarditis is difficult, especially in a patient who previously has undergone unsuccessful antibiotic therapy. Recent dental extractions, intravenous drug abuse, and infection from other areas of the body can precede and cause bacterial endocarditis.

Lung abscesses can result from certain types of pneumonia, from chronic lung disease, or from infection anywhere in the body. Lung cancer that obstructs a bronchus can cause a localized pneumonia and eventually an abscess behind the obstruction.

A pelvic abscess can arise from pelvic inflammatory disease, a ruptured diverticulum of the colon, appendicitis, regional ileitis, or prior surgery. Subdiaphragmatic and intraabdominal abscesses are associated with perforated duodenal ulcers. Even in the antibiotic era, an abscess usually requires surgical drainage. Successful antibiotic treatment of a well-organized abscess might be impossible and can result in organisms resistant to antibiotics; precise localization, therefore, is imperative.

It is especially in the pelvic and abdominal region that gallium's poor diagnostic specificity for abscess has led to its replacement by ^{111}In-labeled leukocytes.

GALLIUM IMAGING

Historic Perspective

Gallium has 14 known isotopes, which range in mass number from 63 to 78. Because of an inappropriate half-life, type of emission, and production problems, only ^{67}Ga, ^{68}Ga, and ^{72}Ga seem likely to be useful in clinical nuclear medicine. Between 1949 and 1951 ^{72}Ga was first investigated by Dudley[14-16,50] as a diagnostic and therapeutic agent for osteogenic sarcoma and metastases to bone. ^{72}Ga was not especially valuable in these situations, but the bone-seeking property of gallium was demonstrated. In the early 1960s Brookhaven National Laboratories developed a germanium-68/gallium-68 generator. Germanium-68 (^{68}Ge) has a long half-life (280 days) and decays to ^{68}Ga, a positron emitter with a half-life of 68 minutes. The long-lived germanium parent and the short-lived gallium daughter looked like a promising combination for clinical use. ^{68}Ga as ethylenediamine tetraacetic acid (EDTA) was used with some success as a brain-imaging agent.[2,57] The citrate was investigated as a bone-imaging agent; however, neither radiopharmaceutical was widely used. By 1965 the technetium generator was commercially available, and pertechnetate quickly became the agent of choice for brain imaging. The early scintillation camera with its 1/2-inch thick sodium iodide crystal was rather inefficient at stopping the 511 keV annihilation photon of ^{68}Ga. A 360 keV collimator was the standard high-energy collimator provided, and resolution was greatly impaired by septal penetration. In 1967 a prototype two-detector positron camera became available but was not mass produced. With the advent of newer positron imaging devices, the ^{68}Ge/^{68}Ga generator may return to nuclear medicine.

In 1965 there was no technetium-labeled phosphate for bone imaging. That year the Medical Division of the Oak Ridge Institute of Nuclear Studies[1] reconfirmed earlier work[9] showing ^{67}Ga administered with carrier gallium to localize in bones within hours. Experiments with carrier-free ^{67}Ga demonstrated concentration in bones much later. Two to 3 days after injection of carrier-free ^{67}Ga, Edwards and Hayes[18] noted intense uptake in the tumor. In this initial report they found that carrier-free ^{67}Ga citrate concentrated in soft tissue tumors, especially in those without prior radiation therapy or chemotherapy. They also found that false-negative results did occur, and they found new tumor sites not previously detected by other modalities. With this evidence of tumor detection, Oak Ridge Associated Universities (ORAU), in a cooperative study with 16 universities, performed nearly 3000 scans between 1970 and 1974, firmly establishing the utility of carrier-free ^{67}Ga citrate in staging and detecting tumors.[12,27,41]

Benign tumors and inflammatory diseases such as sarcoidosis,[66] pneumonia,[13,14] pyelonephritis, active tuberculosis, dermatomyositis,[59] asbestosis, silicosis,[58] inflammation/fibrosis,[47] and fevers of undetermined origin[49] can also be detected by ^{67}Ga imaging. Computers permit calculation of an index of inflammatory activity based on ^{67}Ga lung uptake. This index of ^{67}Ga lung accumulation has been demonstrated to correlate with histopathologic scores of inflammation and fibrosis in lung tissue.[6,47] Gallium has great avidity for all acquired immunodeficiency syndrome (AIDS)-related causes of inflammation, especially *Pneumocystis carinii* pneumonia.

Chemical Toxicity

Gallium toxicity[15] is characterized by vomiting, skin rash, proteinuria, anemia, and leukopenia and results from doses of 71 mg/kg or greater. Toxicity is variable in experimental animals.[8] Six millicuries of ^{67}Ga contains only 10 ng of elemental gallium, providing a substantial chemical toxicity safety factor.[61] Carrier-free gallium citrate is the radiotracer used. In early preparations excess citrate became bound to calcium and caused hypocalcemia.[53] This has not been a problem with the amounts of citrate currently used (2 mg of sodium citrate/2 mCi of ^{67}Ga). In the past, differences in the citrate concentration between manufacturers were found and were thought to account for diagnostic differences reported in the literature.[64] This has not been a problem in the past 10 years.

Production

Carrier-free ^{67}Ga is cyclotron produced by several methods involving proton bombardment of a zinc-oxide target. The reactions are as follows:

$$^{67}Zn(p,n)^{67}Ga$$
$$^{68}Zn(p,2n)^{67}Ga$$

Zinc-67 (^{67}Zn) and ^{68}Zn occur with a natural abundance of 4% and 18%, respectively.

How "free" is carrier free? If natural zinc targets are used, as much as 4 µg of stable gallium can contaminate each milliliter of the final carrier-free gallium, depending on the amount of stable gallium in the target.[37] Ten millicuries of ^{67}Ga contains 15×10^{13} atoms of ^{67}Ga. The 40 µg of stable gallium in 10 ml contains 36×10^{16} atoms, about 2400 stable gallium atoms for each radioactive atom when the target is from natural zinc. Carrier-free gallium made from a natural zinc target is not really carrier free. Recent improvements have been made in enriching the target so that it is 99% ^{68}Zn. ^{67}Ga made from such a target contains no stable gallium in the final injectate.

Additional production methods are available, such as alpha particle bombardment of a zinc target, deuteron bombardment of a zinc target, and alpha particle bombardment of a copper target.

Biodistribution Differences Between Carrier-Free and Carrier-Added Gallium Citrate

When nanograms of carrier-free ^{67}Ga per kilogram of body weight are injected into humans, the percentage of activity per organ is far different from the percentage of activity per organ when the same amount of ^{67}Ga is accompanied with milligram per kilogram body weight quantities of stable gallium.[1] In the carrier-free state, ^{67}Ga concentrates first in the liver, soft tissues, abscesses, and some cancers. After 2 to 3 days it concentrates slightly in bone. With carrier gallium added, ^{67}Ga initially concentrates more heavily in bone.

Distribution of Carrier-Free Gallium Citrate

After intravenous injection of carrier-free ^{67}Ga citrate, binding to serum proteins (probably transferrin)[10,28] and alpha and beta globulins occurs, with little activity in albumin and gamma globulins.[19,29] Blood clearance is fairly rapid initially, with only 25% of the injected dose remaining in the blood at 3 hours, 7% at 24 hours, and 5% at 40 hours; only 2% remains in the intravascular space at 5 days. Once gallium has entered a tissue, it remains there. About 10% to 15% of the injected dose is excreted in the urine in the first 24 hours, whereas approximately 10% of the injected dose is excreted in the stool. Accounting for decay, 65% remains in the body.[5] About 20% of the dose is eliminated, with an effective half-life of 69.5 hours[27] (Figure 20-1).

Attempts have been made in the past to increase the target-to-background ratio of gallium images. These efforts first involved the administration of stable scandium, an element with chemical properties similar to those of gallium. When administered to animals, scandium caused a definite decrease in background gallium. However, scandium administration to humans resulted in a hemolytic anemia. In animals, the administration of iron-dextran complex (Imferon) has been successful in decreasing the blood background and significantly enhancing the target-to-background ratio.[36,52]

From autopsy studies the five organs with the greatest mean percentage of injected dose per kilogram are the spleen (4%), the renal cortex (3.8%), bone marrow (3.6%), liver (2.8%), and bone (1.4%).[51] From patient to patient, there was a tenfold range of activity for each organ. Brain and muscle contained one seventh to one fortieth the activity of the five most active organs.

Several mechanisms of gallium localization have been suggested: (1) involvement of iron-binding molecules,[46,55,65] (2) a unique tumor-specific protein,[34] and (3) gallium exchange with intracellular calcium-binding sites.[3] Data from a variety of experimental techniques[33-35,45,46] plus data in humans[20] suggest that transferrin, the iron-binding protein in serum, is involved in ^{67}Ga delivery to the tissue. At the tumor or abscess site, the ^{67}Ga is transferred into the cell in a manner not totally understood. At this point, calcium-binding components, ferritin, the iron storage protein, or a unique tumor-specific protein could deposit ^{67}Ga into the cell. The ^{67}Ga eventually is deposited in small structures, lysosomes present in the cell's cytoplasm.[61]

Great variations in tumor uptake are seen from one tumor to another in the same patient. In general, tumors with a significant fibrotic or necrotic content accumulate lesser

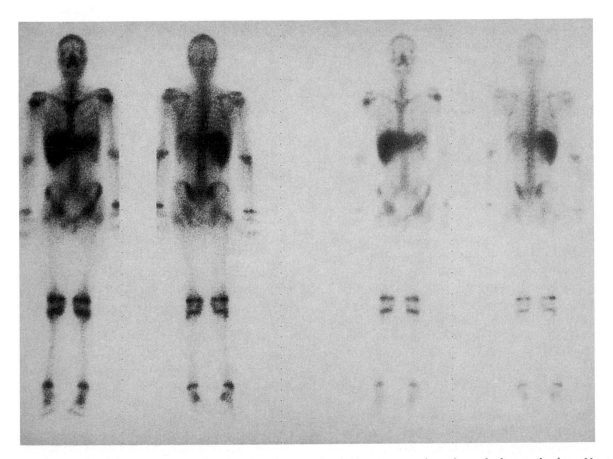

Figure 20-1 Normal whole body anterior and posterior scintigrams of a child. Note normal uptake in the liver and spleen. Normal symmetric uptake is seen in the epiphyses and lacrimal glands.

amounts of gallium. Tumors with less than 5% of injected dose per kilogram are very difficult to visualize, as are tumors less than 2 cm in diameter.

The question of whether gallium concentration by a tumor and the rate of deoxyribonucleic acid (DNA) synthesis are associated was examined in experimental animals with tumors. Small tumors (e.g., Harding-Passey melanomas) showed decreased gallium uptake with increased DNA synthesis; larger tumors, however, showed increased gallium uptake with increased DNA synthesis. Chemotherapy of some experimental tumors caused a sharp reduction in DNA synthesis but no change in gallium uptake.[60] In everyday gallium imaging, loss of gallium uptake by a tumor is an indication of successful radiation therapy or chemotherapy. Continued uptake of ^{67}Ga citrate indicates continued tumor activity.[23,40,42,43]

Technical Considerations

Imaging protocols consist of the establishment of guidelines for dosages, optimum time after injection for imaging, photopeak settings, information density, collimation, and positioning. Certain data, such as decay mode and dosimetry, must be presented as a rationale for these guidelines. Variations of the guidelines depend on the instrumentation available.

Preparation for scanning with ^{67}Ga citrate must be twofold, physical and emotional. Physical preparation primarily concerns elimination of gallium-containing feces from the colon. About 9% to 15% of the gallium is excreted through the bowel, especially in the first 24 hours. At 24 hours, gallium that accumulates in the bowel is seen as areas of increased activity that may be mistaken for cancer, abscess, or inflammation. In the first 24 hours, gallium can attach itself to newly forming colon mucosal cells, which over the course of several days shed into the lumen of the colon. While the gallium is in the mucosa, bowel cleansing is not successful at removing activity from the abdomen.

The more commonly used bowel preparations are a combination of bisacodyl tablets and magnesium citrate or cleansing enemas. Little research has been done on the efficacy of this type of preparation. Zeman and Ryerson[67] reported that patients given bisacodyl tablets and magnesium citrate showed no greater bowel clearance than patients without preparation. Other reports claim bowel preparation to be necessary.[4] The patient's diet is another variable. It is likely, but as yet unproven, that patients on a normal or high-fiber diet have a greater clearance of gallium from the bowel than patients on a low-bulk or liquid diet. If possible, a regular diet should be continued. If the patient has diarrhea, bowel preparation is unnecessary and can aggravate dehydration and electrolyte loss. Accumulation of gallium in the abdomen in patients with diarrhea is almost always indicative of a pathologic condition.

The emotional aspect of gallium scanning is important and often unappreciated. Adequate emotional preparation can yield many benefits: decreased motion, decreased

Table 20-1	^{67}Ga radionuclide characteristics				
Nuclide	**Production**	**Half-life**	**Principal radiations**		
			meV	**%**	
^{67}Ga	^{67}Zn(p,n)^{67}Ga	78 hr	0.093	40	
	^{68}Zn(p,2n)^{67}Ga				
			0.184	24	
			0.296	22	
			0.388	7	

From the Bureau of Radiological Health: *Radiological health handbook,* Washington, DC, 1970, US Department of Health, Education, and Welfare.

imaging time, fewer repeat views, and less time spent explaining the examination after the fact. Credibility is greater when the explanation is initiated by the person performing the test. The nuclear medicine staff should not expect the referring physician or nurse on the ward to explain the test to the patient adequately. Ethically and practically, a technologist should never inform a patient of anything related to the patient's specific condition or supply a patient with any records that the physician has not cleared.

Before injection, the patient should be informed of the duration of the overall gallium study. Depending on the type of equipment and the dose, this ranges from 40 minutes to 3 hours. A longer examination than expected can be a threatening experience that can be prevented by the patient's prior knowledge of the duration of the test. The patient should also know of the need to remain still during the procedure and that various views might be required. The need to take images even 7 days later must be considered.

A camera with a scanning table or its equivalent is used. The patient is placed comfortably supine and is imaged posteriorly from below the table and then anteriorly from above to include all the body from the top of the head to approximately midthigh. If a prone position is used, the head, neck, and perhaps shoulder will be rotated in an undesirable semioblique position that will require static images of the neck so that both right and left cervical areas can be compared. In addition, the prone position usually is painful if the patient recently has undergone abdominal surgery.

Doses for intravenous injection of carrier-free ^{67}Ga citrate range from 6 to 10 mCi for a 70 kg adult. In the selection of an injection site, care should be taken to avoid choosing a possible site of clinical interest. The technologist should always record the date, time, and site of injection.

Radiation Characteristics

^{67}Ga has a half-life of 78 hours (3.25 days) and decays by electron capture. It has four principal gamma ray energies (Table 20-1). The radiation absorbed dose from 5 mCi of ^{67}Ga citrate is shown in Table 20-2.[48]

Table 20-2	Radiation dosimetry for ^{67}Ga citrate
Organ	**^{67}Ga citrate (rad/5 mCi)**
Whole body	1.3
Skeleton	2.2
Liver	2.3
Bone marrow	2.9
Spleen	2.65
Kidney	2.05 (calyx)
Ovary	1.4
Testes	1.2
Stomach	1.1
Small intestine	1.8
Upper colon	4.5

From Medical Internal Radiation Dose (MIRD): Dose estimate report no 2, *J Nucl Med* 14:755, 1973.

Imaging Time after Injection

Imaging of a patient injected with ^{67}Ga citrate can take place from 6 hours to 1 week after injection. Once deposited, gallium remains in tissue, and the target-to-background ratio increases with the passage of time as blood clearance progresses. Considerations other than target-to-background ratios may dictate earlier rather than later imaging, such as the urgency of possible surgery for an abscess, the cost of hospitalization, the fact that imaging time increases with physical decay, and the necessity of delaying other studies that might interfere with the imaging study.

Hopkins and Mende[39] have evaluated ^{67}Ga citrate imaging for subphrenic abscess performed 6 hours after injection. They found no additional positive sites at 24 or 72 hours compared with the 6-hour scans. In another study[38] it was noted that gallium citrate was not yet in the bowel at 6 hours, and in that study focal activity in the abdomen was indicative of a pathologic condition. Beihn and colleagues[5] combined ^{99m}Tc sulfur colloid and ^{67}Ga imaging for abscess detection. They subtracted technetium counts in the liver from gallium counts and showed that increased gallium counts were associated with early detection of intrahepatic abscesses.

Our own results with imaging at 12 to 24 hours have been less than optimal. Although it is true that many abscesses have been demonstrated at this time, we have found that more than half were equivocally detected and that re-imaging at 48 and 72 hours was required.

Kaplan and co-workers[43] have published their extensive experience with 7-day delayed gallium scans. They have found the 7-day delay to be vital to improved sensitivity and specificity of the gallium scan. Our experience fully supports this enthusiasm. The much-reduced body background more than makes up for the reduced count rate. We have obtained clinically important diagnostic information as long as 16 days after injection of 10 mCi of ^{67}Ga citrate.

Kaplan and others[23,40,42,43] have found a negative gallium scan to be an accurate predictor of successful therapy of lymphoma. A normal gallium scan, even with residual radiographic masses, indicates that those masses are tumor free, whereas an abnormal gallium scan provides strong evidence of tumor activity in the area even in the absence of radiographic masses.

Instrumentation and Technique Variations

A variety of equipment can be used for gallium imaging. Initially, rectilinear scanners were used, especially those with whole body and minification capabilities. In recent years the evolution of the scintillation camera with its increase in field size and the introduction of multiple pulse height analyzers have supplanted the rectilinear scanner. Scintillation cameras with whole body and single positron emission computed tomography (SPECT) imaging capabilities are necessary for modern gallium imaging.

For whole body imaging, the patient receives 6 to 10 mCi of ^{67}Ga citrate intravenously. After a 2- to 7-day delay, imaging is performed, and 2 million–count whole body images are obtained. Simultaneous anterior and posterior whole body images require 15 to 30 minutes and usually are obtained with two different analog outputs to film so that the dynamic range of the data can be displayed within the limited gray scale capability of film.

High- to medium-energy collimators (rated at a minimum of 300 keV) must be used because of the physical characteristics of gallium photon emission. If a low-energy collimator is used and the pulse height analyzer is set at the 93 keV peak, scatter and septal penetration from the high-energy photons destroy meaningful resolution. If two photopeaks can be summed, the 93 keV and 184 keV peaks are chosen. Optimally, the 93 keV, 184 keV, and 296 keV peaks are used. Regardless of the photopeak chosen, a high- to medium-energy collimator is needed to collimate the higher energies and reduce septal penetration even if only lower energies are selected for imaging. When three peaks can be used, the imaging time is halved, with a constant information density compared with use of the 93 keV peak alone. With all peaks we use a 20% window centered on each photopeak.

Technically suboptimum images are the major cause of difficulty in confident, accurate interpretation of ^{67}Ga studies. Adequate counts must be acquired, and the intensity of those counts must be distributed over the dynamic range of the film. Ideally the diagnosis should be made from the digital data displayed on a monitor. In whole body scanning sternal activity is made to correspond to a midpoint in the dynamic range of the film. Areas of increased or decreased activity usually remain within the dynamic range of the film. If equivocal areas are noted, additional static images of 300,000 counts for a standard-field camera and 500,000 counts for a large-field camera are adequate. Repeating selected views, especially of the abdomen at 48 hours, and occasionally more delayed views at 72 and 96 hours are important for accurate clinical results.

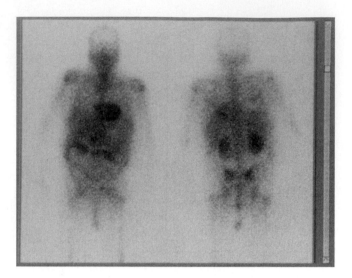

Figure 20-2 ^{67}Ga whole body scan demonstrates uptake by lymphoma with involvement of the heart, right kidney, and intraabdominal lymph nodes.

SPECT imaging with ^{67}Ga can produce exceptional clinical results. Inflammation and gallium-avid tumors, especially Hodgkin's disease and squamous cell carcinoma of the lung, can be detected, and the extent of disease and response to treatment can be accurately estimated.

In the past most SPECT imaging with gallium has been performed with single-head cameras. Dual- and triple-detector cameras with large rectangular fields of view are the current state-of-the-art. Satisfactory imaging can be performed 48 hours after injection. The 184 keV and 296 keV peaks can be summed. A 64×64 acquisition matrix, 64 stops at 35 sec/stop, requires almost an hour. Filtered back-projection reconstruction using a Butterworth filter, cutoff 0.4, order 6, or its equivalent is suggested. Currently, the dual- and triple-detector SPECT systems offer greater count acquisition, better statistics, and better spatial resolution.

Figure 20-2 shows an example case for gallium imaging. The patient was a 35-year-old male who was seen in an infectious disease department for recurrent fevers and night sweats. The chest x-ray was normal as were the computed tomography (CT), magnetic resonance imaging (MRI), sonography, and initial hematologic studies. The patient received an intravenous injection of 10 mCi of gallium citrate. Forty-eight hours later, a whole body scan from head to feet was performed (only head to knees is shown in Figure 20-2). The whole body image contains 2 million counts. The anterior image on the left reveals intense cardiac uptake, best seen in the anterior view, with lesser focal uptake seen in the region of the celiac axis. Colonic uptake in the transverse colon is within normal limits. The spleen was remarkable by its lack of gallium avidity. Asymmetric uptake was noted on the posterior image, with increased gallium retention in the right kidney.

Because of activity in the heart, the celiac nodes and right kidney lymphoma were the primary considerations. Myocarditis could produce such cardiac uptake, but the intraabdominal and right renal uptake and normal cardiac status could not be explained by the diagnosis of myocarditis. Biopsy of the intraabdominal lymph node revealed T-cell lymphoma with involvement of the heart, right kidney, and intraabdominal lymph nodes. SPECT imaging of the abdomen provided definitive localizing information not available by standard diagnostic techniques.

Future Trends

Currently no radiopharmaceutical is available that is specific for cancer. The most extensive clinical experience has been with carrier-free ^{67}Ga citrate. Even so, some nuclear medicine departments find it difficult to produce results that are helpful to clinicians. A nuclear medicine physician must have an optimum image based on standard technical factors. Without a stable technique, the physician's report becomes an expensive "weather report," which points in all directions and does little to aid the clinician. The nuclear medicine physician must develop confidence in the accuracy of his or her interpretation. Without confidence in the ability of gallium imaging to detect abscesses and tumors, the report will be equivocal and nondiagnostic. The typical response of the insecure physician is "let's do CT or MRI instead."

The future of nuclear medicine lies in the development of new radiotracers that demonstrate altered biochemistry and physiology before an anatomic defect develops. To some degree nuclear medicine has this capability now with carrier-free ^{67}Ga citrate. New radiotracers, labeled antibodies, and labeled peptides can dramatically improve the specificity of tumor imaging in the future.

INDIUM-111 WHITE CELL IMAGING

In the early 1970s ^{111}In chloride was used as a tumor and abscess imaging agent. [111]In chloride had the advantage over ^{67}Ga of not concentrating in the gastrointestinal tract,[11] but clinical results of tumor and abscess imaging revealed ^{111}In chloride to be slightly inferior to [67]Ga. [111]In has unusually good imaging characteristics, and interest in its use progressed.

Radiation Characteristics

[111]In has a physical half-life of 67.4 hours. It decays by electron capture, producing two gamma photons with a combined frequency of 1.8 photons for each disintegration. Both photons have excellent energies for external imaging (Table 20-3). The end product of ^{111}In decay is stable cadmium-111.

White Blood Cell as a Complex Imaging Agent

White blood cells are of two general classes, granulocytes and lymphocytes. Neutrophils, the type of granulocyte involved with defense against pyogenic bacteria, can be tagged with ^{111}In oxine or ^{99m}Tc-HMPAO. The ability of the labeled neutrophils to migrate to the area of infection is

Nuclide	Half-life	Principal radiations	
		keV	%
[111]In	67.4 hr	171	90.0
		247	94.2

Table 20-3 ^{111}In radionuclide characteristics

maintained, which provides a specific method of localization of infectious processes. With the development of new diagnostic procedures of medical value, in the future the eosinophil, a granulocyte involved in the allergic response, and the basophil might be selectively tagged.

Lymphocytes can be separated into groups based on specific antibody production. If these selected populations of lymphocytes could be tagged and their location and degree of concentration measured, specific diagnostic information could be developed that could revolutionize medical practice. Currently, most work has been performed with labeled neutrophils to detect localized infectious processes.

Most major advances in nuclear medicine are the result of radiopharmaceutical progress. The diagnostic potential of labeled white cells has been recognized for years, but the development of a nondestructive tag that would not interfere with the cells' biologic properties appeared to be a serious problem. The lipid coating of white cells and the presence of plasma protein prevented a straightforward approach. If plasma proteins were present, the ^{111}In tagged the protein instead of the neutrophil. Removal of the plasma from the white cells causes a loss of cell viability. Labeling with ^{111}In oxine is a balance between efficiency of tagging and cell viability.

Many attempts have been made to label white cells. [99m]Tc sulfur colloid labels granulocytes[20] and has satisfactorily demonstrated experimental abscesses in animals but has not been so successful in humans. When technetium sulfur colloid is incubated with white blood cells, the neutrophils phagocytize some of the colloid. However, the cells recognize this as a signal to activate their own bactericidal mechanisms. During this process the cell enlarges, activates its lysozymal system to digest the colloidal particle, and in the process loses its ability to migrate to an area of infection. It is soon destroyed by its own lysozymal enzymes. Of course, not all the technetium sulfur colloid is phagocytized, and a significant residual remains to be injected and be phagocytized by the Kupffer cells of the liver and spleen, thereby presenting an unwanted background in the exact regions that need to be most critically observed for intraabdominal abscess formation.

[111]In Oxine Complex

In 1977 Thakur and colleagues[62] demonstrated a method for labeling white cells with ^{111}In oxine and showed it to be superior to ^{67}Ga citrate for localizing experimental abscesses

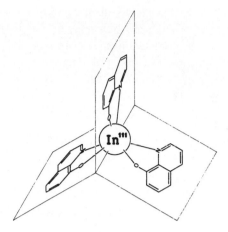

Figure 20-3 ^{111}In oxine complex: three oxine molecules surround the ^{111}In atom.

in dogs. Since these researchers' initial report, numerous other publications have demonstrated the utility of ^{111}In-labeled white cells in the diagnosis of localized infectious processes in the clinical situation. The ability to tag white cells in a clinical setting provides nuclear medicine with a powerful new diagnostic agent.

The structural formula of ^{111}In oxine is shown in Figure 20-3. Three oxine molecules surround the ^{111}In atom, creating a lipophilic complex able to penetrate the lipid cell membrane. In the cell, the ^{111}In-oxine bond is broken, the ^{111}In binds to cytoplasm, and the oxine is released from the cell. The cell's ability to recognize its environment and to migrate to areas of inflammation is associated with its surface. Specialized protein molecules extend through the lipid membrane and provide communication between the external environment and the cell itself. The oxine labeling method seems to spare the surface of the cell.

Labeling Method

The usual labeling method is to take approximately 50 ml of the patient's blood and to use the patient's own white cells. Some patients do not have an adequate number of white cells in the peripheral blood, a condition known as *granulocytopenia*. The absence of granulocytes is called *agranulocytosis*. In this situation a donor, properly typed by the blood bank, can provide the granulocytes to be tagged.

Care must be taken to separate the white cells from the red cells and platelets. Several methods have been proposed for accomplishing this separation, but it is vital that it be performed satisfactorily. The initial separation may remove the bulk of the red cells, but additional means are necessary to eliminate the remainder. Consider the problems. A cubic millimeter usually has 5 million red cells and 5000 white cells. Even if the initial gross separation method is 99.9% complete in eliminating the red cells, the mixture still contains 5000 red cells and 5000 white cells/mm³.

After the initial separation by gravity, red cells may be more thoroughly separated by hypotonic hemolysis, by the addition of ammonium chloride solution, or by the use of methyl cellulose. With hypotonic hemolysis, water is added to the mixture of red and white cells. Because red cells are more sensitive to osmotic changes than white cells, the red cells hemolyze and the red cell fragments are removed, leaving behind the white cells. The specific method we use is the method of Thakur and Gottschalk[63] (Box 20-1). Injection of 500 μCi of ^{111}In-labeled white cells provides an adequate count rate at 24 hours. Local commercial nuclear pharmacies offer the service of tagging an individual's white cells with ^{111}In oxine.

Box 20-1 Preparation of ^{111}In-Labeled White Cells

Materials

- [111]In oxine (from 3.5.1. or purchased commercially)
- Hank's balanced salt solution (HBSS):

  2.00 g NaCl   0.025 g $MgCl_2$.6 H_2O
  0.010 g K CI   0.25 g glucose
  0.035 g $CaCl_2$ 20.065 g Hepes buffer
  0.025 g $MgSO_4$.7 H_2O

  Add 250 ml of H_2O, adjust pH to 7.4, and filter into sterile, pyrogen-free vials.
- Ammonium chloride solution:

  2.07 g NH_4CI
  0.25 g $KHCO_3$
  0.093 g EDTA

  Add 250 ml of H_2O, adjust pH to 7.4, and filter into sterile, pyrogen-free vials.
- 50 ml polypropylene centrifuge tubes
- Oxford Macroset pipette and sterile tips
- 2% (w/v) methylcellulose solution
- Heparin

Method

1. Use sterile technique and supplies.
2. Collect 50 ml of blood in a 60 ml syringe containing 1 to 2 ml of heparin (250 to 1,000 units) and 1.5 ml of 2% methylcellulose solution.
3. Clamp the syringe barrel to a ring stand in an upright position and tilt the syringe about 20 degrees from the perpendicular. This allows the red blood cells (RBCs) to settle and produces a leukocyte-rich plasma (LRP).
4. Remove the needle and replace with a butterfly.
5. Express the LRP into a 50 ml sterile polypropylene centrifuge tube, taking care not to collect RBCs. Remove 0.5 ml for the white blood cell (WBC) count.
6. Centrifuge the LRP at $450 \times G$ for 5 minutes to obtain a WBC button.
7. Remove the leukocyte-poor plasma (LPP) supernatant and save at 37°C.
8. Resuspend the WBCs in 5 ml of ammonium chloride solution (to destroy RBCs) and immediately centrifuge at $450 \times G$ for 5 minutes.
9. Resuspend WBCs in 5 ml of HBSS with gentle agitation and centrifuge at $450 \times G$ for 5 minutes.
10. Resuspend WBCs in 5 ml of HBSS and add about 2 mCi of ^{111}In oxine.
11. Incubate 20 to 30 minutes at 37°C. Gently agitate the mixture three or four times during the incubation to ensure adequate mixing.
12. While the WBCs are incubating with ^{111}In, centrifuge the LPP at $1,000 \times G$ for 15 minutes. Save the supernatant platelet-poor plasma (PPP).
13. After incubation, add 5 ml of PPP obtained in step 12 to WBCs and mix gently. The plasma aids in the removal of loosely bound [111]In.
14. Centrifuge mixture at $450 \times G$ for 5 minutes.
15. Remove the supernatant, add 5 ml of PPP, and repeat step 14. Count the activity in the supernatants and pellet and determine the labeling efficiency. Include the supernatant from the previous spin in the efficiency calculation. At least 500 μCi of activity should be seen in the cells.
16. Add 5 ml of PPP to the WBCs, gently mix, and measure the activity. The WBCs now are ready for injection. Remove 0.5 ml for a count differential cell smear and trypan test.

Modified from Thakur ML, Gottshalk A, editors: *In-111 labeled neutrophils, platelets and lymphocytes,* New York, 1980, Trivirum.

The viability of the cell, after undergoing the stress of labeling, can be measured by its ability to exclude trypan blue dye, which enters and stains a nonviable cell but does not stain a viable cell. Chemotaxis, the granulocyte's ability to migrate in response to an appropriate chemical stimulus, can be measured by special assays described by Boyden.[7] Observation of a portion of the labeled cells by light microscope is a simple procedure that can detect clumping of white cells. Dutcher and co-workers[17] have estimated that their patients were injected with approximately 6 million to 15 million granulocytes, labeled with 360 to 560 µCi of [111]In. Using this method, approximately 95% of the cells were granulocytes. The entire labeling process can be completed in 2 hours or less, and labeling efficiencies of 85% to 90% can be expected.[44] Speed of labeling is important. The life of a neutrophil is about 9 hours. If it takes 6 hours to draw blood, separate cells, transport the blood, and re-inject cells, most of the labeled neutrophils will be nonviable.

Technical Considerations

Slow injection through a large needle (20 gauge or larger) is required. Injection through a small needle causes serious shearing forces at the needle tip, which destroy all cells involved. The larger needle reduces mechanical trauma to the cells during injection. The less plastic tubing the cells must contact, the better. Polypropylene is a satisfactory plastic. Glass syringes should be avoided because blood components can react with it. Silicon lubricant, found in glass and some plastic syringes, interferes with the oxine and labeling.

The optimum time to image is the subject of some debate. Several investigators[54] suggest imaging at 3 to 4 hours and again 24 hours after injection, although one study in granulocytopenic patients found excellent results at 30 minutes.[17] We scan at 4 hours after injection and again at 24 hours. If scans are taken at 1 to 2 hours, excessive labeled neutrophils are present in the lungs; this is a normal event. Labeled white cells are retained in the lungs for the first 1 to 2 hours.

Collimation should be accomplished with a medium- to high-energy collimator. If dual pulse height analyzers are available, they can be set to 173 keV and 247 keV photopeaks. If only one analyzer is available, both peaks can be observed; however, the instrument must have a window capability of at least 60% width (centerline of 208 keV, window of 146 to 270 keV). Some discriminators have a maximum window of only 50%.

Kipper and Williams[44] suggest that the first image be taken of the liver, with an information content of 700 counts/cm[2] over the liver, that time be recorded, and that other views be taken for preset time. If information density is not available on the camera, a preset count of 300,000 counts over the liver, followed by that time for preset time for other views, is suggested. Recording of the images on a nuclear medicine computer is an excellent means of avoiding having to repeat the view because the photographic exposure was not appropriate for the number of counts acquired. If labeling efficiency is low and the count rate is low from the patient, images with fewer counts may have to be accepted. The general rule still holds that febrile and demented patients have great difficulty remaining motionless for longer than 5 minutes; therefore, a maximum time of 5 minutes per view may be a reasonable protocol criterion if adequate counts can be obtained. Both anterior and posterior views of the head, neck, thorax, abdomen, and pelvis should be obtained. The technologist should ask if there are any sites of suspected involvement in the extremities.

A normal pattern of uptake is seen after intravenous injection of the radiotracer (Figure 20-4). In the first minutes after injection, the labeled granulocytes accumulate rapidly in the lungs, liver, and spleen. It is thought that the uptake in the lungs is not the result of simple embolism of aggregates of granulocytes; rather, it is a process called *margination,* in which the granulocytes reside temporarily in the lungs. Clearing of the lungs begins at around 30 minutes. Granulocyte accumulation in the liver and spleen persists for at least 48 hours.

The estimated radiation dose is shown in Table 20-4. The absorbed dose varies with tagging efficiency and regional localization but in general appears to be acceptable, especially considering the serious consequences of failure to diagnose an abscess.

Numerous publications have attested to the clinical utility of ^{111}In white cell imaging (Figure 20-5). Several articles demonstrate a sensitivity (true-positive rate) of greater than 90% and a specificity (true-negative rate) of greater than 90%. One investigator reporting 312 cases found a sensitivity of 95% and a specificity of 97%. When ^{111}In-labeled white cells and ^{67}Ga citrate were compared with an assumed sensitivity of 90%, the ^{111}In white cell specificity was 97%, whereas the ^{67}Ga citrate specificity was 64%.[26] In one report, ^{111}In white cells were superior at detecting focal infections in the first 2 weeks of the infectious process, whereas ^{67}Ga was the superior diagnostic agent for focal infections of longer than 2 weeks' duration.[56] In a comparison of ^{111}In white cells and CT body scans in the diagnosis of intraabdominal abscess, ^{111}In-labeled white cells appeared to be diagnostically superior. Labeling of white cells permits

Table 20-4	Radiation dosimetry for ^{111}In-labeled white cells*		
Organ	**[111]In-labeled white cells (rad/mCi)**
Whole body	0.50-0.53
Liver	1-5
Spleen	18-20.4

From Freeman LM, Weissman HS, editors: *Nuclear medicine annual,* New York, 1982, Raven Press; and Segal AW: *Lancet* 2:1056-1058, 1976.

*Dose distribution depends on the quantity of red cells present.

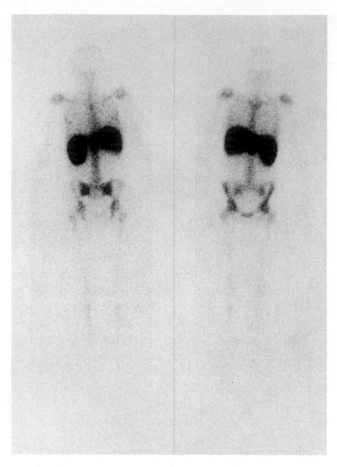

Figure 20-4 Normal posterior and anterior ^{111}In white blood cell whole body scan performed approximately 24 hours after injection of the radiopharmaceutical. Initial images usually are presented with the liver and spleen displayed at maximum film density, because this presentation is good for visualization of the liver and spleen. The initial method of display, scaled to the intense liver and spleen activity, causes the abdomen and pelvis, common sites of pathology, to be presented as areas of such faint activity that mild to moderate inflammation cannot be seen. The images have been windowed so that some minor background in the abdomen and pelvis can be visualized; this is usually necessary for adequate examination of the abdomen and pelvis.

monitoring of important physiologic parameters and offers the promise of significant improvements in patient care.

New methods of labeling are under development. For example, a neutrophil's surface has a specific binding site for specific peptides, and the peptide is labeled with a tracer, ideally [99m]Tc.

Tumor Antibody Imaging

Antigens are large molecules recognized as foreign by the immune system. They are capable of causing the immune system to develop specialized proteins (immunoglobulins) called *antibodies*. Repeated or prolonged exposure to bacteria, viruses, human or animal cells, or certain chemicals can stimulate the immune system to develop antibodies. The development and magnitude of an immune response by an antigen depends on the molecular weight, duration of exposure, and the structure of a specific region called the *epitope*. The same epitope can exist on various tissues. The same epitope existing on multiple tissues reduces the otherwise specific nature of identification of a target tissue. In an imaging situation, if the antigen is released from the surface of the tumor into the blood, localization of the labeled antibody occurs in the blood pool rather than at the site of the tumor. This produces a decreased tumor-to-background ratio and also reduces test sensitivity. Tumor surface antigens that are not shed into the blood are the preferred antigen for making a labeled antibody.

Molecules of less than a certain mass usually are nonantigenic. A molecule too small to cause an immune response by itself may combine with a larger molecule and become capable of producing an immune response. The small molecule is called a *hapten*.

An antigen can sensitize a B lymphocyte. At some later time, when that antigen encounters a B lymphocyte previously sensitized to that antigen, the B lymphocyte is transformed into a plasma cell. Antibodies are produced by plasma cells. A single plasma cell produces many molecules of a single antibody—a monoclonal antibody (Box 20-2). When the antibody meets the precise antigen for which it was created, the antibody adheres to the antigen. During imaging, many labeled antibody molecules that find specific antigens on the tumor cell surface demonstrate the location of the tumor.

A single bacterium, virus, or tumor has many antigenic sites. Each antigen sensitizes a different B lymphocyte. Each B lymphocyte becomes a plasma cell able to produce multiple copies of a single antibody. Multiple monoclonal antibodies result in a polyclonal antibody mixture. In an imaging situation, the mixture of antibodies can aid identification of the tumor target, because each antibody localizes to its specific antigen. Because a particular tumor may or may not express a single specific antigen on its surface, the polyclonal antibody mixture may have a better chance of producing visualization of the tumor.

Antibodies are immune globulins, of which there are several types: IgG, IgD, IgA, IgE, and IgM. The immune globulins can be separated from each other, but it is very difficult to separate IgG into unique purified components. Polyclonal IgG currently is used to image tumors. The IgG molecule has a mass of 150,000 (150 kd).

The IgG molecule has a Y shape (Figure 20-6). IgG is composed of two short and two long chains of protein. One short chain and one long chain are joined by disulfide bonds. At the upper tips of the Y are the sites that react to the particular antigen. This is the variable region, which recognizes its specific target antigen. The lower part of the stem of the Y contains the Fc region, which appears to be rather constant within a species. The Fc region of human antibody is different from a mouse Fc region. The Fc region can be removed from mouse antibody before injection into a human, with a resultant decrease in human antibody production to the mouse antibody.

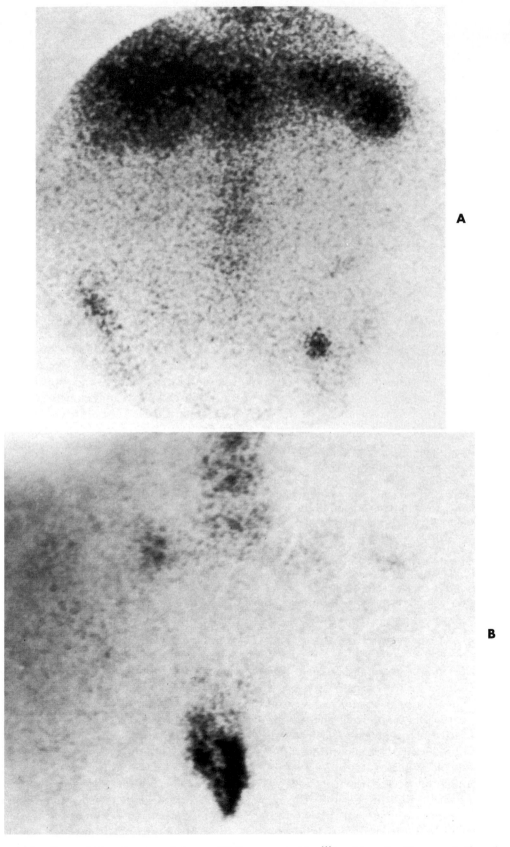

Figure 20-5   Diverticular abscess (**A**) and perirectal abscess (**B**) demonstrated by ^{111}In white cells. Abscesses in these locations are demonstrated with a clarity that gallium cannot provide.

Box 20-2	Monoclonal Antibody Vocabulary
Antigen	A large molecule recognized by the immune system as foreign and capable of stimulating antibody formation
Antibody	Protein (immunoglobulin) synthesized by plasma cells in response to an antigen; the antibody has a specific and precise affinity for the antigen; the antibody locates on a specific site of the antigen, which is called the *antigenic determinate*
Hapten	A small foreign molecule that by itself is not antigenic
Haptenic determinate	The macromolecule to which a hapten binds; the combination of the hapten and the carrier macromolecule can elicit specific antibody formation
Plasma cell	Secretors of antibody molecules; derived from B lymphocytes
T lymphocytes	A type of cell that mediates the cellular immune response, which aids the humoral immune response
Immunoglobulin A (IgA)	Mass of 180 to 500 kd, concentration (3 mg/ml); found in external secretions such as saliva, tears, and mucus
Immunoglobulin D (IgD)	Mass of 175 kd, concentration 0.1 mg/ml; function not yet known
Immunoglobulin E (IgE)	Mass of 200 kd, concentration (0.001 mg/ml); function not yet known, although has a harmful effect in allergic reactions
Immunoglobulin M (IgM)	Mass of 950 kd, concentration (1 mg/ml); first antibody to appear in the serum after stimulation by an antigen
Immunoglobulin G (IgG)	Mass of 150 kd, concentration 12 mg/ml; the shape of the molecule is a flexible Y, which consists of two kinds of polypeptide chains, light (L) and heavy (H); disulfide bonds connect the light chains to the heavy chains, and additional disulfide bonds connect the two heavy chains
Multiple myeloma	Malignant disorder of antibody-producing plasma cells
Hybridoma	Fusion of an antibody-producing cell with a myeloma cell; large amounts of homogeneous antibody can be produced by the hybridoma

Data from Köhler G, Milstein C: Continuous culture of fused cells secreting antibody of predefined specificity, *Nature* 256(5517):485, 1975; and Milstein C: Monoclonal antibodies, *Sci Am* 243:66, 1980.

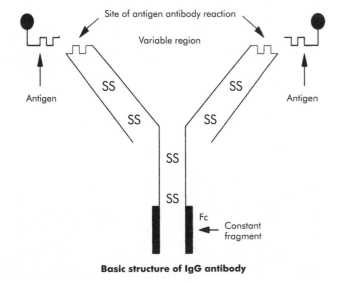

Figure 20-6 Simplified structure of IgG. The antigen-antibody reaction site is restricted to the upper tips of the **Y**.

The IgG molecule is large and relatively immobile compared with smaller molecules. It is not easy for such a large molecule to leave the intravascular space and travel to sites of tumor or infection. The plasma clearance half-time ($t_{1/2}$) of the intact IgG molecule is in the range of 40 hours. An IgG molecule can be divided into small fragments F(ab) by the enzymes pepsin and papain. Pepsin removes the Fc region and produces the $F(ab)_2$ fragment (Figure 20-7), which has a plasma $t_{1/2}$ of approximately 20 hours. Papain also removes the Fc region but in addition divides the molecule into two identical fragments F(ab), each with only one variable site (Figure 20-8). The plasma $t_{1/2}$ of the F(ab) fragment is in the range of 1 hour.[21,22]

As of early 1996, the monoclonal antibodies used in medicine are of mouse origin. The human immune system recognizes mouse antibody as a foreign antigenic substance. Human antibodies are made to mouse antibody. When a human receives a second injection of mouse antibody, the human immune system is activated and creates variable amounts of human antimouse antibodies (HAMA), with resultant rapid removal of mouse antibody from the system. This HAMA reaction could be avoided if human antibodies

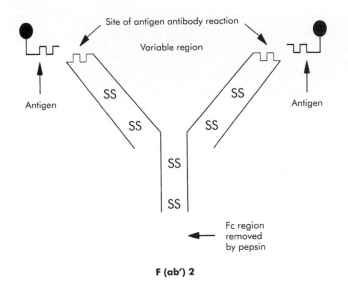

F (ab') 2

Figure 20-7 Removal of the Fc region is associated with a reduction in human antimouse antibodies (HAMA) reaction.

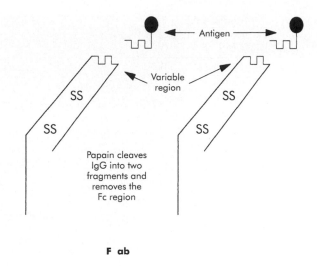

F ab

Figure 20-8 Removal of the Fc region and division into two fragments results in much faster blood clearance.

were used instead of mouse antibodies. At this time, technology is most advanced using the mouse immune system. Techniques must be developed that diminish the intensity of the HAMA reaction. Antibodies of human origin are being developed. Despite the known presence of the HAMA reaction, it is detected in only 50% of humans after administration of a mouse-based radiolabeled antibody tracer. By 6 months mouse antibodies are detected in only 4%.

Clinical trials have demonstrated the ability of radiolabeled antibodies to detect various cancers.[48] Malignant melanoma, small cell carcinoma of the lung, colon cancer, rectal cancer, and ovarian cancer have been detected by both planar and SPECT imaging (Figure 20-9). The labeled antibody approach to colon and rectal cancer has demonstrated the ability to stage the disease in pre-operative patients and to aid in post-operative follow-up and in the management of patients with elevated carcinoma embryonic antigen (CEA). In one study, immunoscintigraphy favorably changed medical management. The sensitivity and specificity are almost twice that of CT and ultrasound of the extrahepatic abdomen and pelvis.

The original concept of nuclear medicine was to cure cancer with radiation. The radiation was to be delivered by molecules, most likely antibodies to the cancer. Because the tagged molecule would be adherent to or within the cancer cell, a beta or alpha emitter could be used. This would provide much improved localization of the dose compared with external beam radiation. In the 1930s and 1940s there was no concept of the scientific and administrative obstructions that would delay accomplishment of this concept. In the past 30 years, more success has been achieved in the development of diagnostic tracers than in molecules suited for therapy.

Some antigens are expressed by more than one cancer; this could cause confusion in identifying the specific cancer of interest. On the other hand, the specific clinical question

to be answered is often answered by the scan, and there may be no confusion in the mind of the clinician. A satisfied clinician is the most powerful advocate for nuclear medicine.

One of the extensively studied of the tumor antigens has been tumor-associated glycoprotein-72 (TAG-72). TAG-72 is found in about 83% of colorectal and 97% of common epithelial ovarian cancers. Most breast, non-small cell lung, pancreatic, and esophageal cancers also express the TAG-72 antigen. For practical clinical purposes, however, minimum cross-reactivity is seen on scans.

A mouse-derived monoclonal antibody, B72.3, binds to the TAG-72 antigenic site. The only normal adult nonmalignant tissue bound is secretory endometrium. The Cytogen Corp. developed this antibody and marketed it as OncoScint after receiving FDA approval. Much investigational work was done with an iodine-131 (^{131}I) label. The current product for humans uses a ^{111}In label. OncoScint is synthesized by linking and chelating ^{111}In with glycyl-tyrosyl-(N, e-diethylenetriaminepentaacetic acid)-lycine hydrochloride (GYK-DTPA*HCl) to an oxidized oligosaccharide component of the B72.3 antibody. The linker chelator structure is fairly good sized even compared with the large antibody. The linker chelator must be placed in a position that does not interfere with the precise contact needed to allow the antigen-antibody reaction to take place.

OncoScint is indicated in the following situations:

1. Post-operative evaluation when local recurrences and post-operative and post-radiation changes cause confusing radiographic changes
2. Detection of occult metastases or synchronous lesions
3. Follow-up of patients at high risk of recurrence
4. Confirmation of the presence of malignancy when biopsy reveals dysplastic changes

OncoScint has a sensitivity in the range of 70%, a specificity of 75%, a positive predictive value of 97%, and a negative

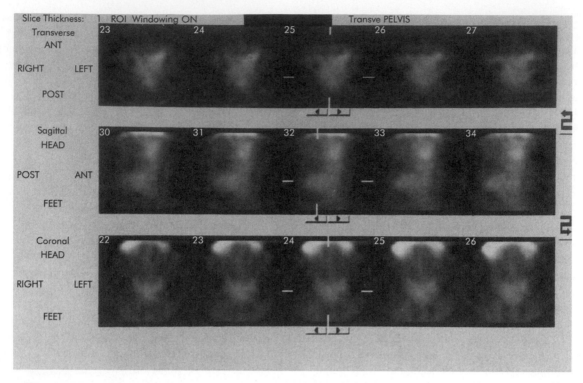

Figure 20-9 [111]In OncoScint (3.5 mCi) SPECT image of the pelvis after a 4-day delay. Acquisition was 360 degrees, 64 × 64 matrix, 64 stops at 35 sec/stop. Reconstruction was performed by filtered back-projection using a Parzen filter. This 55-year-old woman had had colon cancer, which had been resected 3 years ago. Clinical recurrence was seen in the pelvis. The SPECT images show a midline rectal mass approximately 4 inches in diameter. The posterior extent is best seen on the sagittal views. As the tumor extends anteriorly, it extends to the left. This is best seen in the transverse images. These findings were confirmed at surgery. A low-pass filter limits noise but produces a "smooth" image with reduced spatial resolution. However, with a lesion that is 4 inches in diameter, a minor reduction in spatial resolution is of no consequence.

predictive value of 20%. The results of OncoScint scans resulted in a change in patient management in 25% of cases. OncoScint detected occult disease not seen with conventional staging in 10% of cases.

Optimum use of OncoScint is demanding for the technologist. The following is a list of preparation measures and patient instructions given before injection of OncoScint:

1. Explain to the patient the potential for allergic reaction to a foreign protein. Patients who have had a minor reaction to prior iodinated contrast media should have no problem, because no iodine is being injected. Patients who have had a prior anaphylactic reaction may be at higher risk.
2. Ask if the patient has had a barium study in the past week. If so, a kidneys, ureter, and bladder (KUB) radiograph should be taken. The presence of dense barium in the colon will cause difficulties in interpretation and could obscure an active tumor site.
3. Ask about recent healing wounds, recent surgical scars, and the presence and location of ostomy sites. These areas retain OncoScint and cause potential false-positive reports.
4. Determine whether the patient has received other murine-based products and if an allergic response was noted. A recent injection of OncoScint is not a contraindication to its repeat use. A repeat injection may be associated with some minor increase in the probability of an allergic reaction, and the repeat tracer may be swept out of the blood and into the liver a bit faster than the original tracer.
5. Record a baseline temperature, heart and respiratory rate, and blood pressure. If a systemic reaction occurs, the baseline information is always of value.
6. Have epinephrine available to treat anaphylaxis.
7. Have a crash cart and physician in the vicinity to treat anaphylaxis.
8. Slowly inject 4.5 to 5.5 mCi of OncoScint over 5 minutes. Keep the intravenous line open with a heparinized saline flush. Good intravenous access may be lifesaving in the unlikely event of anaphylaxis.
9. Record vital signs at 5, 15, 30, and 60 minutes after injection.
10. Explain to the patient that the injection is just the start of the study. The major information will be obtained 48 and 96 hours later. Diagnostic images may be obtained as long as 144 hours later if needed. Mention that no additional injection will be required. It is very helpful if the injection can be given on a Monday, because the imaging usually can be completed by Friday.
11. Explain the importance of not moving during the scan.

For planar imaging a medium-energy collimator is used, although a high-energy collimator would be satisfactory. The acquisition matrix may be either 128×128 or 256×256, and the energy windows are set at 173 and 247 keV with a 20% window. Colostomy bags are emptied or changed, because the feces in the bag will contain [111]In. The technologist should always be sure to make the patient comfortable! A comfortable, relaxed patient is less likely to move. Ostomy sites and recent healing wounds are marked with either a cold lead or an ^{111}In marker.

Anterior and posterior chest, abdomen, and pelvic images are obtained. Lateral images may be required. At 48 hours, a preset 10-minute image usually is satisfactory, given a normal-size patient and a typical dose. It is important to look at the image; if it is count starved, more counts must be acquired. The technologist should remain with the patient at all times and should talk to the patient about remaining still. Poor statistics in the image and patient motion are the most common causes of nondiagnostic images.

The same positioning is used for all imaging sessions. An effort should be made to present the nuclear medicine physician with anatomically consistent images.

SPECT imaging may be most helpful at 96 to 144 hours after injection. Good images can be obtained with a large-field camera, but a large-crystal, dual-head camera is better. A 360-degree rather than a 180-degree acquisition should be performed. A reasonable time for each projection image is 40 seconds, although this time may have to be increased if the count rate is reduced because of large patient size, administration of a small dose, or partial infiltration of the dose. Because manufacturers do not use identical nomenclature for the filters needed for image reconstruction, the technologist should be familiar with the department's own filters. The acquired statistics usually are small and the projection images noisy. The filters should limit the higher frequencies where noise or poor statistics are found. Uniformity correction and attenuation correction can be used. Despite the apparent count rate limitations, SPECT imaging can provide firm documentation of the presence of active colon cancer.

When OncoScint first came on the market about 1992, an intensive effort was made to educate nuclear medicine physicians and technologists about the clinical and technical aspects of the product. Medical and surgical oncologists have accepted OncoScint only grudgingly, even though it has proved superior to CT in imaging of the extrahepatic abdomen and pelvis. The high cost of OncoScint was given as one drawback. The advent of widespread acceptance of 2[F-18]fluoro-2-deoxy-D-glucose (FDG) PET imaging for colon cancer probably will reduce the use of OncoScint, if not eliminate it entirely.

PET has demonstrated unique capabilities in the detection of cancer.[31] One property of many tumors is an increased metabolic rate. This increase in glucose utilization was discovered by Warberg and earned him a Nobel Prize in the 1930s. Increased glucose utilization can be detected after intravenous administration of the glucose analog FDG.

After intravenous administration, the FDG molecule is phosphorylated by hexokinase and retained in tissue and can be imaged by PET. Increased glucose metabolism is associated with an increased degree of malignancy in many tumors. With some added effort, regional metabolic activity can be calculated. PET imaging for oncology diagnosis is quite sensitive. Metabolically active tumors can be found before they are detected by CT or MRI. Failure of therapy can be identified by a continued increase in regional glucose uptake in the tumor bed or at distant sites. Continued tumor activity can be seen even when anatomic tests, such as CT and MRI, are considered to show cure.[30,32]

The ability of nuclear medicine to examine regional metabolism or antigenic characteristics of potential cancer sites over the entire body is a unique diagnostic capability. CT measures the electron density of tissue, MRI measures the proton density, and ultrasound measures the acoustic properties of tissue. Because cancer begins as a chemical change, long before changes identifiable by CT, MRI, or ultrasound emerge, the potential exists for cancer diagnosis before the development of a mass.

REFERENCES

1. Andrews GA, Knisley RM, Wagner HN: *Radioactive pharmaceuticals,* AEC Symposium Series 6, Washington, DC, 1966, Division of Technical Information, US Atomic Energy Commission.
2. Anger HO, Gottschalk A: Localization of brain tumors with the positron scintillation camera, *J Nucl Med* 4:326-330, 1963.
3. Anghileri LJ, Heidreder M: On the mechanism of ^{67}Ga by tumors, *Oncology* 34(2):74-77, 1977.
4. Bakshi SJ, Parthasarathy KL: Combination of laxatives for cleansing of ^{67}Ga-citrate activity in the bowel, *J Nucl Med* 15:470, 1974.
5. Beihn RM, Damron JR, Hafner T: Subtraction technique for the detection of subphrenic abscess using ^{67}Ga and ^{99m}Tc, *J Nucl Med* 15:371-373, 1974.
6. Bisson G, Drapeau G, Lamourex G et al: Computer-based quantitative analysis of gallium-67 uptake in normal and diseased lungs, *Chest* 84:513-517, 1983.
7. Boyden S: The chemotactic effect of mixtures of antibody and antigen on polymorphonuclear leukocyte, *J Exp Med* 115:453-466, 1962.
8. Bruner HD, Cooper BM, Rehback DJ: A study of gallium. IV. Toxicity of gallium citrate in dogs and rats, *Radiology* 61:550-555, 1953.
9. Bruner HD, Hayes RL, Perkinson JD: Preliminary data on gallium-67, *Radiology* 61:602-612, 1953.
10. Clausen J, Edeling CJ, Fogh J: [67]Ga binding to human serum proteins and tumor components, *Cancer Res* 34:1931-1937, 1974.

11. Coleman RE, Black RE, Welch DM et al: Indium-111 labeled leukocytes in the evaluation of suspected abdominal abscesses, *Am J Surg* 139:99-103, 1980.

12. DeLand FH, Sauerbrunn BJL, Boyd C et al: ^{67}Ga-citrate imaging in untreated primary lung cancer: preliminary report of the cooperative group, *J Nucl Med* 15:408-411, 1974.

13. Dige-Peterson H, Heckscher T, Hertz M: ^{67}Gallium-scintigraphy in nonmalignant lung diseases, *Scand J Resp Dis* 53:314-319, 1972.

14. Dudley HC, Imirie GW Jr, Istock JT: Deposition of radiogallium (Ga^{72}) in proliferating tissues, *Radiology* 55:571-578, 1950.

15. Dudley HC, Levine MD: Studies of the toxic action of gallium, *Exp Ther* 95:487-493, 1949.

16. Dudley HC, Maddox GE, LaRue HC: Studies of the metabolism of gallium, *J Pharm Exp Ther* 96:135-138, 1949.

17. Dutcher JP, Schiffer CA, Johnson GS: Rapid migration of 111-indium–granulocytes to sites of infection, *N Engl J Med* 304:487-589, 1981.

18. Edwards CL, Hayes RL: Tumor scanning with ^{67}Ga citrate, *J Nucl Med* 10:103-108, 1969.

19. Engelstad B, Luk SS, Hattner RS: Altered Ga-67 citrate distribution in patients with multiple red blood cell transfusions, *Am J Radiol* 139:755-759, 1982.

20. Ensslen RD, Jackson FI, Reid AM: Bone and gallium scans in mastocytosis: correlation with count rates, radiography, and microscopy, *J Nucl Med* 24:586-588, 1983.

21. Freeman LM, Blaufox MD, editors: *Seminars in nuclear medicine: monoclonal antibodies I,* Philadelphia, 1989, WB Saunders.

22. Freeman LM, Blaufox MD, editors: *Seminars in nuclear medicine: monoclonal antibodies II,* Philadelphia, 1989, WB Saunders.

23. Front D, Ben-Haim S, Israel O et al: Lymphoma: predictive value of Ga-67 scintigraphy after treatment, *Radiology* 192:349-363, 1992.

24. Ghose T, Nairn RC, Fothergill JE: Uptake of proteins of malignant cells, *Nature* 196:1108-1109, 1962.

25. Goldenberg DM, Preston DF, Primus FJ et al: Photoscan localization of GW-39 tumors in hamsters using radiolabeled anticarcinoembryonic antigen immunoglobulin G, *Cancer Res* 37:1-9, 1974.

26. Goodwin DA, Doherty PW, McDougall IR: *Clinical use of indium-111–labeled white cells: an analysis of 312 cases, neutrophils, platelets and lymphocytes,* New York, 1982, Trivirum.

27. Greenlaw RH, Weinstein MG, Brill AB et al: ^{67}Ga-citrate imaging in untreated malignant lymphoma: preliminary report of the cooperative group, *J Nucl Med* 15:404-407, 1974.

28. Gunasekera SW, King LJ, Lavendar PH: The behavior of tracer gallium-67 towards serum protein, *Clin Chem Acta* 39:401-406, 1972.

29. Hartman RF, Hayes RL: Gallium binding by blood serum, *Fed Proc* 26:780, 1967 (abstract).

30. Hawkins RH, Hoh CR et al: PET-FDG imaging in cancer, *Appl Radiol* 21:51-57, 1992.

31. Hawkins RH, Hoh CK et al: PET cancer evaluation: with FDG, *J Nucl Med* 32:1555-1558, 1991.

32. Hawkins RH, Hoh CK et al: Whole body PET finds promising clinical niche, *Diag Imaging* 14:88, 1992.

33. Hayes RL, Nelson B, Swartzendruber DL et al: Gallium-67 localization in rat and mouse tumors, *Science* 167:289-390, 1970.

34. Hayes RL, Rafter JJ, Byrd BL et al: Studies of the in-vivo entry of Ga-67 into normal and malignant tissue, *J Nucl Med* 22:325-332, 1981.

35. Hayes RL, Rafter JJ, Carlton JE et al: Studies of the in-vivo uptake of Ga-67 by an experimental abscess: concise communication, *J Nucl Med* 23:8-14, 1982.

36. Hill JH, Merz T, Wagner HN Jr: Iron-induced enhancement of ^{67}Ga uptake in a model human leukocyte culture system, *J Nucl Med* 16:1183-1186, 1975.

37. Hirsch JI, Fratkin JM, Sharpe AR Jr: Gallium-67 citrate, drug intell, *Clin Pharm* 7:519-523, 1973.

38. Hopkins GB, Kan M, Mende CW: Early Ga-67 scintigraphy for the localization of abdominal abscesses, *J Nucl Med* 16:990-992, 1975.

39. Hopkins GB, Mende CW: Gallium-67 and subphrenic abscesses: Is delayed scintigraphy necessary? *J Nucl Med* 16:609-611, 1975.

40. Israel O et al: Residual mass and negative gallium scintigraphy in treated lymphoma, *J Nucl Med* 31:365, 1990.

41. Johnston G, Benua RS, Teates CE et al: ^{67}Ga-citrate imaging in untreated Hodgkin's disease: preliminary report of the cooperative group, *J Nucl Med* 15:399-403, 1974.

42. Kaplan WD: *J Nucl Med* 31:369, 1990 (editorial).

43. Kaplan WD et al: Gallium imaging: a predictor of residual tumor viability and clinical outcome in patients with diffuse large cell lymphoma, *J Clin Oncol* 8:1966-1970, 1990.

44. Kipper MS, Williams RJ: Indium-111 white blood cell imaging, *Clin Nucl Med* 8:449-455, 1983.

45. Larson SM, Grunbaum Z, Rarey JS: The role of transferrins in gallium uptake, *Int J Nucl Med Biol* 8:257-266, 1981.

46. Lawless O, Brown DH, Kubner KF et al: Isolation and partial characterization of Ga-67 binding glycoprotein from Morris 5123C rat hepatoma, *Cancer Res* 38:4440-4444, 1978.

47. Line BR, Fulmer JD, Reynolds HY et al: Gallium-67 citrate scanning in the staging of idiopathic pulmonary fibrosis: correlation with physiologic and morphologic features and bronchoalveolar lavage, *Am Rev Resp Dis* 118:355-365, 1978.

48. Medical internal radiation dose (MIRD) report number 2, *J Nucl Med* 14:755-756, 1973.

49. Misami T, Dokoh F, Yagi K et al: Gallium-67 citrate imaging in the detection of focal lesions for anemia, proteinuria, and prolonged fever, *J Nucl Med* 31:512-515, 1990.

50. Mulry WC, Dudley HC: Studies of radiogallium as a diagnostic agent in bone tumors, *J Lab Clin Med* 37:239-252, 1951.

51. Nelson B, Hayes RL, Edwards CL et al: The distribution of gallium in human tissues after intravenous administration, *J Nucl Med* 13:92-100, 1972.

52. Oster ZH, Larson JM, Wagner HN Jr: Possible enhancement of ^{67}Ga-citrate imaging by iron dextran, *J Nucl Med* 17:356-358, 1976.

53. Porter J, Kawana M, Krizek H et al: [67]Ga production with a compact cyclotron, *J Nucl Med* 19:351, 1970 (abstract).

54. Segal AW, Thakur ML, Arnot RN et al: Indium-111–labeled leukocytes for localization of abscess, *Lancet* 2:1056-1058, 1976.

55. Sephton R: Relationship between the metabolism of Ga-67 and iron, *Int J Nucl Med* 8:323-331, 1981.

56. Sfakianakis GN, Al-Shiekha W, Heal A et al: Comparison of scintigraphy with In-111 leukocytes and Ga-67 in the diagnosis of occult sepsis, *J Nucl Med* 23:618-626, 1982.

57. Shealy CN, Aronow S, Brownell GL: Gallium-68 as a scanning agent for intracranial lesions, *J Nucl Med* 5:161-167, 1964.

58. Siemsen JK, Sargent N, Grebe SF et al: Pulmonary concentration of Ga-67 in pneumoconiosis, *Am J Roentgenol* 120:815-820, 1974.

59. Smith WP, Robinson RG, Gobuty AH: Positive whole-body ^{67}Ga scintigraphy in dermatomyositis, *Am J Roentgenol* 133:126-127, 1979.

60. Subramanian G, Rhodes BA, Cooper JF et al, editors: *Radiopharmaceuticals,* New York, 1975, Society of Nuclear Medicine.

61. Swartzendruber DC, Nelson D, Hayes RL: Gallium-67 localization in lysomal-like granules of leukemic and non-leukemic murine tissues, *N Natl Cancer Inst* 46:941-952, 1971.

62. Thakur ML, Coleman RE, Welch MS: Indium-111 labeled leukocytes for the localization of abscess: preparation, analysis, tissue distribution and comparison with gallium-67 citrate in dogs, *J Lab Clin Med* 89:217-218, 1977.

63. Thakur ML, Gottschalk A, editors: *Indium-111 labeled neutrophils, platelets and lymphocytes,* New York, 1980, Trivirum.

64. Waxman AD, Kawada T, Wolf W et al: Are all gallium citrate preparations the same? *Radiology* 117:647-648, 1975.

65. Weiner RE, Schreiber GJ, Hoffer PB: In vitro transfer of Ga-67 from transferrin to ferritin, *J Nucl Med* 24:608-614, 1983.

66. Weiner SN, Patel BP: ^{67}Ga-citrate uptake by the parotid glands in sarcoidosis, *Radiology* 130:753, 1979.

67. Zeman RK, Ryerson TW: Bowel preparation in ^{67}Ga-citrate scanning, *J Nucl Med* 18.886-889, 1977.

SUGGESTED READING

Goswitz FA, Andrews GA, Viamonte M: *Clinical uses of radionuclides,* AEC Symposium Series 27, Washington, DC, 1972, Office of Information Services, US Atomic Energy Commission.

Susan C. Weiss, James J. Conway

chapter **21**

Pediatric Imaging

Objectives

Discuss the considerations involved in dealing with pediatric patients and parents.

List and discuss methods of immobilizing pediatric patients.

Describe techniques for interacting with pediatric patients and their parents.

List the materials needed to perform injections on pediatric patients and list possible injection sites.

Discuss techniques for determining the administered dose of radiopharmaceuticals for pediatric patients.

Describe imaging considerations for bone scintigraphy in pediatric patients.

Discuss renal scintigraphy, renography, cystography, and diuresis studies.

Describe imaging procedures for the pediatric gastrointestinal system, including hepatobiliary conditions, Meckel's diverticulum, gastroesophageal reflux, and gastric emptying.

Describe imaging procedures for pediatric cardiovascular nuclear medicine.

*T*he disease processes of the pediatric age group and the technical requirements of imaging of children differ significantly from those encountered in adults. The nuclear medicine technologist should have an understanding of the differences to perform adequate pediatric nuclear medicine studies. A busy nuclear medicine department that primarily performs procedures on adults may find the occasional pediatric patient to be disruptive to the smooth flow of the day's workload. From the moment the child enters the department, the routine methods of operation must be modified in response to the child's needs. Several factors must be considered, including the equipment and its ability to resolve small structures, patient safety and nursing care, immobilization techniques, patient and parent psychology, the injection technique, and the technical requirements for specific procedures.

TECHNICAL CONSIDERATIONS

Instrumentation

A good rule of thumb is that a pediatric nuclear medicine study should be performed with an imaging instrument that has the highest state-of-the-art resolution. Another good rule is to include only the area of interest in the field of view. For example, when studying the kidneys of an infant, including the entire torso only contributes unnecessary counts and reduces the information from the site of interest. Therefore the instrument should also have the capability to magnify images. Computer zooming is not effective, because it does not enhance resolution. For example, for performing a neonatal bone imaging procedure and given the choice between a large field of view camera with no magnification and a standard field of view camera with magnification, the standard field of view instrument should be chosen. The use of magnifying devices such as converging and pinhole collimators also is recommended for imaging of small parts. The pinhole collimator is particularly useful for imaging the hips during bone imaging for Legg-Calvé-Perthes disease, because the resolution is excellent.

Patient Safety and Care

Safety is essential when dealing with a pediatric patient. The child should never be left alone in an imaging room or on an imaging table. Immobilization devices such as sandbags, Velcro straps, or adhesive tape should be used as a "safety belt." Ideally, two individuals should perform the pediatric study, a technologist to acquire the images and another to remain close to the child. Having two people serves two functions. First, and of primary importance, is safety. The individual, who may or may not be a nuclear medicine technologist, should be close enough to the patient to prevent falls or other catastrophes. Second, the technologist can position the patient while the other person starts the imaging sequence, thus increasing efficiency. Also, the second person can immobilize or entertain the child and may function as the sedation monitor during studies when sedation is required.

Nuclear medicine technologists should be certified in cardiopulmonary resuscitation (CPR) and trained to deal with various intravenous infusion equipment and monitoring devices, such as pulse oximeters. Special emphasis on pediatric resuscitation techniques should be provided during CPR training programs. It may be necessary to request special training from resource groups such as nursing or respiratory therapy to ensure appropriate use of pediatric infusion and monitoring devices. It is recommended that technologists who monitor sedated patients also receive Advanced Cardiac Life Support training.

To produce a high-quality pediatric nuclear medicine study, the technologist should have the attitude that the child deserves only the best that is available. Technologists should embrace the concept that any amount of absorbed radiation dose is significant and that the study therefore must be justified. A repeat study because of technical deficiency is unjustified.

Immobilization Techniques

Immobilization is required if the patient is either unable or unwilling to remain still for the time required. Various immobilization techniques are available, including wrapping, sandbagging, and sedation.[14] In addition, some nuclear medicine technologists become adept at entertaining the child as distraction from the boredom of holding still for long intervals. It is a good practice to ask the parent to bring along a favorite toy, blanket, or object that can provide comfort and reassurance to the child and that may serve as an aid in holding the child's attention. When available, a television with children's programming is a helpful resource,

as are other distractions such as tape recorders with stories or music. Keeping a supply of small toys and books in the nuclear medicine department is a good idea. Sleep deprivation or delaying the patient's normal nap time before the scheduled study might induce sleep. Many younger children are accustomed to having a story read to them just before bedtime, and simulation of that situation might induce calm or even sleep.

Mechanical techniques. Wrapping or swaddling, sandbags, and Velcro straps or adhesive tape immobilization techniques have been advocated. Each technique has its advantages and disadvantages and should be used judiciously. Wrapping effectively immobilizes the child, but monitoring of the respiratory rate, skin tone, pulse, and blood pressure is inhibited by this technique. Overheating can occur as well. If an emergency arises with the patient's condition, the time needed to unwrap the child can be frustrating.

Sandbags are also used to stabilize the patient's arms or legs in an appropriate position. However, in the neonate or infant, sandbags may be too heavy or may cause ischemia, particularly if used for prolonged imaging times. Sandbags also attenuate photons and can create artifacts in the image. They are primarily used as safety devices positioned alongside the body to prevent the child from rolling off the table.

Surgical adhesive tape can be used to help immobilize, but tape should never be applied directly to the skin. Many children are allergic to adhesive tape, and it can stick to the skin or hair and cause pain on removal. Adhesive tape is more practical as a safety device and should be used like a seat belt. Allergy to rubber tourniquets is also a problem. Velcro strap devices attached to the imaging table may be preferable to adhesive tape. Immobilization, particularly with infants, can also be accomplished by the technologist or the parent simply by holding the child in place with gentle pressure on the part being imaged.

Sedation techniques. Sedation is an effective means of achieving immobilization. However, sedation should be used judiciously and with the appropriate monitoring protocol so that complications are minimized and the patient can adequately recover from the effects of the sedation before discharge. Rarely, with idiosyncratic reactions to the sedation, it may be necessary to keep the child in the hospital overnight to ensure complete recovery. Sedation is most often used for patients 1 to 4 years old, especially for bone imaging, single photon emission computed tomography (SPECT) imaging, positron emission tomography (PET) imaging, and for patients with mental retardation or behavior problems. Special consideration must be given to sedating a child with a brain injury, respiratory distress, cyanosis, or a history of an adverse reaction to sedation. The technologist must be aware of all medications the child is receiving and the time of the last dose.

The American Academy of Pediatrics has published guidelines for the sedation and recovery of children.[7] These guidelines emphasize the use of approximate doses to reach various levels of consciousness and appropriate monitoring of vital signs using modern devices such as electronic oxygen saturation monitors. Children with severe systemic disease should be cared for by an anesthesiologist if sedation is required. All personnel monitoring sedated children must be certified in pediatric CPR, and all information regarding the sedative, dose administered, monitoring, and recovery must be permanently documented as part of the patient's record. State or local laws may also govern sedation, such as who can administer it. The responsible physician must be readily available. Finally, the parent must be cautioned that delayed reactions can occur and must be given written instructions and emergency phone numbers to call if any are observed. It is highly preferable that an institutional policy (and procedure) for the use of sedation, which follows the guidelines, be in place before any sedatives are used. The policy should include quality improvement processes and oversight.

Our current pharmaceutical of choice for sedation in a healthy child is chloral hydrate. It is the drug most commonly used for the sedation of children for diagnostic tests.[29] Chloral hydrate can be administered orally or rectally and is usually effective within 20 to 30 minutes. The child usually loses consciousness long enough for a bone scintigram using the multiple-spot image technique. The failure rate of chloral hydrate is relatively high (approximately 13%),[47] but it is also relatively safe. Others have reported using midazolam as a nasal spray to achieve patient cooperation, particularly for studies of the bladder. The drug also produces an amnesia-like effect, which is advocated by some because catheterization of the bladder for some patients is a traumatic event.[30] Lower doses of all sedatives are recommended for children who are debilitated or who have respiratory or neurologic deficits.

The effectiveness of chloral hydrate is variable; some children may require a longer time to go to sleep. Providing a quiet, darkened environment can help. Individual imaging rooms help segregate the patient from the noisy department. Some children never fall asleep completely but are quieted enough to enable the technologist to perform the imaging procedure, particularly when the child is reassured that no further pain is associated with the procedure. An occasional child might exhibit an adverse or opposite effect to the sedation, that is, become more combative and uncontrollable. This is particularly so if the child is allowed to become extremely agitated before sedation. For this reason we recommend to the parents that they not discuss the procedure with the child before coming to the hospital, especially if the child is easily agitated regarding such medical procedures. Frequently, a history of sedative use indicates whether a given pharmaceutical is appropriate to use for sedation. If chloral hydrate is not indicated or if there are other medical reasons, an anesthesiologist should be consulted. Very rarely, the child may need to be admitted to the hospital and be given a general anesthetic for performance of the procedure.

The possible risks and implications of any sedation should be discussed with the parents to allay concern and to prepare for the possibility of the child being admitted to the hospital for adequate recovery. Formal arrangements should be agreed on between the nuclear medicine and anesthesiology departments for the recovery of patients sedated late in the workday or for those who have adverse reactions to the sedation.

Patient-Parent Interaction

A major consideration is the psychologic interaction between the child and the parent.[50] A pediatric study usually necessitates dealing with a family unit, that is, the parent, the child, and at times other members of the family as well. Frequently, either the parent or the child indicates apprehension about the procedure. The examination should be explained to the child as well as the parent. One explanation is given in terms that the parent will understand and another at the level of the child's understanding. The nuclear medicine technologist must assess the situation and determine which of the explanations should be given first. If the patient is under 3 years of age, it is of little value to discuss the study with the child. If the patient is an older child, the parent's explanation becomes secondary.

If the patient is of childbearing age, the importance of inadvertent radiation exposure of a fetus must be considered. The technologist should directly address the issue of possible pregnancy. A girl's sexual activity may begin as early as 10 years of age. It is appropriate to determine the date of the patient's last menstrual cycle and to inquire if the patient is sexually active. The adolescent may deny sexual activity in the presence of the parent or others, therefore the technologist should question the patient privately.[9] That information should be noted in the patient's nuclear medicine record.

Assessment of the patient-parent relationship and interaction is important for successful performance of a nuclear medicine examination of a pediatric patient. The parent may convey apprehension or other emotions to the child in many ways, both verbally and nonverbally. This communication has a direct effect on the child's behavior. The parenting philosophy may have a direct effect on the child's behavior as well. For example, if the parent is permissive, the child might refuse to cooperate, and the parent might not intervene or even perceive a need to intervene to correct the child's behavior. Other parents exhibit strict authoritarian parenting techniques, and the child might be passive.

It might be appropriate for the technologist or the nuclear medicine physician to privately discuss with the parent the effect of the parent's behavior on the child and the technologist's ability to perform a successful examination. Generally, it is preferable to allow the parent to accompany the child into the imaging room to observe the entire procedure.[6] It is usually more comforting to the child to have the parent in attendance. However, if a child is uncooperative and the technologist cannot gain the child's cooperation with the assistance of the parent, it may be necessary to ask the parent to leave the room until the child agrees to cooperate. The technologist must be firm and authoritative in the approach to the child to maintain control of the situation. Patient cooperation should be praised, both to the child and to the parent. Allowing the child to participate in the study, for example, by letting the child control the remote stop-start switch on the gamma camera, enhances further cooperation.

Cooperation is often accomplished by dealing truthfully with the child. For example, if an injection is necessary, it is preferable to tell the child that there will be some discomfort. To do otherwise ensures loss of trust and cooperation. The technologist must also listen to the child's complaints and respond to them appropriately. The technologist should never allow the child to become abusive, either physically or verbally, and the child should be rewarded for good behavior and cooperation. Presenting small toys or other items as gifts to the patient upon completion of the study is a good method of reinforcing the child's perception of the experience as being nontraumatic. The technologists at the Children's Memorial Hospital in Chicago provide the child with a choice of rewards from a "goodie" box before discharging them from the department.

Injection Technique

For successful intravenous administration of a radiopharmaceutical to the pediatric patient, the injection should be performed by individuals whose attributes include a delicate manual dexterity, calmness under stressful conditions, and a capability for empathy. Nuclear medicine technologists might be the most capable for this task, because they receive formal training in phlebotomy and, unless otherwise prohibited by state regulation, are readily available to perform most of the radiopharmaceutical administrations.

It is commonly believed that an intravenous injection in an infant or child is more difficult. However, when proper technique is used, the procedure is successful in the vast majority of cases. The following technique has been used with a very high success rate at the Children's Memorial Hospital.[14] The technique requires an appropriate explanation to the child, ready availability of the required materials, and preferably two individuals, one to insert the needle and the other to assist in immobilizing the patient. The child should be told that the injection will cause a small sensation of pain and that it is appropriate to cry when it hurts. If fact, many times when the child is told to scream "ouch" when it hurts, the child concentrates so heavily on the expectation of pain, that the injection is completed without the child realizing the needle has been inserted.

A tray should be prepared that includes all the necessary items for administration of the radiopharmaceutical. Included on the tray should be scalp vein infusion sets of a variety of sizes, usually 21-, 23-, and 25-gauge needles, and a three-way disposable stopcock with the radionuclide syringe attached to one port and a syringe of normal saline (minimum 10 ml) attached to the side port (Figure 21-1). Alcohol wipes, dry 2 × 2 sterile sponges, a pediatric-size tourniquet, disposable sterile gloves, nonallergenic tape for fixation of the needle, and various sizes of support boards are also needed. The tray is lined with plastic-backed disposable paper to prevent contamination in case the radionuclide spills. The syringe containing the radiopharmaceutical should be enclosed in a lead syringe shield.

The injection should be performed using aseptic technique and universal precautions. The selection of an injection site is of utmost importance. All the preferred injection sites should be examined before an attempt is made to insert the needle. Several sites are objectionable and should be used only under unusual circumstances. The antecubital veins are often deeply situated and are not visible or palpa-

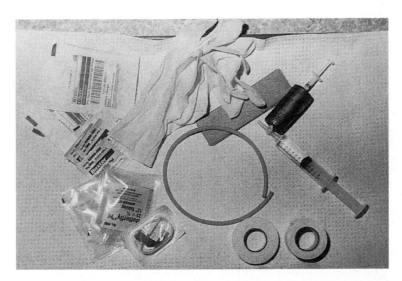

Figure 21-1 Injection tray used to transport all required materials from the preparation area to the injection room. Note that some materials are duplicated in case more than one attempt must be made to insert the IV line.

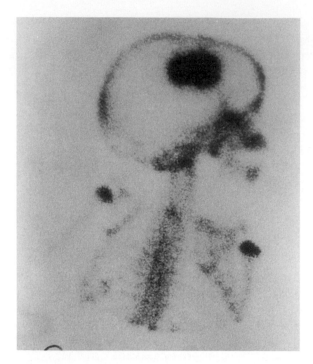

Figure 21-2 Extravasation of a scalp vein injection, which causes an easily recognized artifact on images of the head.

ble in young children. They are often used for blood sampling and, as a consequence, are traumatized before the child reaches the nuclear medicine department. It is possible to infiltrate the entire radiopharmaceutical dose into the antecubital space without observing any indication of extravasation. Scalp veins are not only esthetically objectionable and more frightening to the child, but often trauma to the scalp and extravasation produce significant artifacts on subsequent images (Figure 21-2). Serious complications such as hip joint infection and femoral artery thrombosis have been reported from attempted use of femoral veins.[34] Finally, use of the jugular veins is difficult because of the manipulations necessary to produce venous dilation, such as extending the head and neck and forcibly restraining the child's head to the side. It is also esthetically objectionable to the parents and a very frightening experience for the child.

Preferred sites include the veins on the dorsum of the hand and the foot. The veins in these sites usually are not already traumatized, because they are rarely used for blood sampling, are usually visible because of their superficial location, and are usually oriented in a linear fashion. In addition, during a dynamic study the hands and feet are usually more accessible if the child is beneath the camera, and they are easily immobilized for the injection.[11]

Immobilization of the hand or the foot can easily be accomplished by holding the wrist or the foot between the index and middle finger and holding the patient's fingers or toes down with the thumb (Figure 21-3). Extension of the joint at the elbow and flexion at the wrist further immobilizes the hand veins and reduces the patient's ability to with-

draw the extremity. Extension of the knee and ankle joints helps immobilize the veins on the dorsum of the foot. In older children it is helpful to have a second person gently restrain the arm or leg. If this is done, the technologist must remember to loosen all restraints for a short interval before injecting the radiopharmaceutical so as not to produce a tourniquet effect artifact[52] (Figure 21-4).

The size of the scalp vein needle should be selected to match the caliber of the vein. The needle is connected to the three-way stopcock with the valve on the stopcock positioned such that the saline syringe portal is open to the scalp vein needle. Saline is flushed through the scalp vein needle set before use. The venipuncture should be performed with the bevel of the scalp vein needle in the down position. In this manner the needle bevel enters the vein in a parallel fashion and not at an angle. It is preferable to direct the needle toward the confluence of branching vessels into a single vein. As soon as the needle has entered the vein, blood immediately refluxes into the infusion tubing at the needle hub. Application of suction by drawing back on the saline syringe is unnecessary in children because blood in the needle hub does not appear unless the needle is intravenously located, and it can safely be concluded that the vein has been entered. In adults the larger caliber veins may not exhibit sufficient pressure beyond the tourniquet to reflux blood into the needle hub.

When blood is seen in the tubing, no further manipulation of the needle should be attempted, such as threading the needle into the vein, because further manipulation frequently results in perforation of the opposite venous wall or dislodgment from the vein. The tourniquet should be immediately released and a test injection of saline made to confirm the intravenous placement. Any immediate swelling about the site of the needle tip indicates an extravascular location and necessitates removal of the needle and use of another site. If the test injection of saline confirms appropriate placement of the needle, the stopcock is switched to the radionuclide syringe for administration of the radiopharmaceutical. A short delay before injecting the radiopharmaceutical is suggested to eliminate the tourniquet effect artifact. During the injection, passage of the saline or radiopharmaceutical through the veins over the wrist or foot can be observed and felt beneath the technologist's index finger. Once the radiopharmaceutical syringe is empty, the residual activity within the stopcock and tubing is flushed with the remaining saline.

Radiopharmaceutical Administered Dose

Methods proposed to calculate the amount of radioactivity for a specific study are based on the child's weight and body surface area, estimation of organ volume, percentage of adult dose, and fixed dose. However, these methods tend to underestimate doses at the low end of the scale or to overestimate them at the upper end of the scale. A minimum amount of activity is required for adequate imaging, even in the smallest child. Selection of a method or individual dose

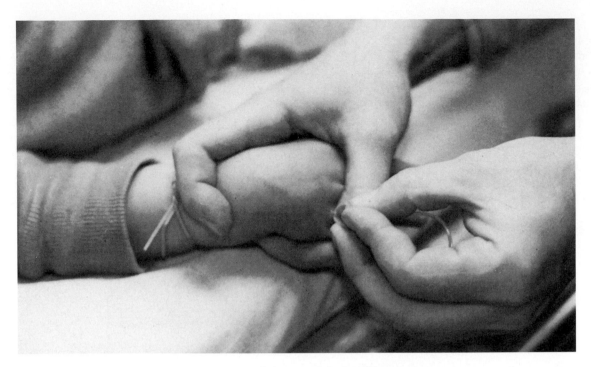

Figure 21-3   Immobilization of the hand for injection.

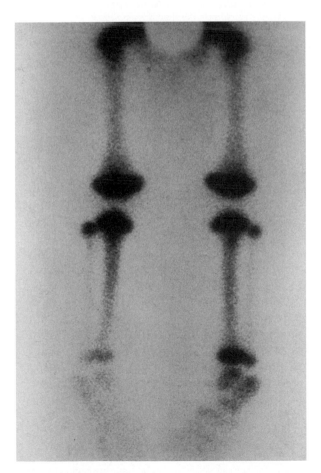

Figure 21-4   Increased localization in the left lower extremity caused by tourniquet effect of the restraint during injection of radionuclide into the foot.

should be based on the principle of "as low as reasonably achievable" (ALARA). Conversely, a maximum limit should be established. The method used for radiopharmaceutical dose determination at the Children's Memorial Hospital is empirically derived. That is, the administered dose and dose ranges are determined by experience based on several factors, including the patient's condition, the imaging technique desired (i.e., static versus dynamic imaging and limited bone imaging versus SPECT imaging), the imaging equipment to be used, the radionuclide energy, the biologic half-life of the radiopharmaceutical, and the percentage of localization in the organ of interest.

The empirically determined radiopharmaceutical dose is primarily based on the interval for which most patients are able to remain still. When they are being fed, most children and even babies are able to remain still for an interval as long as 5 minutes. Based on that assumption, the empiric method estimates the radiopharmaceutical dose required to obtain a specific type of image at the appropriate time interval after injection that can be acquired in 5 minutes for a specific imaging technique; that is, the use of magnification, choice of collimation, and the sensitivity of the camera. Based on the empiric method and experience, recommended radiopharmaceutical dose ranges for common radionuclide studies used at the Children's Memorial Hospital are provided in Table 21-1.

Some radiopharmaceutical package inserts contain information about the recommended administered dose to be used in children. Some do not, however, because many radiopharmaceuticals have not been tested specifically for safety and efficacy in the pediatric population. This is because phase II and III clinical trials are costly and difficult to perform in the pediatric population. The U.S. Food and Drug Administration (FDA), in cooperation with its Radiopharmaceutical Drug Advisory Committee and members of the Pediatric Nuclear Medicine Council of the Society of Nuclear Medicine, has worked to provide labeling information for pediatric radiopharmaceuticals and continues to do so. Most radiopharmaceutical companies provide technical support services to give assistance in cases in which the package insert information is not available. These services maintain information derived from the literature on pediatric administered doses for their products to disseminate to their customers. Other sources of information on recommended pediatric administered doses are the local commercial radiopharmacies.

Positioning

It is preferable to obtain as many images as possible with the gamma camera beneath the patient. This serves two purposes. First, it is a frightening experience for the child to have the massive detector overhead. Second, it is easier to monitor condition and vital signs without the detector obscuring the view of the child. In addition, older children are able to watch television, read a book, or be otherwise distracted. For anterior images the child can be placed prone on the imaging table. In fact, many children sleep in the prone position, and such positioning helps calm them. A small patient can be placed directly on top of the collimator for imaging.

Of paramount importance is appropriate positioning of the child within the gamma camera's field of view. The determination of abnormal radionuclide localization depends on comparison of one site with its contralateral side. This can readily be accomplished only if the patient's position is anatomic and symmetric (Figure 21-5). If it is impossible to position the patient anatomically because of the clinical condition, both sides should be malpositioned identically and symmetrically to allow comparison. Anatomic positioning is even more important for SPECT imaging because a slight

Table 21-1 Pediatric administered doses

Procedure	Radiopharmaceutical	Administered dose*	Minimum	Maximum
Brain scintigram	^{99m}Tc-TPA	400 µCi/lb	10 mCi	20 mCi
Brain SPECT perfusion	^{99m}Tc-HMPAO	285 µCi/kg	5 mCi	20 mCi
Angiogram	^{99m}Tc pertechnetate	200 µCi/lb	2.5 mCi	15 mCi
Liver scintigram	^{99m}Tc sulfur colloid	25 µCi/lb	500 µCi	2 mCi
Lung scintigram	^{99m}Tc-MAA	25 µCi/lb	500 µCi	2 mCi
Renal scintigram	^{99m}Tc-DTPA	50 µCi/lb	2.5 mCi	15 mCi
	or			
	^{99m}Tc glucoheptonate	50 µCi/lb	2.5 mCi	15 mCi
	or			
	^{99m}Tc-MAG3	22 µCi/lb	1 mCi	5 mCi
Renogram	^{131}I hippuran	100 µCi	50 µCi	100 µCi
Bone scintigram	^{99m}Tc diphosphonate	300 µCi/lb	5 mCi	20 mCi
Limited bone scintigram	^{99m}Tc diphosphonate	200 µCi/lb	5 mCi	20 mCi
Cystogram	^{99m}Tc pertechnetate	1 mCi	1 mCi	1 mCi
Thyroid uptake	^{123}I sodium iodide	100 µCi	2 µCi	100 µCi
Thyroid scintigram	^{99m}Tc pertechnetate	1 to 2 mCi	1 mCi	2 mCi
Plasma volume	^{123}I-HAS	3 µCi	1 µCi	3 µCi
Gallium scintigram	^{67}Ga citrate	3 to 10 mCi	3 mCi	10 mCi
Subarachnoid scintigram	^{111}In-DTPA	300 µCi	100 µCi	300 µCi
Dacryoscintigraphy	^{99m}Tc pertechnetate	200 µCi/drop	400 µCi	800 µCi
Gastroesophageal reflux	^{99m}Tc sulfur colloid	150 µCi	150 µCi	150 µCi
MUGA study	^{99m}Tc pertechnetate	350 µCi/lb	10 mCi	20 mCi
Meckel's scintigram	^{99m}Tc pertechnetate	100 µCi/lb	2.5 mCi	15 mCi
Gastrointestinal bleeding	^{99m}Tc sulfur colloid	5 mCi	1 mCi	5 mCi
Hepatobiliary study	^{99m}Tc mebrofenin	100 µCi/kg	1 mCi	8 mCi
Testicular scintigram	^{99m}Tc pertechnetate	200 µCi/lb	5 mCi	15 mCi
MIBG scintigram	^{131}I-MIBG	500 µCi	2 mCi	—

*The nuclear medicine physician might double or increase the dose depending on the clinical situation, such as an uncooperative or retarded child or a critical condition, to expedite the study and optimize results.
MUGA, Multiple gated acquisition; *MIBG,* metaiodobenzylguanidine; *DTPA,* diethylenetriamine pentaacetic acid; *MAG3,* mercaptoacetyl triglycine; *MAA,* microaggregated albumin; *HSA,* human serum albumin.

rotation can cause the appearance of increased or decreased activity on individual tomographic slices as an artifact of positioning. Current state-of-the-art SPECT software can correct some poor positioning rotational artifacts. When using the SPECT imaging table, it might be preferable to place the patient prone, because many children sleep in this

manner and therefore are more comfortable in this position. It also may be advantageous to position the child feet first, rather than head first, in the gantry, so that the patient can look up from that position and see something other than the back of the gantry.

Of particular concern is the safety of the patient on the narrow SPECT imaging table. We devised a patient safety restraint that wraps around the child and the imaging table using Velcro strapping, thus securing the patient to the table to prevent falls (Figure 21-6) and ensure immobilization. The device does not attenuate, because it is made of vinyl and Velcro strapping.

CLINICAL APPLICATIONS

This section reviews the most commonly performed pediatric nuclear medicine procedures, with particular attention to technique. This is not meant to be a comprehensive review of all pediatric nuclear medicine procedures. For specific topics not included in this section, the reader should examine the current literature and the other chapters of this textbook related to specific imaging procedures.

Skeletal System

In our pediatric nuclear medicine practice, bone scintigraphy comprises almost 40% of the studies performed annually. It requires particular attention to technical detail. The technologist should be familiar with the appearance of normal pediatric bone localization and with skeletal anatomy so as to use appropriate positioning and to recognize artifacts.

The development of technetium-99m (^{99m}Tc) phosphate radiopharmaceuticals, as well as improved resolution and instrumentation with increased sensitivity, have made bone scintigraphy a practicality in the pediatric population. Technetium-phosphate radiopharmaceuticals give acceptable

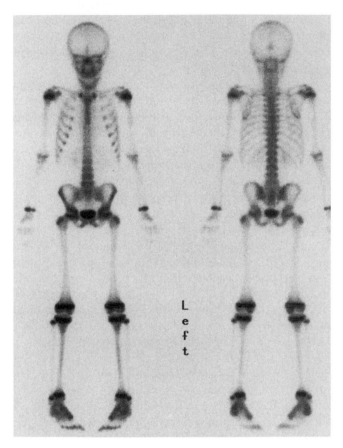

Figure 21-5 Symmetric positioning for a whole body bone scan allows comparison of one side with the other.

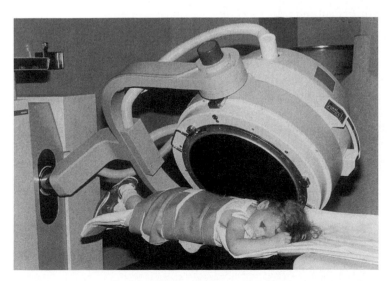

Figure 21-6 Patient restraining device used as a safety belt during SPECT imaging. Note the patient's position, prone and with the feet toward the detector; this position is comforting to some patients.

radiation absorbed dosimetry, and the improved resolving power of the gamma camera over older instrumentation allows adequate bone scintigraphy even in full-term and premature neonates.

Clinical indications for bone scintigraphy include infection, occult trauma, tumor localization, sports injuries, and orthopedic disorders such as avascular necrosis.[12] These conditions often are painful, which can inhibit the patient's ability to cooperate for a lengthy imaging procedure. Sedation or pain medication might be required to obtain adequate images. Because the technique of bone scintigraphy requires a 2- to 3-hour delay between injection of the radiopharmaceutical and acquisition of the static images, the technologist has adequate time to assess the patient's ability to cooperate and to arrange for appropriate medication and monitoring. Chloral hydrate should be administered approximately 30 to 45 minutes before the scheduled imaging time to allow adequate time for the sedation to take effect. If SPECT imaging is to be done, the SPECT image should be obtained as soon as the patient has fallen asleep, if possible, to ensure adequate sedation throughout the SPECT acquisition. At times this is not possible, because the site of the abnormal localization is unknown and routine static images must be acquired first to identify the location.

For specific clinical indications, bone scintigraphy is performed in one, two, or three phases. A one-phase bone scintigram consists of delayed static images acquired at 2 to 3 hours after injection. For a two-phase bone imaging procedure, an immediate extracellular (blood pool) image of a minimum of 500,000 counts of the area of interest is acquired within the first few minutes after injection, and delayed static images are acquired at 2 to 3 hours. The three-phase bone scintigram includes a dynamic acquisition of the area of interest begun immediately after injection at a frame rate of 5 sec/frame for 12 frames. The dynamic acquisition is followed by blood pool images and routine static images at 2 to 3 hours after injection.

Whole body images allow the interpreter to survey the entire skeleton; this is helpful in recognizing patterns of distribution, malposition, and subtle asymmetric localizations. The distribution pattern often defines the disease process, such as in child abuse, in which diaphyseal localization in the extremities is characteristic of a shaken child. A normal distribution pattern in the physes of the child is recognized. The physes at the knees have greater activity than the physes at the ankles, which in turn have greater activity than the physes of the hips. The reverse is true in the upper extremities. The physes at the shoulder have greater activity than the physes at the wrists, which have greater activity than the physes at the elbows. A knowledge of these patterns allows differentiation of abnormalities, increased or decreased, at any given joint.[10] The differences in the various physes are altered if the images are obtained in the anterior or posterior position because of varying distances from the camera. Single spot images of the extremities do not allow detection of subtle differences in localization because exact positioning of the areas of interest is difficult to achieve.

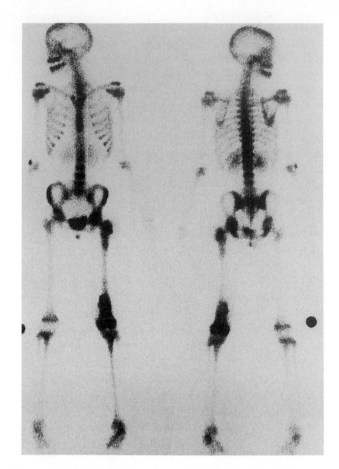

Figure 21-7 Whole body images allowed recognition of abnormal localization of radionuclide in the scapula, which was not recognized on a limited bone scan performed at another institution.

Careful attention should be paid to the statistics of the images acquired. When a whole body imaging device is used, a minimum of 1 million counts per image is required. Both anterior and posterior whole body images with the patient positioned anatomically and symmetrically are necessary for an adequate survey (Figure 21-7). Patients under 5 years of age or older patients of short stature should have survey images done as spot films with magnification as necessary to provide sufficient detail. In addition to the whole body survey images, spot images should be acquired for a minimum of 500,000 counts each. Subsequent spot magnification films of particular areas of interest should have a minimum of 250,000 counts/view. Limited one-phase bone scintigraphy is used only for follow-up examination, such as for Legg-Calvé-Perthes disease. Such a study consists of one posterior total body film, spot films of the pelvis (anterior anatomic projection of the hips and posterior frog-leg lateral of the hips), and pinhole anterior and frog-leg lateral views of the hips. These magnified views should exclude the bladder and include only the acetabulum and hips to the level of the lesser trochanter (Figure 21-8).

Infection. Bone scintigraphy is the most sensitive and specific imaging technique currently available for differentiat-

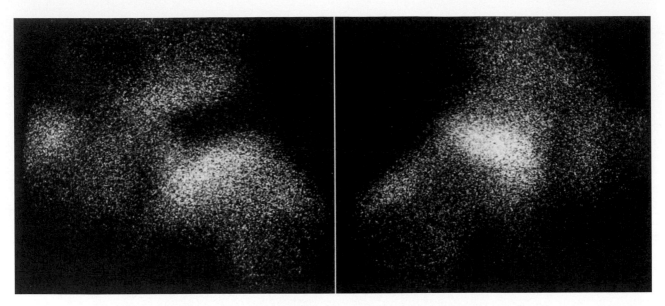

Figure 21-8 Pinhole views of the hips are acquired by positioning the hip in the center of the field of view and lowering the camera until the collimator is pressing on the patient's skin. The left hip demonstrates total avascularity of the epiphysis; the right hip is normal.

ing septic arthritis, cellulitis, and osteomyelitis.[28] Frequently x-ray examinations are completely normal in these disorders. Musculoskeletal infection includes pain and limitation of motion, and the patient usually but not always has an elevated erythrocyte sedimentation rate and frequently fever. In the neonatal population, however, the only clinical finding may be the lack of movement of an extremity. Early identification of septic arthritis or osteomyelitis is imperative to prevent bone or joint destruction and subsequent deformity. For example, in our experience an untreated septic arthritis of the hip of longer than 5 days' duration has a 50% probability of developing avascular necrosis of the proximal femoral epiphysis.[8]

The typical scintigraphic appearance of acute osteomyelitis is a well-defined focus of increased radionuclide localization, or *hot* lesion, seen on all three phases of the bone scan. The lesion is invariably in the metaphysis of the bone. On occasion, however, it presents as a photopenic, or *cold* lesion, when the vascular supply to the bone is compromised by surrounding tissue edema (compartment syndrome) or vascular thrombosis.[3] Detection and identification of ischemic osteomyelitis (which produces a cold area on the bone scintigram) warrant an emergency surgical drainage procedure to reduce the pressure in the tissues and enhance the return of blood flow.

Trauma. Because radionuclide scintigraphy has a high sensitivity for defining bone changes caused by trauma, it is an extremely useful tool for several disorders in the pediatric population. The normal bumps and bruises of childhood play do not produce abnormalities on bone scintigraphy. Significant or repeated trauma is required to produce perfusion and metabolic changes that are evident on bone scintigraphy. Several such conditions are well

recognized, including occult fractures,[46] child abuse,[49] sports injuries,[38,41,42,54] and stress changes in the spine associated with spondylolysis.[24] Other conditions readily obvious on bone imaging and thought to be related to trauma are reflex sympathetic dystrophy[27] and myositis ossificans.[37] It is important to note that all these disorders have a normal x-ray appearance in the early and sometimes even late stages.

A young toddler who is limping or refusing to walk but has a normal x-ray result will demonstrate increased localization of radionuclide at a site of occult trauma. The lesion might be an occult undisplaced fracture or a microtrabecular bone injury. Frequent sites include the calcaneus, cuboid, patella, and metatarsal bones. Identification of abnormal radionuclide localization in the bones of the foot, particularly in a small child, requires magnification images to adequately distinguish the bone involved (Figure 21-9). Because of the prolonged imaging time required to acquire adequate magnification images of the hands or feet, lower count images (50,000) at higher intensity settings are necessary.

Correlative studies of bone scintigraphy versus x-ray survey examinations have documented that scintigraphy has a greater sensitivity (27%) for recognizing bone trauma in child abuse.[49] Although x-rays provide better evidence of healed fractures and undisplaced hairline skull fractures, bone scintigraphy better demonstrates injuries of flat bones, such as the ribs, pelvis, and spine, and of soft tissue injury. X-ray and bone scintigraphy, therefore, are used in a complementary manner to document evidence of child abuse. The technical quality of bone scintigraphy in child abuse is important, because most child abuse occurs in infants and young children under the age of 2. Their small bone structure requires high-resolution magnification

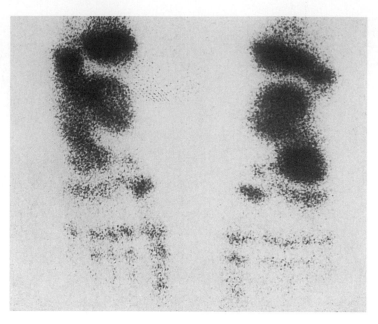

Figure 21-9 Electronically magnified image of both feet, which took 10 minutes of acquisition time and was required to visualize abnormal localization adequately.

imaging to define the appropriate information for interpretation.

Organized competitive sports for children have become more popular in recent years. Because athletic activities require repeated practice of a particular motion or series of motions, a chronic and repetitive stress effect is exerted on the bones. This can produce focal metabolic changes that are evident on bone scintigraphy and that often are related to a particular type of sport. For example, teenagers who train as runners often develop shin splits or stress fractures of the tibia. Speed skaters, because of uneven stress on the feet as a result of the specific direction in which they race, may have a stress injury in one foot and not the other. Baseball pitchers demonstrate hypertrophy of the throwing arm. Frequently an athlete overlooks a specific trauma incident and is brought to the nuclear medicine department because of chronic and persistent bone pain. The information that the child participates in a particular sport frequently is either not conveyed or is not known by the referring physician. Often it is the nuclear medicine technologist who, when seeking a cause for the abnormal appearance on the bone scintigram, finally elicits the history of a specific sports trauma, which explains the scintigraphic findings.

Stress on the pars interarticularis of the vertebrae can cause spondylolysis, which can be evident on bone scintigraphy as a focal area of increased localization. The patient develops back pain without fever. It is common in weight lifters and football and basketball players. SPECT imaging is necessary in this disorder if the routine static images fail to demonstrate an abnormality or are equivocal.[15] SPECT imaging detects approximately one third more abnormalities than planar scintigraphic images. Radionuclide scintigraphy

is much more sensitive than x-ray examinations in recognizing all the forms of sports trauma.

Hip pain. Hip pain in the child may have a variety of causes, including toxic synovitis, septic arthritis, slipped capital femoral epiphysis,[45] and avascular necrosis of the femoral head.[12] Adequate imaging of the hip is achieved with the use of magnification techniques with a pinhole collimator.[39] The technologist initially should position the patient's normal hip with the pinhole collimator raised about 1 to 2 feet above it. Once the hip is visualized in the center of the field of view, the camera is lowered until the pinhole is touching and pressing lightly on the patient's skin. An anterior image is acquired for at least 100,000 counts. Subsequent images of the normal hip in the frog-leg lateral position and the painful hip in the anterior and frog-leg lateral positions are acquired for the same time as for the anterior image of the normal hip. The bladder must be emptied before imaging so that activity from a full bladder does not degrade the images by reducing the number of counts from the area of interest. If the child is unable to void, the bladder should be excluded from the image by a lead shield.

Oncologic disorders. Children with oncologic disorders benefit from bone scintigraphy for the diagnosis, staging, and assessment of disease response to therapy. These patients can also show a variety of focal abnormalities on bone scintigraphy that are unrelated to the neoplastic disease and that might be confusing in their interpretation. Children with oncologic disorders may have osteoporosis from chemotherapy or poor nutrition; their bones are weaker;

furthermore, they may be more susceptible to trauma or injury because of a physical handicap, such as an amputation. Consequently, traumatic bone lesions frequently are detected on bone imaging performed for oncologic reasons. Amputees can display abnormal radionuclide localization at the end of the stump or in the hemipelvis because altered ambulation caused by a prosthetic device induces stress in the bone.[1] The use of crutches frequently causes increased radionuclide localization on the inner aspect of the proximal portion of the humeri. Conversely, diminished radionuclide localization, which appears as an asymmetry in the images, may be related to radiotherapy. It is important that the technologist who performs the bone scintigraphy procedure document such potential causes of abnormal localization to alert the nuclear medicine physician to allow for an appropriate interpretation of the abnormality.

SPECT technique. As mentioned previously, SPECT bone scintigraphy is extremely valuable because of its greater sensitivity in detecting subtle localization abnormalities from occult metastases, occult trauma, or localized early infection. This is especially true in the examination of the spine. The anatomy of the spine is complex, x-ray changes appear late in the disease, and planar scintigraphy defines relatively gross abnormalities. SPECT techniques require stringent quality control that is very time-consuming. In addition to the routine daily quality control procedures for the gamma camera, pediatric SPECT scintigraphy requires generation of flood-correction matrices and centers of rotation (COR) measurements for every possible combination of collimator and magnification factor that might be used. Because of the age range of patients imaged, this may require a 2-week cycle of nightly quality control acquisitions.

When a single-head SPECT instrument is used, data acquisition requires 45 to 60 minutes for statistical adequacy. Younger patients might require sedation or immobilization, sometimes even when they are cooperative.

For studies of the hips and pelvis, artifacts caused by radionuclide accumulation in the bladder can be controlled by catheterization of the bladder with continuous drainage. The upper extremities in the field of view for chest SPECT are an additional problem, which can be controlled by strapping the arms above the head for studies of the thorax.

Data processing is time-consuming, because on many studies, the data are derived from statistically poor frames as a result of limitation of the radionuclide dose or patient motion. Such poor data may require deletion of frames or other manipulation techniques. Standard protocols should not be used for data processing, because the information varies greatly from patient to patient. Computer systems that allow single-slice reconstruction with a variety of filters are helpful in determining the appropriate filter to be used for each individual patient. For SPECT images of the spine, quantification of abnormal localization of the radionuclide can be performed by placing regions of interest over the abnormal area and the contralateral normal site to derive a ratio of activity (Figure 21-10).

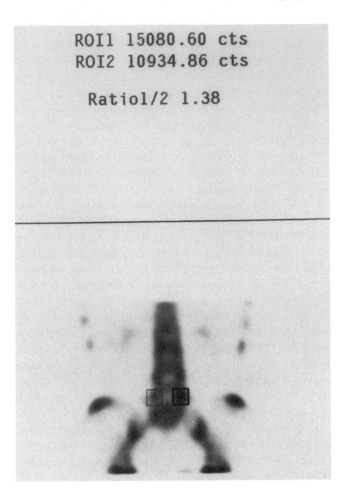

Figure 21-10 Quantitation of localization of radionuclide for bone SPECT imaging. Note the typical hot appearance of spondylolysis.

Genitourinary System

Radionuclide studies of the genitourinary tract account for about 30% of all radionuclide studies performed on the pediatric population. The primary examinations include renography and renal scintigraphy, diuresis renography, direct radionuclide cystography, and scrotal scintigraphy. Radionuclide cystography and frequently renography require placement of a urinary bladder catheter to provide adequate drainage. It is useful for nuclear medicine technologists to develop the skill of bladder catheterization or for the nuclear medicine department to have an identified individual readily available to expedite the procedure and to prevent increased anxiety in the child by unnecessary delays in beginning the study. The technique of catheterization is described in the discussion on radionuclide cystography.

Renal scintigraphy, renography, and diuresis renography. Several disorders in childhood require imaging and function studies of the urinary tract, including infection, ureteropelvic or ureterovesical junction obstruction, neonatal hydronephrosis or hydroureteronephrosis, renal transplantation, renal vein thrombosis, and congenital anomalies in the neonate. Horseshoe kidneys, duplications, hypoplastic kidneys, and ectopic kidneys all can be diagnosed with radionuclide studies.[19]

A variety of radiopharmaceuticals have been developed for scintigraphic imaging and functional evaluation of the kidneys. Most recently ^{99m}Tc mercaptoacetyl triglycine (^{99m}Tc-MAG3) has become the radiopharmaceutical of choice for imaging and functional analysis in pediatric genitourinary nuclear medicine. Renal cortical scintigraphy is performed using either ^{99m}Tc glucoheptonate (^{99m}Tc-GH) or ^{99m}Tc dimercaptosuccinic acid (^{99m}Tc-DMSA). We prefer ^{99m}Tc-GH over ^{99m}Tc-DMSA. The absorbed dose per millicurie is much less with ^{99m}Tc-GH, therefore higher activity angiographic images can be obtained. We have not experienced significant bowel, liver, or collecting system localization to interfere with interpretation of the cortical regions of the kidneys using magnification and oblique projections.

Techniques such as measurement of the glomerular filtration rate (GFR) and effective renal plasma flow (ERPF) are performed occasionally; however, these techniques are time-consuming when performed using multiple blood samples and are considered technically unreliable in the young child when gamma camera techniques are used. Only relative estimates ($\pm 10\%$ to 20%) are realistically derived even with meticulous techniques.

It is well known that the state of hydration significantly affects the excretion of radiopharmaceuticals, particularly with diuretic stimulation.[16] Because of this, it is appropriate to control and monitor the patient's state of hydration for renography. Oral hydration to tolerance for at least 2 hours before the study should be encouraged. An intravenous line, using either a butterfly needle or an intracath, is inserted for administration of dilute normal saline (5% dextrose in 0.3 normal saline) at a rate of 15 ml/kg over a 30-minute interval beginning at least 15 minutes before injection of the radiopharmaceutical. Hydration is continued through the remainder of the study as a maintenance fluid volume at a rate of 200 ml/kg/24 hr.

If the patient is unable to void on demand, the bladder should be catheterized to ensure adequate drainage during the study. Continuous bladder drainage reduces the absorbed radiation dose to the bladder and gonads and precludes patient movement caused by impending urination. If the catheter does not adequately empty the bladder, as observed on the persistence scope, urine should be aspirated using syringe suction.

^{99m}Tc-MAG3 (22 μCi/lb) is injected as a bolus with the patient positioned supine and the lumbar region in the field of view of the gamma camera. Magnification is used as needed to include only the area from the xiphoid to the symphysis pubis. Static images are obtained at intervals for 20 minutes. Digital information is acquired to derive renal function curves. A rate of 15 or 20 sec/frame is acceptable. At the conclusion of the acquisition, background-subtracted time-activity curves are generated on the computer.[16] The choice of an appropriate background region of interest (ROI) is a hotly debated topic among nuclear medicine practitioners;

because each method described has a drawback,[17] the best course of action is to choose one method to be used consistently. We currently prefer a circumferential ROI around the kidney for derivation of the renogram curve. Different background ROIs are preferred for the diuretic phase. ROIs must approximate as closely as possible the organ being monitored (e.g., the renal pelvis during the diuretic phase of renography) to be accurate in reflecting the appropriate activity.

If excretion of the radiopharmaceutical from the collecting system is delayed, furosemide (Lasix)[22] diuresis renography is performed. If a urinary catheter is not in place, the patient should be asked to empty the bladder. Furosemide diuresis is induced using an administered dose of 1 mg/kg. Acquisition is continued using the same parameters as the renogram phase of the study. The background ROI for the Lasix curve should exclude the ureter, and the ROI should closely approximate only the renal pelvis. A separate ROI for the ureter is used with hydroureteronephrosis.

A variety of data analyses, in addition to the generation of time-activity curves for the whole kidney, can be performed. The percent differential renal function is the total counts from the renogram curve for each kidney minus background counts during the interval between 60 seconds and the initial appearance of radioactivity in the calyces. The time is best determined by viewing the computer images sequentially. The significance of the percent differential renal function in the presence of bilateral disease is questionable. Parenchymal transit time has been advocated as an effective means of differentiating obstruction from other causes of hydronephrosis.[53] Cortical renal function is derived from areas of interest over the kidney cortex as opposed to the entire kidney. The clearance half-life ($t_{1/2}$) response for the diuresis phase of the renogram is a simple quantitative calculation of the disappearance half-life. Unfortunately, the $t_{1/2}$ can be measured in at least eight ways,[17] and all have differing $t_{1/2}$ values for the same data. It is no wonder that the correlation of diuresis renography with surgical results and clinical outcomes has been variable. Although computer software programs are commercially available to calculate the $t_{1/2}$, the validity of these automatic programs may not be documented.

Radionuclide cystography. Direct radionuclide cystography (RNC) for the detection of vesicoureteral reflux (VUR) is more advantageous than the conventional x-ray method because the absorbed radiation dose to the patient is reduced by a factor of at least 100,[18] various functional parameters relating to bladder function and reflux can be quantified, and the quantitative data have prognostic significance regarding the spontaneous cessation of reflux. The techniques of direct and indirect RNC have evolved, beginning with the use of iodine-131 (^{131}I)-labeled x-ray contrast agents in early investigations by Winter and colleagues[56] to an indirect method used by Dodge[20] in an attempt to eliminate catheterization. The indirect method depends on the rapid and complete clearance of the radionuclide through the kidneys after intravenous injection of the radiopharmaceutical. Imaging is then performed during and after voiding. A sudden increase in radioactivity in the upper tracts after voiding indicates reflux. Direct radionuclide cystography allows quantification of the bladder volume at which VUR occurs,[36] measurement of the volume of VUR into the upper tracts,[55] determination of the drainage time of refluxed urine after voiding, and quantification of the residual urine volume.[48] The direct radionuclide technique is more advantageous than the indirect method because it provides continuous monitoring during the filling, voiding, and post-voiding phases of bladder function, whereas the indirect technique examines the urinary tract only during voiding. The direct technique therefore is more sensitive in detecting VUR, because a significant percentage of VUR occurs during the filling phase at low bladder pressure and low bladder volume, which is not recognized by the indirect method.

A major consideration for the use of RNC over the conventional x-ray technique is the marked reduction in absorbed radiation dose to the patient. The dose to the bladder wall from a 1 mCi dose of ^{99m}Tc pertechnetate instilled into the bladder for a 30-minute imaging interval is 30 millirem (mrem).[18] The radiation dose to the gonads is much lower, in the range of 2 to 5 mrem to the testes. The absorbed radiation dose from conventional x-ray cystography varies from hundreds of millirem to several rem per examination, depending on how much fluoroscopy is used. Given the increasing use of radiation modalities for diagnosis of urinary tract abnormalities, modalities that provide the same or greater information with a lower absorbed radiation dose should be used. Radionuclide cystography is strongly recommended for follow-up studies to evaluate the efficacy of therapy for VUR.

Radionuclide cystography can be performed at any nuclear medicine facility that has a scintillation camera. A computer is not necessary. The procedure is simple to perform and can be accomplished in less than 45 minutes with a cooperative patient.

The responsibilities of the technologist can be significant, especially if he or she is trained in the technique of catheterization. Catheterization can be a simple and atraumatic experience if performed properly. Both physical and psychologic trauma can occur if the procedure is poorly performed by improperly trained or inexperienced personnel. Our belief is that individuals who regularly perform catheterization become more efficient and less traumatic in their technique. The child should never be held down forcibly to accomplish catheterization. Rather, one person should assist the child in maintaining a frog-leg position and should maintain a conversation with the child during the procedure. Because the child cannot observe the procedure directly, it usually is a good practice to explain everything that is being done as it happens. This usually calms the patient, because it eliminates fear of the unknown.

Whether the technologist performs the catheterization or not, the technique of direct radionuclide cystography requires careful attention to multiple details to achieve an adequate study with clinically useful information. Because VUR is a dynamic process and may appear only fleetingly and in minimal amounts, technologists must constantly monitor the persistence scope to initiate imaging at the appropriate time to document the reflux. Complete filling of the bladder is required for adequate performance of cystography, and a serious urge to void usually is associated with it, which can affect the patient's ability to cooperate. The technologist must be sensitive to the patient's complaints, yet in a calm, authoritative manner maintain control so that the procedure can be accomplished as quickly as possible with minimum discomfort to the patient and with any VUR adequately documented.

To accomplish catheterization, a Foley catheter is inserted into the bladder after aseptic preparation of the glans penis or perineum. The size of the catheter used depends on the sex and age of the child. A soft size 8 French Foley catheter is used for girls up to 1 year of age. For girls between ages 1 and 3, a size 10 French Foley catheter is recommended, and after 3 years of age a size 12 French Foley catheter can be used. Generally, a catheter one size smaller is used in boys for each age group. Nonballoon catheters are not recommended, because patients tend to void around them and eject the catheter from the bladder. Stiff feeding tubes are not recommended because they are more hazardous, and perforation of the urethra or bladder can occur. The Foley balloon is distended carefully, while the child's reaction is observed, to prevent injury in case of urethral or ureteral location of the balloon.

Quantitative data. After catheterization the bladder is emptied of residual urine, which is collected, measured, and recorded. The expected bladder capacity can be estimated based on the patient's age according to the formula developed by Berger and colleagues.[2] Normal bladder capacity in milliliters equals (age + 2) × 30. After 9 years of age, bladder capacities appear to vary from the formula. The formula is used only as rule of thumb, because capacities can also vary according to the health of the bladder. For example, smaller capacities have been documented after surgical procedures on the bladder or after recurrent infections.

A posterior and both posterior oblique images are obtained at a high-intensity setting, which demonstrates background activity throughout the field of view (Figure 21-11). In this manner minimal amounts of VUR are adequately demonstrated. Images are recorded for a total of 300,000 counts. Rarely, a fleeting minimal VUR occurs, which might not be demonstrated on permanent images. The technologist should note any other unusual occurrences to aid correct interpretation of the study. Then, a 2-minute posterior image is obtained, which includes the entire bladder and upper urinary tract. Total counts of the 2-minute image are recorded for use in calculating the residual volume. This image is acquired at a lower intensity setting to visualize any abnormalities of the bladder. The patient is then seated to void into a bedpan or a urinal, and

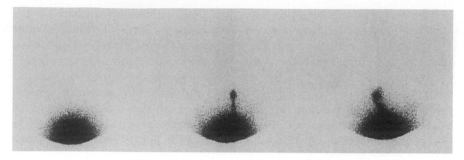

Figure 21-11 Posterior, left posterior oblique, and right posterior oblique images of the bladder and upper urinary tract, demonstrating vesicoureteral reflux on the right.

the gamma camera is positioned against the patient's back. As the balloon of the catheter is deflated, the patient is encouraged to void. As the patient begins to void, the catheter should slide out of the bladder. A voiding image is obtained as the patient empties the bladder. The same high-intensity setting as that used for the pre-void images is set for the voiding image to demonstrate the minimal reflux that can occur only during the higher pressures of voiding. Finally, a 2-minute post-void image, including the bladder and the upper urinary tract, is obtained at a high-intensity setting. The residual volume, total volume at maximum capacity, and the reflux bladder volume for each kidney can be determined according to formulas reported by Weiss and colleagues.[51] It is important to remember that none of the calculated volumes is accurate if urine is lost during the procedure.

The addition of simultaneous recording of bladder pressures during direct radionuclide cystography allows recognition of dysfunctional bladder abnormalities.[31] A physiologic pressure transducer measures intravesical pressure through the drainage port of the Foley catheter. Through the use of this method (the radionuclide cystometrogram), four pressure patterns have been characterized: normal, spastic-reflex, flaccid-paralytic, and uninhibited bladder contraction patterns. Patients with neurologic bladder disorders have the spastic-reflex or flaccid-paralytic pattern. Children with voiding dysfunctions often have evidence of an uninhibited bladder contraction pattern.

Scrotal scintigraphic imaging. Scintigraphic imaging of a painful scrotum provides a useful screening study in determining the need for surgical exploration.[4,5] Torsion of the testis appears as a photopenic (cold) lesion because blood flow to the testicle is impaired by the torsion (Figure 21-12). Inflammatory lesions usually have increased activity in a painful scrotum. In general, ischemic lesions (torsion, abscess, tumor) are managed surgically, whereas hyperemic lesions (epididymitis, orchitis, torsion of the appendix testes) are managed nonsurgically.

Scintigraphy should be performed with a magnification technique such as converging or pinhole collimation. A lead apron shield is placed around and beneath the scrotum and

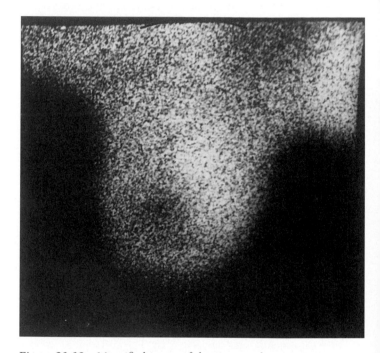

Figure 21-12 Magnified image of the scrotum demonstrates a photopenic (cold) lesion consistent with testicular torsion.

over the thighs. **U**-shaped cutouts of an old lead apron are suitable for the variable sizes of the scrotum at different ages. The penis is gently taped upward on the abdomen with non-allergenic tape. About 5 to 15 mCi of ^{99m}Tc pertechnetate (50 μCi/kg) is injected as a bolus to obtain a radionuclide angiogram of the scrotum so as to evaluate arterial perfusion. Angiographic images are obtained at 4 to 5 sec/image for 60 seconds. Static scintigraphy for a minimum of 1 million counts/view is obtained immediately after the angiogram and 10 minutes after injection. Finally, it is useful to obtain a static scintigram with a lead strip marker on the median raphe of the scrotum, because edema often distorts the size of the side of the scrotum involved, making comparison with the normal side difficult.

Gastrointestinal System

Radionuclide studies of the gastrointestinal tract in children have been a boon to pediatric gastroenterologists in the difficult diagnosis of such conditions as biliary atresia[32] and Meckel's diverticulum.[43,44] Other conditions, such as gastroesophageal reflux and gastrointestinal bleeding, are investigated with radionuclide techniques. Technical considerations for the performance of these studies are different from those for the adult population, depending on the clinical condition in question.

Hepatobiliary scintigraphy. The primary indication for hepatobiliary scintigraphy in the pediatric patient is differentiation of the various causes of neonatal jaundice. Patients with biliary atresia have hyperbilirubinemia and jaundice, which persists or increases in the neonatal period. Left untreated, biliary atresia is a lethal condition at an early age. It is often possible to differentiate an inflammatory liver disease (e.g., neonatal hepatitis) from obstructive biliary tract disease (e.g., biliary atresia) using a ^{99m}Tc iminodiacetic acid (^{99m}Tc-IDA)—derivative radiopharmaceutical. The ^{99m}Tc-IDA radiopharmaceuticals provide diagnostic images even in jaundiced patients with elevated direct serum bilirubin levels. A good hepatocyte extraction efficiency and short parenchymal transit time also are seen with these radiopharmaceuticals. We prefer to use ^{99m}Tc mebrofenin because of its rapid clearance and limited renal excretion. Normal transit times have not been established for children but seem to be less than the normal $t_{1/2}$ for the adult.[25]

Other causes of neonatal jaundice, including neonatal hepatitis, usually are self-limiting conditions not associated with permanent interruption of the biliary drainage system. Differentiation of biliary atresia from other forms of obstruction or inflammatory disease is difficult based only on clinical laboratory tests and other radiologic imaging tests such as ultrasonography. Invasive procedures such as percutaneous transhepatic cholangiography are difficult to perform in children and have associated risks.

Phenobarbital can be used to stimulate biliary excretion of conjugated bilirubin. For this purpose, 5 mg/kg/day is divided into two equal doses 3 to 7 days before hepatobiliary imaging to increase the sensitivity of diagnosis to 90% or greater in distinguishing biliary atresia from other causes of jaundice.[32]

Oral intake is restricted for 2 hours before injection of the radiopharmaceutical. Usually 100 μCi/kg of ^{99m}Tc disofenin is administered intravenously; 140 μCi/kg is administered to patients with a direct bilirubin greater than 5 mg/dl. Scintigraphy is begun immediately, with the patient in a supine position and with the appropriate magnification factor to obtain images that include only the xiphoid to the symphysis pubis within the field of view. Static images are obtained every 5 minutes for 45 to 60 minutes. Lateral images of the abdomen are obtained immediately thereafter. The key image is the left lateral projection. Any activity between the liver edge and the bladder within the abdomen anteriorly is evidence of gastrointestinal activity, which excludes the diagnosis of biliary atresia. Depending on the magnification factor and the collimation, images are obtained from 500,000 to 1 million counts/image. Additional images are obtained at various intervals, typically 3, 6, and 24 hours, or until radioactivity is demonstrated in the gastrointestinal tract.

Meckel's diverticulum imaging. The most common gastrointestinal malformation is Meckel's diverticulum, which occurs in approximately 1% to 3% of the population. Complications develop in about 25% of these individuals. Meckel's diverticulum is the vestigial remnant of the omphalomesenteric duct and usually is found along the antimesenteric border of the distal ileum. Meckel's diverticula often contain gastric mucosa, which leads to complications such as peptic ulceration and hemorrhage. Such complications occur most frequently in children and young adults and require surgical correction.

Routine roentgenographic studies are usually considered of little value. Radionuclide imaging of Meckel's diverticulum is based on the fact that ^{99m}Tc pertechnetate concentrates in gastric mucosa via active transport by the mucous surface cells. Nearly 60% of all Meckel's diverticula contain gastric mucosa and thus can be imaged. Radionuclide imaging has an accuracy of 90% to 98%, making it the optimum examination for identification of Meckel's diverticulum. The clinical presentation varies. Meckel's diverticulum is most often detected as an incidental finding at the time of surgery for other reasons. The patient may develop rectal bleeding as hematochezia (fresh blood tainting the stool), melena, or bright red, symptomless bleeding.

Radionuclide detection of Meckel's diverticulum is technique dependent. False-positive results caused by migration of secreted ^{99m}Tc pertechnetate from the stomach into the distal bowel have been reported. The following scintigraphic technique has been found to enhance the detectability of Meckel's diverticulum.[13]

Radionuclide imaging should be performed before barium sulfate studies or colonoscopy of the bowel. Such procedures can stimulate radionuclide localization as a result of irritation of the mucosa and can cause false-positive interpretation. Barium sulfate attenuates photons and thus theoretically can mask localization of the radionuclide in the diverticulum, causing a false-negative interpretation. Because potassium perchlorate inhibits localization of pertechnetate in ectopic gastric mucosa, this drug should not be given before imaging. Potassium perchlorate should be administered after the radionuclide study to reduce the radiation dose to the thyroid gland. The patient should fast for at least 2 hours before imaging to reduce secretion and migration of ^{99m}Tc pertechnetate from the stomach into the bowel. Occasionally, in the presence of generalized bowel inflammation or irritable bowel, the radionuclide transit time throughout the bowel is rapid, resulting in difficult interpretation. The use of nasogastric suction to reduce transit of secreted nuclide may be helpful during a repeat examination. Premedication with cimetidine, which inhibits secretion of pertechnetate from the cells into the lumen of the bowel, has been used as well. Because a Meckel's diverticulum can be located close to the urinary bladder, the patient should void before and at intervals during the examination to prevent the ^{99m}Tc pertechnetate excreted by the kidneys into the bladder from masking a small diverticulum located adjacent to the bladder.

^{99m}Tc pertechnetate is administered intravenously, and imaging is begun immediately after injection. The usual amount of activity administered is 100 μCi/lb body weight. Anterior gamma camera images are obtained every 5 minutes for 350,000 to 500,000 counts/view for 1 hour. Oblique and lateral views can help isolate the Meckel's diverticulum.

Scintigraphic interpretation criteria. Usually the Meckel's diverticulum appears along with the gastric mucosa 10 to 20 minutes after injection. There might be a delayed appearance, but it rarely occurs after the 1-hour interval. The localization is usually prominent, rounded, and within a small focus. Most diverticula are found in the right lower quadrant of the abdomen, but they can be located anywhere in the abdomen and may be seen to move during the study. The activity should persist on multiple images during the study; however, the potential exists for emptying of the radioactive secretions in a Meckel's lumen or dilution of the radioactivity by blood passing distally into the colon. This is a likely cause of the uncommonly reported false-negative studies. The diverticulum is generally intraabdominal and thus can be distinguished from activity in the retroperitoneal genitourinary tract, particularly on a lateral projection[13] (Figure 21-13).

Gastroesophageal reflux. A common problem facing the pediatric practitioner is the infant or child who constantly "spits up" or vomits. Such findings are a sign of gastroesophageal reflux (GER). It is not unusual for a child occasionally to regurgitate after feedings, but frequent regurgitation indicates a significant pathologic cause. In addition to anatomic abnormalities such as esophageal stricture, tracheoesophageal fistula, and hiatal hernia, GER is associated with brain tumors, mental retardation, recurrent pneumonias, asthma, and sudden infant death syndrome (SIDS). Pediatricians are particularly concerned about the relationship of GER to unexplained recurrent pneumonias.

Clinical indications. Because of the incidence of the aforementioned disorders, a nuclear medicine practice with a busy pediatric component could, if it wanted to, perform many GER studies daily, both as a screening tool and as a confirmatory diagnostic tool. As a screening tool, radionuclide GER studies lack the ability to identify significant abnormalities of the swallowing mechanism, nasopharyngeal reflux, and significant anatomic abnormalities of the esophagus. Therefore it is recommended that in most circumstances, the x-ray esophagram be performed before the radionuclide GER study. If GER is present on the x-ray study, the radionuclide study is unnecessary. The radionuclide GER study is indicated if the x-ray study is normal, because the radionuclide procedure is a more sensitive tech-

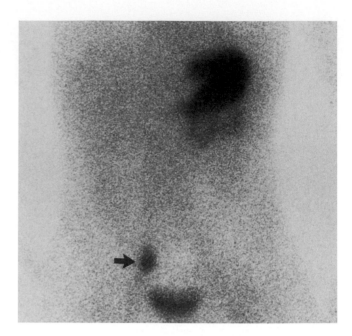

Figure 21-13 Meckel's diverticulum identified by localization in the prominent small, round focus of activity in the lower abdomen (*arrow*).

nique, primarily because it examines the process of GER over a longer interval than is possible with the x-ray study. In addition, the clinician is interested in determining the frequency and magnitude of reflux. These factors help determine the necessity of surgical intervention, such as a Nissen fundoplication. The radionuclide study, therefore, assists in the determination of the significance of GER. No criteria have been established for defining the significance of GER, but it would seem logical that more than three episodes during the examination, reflux that reaches the upper levels of the esophagus or regurgitates into the mouth, and evidence of pulmonary aspiration would have clinical significance.

Factors affecting GER. It is well documented that a number of factors increase the incidence of GER.

1. *Position.* GER is detected most frequently with the patient in the supine position.[40] The incidence of reflux in other positions, such as prone or decubitus, is significantly smaller. If reflux or vomiting occurs with the child in the supine position, the technologist must be prepared to turn the child's face to the side to prevent aspiration of the refluxed gastric contents. This is rare, but it can occur in obtunded or severely retarded children unless preventive measures are taken. The vast majority of incidents of aspiration into the lungs occur during feeding and are caused by abnormal swallowing mechanisms.

2. *Volume.* A direct relationship exists between the volume of the stomach contents and GER. An overdistended stomach is more likely to exhibit GER. Minimal reflux,

which can occur when the stomach is fullest at the initiation of the examination, might be less significant than that which occurs later during the study.

3. *Consistency of stomach contents.* Liquids are more likely to reflux than solids. We prefer to mix the radiopharmaceutical with the patient's normal meal. Milk or milk with cereal assumes a semisolid consistency in the stomach as the milk curdles with stomach acids. To ensure uniformity of mixing, the radiopharmaceutical is placed in the milk or formula and blended or shaken thoroughly before ingestion. A small amount of nonradioactive milk or formula is given last to wash radioactivity out of the mouth and esophagus. If the child is a poor feeder, the radiopharmaceutical should be instilled as an initial bolus to ensure adequate count rates for imaging in the presence of small stomach volumes. If the radiopharmaceutical is instilled into the stomach via an orogastric or nasogastric tube, it is important to ensure that the tip of the tubing is in the fundus of the stomach. Frequently gastric tubes are inserted too far, often into the duodenum or even jejunum. This results in a failed study. We prefer to insert the gastric tubes ourselves. Seldom is tubing longer than the first marker needed when a feeding tube is used. In addition, we instill a small portion of the radiopharmaceutical dose along with some saline to ensure that the tubing has been inserted into the stomach. If the child is crying lustily, the tubing is unlikely to be in the trachea. However, in an obtunded or a severely retarded child, placement of the tubing may be difficult to assess without instillation of a small amount of isotope with saline. The patient's formula or milk should not be used as the bolus in such circumstances.

4. *Abdominal pressure.* The adult technique for studying GER includes application of varying degrees of abdominal pressure with an abdominal band similar to a tourniquet. The GER appears according to the varying degrees of applied abdominal pressure. Caution should be observed in attempting the same manipulation with a child, particularly with an infant, because the abdominal muscles play an important part in pediatric respiration. Abdominal venous return also is compromised by application of tourniquets around the abdomen.

5. *Aspiration of saliva.* Recent studies have demonstrated aspiration of normal saliva in some patients. For that reason, we frequently perform a "salivagram" before instilling radioactivity into the stomach or as a separate study. A drop of the radiopharmaceutical is placed on the patient's tongue, and the patient is monitored during normal swallowing of saliva before the GER study is started. Data are acquired in the dynamic mode. Aspiration is readily recognized as activity in the trachea and bifurcation of the main bronchi (Figure 21-14). Time-activity curves are derived from ROIs over the lungs.[26]

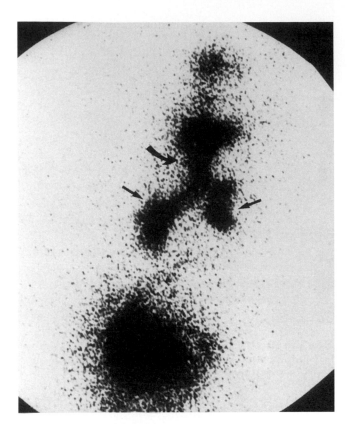

Figure 21-14 Salivagram image demonstrating activity in the trachea (*curved arrow*) and bronchi (*straight arrows*).

Significance of GER. It is difficult to define the significance of GER. Taking into consideration all the influencing factors, it would seem that up to three episodes of GER during an examination, especially if they are minimal and occur at the beginning of the examination, would be of little significance clinically. Multiple episodes throughout the study of a large volume that reaches the level of the patient's mouth, particularly late in the study, would be significant because the contents are potentially aspirable. Be that as it may, the potential for aspiration exists with any episode of GER, and findings should be correlated with the clinical situation, such as failure to thrive and multiple episodes of recurrent pneumonia.

Technical considerations. The radionuclide technique for GER involves instillation of ^{99m}Tc sulfur colloid into the stomach, along with sufficient nonradioactive liquid to fill the stomach. About 150 μCi of ^{99m}Tc sulfur colloid is instilled into the stomach, either by ingestion orally or via an orogastric or a nasogastric tube, along with the infant's normal volume of formula, milk, juice, or glucose water. The patient should have fasted for a minimum of 2 hours before the procedure; when the radiopharmaceutical is given orally, the child usually accepts the radioactive feeding quickly. If the radionuclide is administered via orogastric or nasogastric tube, adequate placement of the tube in the fundus can be ensured by administering half the radiopharmaceutical and, if necessary, repositioning the tube before instillation of the remainder of the feeding and the radiopharmaceutical. The technologist should wear gloves and use absorbent disposable pads around the child's shoulders to protect the clothing and skin from contamination. If contamination occurs, the absorbent pad can be quickly removed even during the examination. The gastric tube is removed immediately after administration of the radionuclide and feeding.

Occasionally an examination is performed on a child who has a gastrostomy tube in place. In such instances the tube should be clamped and its free end secured to the lower abdomen so that any residual radioactivity in the tube is not be confused with reflux or aspirated activity on delayed images. The child is placed supine or in a left lateral decubitus position on top of the gamma camera. A low-energy collimator is used, and magnification imaging is also used, depending on the size of the child. The upper abdomen and thorax should be included in the field of view. A radioactive marker is placed at the level of the upper end of the esophagus or the mouth. Analog images for 25,000 counts are acquired every 5 minutes for 1 hour or intentionally when reflux is recognized on the persistence scope. Digital images are obtained on the computer using 64×64 byte mode matrix at 1 frame/15 sec for the 60-minute interval. After the 60-minute interval, 25,000-count anterior and left lateral images of the entire stomach and bowel are acquired for calculation of emptying percentage at 1 hour. In infants the gastric emptying rate at 1 hour varies considerably (10% to 90%), and standard values have not been defined.

Computer analysis of the data is performed by placing an ROI over the esophagus and a background region. A time-activity curve is generated from the background-subtracted esophageal area. Reflux episodes appear as spikes of increased activity above the background. The emptying percentage is calculated by placing the ROI over the stomach and the bowel for both the anterior and left lateral static images to obtain counts for each area. At a delayed interval of at least 3 hours, an anterior image of the chest for 25,000 counts is obtained, with markers at the shoulders and xiphoid, to seek any evidence of reflux aspiration.

Cardiovascular System

The most common radionuclide studies of the heart in children are those used to detect and quantify cardiac shunts, either left-to-right through a septal defect or patent ductus arteriosus or right-to-left. Surgically produced shunts also are frequently evaluated. All the techniques involve the use of a radioactive tracer such as ^{99m}Tc pertechnetate or macroaggregated albumin (MAA) to document transit of the radionuclide through the cardiovascular system. The major advantages of these techniques are their noninvasive nature, rapidity, and low radiation dose compared with alternative procedures such as cardiac catheterization and contrast angiography.

Left-to-right shunt quantification involves injection of a compact bolus of ^{99m}Tc pertechnetate, preferably through the jugular vein, and digital acquisition of 0.5-second frames to document the transit through the cardiopulmonary circuit. Analog images are also acquired simultaneously. After acquisition the pulmonary time-activity curve is generated and analyzed via the gamma variate analysis to determine the pulmonary-to-systemic flow ratio (QP/QS ratio). This method provides precise quantification of left-to-right shunts with a pulmonary-to-systemic ratio of 1.2 to 3.0, devised by Maltz and Treves.[33]

Right-to-left cardiac shunts are detected using administration of $25\,\mu$Ci/lb of ^{99m}Tc-MAA.[23] After injection of the radioactive particles, the distribution of activity between the systemic circulation and the lungs is determined. If no right-to-left shunt is present, more than 95% of the injected activity is trapped in the pulmonary vascular bed. Activity seen throughout the systemic circulation, including the kidneys, brain, and other organs, is evidence of a right-to-left shunt and can be quantified by acquisition of whole body images and placement of an ROI over the lungs and the rest of the body. The magnitude of the right-to-left shunt is calculated according to the following formula:

Percentage right-to-left shunt $=$

Total body count $-$ Total lung count/Total body count

The examination must be performed immediately after constitution of the radiopharmaceutical to avoid the possibility of radiopharmaceutical breakdown and increased counts from free pertechnetate in the kidneys or bladder.

Positron Emission Tomography (PET) Imaging

Brain imaging in the pediatric population has not been performed frequently in the years since the advent of magnetic resonance imaging (MRI), because this technique provides exquisite anatomic images of the brain. However, with the explosion of PET imaging devices and the widespread availability of fluorodeoxyglucose (FDG), imaging for seizure disorders and other indications has increased significantly. ^{18}F compounds have even been used to measure dopamine dysfunction in children with attention deficit/hyperactivity disorder (ADHD).[21] Other uses are tumor imaging and myocardial blood flow imaging for Kawasaki's disease.[35]

REFERENCES

1. Ami TB et al: Stress fractures after surgery for osteosarcoma: scintigraphic assessment, *Radiology* 163:157-162, 1987.
2. Berger RM et al: Bladder capacity (ounces) equals age (years) plus 2 predicts normal bladder capacity and aids in diagnosis of abnormal voiding patterns, *J Urol* 129:347-349, 1983.

3. Bressler EL, Conway JJ, Weiss SC: Neonatal osteomyelitis examined by bone scintigraphy, *Radiology* 152:685-688, 1984.

4. Chen DCP, Holder LE, Melloul M: Radionuclide scrotal imaging: further experience with 210 patients. I. Anatomy, pathophysiology, and methods, *J Nucl Med* 24:735-742, 1983.

5. Chen DCP, Holder LE, Melloul M: Radionuclide scrotal imaging: further experience with 210 patients. II. Results and discussion, *J Nucl Med* 24:841-853, 1983.

6. Cohen MD, Wood BP, Hodgman CH: The presence of parents with their children during imaging procedures, *Am J Roentgenol Rad Ther Nucl Med* 146:639-641, 1986.

7. Committee on Drugs (American Academy of Pediatrics): Guidelines for monitoring and management of pediatric patients during and after sedation for diagnostic and therapeutic procedures, *Pediatrics* 89:1110-1115, 1992.

8. Conway JJ: Avascular necrosis in septic arthritis of the hip (unpublished work).

9. Conway JJ: Communicating risk information in medical practice, *Radiographics* 12:207-214, 1992.

10. Conway JJ: *Musculoskeletal scintigraphy in children,* Audiovisual program CEL 226, New York, 1992, Society of Nuclear Medicine.

11. Conway JJ: Practical considerations in radionuclide imaging of pediatric patients. In Freeman LM, editor: *Freeman and Johnson's clinical radionuclide imaging,* ed 3, New York, 1984, Grune & Stratton.

12. Conway JJ: Radionuclide bone scintigraphy in pediatric orthopedics, *Pediatr Clin North Am* 33:1313-1334, 1986.

13. Conway JJ: Radionuclide diagnosis of Meckel's diverticulum, *Gastrointest Radiol* 5:209-213, 1980.

14. Conway JJ: Sedation, injection, and handling techniques in pediatric nuclear medicine. In James AE Jr, Wagner HN Jr, Cooke RE, editors: *Pediatric nuclear medicine,* Philadelphia, 1974, WB Saunders.

15. Conway JJ: *SPECT imaging in children: categorical course in nuclear radiology,* Weston, Virginia, 1989, American College of Radiology.

16. Conway JJ: The principles and technical aspects of diuresis renography, *J Nucl Med Technol* 17:208-214, 1989.

17. Conway JJ: "Well-tempered" diuresis renography: its historical development, physiological and technical pitfalls and standardized technique protocol, *Semin Nucl Med* 22:74-84, 1992.

18. Conway JJ et al: Detection of vesicoureteral reflux with radionuclide cystography: a comparison study with roentgenographic cystography, *Am J Roentgenol Rad Ther Nucl Med* 115:720-727, 1972.

19. Conway JJ, Filmer RB: *Nuclear medicine in clinical pediatrics: kidney,* New York, 1975, Society of Nuclear Medicine.

20. Dodge EA: Vesicoureteral reflux: diagnosis with iodine-131 sodium orthoiodohippurate, *Lancet* 1:303-304, 1963.

21. Ernst M et al: High midbrain (F18) DOPA accumulation in children with attention deficit hyperactivity disorder, *Am J Psychol* 156(8):1209-1215, 1999.

22. Furosemide (Lasix). In the *Physician's Desk Reference (PDR),* ed 43, Oradell, New Jersey, 1989, Medical Economics.

23. Gates GF, Orme HW, Dore EK: Cardiac shunt assessment in children with macroaggregated albumin technetium-99m, *Radiology* 112:649-653, 1974.

24. Gelfand MJ, Strife JL, Kereiakes JG: Radionuclide bone imaging in spondylolysis of the lumbar spine in children, *Radiology* 140:191-195, 1981.

25. Gilbert SA, Brown PH, Krishnamurthy GT: Quantitative nuclear hepatology, *J Nucl Med Technol* 15:38-47, 1987.

26. Heyman S, Respondek M: Detection of pulmonary aspiration in children by radionuclide "salivagram," *J Nucl Med* 30:697-699,1989.

27. Holder LE, Cole LA, Myerson MS: Reflex sympathetic dystrophy in the foot: clinical and scintigraphic criteria, *Radiology* 184:531-535, 1984.

28. Howie DW et al: The technetium phosphate bone scan in the diagnosis of osteomyelitis in childhood, *J Bone Joint Surg* 65:431-437, 1983.

29. Keeter S et al: Sedation in pediatric CT: national survey of current practice, *Radiology* 175:745-752, 1990.

30. Ljung B, Andreásson S: Comparison of midazolam nasal spray to nasal drops for the sedation of children, *J Nucl Med Technol* 24:32-34, 1996.

31. Maizels M et al: The cystometric nuclear cystogram, *J Urol* 121:203-205, 1979.

32. Majd M, Reba RC, Altman RP: Effect of phenobarbital on ^{99m}Tc-IDA scintigraphy in the evaluation of neonatal jaundice, *Semin Nucl Med* 9:194-204, 1981.

33. Maltz DL, Treves S: Quantitative radionuclide angiocardiography: determination of Qp:Qs in children, *Circulation* 47:1049-1056, 1973.

34. McKay RJ Jr: Diagnosis and treatment: risks of obtaining samples of venous blood in infants, *Pediatrics* 38:906-908, 1968.

35. Muzik O et al: Quantification of myocardial blood flow reserve in children with a history of Kawasaki disease and normal coronary arteries using positron emission tomography, *J Am Coll Cardiol* 28:757–762, 1996.

36. Nasrallah PF et al: The quantitative nuclear cystogram: an aid in determining the spontaneous resolution of vesicoureteral reflux, *Urology* 12:645-658, 1978.

37. Orzel JA, Rudd TG: Heterotopic bone formation: clinical, laboratory, and imaging correlation, *J Nucl Med* 26:125-132, 1985.

38. Papanicolaou N et al: Bone scintigraphy and radiography in young athletes with low back pain, *Am J Roentgenol Rad Ther Nucl Med* 145:1039-1044, 1985.

39. Paul DJ et al: A better method of imaging the abnormal hips, *Radiology* 113:466-467, 1974.

40. Piepsez A et al: Gastroesophageal scintiscanning in children, *J Nucl Med* 23:631-632, 1982.

41. Rosen PR, Micheli LJ, Treves S: Early scintigraphic diagnosis of bone stress and fractures in athletic adolescents, *Pediatrics* 70:11-15, 1982.

42. Roub LW et al: Bone stress: a radionuclide imaging perspective, *Radiology* 132:431-438, 1979.

43. Sfakianakis GN, Conway JJ: Detection of ectopic gastric mucosa in Meckel's diverticulum and in other aberrations by scintigraphy. I. Pathophysiology and 10-year clinical experience, *J Nucl Med* 22:647-654, 1981.

44. Sfakianakis GN, Conway JJ: Detection of ectopic gastric mucosa in Meckel's diverticulum and in other aberrations by scintigraphy. II. Indications and methods: a 10-year experience, *J Nucl Med* 22:732-738, 1981.

45. Smergel EM et al: Use of bone scintigraphy in the management of slipped capital femoral epiphysis (SCFE), *Clin Nucl Med* 12:349-353, 1987.

46. Starshak RJ, Simons GW, Sty JR: Occult fracture of the calcaneus: another toddler's fracture, *Pediatr Radiol* 14:37-40, 1984.

47. Strain JD et al: Intravenously administered pentobarbital sodium for sedation in pediatric CT, *Radiology* 161:105-108, 1986.

48. Strauss BS, Blaufox MD: Estimation of residual urine and urine flow rates without urethral catheterization, *J Nucl Med* 11:81-84, 1970.

49. Sty JR, Starshak RJ: The role of bone scintigraphy in the evaluation of the suspected abused child, *Radiology* 146:369-375, 1983.

50. Weiss S, Conway JJ: Radionuclide cystography, *J Nucl Med Technol* 15:66-74, 1987.

51. Weiss S, Conway JJ: The technique of direct radionuclide cystography, *Appl Radiol* 4:133-137, 1975.

52. Weiss SC, Conway JJ: An injection technique artifact, *J Nucl Med Technol* 12:10-12, 1984.

53. Whitfield HN et al: The distinction between obstructive uropathy and nephropathy by radioisotope transit times, *Br J Urol* 39:433-436, 1978.

54. Wilcox JR, Moniot AL, Green JP: Bone scanning in the evaluation of exercise-related stress injuries, *Radiology* 123:699-703, 1977.

55. Willi U, Treves S: Radionuclide voiding cystography, *Urol Radiol* 5:161-173, 1983.

56. Winter CC: A new test for vesicoureteral reflux: an external technique using radioisotopes, *J Urol* 81:105-111, 1959.

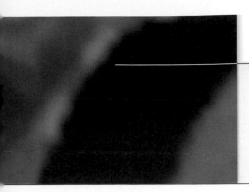

Glossary

A

A number See *atomic mass.*

ablation (1) Separation or detachment. (2) Destruction, that is, by radiation.

abscess Localized collection of pus within tissue.

abscissa The x, or horizontal, axis in a cartesian graph plot.

absorption (μ) coefficient Constant representing the fraction of ionizing radiation absorbed per centimeter thickness of absorbing material.

accelerator Device imparting high kinetic energy to a charged particle, causing it to undergo nuclear or particle reaction.

access time The time required for a computer to locate and retrieve information from a specified location. In the case of memory, this is related to the electronic speed of the address register and read/write circuits. In the case of disks, the access time is the sum of the time taken for the read/write head to locate a particular track plus the time required for information to rotate into the read/write position.

accumulator Register or data buffer used for temporary storage of data.

accuracy Refers to whether a given measurement or set of measurements reflects a true or exact value.

ACE Angiotensin converting enzyme.

achalasia (1) Failure to relax; referring especially to pylorus, cardia, or any other sphincter muscles. (2) Obstruction of the terminal esophagus just proximal to the cardioesophageal junction.

acid Any chemical compound that can either donate a proton or accept a pair of electrons in a chemical reaction.

acidophilic (1) Stains easily with acid dyes. (2) Grows best in acid media.

acinus Smallest lobule of a gland; secretes the product of the gland.

acquisition Intake of data to the computer.

ACTH See *adrenocorticotropin.*

activation analysis Analytical procedure detecting and measuring trace quantities of elements after exposure to a flux of neutrons.

ADC See *analog-digital converters.*

A/D converter See *analog-digital converters.*

address Label, name, or number that designates a location where information is stored.

adduct An addition product, or complex, or one part of the same.

adenohypophysis Anterior lobe of the pituitary.

adenoma Epithelial tumor composed of glandular tissue.

adenosine An endogenously produced nucleoside that causes coronary and systemic vasodilation.

adenylate cyclase Enzyme found in the liver and muscle cell membranes.

adjuvant That which aids or assists.

adrenal cortex Outer portion of the adrenal gland; it produces cortisone.

adrenal medulla Central portion of the adrenal gland; it produces adrenalin.

adrenergic Relating to nerve fibers of the autonomic nervous system that liberate norepinephrine.

adrenocorticotropin Compound isolated from the anterior pituitary having a stimulating effect on the adrenal cortex.

afferent Carrying or conveying toward a center.

affinity (1) Attraction of a specific reactor substance for a ligand. (2) An inherent attraction for substances to undergo reactions with one another.

affinity chromatography Separation of compounds based on differences in their affinities for a given species.

agonist A drug capable of combining with receptors to initiate drug action.

akinesia Abnormal reduction of muscle movement.

ALARA NRC operating philosophy for maintaining occupational radiation exposures "as low as is reasonably achievable."

albumin Class of simple proteins; found in most tissues.

alcohol Organic molecule containing the functional—OH group.

aldehyde Organic molecule containing the

$$\begin{matrix} O \\ \| \\ -C-H \end{matrix}$$

group.

aldosterone Sodium-retaining hormone of the adrenal cortex.

ALGOL (ALGOrithmic Language) High-level compiler language particularly well suited to arithmetic and string manipulations.

algorithm Prescribed set of well-defined rules or processes for the solution of a problem in a finite number of steps.

alimentary canal Food tract starting with the mouth and ending with the rectum and anus.

aliquot Specific measured amount of liquid.

alkane Hydrocarbon with a general formula of C_nH_{2n+2}.

alkene Hydrocarbon that has one double bond and a general formula of C_nH_{2n}.

alkyl Alkane with one hydrogen atom removed.

alkyne Hydrocarbon that contains a triple bond and a general formula of C_2H_{2n-2}.

alpha cells Cells in pancreatic islets containing large granules.

alpha particle (α) Nucleus of a helium atom emitted by certain radioisotopes upon disintegration.

ALU See *arithmetic unit.*

alveoli Terminal air pockets in the lungs.

amelioration Improvement of a disease.

amide Organic molecule with the functional group

$$\begin{array}{c} O \\ \parallel \\ -C-NH_2. \end{array}$$

amine Organic molecule containing the functional group—NH_2.

amino acid Organic acid containing an NH_2 and a COOH group, thus having both basic and acidic properties.

aminophylline A vasodilator and cardiac stimulant.

AMP Adenosine monophosphate; nucleotide containing adenine, a pentose sugar, and one phosphoric acid; product of metabolism.

amphoteric Having two opposite characteristics, especially having the capacity of reacting as either acid or base.

amplifier A device used to linearly increase pulse size.

amplitude The height of a waveform.

ampulla of Vater Dilation of ducts from the liver and pancreas where they enter the small intestine.

AMU See *atomic mass unit.*

amyloidosis A disease characterized by extracellular accumulation of amyloid in various organs and tissues.

analog (1) Representation of a parameter by a signal the magnitude of which voltage, current, or length is proportional to the parameter. (2) Structure with a similar function.

analog computer A computer that parameterizes data in terms of the magnitude of the incoming signals.

analog-digital converters (ADC) Electronic module used to convert an analog signal such as a pulse height into digital information recognizable by a computer.

anastomose To unite an end to another end; to bridge two vessels with a section of a vessel.

androgenic hormone Hormone stimulating male characteristics.

anemia Deficiency of red blood cells.

aneurysm Dilation of part of the wall of an artery.

Anger camera Type of gamma ray scintillation camera, named for its inventor Hal O. Anger.

angiography X-ray photography of the blood vessels with use of a radiopaque substance.

angiotensin Vasoconstrictor substance present in blood.

angstrom A measurement of wavelength (10^{-8} cm).

anion Negatively charged ion.

annihilation Reaction between a pair of particles resulting in their disintegration and the production of an equivalent amount of energy in the form of photons.

anode Positive electrode.

anoxia Deficiency of oxygen.

antecubital Area in front of the elbow.

antibiotics Drugs used to destroy bacteria; extracted from living organisms.

antibody Substance capable of producing specific immunity to a bacterium or virus; found in the blood.

anticholinergic Drugs blocking passage of impulses through the autonomic nerves.

antigen Molecule or particle capable of eliciting an immune response.

antineutrino Neutral nuclear particle emitted in either positron decay or electron capture.

antiserum Serum containing antibodies.

aorta Large artery stemming from the left ventricle.

apatite Crystalline phosphate of lime.

Aplasia Failure of an organ to develop.

aplastic anemia Anemia characterized by absence of red blood cell regeneration.

application program Program that performs a task specific to a particular user's needs.

aqueous Referring to anything dissolved in water.

arachnoid Membrane covering the brain and spinal cord.

arene Hydrocarbon compound that contains an aromatic portion.

arithmetic and logic unit (ALU) See *arithmetic unit.*

arithmetic unit Unit within the computer architecture that performs all mathematical and logical operations. Sometimes called arithmetic and logic unit (ALU).

aromatic compound Chemical compound containing a ring system that has $(4n + 2)\pi$ electrons.

array processor A specially devised high-speed computer that performs computations on image array elements in a parallel fashion.

Arrhenius concept Concept stating that an acid is a compound that acts as a proton donor.

Arrhythmia Variation of the heartbeat.

arterial thrombus Blood clot formed in an artery.

arthrography Radiography after the introduction of opaque contrast material into a joint.

ASCII Abbreviation for American Standard Code for Information Interchange, consisting of 128 seven-bit binary codes for uppercase and lowercase letters, numbers, punctuation, and special communication control characters.

ascites An accumulation of serous fluid in the peritoneal cavity.

ascorbic acid Vitamin C.

asepsis Sterile state.

assembler Programs that assemble symbolic programs into binary form.

assembly language Commands for the minicomputer system written in symbolic or mnemonic form. Typically, three-letter abbreviations, called mnemonics, are used to represent each instruction, and each mnemonic can usually be equaled to one machine-code or binary instruction. An assembly language program is translated to binary code by an assembler.

astrocytoma Central nervous system tumor composed of star-shaped cells.

asynchronous Mode of operation in which an operation is started by a signal that the operation on which it depends is completed. When referring to hardware devices, it is the method in which each character is sent with its own synchronizing information. The hardware operations are scheduled by "ready" and "done" signals rather than by time intervals. In addition, it implies that a second operation can begin before the first operation is complete.

asynchronous transfer Any sequential computer-operational signal that starts an operation when a necessary previous operation is completed.

ataxia Disorder of the neuromuscular system; lacking muscle coordination.

atherosclerosis Arterial hardening.

ATN Acute tubular necrosis.

atom Smallest unit of an element that can exist and still maintain the properties of the element.

atomic mass Mass of a neutral atom usually expressed in atomic mass units.

atomic mass unit Exactly one twelfth the mass of carbon 12; 1.661×10^{-24} g.

atomic number Number of protons in an atom, the symbol of which is Z.

atomic weight Average weight of the neutral atoms of an element.

ATP Adenosine triphosphate.

atrium Cavity of the heart receiving blood.

attenuation Any condition that results in a decrease of radiation intensity.

attenuation correction Compensation for the effects of radiation attenuation in computed tomography which may use mathematical estimate or measured transmission data.

auger electrons Electrons that participate in the production of x rays; pronounced o-zháy.

autofluoroscope A scintillation camera developed by M. Bender and M. Blau.

AV block Impairment of the normal conduction between the atria and the ventricles.

avidity (1) Tendency of a specific reactor substance to hold its ligands. (2) The firmness of a combination of substances in reactions in terms of their dissociation.

Avogadro's number Number of atoms in the gram atomic weight of a given element or the number of molecules in the gram molecular weight of a given substance: 6.022×10^{23} per gram mole.

axion The conducting portion of a nerve fiber.

axis of rotation In SPECT, an imaginary line passing through the center of the gantry about which the camera rotates.

B

background Detected disintegration events not emanating from the sample.

back-projection A computer manipulation of acquired image data back-projected into space.

backscattering Scattering of particulate radiation by more than 90 degrees.

bar phantom See *phantom*.

barn Area unit expressing the area of nuclear cross section; 1 barn = 10^{-24} cm^2.

Barrett esophagus Chronic peptic ulcer of the lower esophagus.

basal ganglia An aggregation of nerve cell bodies of the telencephalon.

base Any compound that either acts as a proton acceptor or an electron pair donor in a chemical process.

baseline Normal evaluation; evaluation before administration of a substance.

BASIC (Beginner's All-purpose Symbolic Instruction Code) High-level interactive, interpreter language for mathematical and string-variable manipulations.

batch mode Automatic computer mode that does not require specific programming instruction.

batch operation Computer operation that runs consecutively without operator intervention.

baud A unit of measurement of transmission speed; bits per second.

bequerel (Bq) The Système Internationale unit of activity, equal to one disintegration per second, 1 Bq = 1 dps.

beta cells Pancreatic cells in the islets of Langerhans.

beta (β^-) particle Electron whose point of origin is the nucleus; electron originating in the nucleus by way of decay of a neutron into a proton and electron (beta particle).

biconcave Having two concave surfaces.

bifunctional chelates Complexing agent with two sites for complexation.

bifunctional drug Drug with ability to attack two types of symptoms or disease.

biliary atresia A congenital absence of bile ducts.

biliary system System including the liver serving both a digestive and an excretory function.

binary Pertaining to the number system with a radix of two.

binary code A code that uses two distinct characters, usually the numbers 0 and 1.

binary digit One of the symbols 1 or 0; called a *bit*.

binder See *specific reactor substance*.

binding constant The equilibrium constant for a reaction between an antibody or binding protein and its antigen or ligand.

binding energy Energy released when a chemical bond is formed; amount of stabilization energy holding a nucleon in the nucleus.

binding sites Sites on a protein where they bind to radionuclides.

bioassay Determination of chemical strength by tests of living tissues.

biochemical Referring to the chemistry of living organisms.

biochemical analogs Chemicals of the living system that resemble one another in function but not in structure.

bioeffects Effects on the biologic system.

biologic distribution Normal distribution of a substance within the living system.

biologic half-life The elapsed time for the biologic elimination of 50% of a material from the body.

biologic matrix Basic materials of living systems.

biopsy Examination of tissue taken from the living body, usually without entirely removing the organ.

BIOS Basic input/output system.

biosynthesis Formation of a compound from other compounds by living organisms.

bisacodyl tablets Drugs used as a laxative.

bit An individual binary digit, either 1 or 0; acronym for *bi*nary digi*t*.

blank scan A daily calibration of PET scanners using the transmission source to measure the count rate and uniformity of each detector with no attenuation material in the scanner. Blank scans are a reference for attenuation correction in addition to providing sinograms for visual evaluation of system uniformity.

bleomycin An antibody substance having antineoplastic properties.

block A group of bytes on a disk or magnetic tape used for data storage.

blood pool Vascular cavity.

bolus Rounded mass or lump quantity; a concentrated radiopharmaceutical given intravenously.

bombardment Exposure of a target to any ionizing radiation.

bootstrap loader Routine whose first instructions are sufficient to load the remainder of itself into memory from an input device and normally start a complex system of programs.

Bowman capsule Sac at the end of uriniferous tubules in the kidneys.

Bragg curve Curve showing specific ionization as a function of distance or energy.

bremsstrahlung x rays Photonic emissions caused by the slowing down of beta particles in matter.

briggsian logarithmic system System of logarithms based on the decimal system, using the base 10.

bromination Chemical addition of bromine to a compound.

bromocryptine A dopamine receptor agonist.

bronchiectasis Dilation of the small bronchial tubes.

bronchioles Small bronchial tubes leading to air cells.

bronchus Large passage carrying air within the lungs.

Brönsted-Lowry concept Concept stating that an acid is a proton donor and a base is a proton acceptor in a chemical process.

brownian movement Motion of minute particles suspended in liquid.

BSP Body substance precautions.

BTU British thermal unit; measurement of heat.

buffer (1) Storage area used to temporarily hold information being transferred between two devices or between a device and memory; often a special register or a designated area of memory. (2) A solution of a weak acid and one of its salts that resists change in pH; usually used to maintain a constant pH for a reaction in solution.

buffer solution Solution that has a specific pH value and is resistant to pH change by addition of acids or bases.

bug Error in a program.

bullous Referring to a bubble or a bladder.

bundle branch block Interventricular block due to interruption of one of the two main branches of the bundle of His.

bus A flat, flexible cable consisting of many transmission lines or wires; it interconnects computer system components to provide communication paths for addresses, data, and control information.

by-product material Radioactive material arising from controlled fission.

byte Group of binary digits usually operated upon as a unit and usually 8 bits long; in ASCII code one character occupies one byte of memory, and the maximum decimal integer that can be stored in an 8-bit byte is 255.

C

C Programming language for computer.

cache memory A high-speed memory, usually part of the CPU.

calyx (*pl. calyces*) Cuplike structure in the kidney that receives urine.

canaliculus Small canal or channel.

carbohydrate Compound consisting of carbon, hydrogen, and oxygen, such as sugars and starches.

carboxylic acids Organic molecules with the

$$\begin{matrix} O \\ \| \\ -C-OH \end{matrix}$$

functional group, which have acidic properties because of this functional group.

carcinogen Substance stimulating the formation of cancer.

carcinoma Malignant tumor consisting of connective tissue enclosing epithelial cells.

cardiac ejection fraction That fraction of the total volume of blood of the left ventricle ejected per contraction.

cardiac output The quantity of blood ejected by the heart over a 1-minute interval.

cardiomyopathy Subacute or chronic disorder of the heart muscle.

carrier Quantity of an element mixed with radioactive isotopes of that element to facilitate chemical operations.

carrier free Adjective describing a nuclide that is free of its stable isotopes.

carrier proteins Macroscopic amounts of nonlabeled proteins present with trace amounts of radiolabeled proteins.

cartesian coordinate system Utilization of numbers to locate a point in relation to two intersecting straight lines.

catabolism The breaking down within the body of complex chemical compounds into simpler ones.

cathode Negative electrode.

cathode ray tube (CRT) Electronic vacuum tube with a display screen where information is displayed.

cation Positively charged ion.

cauda equina End of the spinal cord containing the nerves that supply the rectal area.

CBG Cortisol-binding globulin.

CDC Centers for Disease Control and Prevention.

CEA Carcinoma embryonic antigen.

Celsius (1) Swedish astronomer and inventor. (2) Centigrade, the temperature scale in which there are 100 degrees between ice and boiling water at sea level.

center or rotation (COR) Reference data used for correcting the slight misalignment of SPECT images taken from various projections.

central nervous system That part of the nervous system containing the brain, spinal cord, and nerves.

central processor unit (CPU) Unit of a computing system that includes the circuits controlling the interpretation and execution of instructions—the computer proper, excluding I/O and other peripheral devices.

centrifuge (1) To rotate or spin at high speed for separation. (2) Instrument for rotating or spinning samples at high speed.

cerebral radionuclide angiogram, cerebral radioangiogram Rapid sequential scintiphotos of the blood vessels of the brain.

cerebrospinal fluid (CSF) Fluid found in the cavities of the brain, brainstem, spinal cord, and meninges.

Chagas' disease South American trypanosomiasis.

character A single letter, numeral, or symbol used to represent information.

charged-particle accelerators Device used to electronically accelerate any charged particle. See also *cyclotron* and *electron accelerator*.

chelate Ligand that has two or more potential bonding sites.

chemical equation Symbolic statement describing a process and showing the stoichiometric relationships among the individual species involved in the process.

chemical equilibrium State of lowest energy for a chemical system undergoing a chemical reaction.

chemical reaction Processes that result in chemical change of the participant molecules.

chemistry Study of matter and the changes that matter undergoes.

chi-square test A mathematical procedure applied to a series of observations to determine their amount of variability.

chloramine-T N-chloro-4-methylbenzenesulfonamide sodium salt; an oxidizing agent used in radioiodination of proteins.

chlormerodrin Diuretic containing mercury.

cholecystitis Inflammation of the gallbladder.

cholecystokinin Hormone secreted by the small intestine; stimulates contraction of the gallbladder.

choroid plexus Membrane lining the ventricles of the brain, concerned with formation of cerebrospinal fluid.

chromatography Method of chemical analysis where the solution to be analyzed separates into component parts; some types are gel permeation chromatography, paper chromatography, and affinity chromatography.

cistern Fluid reservoir; enclosed space.

CLIA 88 Clinical Laboratories Improvement Act of 1988.

clock A device within a computer system that keeps time, counts pulses, measures frequency, or generates periodic signals for synchronization.

cloud chamber Chamber where the paths of ionizing radiation can be observed.

COBOL (commercial and business oriented language) High-level incremental compiler language primarily suited to business applications.

cocktail A liquid scintillator.

code A system of symbols representing data or instructions executed by a computer.

coding The writing of instructions for a computer, using a system of symbols meaningful to a computer, an assembler, a compiler, or a language processor.

coefficient Constant by which a variable or other quantity is multiplied in an equation.

coefficient of variation A statistical measurement of the validity of serial observations on a changing parameter.

coincidence counting A means of detecting radiation by two detectors placed in opposition to one another; an event is recorded only when seen by both detectors simultaneously.

coincidence lines Events recorded by detectors placed in opposition.

collagen Protein found in bone and cartilage.

collimators Shielding device used to limit the angle of entry of radiation.

colloid Molecules in a continuous medium that measure between 1 and 100 nm in diameter.

colorimetry Measurement of color.

colostomy Artificial opening in the colon.

column generator Column device using a parent radionuclide absorbed to a support in a column; the daughter radionuclide is usually obtained by elution of the column with a solution that interacts with the daughter but not with the parent.

command A word, mnemonic, or character that, by virtue of its syntax is an input line, causes a computer system to perform a predefined operation.

competitive protein binding Type of competitive binding radioassay in which the specific reactor substance is a native nonimmunologic protein.

compile To produce a binary code program from a program written in source (symbolic) language, by selection of appropriate subroutines from a subroutine library, as directed by the instructions or other symbols of the source program; the linkage is supplied for combining the subroutines into a workable program, and the subroutines and linkage are translated into binary code.

compiler Program used to compile assembly code or source code.

complement A substance normally present in serum that is destructive to certain bacteria and other cells that have been sensitized by specific complement antibody.

complex ions The product resulting from the actions of neutral molecules with either a cation or an anion.

compound Distinct substance formed by a union of two or more elements in definite proportions by weight.

Compton edge See *Compton scatter.*

Compton plateau See *Compton scatter.*

Compton scatter One process by which a photon loses energy through collisions with electrons.

computer Programmable electronic device that can store, retrieve, and process data.

computer program A plan or routine for solving a problem on a computer.

computer system A data processing system consisting of hardware devices, software programs, and documentation that describes the operation of the system.

concentration Strength of substance in a solution.

congener One of two or more things of the same kind.

congenital Existing at birth.

conjugate acid Remainder of a basic compound after it has either accepted a proton or donated an electron pair in a chemical process.

conjugate base Remainder of an acidic compound after it has either donated its acidic proton or accepted an electron pair in a chemical process.

constant A value that remains the same throughout a distinct operation.

conversion electron Orbital electron that has been excited (ionized) by internal conversion of an excited atom.

coordinate covalent bond Covalent bond formed by two atoms in which one atom donates both electrons for the bond.

core memory Main memory storage used by the central processing unit, in which binary data are represented by the switching polarity of magnetic cores.

coronal plane Plane that takes its name from the coronal suture of the skull dividing the body into the front and back portions.

corticosterone Compound isolated from the adrenal cortex.

cortisol Adrenocortical hormone.

Coulomb's law Basic law of electrostatics, which states that

$$F = q_1 q_2/4\pi\varepsilon r^2 \text{ or } F = qq/r^2$$

covalent bond Chemical bond formed by sharing a pair of electrons by two nuclei.

covalent compound Compound held together by covalent bonds.

CPB See *competitive protein binding.*

CPR Cardiopulmonary resuscitation.

CPU See *central processor unit.*

crash *Hardware crash* is the complete failure of a particular device, sometimes affecting the operation of an entire computer system; *software crash* is the complete failure of an operating system characterized by some failure in the system's protection mechanisms.

CRFS Comprehensive renal function study.

critical organ (1) Organ of interest. (2) Organ most affected by a technique.

cross-reactivity Reaction of a molecule with an immunoglobulin directed toward another substance.

CRT See *cathode ray tube.*

crystallography Study of the crystal structure of a molecule.

CSF See cerebrospinal fluid.

CT Computerized tomography.

CU Control unit, a component of a computer's central processing unit.

curie Standard measure of rate of radioactive decay; based on the disintegration of 1 g of radium of 3.7×10^{-10} disintegrations per second.

cutie pie A type of ionization chamber.

CVA Cerebrovascular accident.

cyanocobalamine Vitamin B_{12}.

cyclotron Device for accelerating charged particles to high energies using magnetic and oscillating electrostatic fields, causing the particle to move in a spiral path with increasing energy.

D

data Facts, numbers, letters, and symbols; data are the basic elements of information that can be processed by a computer.

database A computer's compilation of information.

daughter radionuclide Decay product produced by a radionuclide. The element from which the daughter was produced is called the *parent.*

debug Detect, locate, and correct coding or logic errors in a computer program.

debugger Program to assist in tracking down and eliminating errors that occurs in the normal course of program development.

debusser Device used to erase material from a computer or recording tape.

decay Radioactive disintegration of a nucleus of an unstable nuclide.

decay constant Decay rate of a radionuclide based on its half-life.

decay factor Fraction of radionuclei that have decayed in a specified period, according to the following formula:

$$\lambda = 0.693/t_{1/2}$$

decay schemes Diagram showing the decay mode or modes of a radionuclide.

dee A component of a cyclotron in which particle acceleration takes place.

deiodinate Removal of iodine from a compound.

delayed neutrons Neutrons that are emitted in a radioactive process at an appreciable time after fission.

dementia Mental deterioration from disease of the brain.

denaturation Change in chemical and physical properties from the normal state, usually irreversible.

dendrite One of the branching protoplasmic processes of the nerve cell.

densitometry A method of determining bone mineral content from single or dual gamma ray or x ray absorption measurements.

deuterons Nucleus of a deuterium atom (H) containing one proton and one neutron.

device A hardware unit such as an I/O peripheral, magnetic tape drive, or line printer.

device control unit A hardware unit that electronically supervises one or more of the same type of devices; it acts as a link between the computer and the I/O devices.

diabetes mellitus Pathologic condition with an absolute or relative insulin deficiency accompanied by elevated levels of glucose in the blood and urine.

diagnostic (1) Referring to determination of the disease; analysis of symptoms. (2) Pertaining to the detection and isolation of a malfunction (hardware) or mistake (software).

dialysis Process for separating crystalloids and colloids in solution by the difference in their rates of diffusion through a semipermeable membrane.

diastole Relaxation and dilation of the heart.

diethylenetriaminepentaacetic acid (pentetic acid, DTPA) Chelating agent that can be labeled with ^{99m}Tc and used for scintigraphy.

digit Character used to express one of the positive integers.

digital computer Device that operates on discrete data, performing sequences or arithmetic and logical operations in these data.

digitalis Cardiotonic agent from the *Digitalis* plant leaf.

dimer A compound produced by the combination of two like molecules; in the strictest sense, without loss of atoms, usually by elimination of water or similar small molecule between the two, but often by simple covalent bonding.

diphosphonate Organic phosphate compound that can be labeled with ^{99m}Tc and used for scintigraphy.

dipyridamole A potent coronary vasodilator.

direct-memory access Access to data in any location independent of sequential prohibitions.

directory A file in the form of a table containing the names of and pointers to files on a mass storage volume.

DIS Decay in storage.

discriminator An electronic barrier used to eliminate low-amplitude noise pulses.

disintegration General process of radioactive decay, usually measured per unit time; *dps* is disintegrations per second, and *dpm* disintegrations per minute; *dps* is equal to counts per second (*cps*) divided by the efficiency of the detector; *dpm* is equal to counts per minute divided by the efficiency of the detector.

disk Form of rotating memory consisting of a platter of aluminum coated with ferrous oxide that can be magnetized or read by a read/write head in proximity to the surface; most common form of bulk memory device.

display A peripheral device used to represent data graphically; normally refers to some type of cathode ray tube system.

diuretic Substance that promotes the secretion of urine.

diverticulum Blind pouch; usually in the intestine.

DLIS Digoxin-like immunoreactive substance.

DMA See *direct memory access.*

DMSA 2,3-Dimercaptosuccinic acid; a chelating agent that can be labeled with ^{99m}Tc for renal imaging.

DNA Deoxyribonucleic acid.

dopamine An intermediate in tyrosine metabolism and the precursor of norepinephrine and epinephrine; it is present in the central nervous system.

DOS Disk operating system.

dose Amount of ionizing radiation absorbed by a specific area or volume or by the whole body.

dose calibrator An ionization chamber designed to measure radionuclide doses.

dose response curve The graphic relationship between counts bound and amount of standard added in a radioimmunoassay; a standard curve.

dosimetry The accurate determination or calculation of dosage.

DOT Department of Transportation.

DPA (dual photon absorptiometry) A bone mineral content measurement technique using gamma or x-ray absorption with a dual energy photon-emitting source; the dual photons allow for accurate correction of soft tissue interference.

DST Dexamethasone suppression test.

DTPA See *diethylenetriaminepentaacetic acid.*

DVT Deep vein thrombosis.

dynode One of several metal plates with a positive voltage that attracts and accelerates electrons within a photomultiplier tube. There are 8-14 dynodes in a photomultiplier tube, each multiplying the number of electrons by a factor of 3 to 6 times.

dysplasia Abnormality of development.

dyspnea Difficulty in breathing.

E

ECAT Emission computerized axial tomography.

ECG See *electrocardiogram.*

ECT Emission computed tomography.

ED End-diastole.

edema Excess fluid in the body.

edetic acid (ethylenediaminetetraacetic acid, EDTA) Chelating agent.

edge packing An area of increased brightness around the edge of a scintillation camera image.

editor Program to permit data or instructions to be manipulated and displayed. Most commonly used in the preparation of new programs or in the revision and correction of old programs.

EDTA See *edetic acid.*

EEG Electroencephalogram.

EF See *cardiac ejection fraction.*

effective half-life The elapsed time to eliminate a radioactive material from the body by a combination of biologic elimination and radioactive decay; determined from physical and biologic half-lives as $1/t_e = 1/t_p + 1/t_b$.

EI Excretion index.

ejection fraction See *cardiac ejection fraction.*

EKG See *electrocardiogram.*

elastic scattering Scattering caused by elastic collisions between nuclei that result in a conversion of the system's kinetic energy.

electrocardiogram A graphic record of the electrical currents that traverse the heart and initiate its contraction.

electrochemical process Chemical process involving oxidation and reduction of the reaction constituents.

electrolyte Substance that forms ions when dissolved in water.

electrolytic reactions Oxidation-reduction reactions.

electrometer Electrostatic instrument for measuring difference in potential.

electron Elementary particle of an atom with a charge of negative one and a mass of 9.1×10^{-28} g.

electron accelerators Machine used to accelerate electrons using potential differences.

electron capture Method of radioactive decay in which the nucleus captures an orbital electron, which then interacts with a proton, effectively negating the proton and transmuting the nucleus to that of another element.

electron configuration Refers to the space relationships of electrons in an atom.

electronegativity Tendency of a neutral atom to acquire electrons, measured relative to that of fluorine.

electronic structure Structure of the orbital electrons in an atom that satisfies the quantum mechanical Schröl V dinger equation.

electron microscope Microscope that uses an electron beam to form an image on a fluorescent screen.

electron spin resonance (ESR) Spectroscopic technique that determines structural features of a molecule based on electron resonance in a magnetic field.

electron volt (eV) Kinetic energy gained by an electron passing through a potential difference of 1 V.

electrophoresis Liquid paper chromatography carried out under the influence of an electric field.

element Pure substance consisting of atoms of the same atomic number that cannot be decomposed by ordinary chemical means.

eluate The material washed out of a chromatographic column.

elution Separation by solvent extraction.

embolism Matter that blocks a blood vessel.

emission computed tomography See *SPECT.*

empiric, empirical Referring to practical experience.

empirical formula Chemical formula that reflects only the simplest molar ratio of the elements in the compounds, not the actual molar ratio.

EMS Emergency medical system.

emulsion (1) Mixture of two liquids, one suspended within another; colloid system. (2) Suspended mixture in which one of the components is gelatin-like.

endocrine Pertaining to a gland that secretes internally.

endocrinology Study of hormonal secretion and of the endocrine glands.

endogenous Originating or produced within the organism or its parts.

endogonic Intake of energy.

endoscope Instrument, tubular in nature, carrying an illumination source, inserted into a body cavity to permit visual inspection.

endosteum Membrane lining of a hollow bone.

endotoxin Poison from dead bacterial cells; formed while cells are living.

energy levels Quantum levels of an atom satisfying the Schrödinger equation that are allowed levels for electron location.

enzyme Protein catalyzing specific transformation of material.

eosinophil (1) Cell stained readily by eosin. (2) White blood cell characterized by a two- or three-lobed nucleus and cytoplasms containing large granules.

EPA Environmental Protection Agency.

epidemiology Study of disease and its rate of occurrence, manner of spread, and prevalence.

epigastrium Space in the abdomen just below the ribs.

epiphysis (1) Portion of bone between the shaft and the cartilage. (2) Pineal gland.

epithelium Cells of skin and mucous membrane.

equilibrium State of equality between two opposing substances.

equilibrium constant True constant that relates the concentration of products and reactants in a reversible chemical system where no further net change is occurring in those concentrations.

equivalent Weight of chemical species that contains either 1 mol of electrons and 1 mol of replaceable hydrogen, or combines with exactly 8 g of oxygen.

erg A unit of work in the gram-centimeter-second system equal to the amount of work of 1 dyne acting through the distance of 1 cm.

ergometer Instrument used for measuring energy expended.

ERPF Effective renal plasma flow.

error Any discrepancy between a computed, observed, or measured quantity and the specific value or condition.

erythrocyte Red blood cell.

erythrocytosis Increase in red blood cells from a known stimulant.

erythroid Reddish in color.

erythropoiesis Formation of erythrocytes.

ES End-systole.

esters Organic compound formed by the action of an acid with an alcohol; contains the functional group

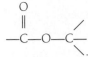

estradiol The most potent, naturally occurring estrogen in mammals.

estrogenic hormone Hormone producing female characteristics.

ether Organic compound containing a C—O—C linkage.

ethylenediaminetetraacetic acid (EDTA) See *edetic acid.*

etiology Study of the causes of disease.

Euler's number The base number (2.718) used in logarithmic calculations named after Leonhard Euler (1701-1783), a Swiss mathematician.

evagination The protrusion of some part or organ from its usual position.

execute To perform an instruction or run a program on a computer.

exergonic Release of energy.

exogenous Originating or produced outside the subject of reference.

exposure rate Rate of exposure to radioactivity usually measured in units of rad per hour.

extirpation Complete removal.

extractor Device that removes something; liquid that removes another substance with it.

extranuclear Referring to the space in an atom outside of the nucleus.

extrinsic testing Scintillation camera uniformity testing done with the collimator in place.

F

families Sets of elements that have the same valence-shell electronic configurations.

fast neutron Neutron that has a minimum energy of 100 keV.

FDA The U.S. Food and Drug Administration.

FDG 2 fluoro-2 deoxy-D-glucose.

ferrokinetics Study of iron within the body.

fibrinolysis Dissolution or splitting of fibrin.

file A logical collection of data that is treated as a unit, occupies one or more blocks on a mass storage volume, and has an associated file name and type.

film badge Photographic film shielded from light; worn by an individual to measure radiation exposure.

filter A computer algorithm applied to projections obtained from an imaging system to eliminate noise and artifacts.

filtered backprojection A reconstruction algorithm to create axial slices from projection information.

fission Splitting of a nucleus accompanied by a release of energy and neutrons.

flat-field collimator See *collimator.*

flood phantom See *phantom.*

flood-field uniformity The ability of a scintillation camera to depict a uniform distribution of activity as uniform.

flow chart A graphic representation for the definition, analysis, or solution of a problem in which symbols are used to represent operations, data flow, and equipment.

fluid thioglycollate Medium that provides conditions for growth of aerobic and anaerobic bacteria; used in microbiologic sterility testing of radiopharmaceuticals.

fluor A liquid scintillation medium.

fluorescence Emission of light by an activated chemical complex.

FOCAL (formula calculation) High-level, conversational, interpreter language for mathematical and string variable manipulations developed for Digital Equipment Corporation (Maynard, Mass.) computers.

folate Salt of folic acid.

follicle Sac or pouchlike depression; cavity.

follicle-stimulating hormone (FSH) Anterior pituitary hormone that stimulates follicle growth in the ovaries and spermatogenesis in the testes.

foramen magnum Large opening in the occipital bone between the cranial cavity and the vertebral canal.

FORTRAN (formula translator) High-level compiler language for mathematical and scientific applications.

Fourier transform A mathematical process that converts matrix information into frequency space.

frame mode A method of computer data collection where x and y positional signals are stored in a single matrix.

free radicals Chemical complexes containing an unpaired electron.

frequency Number of cycles per unit time; normal unit is hertz, or cycles per second.

FSH See *follicle-stimulating hormone.*

F-test A statistical test of the null hypothesis.

FTI Free thyroxine index.

function An algorithm, accessible by name and contained in the system software, that performs commonly used operations; an example is the square root calculation function.

functional group Portion of a molecule responsible for its specific chemical properties.

fundus Base of an organ.

fusion Nuclear process in which two discrete nuclei collide and join together, forming a larger nuclide.

FWHM (full width at half maximum) A measurement of curve peak characteristics by comparing the curve width at half the peak height with the value at which the peak occurs. Used for a variety of applications, it is commonly used to express energy or spatial resolution. Results are expressed as a percentage: energy FWHM (%) = $(\Delta E/E) \times 100\%$.

G

g force Centrifugal force.

GABA Gamma-aminobutyric acid.

gamma camera See *Anger camera.*

gamma decay See *gamma emission.*

gamma emission Nuclear process in which an excited nuclide deexcites by emission of a nuclear photon.

gamma globulin Globulins in plasma having the slowest mobility using electrophoresis in neutral or alkaline solutions.

gastrin Hormone stimulating secretion by the gastric glands.

gastroenteropathy Disease of the stomach and intestine.

gastroparesis A slight degree of stomach paralysis.

gate Electronic device capable of performing logic operations within a digital circuit. In nuclear medicine it implies a device that can provide a timing signal to the computer. This signal is usually associated with the QRS complex of the electrocardiograph.

gauss Unit for measuring magnetic field strength; 10,000 gauss = 1 tesla.

Geiger-Müller tube Ionization chamber measuring radiation in the region where the charge produced per ionizing event is independent of the number of primary ions produced by the initial ionizing event.

gel permeation chromatography Separation of compounds because of differences in their rates of permeation of a gel, especially useful for separation of large biomolecules such as proteins.

generator Device using a parent radionuclide to obtain its product, the daughter radionuclide, usually by addition of a solution that interacts only with the daughter.

genetic effects Dominant or recessive effects on progeny.

genitourinary tract Urinary system and the sex organs.

geometry A term used to denote the relationship of a radioactive source's position in terms of a detector's sensitive surface area.

GER Gastroesophageal reflux.

GFR Glomerular filtration rate.

GH, GHA, glucoheptonate A ^{99m}Tc-labeled carbohydrate used for imaging the renal cortex and collecting system, which may also be used for brain imaging.

globulin Simple protein found in serum and tissue.

glomerulus Small cluster of blood vessels or nerve fibers.

glucagon Pancreatic secretion that increases concentration of the blood sugars.

glucocorticoid Hormone secreted by the adrenal cortex, stimulating the conversion of proteins to carbohydrates.

glucoheptonate Chelating molecule that can bind ^{99m}Tc and be used as an imaging agent.

glycogen Form in which carbohydrates are stored in animal tissue.

glycoprotein Protein and a carbohydrate that does not contain phosphoric acid, purine, or pyrimidine.

glycoside Compound formed between a sugar and another organic substance.

G-M tube See *Geiger-Müller* tube.

gonad Ovary or testicle; the sex gland.

graafian follicle Ovarian follicle where the ovum matures.

gram atomic weight Weight in grams of 1 mol of an element.

gram molecular weight Weight in grams of 1 mol of a chemical compound.

granulocyte White blood cell.

granuloma Tumor or neoplasm consisting of newly formed tissue induced by the presence of a foreign body or of bacteria.

Graves disease Diffuse toxic goiter.

gray (Gy) A unit of absorbed dose equal to 1 joule per kilogram in any medium.

growth hormone (GH) Hormone secreted by the anterior pituitary; stimulates growth.

GTT Glucose tolerance test.

H

half-life (t$_{1/2}$) A term used to describe the time elapsed until some physical quantity has decreased to half of its original value.

half-reaction Term used in an electrochemical reaction to describe either the oxidation process or the reduction process as a separate entity.

half-value layer (HVL) Thickness of absorbing material necessary to reduce the intensity of radiation by half; synonymous with half-thickness.

halide Compound containing a halogen.

halogens Family of chemical elements of similar electron structure (i.e., the valence shell is completely filled except for one electron)—fluorine, chlorine, bromine, iodine, and astatine.

HAMA Human antimouse antibodies.

H and D curve A logarithmic plot that describes a photographic film's response to a given amount of exposure; after Huerter and Deerfield.

hapten Molecule that cannot elicit immunoglobulin response by itself but can when bound to a larger carrier molecule.

hardware Physical equipment, such as mechanical, electrical, or electronic devices.

Hashimoto disease Infiltration of the thyroid gland with lymphocytes resulting in progressive destruction of the parenchyma and hypothyroidism.

haversian system System of canals in the bones where the blood vessels branch out.

HBV Hepatitis B virus.

HCFA Health Care Financing Administration.

HCG Human chorionic gonadotropin.

HDP Hydroxymethylene diphosphonate, a ^{99m}Tc-labeled phosphate complex used in bone imaging.

heat-sensitive printer Type of printer that imprints characters on special sensitized paper by use of heat, without the use of an ink ribbon.

helium-3 (^{3}He) Isotope of helium with an atomic weight of three unified mass units.

hemangioma Tumor of blood vessels that is nonmalignant.

hematocrit Relative percentage of erythrocytes in whole blood.

hematology Study of blood and blood-forming organs.

hematopoietic system The blood system.

hemocytometer Instrument used to count blood cells.

hemoglobin Pigment of the blood that carries oxygen.

hemolysis Red blood cell destruction; escape of hemoglobin within the bloodstream.

hemorrhage Bleeding.

HEPA High-efficiency particulate air (filter).

heparin Mucopolysaccharide acid that occurs in tissues, mainly the liver; used in prevention and treatment of thrombosis, bacterial endocarditis, postoperative pulmonary embolism, repair of vascular injury, and to prevent clotting of blood.

hepatoblastoma Tumor of the liver.

hepatoma Tumor of the liver.

heptasulfide Technetium heptasulfide: $^{99m}Tc_2S_7$; coprecipitates with colloidal sulfur particles stabilized with gelatin in ^{99m}Tc–sulfur-colloid preparation.

hertz Basic unit of frequency; 1 hertz (Hz) = 1 cycle per second.

hexadecimal Pertaining to the number system with a radix of 16.

hexane Alkane with the molecular formula C_6H_{14}.

HIDA N,N-(2,6-dimethylphenyl) carbomolymethyl iminodiacetic acid; can be labeled with ^{99m}Tc and used as an imaging agent.

high-level language A programming language whose statements are translated into more than one machine language instruction; examples are BASIC and FORTRAN.

histochemical Referring to the deposit of chemical components in cells.

histogram A graph.

histology Study of the form and structure of tissues.

histopathology The science or study of diseased tissue.

HIV Human immunodeficiency virus.

HMO Health maintenance organization.

HMPAO Hexamethyl propylene animal oxime.

homeostasis The state of equilibrium in the body with respect to various functions and to the chemical compositions of the fluids and tissues.

hormone Chemical having a specific effect on the activity of a specific organ.

HVL See *half-value layer.*

hydrocarbon Compound containing carbon and hydrogen exclusively.

hydrolysis Processes of decomposition by the addition of water.

hydroxide The ion OH^-.

hydroxyapatite Compound $Ca_{10}(PO_4)_6(OH)_2$; inorganic constituent of bone and teeth.

8-hydroxyquinoline (oxine) Compound that can form a complex with indium and gallium and be used to label blood cells.

hygroscopic Having an affinity for water.

hyperemia Excess blood in an organ or part of the body.

hyperglycemia Excessive sugar (glucose) in the blood.

hyperplasia An increase in the number of cells in a tissue or organ, excluding tumor formation.

hyperthyroidism Overactive thyroid gland.

hypoglycemia Not enough sugar (glucose) in the blood.

hypokinesia Diminished motor function.

hypopituitarism Insufficient secretion of the pituitary.

hypothalamus Part of the forebrain below the cerebrum.

hypothyroidism Insufficient activity of the thyroid.

I

ICRP International Commission on Radiation Protection.

IDA Iminodiacetic acid, a family of ^{99m}Tc-labeled radiopharmaceuticals used to evaluate the hepatobiliary system.

IF See *intrinsic factor.*

iminodiacetic acid Chelating group capable of binding technetium so that it can be attached to biologically active molecules, such as HIDA.

immunoactive Immunity produced by stimulation of antibody-producing mechanisms.

immunoglobulin Type of protein, isolated from the globulin fraction of serum having a characteristic shape and the ability to bind to molecules that are not endogenous to the species producing the immunoglobulin.

immunology Study of resistance to disease or disease agents.

immunoreaction Reaction taking place between an antigen and its antibody.

IMP Iodoamphetamine.

incubate To provide proper conditions for growth or a reaction to occur.

inelastic collision Interaction between two particles resulting in a net loss of kinetic energy in the system.

infarct Area deprived of its blood supply because of an obstruction.

infundibular pulmonic stenosis Obstruction in the outer passage from the right ventricle, restricting blood flow.

inhibition Prevention or interference of a chemical reaction.

inhibitor Substance preventing or interfering with a chemical reaction.

innominate vein Vein receiving blood from the head and neck region.

inoculate To protect against disease by injection of pathogenic microorganisms to stimulate production of antibodies.

inorganic Branch of chemistry having to do with compounds and processes that do not involve carbon.

input Transferal of data from auxiliary or external storage into the internal storage of a computer.

instruction A coded command that tells the computer what to do and where to find the values it is to work with; symbolic instructions must be changed into machine instructions before they can be executed by the computer.

insulin Hormone produced in cells of the pancreas essential for metabolism of carbohydrates.

interface Connection between two systems, such as a scintillation camera and a computer.

internal conversion Nuclear deexcitation process in which the radionuclide deexcites by transferring energy to an orbital electron.

interpreter Computer program that translates and executes each source-language statement before translating and executing the next statement.

interrupts Signals that, when activated, cause a transfer of control to a specific location in memory, thereby breaking the normal flow of control of the routine being executed. An interrupt is normally caused by an external event such as a condition in a peripheral.

interstices Small gaps between tissues or structures.

intrinsic factor (IF) Substance produced by the gastric mucosa and found in the terminal ileum that is necessary for absorption of vitamin B_{12}.

intrinsic testing Scintillation camera uniformity testing with the collimator removed.

intussusception The infolding of one segment of the intestine within another.

inulin Polysaccharide that on hydrolysis yields levulose, which can be used to test kidney function.

inulin clearance test Test of renal function.

inverse square law The radiation intensity of any source decreases inversely as the square of the distance between the source and the detector.

in vitro Outside a living organism.

in vivo Within a living organism.

I/O (input/output) device Computer device that either accepts input or prints out results.

iodination Addition of iodine to a compound.

iodohippuran Agent used for renal imaging.

ion Atom or group of atoms with a net electronic charge.

ion exchange Process involving reversible exchange of ions in a solution and in a solid.

ionic compound Compound held together by purely electrostatic forces.

ionic strength Half the sum of the terms obtained by multiplying the molarity of each ion by the square of its valence.

ionization Process of removing electrons from an atom to create an ion.

ionization chamber A gas-filled radiation detector.

IRMA Immunoradiometric assay.

irradiation Application of radiant energy for therapy or diagnosis.

ischemia Insufficient blood supply because of a spasm or constriction of the artery in an organ or part of the body.

ischemic damage Damage from a constriction of the blood vessel.

islets of Langerhans Pancreatic cells secreting insulin.

isobar Nuclides that have the same total number of neutrons and protons but are different elements.

isoelectric Having uniform electric potential; thus no current is given off.

isomers Two compounds with the same molecular formulas and different structural formulas.

isometric transition Change in the extranuclear portion of an atom from a high-energy level to a lower energy level accompanied by the release of electromagnetic radiation.

isopleth Graph showing frequency of an event as a function of two variables.

isotones Nuclides having the same number of neutrons but a different number of protons.

isotonic Physiologic; compatible with body tissues.

isotopes Nuclides of the same element with the same number of protons but different number of neutrons.

ITLC Instant thin layer chromatography.

ITP Idiopathic thrombocytopenia.

IUPAC International Union of Pure and Applied Chemistry.

J

JCAHO Joint Commission on Accreditation of Healthcare Organizations.

joystick An electronic pointing device for computers.

K

ketone Organic molecule with a carbon-oxygen double bond separating two alkyl portions

$$R-\overset{\overset{\displaystyle O}{\|}}{C}-R$$

kinetic energy That energy of a body due to its motion.

Kupffer cells Part of the reticuloendothelial system; star-shaped cells attached to the wall of the sinu- soids of the liver.

L

lacuna Small hollow cavity.

LAL See *limulus amebocyte lysate*.

lambda Greek letter denoting the decay constant of radioactive species.

language Set of representations, conventions, and rules used to convey information.

Larmor frequency The characteristic frequency at which the resonance of the nucleus is excited in magnetic resonance imaging.

law of constant composition If two (or more) elements combine chemically to form a compound, the relative weights of the constituent elements will always be in a constant proportion to each other.

law of definite proportions If two (or more) elements chemically combine to form a compound, the relative number of moles of each constituent element will be in a proportion of simple whole numbers with each other.

law of mass action The velocity of the chemical reaction is proportional to the masses of the reactants.

law of multiple proportions If two elements form more than one compound, the number of moles of one element in the first compound is proportional to the number of moles of the same element in the second compound.

law of reciprocal proportions Two chemical elements unite with a third element in proportions that are multiples of the union of the first two elements.

Le Chatelier's principle A principle stating that if a system is initially at equilibrium and is forced away from equilibrium when a parameter is changed, the system will spontaneously return to a new equilibrium.

LET See *linear energy transfer*.

leukocyte White blood cell, either granular or nongranular.

leukopenia Less than the normal number of white blood cells.

leukotaxine Crystalline nitrogen substance appearing when tissue is injured.

Lewis concept A concept stating that an acid is an electron-pair accceptor and a base is an electron-pair donor.

LH Luteinizing hormone.

ligand (1) Molecule attached to a central atom using coordinate covalent bonds. (2) In radioimmunoassay an antigen or small molecule that binds to a native carrier protein.

light pen A device resembling a pencil or stylus that is used to input information to a CRT display system.

limulus amoebocyte lysate (LAL) In vitro test for pyrogens; it reacts with gram-negative bacterial endotoxins in nanogram or greater concentrations to form an opaque gel.

linear attenuation coefficient That quantity by which radiation is decreased per unit path length through matter.

linear energy transfer Amount of energy lost by ionizing radiation by way of interaction with matter per centimeter of path length through the absorbing material.

line spread function The profile of counts along a line running perpendicular to a line source.

linear regression A calculation generally performed to show a linear relationship between two variables to predict some y variable based on measurement of some x variable.

lingula Small tonguelike structure.

linker A program that combines many relocatable object modules into an executable module; it satisfies global references and combines program sections.

lipid Fat and fatlike substances.

lipophilic Capable of dissolving, of being dissolved in, or of absorbing lipids.

lipoproteins Combination of a lipid and a protein.

liquid-drop model Theoretical model of the nucleus that assumes a simple continuous nuclear potential and spheroid shape.

liquid scintillation counter A system for detecting beta-emitting radionuclides using a liquid scintillator in which the radioactive source is dissolved.

listing The printed copy generated by a line printer or terminal.

list mode A method of computer data collection where x and y positional signals are stored sequentially in memory in the form of a list.

load To store a program or data in memory; to mount a tape on a device such that the read point is at the beginning of the tape; to place a removable disk in a disk drive and start the drive.

location An address in storage or memory where a unit of data or an instruction can be stored.

logarithm Exponent of the power of a base that equals a given number.

logit Mathematical relationship defined as $\ln y/l - y$.

loop A sequence of instructions executed repeatedly until a terminal condition prevails.

Lugol solution An iodine solution.

LV Left ventricle.

LVEF Left ventricular ejection fraction; see also *cardiac ejection fraction.*

lymphangiography Radiography of the lymph channels.

lymphocyte White blood cell with a single rounded nucleus.

lymphoma Tumor composed of lymph node tissue.

lyophilize To rapidly freeze and dehydrate a substance.

lysis (1) Separation of adhesions binding different structures. (2) Destruction of a cell by a specific agent. (3) Abatement of disease symptoms.

M

MAA Macroaggregated albumin.

machine code See *object code.*

machine language See *language.*

macro (1) Directions for expanding abbreviated text; a boilerplate that generates a known set of instructions, data, or symbols; a macro is used to eliminate the need to write a set of instructions that are used repeatedly. (2) Prefix meaning huge or of large scale.

macroglobulin Protein of high molecular weight.

macrophage Large white blood cell; active in bacterial destruction.

MAG3 Mercaptoacetyl triglycine.

magnetic field Field induced by moving electrical charges.

magnetic quantum number Quantum number (m, m_i, or M) that defines the orientation of an orbital in space.

magnetic tape A plastic-base tape in which data is imprinted magnetically.

malabsorption Inadequate absorption of nutrients in the gastrointestinal tract.

manometer Device used to measure the pressure of liquids.

mass Basic parameter of matter referring to the quantity of matter present. It is independent of the object's weight.

mass attenuation coefficient The quotient of the linear attenuation coefficient divided by the density of the matter through which it passes.

mass defect The difference in mass of an atom's constituent particles and its total mass.

mass storage A device that can store large amounts of data readily accessible to the computer.

matrix A rectangular array of elements; any matrix can be considered an array.

maximum permissible dose (MPD) Dose limitations, in rem, placed on each individual as specified by the Nuclear Regulatory Commission.

MDA Minimum detectable amount.

MDP Methylene diphosphonate, a ^{99m}Tc-labeled phosphate complex used in bone imaging.

mean Average of two or more quantities.

Meckel's diverticulum Saclike pouch on the small intestine.

mediastinum Space behind the breastbone containing the heart.

medulloblastoma Tumor of the brain.

megakaryocyte A cell found in the bone marrow developing into blood platelets.

MEK Methyl ethyl ketone.

melanoma Tumor characterized by dark pigmentation.

memory Any form of data storage including main memory and mass storage in which data can be read and written; memory usually refers to the main memory.

mesenchyme Primitive tissue of the embryo.

metabolism Process for transforming foods into compounds used by the body.

metastable state Excited state of a nucleus or atom that has a measurable lifetime; also known as an isometric state.

metastasis Spreading of a disease process from one part of the body to another.

metathesis Chemical process in which two compounds exchange constituents.

microbiologic testing Any test for bacteria, virus, or other microorganism.

microlysis Destruction of a substance into microscopic size.

micrometer (μm) One millionth of a meter; formerly micron.

microprocessor A silicon chip containing many circuits.

microsphere Round mass of a small size, visible only with a microscope.

microvilli Projections of cell membranes greatly increasing the surface area of the cell.

migrating solvent Chromatographic solvent; used to differentially carry the unknown solute to be separated.

MIP Maximum intensity projection; a translucent 3D volume cinematic image.

MIPS Million instructions per second.

mitral stenosis Deformity of the mitral valve of the heart.

mnemonic Aiding the memory; use of an acronym or other pattern to aid the memory.

mobile phase Phase in chromatography that differentially carries the unknown solutes.

modem From *mo*dulate and *dem*odulate. A device used to transmit computer data over telephone lines.

modulation transfer function A curve depicting the image to object contrast ratio as a function of spatial frequency.

molal Unit of concentration associated with molality equal to the number of moles of solute per kilogram of solvent.

molality Unit of solution concentration defined as the number of moles of solute per weight (kg) of solvent.

molar Concentration unit equal to number of moles of solute per liter of solution.

molarity Measure of solution concentration defined as the number of moles of solute per volume (liter) of solution.

mole See *gram molecular weight*.

molecular formula Chemical formula that states the actual number of atoms of each constituent per molecule of the compound.

molecular imaging Techniques that allow visualization of processing taking place at the molecular level.

molecular weight Weight in unified mass units of one molecule of a particular chemical compound.

molecule Basic unit of a chemical compound.

molybdate Compound containing a MoO_4^{-2} group.

monatomic One atom per molecule, usually referring to elements (such as the noble gases) in their native state.

monitor The master control program that observes, supervises, controls, or verifies the operation of a computer system; the collection of routines that controls the operation of user and system programs, schedules, operations, allocates resources, and performs I/O.

monoclonal antibodies Immunoglobulins, chemically identical in structure, produced by a group of cells that are genetically identical.

monocyte White blood cell having one rounded nucleus that increases in number during certain types of infections.

monoenergetic Having a single energy.

MOPS Manually operated pipetter/samplers.

morphology Study of the structure of tissues.

motility The power of spontaneous movement.

mouse An electronic pointing device for computers.

MPD See *Maximum permissible dose*.

MPST Mean platelet survival time.

MRI (magnetic resonance imaging) Body imaging technique to observe chemical makeup of tissue using magnetic fields and radiofrequency electromagnetic waves.

MTF See *modulation transfer function*.

mucoid (1) Mucuslike substance. (2) An animal conjugated protein.

mucosal biopsy Removal and examination of some of the tissue of the mucous membrane.

MUGA Multiple gated acquisition.

multiformatter A photographic system designed to produce images from a cathode ray tube in various positions and sizes.

multiple gated acquisition Composite heart-imaging technique performed by synchronizing a patient's heartbeat by means of an electrocardiograph to a scintillation camera/computer.

myeloblast A cell in the bone marrow that develops into a white blood cell.

myelofibrosis Replacement of the bone marrow by fibrous tissue.

myeloid (1) Referring to bone marrow. (2) Referring to the spinal cord. (3) Cell resembling a red bone marrow cell that did not originate in the bone marrow.

myocardial infarct Heart muscle damage secondary to loss of its blood supply.

myocardial ischemia Obstruction or constriction in the coronary arteries resulting in a deficiency of blood to the heart muscle.

myocardium Heart muscle.

N

N See *Neutron number*.

naperian logarithmic system Logarithmic system using the base *e*, which is a mathematical constant ($e = 2.71$).

nasopharyngeal Referring to that part of the pharynx above the soft palate.

natural logarithm See *naperian logarithmic system*.

NCRP National Council on Radiation Protection and Measurement.

negatron Negative electron.

NEMA National Electrical Manufacturers Association.

neonate Newborn to 4-week-old infant.

neoplasia Condition characterized by new tumors or growths.

nephrology Study of the kidney.

nephron Part of the kidney that secretes urine.

nephrosis Degeneration of the kidney.

neurinoma Enlargement of a node or tumor on a peripheral nerve.

neuroglia Nonnervous cellular elements of nervous tissue.

neurohormone Hormone stimulating the mechanism of the nerves.

neurohumeral Referring to a chemical secreted by a neutron.

neurohypophysis Main part of the posterior pituitary (hypophysis cerebri).

neuron Nerve.

neuropathology Study of nervous system diseases by examination of those tissues.

neutralization Chemical reaction in which an acid and a base react to form a salt and water.

neutrino Nuclear particle emitted during positron decay.

neutron Nuclear particle that is found in the nucleus, is electrically neutral, and has a mass of one mass unit.

neutron activation Nuclear process in which a nucleus absorbs a thermal neutron and deexcites by way of gamma-ray emission.

neutron flux Measure of neutron intensity defined as the number of neutrons passing through one square centimeter of area per second.

neutron number Number of neutrons in a nucleus (symbol for neutron number is N).

neutrophil White blood cell with three to five lobes connected by chromatin and cytoplasm containing five granules.

nidus (1) Focus of infection. (2) Depression in the brain surface.

NIST National Institute of Standards and Technology. Formerly National Bureau of Standards (NBS).

NMR (nuclear magnetic resonance). See *magnetic resonance imaging (MRI)*.

noble gas Any chemical element that has a completely filled valence-shell configuration in its neutral state–helium, neon, argon, krypton, xenon, and radon.

noise Extraneous interference in an electronic circuit of statistical manipulation.

nomogram Conversion scale.

nonpolar bond Chemical bond in which a pair of electrons is equally shared by two nuclei.

nonspecific binding (NSB) Binding of the radioligand to substances or surfaces other than the specific reactor substance.

normal Concentration unit defined as the number of equivalent weights of solute per liter of solution.

normality Method of expressing concentration defined as the number of equivalent weights of solute per volume of solution.

normalize A term used in association with computer-defined regions of interest to indicate that counts contained in the regions have been converted to the same size region.

NRC See *Nuclear Regulatory Commission*.

NSB See nonspecific binding.

nuclear charge Charge of the nucleus of an atom equal to the number of protons multiplied by the charge of a proton.

nuclear fission Nuclear process in which a nucleus splits into two pieces accompanied by neutron emission and energy release.

nuclear reactor Device that under controlled conditions is used for supporting a self-sustained nuclear reaction.

Nuclear Regulatory Commission (NRC) United States government agency regulating by-product material.

nuclear stability Condition to describe a nucleus that is stable with respect to radioactive decay.

nucleons Any particle commonly contained in the nucleus of an atom.

nucleus (1) Portion of an atom containing the neutrons and the protons. (2) Spheric body that is the core of a cell. (3) Mass of gray matter in the central nervous system.

NUTRAN High-level computer language.

Nyquist frequency the highest frequency that can be represented in an image.

O

object code Relocatable machine language code.

obtund To dull or blunt, especially to blunt sensation or deaden pain.

occipital Referring to the back of the head or occiput.

Occupational Safety and Health Administration (OSHA) United States government agency regulating health standards in the workplace.

octal The number system with a radix of 8; for example, octal 100 is decimal 64.

OIH See *ortho-iodohippurate*.

oleic acid (octadecanoic acid) Straight-chained organic acid with the molecular formula $C_{18}H_{36}O_2$.

oncocytoma Granular cell adenoma of the parotid gland.

op code See *operation code*.

operand That which is affected, manipulated, or operated upon.

operating systems Collection of programs, including a monitor or executive and system programs, that organizes a central processor and peripheral devices into a working unit for the development and execution of application programs.

operation code Code used to start the operation of a program.

optic chiasma The point of crossing of the fibers of the optic nerve.

orbital Energy sublevels occupied by electrons in an atom.

ordinate The y, or perpendicular, axis in a cartesian graph or plot.

organic chemistry Branch of chemistry dealing with the study of compounds of carbon.

organic compounds Any of the class of chemical compounds that contain carbon.

organomegaly Abnormal enlargement of an organ.

ortho-iodohippurate (OIH) Iodinated renal imaging agent.

OSHA See *Occupational Safety and Health Administration.*

osmoreceptor Specialized sensory nerve ending that (1) gives rise to sense of smell and (2) is stimulated by changes in osmotic pressures of the surrounding medium.

osseous Composed of bone.

osteoblast Immature bone-producing cell.

osteoclast Large multinuclear cell associated with destruction of bone.

osteocyte Cell lodged in flat oval cavities of the bone.

osteogenesis Bone development.

osteomyelitis Infection of the bone.

output Information transferred from the internal storage of a computer to output devices or external storage.

ovary Female reproductive gland.

oxidation Process by which a substance loses electrons in an oxidation-reduction reaction.

oxidation-reduction Chemical reaction in which electrons are transferred from one substance to another substance.

oxidizing agent Substance in an oxidation-reduction reaction that causes another substance to lose electrons.

oxine See *8-hydroxyquinoline.*

P

P wave The first complex of the electrocardiogram representing depolarization of the atria.

Paget's disease Osteitis deformans.

PAH Paraaminohippuric acid.

pair production Photonic deexcitation process in which a photon disintegrates into an electron-positron pair, each of which gains an equal amount of kinetic energy.

pancreas Large gland secreting enzymes into the intestines for digestion and manufacturing and secreting insulin.

papilla of Vater Prominent tissue in the duodenum where the bile duct enters the intestine.

parathormone Hormone secreted by the parathyroid gland.

parathyroid glands Four small endocrine glands on the lateral lobe of the thyroid that control calcium and phosphorus metabolism.

parenchyma Essential elements of an organ as distinguished from its framework.

parent radionuclide Radionuclide that decays to a specific daughter nuclide either directly or as a member of a radioactive series.

parotid gland Salivary gland.

Pascal A computer programming language.

PAS Paraaminosalicylic acid.

pathology Study of disease based on examination of diseased tissue.

pathophysiology Study of disordered function of organs.

Pauli exclusion principle Two electrons in the same atom cannot have the exact same set of quantum numbers.

Pauling scale A measure of electronegativity with fluorine arbitrarily assigned a value of 4.

pedicle Stemlike part of attaching structure.

PEG Poyethylene glycol.

pellet (1) Small pill. (2) A granule.

pentetic acid (diethylenetriaminepentaacetic acid, DTPA) Chelating agent that can be labeled with ^{99m}Tc and used for scintigraphy.

peptide Low molecular weight compound containing two or more amino acids.

peptide hormone Hormones excreted by the pituitary, parathyroid, and pancreas.

percent trace binding The amount of radioactivity bound by a specific reactor substance in a solution containing the substance of interest, divided by the amount of radioactivity bound by a solution where the substance of interest is undetectable, times 100.

perchlorate Any chemical compound that contains the CIO_4 group.

perfusion Passage of a fluid into an organ to thoroughly permeate it.

pericardium Tissue sheath encasing the heart.

perineal region Floor of the pelvis.

period (1) In wave motion phenomena it is the time required to complete one cyclic motion, equalizing the reciprocal of the frequency. (2) Elements in a horizontal line on the periodic chart.

periodic chart Chart of the elements depicting the interrelationships among them based on their electronic configurations.

periosteal bone Bone that develops directly from and beneath the periosteum.

periosteum Thin tissue encasing bones that possesses bone-forming potential.

peripheral (1) Near the surface, distant; distal, opposite of proximal. (2) Any device distinct from the central processor that can provide input or accept output from the computer.

peripheral blood Blood that circulates in the vessels remote from the heart.

peripheral vessels Blood vessels that are remote from the heart.

pernicious anemia Anemia from lack of secretion by the gastric mucosa of intrinsic factor, which is important to blood formation.

pertechnetate Any chemical compound containing the TcO_4> group.

PET Positron emission tomography.

PGA Pteroyglutamic (folic) acid.

pH Measure of the hydrogen ion concentration in a solution; equals the negative logarithm of the hydrogen ion concentration.

pH meter Device used to measure the pH of a solution based on the potential difference between the solution and a standard calomel electrode.

phagocyte Cell that destroys bacteria or other foreign bodies.

phagocytize To ingest cells or microorganisms by a cell (a phagocyte).

phagocytosis Destruction of bacteria or other foreign bodies by phagocytes.

phantom (1) Model of some part of the body in which radioactive material can be placed to simulate conditions in vivo. (2) A device that yields information concerning the performance of a medical imaging system.

pharmacokinetics Study of the activity of drugs and medicines.

pharmacology Study of drugs and medicine.

pharynx Back of the nasal passages and mouth; the throat.

phase The time relationship between two events.

phenols Organic compounds with the functional group OH⁻ attached to an aromatic ring.

phosphor Chemical compound that upon photonic absorption will deexcite slowly by emitting light.

phosphorylation Chemical process in which a molecule acquires a PO_4^{-3} group.

photocathode Negative electrode of a photomultiplier tube.

photodisintegration Disintegration event triggered by photonic interactions.

photoelectric effect Process by which photons deexcite through absorption by electrons, resulting in ionization phenomena.

photomultiplication Multiplication of the signal given off by the interaction of a photon in a scintillation detector.

photomultiplier tube An electronic tube that converts light photons to electric pulses.

photon Discrete packet of electromagnetic energy.

photopeak A peak or increase in a graphic representation of a radioactive spectrum characteristic of the radionuclide under study.

phrenic artery Artery in the diaphragm.

phylogenetic, phylogenic Referring to the developmental history of an organism or race.

physical half-life The elapsed time to reach half of the original quantity of radioactivity by decay.

physiology Study of the function of tissues or organs.

pipeline processing Computer instructions carried out in an assembly line fashion.

pipet (or pipette) (1) Device used to deliver a precise amount of a liquid. (2) The act of using such a device.

pituitary Endocrine gland located at the base of the brain; regulates growth and secretions of other endocrine glands.

pixel From *picture el*ement; a single image element.

PL/1 (programming language 1) High-level computer language.

placenta Organ attaching the embryo to the uterus; the afterbirth.

placental barrier Term used to describe the semipermeable barrier interposed between the maternal and fetal blood by the placental membrane.

Planck's constant 6.626186×10^{-27} erg-seconds.

planimetry Measurement of plane surfaces.

plasma Fluid of the blood not including the red and white blood cells.

platelet, blood platelet, thrombocyte Small, colorless disks that aid in blood clotting found in circulating blood.

plethysmography Measurement of changes in volume using a plethysmograph.

pleura Membrane lining of the chest cavity and lungs.

pleural effusion Fluid in the space that contains the lungs and the thoracic cavity.

PnAO Propylene amine oxime, a ^{99m}Tc-labeled complex that crosses the blood-brain barrier and is used to image regional cerebral perfusion.

point spread function The profile of counts along a line through a point source of radioactivity.

Poisson distribution A statistical distribution of events.

polar covalent bond Covalent bond formed by the unequal sharing of a pair of electrons between two atoms.

polarization The development of differences in potential between two points in living tissues.

polar map a concentric plot of cardiac short axis slices from apex at the center to basal slices on the outside.

polyatomic ion Ion composed of more than one atom.

polycythemia Disease characterized by an overabundance of red blood cells.

polycythemia vera (p. vera) Inherited disease characterized by increase of red blood cells and total blood volume accompanied by splenomegaly, leukocytosis, thrombocytosis, and bone marrow hyperactivity.

polymer Compound formed of simpler molecules, usually of high molecular weight.

polymerization Formation of a polymer.

polypeptide Compound containing two or more amino acids linked by a peptide bond.

polyphosphate Any molecule containing the $(PO_3)_n$ group.

pons (1) Slip of tissue connecting two parts of an organ. (2) Part of the base of the brain.

popliteal fossa Depression at the back of the knee.

porcine From a pig.

porta hepatis Part of the liver receiving the major blood vessels.

positron (β^+) Transitory nuclear particle with a mass equal to that of an electron and a charge equal to that of a proton.

potentiometer See *voltmeter*.

preamplifier A device placed between a detector and an amplifier used to shape and increase pulse size.

precipitate Solid compound that is produced in a chemical reaction between two soluble compounds in a solution.

precision Refers to the variations of individual measurements.

precordium Upper abdominal region.

pressure Force per unit area.

primary fluor A liquid scintillator.

primordial Formed early in the course of development.

principal quantum number (n or n_i) Relative distance from the nucleus at which the electron will be found and also its relative energy.

processor See *central processor unit*.

proerythroblast Primitive erythrocyte.

progesterone Hormone secreted by the ovaries.

program Complete sequence of instructions and routines necessary to solve a problem.

program development Process of writing, entering, translating, and debugging source programs.

prolactin Hormone secreted by the anterior pituitary.

promonocyte Intermediate cell between the monoblast and monocyte.

prompt neutrons Neutrons from a fission event that are emitted immediately after or during the event.

proportional counter A gas-filled radiation detector.

proprioception Process of receiving stimulation within the tissue.

prostaglandins Substance causing strong contractions of smooth muscle and dilation of the vascular bed.

prostatic hypertrophy Enlargement of the prostate because of an increase in the size of its cells.

protease Enzyme that digests protein.

protein High molecular weight compound of many amino acids linked by peptide bonds.

proteinuria Protein in the urine.

prothrombin Protein combining with other proteins to form thrombin, a clotting agent.

proton Nuclear particle with a mass of one unified mass unit and a charge of $+1.6 \times 10^{-9}$ coulomb.

psi Pounds per square inch; unit of pressure.

PTH Parathyroid hormone; parathyrin.

PTHrP Parathyroid hormone-related peptide.

ptosis Denotes a falling or downward displacement of an organ.

pulmonary Referring to the lungs.

pulmonic stenosis Obstruction from the right ventricle, restricting the outflow of blood.

pulse height analysis See *pulse height analyzer (PHA)*.

pulse height analyzer (PHA) Instrument that accepts input from a detector and categorizes the pulses on the basis of signal strength.

pulse height window See *window*.

PVC Premature ventricular contraction.

pyelonephritis Inflammation of the kidney and the pelvis of the kidney.

pylorus Part of the stomach just before the duodenum.

pyogenic Pus forming; bacterial.

pyrogen Fever-inducing substance.

pyrophosphate Chemical compound containing a $P_2O_7^{-4}$.

Q

QF See *quality factor.*

QMP Quality management program.

QRS complex The principal deflection in the electrocardiogram representing ventricular depolarization.

qualitative chemical analysis Determination of the identity of each constituent in a chemical system.

quality control serum A serum sample that is analyzed many times to yield data about the statistical reproducibility of a radioassay.

quality factor (QF) Linear energy transfer—dependent factor by which absorbed doses are to be multiplied to account for the varying effectiveness of different radiations.

quantitative chemical analysis Branch of chemical analysis dealing with the determination of how much of a constituent there is in a chemical compound.

quantum mechanics Branch of physics dealing with the mathematical description of the wave properties of atomic and nuclear particles.

quantum number Value describing the location of an electron in the electron configuration of an atom.

quenching (1) Action of a gas added to a Geiger-Müller detector, allowing it to resolve. (2) An undesirable reduction of light output from a liquid scintillator.

R

R wave A portion of the QRS electrocardiographic signal denoting ventricular contraction and relaxation.

rad See *radiation absorbed dose.*

radial immunodiffusion Immunochemical method used for the determination of serum concentrations of physiologically important substances.

radiation absorbed dose (rad) Quantity of radiation that deposits 100 ergs of energy per gram of absorbing material.

radiation dose Quantity of radiation absorbed by some material.

radiation exposure Exposure to ionizing radiation.

radiation safety Methods of protecting workers and the general population from the deleterious effects of radiation.

radiochemistry Study of the chemistry of radioactive elements.

radiochromatography Chromatography using NaI crystal for detection of substances labeled with a radioisotope.

radiocolloids Colloid of a solid in a liquid where the solid phase contains a radioisotope.

radiograph Image of the internal structure of objects by exposure of film to x rays; roentgenogram.

radioimmunoassay Assay by immunologic procedures using radioactive antigens.

radionuclide Unstable nucleus that transmutes by way of nuclear decay.

radionuclidic purity Amount of total radioactive species in a sample that is the desired radionuclide.

radiopharmaceutical Radioactive drug used for therapy or diagnosis.

radiopharmacology Study of radioactive drugs and their therapeutic and diagnostic uses.

radiopharmacy Laboratory producing and dispensing solutions labeled with radioisotopes for therapeutic and diagnostic purposes.

radioreceptor Sensory nerve terminal stimulated by radiant energy.

RAM (random access memory) Memory accessed in such a way that the next location from which data are obtained is not dependent on the location of the previously obtained data.

raphe A seam; the line of union of two contiguous and similar structures.

RAS Renal artery stenosis.

RAST Radioallergosorbent test.

rate meter Device, used in conjunction with a detector, that measures the rate of activity of a radioisotope; usually in units of counts per minute or counts per second.

RBE See *relative biologic effectiveness.*

reaction Any process resulting in a net change to the constituents of the system.

reactor See *nuclear reactor.*

read-only input (ROI) Input only from the memory or from an internal source. (Contrast *regions of interest [ROI].*)

read-only memory Internal acquisition of data from the memory in computers.

reagent Any chemical used in a process.

real time In computer terminology the actual time elapsed during the program.

real-time system System in which the computation is performed while a related physical activity is occurring; the program results are used in guiding the physical process.

receptor Sensory nerve terminal responding to stimulation by transmission of impulses to the central nervous system.

rectilinear scanner An imaging device that passes over the area of interest in a rectilinear fashion.

red blood cells (RBC) Any blood cells containing hemoglobin.

redox Abbreviation for an oxidation-reduction reaction.

reducing agent Substance that donates electrons in an oxidation-reduction reaction.

reduction In an oxidation-reducing reaction it is the process by which one substance gains electrons.

reflex A reaction or involuntary movement.

regions of interest (ROI) Portion of the data field that is to be studied. (Contrast *read-only input [ROI].*)

register A device capable of storing a specified amount of data such as a word. See also *accumulator.*

regression analysis See *linear regression.*

relative biologic effectiveness (RBE) Ratio of the biologic response derived from a particular radiation as compared with another radiation exposure.

rem See *roentgen equivalent man.*

renal cortex Smooth outer layer of the kidney.

replacement reaction Chemical process in which an ion is replaced by another species in a compound.

resolution The ability of a counting or imaging system to accurately depict two separate events in space, time, or energy as separate.

resolving time The length of time taken by a detector to sense and process a nuclear event.

resorption A loss of substance by lysis.

rest mass Mass that is not in motion.

reticuloendothelial cells Phagocytes.

RFQ Radiofrequency quadripole accelerator.

RIA See *radioimmunoassay.*

RISC Reduced instruction set computer.

RNA Ribonucleic acid; responsible for transmission of inherited traits.

RNC Radionuclide cystography.

ROC curve Receiver operating characteristic curve: a graphic representation of sensitivity and specificity.

roentgen (R) Quantity of x or gamma radiation per cubic centimeter of air that produces one electrostatic unit of charge.

roentgen equivalent man (rem) Unit of radiation dose defined as the product of rad and RBE.

ROI See *read-only input* and *regions of interest.*

ROM See *read-only memory.*

RSO Radiation safety office(r).

run A single continuous execution of a program.

Rutherford scattering See *elastic scattering.*

RV Right ventricle.

RVG Radionuclide ventriculogram.

S

saccule Small sac or pouch.

sagittal (1) Plane or section parallel to the long axis of the body. (2) Arrowlike shape.

saline Sodium chloride in water.

saline solution, physiologic Salt solution compatible with body tissues.

salivary glands Glands secreting saliva, connected to the mouth by ducts; the three glands are the parotids, submaxillaries, and sublinguals.

saturation analysis A type of competitive binding assay where the specific reactor substance-binding sites are all occupied (saturated) by ligand; RIA is a type of saturation analysis.

scaler An electronic pulse counter.

Schilling test Test for primary pernicious anemia.

scientific notation A system of utilizing signs or numbers to represent numbers of greater and lesser magnitudes.

scintigraphic agent Substance injected to produce images of internal organs; usually a radioactive solution.

scintigraphy Imaging the distribution of a radionuclide with scintillation detection.

scintillation Flash of light produced in a phosphor by radiation.

scleroderma (1) Thickening of the skin by swelling. (2) Thickening of the fibrous tissue.

secondary fluor (waveshifter) A liquid scintillator.

secretin Hormone-stimulating secretion of pancreatic juice and bile secreted by the duodenal mucous membrane.

secular equilibrium Parent-daughter radioisotope pair in which the parent has a much longer half-life than does the daughter radionuclide.

semiconductor Substance whose conductivity is enhanced by the addition of another substance or through the application of heat, light, or voltage.

senescent Growing old; characteristic of old age.

sensitivity (1) Pertains to the ability of a given test to determine what fraction or percentage of ill patients will have a positive test result. (2) Efficiency of a given detector system.

septal Referring to a wall or partition.

septum A wall or partition.

serous Referring to serum.

serum Liquid remaining after blood has clotted.

shells Energy levels in electronic configuration.

shielding Absorbing material used to attenuate ionizing radiation.

shunt Bypass; an alternate course.

SI Serum iron, see also *specific ionization*.

SIDS Sudden infant death syndrome.

sievert (Sv) Unit for dose equivalent. For a quality factor (QA) = 1, one sievert is the dose equivalent of one gray (100 rad); 1 Sv = 100 rem.

signal-to-noise ratio A ratio describing the relationship between desired and unwanted information.

sinogram A two-dimensional plot of SPECT or PET projection count profiles on the horizontal axis versus angle of the projection on the vertical axis.

sinusoid Beginning of the venous system in the spleen, liver, bone marrow, and so on, that has an irregularly shaped, thin-walled space.

sinusoidal (1) Referring to a recess or cavity. (2) Referring to an abnormal channel that permits the escape of pus.

Sjögren syndrome An aggregate of signs and symptoms including dryness of mucous membranes, purpuric spots on the face, and bilateral parotid enlargement.

SNR Signal-to-noise ratio.

software Collection of programs and routines associated with a computer.

software bootstrap A bootstrap activated by loading the instructions and specifying the appropriate load and start address.

sol Liquid colloid solution.

solid phase antibody An antibody chemically linked to a solid surface.

solute Material dissolved into a solution.

solution Physical system consisting of one or more substances dissolved in another substance.

solvent Substance that acts as the dissolving agent in a solution.

solvent extraction Use of a second solvent to preferentially dissolve a compound out of another solution.

sorption Adsorption or absorption.

SPA (single photon absorptiometry) Bone mineral content measurement technique using gamma-ray or x-ray absorption with a single energy photon-emitting source.

spallation To chip or flake off.

specific activity Unit pertaining to the disintegrations per gram of a radioisotope.

specific ionization (SI) Linear rate of energy attenuation of ionizing radiation measured in terms of the number of ion pairs produced per unit distance traveled.

specificity The ability of a given test to determine what fraction or percentage of well patients will have a negative test result. Ability of a substance to recognize and bind to only one other molecule.

specific reactor substance Material capable of specifically and reversibly reacting with another molecule.

SPECT (single photon emission computed tomography) An imaging technique associated with single gamma-ray–emitting radiopharmaceuticals obtained using a scintillation camera that moves around the patient to obtain images from multiple angles for tomographic image reconstruction.

spectrometer Device measuring electromagnetic radiation characteristics in a spectrum.

spectrophotometry Use of an instrument that measures light or color by photonic transmission.

spermatogenesis Process of forming sperm.

sphincter Muscle controlling a body opening.

splanchnic Pertaining to the interior organs in any of the four great body cavities.

splenic hilum Fissure where vessels and nerves enter the spleen.

spondylolysis Breaking down or dissolution of the body of the vertebra.

SRS See *specific reactor substance*.

SSKI Saturated solution of potassium iodide.

stable electron configuration Configuration of electrons about an atom in the atom's lowest energy state.

standard A solution of pure substance of known concentration to which unknown substances may be compared.

standard deviation The square root of the average of the squares of the deviation of the value of a set of measurements from each of the individual measurements.

stannous ion Ion of tin in the +2 valence state.

stationary phase Chromatographic phase that does not move with the solvent front.

steatorrhea Excess fat in the feces.

stellate Star shaped.

stenosis A narrowing of a canal or vessel.

Stenson ducts Canals that empty the parotid gland.

steroid Complex molecular structure containing four interlocking rings—three contain six carbon atoms each and the fourth contains five carbon atoms.

stoichiometry Study of numeric interrelationships between chemical elements and compounds and the mathematical laws governing such relationships.

storage Device into which data can be entered and held and from which it can be retrieved.

stroke volume The quantity of blood ejected by the heart in a single beat.

student's *t-test* A test of statistical significance of a deviation.

subarachnoid Below the membrane between the dura mater and the pia mater.

subendocardial Below the endocardium.

subphrenic Below the diaphragm.

subprogram A program or a sequence of instructions that can be called to perform the same task (although perhaps on different data) at different points in a program or in different programs.

sulcus Any of the grooves or furrows on the surface of the brain.

supernatant, supernate Liquid lying above or floating on a precipitated material.

survey meter Meter that measures rate of radioactive exposure, usually in units of milliroentgens per hour.

SVC Superior vena cava.

synapse The place where a nerve impulse is transmitted from one neuron to another.

synarthrosis Immovable joint, where bones lock within one another.

synchronous Performance of a sequence of operations controlled by an external clocking device; implies that no operation can take place until the previous operation is complete.

synchronous transfer Sequenced computer program operated by an external clock that does not permit a step to proceed until the previous step is completed.

syncope Fainting.

synovia Transparent fluid found in joint cavities.

synovitis Inflammation of joint-lining membrane.

Système Internationale (SI) International system of units used to replace traditional units as a result of U.S. metrication laws PL 93-380 and PL 94-168.

systole Contraction and expelling of blood from the heart.

T

T_3 Triiodothyronine.

T_4 Tetraiodothyronine; thyroxine.

T wave The next deflection in the electrocardiogram following the QRS complex; it represents ventricular repolarization.

target Object to be bombarded by ionizing radiation, usually in an accelerator or cyclotron.

TBG See *thyroid-binding globulin*.

TBPA Thyroxine-binding prealbumin.

terminal An I/O device such as an LA120 terminal that includes a keyboard and a display mechanism; in PDP11 systems a terminal is the primary communication device between a computer and a user.

tentorium Fibrous tissue shelf separating the cerebrum from the cerebellum.

tesla Unit for measuring magnetic field strength; 1 tesla = 10,000 gauss.

testosterone Hormone produced by the testes, influencing the male characteristics.

tetrahedron Molecular geometry in which the central atom is attached to four other atoms and the bond axes are directed along the diagonals of a cube.

tetralogy of Fallot Birth defect involving deformities of the blood vessels and walls of the heart chamber.

therapeutic Referring to the treatment of disease.

therapeutic window Range of dosage of a pharmaceutical that produces a beneficial effect.

thermal neutrons Neutrons with a maximum kinetic energy of 100 keV.

thermionic emission Electrons freed from an atom by heat.

thermodynamics Study of processes based on energy changes in the system.

thermoluminescent detector (TLD) Type of crystal used to monitor radiation exposure by emitting light; used in a film badge or ring badge.

thiols Family of organic compounds containing the functional group—SH.

thoracic cage Chest cavity.

thrombin Enzyme used as a clotting agent.

thrombocyte See *platelet*.

thrombosis Formation of a blood clot.

thyroid-binding globulin (TBG) Serum protein that is the primary agent for transport for thyroid hormone.

thyroid gland Endocrine gland that regulates metabolism.

thyrotropin (TSH) Hormone stimulating the thyroid secreted by the anterior pituitary.

thyroxine Hormone of the thyroid gland; 3,5,3,5-tetraiodothyronine.

time constant The speed of response of a rate meter.

time sharing Method of allocating central processor time and other computer services to multiple uses so that the computer, in effect, processes a number of programs simultaneously.

titer (1) Aliquot of titrant (solution of known concentration). (2) The quantity of a substance required to produce a reaction with a given amount of another substance.

Title 10 of the Code of the Federal Regulations, Part 20 (10 CFR, Part 20) *United States Nuclear Regulatory Commission Rules and Regulations, Standards for Protection against Radiation;* Title 10 of the CFR pertains to atomic energy.

titration Method of quantitative analysis in which one substance is volumetrically added to another substance with which it quantitatively reacts.

titrimetric procedures Chemical laboratory procedure for quantitative analysis by addition of solution of a known concentration to a solution of unknown concentration.

TLD See *thermoluminescent detectors*.

torcula Hollow, expanded area.

tomograph Any image representing three-dimensional information.

total count tube A tube in an RIA to which an aliquot of labeled ligand only has been added to serve as a check on the delivery of that material.

TQM Total quality management.

trabeculae Fibrous tissue supporting the structure of an organ.

tracer study Examination either in vivo or in vitro using a small amount of radionuclide-labeled substance to follow its path.

trackball An electronic pointing device for a computer.

transcobalamin Derivative of the cobalt-containing complex common to all members of the vitamin B_{12} group.

transferrin Serum globulin binding and transporting iron.

transient equilibrium Equilibrium reached by a parent-daughter radioisotope pair in which the half-life of the parent is longer than the half-life of the daughter.

transmittance The fraction of light that passes through photographic film.

transmutation Nuclear process by which one element is changed into another element.

transudate Term given to solvents and solutes that pass through a membrane.

transverse tomography Transverse scanning of a cross section of an organ, done from multiple directions, and then superimposed in a specific manner.

trauma Injury; wound.

TRH Thyrotropin-releasing hormone.

tritium Isotope of hydrogen with a mass of three unified mass units, consisting of one proton and two neutrons.

TSH Thyroid-stimulating hormone; See *thyrotropin*.

turnkey Computer system sold in a ready-to-use state.

Tyndall effect Light reflected or dispersed by particles suspended in a gas or liquid.

tyrosine Amino acid present in proteins that are susceptible to radioiodination.

U

UIBC See *unsaturated iron-binding capacity*.

ultrasonic nebulizer Device used for dispersing liquids in a fine mist through the use of sound waves.

ultrasonography Use of sound waves to image an internal structure of the body.

uniformity correction Compensation for detector non-uniformity.

United States Pharmacopeia (USP) Official listing of all drugs and medications.

UNIX A computer operating system.

unsaturated iron-binding capacity (UIBC) Amount of serum transferrin that is not saturated with iron.

USP See *United States Pharmacopeia*.

V

vaccine Dead bacteria given to build specific immunity against disease.

valence electrons Electrons in the outermost energy level.

valence state Ionization state of an element in an ionic compound.

van der Waals bond Attraction between the charged portions of two molecules, known as dipoles.

variable The symbolic representation of a logical storage location that can contain a value that changes during a processing operation.

variance Degree of change.

vascular Referring to the vessels.

vascular bed Entire blood supply of an organ or structure.

vascular lesion Lesion that affects the vessels.

vasculature (1) Supply of vessels to a region. (2) Vascular system.

vasculitis Inflammation of a vessel.

vasoconstrictor Something that causes the constriction of blood vessels.

vasodilator Something that causes the dilation of blood vessels.

VDT Video display terminal.

venipuncture Placement of a needle within a vein.

venography Radiography of the veins using a contrast medium; phlebography.

venous thrombi Blood clots within the veins.

ventilation Process of supplying air.

ventilation-perfusion ratio (V/Q) Comparison of functioning ventilatory space and perfused tissue within the lung; ratio of minute flow of air through alveoli to minute flow of blood through pulmonary capillaries.

ventricular Referring to a small cavity or chamber.

ventriculography Radiography of the ventricles of the brain.

vesicoureteral reflux Backward flow of urine through the bladder and into a ureter.

vitamin Organic compound necessary to maintain normal growth or function; found in some amounts in plants and animals.

volt Basic unit of electrical potential equal to one joule per coulomb.

voltmeter Device used to measure potential difference in electric circuits; potentiometer.

volume (1) Amount of space occupied in three dimensions. (2) A mass storage medium that can be treated as file-structured data storage.

volume dilution Dilution of a solution by addition of pure liquid solvent.

volume rendering Surface or MIP display of 3D tomographic data.

V/Q See *ventilation-perfusion ratio*.

VUR See *vesicoureteral reflux*.

W

wavelength Length per cycle in wave-motion mechanics.

well counter A thallium-activated sodium iodide crystal scintillation detector with a hole in the crystal to accommodate a sample vial.

white blood cell (WBC) Blood cell whose nucleus determines the type of cell: lymphocyte, monocyte, neutrophil, eosinophil, basophil.

window (1) Region of interest. (2) Limits of energy radiation accepted by a pulse-height analyzer.

wipe test Testing for removable contamination.

word Unit of data that may be stored in one addressable location (most microcomputers use 16-bit words).

WORM A type of optical disk drive; *write once read many*.

X

xerostomia Dryness of the mouth.

x-pulse In an Anger scintillation camera, those pulses emanating from the resistor/capacitor network positioned in a horizontal manner.

x ray Photonic radiation originating from electronic deexcitation.

x-ray diffraction Spectroscopic method for determining crystal structure by the interaction of x rays with the atoms involved in the crystalline structure.

xiphisternum Inferior tip of the sternum.

Y

y pulse In an Anger scintillation camera those pulses emanating from the resistor/capacitor network positioned in a vertical manner.

Z

Z number See *atomic number.*

zipper effect Overlap of two or more images.

Zollinger-Ellison syndrome Familial polyendocrine adenomatosis.

z pulse In an Anger scintillation camera it represents the sum of the x and y pulses.

Answers to Mathematics and Statistics Review

1. b
2. c
3. c
4. a
5. d
6. c
7. b
8. a
9. d
10. a

11. b
12. d
13. c
14. b
15. d
16. c
17. b
18. c
19. a
20. b

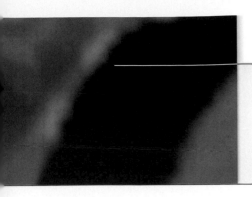

Illustration Credits

Figure 3-6—From Bushberg JT, Seibert JA, Leidholdt EM, and Boone JM: *The Essential Physics of Medical Imaging,* ed 2, Philadelphia, 2002, Lippincott Williams & Wilkins.

Figures 3-7, 3-35—From Rollo FD: *Nuclear medicine physics, instrumentation, and agents,* St. Louis, 1977, Mosby.

Figures 3-17, 3-20—From Boyd CM, Dalrymple GV: *Basic principles of nuclear medicine,* St. Louis, 1974, Mosby.

Figure 3-24—From Ter-Pogossian M et al: *Sci Am* 243(4), 1980.

Figures 3-41, 3-44—From Greer K et al: *J Nucl Med Technol* 13:76-85, 1985.

Figure 6-3—From Kowalsky RJ, Perry JR: *Radiopharmaceuticals in nuclear medicine practice,* Norwalk, Conn, 1987, Appleton & Lange.

Figure 7-1—From Ionizing radiation exposure of the population of the United States, *National Council on Radiation Protection Report No. 93,* Washington, DC, 1987, The Council.

Figures 8-2, 8-3, 8-4, 8-6, 8-7, 8-8, 8-9, 8-10, 8-14 through 8-26, 8-28, 8-29—From Kowalczyk N, Donnett K: *Integrated patient care for the imaging professional,* St. Louis, 1996, Mosby.

Figures 8-5, 8-27—Modified from Potter PA, Perry AG: *Fundamentals of nursing: concepts, process, and practice,* ed 3, St. Louis, 1994, Mosby.

Figures 12-3, 12-4—From Agur AMR: *Grant's atlas of anatomy,* ed 9, Baltimore, 1991, Williams & Wilkins.

Figures 12-5, 12-7, 12-8, 18-1, 18-2—From Anthony CP, Thibodeau GA: *Textbook of anatomy and physiology,* ed 10, St. Louis, 1979, Mosby.

Figure 12-6—From Netter FH: *The CIBA collection–nervous system,* vol 1, West Caldwell, NJ, 1983, CIBA Pharmaceutical.

Figure 12-9—From Maisey M, Britton KE, Gilday DL, eds: *Clinical nuclear medicine,* ed 2, London, 1992, Chapman & Hall.

Figure 12-10—From Gilman S, Newman SW: *Manter and Gatz's essentials of clinical neuroanatomy and neurophysiology,* ed 7, Philadelphia, 1987, FA Davis.

Figure 12-19, *left* (drawing)—From Stark D, Bradley W: *Magnetic resonance imaging,* ed 2, St. Louis, 1992, Mosby.

Figures 13-1, 13-2, 16-1, 16-18, 16-25, 18-3, 18-4, 18-5—From Thibodeau GA: *Anthony's textbook of anatomy and physiology,* ed 13, St. Louis, 1990, Mosby.

Figure 13-3—From Goldsmith SJ: Thyroid: in vivo tests of function and imaging. In Rothfeld B: *Nuclear medicine: endocrinology,* Philadelphia, 1978, JB Lippincott.

Figure 13-13—From Becker DV, Hurley JR: Current status of radioiodine (^{131}I) treatment of hyperthyroidism. In Freeman L, Weissman HS, eds: *Nuclear medicine annual 1982,* New York, 1982, Raven Press.

Figure 13-21—Redrawn from data reported by Melicow MM: *Cancer* 40:1987-2004, 1977.

Figures 14-2, 14-4—From Hammond EC: The effects of smoking, *Sci Am* 39:207, 1962. Copyright 1962 by Scientific American, Inc. All rights reserved.

Figures 15-31, 15-32—From Gropler RJ et al: *J Am Coll Cardiol* 19:989, 1992.

Figures 16-26, 18-6—From Hamilton WJ: *Textbook of human anatomy,* ed 2, St. Louis, 1979, Mosby; courtesy The Macmillan Press Ltd, Houndsmill Basingstoke, Hampshire, England.

Figure 17-20—From Henkin RE, Boles MA, Dillehay GL et al: *Nuclear medicine,* St. Louis, 1996, Mosby.

Figure 20-5—From Kipper MS, Williams RJ: Indium-111 white blood cell imaging, *Clin Nucl Med* 8:449-455, 1983.

Index

A

Abacus, invention of, 99
Absolute activity calibration, 301-302
Absorbed dose, 185
Accelerator-produced radionuclides, 159-160
Accidents, 202-203
Accuracy, 22, 32, 80
ACEI. *See* Angiotensin converting enzyme inhibitor (ACEI)
Acetazolamide (Diamox), 218t
Acetylcholine, 333
Achalasia, 452f
Acid-citrate-dextrose, 166
Acidophils, 351
Acids, 146, 147-148
Acoustical stethoscope, 228f
Acquired immunodeficiency syndrome (AIDS), 538
Acquisition, 312-313
  2nd, 296f
  software, 294
Acromegaly, 353
ACTH. *See* Adrenal cortex-stimulating hormone (ACTH)
Activity control chart, 80f
Acute renal failure, 485
Acute tubular necrosis (ATN), 483
Adaptive filters, 119, 120f
ADC. *See* Analog-to-digital converters (ADC)
Adenocard. *See* Adenosine (Adenocard)
Adenomas, 356
  adrenal, 131I NP-59, 380, 380f
  functioning, 363-364
  parathyroid
    99mTc-methoxyisobutyl-isonitrile (MIBI), 371, 372f
    99mTc pertechnetate, 371
Adenosine (Adenocard), 171, 218t, 430
ADH. *See* Vasopressin
Adrenal adenomas, 380, 380f
Adrenal cortex, 377-380
  anatomy and physiology of, 377-378
  nuclear medicine procedures, 378-380
Adrenal cortex-stimulating hormone (ACTH), 351, 378
Adrenal glands, 217t, 377
  metastases, FDG PET, 318
Adrenal medulla, 380-382
  131I-MIBG, 381
Adrenergic blockers affecting exercise test, 428t
Adrenergics, 216t
Adrenocorticotropin, 351
Adult cardiopulmonary arrest (CPR), 231f
Aerosol ventilation imaging, 397-398
Affinity diagram, 235
Agranulocytosis, 543
AIDS. *See* Acquired immunodeficiency syndrome (AIDS)
Airborne activity
  control and evaluation, 200-201
  samplers, 191
Airborne transmission, 226
Air flow measuring devices, 191
Airways, 387f, 388f
  anatomy and physiology, 387
  obstructed, 229-230
ALARA. *See* As low as reasonably achievable (ALARA)
Albumin particles injection site, 394f
Alcohols, 152t, 155
  effect on lower esophageal sphincter, 453

Aldehydes, 152t
Aldesleukin (Proleukin), 423t
Aldosterone, 481
Algebraic equations, 3-4
Alkanes, 152t, 153, 154t
Alkenes, 152t, 153-154
Alkyl groups, 155t
Alkynes, 152t
Alpha decay, 43, 158
Alpha particles, 51
Aluminum, 180
Alveoli, 388, 388f
Alzheimer's disease, 340, 341
American Association of Physicists in Medicine standards, 280
American Society of Nuclear Cardiology standards, 280
American Standard Code for Information Interchange (ASCII), 101
Amides, 153t, 156
Amines, 153t
Amplitude images, 420, 421f
Ampule, preparing medication from, 220f
Amyloidosis, 459
Analgesics, 217t
Analog-to-digital converters (ADC), 106
Analysis of variance (ANOVA), 29
Analytical engine, 99
Analytic balance, 127, 129f
Anatomic dead space, 389
Androgens, 355
Anemia, 522
Anemometers, 191, 191f
Aneroid manometers, 228f
Aneurysmal bone cyst of tibia, 507f
Anger positioning logic, 70f
Anger scintillation cameras, 64-73, 68, 71, 74
  for bone imaging, 501-502
  collimators for, 66f
    arrangement of, 70f
  dual detector, 65f
Angiotensin converting enzyme inhibitor (ACEI), 481
  augmented renal scintigraphy, 485-486
Angiotensin II, 481
Anion, 135
Annihilation, 51
Annihilation photons, 298f
Annual effective dose equivalent in United States, 188t
Antecubital vein, 220
Anterior pituitary gland, 351, 352t
Anterior spinal muscles, FDG accumulations, 314
Antiarrhythmics affecting exercise test, 428t
Antibiotics, 216t
Antibodies
  antiintrinsic factor-blocking, 534
  defined, 548b
  human antimouse, 548, 549
  monoclonal, 171
    vocabulary of, 548b
Anticholinergics, 216t
Anticoagulants, 216t
Anti-coincidence circuit, 63
Anticonvulsants, 217t
Antidiabetics, 217t
Antidiuretic hormone (ADH). *See* Vasopressin
Antiemetics, 217t
Antifungals, 216t

Quantitative chemical analysis, 138-139
Quantitative image information, 303-304
Quantum number, 131, 132t
Quenching, 63
Quimby-Marinelli-Hine formula, 368

R

Rad, 6t, 185
Radial pulse, 228f
Radiation
  absorbed dose, 368, 368t, 369f
  attenuation of, 14-16, 15f
  braking, 53-54
  Bremsstrahlung, 53-54
  cosmic, 187
  detection of, 57-64
  dose, recommendations and regulations, 188
  electromagnetic, 38
    interactions with matter, 51t
  exposure, 185
    external personnel, 194-195
    medical, 187
    sources of, 187
  gamma, 158, 246
    intensity, 185
    scattering of, 52-53
  internal, 187
  ionizing
    biologic effects of, 206-209
    quality factor values for, 186t
  percent transmitted, 195t
  workers, occupational exposure, 189t
Radiation safety, 184-209
  audit, 203-204
  committee, 195-196
  laboratory instrumentation, 189-190
  officer, 193, 195-196
  practices and training, 195-196
  program, 195-200
Radioactive decay, 11-13, 41
  equations, 6
  linear plot of, 17f
  schematics of, 46-49
Radioactive gases, 191
  storing and using, 201-202
Radioactive materials
  control of, 196-200
  opening packages, 196
  ordering and receiving, 196
Radioactive pharmaceuticals, withdrawal of, 219-220
Radioactive tracers, 330
Radioactive waste disposal, 203-204
Radioactive xenon, 392. See also Xenon-133 (Xe133)
Radioactivity
  computation as, 11
  measurement of, 190
  semilog plot of, 17f
Radioactivity units, 49-50
Radiochemical purity, 175-180
  calculation of, 178
  for 18F-FDG, 181
  99mTc-exametazime, 179f
  99mTc-mertiatide, 179, 180f
Radiochemistry, 157-183
Radiochromatogram scanner, 177f
Radiogenic increment, 207
Radioimmunoassay
  pancreas, 373
  thyroid gland, 357
Radiolabeled aminopyrine breath test, 472
Radionuclide cisternogram, 342
Radionuclide cystography (RNC), 566-568
Radionuclide dose calibrator, 190
Radionuclide generator testing, 199
Radionuclide imaging
  cardiovascular system, 410-413
  skeletal system, 497-501
Radionuclides, 41
  accelerator-produced, 159-160
  daughter, 162f
  decay properties of, 161t, 172t
  evaluation of ventricular function, 413-424
  for painful bone metastases, 511-512
  for positron emission tomography (PET), 286t

Radionuclides (*Continued*)
  production of, 157-164
  purity of, 175
  thyroid imaging, 361t
Radionuclide shuntogram, 342
Radionuclide therapy for thyroid gland, 366-370
Radionuclide ventriculogram (RVG), 112, 166
Radionuclide vesicoureteral reflux (VUR), 488
Radiopharmaceuticals, 172-174
  administration of, 199f
  for cardiac imaging, 411b
  central nervous system, 342-344
  genitourinary system, 481-482
  intrathecal administration of, 343f
  quality assurance, 175-182
  renal, 482t
  technetium, 164-169
  used for blood pool imaging, 417-422
  used for myocardial perfusion imaging, 425-426
  used for ventilation lung imaging, 394t
  use measurement, 199
Radiopharmacology, 157-183
Radiotracers, new, 327
Radio waves, 38
Radon, estimated whole body dose equivalent, 187
RAM. See Random access memory (RAM)
Ramp filter, 74, 119, 119f, 257, 257f
Random access memory (RAM), 101
Random decay affecting count rate, 64
Random labels, 523-524
Ratemeter, 59
Ratios, 3-4
81Rb. See Rubidium-81 (81Rb)
82Rb. See Rubidium-82 (82Rb)
RBC. See Red blood cells (RBC)
RBE. See Relative biologic effect (RBE)
Reactor-produced radionuclides, 159
Read-only memory (ROM), 101
Rebreathing apparatus, 396f
Receiver operating characteristic (ROC) curve, 33, 33f
Recessive genes, 209
Recombinant human TSH (rTSH), 364
Reconstruction, 74
  algorithms, 296-297
Recordable event, 204
Rectum, barium in, 480f
Red blood cell mass, measurement of, 525
Red blood cells (RBC), 522, 522t
  51Cr ascorbic acid labeling of, 525-526
  survival graph, 528f
Red blood cells (RBC) survival study, 527-529
Redistribution, 425
Reduced-instruction set computer (RISC), 102
Reduced technetium complexes, 166-169
Reflectance, 262
Region of interest (ROI), 319
Regression analysis, 20f
Regression equation, 21
Regression line, calculation of, 19-20
Reimbursement, payor, 310
Relative biologic effect (RBE), 185
Rem, 6t
Remaining activity, 12
Renal artery stenosis, 485-486
Renal failure, acute, 485
Renal imaging
  agents, 167, 167f
  morphologic, 486-488
Renal parenchyma, 483f
Renal radiopharmaceuticals, 482t
Renal scintigraphy in children, 565-566
Renal transplant patients, renal imaging, 485
Renography, 484f
  in children, 565-566
Reporting after spills, 202
Reproducibility of nonimaging scintillation detectors, 82
Rescue breathing, 230f
Residual volume, 389
Resolution, 68, 245
  for cameras, 89, 91
  effect on emission computed tomography (ECT), 78-79
  recovery
    single photon emission computed tomography (SPECT), 266-267
Resolving time, 63-64
Respirations, 228